Nursing Care Plans

Diagnoses, Interventions, and Outcomes

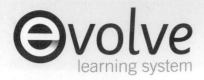

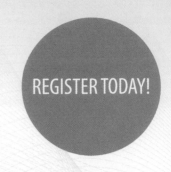

To access your Student resources, visit:

http://evolve.elsevier.com/Gulanick/

Care Plan Constructor

- Build, edit, and print a customized care plan by choosing from 68 nursing diagnoses from the 7th edition of *Nursing Care Plans: Diagnoses, Interventions, and Outcomes.* Select each diagnosis, intervention, and outcome you wish to include in your care plan.

Additional Care Plans

Choose from 24 additional medical-surgical care plans for further study and guidance:

- Adrenal Insufficiency (Addison's Disease)
- Amyotrophic Lateral Sclerosis (ALS)
- Anorexia Nervosa
- Blood Component Therapy
- Bulimia
- Central Venous Access Devices
- Common Mood Disorders: Depression and Bipolar Disorder
- Dermatitis
- Diabetes Insipidus
- Diabetic Ketoacidosis (DKA) and Hyperglycemic Hyperosmolar Nonketotic Syndrome (HHNS)
- Erectile Dysfunction (ED)
- Hematopoietic Stem Cell Collection
- Hemophilia
- Hemorrhoids/Hemorrhoidectomy
- Lyme Disease
- Myasthenia Gravis
- Near-Drowning
- Plastic Surgery for Wound Closure
- Premenstrual Syndrome (PMS)
- Severe Acute Respiratory Syndrome (SARS)
- Suicide
- Syndrome of Inappropriate Antidiuretic Hormone (SIADH)
- Traction
- West Nile Virus

7th Edition

Nursing Care Plans

Diagnoses, Interventions, and Outcomes

Meg Gulanick, PhD, APRN, FAAN
Professor, Marcella Niehoff School of Nursing
Loyola University Chicago
Chicago, Illinois

Judith L. Myers, RN, MSN
Assistant Professor of Nursing
Grand View University
Des Moines, Iowa

ELSEVIER
MOSBY

3251 Riverport Lane
St. Louis, Missouri 63043

NURSING CARE PLANS: DIAGNOSES, INTERVENTIONS, AND OUTCOMES   ISBN: 978-0-323-06537-5
Copyright © 2011, 2007, 2003, 1998, 1994, 1990, 1986 by Mosby, Inc., an affiliate of Elsevier Inc.

Library of Congress Cataloging-in-Publication Data

Nursing care plans : diagnoses, interventions, and outcomes / [edited by] Meg Gulanick, Judith L. Myers. — 7th ed.
    p. ; cm.
  Includes bibliographical references and index.
  ISBN 978-0-323-06537-5 (pbk. : alk. paper)
  1. Nursing care plans—Handbooks, manuals, etc. I. Gulanick, Meg. II. Myers, Judith L.
  [DNLM: 1. Patient Care Planning—Handbooks. 2. Nursing Care—Handbooks. 3. Nursing Diagnosis—Handbooks. 4. Outcome Assessment (Health Care)—Handbooks. WY 49]
  RT49.N87 2011
  610.73—dc22

2010036379

Vice President and Publisher: Loren Wilson
Acquisitions Editor: Robin Carter
Developmental Editor: Deanna Dedeke
Publishing Services Manager: Jeff Patterson
Senior Project Manager: Anne Konopka
Design Direction: Maggie Reid

Printed in the United States of America

Last digit is the print number: 9 8 7 6 5 4 3

Contributors to seventh edition

Virginia B. Bowman, MSN, RN, CNS, AOCNS, CORLN
Advanced Practice Nurse
Head and Neck Reconstructive Surgery
University of Texas M. D. Anderson Cancer Center
Houston, Texas

Judy Lau Carino, MSN, CNP
Clinical Instructor
Adjunct Faculty
Niehoff School of Nursing
Loyola University Chicago
Chicago, Illinois

Debra L. Cason, MSN, RNCS
Assistant Professor of Nursing
Grand View University
Des Moines, Iowa

Sandra Coslet, RN, MSN, MBA
Pulmonary Hypertension Program
University of Chicago Medical Center
Chicago, Illinois

Paula Cox-North, MN, NP-C
Advanced Registered Nurse Practitioner
Pacific Medical Center
Harborview Medical Center
Seattle, Washington

Jennifer L. Crosby, APN, MSN, CCRN, CCNS-CSC
Cardiac Surgery
Advocate Christ Medical Center
Oak Lawn, Illinois

Gail DeLuca, MSN, APRN
Family Nurse Practitioner
University of Chicago
Chicago, Illinois

Lisa C. Dobogai, MS, APN, AOCNP
Acute Care Nurse Practitioner
Stem Cell Transplant
University of Illinois Medical Center
Chicago, Illinois

Amy Dolce, APN, MS, AOCN, CHPN
Clinical Nurse Specialist
Northwest Community Hospital
Arlington Heights, Illinois

Nadia Goraczkowski-Jones, RN, BSN
Nurse Coordinator
Iowa Health Des Moines
Des Moines, Iowa

Rebecca Hagensee, RN, MSN
Cardiology Clinical Coordinator
Elmhurst Clinic
Elmhurst, Illinois

Mary Ellen Hand, RN, MSN
Nurse Coordinator
Head and Neck Cancer
Rush University Hospital
Chicago, Illinois

Margo S. Henderson, DNP, FNP-BC
Assistant Professor of Nursing
Medical College of Georgia
School of Nursing
Augusta, Georgia

Linda Kamenjarin, APN
Advanced Practice Nurse
Cardiovascular Surgery
Advocate Christ Medical Center
Oak Lawn, Illinois

Tamara M. Kear, RN, MSN, CNN
Assistant Professor
Gwynedd-Mercy College
School of Nursing
Gwynedd Valley, Pennsylvania

Lucina Kimpel, RN, PhD
Assistant Professor of Nursing
Grand View University
Des Moines, Iowa

Katherine T. Leslie, RN, BSN
Cardiovascular Surgery
Advocate Christ Medical Center
Oak Lawn, Illinois

Mary Jo Mikottis, RN, MSN
Nurse Clinician
Elmhurst Memorial Healthcare
Elmhurst, Illinois

Linda Denise Oakley, RN, PhD
Professor
School of Nursing
University of Wisconsin—Madison
Madison, Wisconsin

Linda Ohler, RN, MSN, CCTC, FAAN
Editor
Progress in Transplantation
Program Manager
CUF and Heart Transplantation
Medical College of Virginia
Commonwealth University Health System
Richmond, Virginia

Judy K. Orth, RN, CHPN, BSN, MA
Adjunct Professor
Grand View University
Des Moines, Iowa

Joanne Pfeiffer, BSN, MEd, CHTP
Professor Emeritus
Grand View University
Des Moines, Iowa

Dottie Roberts, MSN, MACI, RN, CMSRN, OCNS-C
Clinical Nurse Specialist
Palmetto Health Baptist
Columbia, South Carolina

Kathy G. Supple, MSN, APN-BC, CCRN
Acute Care Nurse Practitioner
Burn Center
Loyola University Medical Center
Maywood, Illinois

Terry D. Takemoto, PhD, RN, BC, PCCN, AE-C
Supervisor
Educational Consultant
Kindred Chicago Lakeshore
Chicago, Illinois

Geraldine Tansey, RN, APN, MS
Clinical Nurse Specialist
Cardiovascular Surgery
Advocate Christ Medical Center
Oak Lawn, Illinois

Stacy VandenBranden, RN, MS, CPNP
Pediatric Nurse Practitioner
Division of Pulmonary Medicine
Children's Memorial Medical Center
Chicago, Illinois

Jeffrey Zurlinden, RN, MS
Clinical Coordinator
Northwestern Memorial Hospital
Chicago, Illinois

Contributors to sixth edition

Pamela Cianci
Marianne T. Cosentino
Linda Flemm
Patricia J. Friend
Katrina Gallagher
Connie Huberty
Judi Jennrich
Catherine A. Kefer
Vicki A. Keough
MariJo Letizia
Shelby J. Neel
Kelly Oney
Sue Penckofer
Carol White

We also want to acknowledge the prior editors of this classic book: Deidra Gradishar, Susan Galanes, Audrey Klopp, and Michele Knoll Puzas, along with the team of nurse contributors from the five earlier editions who provided the foundation for *Nursing Care Plans: Diagnoses, Interventions, and Outcomes* as it is known today.

Nursing Faculty Reviewers

Tim J. Bristol, PhD, RN, CNE
Nursing Education Consultant
Waconia, Minnesota

Jeanne Burnkrant, MS, RN
Instructor of Nursing
Loretto Heights School of Nursing
Regis University
Denver, Colorado

Mariann Montgomery, MSN, RN, CNE
Assistant Professor of Nursing
Kent State University Tuscarawas
New Philadelphia, Ohio

Kathleen S. Whalen, PhD, RN
Assistant Professor
Loretto Heights School of Nursing
Regis University
Denver, Colorado

Student Reviewers

Rhonda Berenz
Goldfarb School of Nursing
Barnes-Jewish College
St. Louis, Missouri

Debra Harris
Goldfarb School of Nursing
Barnes-Jewish College
St. Louis, Missouri

Sarah Hollenberg
Nursing Program
University of Missouri–St. Louis
St. Louis, Missouri

Natasha Jones
Goldfarb School of Nursing
Barnes-Jewish College
St. Louis, Missouri

Joseph Linville
Goldfarb School of Nursing
Barnes-Jewish College
St. Louis, Missouri

Sara Olsen
Goldfarb School of Nursing
Barnes-Jewish College
St. Louis, Missouri

Natalie Schapiro
Goldfarb School of Nursing
Barnes-Jewish College
St. Louis, Missouri

Jennifer Triefenbach
Goldfarb School of Nursing
Barnes-Jewish College
St. Louis, Missouri

Lindsay Walsh
Nursing Program
Truman State University
Kirksville, Missouri

Our primary goal for this edition of *Nursing Care Plans: Diagnoses, Interventions, and Outcomes* has been to build on the quality of the premier resource used by nurses to plan care for an increasingly diverse population of patients. This work is the most comprehensive care planning book on the market, with over 200 care plans covering the most common nursing diagnoses and clinical problems in medical-surgical nursing patients. The care plans focus on patients with both acute and chronic medical conditions in the acute care, ambulatory, and home care setting. Growing attention has been given to health promotion–focused concerns, while continuing to provide updated content incorporating the latest evidence-based data and best practice guidelines to help the reader provide the highest-quality nursing care.

Nursing Care Plans: Diagnoses, Interventions, and Outcomes continues to offer "two books in one." Besides including an **introductory chapter on how to use care plans** to provide safe, individualized, and quality care (Chapter 1), the book contains **68 of the most commonly used nursing diagnoses** in Chapter 2 and **143 of the most commonly used medical-surgical adult health care plans** in Chapters 3 to 14. Expanded information has been added to the introductions for the nursing diagnosis care plans in Chapter 2 and for the medical disorder care plans in the remaining chapters. This information provides a foundation for understanding the nursing care for a specific nursing diagnosis or medical disorder. **New content on patient safety and preventable complications** addresses national initiatives and discusses the nurse's responsibility in preventing complications such as falls, pressure ulcers, infections, and the like.

In Chapter 2, **new care plans have been added for the NANDA International (NANDA-I) diagnoses** of *impaired dentition, disturbed energy field, readiness for enhanced immunization status (adult), sedentary lifestyle, post-trauma syndrome,* and *relocation stress syndrome.* In the remainder of the book, **new medical disorder care plans** added to this edition include pulmonary arterial hypertension, cystic fibrosis, carpal tunnel syndrome, peptic ulcer disease, fibromyalgia, solid organ transplant, hemodialysis, pelvic relaxation disorder, hyperthyroidism, and psoriasis.

The essential format for the book and for the individual care plans has not changed from the sixth edition. These care plans include **assessments and therapeutic interventions** across the continuum of care. Chapter 2 also contains a section on **patient education and continuity of care** for each nursing diagnosis. **Ongoing Assessments** throughout this book contain the latest information on methods of assessment and for laboratory and diagnostic tests. **Revised and expanded outcomes** include new measurable and specific terms for each nursing diagnosis. **Therapeutic Interventions** include up-to-date information on **independent and collaborative clinical management** and on **drug therapy** related to nursing diagnoses and medical disorders. The **rationales** for the Ongoing Assessments and Therapeutic Interventions have been thoroughly updated and expanded to include current care and patient safety standards and clinical practice guidelines in nursing and other health care disciplines. **Related care plans** are referenced where applicable, making it easy to cross reference content throughout the book. We continue to include the latest editions of **Nursing Interventions Classification (NIC) and Nursing Outcomes Classification (NOC) labels** at the beginning of each care plan. The index includes entries for all nursing diagnoses, all medical diagnoses, and all synonyms for the medical diagnoses, providing an easy-to-use, practical tool for accessing the book's content.

We continue to use the Evolve website as an adjunct to the printed book. The **expanded website now includes 24 additional care plans** on a wide range of disorders (see the inside front cover of this book for a full list). The **revised Online Care Plan Constructor** on the Evolve website contains all nursing diagnosis care plans from Chapter 2. It enables the user to **customize care plans** for an individual patient, select from NANDA-I diagnoses, and list specific related factors, NOC outcomes, NIC interventions and rationales, home care interventions, and specific patient/family teaching. This tool has been updated to reflect the additional nursing diagnosis care plans added to the text and is enhanced to allow the user to save customized data. An additional enhancement is the ability to export saved care plans to a word processing program.

We are grateful to the many contributors to previous editions of this book. Their work continues to be the foundation for the nurses who have contributed to the revisions for this edition.

Meg Gulanick, PhD, APRN, FAAN
Judith L. Myers, RN, MSN

CONTENTS

Using Nursing Care Plans to Provide Individualized, Safe, and Quality Care

Introduction

According to the American Nurses Association (ANA), nursing is the diagnosis and treatment of human responses to actual and potential problems. A broad foundation of scientific knowledge, including the biological and behavioral sciences, combined with the ability to assist patients, families, and other caregivers in managing their own health needs, defines the scope of nursing practice. Nursing care in this context transcends settings, crosses the age continuum, and supports a wellness philosophy focused on self-care. In many ways, the roles of nurses are enhanced by opportunities to provide nursing care in the more natural, less institutional paradigms that are demanded by restructured health care financing. Studies continue to document that society places its highest trust in nurses. To deserve this trust, nurses will need to continuously strive to improve health care quality. The current challenges in seizing these opportunities include the following: (1) recognition of the growing chasm between what currently "exists" in health care and what "should be" to achieve the safe, quality care that every patient deserves; (2) the importance of working effectively in interdisciplinary teams to deliver patient-centered care; (3) the need for more effective professional communication; (4) the need to help patients better navigate through difficult acute and chronic care issues; (5) the ability of the nursing educational system to increasingly prepare nurses for settings outside the hospital environment, as well as within the complex hospital setting; (6) the ability of nurses themselves to be comfortable with the responsibility of their roles; (7) the need to increase the recruitment and retention of nurses from diverse backgrounds to meet the needs of an increasingly diverse population; and (8) the availability of tools to assist nurses in assessing, planning, and providing care. *Nursing Care Plans: Diagnoses, Interventions, and Outcomes* is such a tool.

Components of These Nursing Care Plans

Each care plan in this book begins with an expanded definition of the title problem or diagnosis (Figure 1-1). These definitions include enough information to guide the user

in understanding what the problem or diagnosis is, information regarding the incidence or prevalence of the problem or diagnosis, a brief overview of the typical management and/or the focus of nursing care, and a description of the setting in which care for the particular problem or diagnosis can be expected to occur.

Each problem or diagnosis is accompanied by one or more cross-references, some of which may be synonyms (see Figure 1-1). These cross-references assist the user in locating other information that may be helpful in deciding whether this particular care plan is indeed the one the user needs.

For each care plan, appropriate nursing diagnoses are developed, each with the following components:
- Common related factors (those etiologies associated with a diagnosis for an actual problem) (Figure 1-2)
- Defining characteristics (assessment data that support the nursing diagnosis) (see Figure 1-2)
- Common risk factors (those situations or conditions that contribute to the person's potential to develop a problem or diagnosis) (Figure 1-3)
- Common expected outcomes (see Figure 1-3)
- Ongoing assessment (see Figure 1-3)
- Therapeutic interventions (both independent and collaborative) (Figure 1-4)

Each nursing diagnosis developed is based on the NANDA International (NANDA-I) label unless otherwise stated. Wherever possible, expanded rationales assist the

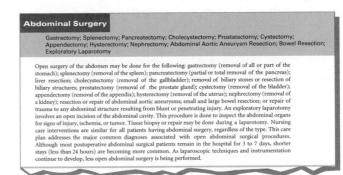

Abdominal Surgery

Gastrectomy; Splenectomy; Pancreatectomy; Cholecystectomy; Prostatectomy; Cystectomy; Appendectomy; Hysterectomy; Nephrectomy; Abdominal Aortic Aneurysm Resection; Bowel Resection; Exploratory Laparotomy

Open surgery of the abdomen may be done for the following: gastrectomy (removal of all or part of the stomach); splenectomy (removal of the spleen); pancreatectomy (partial or total removal of the pancreas); liver resection; cholecystectomy (removal of the gallbladder); removal of biliary stones or resection of biliary structures; prostatectomy (removal of the prostate gland); cystectomy (removal of the bladder); appendectomy (removal of the appendix); hysterectomy (removal of the uterus); nephrectomy (removal of a kidney); resection or repair of abdominal aortic aneurysms; small and large bowel resection; or repair of trauma to any abdominal structure resulting from blunt or penetrating injury. An exploratory laparotomy involves an open incision of the abdominal cavity. This procedure is done to inspect the abdominal organs for signs of injury, ischemia, or tumor. Tissue biopsy or repair may be done during a laparotomy. Nursing care interventions are similar for all patients having abdominal surgery, regardless of the type. This care plan addresses the major common diagnoses associated with open abdominal surgical procedures. Although most postoperative abdominal surgical patients remain in the hospital for 3 to 7 days, shorter stays (less than 24 hours) are becoming more common. As laparoscopic techniques and instrumentation continue to develop, less open abdominal surgery is being performed.

Figure 1-1 Expanded definition and cross-references of a care plan.

NANDA-I NDx Ineffective Breathing Pattern

Common Related Factors	Defining Characteristics
Abdominal incision pain Abdominal distention compromising lung expansion Sedation	Dyspnea, tachypnea/bradypnea Poor coughing effort Shallow breathing Splinting respirations Altered chest excursion Refusal/inability to use incentive spirometer

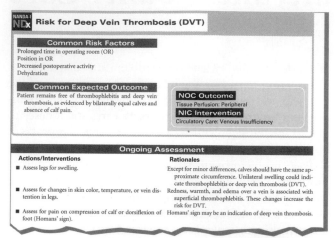

Figure 1-2 Common related factors and defining characteristics of the nursing diagnosis.

NANDA-I NDx Risk for Deep Vein Thrombosis (DVT)

Common Risk Factors

Prolonged time in operating room (OR)
Position in OR
Decreased postoperative activity
Dehydration

Common Expected Outcome

Patient remains free of thrombophlebitis and deep vein thrombosis, as evidenced by bilaterally equal calves and absence of calf pain.

NOC Outcome

Tissue Perfusion: Peripheral

NIC Intervention

Circulatory Care: Venous Insufficiency

Ongoing Assessment

Actions/Interventions	Rationales
■ Assess legs for swelling.	Except for minor differences, calves should have the same approximate circumference. Unilateral swelling could indicate thrombophlebitis or deep vein thrombosis (DVT).
■ Assess for changes in skin color, temperature, or vein distention in legs.	Redness, warmth, and edema over a vein is associated with superficial thrombophlebitis. These changes increase the risk for DVT.
■ Assess for pain on compression of calf or dorsiflexion of foot (Homans' sign).	Homans' sign may be an indication of deep vein thrombosis.

Figure 1-3 Common risk factors, common expected outcomes, and ongoing assessment of the nursing diagnosis.

Therapeutic Interventions

Actions/Interventions	Rationales
■ Reinforce or encourage leg exercises taught preoperatively; strive for 10 repetitions each hour until fully ambulatory.	Contracting the leg muscles decreases venous stasis and encourages good venous return; both decrease the opportunity of thromboembolic developments.
▲ Use antiembolic stockings or sequential compression devices while the patient is in bed.	Both interventions promote venous blood flow and reduce venous stagnation.
■ Discourage gatching of the bed at the knee. Encourage the patient not to cross legs at the knee or ankle while in bed.	Compression on veins contributes to venous pooling in the legs and decreased venous return.
▲ Encourage ambulation by the patient as soon as possible according to physician's prescription.	Being fully upright is preferable to "dangling" or sitting in a chair because contracted muscles push against the leg vessels and improve venous return most effectively when the patient is upright and legs are straight.
▲ Administer prophylactic anticoagulant therapy as prescribed.	Low-dose or low-molecular-weight heparin are used to prevent thrombus formation.
▲ Administer IV fluids; encourage oral fluid intake as prescribed.	Adequate hydration reduces hemoconcentration, and reduces the risk for deep vein thrombosis.
■ Before discharge, instruct the patient and family about guidelines for resuming normal activity.	Providing guidelines promotes the return of activity at an appropriate level, which will help reduce the complications of immobility and promote a sense of well-being.

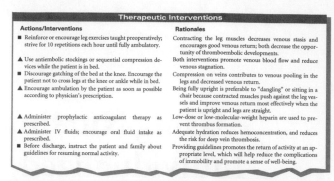

Figure 1-4 Therapeutic interventions of the nursing diagnosis.

user in understanding the information presented; this allows for use of *Nursing Care Plans: Diagnoses, Interventions, and Outcomes* as a singular reference tool. The interventions and supporting rationales for each care plan represent current research-based knowledge and evidence-based clinical practice guidelines for nursing and other health care professionals. Many care plans also refer the user to additional diagnoses that may be pertinent and would assist the user in further developing a care plan. Each diagnosis developed in these care plans also identifies the Nursing Interventions Classification (NIC) interventions and the Nursing Outcomes Classifications (NOC) outcomes.

Nursing Diagnoses Taxonomy, and Interventions and Outcomes Classifications

As *Nursing Care Plans: Diagnoses, Interventions, and Outcomes* continues to mature and reflect the changing times and needs of its readers, as well as the needs of those for whom care is provided, nursing diagnoses continue to evolve. The body of research to support diagnoses, their definitions, related and risk factors, and defining characteristics is ever increasing and gaining momentum. Nurses continue to study both independent and collaborative interventions for effectiveness and desirable outcomes.

The taxonomy of nursing diagnoses as a whole continues to be refined; its use as an international tool for practice, education, and research is testament to its importance as an organizing framework for the body of knowledge that is uniquely nursing. As a taxonomy, nursing diagnosis and all its components are standardized. Nurses must remember that care plans developed for each diagnosis or cluster of diagnoses for particular patients must be individualized. The tailoring of the care plan is the hallmark of nursing practice.

Nursing Interventions Classification (NIC) presents an additional opportunity for clarifying and organizing what nurses do. With NIC, nursing interventions have been systematically organized to help nurses identify and select interventions. In this seventh edition, NIC information continues to be presented along with each nursing diagnosis within each care plan, giving the user added ability to use NIC taxonomy in planning for individualized patient care. According to the developers of NIC, nursing interventions are "any treatment, based upon clinical judgment and knowledge, that a nurse performs to enhance patient/client outcomes" (Bulechek, Butcher, and Dochterman, 2008, p. 3). These interventions may include direct or indirect care and may be initiated by a nurse, a physician, or another care provider. Student nurses, practicing nurses, advanced practice nurses, and nurse executives can use nursing diagnoses and NIC as tools for learning, organizing, and delivering care; managing care within the framework of redesigned health care and within financial constraints through the development of critical paths; identifying research questions; and monitoring the outcomes of nursing care both at an individual level and at the level of service provision to large populations of patients.

Nurse investigators at the University of Iowa have developed Nursing Outcomes Classification (NOC), a taxonomy of patient outcomes that are sensitive to nursing interventions. The authors of this outcomes taxonomy state, "For the nursing profession to become a full participant in clinical evaluation research, policy development, and interdisciplinary work, it is essential that patient outcomes influenced by nursing care be identified and measured" (Moorhead and others, 2008, p. 9). In this context, an outcome is defined as the status of the patient or family that follows and is directly influenced by nursing interventions.

The following portion of this chapter guides the user of this text through the steps of individualized care plan development. It also contains recommendations about how this book can be used to ensure safe and quality care, as a tool for quality improvement work and creating seamless nursing care delivery regardless of where in the continuum of health care the patient happens to be, for the development of patient education materials, and as the basis of critical path development.

Using *Nursing Care Plans: Diagnoses, Interventions, and Outcomes*

Developing an Individualized Care Plan

The nursing care plan is best thought of as a written reflection of the nursing process: What does the assessment reveal? What should be done? How, when, and where should these planned interventions be carried out? What is the desired outcome? That is, will the delivery of planned interventions result in the desired goal? The nurse's ability to carry out this process in a systematic fashion, using all available information and resources, is the fundamental basis for nursing practice. This process includes correctly identifying existing needs, as well as recognizing potential needs and/or risks. Planning and delivering care in an individualized fashion to address these actual or potential needs, as well as evaluating the effectiveness of that care, is the basis for excellence in nursing practice. Forming a partnership with the patient and/or caregiver in this process and humanizing the experience of being a care recipient is the essence of nursing.

The Assessment

All the information that the nurse collects regarding a particular patient makes up the assessment. This assessment allows a nursing diagnosis, or clinical judgment, to be made. This, in turn, drives the identification of expected outcomes (i.e., what is desired by and for this particular patient in relation to this identified need) and the care plan. Without a comprehensive assessment, all else is a "shot in the dark."

Nurses have always carried out the task of assessment. As science and technology progress, information is more abundant than at any other time in history; however, length of contact with each patient becomes shorter, so astute assessment skills are essential to a nurse's ability to plan and deliver effective nursing care.

Assessment data are abundant in any clinical setting. What the nurse observes, what a history (written or verbal) reveals, what the patient and/or caregiver reports (or fails to report) about a situation, problem, or concern, and what laboratory and other diagnostic information is available are all valid and important data.

Methods useful in gathering these diverse data include interview, direct and indirect observation, physical assessment, medical records review, and analysis and synthesis of available laboratory and other diagnostic studies. The sum of all information obtained through any or all of these means allows the nurse to make a nursing diagnosis.

Gordon's (1976) definition of a nursing diagnosis includes only those problems that nurses are capable of treating, whereas others have expanded the definition to include any health-related issue with which a nurse may interface. In *Nursing Care Plans: Diagnoses, Interventions, and Outcomes* the nursing diagnosis terminology conforms to the NANDA International *Nursing Diagnoses: Definitions & Classification, 2009-2011* unless otherwise stated.

Performing the Assessment

A nurse has knowledge in the physical and behavioral sciences, is a trusted member of the health care team, and is the interdisciplinary team member who has the most contact with a patient. Because of these qualities, a nurse is in a key position to collect data from the patient and/or caregiver at any point at which the patient enters the health care continuum, whether in the home, in a hospital, in an outpatient clinic, or in a long-term care facility.

Interviewing is an important method of gathering information about a patient. The interview has the added dimensions of providing the nurse with the patient's subjective input on not only the problem but also what the patient may feel about the causes of the problem, how the problem has affected the patient as an individual, what outcomes the patient wants in relation to the particular problem, as well as insight into how the patient and/or caregiver may or may not be capable of participating in management of the problem.

Good interviewing skills are founded on rapport with the patient, the skill of active listening, and preparation in a systematic, thorough format with comprehensive attention given to specific health-related problems. The nurse as the interviewer must be knowledgeable of the patient's overall condition and the environment in which the interview will take place. A comprehensive interview that includes exploration of all the functional health patterns is ideal and will provide the best overall picture of the patient. When time is a limiting factor, the nurse may review existing medical records or other documents before the interview so that the interview can be focused. Care must be taken, however, to not "miss the forest for the trees" by conducting an interview in a fashion that precludes the discovery of important information the patient may have to share.

During an interview the patient may report the following types of information:
- Bothersome or unusual signs and symptoms (e.g., "I have been having cramps and bloody diarrhea for the past month.")
- Changes noticed (e.g., "It's a lot worse when I drink milk.")

- The impact of these problems on his or her ability to carry out desired or necessary activities (e.g., "I know every washroom at the mall. It's tough having lunch with friends.")
- Issues associated with the primary problem (e.g., "It's so embarrassing when my stomach starts to rumble loudly.")
- The impact of these problems on significant others (e.g., "My daughter cannot understand why a trip to the zoo feels like a challenge.")
- What specifically caused the patient to seek attention (e.g., "The amount of blood in the past couple of days really has me worried, and the pain is getting worse.")

In addition, the patient may share the following:

- Previous experiences or history (e.g., "My brother has had Crohn's disease for several years; this is how he started out.")
- Health beliefs and feelings about the problem (e.g., "I have always figured it would catch up with me sooner or later, with all the problems like this in our family.")
- Thoughts on what would help solve the problem (e.g., "Maybe I should watch my diet better.")
- What has been successful in the past in solving similar problems (e.g., "They kept my brother out of surgery for years with just a diet and medicine.")

From this scenario, it is clear that the interviewing nurse would want to explore issues of elimination, pain, nutrition, knowledge, and coping.

Information necessary to begin forming diagnoses has been provided, along with enough additional information to guide further exploration. In this example, the nurse may choose diarrhea as the diagnosis. Using NANDA-I–approved related factors for diarrhea, the nurse will want to explore stress and anxiety, dietary specifics, medications the patient is taking, and the patient's personal and family history of bowel disease.

The defining characteristics for diarrhea (typical signs and symptoms) have been provided by the patient to be cramping; abdominal pain; increased frequency of bowel movements and sounds; loose, liquid stools; urgency; and changes in the appearance of the stool. These defining characteristics support the nursing diagnosis *diarrhea*.

To explore related concerns such as pain, nutrition, knowledge, and coping, the nurse should refer to defining characteristics for *imbalanced nutrition: less than body requirements; deficient knowledge; acute pain;* and *ineffective coping*. The nurse should then interview the patient further to determine the presence or absence of defining characteristics for these additional diagnoses.

To continue this example, the nurse might ask the patient the following questions: Have you lost weight? Of what does your typical breakfast/lunch/dinner consist? How is your appetite? Describe your abdominal cramping. How frequent is the discomfort? Does it awaken you at night? Does it interfere with your daily routine? On a scale of 1 to 10, with 10 being the worst pain you have

ever had, how bad is the cramping? Can you tell me about your brother's Crohn's disease? Have you ever been told by a doctor that you have Crohn's or a similar disease? How are you handling these problems? Have you been able to carry out your usual activities? What do you do to feel better? In asking these questions, the nurse can decide whether the four additional diagnoses (*imbalanced nutrition: less than body requirements; deficient knowledge; acute pain;* and *ineffective coping*) are supported as actual problems or are problems for which the patient may be at risk.

Family, caregivers, and significant others can also be interviewed. When the patient's condition makes him or her incapable of being interviewed, these may be the nurse's only sources of interview information.

Physical assessment provides the nurse with objective data regarding the patient and includes a general survey followed by a systematic assessment of the physical and mental conditions of the patient. Findings of the physical examination may support subjective data already given by the patient or may provide new information that requires additional interviewing. In reality, the interview continues as the physical assessment proceeds and as the patient focuses on particulars. The patient is then able to enhance earlier information, remember new information, become more comfortable with the nurse, and share additional information.

Patient comfort and cooperation are important considerations in performing the physical examination, as is privacy and an undisturbed environment. Explaining the need for assessment and what steps are involved is helpful in putting the patient at ease and gaining cooperation.

Methods used in physical assessment include inspection (performing systematic visual examination), auscultation (using a stethoscope to listen to the heart, lungs, major vessels, and abdomen), percussion (tapping body areas to elicit information about underlying tissues), and palpation (using light or heavy touch to feel for temperature, normal and abnormal structures, and any elicited subjective responses). The usual order of these assessment techniques is inspection, palpation, percussion, and auscultation, except during the abdominal portion of the physical examination. Percussion and palpation may alter a finding by moving gas and bowel fluid and changing bowel sounds. Therefore percussion and palpation should follow inspection and auscultation when the abdomen is being examined.

To continue the example, the nurse may note, through inspection, that the patient is a thin, pale, well-groomed young woman who is shifting her weight often and has a strained facial expression. When asked how she feels at the present, the patient gives additional support to the diagnoses *ineffective coping* and *deficient knowledge* ("I don't understand what is wrong with me; I feel tired and stressed out all the time lately"). Physical examination reveals a 10-pound weight loss, hyperactive bowel sounds, and abdominal pain, which is expressed when the nurse palpates the right and left lower quadrants of the patient's abdomen. These findings further support the nursing diagnoses *diarrhea; imbalanced nutrition: less than body requirements;* and *acute pain.*

Using General Versus Specific Care Plan Guides

General

At this point, the nurse has identified five nursing diagnoses: *diarrhea, imbalanced nutrition: less than body requirements, acute pain, deficient knowledge,* and *ineffective coping. Nursing Care Plans: Diagnoses, Interventions, and Outcomes* is organized to allow the nurse to build a care plan by using the primary nursing diagnoses care plans in Chapter 2. A nurse can also select, by medical diagnosis, a set of nursing diagnoses that have been clustered to address a specific medical diagnosis and then further individualize it for a particular patient.

Using the first method from Chapter 2, the nurse had every possible related factor and defining characteristic from which to choose to tailor the care plan to the individual patient. It is important to individualize these comprehensive care plans by highlighting those related factors, defining characteristics, assessment suggestions, and interventions that actually pertain to specific patients. Nurses should add any that may not be listed, customize frequencies for assessments and interventions, and specify realistic time frames for outcome achievement. (The blanket application of these standard care plans negates the basic premise of tailoring care to meet individual needs.) To complete the example used to demonstrate individualizing a care plan using this text, the nurse should select the nursing interventions based on the assessment findings, proceed with care delivery, and evaluate whether selected patient outcomes have been achieved.

Specific

Using the clustered diagnoses usually labeled by a medical diagnosis found in Chapters 3 to 14 (e.g., inflammatory bowel disease), the nurse has the added benefit of a brief definition of the medical diagnosis; an overview of typical management, including the setting (home, hospital, outpatient); synonyms that are useful in locating additional information through cross-referencing; and associated nursing diagnoses with related factors and defining characteristics. Again, it is important that aspects of these care plans be selected and applied (i.e., individualized) based on specific assessment data for a particular patient.

As a tool that guides nursing care delivery, the care plan must be updated and revised periodically to remain useful in care provision. Revisions are based on goal attainment, changes in the patient's condition, and response to interventions. In today's fast-paced, outpatient-oriented health care system, revision will be required often.

As the patient moves through the continuum of care, a well-developed care plan can enhance the continuity of care and contribute to seamless delivery of nursing care, regardless of the setting in which the care is provided. This will serve to replace replication with continuity and ultimately increase the patient's satisfaction with care delivery.

Ensuring Quality and Safety

Ever since the 1999 Institute of Medicine published its landmark report, *To Err Is Human: Building a Safer Health System*, there has been a major focus on transforming the health care environment. With nurses as the largest provider of health care in this country, quality and safety must be "their job."

Nurses are well positioned to positively influence patient outcomes. These efforts are in concert with physicians and hospital administrators in pursuit of high-quality, safe care. Accreditation and regulatory bodies, professional nursing and medical societies, and quality improvement organizations alike are partnering to provide a culture of safety for patients and families. For example, in 2002 The Joint Commission (TJC) established its National Patient Safety Goals (NPSG) program to help accredited organizations address specific areas of concern in regard to patient safety. Some of the general performance measures identified as a means of reducing errors included "do not use" abbreviations, hand-off communication, standardized drug concentrations, infusion-pump free-flow protection, Centers for Disease Control and Prevention (CDC) hand hygiene guidelines, surgical site marking, "time-out" before surgery, and medication reconciliation. Although an extremely important part of medical and nursing practices, these procedures would not be described in a typical nursing care plan. Similarly, general guidelines for implementing evidence-based practices to prevent health care–associated infections caused by multiple-drug–resistant organisms, to prevent central line–associated bloodstream infections, and to prevent surgical site infections, although critical to patient safety, are also not routinely found in a typical care plan.

In contrast, the Patient Safety Indicators recommended by the Agency for Healthcare Research and Quality (AHRQ) provide information about potentially preventable complications and adverse events for a variety of diagnoses or procedures, and these are incorporated into relevant care plans in *Nursing Care Plans: Diagnoses, Interventions, and Outcomes*. Some examples include attention to fall assessment and prevention, pressure ulcer assessment and prevention, pain management, prevention of pulmonary embolism or deep vein thrombosis, prevention of postoperative sepsis, prevention of hospital-acquired pneumonia, and avoidance of selected infections as a result of medical care. Moreover, TJC provides National Quality Improvement Goals and Guidelines that when followed by health care providers have resulted in faster patient recoveries with fewer complications. Some of these include pneumonia care, acute myocardial infarction care, heart failure care, blood clot prevention, and surgical infection prevention care. These measures are highlighted in the respective care plans.

Finally, when evidence-based practice and clinical practice guidelines are used to guide health care decisions and deliver care, the best patient outcomes are achieved. Such guidelines, when available, are well integrated into the plans of care in *Nursing Care Plans: Diagnoses, Interventions, and Outcomes.* Nurses are reminded that a key element in evidence-based clinical decision making is the responsibility to personalize the evidence to apply to a specific patient's values and circumstances. Even the best research evidence cannot be followed blindly.

Tools for Performance Improvement

This book can also be used to identify outcome criteria in quality improvement projects and in the development of monitoring tools. For example, a nursing department, home health agency, or interdisciplinary pain management team may be interested in monitoring and improving its pain management outcomes. Using the Chapter 2 care plan for *acute pain,* the process of pain management can be monitored simply by using each assessment and intervention as a measurable indicator. The outcome of pain management assessment and intervention can also be studied through direct observation, records review, and/or patient satisfaction measures. There has been increasing focus on the interrelatedness of services and systems. The care plans in this text include independent and collaborative assessment suggestions and interventions, which facilitate use of the care plans as tools for quality improvement activities. Nurses, other health care professionals, clinical managers, and risk management and quality improvement staff will find that the care plans in this text provide specific, measurable detail and language. This aids in the development of monitoring tools for a broad scope of clinical issues.

Finally, when benchmarks are surpassed and there is desire to improve an aspect of care, the plans of care in *Nursing Care Plans: Diagnoses, Interventions and Outcomes* contain state-of-the-art information that will be helpful in planning corrections or improvements. These outcomes can be measured after implementation. The similarities between the nursing process (assess, plan, intervene, and evaluate) and accepted methods for quality improvement (measure, plan improvements, implement, and remeasure) make these care plan guides natural tools for use in performance improvement activities.

Development of Patient Education Materials

Education of patients and their families/significant others has always been a priority role for nurses. *Nursing Care Plans: Diagnoses, Interventions, and Outcomes* is an excellent source book for key procedural and self-care information to share with patients for over 200 medical problems. It also provides guidance for teaching both the population of ill patients and healthier clients seeking health promotion and disease prevention strategies. Educational content is provided using two formats. For the Chapter 2 general nursing diagnoses, a separate section on Education/Continuity of Care is found near the end of each plan of care. This chapter also provides a more general overview of key educational assessments and interventions pertaining to all learners, as found in the *deficient knowledge* and the *health-seeking behaviors* care plans. The subsequent chapters using the clustered medical diagnoses have the patient education material integrated throughout the care plan, rather than in a separate section at the end. These interventions, along with associated rationales, follow the Ask Me 3 directive on health literacy, which recommends that patient education sessions provide answers to the following questions: What is my main problem? What do I need to do? Why is it important for me to do this? For some medical problems that require a larger focus on education and self-management, a separate nursing diagnosis of *deficient knowledge* may be found within the care plan.

A Basis for Clinical Paths

Clinical paths (also called critical paths or pathways, or care maps) are interdisciplinary care plans to which time frames have been added. The clinical path is designed to track the care of a patient based on average and expected lengths of stay in an acute care setting. Clinical paths can also be developed for the home care and long-term care settings. The path provides guidelines about the sequence of care provided by the various members of the health care team responsible for the care of the patient. Interventions in a specific clinical path may include patient education, diet therapy progression, medications, consultations and referrals to other members of the health care team, activity progression, and discharge planning. The nurse is usually responsible for implementing and monitoring the patient's progress and noting deviations from the suggested time frame.

Clinical paths are useful in organizing care delivered to a specific population of patients for whom a measurable sequence of outcomes is readily identifiable. For example, most patients having total hip replacement sit on the edge of their beds by the end of the operative day and are up in a chair by noon on the first postoperative day. They also resume a regular diet intake and stand by the end of the first postoperative day. They progress to oral analgesics by the third postoperative day and are ready for discharge on the fifth postoperative day. Every patient with total hip replacement may not progress according to this path because of individual factors such as other medical diagnoses, development of complications, or simple individual variation. However, most will, and as such, a clinical path can be a powerful tool not only in guiding care but also in monitoring use of precious resources and making comparative judgments about outcomes of one physician group, hospital unit, or facility against external benchmarks. This may facilitate consumer decision making and enable those who finance health care to base judgments about referrals on outcome measures of specific physicians, hospitals, surgical centers, and other places.

The care plan forms the basis of a clinical path. *Nursing Care Plans: Diagnoses, Interventions, and Outcomes* can be used as the clinical basis from which to begin the development of the clinical path. Because nursing care plans in this text are organized by nursing diagnoses, adaptation of these care plans into clinical paths may require organizing the information differently.

References

Bulechek G, Butcher H, Dochterman J, editors: *Nursing Interventions Classification (NIC)*, ed 5, St. Louis, 2008, Mosby.

Gordon M: Nursing diagnosis and the diagnostic process, *American Journal of Nursing* 76:1298, 1976.

Moorhead S, Johnson M, Maas M, Swanson E, editors: *Nursing Outcomes Classification (NOC)*, ed 4, St. Louis, 2008, Mosby.

CHAPTER

2

Nursing Diagnosis Care Plans

 NANDA-I NDx **Activity Intolerance**

Definition: Insufficient physiological or psychological energy to endure or complete required or desired daily activities

Most activity intolerance is related to generalized weakness and debilitation secondary to acute or chronic illness and disease. This is especially apparent in older patients with a history of orthopedic, cardiopulmonary, diabetic, or pulmonary-related problems. The aging process itself causes reduction in muscle strength and function, which can impair the ability to maintain activity. Activity intolerance may also be related to factors such as obesity, malnourishment, anemia, side effects of medications (e.g., β-blockers), or emotional states such as depression or lack of confidence to exert oneself. Nursing goals are to reduce the effects of inactivity, promote optimal physical activity, and assist the patient with maintaining a satisfactory quality of life.

Common Related Factors

Generalized weakness
Deconditioned state
Sedentary lifestyle
Insufficient sleep or rest periods
Depression or lack of motivation
Prolonged bed rest
Imposed activity restriction
Imbalance between oxygen supply and demand
Pain
Side effects of medications

Defining Characteristics

Verbal report of fatigue or weakness
Unable to endure or complete desired activities
Abnormal heart rate, BP, or respiratory response to activity
Exertional discomfort or dyspnea

Common Expected Outcomes

Patient exhibits activity tolerance as evidenced by rating of perceived exertion of 3 or less (0 to 10 scale), heart rate less than or equal to 120 beats/min (or within 20 beats/min of resting heart rate), systolic blood pressure (BP) within 20 mm Hg increase over resting systolic BP, respiratory rate less than 20 breaths/min, absence of chest pain or dyspnea.
Patient reports ability to perform required activities of daily living.
Patient verbalizes and uses energy-conservation techniques.

NOC Outcomes
Activity Tolerance; Energy Conservation; Knowledge: Treatment Regimen; Self Care: Activities of Daily Living

NIC Interventions
Energy Management; Teaching: Prescribed Activity/Exercise

Ongoing Assessment

Actions/Interventions

- Determine the patient's perception of causes of activity intolerance.
- Assess the patient's level of mobility.

- Assess nutritional status.
- Monitor the patient's sleep pattern and amount of sleep achieved over the past few days.
- Assess the need for ambulation aids: bracing, cane, walker, equipment modification for ADLs.

- Assess the patient's baseline cardiopulmonary status before initiating activity using the following measures:
  - Heart rate
  - Orthostatic BP changes

- Assess patient's perception of effort required to perform each activity.

- Observe and document response to activity. Signs of abnormal responses to be reported include the following:
  - Increased heart rate of 20 to 30 beats/min over resting rate, or 120 beats/min
  - Palpitations/noticeable change in heart rhythm
  - Significant increase in systolic BP (greater than 20 mm Hg)
  - Significant decrease in systolic BP (greater than 10 mm Hg)
  - Dyspnea, labored breathing, wheezing
  - Excessive weakness, fatigue
  - Light-headedness, dizziness, pallor, diaphoresis
  - Chest discomfort
- Assess emotional response to limitations in physical abilities.
- Evaluate the need for oxygen with increased activity.

Rationales

Causative factors may be temporary or permanent, physical or psychological. Assessment guides treatment.

This information will serve as a basis for formulating realistic short- and long-term goals.

Adequate energy reserves are required for activity.

Difficulties sleeping need to be addressed before activity progression can be achieved.

Some aids may require more energy expenditure for patients who have reduced upper arm strength (e.g., walking with crutches). Adequate assessment of energy requirements is indicated.

Close monitoring serves as a guide. Heart rate should not increase more than 20 to 30 beats/min above resting with routine activities. This number will change depending on the intensity of activity the patient is attempting (e.g., climbing one flight of stairs versus walking on a flat surface). Older patients are more susceptible to orthostatic drops in blood pressure with position changes.

The Borg Scale uses ratings from 0 to 10 to determine rating of perceived exertion. A rating of 2 (light) to 3 (moderate) is an acceptable level for most people performing activities of daily living. Higher ratings are used for high-intensity physical exercise.

Close monitoring serves as a guide for optimal progression of activity.

Depression over inability to perform desired/required activities can be a source of stress and aggravation.

Portable pulse oximetry can be used to assess for oxygen desaturation. Supplemental oxygen may help compensate for the increased oxygen demands.

Therapeutic Interventions

Actions/Interventions

- Establish guidelines and goals of activity with the patient and caregiver.

Rationales

Motivation is enhanced if the patient participates in goal setting. Depending on the etiological factors of the activity intolerance, some patients may be able to live independently and work outside the home. Other patients with chronic debilitating disease may remain homebound.

■ = Independent   ▲ = Collaborative

Actions/Interventions	Rationales
■ Evaluate need for additional help at home (e.g., housekeeper, neighbor to shop, family assistance).	Coordinated efforts are more meaningful and effective in assisting patient in conserving energy.
■ Encourage adequate rest periods, especially before meals, other ADLs, exercise sessions, and ambulation.	Rest between activities provides time for energy conservation and recovery. Heart rate recovery following activity is greatest at the beginning of a rest period.
■ Refrain from performing nonessential procedures.	Patients with limited activity tolerance need to prioritize tasks.
■ Anticipate the patient's needs (e.g., keep telephone and tissues within reach).	Attention to placement of commonly used supplies can reduce the risk for falling while reaching.
■ Assist with ADLs as indicated; however, avoid doing for patients what they can do for themselves.	Assisting the patient with ADLs allows for conservation of energy. Caregivers need to balance providing assistance with facilitating progressive endurance that will ultimately enhance the patient's activity tolerance and self-esteem.
■ Provide bedside commode as indicated.	Commode requires less energy expenditure than using a bedpan.
■ Encourage physical activity consistent with the patient's energy resources.	This promotes a sense of autonomy while being realistic about capabilities.
■ Assist patients with planning activities for times when they have the most energy.	Activities should be planned to coincide with the patient's peak energy level. Not all self-care and hygiene activities need to be completed in the morning. Likewise, not all housecleaning needs to be completed in one day.
■ Encourage verbalization of feelings regarding limitations.	Acknowledgment that living with activity intolerance is both physically and emotionally difficult aids coping.
■ Progress activity gradually, as with the following: • Active range-of-motion (ROM) exercises in bed, progressing to sitting and standing • Dangling the legs 10 to 15 minutes three times daily • Deep-breathing exercises three or more times daily • Sitting up in chair 30 minutes three times daily • Walking in room 1 to 2 minutes three times daily • Walking in the hall 25 feet or walking through the house, then slowly progressing to walking outside the house, saving energy for return trip	Appropriate progression prevents overexerting the heart while promoting attainment of short-range goals. Duration and frequency should be increased before intensity.
■ Encourage active ROM exercises. If further reconditioning is needed, confer with rehabilitation personnel.	Exercise maintains muscle strength, joint ROM, and exercise tolerance.
■ Encourage patient to choose activities that gradually build endurance.	Physically inactive patients need to improve functional capacity through repetitive exercises over a longer period of time. Strength training is valuable in enhancing endurance for many ADLs.
■ Provide emotional support while increasing activity. Promote a positive attitude regarding abilities.	Patients may be fearful of overexertion and potential damage to the heart. Appropriate supervision during early efforts can enhance confidence.
■ Provide the patient with the adaptive equipment needed for completing ADLs.	Appropriate aids will enable the patient to achieve optimal independence for self-care and reduce energy consumption during activity.

Education/Continuity of Care

Actions/Interventions	Rationales
■ Teach the patient and caregivers to recognize signs of physical overactivity.	Knowledge promotes awareness of when to reduce activity.
■ Involve the patient and caregivers in goal setting and care planning.	Setting small, attainable goals can increase self-confidence and self-esteem.

Nursing Diagnosis Care Plans

Actions/Interventions

▲ When the patient is hospitalized, arrange for a physical therapist to assess the need for family or significant others to bring in an ambulation aid (e.g., walker, cane) from home.

■ Teach the importance of continued activity at home.

■ Assist in assigning priority to activities to accommodate energy levels.

■ Teach energy-conservation techniques, such as the following:
  - Sitting to do tasks
  - Changing positions often
  - Pushing rather than pulling
  - Sliding rather than lifting
  - Working at an even pace
  - Placing frequently used items within easy reach
  - Resting for at least 1 hour after meals before starting a new activity
  - Using wheeled carts for laundry, shopping, and cleaning needs
  - Organizing a work-rest-work schedule

■ Teach appropriate use of environmental aids (e.g., bed rails, elevating head of bed while patient gets out of bed, chair in bathroom, hall rails).

■ Teach ROM and strengthening exercises.

■ Encourage patient to verbalize concerns about discharge and home environment.

■ Refer to community resources as indicated.

Rationales

The patient can begin to make connection/transition to home, and the staff can assess proper functioning and use of assistive devices.

Consistent activity maintains strength, ROM, and endurance gain.

With a reduced functional capacity, pacing of priority tasks first may better meet the patient's needs.

Energy-conservation techniques reduce oxygen consumption, allowing more prolonged activity. For example, standing requires more work than sitting, evenly paced work allows enough time so not all work is completed in a short period.

These aids conserve energy and reduce the risk for falls.

Exercise promotes increased venous return, prevents contractures, and maintains/increases muscle strength and endurance.

Verbalization can reduce feelings of anxiety and fear and open doors for ongoing communication.

Continuity of care is facilitated through the use of community resources. Supervised programs in a structured environment may be beneficial.

Ineffective Airway Clearance

Definition: Inability to clear secretions or obstructions from the respiratory tract to maintain a clear airway

Maintaining a patent airway is vital to life. Coughing is the main mechanism for clearing the airway. However, the cough may be ineffective in both normal and disease states secondary to factors such as pain from surgical incisions or trauma, respiratory muscle fatigue, or neuromuscular weakness. Other mechanisms that exist in the lower bronchioles and alveoli to maintain the airway include the mucociliary system, macrophages, and the lymphatics. Factors such as anesthesia and dehydration can affect function of the mucociliary system. Likewise, conditions that cause increased production of secretions (e.g., pneumonia, bronchitis, and chemical irritants) can overtax these mechanisms. Ineffective airway clearance can be an acute (e.g., postoperative recovery) or chronic (e.g., from cerebrovascular accident [CVA] or spinal cord injury) problem. Older patients, who have an increased incidence of emphysema and a higher prevalence of chronic cough or sputum production, are at high risk.

Common Related Factors

Decreased energy and fatigue
Tracheobronchial infection
Tracheobronchial obstruction (including foreign body aspiration)
Copious and tenacious tracheobronchial secretions
Impaired respiratory muscle function
Presence of artificial airway
Airway spasm/asthma
Neuromuscular dysfunction

Defining Characteristics

Abnormal breath sounds (crackles, rhonchi, wheezes)
Changes in respiratory rate or depth
Hypoxemia/cyanosis
Dyspnea
Ineffective cough
Excessive secretions
Orthopnea

Common Expected Outcome

Patient will maintain clear open airways as evidenced by normal breath sounds, normal rate and depth of respirations, and ability to effectively cough up secretions after treatments and deep breaths.

NOC Outcome
Respiratory Status: Airway Patency
NIC Interventions
Cough Enhancement; Airway Management; Airway Suctioning

Ongoing Assessment

Actions/Interventions	Rationales
■ Assess airway for patency.	Maintaining the airway is always the first priority, especially in cases of trauma, acute neurological decompensation, or cardiac arrest.
■ Auscultate lungs after coughing for presence of adventitious breath sounds, as in the following:	Diminished breath sounds or the presence of adventitious sounds may indicate an obstructed airway.
• Decreased or absent breath sounds	These may indicate presence of a mucous plug or other major airway obstruction.
• Wheezing	Wheezing may indicate partial airway obstruction or resistance.
• Coarse crackles	Crackles may indicate presence of secretions along larger airways.
■ Assess respirations; note quality, rate, rhythm, depth, flaring of nostrils, dyspnea on exertion, evidence of splinting, use of accessory muscles, and position for breathing.	Abnormality indicates respiratory compromise. An increase in respiratory rate and rhythm may be a compensatory response for airway obstruction.
■ Assess changes in level of consciousness.	Increasing confusion, restlessness, and/or irritability can be early signs of cerebral hypoxia. Lethargy and somnolence are late signs.
■ Assess changes in HR, BP, and temperature.	Tachycardia and hypertension may be related to increased work of breathing or hypoxia. Fever may develop in response to retained secretions or atelectasis or may be a manifestation of an infectious or inflammatory process.
■ Assess cough for effectiveness and productivity.	Coughing is the most helpful way to remove secretions. Possible causes of ineffective cough may be respiratory muscle fatigue, severe bronchospasm, or thick and tenacious secretions.
■ Assess secretions, noting color, viscosity, odor, and amount.	Abnormalities may be a result of infection, bronchitis, chronic smoking, or other condition. A sign of infection is discolored sputum (no longer clear or white); an odor may be present. Thick, tenacious secretions increase airway resistance and work of breathing and may be indicative of dehydration.
▲ Send a sputum specimen for culture and sensitivity testing, as appropriate.	Respiratory infections increase the work of breathing; antibiotic treatment is indicated.

Actions/Interventions

▲ Use pulse oximetry to monitor oxygen saturation; assess arterial blood gases (ABGs).

■ Assess hydration status: skin turgor, mucous membranes, tongue.
■ Assess for abdominal or thoracic pain.
▲ If the patient is on mechanical ventilator, monitor for peak airway pressures and airway resistance.
■ Assess use of herbal remedies (e.g., echinacea for upper respiratory infections, goldenseal for pneumonia, ma huang for bronchospasm).

■ Assess the patient's knowledge of disease process.

Rationales

Pulse oximetry is a useful tool to detect chages in oxygenation. Oxygen saturation should be maintained at 90% or greater. Increasing $Paco_2$ and decreasing Pao_2 and pulse oximetry readings can result from increased pulmonary secretions and respiratory fatigue.

Airway clearance is impaired with inadequate hydration and subsequent secretion thickening.

Pain can result in shallow breathing and an ineffective cough.

Increases in these parameters signal accumulation of secretions or fluid and potential for ineffective ventilation.

Drug interactions with prescribed medications and contraindications need to be evaluated (e.g., ma huang contains ephedrine, which should not be used by patients with hypertension, heart disease, prostatic hyperplasia, or diabetes).

Patient education will vary depending on the acute or chronic disease state as well as the patient's cognitive level.

Therapeutic Interventions

Actions/Interventions

■ Assist the patient in performing coughing and breathing maneuvers.
■ Instruct the patient in the following:
  • Optimal positioning (sitting position)
  • Use of pillow or hand splints when coughing
  • Use of abdominal muscles for more forceful cough
  • Use of quad and huff techniques
  • Use of incentive spirometry
  • Importance of ambulation and frequent position changes
■ Use upright position (if tolerated, head of bed at 45 degrees; sitting in chair). If patient is bedridden, routinely check the patient's position so he or she does not slide down in bed.
▲ If cough is ineffective, use nasotracheal suctioning as needed based on presence of adventitious lung sounds and/or increased ventilatory pressure.
  • Explain procedure to patient.

  • Use well-lubricated soft catheters.

  • Use curved-tip catheters and head positioning (if not contraindicated).
  • Instruct the patient to take several deep breaths before and after each nasotracheal suctioning procedure and use supplemental oxygen, as appropriate.
  • Stop suctioning and provide supplemental oxygen (assisted breaths by resuscitation bag as needed) if the patient experiences bradycardia, an increase in ventricular ectopy, and/or significant desaturation.
  • Use universal precautions: gloves, goggles, and mask, as appropriate.

Rationales

Coughing is the most helpful way to remove most secretions. The patient may be unable to perform independently.

Controlled coughing techniques help mobilize secretions from smaller airways to larger airways because the coughing is done at varying times. The sitting position and splinting the abdomen promote more effective coughing by increasing abdominal pressure and upward diaphragmatic movement. Ambulation helps maintain adequate lung expansion, mobilizes secretions, and reduces atelectasis.

Upright position prevents abdominal contents from pushing upward and inhibiting lung expansion. This position promotes better lung expansion and improved air exchange.

Suctioning is indicated when patients are unable to remove secretions from the airways by coughing because of weakness, thick mucous plugs, or excessive or tenacious mucus production. It can also stimulate a cough. Frequency of suctioning should be based on patient's clinical status, not on preset routine, such as every 2 hours. Oversuctioning can cause hypoxia and injury to bronchial and lung tissue.

Suctioning with a well-lubricated catheter minimizes irritation and prevents trauma to mucous membranes.

These facilitate secretion removal from a specific side (right versus left lung).

Hyperoxygenation before, during, and after suctioning decreases hypoxia related to suctioning procedure.

Oxygen therapy is indicated to increase oxygen saturation and reduce potential complications.

These precautions prevent transmission of pathogenic microorganisms.

■ = Independent ▲ = Collaborative

Actions/Interventions	Rationales
▲ Institute appropriate isolation precautions for positive cultures (e.g., methicillin-resistant *Staphylococcus aureus* [MRSA] or tuberculosis).	These precautions prevent transmission of pathogenic microorganisms.
■ Maintain humidified oxygen as prescribed.	Increasing humidity of inspired air will decrease viscosity of secretions and facilitate their removal.
■ Encourage increased fluid intake within the limits of cardiac reserve and renal function.	Maintaining hydration increases ciliary action to remove secretions and reduces viscosity of secretions. It is easier for the patient to mobilize thinner secretions with coughing.
▲ Administer medications (e.g., antibiotics, inhaled steroids, mucolytic agents, bronchodilators, expectorants) as ordered, noting effectiveness and side effects.	A variety of medications are available to treat specific problems. Most promote clearance of airway secretions and may reduce airway resistance.
▲ Consult a respiratory therapist for chest physiotherapy and nebulizer treatments as indicated (hospital and home care or rehabilitation environments).	Chest physiotherapy includes the techniques of postural drainage and chest percussion to loosen and mobilize secretions smaller airways that cannot be removed by coughing or suctioning. A nebulizer may be used to humidify the airway to thin secretions to facilitate their removal; it may also be used to deliver bronchodilators and mucolytic agents.
▲ Coordinate optimal time for postural drainage and percussion (i.e., at least 1 hour after eating).	This measure reduces aspiration.
■ For patients with reduced energy, pace activities. Maintain planned rest periods. Promote energy-conservation techniques.	Fatigue is a contributing factor to ineffective coughing. Effective coughing is hard work and may exhaust an already compromised patient.
▲ For acute problems, anticipate bronchoscopy.	Bronchoscopy obtains lavage samples for culture and sensitivity testing and removes mucous plugs.
▲ If secretions cannot be cleared, anticipate the need for an artificial airway (intubation). After intubation, do the following: • Institute suctioning of the airway as determined by the presence of adventitious sounds, increased peak airway pressures, and visible secretions in the tubing.	Being prepared for an emergency helps prevent further complications. Intubation may be needed to facilitate removal of tenacious or copious amounts of secretions and provide source for augmenting oxygenation.
■ For patients with complete airway obstruction, institute appropriate basic life support measures.	These measures are used to relieve airway obstructions and to sustain life until definitive treatment can be provided.

Education/Continuity of Care

Actions/Interventions	Rationales
■ Teach coughing, breathing, and splinting techniques.	These techniques facilitate clearance of secretions and prevent atelectasis. Dyspnea may be reduced by pursed-lip or diaphragmatic breathing.
■ Instruct the patient in how to use prescribed medications and inhalers, as appropriate.	Instruction promotes safe and effective medication administration.
■ In the home setting, instruct caregivers regarding the need for humidification and adequate hydration.	Thin secretions are easier to clear from the airway.
■ Instruct caregivers in suctioning techniques. Provide opportunity for return demonstration. Adapt techniques for the home setting.	Instruction promotes safe and effective removal of secretions from the airway.
■ For patients with debilitating disease (e.g., CVA, neuromuscular impairment) being cared for at home, instruct caregivers in chest physiotherapy, as appropriate.	Chest physiotherapy loosens and mobilizes secretions.
■ Teach the patient about environmental factors that can precipitate respiratory problems.	Chemical irritants and allergens can increase mucus production and bronchospasm.
■ Explain effects of smoking, including secondhand smoke. Refer the patient and/or significant others to smoking-cessation group, as appropriate.	Chemical irritants and allergens can increase mucus production and bronchospasm.

Actions/Interventions

▲ Refer to the pulmonary clinical nurse specialist, home health nurse, or respiratory therapist as indicated.

■ Refer to the American Lung Association Call Center and support groups (e.g., Better Breathers Club).

Rationales

Use of consultants may be required to ensure that patient needs are met and outcomes achieved.

Support groups provide emotional support and information that may assist patients in coping with chronic illness.

Related Care Plans

Pneumonia, p. 429
Tracheostomy, p. 461
Tuberculosis, p. 468

NANDA-I

Latex Allergy Response

Definition: A hypersensitive reaction to natural latex rubber products

Latex allergy is a hypersensitivity reaction to the proteins in natural rubber latex derived from the sap of the rubber tree, *Hevea brasiliensis.* Products made from synthetic rubber may be called *latex* but do not contain the proteins known to cause an allergic response. The incidence of latex allergy increased after 1985 with the introduction of standard precautions to prevent the spread of bloodborne pathogens such as the human immunodeficiency virus. Soft rubber products such as gloves have the highest content of latex protein and the most potential to cause an allergic response. The people at highest risk for latex allergy include those who wear latex gloves as part of their jobs, such as health care workers, food service workers, housekeepers, and hairdressers. People employed in industries that manufacture latex rubber products are at risk, too. Another group of people at risk are those who undergo repeated surgeries, especially if the surgeries begin in childhood. Evidence indicates a high incidence of latex allergy in people with spina bifida who have had multiple surgeries in childhood. People with a variety of food allergies and sensitivities also have increased risk for latex allergy. Natural latex rubber allergies are IgE-mediated reactions to at least 10 different low–molecular-weight water-soluble proteins contained in the rubber tree sap. The range of hypersensitivity reactions to latex rubber include mild to severe contact dermatitis, respiratory allergic symptoms, and anaphylaxis.

Common Related Factor

Hypersensitivity to natural latex rubber protein

Defining Characteristics

Life-threatening reactions occurring less than 1 hour after exposure to latex protein:
- Bronchospasm
- Dyspnea
- Wheezing
- Respiratory arrest
- Hypotension
- Cardiac arrest
- Contact urticaria progressing to generalized symptoms
- Orofacial edema
- Abdominal pain
- Flushing and erythema
- Restlessness

■ = Independent   ▲ = Collaborative

Type IV hypersensitivity reactions:
Delayed reactions
- Eczema
- Redness
- Irritation
Irritant reactions
- Erythema
- Chapped, cracked skin
- Blisters

Common Expected Outcomes

Patient implements strategies to avoid exposure to sources of latex rubber.
Patient seeks immediate treatment for symptoms of latex allergy response.

NOC Outcomes
Allergic Response: Localized; Immune Hypersensitivity Response; Tissue Integrity: Skin and Mucous Membranes

NIC Interventions
Latex Precautions; Allergy Management

Ongoing Assessment

Actions/Interventions	Rationales
■ Assess for history of myelomeningocele or urogenital abnormalities in childhood.	Multiple surgeries to correct congenital neural tube defects or urinary tract abnormalities in childhood are associated with increased risk for latex allergy.
■ Assess for history of food allergies to bananas, avocados, tomatoes, kiwi, mangos, and chestnuts.	These foods have proteins similar to latex rubber. People with these specific food allergies may have a cross sensitivity to latex. These foods are associated with anaphylactic reactions in people with latex sensitivity.
■ Assess for a history of allergic reactions to figs, apples, celery, melon, potatoes, papayas, cherries, and peaches.	People with sensitivity to these foods have been found to be at higher risk for developing latex allergy.
■ Assess for allergic reactions after contact with products containing latex such as blowing up a balloon, using a condom or diaphragm, undergoing a vaginal or rectal examination, wearing latex gloves, or doing other work-related activities that involved exposure to latex.	People may not be aware of latex allergy. Symptoms may have developed after blowing up a balloon, medical or dental procedures where latex products were used, or in the work environment. The person may not have associated the symptoms with exposure to latex. The symptoms may have included skin rash, itching, swelling, hives, shortness of breath, runny nose, or cough.
▲ Refer the patient for immunological testing for latex sensitivity.	Diagnostic tests are available to detect IgE immunoglobulins specific to latex and related compounds. Skin prick testing also may be used to identify latex allergy.

Therapeutic Interventions

Actions/Interventions	Rationales
For the hospitalized patient:	
■ Place allergy band on the patient.	All health care providers need to be notified of the patient's latex allergy.
■ Record latex allergy in the patient's medical record and post a sign over the patient's bed about latex allergy.	Visible signs are used to increase the awareness of all providers and reduce possible exposure to latex.
■ Remove latex products from the patient's immediate environment.	All latex products need to be removed from the patient's environment to reduce exposure. These products include blood pressure cuffs, gloves, adhesive tape, tourniquets, injection ports, electrode pads, stethoscope tubing, rubber syringe stoppers, and medication vial stoppers.

Actions/Interventions	**Rationales**
■ Place latex-free equipment in the patient's room.	Most hospitals have latex-free equipment available from the central supply department. It may be necessary to have an emergency crash cart available with latex-free equipment.
■ Use powder-free, nonlatex gloves for any care activities requiring glove use.	Cornstarch powder is added to latex gloves during manufacturing. The powder reduces the stickiness of the latex to increase ease of putting on and removing gloves. Research shows that latex protein adheres to the powder. When the gloves are removed, the powder with the attached latex protein is aerosolized. Inhalation of the particles in the air accounts for the respiratory symptoms experienced by the person with a latex allergy.
■ If latex products must be used (tubing, blood pressure cuffs, tourniquets), wrap the patient's extremity with cotton gauze before applying the equipment.	This measure will reduce direct contact between the patient's skin and the latex protein.
▲ Administer medications as prescribed.	Antihistamines, corticosteroids, and H_2-histamine blockers are used as premedications if the patient is undergoing procedures in which latex exposure may occur. Steroids and antihistamines can be used topically or orally to control local allergic reactions such as contact dermatitis.
▲ Initiate appropriate emergency care if the patient shows signs of an acute systemic reaction.	Measures to maintain airway patency, breathing effectiveness, and circulation are priorities. Drug therapy may include epinephrine and steroids to reverse the allergic reaction.

Education/Continuity of Care

Actions/Interventions	**Rationales**
■ Educate the patient and family members about signs and symptoms of latex allergy reaction: skin rash; hives; flushing; itching; nasal, eye, or sinus symptoms; asthma; and shock.	Recognition of a latex allergy reaction is necessary for prompt treatment, especially to prevent progression of the reaction to anaphylaxis.
■ Educate the patient and family members about emergency treatment, as appropriate.	Patients with a high level of latex sensitivity and their families need to learn to use injectable epinephrine at the onset of respiratory symptoms. This action is necessary to reduce the risk for anaphylaxis.
■ Educate the patient and family about sources of latex in the home and work environment.	Patients and family members need to learn about sources of latex in the home and workplace. Sources of latex include balloons, condoms and diaphragms, rubber bands, adhesive tape, erasers, toys, sports equipment, carpet backing, elastic on clothing, computer mouse pads, buttons on electronic equipment, and shoe soles.
■ Encourage the patient to wear a medical alert tag, carry identification, and notify all health care providers about latex allergy.	Proper identification is necessary to reduce accidental exposure to latex during health care procedures.
■ Encourage the patient to notify his or her employer about latex allergy and ways to reduce workplace exposure.	Modifications in the workplace are necessary to reduce exposure to latex. The National Institute for Occupational Safety and Health has educational material about latex allergy and prevention.

■ = Independent ▲ = Collaborative

Anxiety

Definition: Vague uneasy feeling of discomfort or dread accompanied by an autonomic response (the source often nonspecific or unknown to the individual); a feeling of apprehension caused by anticipation of danger. It is an alerting signal that warns of impending danger and enables the individual to take measures to deal with the threat.

Anxiety is probably present at some level in every individual's life, but the degree and the frequency with which it manifests differ broadly. Each individual's response to anxiety is different. Some people are able to use the emotional edge that anxiety provokes to stimulate creativity or problem-solving abilities; others can become immobilized to a pathological degree. The feeling is generally categorized into four levels for treatment purposes: mild, moderate, severe, and panic. Mild anxiety can enhance a person's perception of the environment and his or her readiness to respond. Moderate anxiety is associated with a narrowing of the person's perception of the situation. The person with moderate anxiety may be more creative and more effective solving problems. Severe anxiety is associated with increasing emotional and physical feelings of discomfort. Perceptions are further narrowed. The person with severe anxiety begins to manifest excessive autonomic nervous system signs of the fight-or-flight stress response. The person in a panic stage of anxiety has distorted perceptions of the situation. His or her thinking skills become limited and irrational. The person may be unable to make decisions. In the severe and panic stages of anxiety, the nurse needs to intervene to promote patient safety. The nurse can encounter the anxious patient anywhere in the hospital or community. The presence of the nurse may lend support to the anxious patient and provide some strategies for traversing anxious moments or panic attacks.

Common Related Factors

Changes in or threats to:
- Economic status
- Environment
- Health status
- Interaction patterns
- Interpersonal relationships
- Role function or status
- Self-concept

Maturational or situational crises

Stress

Substance abuse

Unconscious conflict about essential life goals or values

Unmet needs

Defining Characteristics

Behavioral:
- Diminished productivity
- Expressed concerns about changes in life events
- Insomnia
- Restlessness

Affective:
- Apprehensive
- Feelings of inadequacy
- Focus on self
- Irritability
- Painful or persistent increased helplessness

Cognitive:
- Confusion
- Difficulty concentrating
- Diminished ability to learn or solve problems
- Fear of unspecified consequences

Physiological, sympathetic:
- Anorexia
- Diarrhea
- Dry mouth
- Facial flushing
- Increased blood pressure, pulse, respirations
- Twitching, increased reflexes

Physiological, parasympathetic:
- Abdominal pain
- Faintness
- Fatigue
- Nausea
- Urinary frequency, urgency

Common Expected Outcomes

Patient monitors signs and intensity of anxiety.

Patient uses effective coping mechanisms.

Patient describes a reduction in the level of anxiety experienced.

Patient maintains a desired level of role function and problem solving.

NOC Outcomes
Anxiety Self-Control; Coping
NIC Interventions
Anxiety Reduction; Presence; Calming Technique; Emotional Support

Ongoing Assessment

Actions/Interventions	Rationales
■ Assess patient's level of anxiety.	The person with mild anxiety will have minimal or no physiological symptoms of anxiety. Vital signs will be within normal ranges. The person will appear calm but may report feelings of nervousness such as "butterflies in the stomach." The person with moderate anxiety may appear energized with more animated facial expressions and tone of voice. Vital signs may be normal or slightly elevated. The person may report feeling tense. With severe anxiety, the person will have symptoms of increased autonomic nervous system activity, such as elevated vital signs, diaphoresis, urinary urgency and frequency, dry mouth, and muscle tension. The person may be agitated, irritable, and report feeling overloaded or overwhelmed by new stimuli. In the panic level of anxiety, the autonomic nervous system increases to the level of sympathetic neurotransmitter release. The person becomes pale, hypotensive, and experiences poor muscle coordination. The person reports feeling completely out of control and may display extremes of behavior from combativeness to withdrawal.
■ Use the State-Trait Anxiety Inventory to differentiate between the person's anxiety level as a temporary response state and a long-standing personality trait.	The State-Trait Anxiety Inventory, developed by Spielberger, is considered a definitive tool for measuring anxiety in adults. The tool is written at the sixth-grade reading level and is available in over 40 languages.
■ Determine how the patient uses defense mechanisms to cope with anxiety.	Interviewing the patient helps determine the effectiveness of coping strategies currently used by the patient. Defense mechanisms are used by people to preserve the ego and manage anxiety. Some defense mechanisms are highly adaptive in managing anxiety, such as humor, sublimation, or suppression. Other defense mechanisms may lead to less-adaptive behavior, especially with long-term use. These defense mechanisms include displacement, repression, denial, projection, and self-image splitting.
■ Suggest that the patient keep a log of episodes of anxiety. Instruct the patient to describe what is experienced and the events leading up to and surrounding the event. The patient should note how the anxiety dissipates.	The patient may use these notes to begin to identify trends that manifest anxiety. If the patient is comfortable with the idea, the log may be shared with the care provider, who may be helpful in problem solving. Symptoms often provide the care provider with information regarding the degree of anxiety being experienced. Physiological symptoms and/or complaints intensify as the level of anxiety increases.

■ = Independent   ▲ = Collaborative

Nursing Diagnosis Care Plans

Therapeutic Interventions

Actions/Interventions	Rationales
■ Acknowledge awareness of the patient's anxiety.	Because a cause for anxiety cannot always be identified, the patient may feel as though the feelings being experienced are counterfeit. Acknowledgment of the patient's feelings validates the feelings and communicates acceptance of those feelings.
■ Reassure the patient that he or she is safe. Stay with the patient if this appears necessary.	The presence of a trusted person may help the person feel less threatened. Anxiety may escalate to a panic level if the patient feels threatened and unable to control environmental stimuli.
■ Maintain a calm manner while interacting with the patient.	The health care provider can transmit his or her own anxiety to the hypersensitive patient. The patient's feeling of stability increases in a calm and nonthreatening atmosphere.
■ Establish a working relationship with the patient through continuity of care.	An ongoing relationship establishes a basis for comfort in communicating anxious feelings.
■ Orient the patient to the environment and new experiences or people as needed.	Orientation and awareness of the surroundings promote comfort and may decrease anxiety.
■ Use simple language and brief statements when instructing the patient about self-care measures or about diagnostic and surgical procedures.	When experiencing moderate to severe anxiety, patients may be unable to comprehend anything more than simple, clear, and brief instructions.
■ Reduce sensory stimuli by maintaining a quiet environment; keep "threatening" equipment out of sight.	Anxiety may escalate to a panic state with excessive conversation, noise, and equipment around the patient. Increasing anxiety may become frightening to the patient and others.
■ Encourage the patient to seek assistance from an understanding significant other or from the health care provider when anxious feelings become difficult.	The presence of significant others reinforces feelings of security for the patient.
■ Encourage the patient to talk about anxious feelings and examine anxiety-provoking situations if they are identifiable. Assist patient in assessing the situation realistically and recognizing factors leading to the anxious feelings. Avoid false reassurances.	Talking about anxiety-producing situations and anxious feelings can help the person perceive the situation in a less-threatening manner. Expressing emotions can enhance the patient's coping strategies.
■ As the patient's anxiety subsides, encourage exploration of specific events preceding both the onset and reduction of the anxious feelings.	Recognition and exploration of factors leading to or reducing anxious feelings are important steps in developing alternative responses. The patient may be unaware of the relationship between emotional concerns and anxiety.
■ Support the patient's use of coping strategies that the patient has found effective in the past.	Using anxiety-reduction strategies enhances the patient's sense of personal mastery and confidence.
■ Assist the patient in developing new anxiety-reducing skills (e.g., relaxation, deep breathing, positive visualization, and reassuring self-statements).	Learning new coping methods provides the patient with a variety of ways to manage anxiety.
■ Assist the patient in developing problem-solving abilities. Emphasize the logical strategies that the patient can use when experiencing anxious feelings.	Learning to identify a problem and to evaluate the alternatives to resolve that problem helps the patient cope.
■ Instruct the patient in the appropriate use of antianxiety medications.	Short-term use of antianxiety medications can enhance patient coping and reduce physiological manifestations of anxiety.
■ Teach the patient to limit use of central nervous system stimulants.	Stimulants, such as caffeine and nicotine, can increase physical symptoms of anxiety.

Education/Continuity of Care

Actions/Interventions	Rationales

■ Assist the patient in recognizing symptoms of increasing anxiety; explore alternatives to use to prevent the anxiety from immobilizing him or her.

The ability to recognize anxiety symptoms at lower intensity levels enables the patient to intervene more quickly to manage his or her anxiety. The patient will be able to use problem-solving abilities more effectively when the level of anxiety is low. Knowledge of anxiety and effective coping strategies can help the patient's feelings of control over anxiety-producing situations.

■ Remind the patient that anxiety at a mild level can encourage growth and development and is important in mobilizing changes.

Cognitive appraisal of mild anxiety can help the patient perceive the anxiety as an opportunity to develop new strengths that enhance coping.

■ Instruct the patient in the proper use of medications and educate him or her to recognize adverse reactions.

Medication may be used if the patient's anxiety continues to escalate and the anxiety becomes disabling.

▲ Refer the patient for psychiatric management of anxiety that becomes disabling for an extended period.

Additional, long-term professional care may be needed when anxiety becomes severe and interferes with daily functioning.

Risk for Aspiration

Definition: At risk for entry of gastrointestinal secretions, oropharyngeal secretions, solids, or fluids into tracheobronchial passages

Aspiration is the entry of secretions or materials such as foods/liquids into the trachea and lungs and occurs when protective reflexes are decreased or compromised. Aspiration from the oropharynx into the lungs can result in aspiration pneumonia. Depending on the acidity of the aspirate, even small amounts of gastric acid contents can damage lung tissue, resulting in chemical pneumonitis. Both acute and chronic conditions can place patients at risk for aspiration. Acute conditions, such as postanesthesia effects from surgery or diagnostic tests, occur predominantly in the acute care setting. Chronic conditions, including altered consciousness from head injury, spinal cord injury, neuromuscular weakness, hemiplegia and dysphagia from stroke, use of tube feedings for nutrition, and artificial airway devices such as tracheostomies, may be encountered in the home, rehabilitative, or hospital setting. Older and cognitively impaired patients are at high risk. Aspiration is a common cause of death in comatose patients. The National Quality Forum recommends that every patient should be evaluated for aspiration risk upon admission and periodically during the patient's stay.

Common Risk Factors

Reduced level of consciousness
Depressed cough or gag reflexes
Impaired swallowing
Presence of tracheostomy or endotracheal tube
Presence of gastrointestinal tubes
Tube feedings
Increased gastric residual
Anesthesia or medication administration
Decreased gastrointestinal motility
Drug or alcohol intoxication
Facial, oral, or neck surgery or trauma
Situations hindering elevation of upper body
Seizure activity
Advanced age

■ = Independent   ▲ = Collaborative

Common Expected Outcome

Patient maintains a patent airway as evidenced by normal breath sounds, absence of coughing, no shortness of breath, and no aspiration.

NOC Outcomes
Aspiration Control; Respiratory Status: Ventilation

NIC Interventions
Aspiration Precautions; Respiratory Monitoring

Ongoing Assessment

Actions/Interventions	Rationales
■ Monitor level of consciousness.	A decreased level of consciousness is a prime risk factor for aspiration.
■ Assess presence or absence of cough and gag reflexes.	The lungs are normally protected against aspiration by reflexes such as cough and gag. When these reflexes are absent or reduced, the patient is at increased risk.
■ Evaluate swallowing ability by assessing for the following: • Coughing, choking, throat clearing, gurgling or "wet" voice during or after swallowing • Residual food in mouth after eating • Regurgitation of food or fluid through the nares	Impaired swallowing increases the risk for aspiration. There remains a need for valid and easy-to-use methods to screen for aspiration risk.
▲ Assess results of swallowing studies as ordered.	For high-risk patients, performance of a videofluoroscopic swallowing study may be indicated to determine the nature and extent of any swallowing abnormality.
■ In patients with tracheostomies, observe for food particles in tracheal secretions.	Food is not normal in the tracheobronchial passages. It signifies aspirated material.
■ Auscultate bowel sounds to evaluate bowel motility, and assess for abdominal distention and firmness.	Decreased gastrointestinal motility increases the risk for aspiration because food or fluids accumulate in the stomach. Older patients have a decrease in esophageal motility, which delays esophageal emptying. When combined with the weaker gag reflex of older patients, aspiration is a higher risk.
■ Assess for presence of nausea or vomiting.	Nausea or vomiting places patients at great risk for aspiration, especially if the level of consciousness is compromised. Antiemetics may be required to prevent aspiration of regurgitated gastric contents.
▲ Assess pulmonary status for clinical evidence of aspiration. Auscultate breath sounds for development of crackles and/or wheezes. Monitor chest x-ray results as ordered.	Aspiration of small amounts can occur without coughing or sudden onset of respiratory distress, especially in patients with a decreased level of consciousness. Pulmonary infiltrates on chest x-ray results indicate some level of aspiration has already occurred.
■ In patients with endotracheal or tracheostomy tubes, monitor the effectiveness of the cuff. Collaborate with the respiratory therapist, as needed, to determine cuff pressure.	An ineffective or overinflated cuff can increase the risk for aspiration. Properly inflated cuffs are the best protection.

Therapeutic Interventions

Actions/Interventions	Rationales
■ Keep suction setup available (in both hospital and home settings), and use as needed.	Tracheal suction may be necessary to maintain a patent airway. Secretions can rapidly accumulate in the posterior pharynx and upper trachea, increasing risk for aspiration.
■ Notify the physician or other health care provider immediately of noted decrease in cough and/or gag reflexes or difficulty in swallowing.	Early intervention protects the patient's airway and prevents aspiration. Anyone identified as being at high risk for aspiration should be kept NPO (nothing by mouth) until further evaluation is completed.

Actions/Interventions

■ Position patients with a decreased level of consciousness supine on their side.

■ Supervise or assist the patient with oral intake. Never give oral fluids to a comatose patient.

■ Offer foods with consistency that the patient can swallow. Use thickening agents if recommended by a speech pathologist.

■ Encourage the patient to chew thoroughly and eat slowly during meals.

■ For patients with reduced cognitive abilities, remove distracting stimuli during mealtimes. Instruct the patient not to talk while eating.

■ Place whole or crushed pills in soft foods (e.g., custard). Verify with a pharmacist which pills should not be crushed. Substitute medication in elixir form as indicated.

■ Place medication and food on the strong side of the mouth when unilateral weakness or paresis is present.

■ Offer liquids *after* food is eaten.

■ Position the patient at a 90-degree angle, whether in bed or in a chair or wheelchair. Use cushions or pillows to maintain position. Maintain the patient in an upright position for 30 to 45 minutes after feeding.

■ Provide oral care before and after meals.

▲ In patients with artificial airways:
  • Perform oral suctioning as needed.

  • Brush teeth twice a day, and swab mouth with sponge applicators every 2 to 4 hours between brushing.

▲ In patients with nasogastric (NG) or gastrostomy tubes:
  • Check placement before feeding, using tube markings, x-ray study (most accurate), pH of gastric fluid, and color of aspirate as guides.

  • Check residuals before feeding, or every 4 hours if feeding is continuous. Hold feedings if amount of residuals is large, and notify the physician.

  • Test sputum with glucose oxidase reagent strips.

Rationales

This positioning (rescue positioning) decreases the risk for aspiration by promoting the drainage of secretions out of the mouth instead of down the pharynx, where they could be aspirated.

Supervision helps detect abnormalities early and enables implementation of strategies for safe swallowing. Withholding fluids/foods as needed prevents aspiration.

Thickened semisolid foods like pudding and hot cereal are most easily swallowed and less likely to be aspirated. Liquids and thin foods like creamed soups are most difficult for patients with dysphagia.

Well-masticated food is easier to swallow; food cut into small pieces may also be easier to swallow.

Concentration must be focused on chewing and swallowing. When talking and eating/drinking at the same time, there is higher risk for the airway being opened while food is in the pharynx.

Mixing pills with food helps reduce risk for aspiration.

Careful food placement facilitates chewing and successful swallowing.

Ingesting food and fluids together increases swallowing difficulties.

The upright position facilitates the gravitational flow of food or fluid through the alimentary tract. If the head of the bed cannot be elevated because of the patient's condition, use a right side-lying position after feedings to facilitate passage of stomach contents into the duodenum.

Oral care before meals reduces bacterial counts in the oral cavity. Oral care after eating removes residual food that could be aspirated at a later time.

Suctioning reduces the volume of oropharyngeal secretions and reduces aspiration risk.

Oral care reduces the risk for ventilator-associated pneumonia by decreasing the number of microorganisms in aspirated oropharyngeal secretions.

A displaced tube may erroneously deliver tube feeding into the airway. Chest x-ray verification of accurate tube placement is most reliable. Gastric aspirate is usually green, brown, clear, or colorless with a pH between 1 and 5.

Large amounts of residuals indicate delayed gastric emptying and can cause distention of the stomach, leading to reflux emesis. The amount of residuals may vary depending on the volume and rate of infusion; however, the evaluation can be unreliable. Feedings are often held if residual volume is greater than 50% of the amount to be delivered in 1 hour.

Significant amounts of glucose in sputum may be indicative of aspiration.

■ = Independent   ▲ = Collaborative

Actions/Interventions	Rationales
• Place dye (e.g., methylene blue) in NG feedings only with physician's order.	Detection of the color in pulmonary secretions would indicate aspiration. However, regular amounts of some dyes may discolor skin, body fluids, and tissues and increase morbidity and mortality, especially in patients with increased intestinal permeability or metabolic disorders such as sepsis. Thus routine use is discouraged without physician's order.
• Elevate the head of the bed to 30 to 45 degrees while feeding the patient and for 30 to 45 minutes afterward if feeding is intermittent. Turn off the feeding before lowering the head of the bed. Patients with continuous feedings should be in an upright position.	Upright positioning reduces aspiration by decreasing reflux of gastric contents.
▲ Consult a speech pathologist, as appropriate.	A speech pathologist can be consulted to perform a dysphagia assessment that helps determine the need for videofluoroscopy or modified barium swallow and to establish specific techniques to prevent aspiration in patients with impaired swallowing.

Education/Continuity of Care

Actions/Interventions	Rationales
■ Explain to the patient and caregiver the need for proper positioning.	Upright positioning decreases the risk for aspiration.
■ Instruct in proper feeding techniques.	Both the patient and caregiver need to be active participants in implementing the treatment plan to optimize safe nutritional intake.
■ Instruct in upper airway suctioning techniques to prevent accumulation of secretions in the oral cavity.	Patient safety is a priority.
■ Instruct in signs and symptoms of aspiration.	Information aids in appropriate assessment of high-risk situations and determination of when to call for further evaluation.
■ Instruct the caregiver in what to do in case of emergency.	Instruction facilitates appropriate management of potentially life-threatening situations. Respiratory aspiration requires immediate action by the caregiver to maintain the airway and promote effective breathing and gas exchange.
▲ Refer the patient to a home health nurse, rehabilitation specialist, or occupational therapist as indicated.	Use of consultants may be required to ensure that outcomes are achieved.

Disturbed Body Image

Definition: Confusion in mental picture of one's physical self

Body image is the attitude a person has about the actual or perceived structure or function of all or parts of his or her body. This attitude is dynamic and is altered through interaction with other persons and situations, and it is influenced by age and developmental level. As an important part of one's self-concept, body image disturbance can have a profound impact on how individuals view their overall selves.

Throughout the life span, changes in a person's body related to normal growth and development can result in changes in the person's body image. For example, a woman may experience disturbed body image during pregnancy. Physical changes associated with aging may result in body image disturbance for the older adult.

Societal and cultural norms for ideal body shape, size, and appearance have a significant influence on a person's body image. Variations from the norm can result in body image disturbance. The value that an individual places on a body part or function may be more important in determining the degree of disturbance than the actual alteration in the structure or function. Therefore the loss of a limb may result in a greater body image disturbance for an athlete than for a computer programmer. The loss of a breast to a fashion model or a hysterectomy in a nulliparous woman may cause serious body image disturbances even though the overall health of the individual has been improved. Removal of skin lesions, altered elimination resulting from bowel or bladder surgery, and head and neck resections are other examples that can lead to body image disturbance.

The nurse's assessment of the perceived alteration and importance placed by the patient on the altered structure or function will be very important in planning care to address body image disturbance.

Common Related Factors

Situational changes (e.g., pregnancy; temporary presence of a visible drain or tube, dressing, attached equipment)

Permanent alterations in structure and/or function (e.g., mutilating surgery, removal of body part [internal or external])

Malodorous lesions

Change in voice quality

Defining Characteristics

Verbalization about altered structure or function of a body part

Verbal preoccupation with changed body part or function

Naming changed body part or function

Refusal to discuss or acknowledge change

Focusing behavior on changed body part and/or function

Actual change in structure or function

Refusal to look at, touch, or care for altered body part

Change in social behavior (e.g., withdrawal, isolation, flamboyance)

Compensatory use of concealing clothing or other devices

Common Expected Outcome

Patient demonstrates enhanced body image and self-esteem as evidenced by ability to look at, touch, talk about, and care for actual or perceived altered body part or function.

NOC Outcomes
Body Image; Self-Esteem

NIC Interventions
Body Image Enhancement; Grief Work Facilitation; Coping Enhancement

Ongoing Assessment

Actions/Interventions

■ Assess perception of change in structure or function of body part (also proposed change).

■ Assess perceived impact of change on activities of daily living (ADLs), social behavior, personal relationships, and occupational activities.

Rationales

The extent of the response is more related to the value or importance the patient places on the part or function than the actual value or importance. Even when an alteration improves the overall health of the individual (e.g., an ileostomy for an individual with precancerous colon polyps), the alteration may result in a body image disturbance.

Changes in body image can have an impact on the person's ability to carry out daily roles and responsibilities.

■ = Independent   ▲ = Collaborative

Actions/Interventions	Rationales
■ Assess impact of body image disturbance in relation to the patient's developmental stage.	Adolescents and young adults may be particularly affected by changes in the structure or function of their bodies at a time when developmental changes are normally rapid and at a time when developing social and intimate relationships is particularly important.
■ Note the patient's behavior regarding the actual or perceived changed body part or function.	There is a broad range of behaviors associated with body image disturbance, ranging from totally ignoring the altered structure or function to preoccupation with it.
■ Note the frequency of the patient's self-critical remarks.	Negative statements about the affected body part indicate limited ability to integrate the change into the patient's self-concept.

Therapeutic Interventions

Actions/Interventions	Rationales
■ Acknowledge normalcy of emotional response to actual or perceived change in body structure or function.	Experiencing stages of grief over loss of a body part or function is normal and typically involves a period of denial, the length of which varies between individuals.
■ Help the patient identify actual changes.	Patients may perceive changes that are not present or real, or they place an unrealistic value on a body structure or function.
■ Encourage verbalization of positive or negative feelings about the actual or perceived change.	It is worthwhile to encourage the patient to separate feelings about changes in body structure and/or function from feelings about self-worth. Expression of feelings can enhance the person's coping strategies.
■ Assist the patient in incorporating actual changes into ADLs, social life, interpersonal relationships, and occupational activities.	Opportunities for positive feedback and success in social situations may hasten adaptation.
■ Demonstrate positive caring in routine activities.	Professional caregivers represent a microcosm of society, and their actions and behaviors are scrutinized as the patient plans to return to home, work, and other activities.

Education/Continuity of Care

Actions/Interventions	Rationales
■ Teach the patient about the normalcy of body image disturbance and the grief process.	The person experiencing a body image change needs new information to support cognitive appraisal of the change.
■ Teach the patient adaptive behavior (e.g., use of adaptive equipment, wigs, cosmetics, clothing that conceals the altered body part or enhances remaining part or function, use of deodorants).	Adaptive behaviors compensate for the actual changed body structure and function.
■ Help the patient identify ways of coping that have been useful in the past.	Asking patients to remember other body image issues (e.g., getting glasses, wearing orthodontics, being pregnant, having a leg cast) and how they were managed may help the patient adjust to the current issue.
■ Refer the patient and caregivers to support groups composed of individuals with similar alterations.	Lay persons in similar situations offer a different type of support, which is perceived as helpful (e.g., United Ostomy Association, Y Me?, I Can Cope, Mended Hearts).

NANDA-I NDx Bowel Incontinence

Definition: Change in normal bowel habits characterized by involuntary passage of stool

Bowel incontinence, also called fecal incontinence, may occur as a result of injury to nerves and other structures involved in normal defecation or as the result of diseases that alter the normal function of defecation. Treatment of bowel incontinence depends on the cause. Injury to rectal, anal, or nervous tissue, such as from trauma, childbirth, radiation, or surgery, can result in bowel incontinence. Infection with resultant diarrhea or neurological disease such as stroke, multiple sclerosis, and diabetes mellitus can also result in bowel incontinence. In older patients, dementia can contribute to bowel incontinence when the individual cannot respond to normal physiological cues. Normal aging causes changes in the intestinal musculature that may contribute to bowel incontinence. Fecal impaction, as a result of chronic constipation and/or denial of the defecation urge, can result in involuntary leakage of stool past the impaction. Loss of mobility can result in functional bowel incontinence when the person is unable to reach the toilet in a timely manner. Loss of bowel continence is an embarrassing problem that leads to social isolation, and it is one of the most common reasons that older patients are admitted to long-term care facilities. Goals of management include reestablishing a continent bowel elimination pattern, preventing loss of skin integrity, and/or planning management of fecal incontinence in a manner that preserves the individual's self-esteem.

Common Related Factors

Neuromuscular problems:
- Stroke
- Multiple sclerosis
- Muscular dystrophy
- Myasthenia gravis
- Diabetes
- Dementia
- Lower motor nerve trauma
- Spinal cord injury

Musculoskeletal problems:
- Pelvic floor relaxation
- Nerve trauma
- Damage to sphincters
- Radiation to pelvis
- Infection
- Postoperative injuries
- Fecal impaction
- Medications
- Hyperosmolar food or fluid intake
- Immobility
- Lack of accessible toileting facilities

Defining Characteristics

Passive incontinence (involuntary passage of feces and flatus without any awareness)

Urge incontinence (discharge of feces and flatus in spite of active attempts to retain these contents)

Fecal seepage (undesired leakage of stool after a bowel movement with otherwise normal continence and evacuation)

Common Expected Outcome

Patient is continent of stool or reports decreased episodes of bowel incontinence.

NOC Outcomes

Bowel Continence; Self-Care: Toileting

NIC Interventions

Bowel Incontinence Care; Bowel Management; Bowel Training; Self-Care Assistance: Toileting

■ = Independent ▲ = Collaborative

Ongoing Assessment

Actions/Interventions	Rationales
■ Assess the patient's normal bowel elimination pattern.	There is a wide range of "normal" for bowel elimination; some patients have two bowel movements per day, whereas others may have a bowel movement as infrequently as every third or fourth day.
■ If there is current pathology that may affect bowel elimination, determine the premorbid bowel elimination pattern.	Most people feel the urge to defecate shortly after the first oral intake (e.g., coffee or breakfast) of the day; this is a result of the gastrocolic reflex.
■ Determine the cause of incontinence (i.e., review related factors).	Knowledge of causative factors provides direction for subsequent interventions. Often there are multiple contributory factors.
■ Perform manual check for fecal impaction.	When the patient has a fecal impaction (hard, dry stool that cannot be expelled normally), liquid stool may leak past the impaction.
■ Assess whether current medications or treatments may be contributing to bowel incontinence.	Hyperosmolar tube feedings, bowel preparation agents, pelvic and/or abdominal irradiation, some chemotherapeutic agents, and certain antibiotic agents may cause explosive diarrhea that the patient cannot control.
■ Assist in preparing the patient for diagnostic measures.	These determine the causes of bowel incontinence. Tests include flexible sigmoidoscopy, barium enema, colonoscopy, and anal manometry (study to determine function of rectal sphincters).
■ Assess the degree to which the patient's daily activities are altered by bowel incontinence.	Patients may restrict their own activity or become isolated from work, family, and friends because they fear odor and embarrassment.
■ Assess the use of diapers, sanitary napkins, incontinence briefs, fecal collection devices, and underpads.	Patients or caregivers may substitute familiar products (e.g., sanitary napkins) for more appropriate incontinence products out of ignorance or embarrassment.
■ Assess perineal skin integrity.	Stool can cause chemical irritation to the skin, which may be exacerbated by the use of diapers, incontinence briefs, and underpads.
■ Assess the patient's ability to go to the bathroom independently.	Soiling accidents that occur as a result of the patient's inability to get to the bathroom may be solved by rearranging the environment, planning for trips to the bathroom, or by providing a bedside commode.
■ Assess the patient's environment for availability of an accessible toilet facility.	Inadequate access to toileting facilities in the home (e.g., bathroom on upper level), in the work environment, at the shopping mall, and the like can aggravate the incontinence experience.
■ Assess fluid and fiber intake.	Fiber and fluids are related to normal bowel evacuation.

Therapeutic Interventions

Actions/Interventions	Rationales
■ Ensure fluid intake of at least 3000 mL/day, unless contraindicated.	Moist stool moves through the bowel more easily than hard, dry stool and prevents impaction. If the patient has a significant amount of diarrhea, fluids provide important volume replacement.
▲ Provide high-fiber diet under the direction of a dietitian, unless contraindicated.	Fiber aids in bowel elimination because it is insoluble and absorbs fluid as the stool passes through the bowel; this creates bulk. Bulky stool stimulates peristalsis and expulsion of stool from the bowel.
■ Encourage intake of natural bulking agents to thicken stools, for example, foods such as banana, rice, and yogurt.	If bowel incontinence is related to diarrhea, these foods help provide bulk to the stool by absorbing fluids from the stool.

Actions/Interventions

- Manually remove the fecal impaction, if present.

- Encourage mobility or exercise if tolerated.

- Provide a bedside commode and assistive devices (e.g., cane, walker) or assistance in reaching the commode or toilet.
- ▲ Institute a bowel program.

  - Encourage bowel elimination at the same time every day.

  - After breakfast (or a warm drink), administer a suppository and perform digital stimulation every 10 to 15 minutes until evacuation occurs.
  - Place patient in an upright position for defecation.

- Wash the perineal area after each evacuation with soap and water. Dry thoroughly.
- Treat any perianal irritation with a moisture barrier ointment.

- Discourage the use of pads, diapers, or collection devices as soon as possible.
- Use fecal collection systems selectively over pads, diapers, and rectal tubes.

Rationales

Presence of fecal impaction can interfere with establishment of a regular bowel routine.
Increasing mobility stimulates peristalsis and aids in bowel evacuation.
Immediate access reduces unnecessary "accidents."

Facilitating regular time for bowel evacuation prevents the bowel from emptying sporadically (i.e., decreases incontinence).
Shortly after breakfast is a good time because the gastrocolic reflex is stimulated by food or fluid intake.
For some etiologies, direct stimulation of the renal sphincter and lower colon may be required to initiate peristalsis.

Flexion of the thighs (e.g., sitting upright with feet flat on floor) facilitates muscular movement that aids in defecation.
Any fecal material left on the skin can cause skin excoriation and pain.
Perineal or perianal pain from irritation may result in fear of defecating and cause the patient to deny the urge to defecate. Repeated denial of the urge to defecate results in impaction, and eventually in bowel incontinence.
Fecal containment devices can be useful in the short term to prevent soiling.
These devices (fecal collectors—pouches that adhere to the skin around the rectum—or rectal tube collection systems—rectal tubes that stay in the rectum via inflated balloons and drain liquid stool into a collection bag) allow for collection and disposal of stool without exposing the perianal skin to stool; odor and embarrassment are controlled because the stool is contained. These devices work best for individuals who are in bed the majority of time.

Education/Continuity of Care

Actions/Interventions

- Teach the patient or caregiver the causes of bowel incontinence.
- Teach the patient or caregiver the importance of fluid and fiber in maintaining soft, bulky stool.

- Teach the patient the importance of establishing a regular time for bowel evacuation.
- Teach the caregiver the use of a fecal incontinence device, if appropriate.
- Teach the patient to manage perianal irritation prophylactically by washing with soap and water, drying thoroughly after each bowel movement, and applying a moisture barrier ointment containing zinc oxide or dimethicone.

Rationales

Knowledge of causative factors can clarify appropriate treatment approach.
Teaching the patient or caregiver methods to manage bowel incontinence improves personal efficacy and can enhance compliance with the therapeutic regimen.
Information provides rationale for therapy and aids the patient in assuming responsibility for self-care later.
Supportive caregiving may be required. Use of specific devices may be challenging.
Patients and caregivers need to prevent skin irritation and pain that can result from fecal incontinence.

■ = Independent   ▲ = Collaborative

NANDA-I NDx Ineffective Breathing Pattern

Definition: Inspiration and/or expiration that does not provide adequate ventilation

Ineffective breathing patterns are considered a state in which the rate, depth, timing, rhythm, or chest/abdominal wall excursion during inspiration, expiration, or both do not maintain optimum ventilation for the individual. Most acute pulmonary deterioration is preceded by a change in breathing pattern. Respiratory failure may be associated with changes in respiratory rate, abdominal and thoracic patterns for inspiration and expiration, and in depth of ventilation. Breathing pattern changes may occur in a multitude of conditions: heart failure, diaphragmatic paralysis, airway obstruction, respiratory infection, neuromuscular impairment, trauma or surgery resulting in musculoskeletal impairment and/or pain, cognitive impairment and anxiety, metabolic abnormalities (e.g., diabetic ketoacidosis, uremia, or thyroid dysfunction), peritonitis, drug overdose, pleural inflammation, and chronic respiratory disorders such as asthma or chronic obstructive pulmonary disease (COPD).

Common Related Factors

Neuromuscular impairment
Spinal cord injury
Musculoskeletal impairment
Tracheobronchial obstruction
Inflammatory process: viral or bacterial
Perception or cognitive impairment
Decreased energy and fatigue
Pain
Anxiety

Defining Characteristics

Dyspnea
Tachypnea/bradypnea
Orthopnea
Assumption of three-point position to breathe
Nasal flaring
Respiratory depth changes
Altered chest excursion
Use of accessory muscles
Pursed-lip breathing or prolonged expiratory phase
Increased anteroposterior chest diameter
Irregular or paradoxical breathing

Common Expected Outcome

The patient will maintain an effective breathing pattern, as evidenced by relaxed breathing at normal rate and depth and absence of dyspnea.

NOC Outcomes
Respiratory Status: Ventilation; Vital Sign Status
NIC Interventions
Airway Management; Respiratory Monitoring

Ongoing Assessment

Actions/Interventions

- Assess respiratory rate, rhythm, and depth.

- Monitor breathing patterns:
  - Bradypnea (slow respirations)
  - Tachypnea (increase in respiratory rate)
  - Hyperventilation (increase in respiratory rate or tidal volume, or both)
  - Kussmaul's respirations (deep respirations with fast, normal, or slow rate)

Rationales

Respiratory rate and rhythm changes are early warning signs of impending respiratory difficulties.
Specific breathing patterns may indicate an underlying disease process or dysfunction. Cheyne-Stokes respiration usually represents bilateral dysfunction in the deep cerebral hemispheres associated with brain injury or metabolic abnormalities. Apneusis and ataxic breathing and Biot's respirations are associated with failure of the respiratory centers in the pons or medulla.

Actions/Interventions

- Cheyne-Stokes respiration (waxing and waning with periods of apnea between a repetitive pattern)
- Apneusis (sustained maximal inhalation with pause)
- Biot's respirations (irregular periods of apnea alternating with periods in which four or five breaths of identical depth are taken)
- Ataxic patterns (irregular and unpredictable pattern with periods of apnea)

■ Assess for use of accessory muscles (scalene and sternocleidomastoid).

■ Monitor for diaphragmatic muscle fatigue or weakness (paradoxical motion).

■ Note retractions or flaring of nostrils.

■ Assess the position that the patient assumes for breathing.

■ Inquire about precipitating and alleviating factors.

■ Assess ability to clear secretions.

■ Assess sputum for quantity, color, consistency, and odor.

■ If the sputum is discolored (no longer clear or white), send the specimen for culture and sensitivity testing, as appropriate.

■ Assess level of anxiety.

■ Monitor for changes in level of consciousness.

■ Assess skin color and temperature.

■ Monitor pulse oximetry and arterial blood gases (ABGs) as appropriate. Note changes.

■ Assess for thoracic or upper abdominal pain.
■ Monitor vital capacity in patients with neuromuscular weakness, and observe trends.
▲ Assess nutritional status (e.g., weight, albumin and electrolyte levels).

Rationales

Work of breathing increases greatly as lung compliance decreases. As moving air in and out of the lungs becomes more and more difficult, the breathing pattern alters to include use of accessory muscles to increase chest excursion to facilitate effective breathing.

Paradoxical movement of the abdomen (an inward versus outward movement during inspiration) is indicative of respiratory muscle fatigue and weakness.

These signify an increase in respiratory effort.

A three-point position or orthopnea is associated with breathing difficulty.

Knowledge of these factors is useful in planning interventions to prevent or manage future episodes of dyspnea.

An obstructed airway may cause a change in breathing pattern.

These may be indicative of an etiology for the alteration in breathing pattern.

An infection may be present. Respiratory infections increase the work of breathing, resulting in fatigue and changes in breathing pattern. Antibiotic treatment may be indicated.

Hypoxia and the sensation of "not being able to breathe" is frightening and may cause worsening hypoxia.

Restlessness, confusion, and/or irritability can be early indicators of insufficient oxygen to the brain. Lethargy and somnolence are late signs of hypoxia.

Pale or cyanotic color indicates increased concentration of deoxygenated blood and indicates that the breathing pattern is no longer effective to maintain adequate oxygenation of tissues. Cool, pale skin may be secondary to a compensatory/vasoconstrictive response to hypoxemia.

Pulse oximetry is a useful tool to monitor oxygen saturation and detect early changes in oxygenation. Increasing $Paco_2$ and decreasing Pao_2 are signs of respiratory failure. As the patient's condition begins to fail, the respiratory rate decreases and $Paco_2$ begins to increase.

Pain can result in shallow breathing.

Monitoring detects changes early so ventilatory support may be initiated before full decompensation occurs.

Malnutrition may result in premature development of respiratory failure because it reduces respiratory mass and strength. It blunts ventilatory responses to hypoxia and impairs pulmonary and systemic immunity. Overfeeding increases production of CO_2, which increases respiratory drive and respiratory muscle fatigue.

■ = Independent ▲ = Collaborative

Nursing Diagnosis Care Plans

Actions/Interventions

- Assess use of herbal remedies (e.g., ma huang for broncho-spasm, or licorice and hyssop for reducing cough and pro-moting expectoration).

- ▲ Avoid high concentration of oxygen in patients with COPD unless ordered.

Rationales

Drug interactions with prescribed medications and contraindi-cations need to be evaluated (e.g., ma huang contains ephedrine, which should not be used by patients with hypertension, heart disease, prostatic hyperplasia, or diabetes).

Hypoxia stimulates the drive to breathe in the chronic CO_2 retainer patient. When applying oxygen, close monitoring is imperative to prevent unsafe increases in the patient's Pao_2, which could result in apnea.

Therapeutic Interventions

Actions/Interventions

- Position the patient with proper body alignment for optimal breathing pattern.
- ▲ Maintain oxygen saturation at or above 90%.

- Encourage sustained deep breaths by:
  - Using demonstration (emphasizing slow inhalation, holding end inspiration for a few seconds, passive exha-lation, and pursed-lip breathing).
  - Using incentive spirometer (place close for convenient patient use)
  - Asking the patient to yawn
- Evaluate appropriateness of inspiratory muscle training.

- Encourage the patient to clear his or her own secretions with effective coughing. If secretions cannot be cleared, suction as needed.

- Use universal precautions (e.g., gloves, goggles, and mask) as appropriate. If secretions are purulent, precautions should be instituted before receiving the culture and sensi-tivity final report. Institute appropriate isolation proce-dures for positive cultures (e.g., methicillin-resistant *Staphylococcus aureus* or tuberculosis).
- Plan activity and rest to maximize the patient's energy.

- Provide reassurance and allay anxiety by staying with the patient during acute episodes of respiratory distress.

- Encourage diaphragmatic breathing for the patient with chronic disease.
- ▲ Use pain management as appropriate.
- ▲ Administer respiratory medications as ordered.

Rationales

If not contraindicated, a sitting position allows adequate dia-phragmatic and lung excursion and chest expansion.

An oxygen saturation of less than 90% leads to tissue hypoxia, acidosis, dysrhythmias, and decreased level of conscious-ness.

These techniques promote deep inspiration, which increases oxygenation and prevents atelectasis. Controlled breath-ing techniques may also help slow respirations in patients who are tachypneic. Prolonged expiration prevents air trapping.

This training improves conscious control of respiratory mus-cles and inspiratory muscle strength.

Productive coughing is the most effective way to remove most secretions. If patient is unable to perform indepen-dently, suctioning may be needed to promote airway patency and reduce work of breathing.

These measures prevent transmission of pathogenic microor-ganisms.

Fatigue is common with the increased work of breathing. Activity increases metabolic rate and oxygen require-ments. Rest helps mobilize energy for more effective breathing and coughing efforts.

The presence of a trusted person may help the patient feel less threatened and can reduce anxiety, thereby reducing oxygen requirements.

This breathing technique relaxes muscles and increases the patient's oxygen level.

Pain relief enhances the ability to deep breathe and cough.

β-Adrenergic agonist medications relax airway smooth mus-cles and cause bronchodilation to open air passages. Cor-ticoid steroids are effective antiinflammatory drugs for treatment of reversible airflow obstruction.

Actions/Interventions

- Anticipate the need for intubation and mechanical ventilation if the patient is unable to maintain adequate gas exchange with the present breathing pattern.

Rationales

Early intubation and mechanical ventilation are recommended to prevent full decompensation of the patient and a potentially life-threatening situation. Mechanical ventilation provides supportive care to maintain adequate oxygenation and ventilation.

Education/Continuity of Care

Actions/Interventions

- Teach the patient or caregivers appropriate breathing, coughing, and splinting techniques.

- Teach patients to pace activities and to avoid unnecessary tasks when dyspneic.
- Instruct about medications: indications, dosage, frequency, and potential side effects. Include review of metered-dose inhaler and nebulizer treatments, as appropriate.
- Explain use of oxygen therapy, including the type and use of equipment and why its maintenance is important.
- Assist the patient or caregiver in learning signs of respiratory compromise. Refer significant others or caregivers to participate in basic life support class for cardiopulmonary resuscitation, as appropriate. Provide emergency phone numbers.

Rationales

These techniques facilitate adequate clearance of secretions and prevent atelectasis. Dyspnea also may be reduced by techniques such as pursed-lip or diaphragmatic breathing.

Energy-conserving methods reduce fatigue, dyspnea, and oxygen consumption.

This information promotes safe and effective medication administration.

Issues related to home oxygen use, storage, and precautions need to be addressed for safe and effective treatment.

This instruction prevents delays in seeking help and facilitates appropriate management in life-threatening situations. Patient and family members may not remember phone numbers in an emergency situation.

Related Care Plans

Ineffective airway clearance, p. 11
Pneumonia, p. 429
Tuberculosis, p. 468

Decreased Cardiac Output

Definition: Inadequate blood pumped by the heart to meet the metabolic demands of the body

Common causes of reduced cardiac output include myocardial infarction, hypertension, valvular heart disease, congenital heart disease, cardiomyopathy, pulmonary disease, arrhythmias, drug effects, fluid overload, decreased fluid volume, and electrolyte imbalance. Older patients are especially at risk because the aging process causes reduced compliance of the ventricles, which further reduces contractility and cardiac output. Patients may have acute, temporary problems or experience chronic, debilitating effects of decreased cardiac output. Patients may be managed in an acute, ambulatory care, or home care setting. This care plan focuses on the acute management.

Common Related Factors

Increased or decreased ventricular filling (preload)
Increased afterload
Impaired contractility
Alteration in heart rate, rhythm, and conduction
Decreased oxygenation
Cardiac muscle disease

Defining Characteristics

Variations in hemodynamic parameters (blood pressure [BP], heart rate, central venous pressure [CVP], pulmonary artery pressures, venous oxygen saturation [SvO_2], cardiac output)
Dysrhythmias, electrocardiogram (ECG) changes
Crackles, tachypnea, dyspnea, orthopnea, cough, abnormal arterial blood gases (ABGs), frothy sputum
Weight gain, edema, decreased urine output
Anxiety, restlessness

■ = Independent   ▲ = Collaborative

Syncope, dizziness

Decreased activity tolerance/fatigue

Abnormal heart sounds (S_3, S_4)

Decreased peripheral pulses; cold, clammy skin/poor capillary refill

Confusion

Change in level of consciousness

Angina

Ejection fraction less than 40%

Pulsus alternans

Common Expected Outcome

Patient has adequate cardiac output as evidenced by systolic BP within 20 mm Hg of baseline; heart rate 60 to 100 beats/min with regular rhythm; urine output greater than or equal to 30 mL/hr; strong peripheral pulses; warm, dry skin; eupnea with absence of pulmonary crackles; and orientation to person, time, and place.

NOC Outcomes
Cardiac Pump Effectiveness; Circulation Status; Knowledge: Disease Process; Knowledge: Treatment Program
NIC Interventions
Cardiac Care; Hemodynamic Regulation; Teaching: Disease Process

Ongoing Assessment

Actions/Interventions	Rationales
■ Assess for any changes in level of consciousness.	Hypoxia and reduced cerebral perfusion are reflected in restlessness, irritability, and difficulty concentrating. Older patients are especially susceptible to reduced perfusion.
■ Assess heart rate and blood pressure.	Sinus tachycardia and increased arterial BP are seen in the early stages; BP drops as the condition deteriorates. Older patients have reduced response to catecholamines; thus their response to reduced cardiac output may be blunted, with less increase in heart rate. Pulsus alternans (alternating strong-then-weak pulse) is often seen in heart failure patients.
■ Assess skin color, temperature, and moisture.	Cold, pale, clammy skin is secondary to compensatory increase in sympathetic nervous system stimulation and low cardiac output and desaturation.
■ Assess peripheral pulses, including capillary refill.	Pulses are weak with reduced stroke volume and cardiac output. Capillary refill is slow, sometimes absent.
■ Assess fluid balance and weight gain.	Compromised regulatory mechanisms may result in fluid and sodium retention. Body weight is a more sensitive indicator of fluid or sodium retention than intake and output.
■ Assess urine output. Determine how often the patient urinates.	The renal system compensates for low BP by retaining water. Oliguria is a classic sign of decreased renal perfusion. Diuresis is expected with diuretic therapy.
■ Assess heart sounds for gallops (S_3, S_4).	S_3 denotes reduced left ventricular ejection and is a classic sign of left ventricular failure. S_4 occurs with reduced compliance of the left ventricle, which impairs diastolic filling.
■ Assess respiratory rate, rhythm, and breath sounds. Determine any occurrence of paroxysmal nocturnal dyspnea (PND) or orthopnea.	Rapid shallow respirations are characteristic of reduced cardiac output. Crackles reflect accumulation of fluid secondary to impaired left ventricular emptying. They are more evident in the dependent areas of the lung. Orthopnea is difficulty breathing when supine; PND is difficulty breathing at night.
▲ Assess B-type natriuretic peptide (BNP).	B-type natriuretic peptide (BNP) is elevated with left ventricular failure and serves as a "white count" for heart failure. This test aids in differentiating causes of symptoms.

Actions/Interventions

▲ If hemodynamic monitoring is in place:
  - Monitor CVP, right arterial pressure (RAP), pulmonary artery pressure (PAP) (systolic, diastolic, and mean), and pulmonary capillary wedge pressure (PCWP).
  - Perform cardiac output determination.

  - Monitor SvO₂ continuously.

■ Monitor ECG for rate; rhythm; ectopy; and change in PR, QRS, and QT intervals.

■ Assess for complaints of fatigue and reduced activity tolerance.

■ Assess for chest pain.

■ Assess contributing factors so appropriate care plan can be initiated.

Rationales

Hemodynamic parameters provide information aiding in differentiation of decreased cardiac output secondary to fluid overload versus fluid deficit.

Cardiac output measurement provides objective numbers to guide therapy.

Change in oxygen saturation of mixed venous blood is one of the earliest indicators of reduced cardiac output.

Cardiac dysrhythmias may occur from low perfusion, acidosis, or hypoxia. Tachycardia, bradycardia, and ectopic beats can further compromise cardiac output. Older patients are especially sensitive to the loss of atrial kick in atrial fibrillation.

Physical activity increases the demands placed on the heart; fatigue and exertional dyspnea are common problems with low cardiac output states. Close monitoring of the patient's response serves as a guide for optimal progression of activity.

Chest pain indicates an imbalance between myocardial oxygen supply and demand.

Specific etiologies guide treatment.

Therapeutic Interventions

Actions/Interventions

▲ Maintain optimal fluid balance. For patients with decreased preload, administer fluid challenge as prescribed, closely monitoring effects.

▲ For patients with increased preload, restrict fluids and sodium as ordered.

▲ Administer medication as prescribed, noting response and watching for side effects and toxicity. Clarify with physician parameters for withholding medications.

▲ Maintain hemodynamic parameters at prescribed levels.

▲ Maintain adequate ventilation and perfusion, as in the following:
  - Place patient in semi- to high-Fowler's position.

  - Place patient in supine position.

  - Administer oxygen therapy as prescribed.

■ Maintain physical and emotional rest, as in the following:
  - Restrict activity.
  - Provide quiet, relaxed environment.
  - Organize nursing and medical care.
  - Monitor progressive activity within limits of cardiac function.

▲ Administer stool softeners as needed.

▲ Monitor sleep patterns; administer sedative.

Rationales

Volume therapy may be required to maintain adequate filling pressures and optimize cardiac output.

Fluid restriction decreases extracellular fluid volume and reduces demands on the heart.

Depending on etiological factors, common medications include digitalis therapy, diuretics, vasodilator therapy, antidysrhythmics, angiotensin-converting enzyme inhibitors, and inotropic agents.

For patients in the acute setting, close monitoring of these parameters guides titration of fluids and medications.

When fluid overload is an etiology, upright positioning reduces preload and ventricular filling.

For hypovolemia, supine positioning increases venous return and promotes diuresis.

The failing heart may not be able to respond to increased oxygen demands. Oxygen saturation needs to be greater than 90%.

Activity restriction and a quiet environment reduce oxygen demands. Attention to priority care delivery optimizes use of the patient's limited energy resources. Careful activity progression prevents overexertion and stress on the cardiopulmonary system.

Straining for a bowel movement further impairs cardiac output.

Rest is important for conserving energy.

■ = Independent   ▲ = Collaborative

Actions/Interventions

▲ If dysrhythmia occurs, determine patient response, document, and report if significant or symptomatic.
  • Have antidysrhythmic drugs readily available.
  • Treat dysrhythmias according to medical orders or protocol, and evaluate response.

▲ If invasive adjunct therapies are indicated (e.g., intraaortic balloon pump, pacemaker), maintain within prescribed protocol.

Rationales

Both tachydysrhythmias and bradydysrhythmias can reduce cardiac output and myocardial tissue perfusion.

Electrical/mechanical assist devices may be indicated to support cardiac output when more basic therapies fail. Nurse needs to follow protocols for managing each device.

Education/Continuity of Care

Actions/Interventions

■ Explain symptoms and interventions for decreased cardiac output related to etiological factors.

■ Explain drug regimen, purpose, dose, and side effects.

■ Explain diet restrictions (fluid, sodium).

■ Explain progressive activity schedule and signs of overexertion.

Rationales

Thorough understanding of specific causes for each patient's disease is necessary for appropriate follow-through of treatment plan.

Information provides rationale for therapy and aids the patient in assuming responsibility for self-care later.

Diet changes and restrictions can be especially challenging to patients and may require ongoing monitoring.

Close monitoring of one's response to progressive activity reduces the risk for overexertion.

Related Care Plans

Dysrhythmias, p. 249
Shock, Cardiogenic, p. 331
Chest trauma, p. 375
Deficient fluid volume, p. 72
Acute coronary syndromes/Myocardial infarction, p. 209

NANDA-I
NDx **Caregiver Role Strain**

Definition: Difficulty in performing family caregiver role

The focus of this care plan is on the supportive care rendered by family, significant others, or caregivers responsible for meeting the physical and/or emotional needs of the patient. With limited access to health care for many people, most diseases are diagnosed and managed in the outpatient setting. Rapid hospital discharges for even the most complex health problems result in the care of acute and chronic illnesses being essentially managed in the home environment. Today's health care environment places high expectations on the designated caregiver, whether a family member or someone for hire. For many older patients, the only caregiver is a fragile spouse overwhelmed by his or her own health problems. Even in cultures in which care of the ill is the anticipated responsibility of family members, the complexities of today's medical regimens, the chronicity of some disease processes, and the burdens of the caregiver's own family or environmental milieu provide an overwhelming challenge. Caregivers have special needs for knowledge and skills in managing the required activities, access to affordable community resources, and recognition that the care they are providing is important and appreciated. Moreover, caregivers can be considered "secondary patients" who are at high risk for injury and adverse events. Nurses can assist caregivers by providing the requisite education and skill training and offering support through home visits; special clinic sessions; telephone access for questions and comfort; innovative strategies such as telephone or computer support, or "chat groups"; opportunities for respite care; and guidance in engaging in activities that promote their own health (nutrition, exercise, sleep, stress management).

Common Related Factors

Illness severity of care receiver
Unpredictable illness course
Discharge of family member with significant home care needs
Caregiver has health problems
Caregiver has knowledge deficit regarding management of care
Caregiver's personal and social life is disrupted by demands of caregiving
Caregiver has multiple competing roles
Caregiver's time and freedom is restricted because of caregiving
Past history of poor relationship between caregiver and care recipient
Caregiver feels care is not appreciated
Social isolation from others
Caregiver has no respite from caregiving demands
Caregiver is unaware of or reluctant to use available community resources
Community resources are not available or not affordable
Economic hardship

Defining Characteristics

Caregiver expresses difficulty in performing patient care
Caregiver expresses apprehension about future regarding own ability to provide care
Caregiver verbalizes anger with responsibility of patient care
Caregiver worries that own health will suffer because of caregiving
Caregiver states that formal and informal support systems are inadequate
Caregiver regrets that caregiving responsibility does not allow time to meet personal needs
Caregiver expresses problems in coping with patient's behavior
Caregiver expresses negative feeling about patient or relationship
Caregiver neglects patient care
Caregiver abuses patient
Caregiver expresses change in own health status (e.g., fatigue, gastrointestinal upset, headache, weight changes, anger, disturbed sleep, frustration, stress)

Common Expected Outcomes

Caregiver expresses satisfaction with caregiver role.
Caregiver demonstrates competence and confidence in performing the caregiver role by meeting care recipient's physical and psychosocial needs.
Caregiver reports that formal and informal support systems are adequate and helpful.
Caregiver demonstrates flexibility in dealing with problem behavior of care recipient.

NOC Outcomes
Caregiver Well-Being; Caregiver-Patient Relationship
NIC Intervention
Caregiver Support

Ongoing Assessment

Actions/Interventions

■ Assess caregiver–care recipient relationship.

■ Assess family communication pattern.

■ Assess family resources and support systems.

■ Determine the caregiver's knowledge and ability to provide patient care, including bathing, skin care, safety, nutrition, medications, and ambulation.
■ Assess the caregiver's appraisal of the caregiving situation, level of understanding, and willingness to assume caregiver role.

Rationales

Mutually rewarding relationships foster a therapeutic caregiving experience. Dysfunctional relationships can result in ineffective, fragmented care or even lead to neglect or abuse.
Open communication in the family creates a positive environment, whereas concealing feelings creates problems for caregiver and care recipient.
Family and social support is related positively to coping effectiveness. Some cultures are more accepting of this responsibility. However, factors such as blended family units, aging parents, geographical distances between family members, and limited financial resources may hamper coping effectiveness.
Basic instruction may reduce caregiver's anxiety and improve the relationship.

Caregivers need to have a realistic perspective of the situation and the scope of responsibility. Individual responses to caregiving situations are mediated by an appraisal of the personal meaning of the situation. For some, caregiving is viewed as "a duty"; for others it may be an act of love.

■ = Independent ▲ = Collaborative

Actions/Interventions

- Assess for neglect and abuse of the care recipient.

- Assess the caregiver's health.

Rationales

Safe and appropriate care are priority nursing concerns. The nurse must remain a patient advocate to prevent injury to the care recipient and strain on the caregiver.

Even though strongly motivated to perform the role of caregiver, the person may have physical impairments (e.g., vision problems, musculoskeletal weakness, limited upper body strength) or cognitive impairments that affect the quality of the caregiving activities.

Therapeutic Interventions

Actions/Interventions

- Encourage the caregiver to identify available family and friends who can assist with caregiving.

- Encourage involvement of other family members to relieve pressure on the primary caregiver.

- Suggest that the caregiver use available community resources such as respite, home health care, adult day care, geriatric care, housekeeping services, home health aides, Meals On Wheels, companion services, and others, as appropriate.
- Encourage the caregiver to set aside time for self.

- Teach the caregiver stress-reducing techniques.

- Encourage the caregiver in support group participation.

- Encourage the care recipient to thank the caregiver for care given.
- Acknowledge to the caregiver his or her role and its value.

- Provide time for the caregiver to discuss problems, concerns, and feelings. Ask the caregiver how he or she is managing.
- Inquire about the caregiver's health. Provide suggestions for ways to adjust the daily routines to meet the physical limitations of the caregiver.

Rationales

Successful caregiving should not be the sole responsibility of one person. Respite care helps family members cope with the burden of care. In some situations there may be no readily available resources; however, often family members hesitate to notify other family members or significant others because of unresolved conflicts in the past.

Caring for a family member can be a mutually rewarding and satisfying family experience. However, as typical family sizes become smaller because of postponing having children until later in life, future generations will have fewer nuclear family members to provide assistance.

Resources provide opportunity for multiple competent providers and services on a temporary basis or for a more extended period.

The caregiver may need reminders to attend to own physical and emotional needs. Having own "respite" time helps conserve physical and emotional energy. Simple activities such as a relaxing bath, time to read a book, or going out with friends help to maintain physical and mental well-being.

It is important that the caregiver has the opportunity to relax and reenergize emotionally throughout the day to be able to emotionally and physically assume care responsibilities.

Groups that come together for mutual support can be quite beneficial in providing education and anticipatory guidance. Groups can meet in the home, social setting, by telephone, or even through the Internet.

Feeling appreciated decreases feelings of strain.

Caregivers have identified how important it is to feel appreciated for their efforts. The patient may not be able to express this himself or herself.

As a caregiver, the nurse is in an excellent position to provide emotional support and provide guidance throughout this challenging period.

The caregiver may have his or her own health challenges that can become aggravated during the caregiving process.

Education/Continuity of Care

Actions/Interventions	Rationales
■ Provide information on disease process and management strategies.	Accurate information increases understanding of the care recipient's condition and behavior. Caregivers may have an unrealistic picture of the extent of care required at the present time. Home care therapies are becoming increasingly complex (e.g., home dialysis, ventilator care, terminal care, and Alzheimer's care) and require careful attention to the educational process.
■ Instruct the caregiver in management of the care recipient's nursing diagnoses. Demonstrate necessary caregiving skills, and allow sufficient time for learning before return demonstration.	Increased knowledge and skills increase the caregiver's confidence and decrease strain.
■ Refer the caregiver to a social worker for referral for community resources and/or financial aid, if needed.	Grants or special funds can sometimes be used to assist with physical needs.

NANDA-I
NDx Impaired Verbal Communication

Definition: Decreased, delayed, or absent ability to receive, process, transmit, and use a system of symbols

Human communication takes many forms. Persons communicate verbally through the vocalization of a system of sounds that has been formalized into a language. They communicate using body movements to supplement, emphasize, or even alter what is being verbally communicated. In some cases, such as American Sign Language (the formal language of the deaf community) or Signed English, communication is conducted entirely through hand gestures that may or may not be accompanied by body movements and pantomime. Language can be read by watching an individual's lips to observe words as they are shaped. Humans communicate through touch, intuition, written means, art, and sometimes a combination of all of the mechanisms. Communication implies the sending of information as well as the receiving of information. When communication is received, it ceases to be the sole product of the sender as the entire experiential history of the receiver takes over and interprets the information sent. At its best, effective communication is a dialogue that not only involves the transmission of information but also clarification of points made, expansion of ideas and concepts, and exploration of factors that fall out of the original thoughts transmitted. Communication is a multifaceted, kinetic, reciprocal process. Communication may be impaired for any number of reasons, but rarely are all avenues for communication compromised at one time. The task for the nurse, whether encountering the patient in the hospital or in the community, becomes recognizing when communication has become ineffective and then using strategies to improve transmission of information.

Common Related Factors

Brain injury or tumor that adversely affects the transmission, reception, or interpretation of language or other forms of communication
Structural problem (e.g., cleft palate, laryngectomy, tracheostomy, intubation, or wired jaws)
Cultural difference (e.g., speaks different language)
Dyspnea
Fatigue
Sensory challenge involving hearing or vision

Defining Characteristics

Inability to find, recognize, or understand words
Difficulty vocalizing words
Inability to recall familiar words, phrases, or names of known persons, objects, and places
Unable to speak dominant language
Problems in receiving the type of sensory input being sent or sending the type of input necessary for understanding

■ = Independent   ▲ = Collaborative

Nursing Diagnosis Care Plans

Patient uses a form of communication to get needs met and to relate effectively with persons and his or her environment.

NOC Outcomes

Communication: Expressive Ability; Communication: Receptive Ability; Information Processing

NIC Interventions

Active Listening; Communication Enhancement: Hearing Deficit; Communication Enhancement: Speech Deficit

Ongoing Assessment

Actions/Interventions	Rationales
■ Assess the following: 　• The patient's primary and preferred means of communication (e.g., verbal, written, gestures) 　• Ability to understand spoken word	Patients may have skill with many forms of communication, yet they will prefer one method for important communication. It is important for health care workers to understand that the construct of gestured language has an entirely different structure from verbal and written English. Signed English is not the true language of the deaf community but an instructional mechanism developed to teach the structure of English so that individuals with hearing impairments may read and write it. Some members of the deaf community learn to do so effectively. American Sign Language is the true language of the deaf community. U.S. federal law requires the use of an official interpreter to communicate with persons who choose to receive informed consent and other important medical information in their own language.
• The patient's preferred language for verbal and written communication	Patients may speak a language quite well without being able to read it effectively. Discharge self-care and follow-up information must be communicated and reinforced with written information that the patient can use. The nurse can no longer assume that it is the patient's responsibility to grasp the information that is being provided. In recognition of the vast array of cultures and physical challenges that patients face, it is the nurse's responsibility to communicate effectively.
• Ability to understand written words, pictures, gestures	In some cases, the only way to be certain that communication has been effective is to arrange for a certified interpreter to validate information from both sides of the dialogue.
■ Assess conditions or situations that may hinder the patient's ability to use or understand language, such as the following: 　• Alternate airway (e.g., tracheostomy, oral or nasal intubation) 　• Orofacial/maxillary problems (e.g., wired jaws)	When air does not pass over vocal cords, sounds are not produced. Words are articulated by coordinated movement of mouth and tongue; when movement is impinged, communication may be ineffective.
■ Assess for presence of expressive dysphasia (inability to convey information verbally) and receptive dysphasia (word meaning may be scrambled during the processing of information by the patient's brain).	The person with expressive dysphagia has nonfluent speech; however, his or her verbal comprehension is often intact. The ability to read and write may be impaired with this type of dysphagia. The person with receptive dysphagia has fluent speech, but the content of his or her communication is often meaningless. The primary disturbance is an inability to understand all forms of language.

Actions/Interventions

■ Assess for presence and history of dyspnea.

■ Assess energy level.

■ Assess knowledge of patient's, family's, or caregiver's understanding of sign language, as appropriate.

Rationales

Patients who are experiencing breathing problems may reduce or cease verbal communication that may complicate their respiratory efforts.

Fatigue and/or shortness of breath can make communication difficult or impossible.

Individuals who have no formal training in sign language usually develop mechanisms for communication, but because communication is such a critical aspect of everyone's life, consider formal training for patients and caregivers to enhance communication.

Therapeutic Interventions

Actions/Interventions

■ Assist the patient in seeking an evaluation of his or her home and work settings.

■ Anticipate patient needs, and pay attention to nonverbal cues.

■ Place important objects within reach.

■ Provide alternate means of communication for times when interpreters are not available (e.g., a phone contact who can interpret the patient's needs).

■ Encourage the patient's attempts to communicate; praise attempts and achievements.

■ Listen attentively when the patient attempts to communicate. Clarify your understanding of the patient's communication with the patient or an interpreter.

■ Never talk in front of the patient as though he or she comprehends nothing.

■ Keep distractions such as television and radio at a minimum when talking to the patient.

■ Do not speak loudly unless the patient is hearing impaired.

■ Avoid use of medical jargon.

■ Maintain eye contact with the patient when speaking. Stand close, within the patient's line of vision (generally midline).

■ Give the patient ample time to respond. Avoid finishing sentences for the patient. Allow the patient to complete his or her sentence and thought, but if the patient appears to be having difficulty, ask the patient for permission to help. Say the word or phrase slowly and distinctly if help is requested. Be calm and accepting during attempts; do not say you understand if you do not.

Rationales

This information will identify the need for assistive devices such as talking computers, telephone typing device, and interpreters.

The nurse should set aside enough time to attend to all of the details of patient care. Care measures may take longer to complete when there is a communication deficit.

Convenient placement maximizes the patient's sense of independence.

Alternative means of communication (e.g., flash cards, symbol boards, or electronic messaging) can help the person express ideas and communicate needs.

Positive feedback enhances the patient's efforts to overcome communication barriers.

Patients need feedback about the success of their communication attempts. Feedback promotes effective communication by allowing the sender of the message to verify that the message sent was the message received.

Excluding the patient from an interaction increases the patient's sense of frustration and feelings of helplessness.

Removing environmental distractions keeps the patient focused, decreases stimuli going to the brain for interpretation, and enhances the nurse's ability to listen.

Loud talking does not improve the patient's ability to understand if the barriers are primarily language, dysphasia, or a sensory deficit.

Technical terminology used by health care providers can sound like a foreign language to patients and family.

Patients may have a defect in their field of vision or may need to see the nurse's face or lips to enhance understanding of what is being communicated.

This approach may reduce frustration and enhance trust. It may be difficult for patients to respond under pressure; they may need extra time to organize responses, find the correct word, or make necessary language translations.

■ = Independent   ▲ = Collaborative

Actions/Interventions	Rationales
■ If the patient's ability to speak is limited to "yes" and "no" answers, try to phrase questions so that the patient can use these responses.	Patients can become easily frustrated when they cannot communicate in a simple manner.
■ Use short sentences, and ask only one question at a time.	This technique allows the patient to stay focused on one thought. Sudden shifts from one subject to another do not allow time for the brain to keep pace with the messages.
■ Speak slowly and distinctly, repeating key words to prevent confusion. Supplement verbal communication with meaningful gestures.	This approach provides the patient with more channels through which information can be communicated.
■ Give concrete directions that the patient is physically capable of doing (e.g., "point to the pain," "open your mouth," and "turn your head").	Simple, one-action directions enhance comprehension for the patient with language impairment.
■ When the patient has difficulty with verbal expressions, support the work the patient is doing in speech therapy by providing practice sessions often throughout the day. Begin with simple words (e.g., "yes," "no," "this is a cup"), then progress.	Practice with language skills in a supportive environment will increase the patient's communication. Reinforcement by repetition and practice enhances learning.
■ When the patient cannot identify objects by name, give practice in receiving word images (e.g., point to an object, and clearly enunciate its name: "cup" or "pen").	Visual cueing reinforces language comprehension.
■ Correct errors.	Not correcting errors reinforces undesirable performance and makes correction more difficult later.
■ Provide a list of words that the patient can say; add new words to it. Share this list with family, significant others, and other care providers.	Sharing information with others broadens the group of people with whom the patient can communicate.
■ Provide the patient with word-and-phrase cards, writing pad and pencil, or picture board. Use eye blinks or finger movements for "yes" or "no" responses.	Supplemental communication devices are especially helpful for intubated and tracheal patients or those whose jaws are wired.
■ Carry on a one-way conversation with a totally dysphasic patient.	It may not be possible to determine what information is understood by the patient, but it should not be assumed that the patient understands nothing about his or her environment.
▲ Consult a speech therapist for additional help. See that the patient is well rested before each session with the speech therapist.	Fatigue may have an adverse effect on learning ability.
▲ Consider use of an electronic speech generator in postlaryngectomy patients.	Adaptive devices can facilitate communication with patients who cannot produce vocal speech.

Education/Continuity of Care

Actions/Interventions	Rationales
■ Inform the patient, significant others, or caregiver of the type of dysphasia the patient has and how it affects speech, language skills, and understanding.	Many family members assume that a patient's mentation has been affected by a brain injury or tumor; this may or may not be true, and if true, some of the effects may be amenable to remediation.
■ Offer significant others the opportunity to ask questions about the patient's communication problem.	It is important for the family to know that there are many ways to send information to someone and that time may be needed to understand the special needs of the patient.
■ Encourage family members and caregivers to talk to the patient even though the patient may not respond. Suggest that the family engage the patient often throughout the day for short periods. Encourage the family to look for cues that the patient is overstimulated or fatigued.	Meaningful interactions with others decrease the patient's sense of isolation and may assist in recovery from dysphasia. Overstimulation and fatigue hinder effective communication.

Actions/Interventions	Rationales
■ Encourage the patient to socialize with family and friends.	Communication should be encouraged despite impairment.
■ Explain that brain injury decreases attention span.	Changes in cognitive function often accompany language dysfunction in the patient with a brain injury. A decreased attention span limits the patient's ability to concentrate during a long conversation.
▲ Provide the patient with an appointment with a speech therapist, if not already done.	Outpatient speech therapy can support the patient's efforts to recover language skills.
■ Inform the patient and significant others to seek information about dysphasia from the American Speech-Language-Hearing Association, 10810 Rockwell Pike, Rockville, MD 20852.	Community resources can offer additional information and support to patients and families coping with impaired language and communication skills.
■ Refer deaf patients and their families to their local hearing society for community support, education, and sign language training.	Specialized services may be required to meet needs.

Chronic Confusion

Definition: An irreversible, long-standing, and/or progressive deterioration of intellect and personality characterized by decreased ability to interpret environmental stimuli, decreased capacity for intellectual thought processes, and manifested by disturbances of memory, orientation, and behavior

Chronic confusion is not limited to any one age-group, gender, or clinical problem. Chronic confusion can occur in a variety of settings, including the home, hospital, and long-term care facilities. Although often associated with older adults with dementia, younger adults with chronic illnesses may also be affected. Depression, multiple sclerosis, brain infections and tumors, repeated head trauma (as seen in athletes), abnormalities resulting from hypertension, diabetes, anemia, endocrine disorders, malnutrition, and vascular disorders are examples of illnesses that may be associated with chronic confusion. The person with chronic confusion experiences a gradual but progressive decline in cognitive function. Over months or years, the person has increasing problems with memory, comprehension, judgment, abstract thinking, and reasoning. The loss of cognitive ability may result in problems for the person with communication, activities of daily living, and emotional stability. Chronic confusion can have a profound impact on family members and family processes as the patient requires more direct supervision and care. This care plan discusses the management of chronic confusion in any setting. It also identifies the importance of addressing the needs of the caregivers.

Common Related Factors	Defining Characteristics
Alzheimer's disease (dementia of the Alzheimer's type)	Clinical evidence of organic impairment
Multiinfarct dementia	Altered interpretation/response to stimuli
Cerebrovascular accident (CVA)	Progressive/long-standing cognitive impairment
Acquired immunodeficiency disease	No change in level of consciousness
Chronic hepatic encephalopathy	Impaired memory (short-term, long-term)
Chronic drug intoxication	Altered personality
Chronic subdural hematoma	
Parkinson's disease	
Huntington's chorea	
Creutzfeldt-Jakob disease	

■ = Independent   ▲ = Collaborative

Common Expected Outcomes

Patient will remain safe and free from harm.

Family or significant others will verbalize understanding of disease process/prognosis and the patient's needs, identify and participate in interventions to deal effectively with the situation, and provide for maximal independence while meeting safety needs of the patient.

NOC Outcomes

Cognitive Orientation; Decision Making; Distorted Thought Control; Safety Behavior: Home Physical Environment

NIC Interventions

Dementia Management; Environmental Management: Safety; Family Involvement Promotion

Ongoing Assessment

Actions/Interventions	Rationales
■ Assess degree of impairment:	The degree of confusion will determine the amount of reorientation and intervention the patient will need to evaluate reality accurately. The person may be awake and aware of his or her surroundings.
• Evaluate responses on diagnostic examinations (e.g., memory impairments, reality orientation, attention span, calculations).	Decreased attention span and memory loss can contribute to the person's inability to accurately respond to environmental stimuli. A common screening tool is the Mini-Mental State Examination. The Confusion Assessment Method (CAM) is a valid and reliable instrument that can help monitor changes in the person's cognitive function. This tool is effective when assessing older adults.
• Test ability to receive and send effective communications.	Ability and/or willingness to respond to verbal direction and/or limits may vary with degree of reality orientation.
• Note deterioration and changes in personal hygiene or behavior.	This information assists in developing a specific plan for grooming and hygiene activities.
• Talk with significant others regarding baseline behaviors, length of time since onset or progression of the problem, their perception of the prognosis, and other pertinent information and concerns for the patient.	Assessment can identify areas of physical care in which the patient needs assistance. These areas include nutrition, elimination, sleep, rest, exercise, bathing, grooming, and dressing. It is important to distinguish ability and motivation in the initiation, performance, and maintenance of self-care activities. Patients may either have the ability and minimal motivation, or motivation and minimal ability.
■ Evaluate response to care providers and receptiveness to interventions.	A patient who has developed trust in a care provider, as well as a relationship with him or her, may be able to accept direction.
■ Determine anxiety level in relation to the situation. Note behavior that may be indicative of potential for violence.	Confusion, disorientation, impaired judgment, suspiciousness, and loss of social inhibitions may result in socially inappropriate and/or harmful behaviors to self or others. The patient may have poor impulse behavior control.
■ Assess for sundown syndrome.	This phenomenon associated with confusion occurs in the late afternoon. The patient exhibits increasing restlessness, agitation, and confusion. Sundowning may be related to sleep disorders, hunger, thirst, or unmet toileting needs.

Therapeutic Interventions

Actions/Interventions	Rationales
■ Prevent further deterioration and maximize level of function: • Provide calm environment; eliminate extraneous noise and stimuli.	Increased levels of visual and auditory stimulation can be misinterpreted by the confused patient. Pictures on walls or even shadows can be perceived by the confused patient as threatening. High noise levels can disrupt sleep and add to levels of anxiety and stress.

Actions/Interventions

- Communicate using simple, concrete nouns in positive terms.

- Maintain consistency in the person's environment and daily schedule.

- Avoid challenging illogical thinking because defensive reactions may result.

- Encourage the family and significant others to provide ongoing orientation and input about current news and family happenings.

- Maintain reality-oriented relationships and environment (e.g., display clocks, calendars, personal items, seasonal decorations).

- Encourage participation in resocialization groups.

- Allow the patient to reminisce, existing in his or her own reality if not detrimental to the patient's well-being.
- Provide safety measures (e.g., close supervision, identification bracelet, medication lockup, lower temperature on hot water tank).
- ■ Provide repetitive hand activities.

Rationales

This communication technique can reduce anxiety experienced in unfamiliar surroundings. For example, asking the confused person to "Stay sitting in the chair" is more positive than saying "Don't get up."

Consistency in placement of furnishings promotes orientation and memory. Following the same schedule each day reduces stress and anxiety caused by change.

Challenges to the patient's thinking can be perceived as threatening. The confused patient will become more anxious and even combative.

Increased orientation ensures a greater degree of safety for the patient. The confused patient may not completely understand what is happening. The caregiver's facial expression and tone of voice may enhance the patient's level of comfort.

Orientation to one's environment increases one's ability to trust others. Encourage the patient to check the calendar and clock often to orient himself or herself. Familiar personal possessions increase the patient's comfort level and decrease the sense of alienation that the patient may feel in a strange environment.

Encouraging the patient to assume responsibility for his or her own behavior will increase his or her sense of independence. It is important for the patient to learn socially appropriate behavior through group interactions. This approach provides an opportunity for the patient to observe the impact his or her behavior has on those around him or her. It also facilitates the development of acceptable social skills.

Depending on etiology, long-term memory is usually retained longer than short-term; reminiscing can be enjoyable to the patient.

These measures promote patient safety.

Engaging in safe, repetitive activities occupies the patient's mind and hands. The activities may reduce agitation and provide a release of energy. The confused person may find it calming to fold and refold towels and washcloths. A box filled with pieces of cloth, balls of yarn, and stuffed animals can promote contentment as the patient removes items from the box and replaces them.

Education/Continuity of Care

Actions/Interventions

- ■ Assist family and significant others in developing coping strategies.
  - Determine family members' resources and their availability and willingness to participate in meeting the patient's needs.
  - Identify appropriate community resources (e.g., Alzheimer's or brain injury support groups, respite care).
  - Evaluate attention to own needs, including the grieving process.

Rationales

Referral of the family for often-needed legal and financial guidance may be necessary.

Community resources provide support, assist with problem solving, and help the family cope with the long-term stress in caring for the patient.

Caregiver strain can lead to increasing frustration with the confused person. The frustration can precipitate anger and abuse.

■ = Independent ▲ = Collaborative

Actions/Interventions

- Provide written information for significant others on living with chronic confusion.
- Promote wellness (teaching and discharge considerations).
■ Determine ongoing treatment needs and appropriate resources.

- Develop a care plan with the family to meet the patient's and the family's individual needs.
- Provide appropriate referral (e.g., Meals On Wheels, adult home care, home care agency, respite care).

Rationales

This information assists significant others with understanding the disorder and its impact on their lives.

All these interventions should maximize the patient's level of functioning and quality of life for both the family and the caregivers.

The family needs to let the patient do all that he or she is able to do.

Community resources can support the family and reduce the demands associated with caregiving.

Related Care Plan

Alzheimer's disease/Dementia, p. 475

Constipation

Definition: Decrease in normal frequency of defecation accompanied by difficult or incomplete passage of stool and/or passage of excessively hard, dry stool

Constipation is a common, yet complex problem; it is especially prevalent among older patients. Diet, exercise, and daily routine are important factors in maintaining normal bowel patterns. Too little fluid, too little fiber, inactivity or immobility, and disruption in daily routines can result in constipation. Use of medications, particularly narcotic analgesics or overuse of laxatives, can cause constipation. Overuse of enemas can cause constipation, as can ignoring the need to defecate. Psychological disorders such as stress and depression can cause constipation. Because privacy is an issue for most, being away from home, hospitalized, or otherwise being deprived of adequate privacy can result in constipation. Because "normal" patterns of bowel elimination vary so widely from individual to individual, some people believe they are constipated if a day passes without a bowel movement; for others, every third or fourth day is normal. Chronic constipation can result in the development of hemorrhoids; diverticulosis (particularly in older patients who have a high incidence of diverticulitis); straining at stool, which can cause sudden death; and although rare, perforation of the colon. Constipation is usually episodic, although it can become a lifelong, chronic problem. Because tumors of the colon and rectum can result in obstipation (complete lack of passage of stool), it is important to rule out these possibilities. Dietary management (increasing fluid and fiber) remains the most effective treatment for constipation.

Common Related Factors

Inadequate fluid intake
Low-fiber diet
Inactivity, immobility
Medication use
Lack of privacy
Fear of pain with defecation
Habitual denial and ignoring of urge to defecate
Laxative abuse
Stress and/or depression
Tumor or other obstructing mass
Neurogenic disorders

Defining Characteristics

Infrequent passage of stool
Passage of hard, dry stool
Straining at stools
Passage of liquid fecal seepage
Frequent but nonproductive desire to defecate
Anorexia
Abdominal distention
Nausea and vomiting
Dull headache
Verbalized pain or fear of pain with defecation

Common Expected Outcomes

Patient passes soft, formed stool at a frequency perceived as "normal" by the patient.

Patient or caregiver verbalizes measures that will prevent recurrence of constipation.

NOC Outcomes
Bowel Elimination; Medication Response; Self-Care Toileting

NIC Interventions
Constipation/Impaction Management; Bowel Training; Teaching: Prescribed Medication

Ongoing Assessment

Actions/Interventions	Rationales
■ Assess usual pattern of elimination; compare with present pattern. Include size, frequency, color, and quality of stool.	"Normal" frequency of passing stool varies from twice daily to once every third or fourth day. It is important to ascertain what is "normal" for each individual.
■ Evaluate laxative use, type, and frequency.	Chronic use of laxatives causes the muscles and nerves of the colon to function inadequately in producing an urge to defecate. Over time, the colon becomes atonic and distended.
■ Evaluate reliance on enemas for elimination.	Abuse or overuse of cathartics and enemas can result in dependence on them for evacuation, because the colon becomes distended and does not respond normally to the presence of stool.
■ Evaluate usual dietary habits, eating habits, eating schedule, and liquid intake.	Change in mealtime, type of food, and disruption of usual schedule can lead to constipation.
■ Assess activity level.	Prolonged bed rest, lack of exercise, and inactivity contribute to constipation.
■ Evaluate current medication usage that may contribute to constipation.	Drugs that can cause constipation include the following: narcotics, antacids with calcium or aluminum base, antidepressants, anticholinergics, antihypertensives, general anesthetics, hypnotics, and iron and calcium supplements.
■ Assess the need for privacy for elimination (e.g., use of bedpan, access to bathroom facilities with privacy during work hours).	Many individuals report that being away from home limits their ability to have a bowel movement. Those who travel or require hospitalization may have difficulty having a bowel movement away from home.
■ Evaluate fear of pain with defecation.	Hemorrhoids, anal fissures, or other anorectal disorders that are painful can cause the patient to ignore the urge to defecate, which over time results in a dilated rectum that no longer responds to the presence of stool.
■ Assess degree to which the patient's procrastination contributes to constipation.	Ignoring the defecation urge eventually leads to chronic constipation, because the rectum no longer senses, or responds to, the presence of stool. The longer the stool remains in the rectum, the drier and harder (and more difficult to pass) it becomes.
■ Assess for history of neurogenic diseases, such as multiple sclerosis or Parkinson's disease.	Neurogenic disorders may alter the colon's ability to perform peristalsis.

Therapeutic Interventions

Actions/Interventions	Rationales
■ Encourage daily fluid intake of 2000 to 3000 mL/day, if not contraindicated medically.	Adequate fluid is necessary to keep the fecal mass soft. However, patients, especially older patients, may have cardiovascular limitations that require that less fluid be taken.
■ Encourage increased fiber in diet (e.g., raw fruits, fresh vegetables, whole grains); a minimum of 20 g of dietary fiber per day is recommended.	Fiber passes through the intestine essentially unchanged. When it reaches the colon, it absorbs water and forms a gel, which adds bulk to the stool and makes defecation easier.

■ = Independent   ▲ = Collaborative

Actions/Interventions	Rationales
■ Encourage the patient to consume prunes, prune juice, cold cereal, and bean products.	These foods are "natural" cathartics because of their high fiber content.
■ Encourage physical activity and regular exercise. Encourage isometric abdominal and gluteal exercises.	Ambulation and/or abdominal exercises strengthen abdominal muscles that facilitate defecation.
■ Encourage a regular time for elimination.	Many persons defecate following the first daily meal or coffee, as a result of the gastrocolic reflex; depending on the person's usual schedule, any time, as long as it is regular, is fine.
■ Digitally remove fecal impaction.	Stool that remains in the rectum for long periods becomes dry and hard; debilitated patients, especially older patients, may not be able to pass these stools without manual assistance.
■ Suggest the following measures to minimize rectal discomfort:	
• Warm sitz bath	The warmth of the water relaxes muscles before defecation attempts.
• Hemorrhoidal preparations	These over-the-counter preparations shrink swollen hemorrhoidal tissue.
■ For hospitalized patients, the following should be employed:	
• Orient patient to location of bathroom, and encourage use, unless contraindicated.	A sitting position with knees flexed straightens the rectum, enhances use of abdominal muscles, and facilitates defecation.
• Offer a warmed bedpan to bedridden patients; assist patient in assuming a high-Fowler's position with knees flexed.	This position best uses gravity and allows for effective Valsalva maneuver.
• Curtain off the area.	Providing privacy helps the person relax for defecation.
■ For patients with neurogenic bowel problems:	
• Abdominal massage—Using heel of hand or a tennis ball, apply and release pressure firmly but gently around abdomen in a clockwise direction.	Abdominal massage has been reported to be useful in neurogenic bowel disorder but not for constipation in older adults.
• Digital anorectal stimulation—A gloved lubricated finger is gently inserted into rectum and slowly rotated in a circular motion. This is done for about 15 to 20 seconds until flatus and/or stool is passed.	Digital stimulation increases muscular activity in rectum by raising rectal pressure to aid in expelling fecal matter.

Education/Continuity of Care

Actions/Interventions	Rationales
▲ Consult dietitian regarding dietary sources of fiber.	A person unaccustomed to a high-fiber diet may experience abdominal discomfort and flatulence; a gradual increase in fiber intake is recommended.
■ Explain or reinforce to the patient and caregiver the importance of the following:	These steps lead to reestablishing regular bowel habits.
• A balanced diet that contains adequate fiber, fresh fruits, vegetables, and grains	Twenty grams of fiber per day is recommended.
• Adequate fluid intake (8 glasses per day or 2000 to 3000 mL/day).	Increased hydration promotes a softer fecal mass.
• Regular meals	Successful bowel training relies on routine.
• Regular time for evacuation and adequate time for defecation	Facilitating regular time prevents the bowel from emptying sporadically.
• Regular exercise and activity	Exercises strengthen abdominal muscles and stimulate peristalsis.

Actions/Interventions	Rationales
• Privacy for defecation	Privacy allows the patient to relax, which can help promote defecation.
■ Teach patients and caregivers to read product labels.	It is important for patients and caregivers to determine the fiber content per serving.
▲ Teach use of pharmacological agents as ordered, as in the following:	
• Bulk fiber (Metamucil and similar fiber products)	These laxatives increase fluid, gaseous, and solid bulk of intestinal contents.
• Stool softeners (e.g., Colace)	These laxatives soften stool and lubricate intestinal mucosa.
• Chemical irritants (e.g., castor oil, cascara, Milk of Magnesia)	These laxatives irritate the bowel mucosa and cause rapid propulsion of contents of small intestine.
• Suppositories	These laxatives aid in softening stools and stimulate rectal mucosa; best results occur when given 30 minutes before usual defecation time or after breakfast.
• Oil retention enema	This intervention softens stool.

Ineffective Coping

Definition: Inability to form a valid appraisal of the stressors, inadequate choices of practiced responses, and/or inability to use available resources

For most persons, everyday life includes its share of stressors and demands, ranging from family, work, and professional role responsibilities to major life events such as divorce, illness, and the death of loved ones. How one responds to such stressors depends in part on the person's coping resources. Such resources can include optimistic beliefs, social support networks, personal health and energy, problem-solving skills, and material resources. Sociocultural and religious factors may influence how people view and handle their problems. Some cultures may prefer privacy and avoid sharing their fears in public, even to health care providers. As resources become limited and problems become more acute, this strategy may prove ineffective. Vulnerable populations such as older patients, those in adverse socioeconomic situations, those with complex medical problems such as substance abuse, or those who find themselves suddenly physically challenged may not have the resources or skills to cope with their acute or chronic stressors. Such problems can occur in any setting (e.g., during hospitalization for an acute event, in the home or rehabilitation environment as a result of chronic illness, or in response to another threat or loss).

Common Related Factors

High degree of threat
Disturbance in pattern of appraisal of threat or pattern of tension release
Inadequate support system
Inadequate available resources
Inadequate preparation for stressors
Inadequate level of confidence in ability to cope
Situational crises
Maturational crises

Defining Characteristics

Verbalization of inability to cope
Inability to make decisions
Inability to ask for help
Lack of goal-directed behavior
Inadequate problem solving
Inability to meet role expectations
Abuse of chemical agents
Poor concentration
Fatigue
Destructive behavior toward self or others
Inappropriate use of defense mechanisms
High illness rate
Insomnia

■ = Independent ▲ = Collaborative

Common Expected Outcomes

Patient uses available resources and support systems.
Patient describes and initiates effective coping strategies.
Patient describes positive results from new behaviors.

NOC Outcomes
Coping; Decision Making; Information Processing
NIC Intervention
Coping Enhancement

Ongoing Assessment

Actions/Interventions	Rationales
■ Assess for presence of defining characteristics.	Behavioral and physiological responses to stress can be varied and provide clues to the level of coping difficulty.
■ Assess specific stressors.	Accurate appraisal can facilitate development of appropriate coping strategies. Because a patient has an altered health status does not mean the coping difficulties he or she exhibits are only (if at all) related to that. Persistent stressors may exhaust the patient's ability to maintain effective coping.
■ Determine the patient's perception of the stressful situation.	The patient's cultural heritage and previous experiences may affect the patient's understanding of and response to the current situation. This information provides a foundation for planning care and selecting appropriate interventions.
■ Assess available or useful past and present coping mechanisms.	Successful adjustment is influenced by previous coping success. Patients with a history of maladaptive coping may need additional resources. Likewise, previously successful coping skills may be inadequate in the present situation.
■ Evaluate resources and support systems available to patient.	Patients may have support in one setting, such as during hospitalization, yet be discharged home without sufficient support for effective coping. Resources may include significant others, health care providers such as home health nurses, community resources, and spiritual counseling.
■ Assess level of understanding and readiness to learn needed lifestyle changes.	Appropriate problem solving requires accurate information and understanding of options. Often patients who are ineffectively coping are unable to hear or assimilate needed information.
■ Assess decision-making and problem-solving abilities.	Patients may feel that the threat is greater than their resources to handle it and feel a loss of control over solving the threat or problem.

Therapeutic Interventions

Actions/Interventions	Rationales
■ Establish a working relationship with the patient through continuity of care.	An ongoing relationship establishes trust, reduces the feeling of isolation, and may facilitate coping.
■ Provide opportunities to express concerns, fears, feelings, and expectations.	Verbalization of actual or perceived threats can help reduce anxiety and open doors for ongoing communication.
■ Convey feelings of acceptance and understanding. Avoid false reassurances.	An honest relationship facilitates problem solving and successful coping. False reassurances are never helpful to the patient and only serve to relieve the discomfort of the care provider.
■ Encourage the patient to identify his or her own strengths and abilities.	During crises, patients may not be able to recognize their strengths. Fostering awareness can expedite use of these strengths.
■ Assist patients with accurately evaluating the situation and their own accomplishments.	It can be helpful to recognize that the patient has the skills and reserves of strength to do the emotional work required. The patient may need help coming to a realistic perspective of the situation.

Actions/Interventions

- Explore attitudes and feelings about required lifestyle changes.
- Encourage the patient to seek information that increases coping skills.
- Provide information the patient wants and needs. Do not provide more than the patient can handle.
- Encourage the patient to set realistic goals.

- Assist the patient with problem solving in a constructive manner.
- Reduce stimuli in an environment that could be misinterpreted as threatening.

- Provide outlets that foster feelings of personal achievement and self-esteem.
- Point out signs of positive progress or change.

- Encourage the patient to communicate feelings with significant others.
- Help the patient recognize maladaptive behaviors.

Rationales

Each patient is unique. Cultural, religious, ethnic, and individual differences affect attitudes.

Patients who are not coping well may need more guidance initially.

Patients who are coping ineffectively have reduced ability to assimilate information.

Setting realistic goals helps the patient gain control over the situation. Guiding the patient to view the situation in smaller parts may make the problem more manageable.

Constructive problem solving can promote independence and a sense of autonomy.

In the acute hospital setting, patients are often exposed to new equipment and environments. This can increase anxiety and make coping more challenging.

Opportunities to role-play or rehearse appropriate actions can increase confidence for behavior in actual situations.

Patients who are coping ineffectively may not be able to assess progress.

Unexpressed feelings can increase stress.

Pointing out observed behaviors helps the patient focus on more appropriate strategies.

Education/Continuity of Care

Actions/Interventions

- Instruct in need for adequate rest and balanced diet.
- Teach use of relaxation, exercise, and diversional activities as methods to cope with stress.
- ▲ Involve social services, psychiatric liaison, and pastoral care for additional and ongoing support resources.
- Assist in development of an alternative support system. Encourage participation in self-help groups, if available.

Rationales

Inadequate diet and fatigue can themselves be stressors.

A variety of brief interventions can be used toward assisting patients with reducing their level of stress.

Specialized services may be required to meet specific needs.

Relationships with persons with common interests and goals can be beneficial.

NANDA-I NDx **Impaired Dentition**

Definition: Disruption in tooth development/eruption patterns or structural integrity of individual teeth

Good oral health can affect a person's quality of life through such aspects as appearance, self-esteem, enjoyment from food, absence from dental pain and infections, and overall improved health status. Recent studies have examined the relationship between dentition status and dietary habits. It has been shown that many of the foods avoided by people with poor dentition status (such as high-fiber fruits and vegetables) are the ones found to be protective against cardiovascular disease, stroke, metabolic syndrome, and some cancers. Similarly, many people with tooth loss choose easier-to-eat foods containing more saturated fat and refined carbohydrates, putting them at great health risk. Preventative oral health measures to prevent dental caries and tooth loss need to be addressed throughout one's life, especially among older adults, who are at the greatest risk for systemic health problems related to impaired dentition.

■ = Independent ▲ = Collaborative

Common Related Factors

Ineffective oral hygiene
Barriers to self-care
Deficient knowledge regarding dental health
Dietary habits/nutritional deficits
Economic factors/lack of access to professional care
Chronic use of coffee/tea/red wine
Chronic use of tobacco
Chronic vomiting
Excessive use of abrasive cleaning agents
Excessive intake of fluorides
Genetic disposition
Selected prescription medications
Sensitivity to heat or cold

Defining Characteristics

Crown or root caries
Erosion of enamel
Excessive plaque or calculus
Halitosis
Loose teeth
Malocclusion
Missing teeth/absence of teeth
Root caries
Tooth enamel discoloration
Tooth misalignment
Toothache
Worn down or abraded teeth

Common Expected Outcomes

Patient demonstrates ability to care for own teeth and mouth independently as evidenced by a regular routine of brushing and flossing, and using mouthwash and fluoridation appropriately.

Upon examination, patient has clean teeth, healthy gums, and mouth with pleasant odor.

Patient performs regular and complete denture cleaning and care.

Patient obtains regular dental checkups as feasible.

NOC Outcomes
Self-Care: Oral Hygiene; Oral Hygiene

NIC Interventions
Oral Health Promotion; Oral Health Restoration; Oral Heath Maintenance; Nutritional Management

Ongoing Assessment

Actions/Interventions	Rationales
■ Assess oral hygiene practices.	Information provides direction on possible causative factors and guidance for subsequent education. Long-standing habits may be difficult to break.
■ Assess status of teeth (color, presence of debris), gums, mucous membranes, and tongue (color, moisture, texture, irritation, presence of infection). Use moist, padded tongue blade to gently pull back the cheeks, lips, and gums. Use good lighting.	Tongue blades expose areas of oral cavity for inspection. Early assessment facilitates prompt treatment. Specific manifestations guide accurate treatment.
■ Assess nutritional status.	Dental health is closely related to nutritional status, and poor food choices can be a contributing cause for dentition problems. Likewise, poor dentition can affect one's nutrient consumption, with people with loss of teeth consuming fewer fruits and vegetables but more saturated fat. These dietary changes put the patient at increased risk for systemic diseases.
■ Assess mouth for dryness and breath for odor.	A normal flow of saliva is important in keeping the teeth clean. Halitosis can be due to dry mouth, impaired dentition, or a variety of medical problems.
■ Assess use of dental appliances, noting fit. Remove to more completely visualize oral cavity. Determine patient's practice of removing dentures at night.	Information provides direction on possible causative factors and guidance for subsequent education or assistance as needed. Dentures should be removed and cleaned every night.
■ Assess patient's physical and cognitive ability to complete daily oral care routines.	Patients, especially geriatric or acutely ill patients, may need assistance in completing an oral care routine. Perception handicaps may impair an individual's ability to maintain good health practices.

Actions/Interventions	**Rationales**
■ Assess whether economic problems present a barrier to maintaining improved dental hygiene.	Patients may be too proud to ask for assistance or may be unaware of community services available to them. The growing number of uninsured and underinsured Americans, especially as related to dental care, is compounding this problem.
■ Assess for any complaint of tooth ache.	As dental caries progress to the pulp of the tooth, abscess development is common and painful, requiring dental evaluation.
■ Assess to what degree "fear of dentists" plays a role in avoidance of dental care.	Patients may have had prior personal negative experiences or may just be expecting the dental process to be uncomfortable based on misconceptions and exaggerated stories. Providing accurate information about the many "pain-free" treatments available may help to reduce this fear.

Therapeutic Interventions

Actions/Interventions	**Rationales**
■ Establish a mouth care routine including toothbrushing at regular intervals with a soft-bristle toothbrush using a fluoride-containing toothpaste. • Brushing teeth in an up-and-down manner. • Brushing of teeth at least twice a day • Including the gums and tongue in oral care. • Replacing toothbrush as bristles wear down. • Suggest an ultrasonic toothbrush as an alternative for patients with dexterity issues.	Mechanical cleansing of the teeth using a toothbrush is key in effective dental care to prevent plaque buildup.
■ Encourage the patient to rinse mouth with warm saline or an antiplaque mouth rinse.	These measures help promote oral hygiene. Many older patients taking certain medications have dry mouth.
■ Encourage or assist the patient in performing oral hygiene after each meal and as often as needed.	Meticulous oral hygiene reduces buildup of bacteria.
■ Encourage gentle flossing of teeth with unwaxed dental floss as able.	Flossing promotes gum health and reduces buildup of plaque. Correct techniques need to be reinforced.
■ Assist with denture care as needed.	Dentures should be removed and cleaned every night. Often patients do not have the manual dexterity to accomplish this on their own.
■ Apply lubricant to lips and oral mucosa as needed.	Lubrication promotes comfort and prevents cracking.
■ Assist with identifying meal plans tolerated with any special dental problems. Instruct to avoid high-sugar foods that can promote caries.	Adequate nutrition is key to promoting good oral health and tissue healing.

Education/Continuity of Care

Actions/Interventions	**Rationales**
■ Instruct patient (and caregivers as appropriate) in the preventive oral hygiene regimen: brushing, flossing, mouth rinsing, denture care.	Not all patients view dental health as a priority. Information enables the patient to take better control in selecting and implementing required changes in behavior.
▲ Instruct patient in the importance of maintaining a healthy diet despite dentition problems. Refer to dietitian as needed.	Adequate nutrition is key to healthy teeth and body. Depending on the patient's dentition problems, it may not be easy to eat foods high in fiber, such as raw fruits and vegetables. Dietary consultation can provide guidance on any changes required.
■ Instruct patient to avoid abrasive food products such as coffee tea/ red wine, and discourage smoking and tobacco chewing.	These products can cause dental erosion.
■ Instruct patient in importance of regular dental checkups.	Checkups identify and treat problems early.
■ Assist patient in finding access to affordable dental services.	Economic barriers are a huge deterrent to regular dental care for many patients. Potential community resources should be identified as available.

■ = Independent　▲ = Collaborative

Nursing Diagnosis Care Plans

Diarrhea

Definition: Passage of loose, unformed stools

Diarrhea may result from a variety of factors, including intestinal absorption disorders, increased secretion of fluid by the intestinal mucosa, and hypermotility of the intestine. Problems associated with diarrhea, which may be acute or chronic, include fluid and electrolyte imbalance and altered skin integrity. In older patients, or those with chronic disease (e.g., acquired immunodeficiency syndrome), diarrhea can be life threatening. Diarrhea may result from infectious (i.e., viral, bacterial, or parasitic) processes; inflammatory bowel diseases (e.g., Crohn's disease); drug therapies (e.g., antibiotics); increased osmotic loads (e.g., tube feedings); radiation; or increased intestinal motility such as with irritable bowel disease. Treatment is based on addressing the cause of the diarrhea, replacing fluids and electrolytes, providing nutrition (if diarrhea is prolonged and/or severe), and maintaining skin integrity. Health care workers and other caregivers must take precautions (e.g., diligent hand washing between patients) to avoid spreading diarrhea from person to person, including self.

Common Related Factors

Stress
Anxiety
Side effects of medication use
Laxative abuse
Gastrointestinal disorders
Motor disorders: irritable bowel
Mucosal inflammation: Crohn's disease or ulcerative colitis
Malabsorption
Increased secretion
Enteric infections: viral, bacterial, or parasitic
Disagreeable dietary intake
Tube feedings
Radiation
Chemotherapy
Surgical procedures: bowel resection, gastrectomy
Short bowel syndrome
Lactose intolerance
Alcohol abuse

Defining Characteristics

Abdominal pain
Cramping
Frequency of stools (more than 3/day)
Loose or liquid stools
Urgency
Hyperactive bowel sounds or sensations

Common Expected Outcomes

Patient passes soft, formed stool no more than three times per day.
Patient has negative stool cultures.

NOC Outcomes
Bowel Elimination; Fluid Balance; Medication Response
NIC Interventions
Diarrhea Management; Enteral Tube Feeding; Teaching: Prescribed Medications

Ongoing Assessment

Actions/Interventions	Rationales
■ Assess for abdominal pain, cramping, frequency, urgency, loose or liquid stools, and hyperactive bowel sensations.	These are findings associated with diarrhea.
▲ Culture stool.	Testing will identify causative organisms.

Actions/Interventions	Rationales
■ Inquire about the following:	
• Tolerance to milk and other dairy products	Patients with lactose intolerance have insufficient lactase, the enzyme that digests lactose. The presence of lactose in the intestines increases osmotic pressure and draws water into the intestinal lumen.
• Medications the patient is or has been taking	Laxatives and antibiotics may cause diarrhea. *C. difficile* can colonize the intestine following antibiotic use and lead to pseudomembranous enterocolitis: *C. difficile* is a common cause of nosocomial diarrhea in health care facilities. Magnesium and calcium supplements can also cause diarrhea.
• Food intolerances	Spicy, fatty, or high-carbohydrate foods; caffeine; sugar-free foods with sorbitol; or alcohol may cause diarrhea.
• Method of food preparation	Fried food, food contaminated with bacteria during preparation, or contaminated tube feedings may cause diarrhea.
• Osmolality of tube feedings	Hyperosmolar food or fluid draws excess fluid into the gut, stimulates peristalsis, and causes diarrhea.
• Change in eating schedule	Changes in eating pattern can result in gastrointestinal manifestations.
• Current stressors	Some individuals respond to stress with hyperactivity of the gastrointestinal tract.
■ Check for history of the following:	
• Previous gastrointestinal surgery	Following bowel resection, a period (1 to 3 weeks) of diarrhea is normal.
• Gastrointestinal diseases	Diseases such as IBS and gastroenteritis can result in malabsorption and lead to chronic diarrhea.
• Abdominal radiation	Radiation causes sloughing of the intestinal mucosa, decreases usual absorption capacity, and may result in diarrhea.
■ Assess for fecal impaction.	Liquid stool (apparent diarrhea) may seep past a fecal impaction.
■ Assess the impact of therapeutic or diagnostic regimens on diarrhea.	Preparation for radiography or surgery, and radiation or chemotherapy predispose to diarrhea by altering the mucosal surface and transit time through the bowel.
■ Assess hydration status, as in the following:	
• Input and output	Diarrhea can lead to profound dehydration.
• Skin turgor	Decreased skin turgor and tenting of the skin occur in dehydration.
• Moisture of mucous membranes	Dehydration causes dry mucous membranes.
■ Assess condition of perianal skin.	Diarrheal stools may be highly corrosive as a result of increased enzyme content.
■ Explore emotional impact of illness, hospitalization, and/ or soiling accidents.	Loss of control of bowel elimination that occurs with diarrhea can lead to feelings of embarrassment.

Therapeutic Interventions

Actions/Interventions	Rationales
▲ Give antidiarrheal drugs as ordered.	Most antidiarrheal drugs suppress gastrointestinal motility, thus allowing for more fluid absorption. Supplements of beneficial bacteria ("probiotics") or yogurt may reduce symptoms.
■ Provide the following dietary alterations:	
• Bulk fiber (e.g., cereal, grains, Metamucil)	Bulking agents and dietary fibers absorb fluid from the stool and help thicken the stool.
• "Natural" bulking agents (e.g., rice, apples, matzos, cheese)	
• Avoidance of stimulants (e.g., caffeine, carbonated beverages)	Stimulants may increase gastrointestinal motility and worsen diarrhea.

■ = Independent   ▲ = Collaborative

Actions/Interventions

- Encourage fluids to 1.5 to 2 L/24 hr plus 200 mL for each loose stool in adults unless contraindicated; consider nutritional support.
- Evaluate appropriateness of physician's radiograph protocols for bowel preparation on basis of age, weight, condition, disease, and other therapies.
- Assist with or administer perianal care after each bowel movement. Barrier creams can be used to protect the skin.
- For patients with enteral tube feeding, employ the following:
  - Change feeding tube equipment according to institutional policy, but no less than every 24 hours.
  - Administer tube feeding at room temperature.
  - Initiate tube feeding slowly.

  - Decrease rate or dilute feeding if diarrhea persists or worsens.
- ▲ For patients with diarrhea from intestinal infection, anticipate the need for contact precautions.

Rationales

Fluids compensate for malabsorption and loss of nutrients.

Older, frail patients or those patients already depleted may require less bowel preparation or additional intravenous fluid therapy during preparation.
This measure prevents perianal skin excoriation.

Contaminated equipment can cause diarrhea.

Extremes of temperature can stimulate peristalsis.
Starting a tube feeding at a slow infusion rate allows the gastrointestinal system to accommodate intake.
Decreasing the rate of infusion or osmolarity of the feeding prevents hyperosmolar diarrhea.
Contact precautions are necessary to prevent the transmission of microorganisms to others.

Education/Continuity of Care

Actions/Interventions

- Teach the patient or caregiver the following dietary changes that can be controlled:
  - Avoid spicy, fatty foods, alcohol, and caffeine.
  - Broil, bake, or boil foods; avoid frying.
  - Avoid foods that are disagreeable.
- Encourage reporting of diarrhea that occurs with prescription drugs.

- Teach the patient or caregiver to use antidiarrheal medications as ordered.
- Teach the patient or caregiver the importance of fluid replacement during diarrheal episodes.
- Teach the patient or caregiver the importance of good perianal hygiene after each bowel movement.
  - Wet wiping or cleansing is most effective.
  - Do not use wipes that contain alcohol or perfumes.
  - Dry perianal area thoroughly by patting and not rubbing area.
  - Use barrier creams to prevent excoriation.
- Teach the patient and caregiver the importance of hand washing following toileting or perianal hygiene.

- Explain the need to avoid unnecessary use of antibiotics.

Rationales

These dietary changes can slow the passage of stool through the colon and reduce or eliminate diarrhea.

There are usually several antibiotics with which the patient can be treated; if the one prescribed causes diarrhea, this should be reported promptly.
Appropriate use of antidiarrheal medications can promote effective bowel elimination.
Fluids prevent dehydration.

Hygiene controls perianal skin excoriation and minimizes risk for spread of infectious diarrhea.

Most acute diarrhea is caused by enteric infection. Good hand washing will prevent the spread of the infectious agents.
Many antibiotics reduce the normal bacterial flora in the intestinal tract causing more harmful bacteria to multiply. Supplements of beneficial bacteria (e.g., yogurt) can reduce antibiotic-associated diarrhea and symptoms.

NANDA-I NDx Disturbed Energy Field

Definition: Disruption of the flow of energy surrounding a person's being that results in a disharmony of the body, mind, or spirit

Each person is an open energy system. The energy field is one aspect of the human energy system, the other parts being the chakras and meridians. This threefold system is vibrational in nature and continuously interactive within itself and all other systems of the body. In energy field disruption the patient may present any number of concerns indicating disharmony and imbalance in one or more of these energy systems (e.g., pain, fatigue, stress, depression, addiction, nausea, also side effects from anesthesia and various therapies).

In many cases the patient has tried several avenues of Western medicine and is not satisfied with the results. Treatment of the physical problem by surgical procedure or medication is often not adequate to bring balance and harmony to the person. The integration of energy work (Eastern medicine) with Western medicine is ideal. Energy-based therapies may find problems before symptoms develop in the body. Nurses can help patients heal in body, mind, and spirit by using energy techniques grounded in traditions thousands of years old (i.e., Reiki, Therapeutic Touch, Healing Touch, and other energy therapies). Nurses acquainted with energy work can assist the patient with healing and restoring energy field balance in any patient care setting, including hospital, home, long-term care, or ambulatory care. This care plan is limited to the most basic energy therapy techniques.

Common Related Factors

Maturational
- Age-related developmental crises
- Age-related developmental difficulties

Physiological
- Illness
- Fatigue
- Depleted nutritional state
- Pain
- Injury
- Sleep deprivation
- Minimal exercise

Psychological
- Anxiety
- Fear
- Grieving
- Pain
- Stress
- Depression

Spiritual
- Minimal spiritual nourishment

Treatment related
- Chemotherapy
- Radiation therapy
- Immobility
- Perioperative experience

Defining Characteristics

A visual healer will see changes in shadings around the person's body.

An auditory healer may pick up sounds of disharmony in the energy field.

A kinesthetic healer may sense tingling, temperature changes, and degree of waves.

■ = Independent   ▲ = Collaborative

Common Expected Outcome

Patient verbalizes decreased pain, improved mood, increased sleep, increased energy, decreased anxiety, and/or decreased stress.

NOC Outcome

Comfort Level; Pain Level; Personal Well-Being; Spiritual Health

NIC Interventions

Therapeutic Touch; Energy Management; Hope; Instillation; Simple Guided Imagery

Ongoing Assessment

Actions/Interventions	Rationales
■ Assess lifestyle.	
■ Assess personal and work stress level (scale of 0 to 10).	Patient reports of changes in personal and work-related situations indicates the cause and severity of stress.
• Activities to promote relaxation	Energy therapy techniques will be implemented based on the patient's coping skills to deal with stress.
• Meditation	The patients use of meditation indicates an ability to quiet the mind and allow the wisdom of the soul to be heard.
• Sleep pattern	The quantity and quality of sleep is essential for promoting body-mind-spirit repair nightly.
• Nutrient intake	Intake of necessary nutrients is essential to promoting healing of energy fields. Nutritional deficiencies contribute to energy field disturbances.
• Duration, frequency, and type of exercise	Exercise and physical activity is a basic contributor in healing of body-mind-spirit. Inadequate physical activity may be a factor in the energy field disturbance.
■ Assess medication use.	Determining the therapeutic benefits and side effects of all medications taken by the patient is important in assessing the energy field disturbance.
■ Assess significant past medical history.	The patient's previous health status provides a window into patterns of health issues experienced in body-mind-spirit and how the patient has coped with them.
■ Discuss patient's key complaints and willingness to begin working on one or two issues at a time.	The patient is the main resource for his or her healing. The nurse is the facilitator, putting the patient in the best possible position for healing.
■ Perform energetic assessment.	The healer starts with both hands, palms open above the patient's head, 1 to 6 inches away from the body, and continues scanning the entire body for lack of symmetry, areas of heat or cold, tingling, ruffles, fullness, or depletion of energy.

Therapeutic Interventions

Actions/Interventions	Rationales
■ Prepare patient and environment.	The nurse begins energy field therapy with an explanation of energy work. The environment for energy therapy needs to provide privacy and a quiet ambiance. Help the patient to the most comfortable position (sitting or lying).
■ Begin every energetic intervention with time for the healer to center.	Centering is the most vital part of energy work and leads to a state of deep peace and inner harmony. The healer's vibrations are in harmony and balance with the universe and thus influence the patient's vibrations to be in harmony and balance, thus promoting healing.

Actions/Interventions	Rationales
■ Identify the healing intention for the patient's highest good, aligned with the Divine will.	Intentionality is of the utmost importance and cocreates the intended outcome. Attuning to the patient and sending unconditional love helps the healer sense the patient's energy field and follow with caring interventions.
■ Unruffle or smooth the energy field by placing hands, palms open, 1 to 6 inches above the patient's body, smoothing the field from head to toe or over the area needing to be cleared. The healer uses short or long graceful strokes in calm rhythmic hand movements.	Unruffling unblocks the stagnated energy and reestablishes a more balanced flow. This change in energy flow allows the patient to relax and obtain relief of pain, discomfort, and/or anxiety.
■ Modulate energy by resting hands on or above the specific area of the body and holding them in place 3 to 5 minutes. The healer observes when the energy change occurs and the area becomes symmetrical and smooth. The patient may comment on changes he or she is feeling.	Modulation of energy brings balance and harmony to the areas of the field that were blocked or congested. Energy change can be subtle, such as cool to warm or hot to cool. The patient may report that throbbing stops, pulsation begins, or that pain may intensify then gradually subside.
■ Reassess the energy field after unruffling or modulating energy, and repeat either process if necessary.	The patient may need more than one attempt to shift energy to a flow of harmony or balance.
■ Ground by holding the patient's feet for several seconds upon completion of session and allowing patient to rest quietly.	This technique allows the patient to connect to the earth's energy and allow the changes to integrate throughout the energy field.
■ Take time to share the experience with the patient, and ensure that the patient is fully conscious.	This sharing allows the patient to hear the healer's report of the session. The healer receives the response of the patient and validates the changes in energy field harmony and balance.
■ Document the result of the intervention along with symptoms, procedure used, observations, and patient feedback.	Ongoing notes are essential for determining goal achievement and planning additional sessions.

Education/Continuity of Care

Actions/Interventions	Rationales
■ Teach the patient the importance of working with the main concern or problem in a manner that involves body, mind, and spirit.	It is important to work with the patient's major concerns holistically. The patient needs to recognize the benefit of exercise, nutrition, relaxation, meditation, sleep promotion, and positive thinking as part of energy field therapy.
■ Give the patient one to two assignments to promote wellness.	The patient needs to assume responsibility for his or her healing and continue to implement wellness activities between energy therapy sessions.
▲ Refer the patient to his or her usual health care provider.	Interprofessional collaboration through integration of Western and Eastern medicine interventions promotes better patient-centered care and restoration of energy field balance.

■ = Independent   ▲ = Collaborative

NANDA-I NDx Risk for Falls

Definition: Increased susceptibility to falling that may cause physical harm

Falls are a major safety risk for adults, especially older adults. According to the Centers for Disease Control and Prevention (CDC), approximately one in three community-dwelling adults over age 65 fall each year, and women fall more frequently than men in this age-group. This number increases to approximately 75% of nursing home residents because of their older age, frailty, chronic medical conditions, and cognitive impairments. Fall-related injuries are the most common cause of accidental death in individuals over 65 years. Injuries sustained as a result of a fall include soft tissue injury, fractures (hip, spine, and wrist), and traumatic brain injury. Fall-related injuries are associated with prolonged hospitalization for older adults. For those surviving a fall, the quality of life is significantly changed following a fall-related injury.

The morbidity, mortality, and economic burdens resulting from patient falls pose serious risk management issues facing the health care industry. Patient falls are caused by multiple factors. Prevention of falls is an important dimension of the nursing care of patients in hospitals and long-term care settings. In 2005, The Joint Commission added the requirement for fall risk assessment and periodic reassessment as a National Patient Safety Goal in the acute care setting, and in 2006 added the requisite of implementing and evaluating a fall prevention program. The Nursing Home Quality Initiative project has a similar focus for that population. Implementation of successful fall prevention programs is an essential part of nursing care in any health care setting and requires a multifaceted approach. The Agency for Healthcare Research and Quality (AHRQ) provides a comprehensive review of risk assessment instruments for various settings, selected prevention strategies, and recommendations from evidence-based practice and research implications. Nurses also have a major role in educating patients, families, and caregivers about the prevention of falls across the care continuum.

Common Risk Factors

History of falls
Wheelchair use
65 years of age or older
Female (if older)
Lives alone
Use of assistive devices for mobility
Presence of acute illness
Orthostatic hypotension
Visual and/or hearing difficulties
Urinary or bowel incontinence
Impaired physical mobility
Diminished mental status
Polypharmacy
Cluttered environment
Unfamiliar, dimly lit room
Weather conditions (wet floors, ice)
Difficulty with gait
Impaired balance
Neuropathy
Decreased lower extremity strength
Sleeplessness
Visual difficulties

Common Expected Outcomes

Patient will not sustain a fall.

Patient and caregiver will implement strategies to increase safety and prevent falls in the home.

NOC Outcomes
Fall Prevention Behavior; Knowledge: Fall Prevention; Risk Control; Risk Detection

NIC Interventions
Fall Prevention; Environmental Management Safety; Teaching: Prescribed Activity/ Exercise; Medication Management; Surveillance: Safety

Ongoing Assessment

Actions/Interventions	Rationales
■ Assess for factors known to increase level of fall risk on admission, after any change in the patient's physical or cognitive status, whenever a fall occurs, periodically during a hospital stay, or at defined times in long-term care settings:	The level of risk and subsequent fall precautions can be determined using standard risk assessment tools that incorporate these intrinsic and extrinsic factors.
• History of falls	Evidence indicates that a person who has sustained one or more falls in the past 6 months is more likely to fall again.
• Mental status changes	Confusion and impaired judgment increase the person's risk for falls.
• Age-related physical changes	Normal changes associated with aging increase the person's risk for falling. These changes include decreased visual capacity, impaired color perception, change in center of gravity, unsteady gait, decreased muscle strength, decreased endurance, altered depth perception, and delayed response and reaction times.
• Sensory deficits	Impaired vision and hearing limit the person's ability to recognize hazards in the environment.
• Use of mobility assistive devices	Improper use and maintenance of mobility aids such as canes, walkers, and wheelchairs increases the person's risk for falls.
• Disease-related symptoms	Increased incidence of falls has been demonstrated in persons with symptoms such as orthostatic hypotension, urinary incontinence, reduced cerebral blood flow, edema, dizziness, weakness, fatigue, and confusion.
• Medications	Side effects of drugs and the drug interactions that occur with polypharmacy increase the person's risk for falls. Drugs that affect blood pressure and level of consciousness are associated with the highest fall risk. Specific drug groups associated with falls include antihypertensives, sedatives, opioid analgesics, tranquilizers, and diuretics.
• Unsafe clothing	Poor-fitting shoes, long robes, or long pants legs can limit a person's ambulation and increase fall risk.
■ Assess the person's environment for factors known to increase fall risk such as unfamiliar setting, inadequate lighting, wet surfaces, waxed floors, clutter, and objects on floor.	Patients who are not familiar with the placement of furniture and equipment in their room are more likely to experience a fall. Anything that blocks or limits a clear, straight path for ambulation can contribute to a person's fall risk.
▲ Refer the person with musculoskeletal problems for diagnostic evaluation.	Patients with musculoskeletal problems such as osteoporosis are at increased risk for serious injury from falls. Bone mineral density testing will help identify the risk for fractures from falls. Physical therapy evaluation can identify problems with balance and gait that can increase a person's fall risk.

■ = Independent ▲ = Collaborative

Therapeutic Interventions

Actions/Interventions	Rationales
■ For the patient in the hospital or long-term care setting:	
• Post signs or use wristband identification to identify the patients at risk for falls and to remind health care providers to implement fall precaution behaviors.	All health care providers need to recognize the patient who is at risk for falls. All care providers are responsible for implementing actions to promote patient safety and prevent falls.
• Move patient to room close to nurses' station.	Nearby location provides for more frequent observation and faster response to call needs.
• Place items used by the patient within easy reach, such as call light, urinal, water, telephone.	Stretching to get items from bedside tables that are out of reach can disrupt the patient's balance and contribute to falls.
• Answer call lights immediately.	Patients who experience delay in having their call lights answered are more likely to get out of bed without assistance. This behavior, especially if they need to go to the bathroom, will increase their risk for falls.
• Place mechanical beds in the lowest possible position. If needed, place the patient's sleeping surface as close to the floor as possible.	Keeping beds in the lowest position reduces the risk for falls and serious injury. In some health care settings, placing the mattress on the floor significantly reduces fall risk.
• Use side rails on beds, as needed. For beds with split side rails, leave at least one of the rails at the foot of the bed down.	Patients who are disoriented or confused have been known to climb over side rails and fall. Research demonstrates that when one of four rails is left down, the patient is less likely to fall.
• Avoid use of restraints to reduce falls.	Studies support that routine use of restraints does not reduce incidence of falls.
• Ensure appropriate room lighting, especially at night.	Older adults with reduced visual capacity will benefit from adequate lighting, especially in an unfamiliar environment. Using a night-light helps increase visibility if the patient must get up at night.
• Encourage the patient to wear shoes or slippers with nonskid soles when ambulating.	Nonskid footwear provides sure footing for the patient with diminished foot and toe lift when walking.
• Orient the patient to the layout of the room. Limit rearranging the furniture in the room.	The more familiar the patient is with the layout of the room, the less likely the patient is to trip over furniture.
• Provide heavy furniture that will not tip over if used for support by the patient when ambulating. Keep primary ambulation path clear and as straight as possible. Avoid clutter on the floor surface.	Patients with balance and gait problems are not as skilled at ambulating around objects that obstruct a straight path.
• Use bed and chair alarms to alert staff when the patient gets up without assistance.	Audible alarms can remind the patient not to get up alone. The use of alarms can be a substitute for physical restraints.
• Provide the patient with a chair that has a firm seat and arms on both sides. Consider locked wheels as appropriate.	This chair style is easier to get out of, especially when the patient experiences weakness and impaired balance when transferring from bed to chair.
▲ Collaborate with other health care team members to evaluate the patient's medications that contribute to falling. Consider peak effects for prescribed medications that affect level of consciousness.	A review of the patient's medications by the prescribing health care provider and the pharmacist can identify side effects and drug interactions that increase the patient's fall risk. The more medications a patient takes, the greater the risk for side effects and interactions such as dizziness, orthostatic hypotension, drowsiness, and incontinence. Polypharmacy in the older adult is a significant risk factor for falls.
■ For patients or residents with impaired ability to follow direction who are at risk for falls, consider use of a sitter to provide continuous one-on-one observation.	Sitters are responsible for ensuring a safe environment.

Nursing Diagnosis Care Plans

Actions/Interventions

■ Encourage the patient to participate in a program of regular exercise and gait training.

■ Encourage the patient to wear eyeglasses and hearing aids and to have these checked routinely.

■ Collaborate with physical therapy and occupational therapy to assist with gait techniques and to provide the patient with assistive devices for transfer and ambulation. Initiate home safety evaluation as needed.

■ Provide high-risk patients with a hip pad.

■ Participate in national reporting initiatives, such as the American Nurses Association National Database of Nursing Quality Indicators.

Rationales

Evidence suggests that people who engage in regular exercise and activity will strengthen muscles, improve balance, and increase bone density. Increased physical conditioning reduces the risk for falls and limits injury that is sustained when a fall occurs.

Fall risk can be reduced if the patient uses appropriate aids to promote visual and auditory orientation to the environment. Poor vision can greatly increase fall risk.

The use of gait belts by all health care providers can promote safety when assisting patients with transfers from bed to chair. Canes, walkers, and wheelchairs can provide the patient with improved stability and balance when ambulating. Raised toilet seats can facilitate safe transfer on and off the toilet.

These pads when properly worn may reduce a hip fracture should a fall occur.

These databases provide hospitals with the ability to view their fall and injury rates in relation to similar hospitals.

Education/Continuity of Care

Actions/Interventions

■ Educate the patient and family caregivers about risk factors for falls in the home. Suggest home adaptations to increase safety.

• Place bright, nonskid strips on the edge of stair treads. Install handrails on both sides of the stairs from top to bottom.

• Ensure that all rugs are securely fastened to the floor or removed.
• Install nonslip surfaces in tubs and showers. Place grab bars near the tub or shower and toilet. Consider use of a shower chair. Use soap on a rope to prevent dropping it.
• Rearrange furniture to have a clear pathway between rooms, especially to the bathroom. Keep traffic patterns free of clutter and electrical cords.
• Increase lighting at the top and bottom of stairs. Use night-lights in bathrooms, bedrooms, and hallways.
• Secure all handrails.

• Rearrange items in kitchen so frequently used ones are in easy reach (waist level).
• Instruct to wear shoes both inside and outside the house.
▲ Refer the family to community resources for assistance in making home safety modifications.

■ Educate the patient and family caregivers about the correct use and maintenance of mobility assistive devices.

■ Suggest patient wear an alarm device in case of fall.

Rationales

Approximately 40% of older adults living in the community sustain at least one fall per year. Falls are the leading cause of accidental death in the home setting. Falls are frequently caused by hazards that are easy to fix.

Older adults have problems differentiating shades of the same color and have diminished depth perception. These physiological changes make it difficult to see the edge of a stair tread that is a uniform color.

Loose throw rugs increase the risk for slipping and falling.

Wet surfaces in bathrooms increase the risk for falls. Grab bars provide support when moving.

People with diminished strength or who use mobility devices are less able to negotiate around obstacles in their path.

Older adults have poor vision at night and in dimly lit areas. Improved lighting reduces fall risk.

Handrails should be on both sides of the stairs and as long as the stairs.

Easy access reduces temptation to stand on stools or chairs to secure needed items.

Wearing slippers or going barefoot increases fall risk.

Many community service organizations provide financial assistance to help older adults make safety improvements in their homes.

Incorrect use or improper maintenance of canes, walkers, and wheelchairs can increase the risk for falls. The devices need to be properly fitted to the individual. Falls can occur if brakes on wheelchairs are not used correctly.

A variety of devices are available to alert providers to come to the scene to assist a patient who falls and cannot get up.

■ = Independent   ▲ = Collaborative

Nursing Diagnosis Care Plans

Actions/Interventions	Rationales
■ Instruct patient and families in what to do after a fall. • If obvious injury, notify medical assistance immediately. • If significant blow to head or any loss of consciousness, initiate immediate medical assistance. • If on anticoagulant therapy but no signs of active bleeding, notify health care provider. • If on anticoagulant therapy and is actively bleeding after fall, call 9-1-1.	Prompt evaluation of the consequences of a fall will facilitate early treatment.

NANDA-I NDx Interrupted Family Processes

Definition: Change in family relationships and/or functioning

Interrupted family processes occur as a result of the inability of one or more members of the family to adjust or perform, resulting in family dysfunction and interruption or prevention of development of the family. Family development is closely related to the developmental changes experienced by adult members. Over time, families must adjust to change within the family structure brought on by both expected and unexpected events, including illness or death of a member, and/or changes in social or economic strengths precipitated by divorce, retirement, and loss of employment. The addition of new family members through birth or adoption may require adaptation to new roles and status for existing family members. Health care providers must also be aware of the changing constellation of families: gay couples raising children, single parents with children, older grandparents responsible for grandchildren or foster children, and other situations.

Common Related Factors

Developmental transitions or crises
Modification in family finances
Modification in family social status
Power shift of family members
Shift in health status of a family member
Shift in family roles
Situational transitions or crises

Defining Characteristics

Changes in communication patterns
Changes in participation in problem solving or decision making
Changes in availability for emotional support
Changes in assigned tasks or effectiveness in completing assigned tasks
Changes in expressions of conflict within family
Changes in expressions of conflict with or isolation from community resources
Changes in satisfaction with family
Changes in intimacy or mutual support

Common Expected Outcomes

Family develops improved methods of communication.
Family uses resources available for problem solving.
Family expresses understanding of mutual problems.

NOC Outcomes

Family Coping; Family Functioning; Family Normalization

NIC Interventions

Family Process Maintenance; Normalization Promotion

Ongoing Assessment

Actions/Interventions	Rationales
■ Assess for precipitating events (e.g., divorce, illness, life transition, crisis).	The Family Inventory of Life Events (FILE) is an assessment tool to identify recent family events. The data from this assessment may suggest the level of family stress. Depending on the stressor, a variety of strategies may be required to facilitate coping.
■ Assess family members' perceptions of the problem.	Resolution of family problems is possible if each person's perceptions are understood. Understanding another's perceptions can lead to clarification and problem solving. A variety of standardized assessment tools are available to gather data about the perceptions of family members.
■ Evaluate strengths, coping skills, and current support systems.	Genograms and ecomaps can be used as tools to help the family identify family structure, the strength of family relationships, sources of support, and use of community resources.
■ Assess developmental level of family members.	The developmental stage of family members will influence family functioning. Developmental transitions may be a source of stress within the family.

Therapeutic Interventions

Actions/Interventions	Rationales
■ Provide opportunities to express concerns, fears, expectations, or questions.	Providing such opportunities promotes communication and support, and may facilitate coping.
■ Explore feelings: identify loneliness, anger, worry, and fear.	The feelings of one family member influence others in the family system.
■ Phrase problems as "family" problems.	This approach promotes a sense of connectedness and reduces the tendency to blame individual family members.
■ Encourage members to empathize with other family members.	Empathy can increase understanding of others' feelings and fosters mutual respect and support.
■ Assist the family in setting realistic goals.	Setting realistic goals helps the family gain control over the situation.
■ Assist the family in breaking down problems into manageable parts.	Guiding them to view the problems in smaller parts may make the situation more tolerable.
■ Assist with problem-solving process, with delineated responsibilities and follow-through.	This method can promote independence and a sense of autonomy.
■ Tailor interventions according to family members' abilities.	This approach enhances self-efficacy and increases chance for successful resolution.
■ Encourage family members to seek information and resources that increase coping skills.	Practical information and positive role models can be very effective.
▲ Refer the family to social services or counseling.	Long-term intervention or assistance may be required to develop new patterns of family interactions and problem solving.

Education/Continuity of Care

Actions/Interventions	Rationales
■ Provide information regarding stressful situations, as appropriate (e.g., pattern of illness, time frames for recovery, and expectations).	Information helps the family understand what they are experiencing and gives them a window to future expectations.
■ Identify community resources that may be helpful in dealing with particular situations (e.g., telephone hotlines, self-help groups, educational opportunities, social services agencies, and counseling centers).	Groups that come together for mutual support or information exchange can be beneficial in helping the family reach goals.

■ = Independent   ▲ = Collaborative

Fatigue

Definition: An overwhelming sustained sense of exhaustion and decreased capacity for physical and mental work at usual level

Fatigue is a subjective complaint with both acute and chronic illnesses. In an acute illness, fatigue may have a protective function that keeps the person from sustaining injury from overwork in a weakened condition. As a common symptom, fatigue is associated with a variety of physical and psychological conditions. Fatigue is a prominent finding in many viral infections such as hepatitis. Patients with rheumatoid arthritis, fibromyalgia, systemic lupus erythematosus, myasthenia gravis, and depression report fatigue as a profound symptom that reduces their ability to participate in their own care and fulfill role responsibilities. The patient with a chronic illness experiencing fatigue may be unable to work full-time and maintain acceptable performance on the job. The economic impact on the individual and the family can be significant. The social effects of fatigue occur as the person decreases his or her participation in social activities. Recently, attention has focused on sleep-disordered breathing as a cause for daytime somnolence, fatigue, and decreased alertness. Common screening methods are available.

Chronic fatigue syndrome is a poorly understood condition that is characterized by prolonged, debilitating fatigue, neurological problems, general pain, gastrointestinal problems, and flulike symptoms. Although the exact cause of chronic fatigue syndrome is not known, one theory suggests that the disorder may represent an abnormal response of the immune system to highly stressful physiological or psychological events.

Common Related Factors

Physiological:
- Sleep deprivation
- Poor physical condition
- Disease states
- Increased physical exertion
- Malnutrition
- Anemia
- Pregnancy
- Chemotherapy/radiation therapy

Psychological:
- Boring lifestyle
- Stress
- Anxiety
- Depression

Environmental:
- Humidity
- Lights
- Noise
- Temperature

Situational:
- Negative life event
- Occupation

Defining Characteristics

Inability to restore energy, even after sleep
Lack of energy or inability to maintain usual level of physical activity
Increased rest requirements
Tired
Verbalization of an unremitting and overwhelming lack of energy
Inability to maintain usual routines
Lethargic or listless
Increased physical complaints
Perceived need for additional energy to accomplish routine tasks
Compromised concentration
Feelings of guilt for not keeping up with responsibilities

Common Expected Outcomes

Patient verbalizes reduction of fatigue as evidenced by reports of increased energy and ability to perform desired activities. Patient demonstrates use of energy-conservation principles.

NOC Outcomes

Activity Tolerance; Endurance; Energy Conservation; Self-Care: Activities of Daily Living

NIC Interventions

Energy Management; Exercise Promotion; Nutrition Management; Sleep Enhancement

Ongoing Assessment

Actions/Interventions	Rationales
■ Assess the patient's description of fatigue: timing (afternoon versus all day), severity, relationship to activities and aggravating/alleviating factors.	Specific information about the patient's experience of fatigue can help the nurse develop an individualized approach. A quantitative rating scale (e.g., 0 to 10) can help the patient describe the amount of fatigue experienced. This method allows the nurse to compare changes in the patient's fatigue level over time. It is important to determine if the patient's level of fatigue is constant or if it varies over time.
■ Assess for possible causes of fatigue, such as: • Recent physical illness • Emotional stress • Depression • Medication side effects • Anemia • Sleep disorders • Imbalanced nutritional intake • Increased responsibilities and demands at home or work	Causative factors may be temporary or permanent, physical or psychological. Identifying the related factors with fatigue can aid in determining possible causes and establishing a collaborative care plan.
■ Assess the patient's ability to perform activities of daily living (ADLs), instrumental activities of daily living (IADLs), and demands of daily living (DDLs).	Fatigue can limit the person's ability to participate in self-care and perform his or her role responsibilities in the family and society, such as working outside the home.
■ Assess the patient's emotional response to fatigue.	Fatigue is a very distressing symptom that significantly affects quality of life. Depending on the acute or chronic nature of the fatigue, anxiety and depression are common emotional responses associated with fatigue. These emotional states can add to the person's fatigue level and create a vicious cycle.
■ Evaluate the patient's routine prescription and over-the-counter medications.	Fatigue may be a medication side effect or an indication of a drug interaction. The nurse should give particular attention to the patient's use of β-blockers, calcium channel blockers, tranquilizers, alcohol, muscle relaxants, and sedatives.
■ Assess the patient's nutritional intake of calories, protein, minerals, and vitamins.	Fatigue may be a symptom of protein-calorie malnutrition, vitamin deficiencies, or iron deficiencies.
■ Evaluate the patient's sleep patterns for quality, quantity, time taken to fall asleep, and feeling upon awakening. Also assess for sleep apnea.	Changes in the person's sleep pattern may be a contributing factor in the development of fatigue. The cycle of interrupted sleep results in reduced REM sleep, which the body requires for rest and to replenish itself. Screening for sleep-disordered breathing may be indicated.
■ Assess the patient's usual level of exercise and physical activity.	Both increased physical exertion and limited levels of exercise can contribute to fatigue.

■ = Independent ▲ = Collaborative

Actions/Interventions

- Evaluate laboratory/diagnostic test results:
  - Blood glucose
  - Hemoglobin and hematocrit
  - Blood urea nitrogen
  - Oxygen saturation, resting and with activity
  - Thyroid-stimulating hormone
- Assess the patient's expectations for fatigue relief, willingness to participate in strategies to reduce fatigue, and level of family and social support.

Rationales

Changes in these physiological measures can be compared with other assessment data to understand possible causes of the patient's fatigue.

The patient will need to be an active participant in planning, implementing, and evaluating realistic therapeutic interventions to relieve fatigue. Social support will be necessary to help the patient implement changes to reduce fatigue.

Therapeutic Interventions

Actions/Interventions

- Encourage the patient to keep a 24-hour fatigue/activity log for at least 1 week.

- Assist the patient with developing a schedule for daily activity and rest. Stress the importance of frequent rest periods.

- ▲ Refer the patient and family to an occupational therapist.

- Implement use of assistive and adaptive devices for ADLs and IADLs:
  - Long-handled sponge for bathing
  - Long shoehorn
  - Sock-puller
  - Long-handled grabber
- Assist the patient with setting priorities for desired activities and role responsibilities. Refrain from performing nonessential activities.

- Promote adequate nutritional intake.

- Encourage an exercise conditioning program as appropriate.

- Encourage the patient to identify tasks that can be delegated to others.

Rationales

Recognizing relationships between specific activities and levels of fatigue can help the patient identify excessive energy expenditure. The log may indicate times of day when the person feels the least fatigued. This information can help the patient make decisions about arranging his or her activities to take advantage of periods of higher energy levels.

A plan that balances periods of activity with periods of rest can help the patient complete desired activities without adding to levels of fatigue. Not all self-care activities need to be completed at one time, such as the morning. Likewise, not all housework needs to be completed in a day.

The occupational therapist can provide the patient with assistive devices and teach the patient energy-conservation techniques. The therapist can also help evaluate the need for additional energy-conservation measures in the home setting.

The use of assistive devices can minimize energy expenditure and prevent injury with activities.

Setting priorities is one example of an energy-conservation technique that allows the patient to use available energy to accomplish important activities. Achieving desired goals can improve the patient's mood and sense of emotional well-being.

The patient will need properly balanced intake of carbohydrates, fats, protein, vitamins, and minerals to provide energy resources.

Fatigue caused by deconditioning and prolonged bed rest can be reduced through improved functional capacity using muscle-strengthening exercise.

Patient and caregiver may need to learn skills for delegating tasks to others to conserve available energy.

Actions/Interventions

- Encourage the patient and family to verbalize feelings about the impact of fatigue.

- Minimize environmental stimuli, especially during planned times for rest and sleep.

Rationales

Acknowledgment that living with fatigue is both physically and emotionally difficult aids in coping. Fatigue can have a profound negative influence on family processes and social interaction. The type or duration of the fatigue experience (acute/temporary versus more chronic fatigue syndrome) affects the significance of any changing roles and responsibilities within the family unit.

Bright lighting, noise, visitors, frequent distractions, and clutter in the patient's physical environment can inhibit relaxation, interrupt rest/sleep, and contribute to fatigue.

Education/Continuity of Care

Actions/Interventions

- Teach the patient and family energy-conservation techniques and time-management strategies.
- Help the patient engage in increasing levels of physical activity and exercise.
- Teach the patient signs and symptoms of overexertion with activity.
- Help the patient develop habits to promote effective rest/sleep patterns.

Rationales

Organization and time management can help the patient conserve energy and prevent fatigue.

Exercise can help the patient build endurance for physical activity and subsequently reduce fatigue.

Changes in heart rate, oxygen saturation, and respiratory rate will reflect the patient's tolerance for activity.

Promoting relaxation before sleep and providing for several hours of uninterrupted sleep can contribute to energy restoration.

Related Care Plan

Sleep disordered breathing, p. 451

NANDA-I NDx Fear

Definition: Response to perceived threat that is consciously recognized as a danger

Fear is a strong and unpleasant emotion caused by the awareness or anticipation of pain or danger. This emotion is primarily externally motivated and source-specific; that is, the individual experiencing the fear can identify the person, place, or thing precipitating this feeling. The factors that precipitate fear are, to some extent, universal; fear of death, pain, and bodily injury are common to most people. Other fears are derived from the life experiences of the individual person. How fear is expressed may be strongly influenced by the culture, age, or gender of the person under consideration. In some cultures it may be unacceptable to express fear regardless of the precipitating factors. Rather than manifesting outward signs of fear as described in the defining characteristics, responses may range from risk-taking behavior to expressions of bravado and defiance of fear as a legitimate feeling. In other cultures fear may be freely expressed and manifestations may be universally accepted. In addition to one's own individual ways of coping with the feeling of fear, there are aspects of coping that are cultural as well. Some cultures control fear through the use of magic, mysticism, or religiosity. Whatever one's mechanism for controlling and coping with fear, it is a normal part of everyone's life. The nurse may encounter the fearful patient in the community, during the performance of diagnostic testing in an outpatient setting, or during hospitalization. The nurse must learn to identify when patients are experiencing fear and must find ways to assist them in a respectful way to negotiate these feelings. The nurse must also learn to identify when fear becomes so persistent and pervasive that it impairs an individual's ability to carry on his or her activities of daily living. Under these circumstances, referral can be made to programs designed to assist the patient in overcoming phobias and other truly debilitating fears.

■ = Independent   ▲ = Collaborative

Common Related Factors

Anticipation of pain
Anticipation or perceived physical threat or danger
Fear of an event
Unfamiliar environment
Environmental stimuli
Separation from support system
Treatments and invasive procedures
Threat of death
Language barrier
Knowledge deficit
Sensory impairment
Specific phobias

Defining Characteristics

Identifies fearful feelings or object of fear
Increased respirations, heart rate, and respiratory rate
Tension
Jitteriness
Apprehension
Impulsivity
Alertness
Avoidance behavior

Common Expected Outcomes

Patient uses effective coping behaviors to reduce fear response.
Patient verbalizes or manifests a reduction or absence of fear.

NOC Outcomes
Fear Self-Control; Coping
NIC Interventions
Anxiety Reduction; Emotional Support

Ongoing Assessment

Actions/Interventions	Rationales
■ Determine what the patient is fearful of by careful and thoughtful questioning.	The external source of fear can be identified, and current responses can be assessed.
■ Create an atmosphere that facilitates trust through active listening.	Patients who find it unacceptable to express fear may find it helpful to know that someone is willing to listen if they decide to share their feelings at some time in the future.
■ Assess the degree of fear and the measures the patient uses to cope with that fear. (This can be done by interviewing the patient and significant others.)	This information helps determine the effectiveness of coping strategies used by the patient.
■ Document behavioral and verbal expression of fear.	Physiological symptoms and/or complaints intensify as the level of fear increases. Note that fear differs from anxiety in that it is a response to a recognized and usually external threat. Manifestations of fear are similar to those of anxiety.
■ Determine to what degree the patient's fears may be affecting his or her ability to perform activities of daily living (ADLs).	Persistent, immobilizing fears may require treatment with antianxiety medications or referral to specially designed treatment programs. Patient safety must always be a priority.

Therapeutic Interventions

Actions/Interventions	Rationales
■ Acknowledge your awareness of the patient's fear	This approach validates the feelings the patient is having and communicates an acceptance of those feelings.
■ Stay with the patient to promote safety, especially during frightening procedures or treatments.	The presence of a trusted person increases the patient's sense of security and safety during a period of fear.
■ Maintain a calm and tolerant manner while interacting with the patient.	The patient's feeling of stability increases in a calm and nonthreatening atmosphere.
■ Establish a working relationship through continuity of care.	An ongoing relationship establishes trust and a basis for communicating fearful feelings.
■ Orient to the environment as needed.	Familiarity with the environment promotes comfort and a decrease in fear.

Actions/Interventions

■ Use simple language and brief statements when instructing the patient regarding diagnostic and surgical procedures. Explain what physical or sensory sensations will be experienced.
■ Reduce sensory stimulation by maintaining a quiet environment, whether in the hospital or home situation. Remove unnecessary threatening equipment.

■ Provide safety measures within the home when indicated (e.g., alarm system, safety devices in showers or bathtubs).
■ Assist the patient in identifying strategies used in the past to deal with fearful situations.

■ As the patient's fear subsides, encourage him or her to explore specific events preceding the onset of the fear.
■ Encourage rest periods.
■ When the patient must be hospitalized or away from home, suggest bringing in comforting objects from home (e.g., music, pillow, blanket, pictures).
■ Access appropriate resources to meet the fearful needs of the patient and family (e.g., spiritual counselor or social worker).

Rationales

When experiencing excessive fear or dread, the patient may be unable to comprehend more than simple, clear, and brief instructions. Repetition may be necessary.

Fear may escalate with excessive conversation, noise, and equipment around the patient. Even though the staff or caregiver may be comfortable around "high-tech" or medical equipment, the patient may not be.
If the home environment is unsafe, the patient's fears are not resolved and fear may become disabling.
This measure helps the patient focus on fear as a real and natural part of life that has been and can continue to be dealt with successfully.
Recognition and explanation of factors leading to fear are significant in developing alternative responses.
Rest improves ability to cope.
Familiar objects in a new environment can enhance feelings of security.

Using community resources provides coordinated patient care that emphasizes supportive health care services.

Education/Continuity of Care

Actions/Interventions

■ Reinforce the idea that fear is a normal and appropriate response to situations when pain, danger, or loss of control is anticipated or experienced.
■ Instruct the patient in the performance of the following self-calming measures that may reduce fear or make it more manageable:

• Breathing modifications

• Exercises in relaxation, meditation, or guided imagery

• Exercises in the use of affirmations and calming self-talk

■ Instruct the patient in the use of physician-ordered antianxiety medications.
▲ Initiate alternative therapies or hands-on comfort.

■ Caution the patient against the use of illicit drugs or the overuse of alcohol to deal with fearful feelings.
■ Encourage an increase in patient and family participation in care.

Rationales

Knowledge serves to reduce unrealistic expectations.

Educating the patient and significant others about anticipatory coping mechanisms will focus energy on prevention with opportunity for growth rather than reaction to the identified fear.
Controlled, rhythmic breathing can promote relaxation and feelings of being in control.
Exercise reduces the physiological response to fear (i.e., increased blood pressure, pulse, respiration).
These enhance the patient's sense of confidence and reassurance.
Short-term use of antianxiety medications can relieve unpleasant feelings.
Measures such as meditation, prayer, music, and Therapeutic Touch may help alleviate fear and promote calm.
Abuse of drugs and alcohol limits the effectiveness of the person's coping ability.
Participation in care assists in coping and may increase a sense of control. (NOTE: Cultures vary in expectations of caregiving based on gender or family position.)

Related Care Plan

Anxiety, p. 18

■ = Independent ▲ = Collaborative

NANDA-I NDx Deficient Fluid Volume

Definition: Decreased intravascular, interstitial, and/or intracellular fluid. This refers to dehydration, water loss alone without change in sodium

Fluid volume deficit, or hypovolemia, occurs from a loss of body fluid or the shift of fluids into the third space, or from a reduced fluid intake. Common sources for fluid loss are the gastrointestinal tract, polyuria, and increased perspiration. Fluid volume deficit may be an acute or chronic condition managed in the hospital, outpatient center, or home setting. The therapeutic goal is to treat the underlying disorder and return the extracellular fluid compartment to normal. Treatment consists of restoring fluid volume and correcting any electrolyte imbalances. Early recognition and treatment are paramount to prevent potentially life-threatening hypovolemic shock. Older patients are more likely to develop fluid imbalances.

Common Related Factors

Inadequate fluid intake
Active fluid loss (diuresis, abnormal drainage or bleeding, diarrhea)
Failure of regulatory mechanisms
Electrolyte and acid-base imbalances
Increased metabolic rate (fever, infection)
Fluid shifts (edema or effusions)

Defining Characteristics

Decreased urine output (less than 30 mL/hr)
Concentrated urine
Output greater than intake
Sudden weight loss
Decreased venous filling pressures (preload)
Hemoconcentration
Increased serum sodium
Hypotension/orthostasis
Thirst
Tachycardia/weak, rapid heart rate
Decreased skin turgor
Dry mucous membranes
Weakness
Changes in level of consciousness

Common Expected Outcome

Patient is normovolemic as evidenced by systolic blood pressure (BP) greater than or equal to 90 mm Hg (or patient's baseline), absence of orthostasis, heart rate 60 to 100 beats/min, urine output greater than 30 mL/hr, and normal skin turgor.

NOC Outcomes
Fluid Balance; Hydration
NIC Interventions
Fluid Monitoring; Fluid Management; Fluid Resuscitation

Ongoing Assessment

Actions/Interventions

- Obtain patient history to ascertain the probable cause of the fluid disturbance.

- Assess, or instruct the patient to monitor, weight daily and consistently, with the same scale and preferably at the same time of day and wearing the same amount of clothing.
- Evaluate fluid status in relation to dietary intake. Determine whether the patient has been on fluid restriction.

Rationales

Such information can help guide interventions. Causes may include acute trauma and bleeding, reduced fluid intake from changes in cognition, large amount of drainage after surgery, or persistent diarrhea.
Instruction facilitates accurate measurement and helps in following trends.

Most fluid enters the body through drinking, water in foods, and water formed by oxidation of foods. For some older adult patients fluids may be purposely restricted to avoid problems with incontinence.

Actions/Interventions

■ Monitor and document vital signs.

■ Monitor blood pressure for orthostatic changes (from patient lying supine to high-Fowler's).

■ Assess skin turgor and mucous membranes for signs of dehydration.

■ Assess color and amount of urine. Report urine output less than 30 mL/hr for 2 consecutive hours.

■ Monitor temperature.

■ Monitor active fluid loss from wound drainage, tubes, diarrhea, bleeding, and vomiting; maintain accurate input and output record.

▲ Monitor serum electrolytes and urine osmolality, and report abnormal values.

■ Monitor for changes in level of consciousness.

■ Evaluate whether the patient has any related heart problem before initiating parenteral therapy.

■ Determine the patient's fluid preferences: type, temperature (hot or cold).

■ During treatment, monitor closely for signs of circulatory overload (headache, flushed skin, tachycardia, venous distention, elevated central venous pressure [CVP], shortness of breath, increased BP, tachypnea, cough).

▲ If hospitalized, monitor hemodynamic status, including CVP, pulmonary artery pressure, pulmonary capillary wedge pressure, and cardiac output/cardiac index if available.

Rationales

Reduction in circulating blood volume can cause hypotension and tachycardia. The change in heart rate is a compensatory mechanism to maintain cardiac output. Usually the pulse is weak and may be irregular if electrolyte imbalance also occurs. Hypotension is evident in hypovolemia.

Postural hypotension is a common manifestation in fluid loss. Note the following orthostatic hypotension significance:
- Greater than 10 mm Hg drop: circulating blood volume is decreased by 20%.
- Greater than 20 to 30 mm Hg drop: circulating blood volume is decreased by 40%.

Loss of interstitial fluid causes loss of skin turgor. Assessment of skin turgor in older adults is less accurate because the skin normally loses its elasticity. Therefore skin turgor assessed over the sternum or the forehead is best. Several longitudinal furrows and coating may be noted along the tongue.

Concentrated urine denotes fluid deficit.

Febrile states decrease body fluids through perspiration and increased respiration.

The most serious problems are related to reduced plasma volume.

Elevated blood urea nitrogen suggests fluid deficit. Urine specific gravity is likewise increased.

Dehydration may alter mental status, especially among older adults. Manifestations may include restlessness, anxiety, lethargy, and confusion.

Cardiac and older patients often have precarious fluid balances and are susceptible to development of pulmonary edema.

Selecting those fluids that the patient enjoys drinking can facilitate replacement therapy.

Close monitoring for responses during therapy reduces complications associated with fluid replacement.

CVP measurements provide information on filling pressures of the right side of the heart. Pulmonary capillary wedge pressure reflects left-sided fluid volume. Cardiac output/cardiac index provides an objective number to guide therapy.

Therapeutic Interventions

Actions/Interventions

▲ Encourage the patient to drink prescribed fluid amounts:
- Place fluids at bedside within easy reach.
- Provide fresh water and a straw.
- Be creative in selecting fluid sources (e.g., flavored gelatin, frozen juice bars, sports drink).
- Provide oral hydrating solutions (e.g., Rehydralyte).

Rationales

Oral fluid replacement is indicated for mild fluid deficit and is a cost-effective method for replacement treatment. Older patients have a decreased sense of thirst and may need ongoing reminders to drink.

■ = Independent ▲ = Collaborative

Actions/Interventions

■ Assist the patient if he or she is unable to feed self, and encourage the caregiver to assist with feedings, as appropriate.
■ Provide oral hygiene.

For more severe hypovolemia:

▲ Obtain and maintain a large-bore intravenous (IV) catheter.
▲ Administer parenteral fluids as ordered. Anticipate the need for an IV fluid challenge with immediate infusion of fluids for patients with abnormal vital signs.
▲ Administer blood products as prescribed.

▲ Assist the physician with insertion of a central venous line and arterial line, as indicated.
▲ Maintain IV flow rate. If signs of fluid overload occur, stop the infusion and have the patient sit up or dangle the legs.

▲ Institute measures to control excessive electrolyte loss (e.g., resting the gastrointestinal tract, administering antipyretics, as ordered). For hypovolemia due to severe diarrhea or vomiting, administer antidiarrheal or antiemetic medications as prescribed, in addition to IV fluids.
▲ Once ongoing fluid losses have stopped, begin to advance the diet in volume and composition.

Rationales

Dehydrated patients may be weak and unable to meet prescribed intake independently.

Fluid deficit can cause a dry, sticky mouth. Attention to mouth care promotes interest in drinking.

Parenteral fluid replacement is indicated to prevent or treat hypovolemic complications.

Fluids are needed to maintain hydration states. Determination of the type and amount of fluid to be replaced and infusion rates will vary depending on clinical status.

Blood transfusions may be required to correct fluid loss from active gastrointestinal bleeding.

These interventions allow more effective fluid administration and monitoring.

Close monitoring of fluid prevents iatrogenic volume overload. Older patients are especially susceptible to fluid overload. Upright positioning decreases venous return and optimizes breathing.

Fluid losses from diarrhea should be concomitantly treated with antidiarrheal medications, as indicated. Antipyretics can reduce fever and associated fluid losses from diaphoresis.

Addition of fluid-rich foods can enhance continued interest in eating.

Education/Continuity of Care

Actions/Interventions

■ Describe or teach causes of fluid losses or decreased fluid intake.
■ Explain or reinforce rationale and intended effect of treatment program. Inform the patient or caregiver of importance of maintaining prescribed fluid intake and special diet.
■ Teach interventions to prevent future episodes of inadequate intake.

■ If patients are to receive IV fluids at home, instruct the caregiver in managing IV equipment. Allow sufficient time for return demonstration.

▲ Refer to home health agency as appropriate.

Rationales

Information is key to managing the problem.

Follow-up care will be the patient's and/or caregiver's responsibility. Information is needed for making correct choices.

Patients need to understand the importance of drinking extra fluid during bouts of diarrhea, fever, and other conditions causing fluid deficits.

Responsibility for maintaining venous access sites and IV supplies may be overwhelming for the caregiver. In addition, older caregivers may not have the cognitive ability or manual dexterity required for this therapy.

Continuity of care is facilitated through the use of community resources.

Related Care Plan

Shock, Hypovolemic, p. 337

Excess Fluid Volume

Definition: Increased isotonic fluid retention

Fluid volume excess, or hypervolemia, occurs from an increase in total body sodium content and an increase in total body water. This fluid excess usually results from compromised regulatory mechanisms for sodium and water as seen in congestive heart failure (CHF), kidney failure, and liver failure. It may also be caused by excessive intake of sodium from foods, intravenous (IV) solutions, medications, or diagnostic contrast dyes. Hypervolemia may be an acute or chronic condition managed in the hospital, outpatient center, or home setting. The therapeutic goal is to treat the underlying disorder and return the extracellular fluid compartment to normal. Treatment consists of fluid and sodium restriction and the use of diuretics. For acute cases, ultrafiltration or dialysis may be required.

Common Related Factors

Excessive fluid intake
Excessive sodium intake
Compromised regulatory mechanisms
Renal insufficiency or failure
Steroid therapy
Low protein intake or malnutrition
Decreased cardiac output; chronic or acute heart disease
Head injury
Liver disease
Severe stress
Hormonal disturbances

Defining Characteristics

Weight gain
Edema
Intake greater than output
Specific gravity changes
Tachycardia
Oliguria
Shortness of breath; orthopnea/dyspnea
Pulmonary congestion on x-ray
Abnormal breath sounds: crackles
Change in respiratory pattern
Third heart sound (S_3)
Increased blood pressure
Jugular vein distention
Increased central venous pressure (CVP)
Increased pulmonary artery pressure (PAP)
Change in level of consciousness
Azotemia
Change in electrolytes
Decreased hemoglobin or hematocrit
Restlessness and anxiety

Common Expected Outcome

Patient is normovolemic as evidenced by urinary output greater than or equal to 30 mL/hr, balanced intake and output, stable weight (or loss attributed to fluid loss), absence or reduction of edema, heart rate less than 100 beats/min, absence of pulmonary congestion (crackles).

NOC Outcome
Fluid Balance
NIC Interventions
Fluid Monitoring; Fluid Management

Ongoing Assessment

Actions/Interventions

■ Obtain patient history to ascertain the probable cause of the fluid disturbance.

Rationales

Such information can help guide interventions. History may include increased fluids or sodium intake, or compromised regulatory mechanisms.

■ = Independent   ▲ = Collaborative

Nursing Diagnosis Care Plans

Actions/Interventions	Rationales
■ Assess, or instruct the patient to monitor weight daily and consistently with the same scale, preferably at the same time of day and wearing the same amount of clothing.	Instruction facilitates accurate measurement and helps follow trends. Sudden weight gain may indicate fluid retention. Different scales or heavier/lighter clothing may show false weight fluctuations.
■ Monitor for a significant weight change (2 pounds in 1 day).	Body weight is a more sensitive indicator of fluid or sodium retention than intake and output. A 2- to 3-pound increase in weight normally indicates a need to adjust fluid or diuretic therapy; 2.2 pounds (1 kg) is equivalent to 1 L of fluid.
■ Monitor input and output closely.	Although overall fluid intake may be adequate, shifting of fluid out of the intravascular to the extravascular spaces may result in dehydration. The risk of this occurring increases when diuretics are given. Patients may use diaries for home assessment.
■ Evaluate weight in relation to nutritional status.	In some heart failure patients, weight may be a poor indicator of fluid volume status. Poor nutrition and decreased appetite over time result in a decrease in weight, which may be accompanied by fluid retention even though the net weight remains unchanged.
■ If the patient is on fluid restriction, review the daily log or chart for recorded intake.	Patients should be reminded to include items that are liquid at room temperature such as gelatin, sherbet, soup, and frozen juice pops.
■ Monitor and document vital signs.	Sinus tachycardia and increased blood pressure are seen in early stages. Older patients have a reduced response to catecholamines; thus their response to fluid overload may be blunted, with less increase in heart rate.
■ Monitor for distended neck veins and ascites. Monitor abdominal girth to follow any ascites accurately.	Patients with hypotonic overhydration exhibit cellular swelling. Distended neck veins are caused by elevated CVP. Ascites occurs when fluid accumulates in extravascular spaces.
■ Auscultate for a third heart sound, and assess for bounding peripheral pulses.	These assessment findings are signs of fluid overload.
■ Assess for crackles in lungs, changes in respiratory pattern, shortness of breath, and orthopnea.	These signs are caused by accumulation of fluid in the lungs.
■ Assess for presence of edema by palpating over the tibia, ankles, feet, and sacrum.	Edema occurs when fluid accumulates in the extravascular spaces. Dependent areas more readily exhibit signs of edema formation. Edema is graded from trace (indicating barely perceptible) to 4 (severe edema). Pitting edema is manifested by a depression that remains after one's finger is pressed over an edematous area and then removed. Measurement of an extremity with a measuring tape is another method of following edema.
▲ Monitor chest x-ray reports.	As interstitial edema accumulates, the x-ray studies show cloudy white lung fields.
■ Evaluate urine output in response to diuretic therapy.	Focus is on monitoring the response to the diuretics, rather than the actual amount voided. At home, it is unrealistic to expect patients to measure each void. Therefore recording two voids versus six voids after a diuretic medication may provide more useful information. NOTE: Fluid volume excess in the abdomen may interfere with absorption of oral diuretic medications. Medications may need to be given intravenously by a nurse in the home or outpatient setting.

Nursing Diagnosis Care Plans

Actions/Interventions

- ■ Monitor for excessive response to diuretics: 2-pound loss in 1 day, hypotension, weakness, blood urea nitrogen elevated out of proportion to serum creatinine level.
- ■ During therapy, monitor for signs of hypovolemia.
- ▲ Monitor serum electrolytes, urine osmolality, and urine-specific gravity.

- ■ Assess the need for an external or indwelling urinary catheter.

- ▲ If hospitalized, monitor hemodynamic status, including CVP, PAP, and pulmonary capillary wedge pressure, if available.

Rationales

Significantly increased response to diuretic therapy can result in fluid deficit and electrolyte imbalances that can cause significant complications.

Monitoring prevents complications associated with therapy.

Specific changes will occur depending on whether hypotonic, isotonic, or hypertonic overhydration is present; specific changes guide treatment therapy.

Treatment focuses on diuresis of excess fluid. Urinary catheters can make measurement of response to diuretic therapy more accurate.

These direct measurements serve as optimal guides for therapy.

Therapeutic Interventions

Actions/Interventions

- ▲ Institute and instruct the patient and/or caregiver regarding fluid restrictions, as appropriate.

- ■ Provide innovative techniques for monitoring fluid allotment at home. For example, suggest that patients measure out and pour into a large pitcher the prescribed daily fluid allowance (e.g., 1000 mL); then every time the patient drinks some fluid, he or she is to remove that amount from the pitcher.
- ▲ Restrict sodium intake as prescribed.

- ▲ Administer or instruct the patient to take diuretics as prescribed.

- ■ Instruct the patient to avoid medications that may cause fluid retention, such as over-the-counter nonsteroidal anti-inflammatory agents, certain vasodilators, and steroids.
- ■ Elevate edematous extremities, and handle with care.

- ■ Reduce constriction of vessels (e.g., use appropriate garments, avoid crossing of legs or ankles).
- ■ Instruct in need for antiembolic stockings or bandages, as ordered.
- ■ Provide interventions related to specific etiological factors (e.g., inotropic medications for heart failure, paracentesis for liver disease).

For acute cases:

- ▲ Consider admission to an acute care setting for hemofiltration or ultrafiltration.
- ▲ Collaborate with the pharmacist to maximally concentrate IV fluids and medications.
- ■ Apply saline lock on IV line.

Rationales

Fluid restrictions help reduce extracellular volume. For some patients, fluids may need to be restricted to 1000 mL per day. Information is key for patients who will be comanaging fluids.

These measures provide a visual guide for how much fluid is still allowed throughout the day, enhancing compliance with the regimen.

Restriction decreases extracellular fluid volume. Diets containing 2 to 3 g of sodium are usually prescribed.

Diuretics aid in the excretion of excess body fluids. Diuretic therapy may include several different types of agents for optimal therapy, depending on the acuteness or chronicity of the patient's problem. For patients with chronic complaints, compliance is often difficult when trying to maintain a normal lifestyle.

Thorough understanding of specific causes, such as medication side effects, is necessary for appropriate follow-up of treatment.

Elevation increases venous return and, in turn, decreases edema. Edematous skin is more susceptible to injury and breakage.

These techniques prevent venous pooling.

These aids help promote venous return and minimize fluid accumulation in the extremities.

Knowledge of causative factors provides direction for subsequent interventions.

These therapies are very effective methods to draw off excess fluid.

Concentration decreases use of unnecessary fluids.

This device maintains patency but decreases fluid delivered to the patient in a 24-hour period.

■ = Independent   ▲ = Collaborative

Actions/Interventions

▲ Administer IV fluids through infusion pump, if possible.

■ Position the patient in a semi-Fowler's or high-Fowler's position.

■ Assist with repositioning every 2 hours if the patient is not mobile.

Rationales

Pumps ensure accurate delivery of IV fluids.

Elevating the head of the bed allows for ease in breathing. This position promotes pooling of fluid in the bases and makes more lung tissue available for gas exchange.

Repositioning prevents fluid accumulation in dependent areas.

Education/Continuity of Care

Actions/Interventions

■ Teach causes of fluid volume excess and/or excess intake to the patient or caregiver.

■ Provide information as needed regarding the individual's medical diagnosis (e.g., CHF, renal failure).

■ Explain or reinforce rationale and intended effect of the treatment program.

■ Identify signs and symptoms of fluid volume excess and symptoms to report.

■ Explain importance of maintaining proper nutrition, hydration, and diet modifications.

Rationale

Information is key to managing problems.

Patients are better able to ask questions and seek assistance when they know basic information about their condition.

Follow-up care will be the patient's and/or caregiver's responsibility. Information is needed for making correct choices.

Patients must have information to make correct choices regarding future treatments.

Knowledge enhances compliance with the treatment plan.

NANDA-I NDx Impaired Gas Exchange

Definition: Excess or deficit in oxygenation and/or carbon dioxide elimination at the alveolar-capillary membrane

By the process of diffusion, the exchange of oxygen and carbon dioxide occurs in the alveolar-capillary membrane area. The relationship between ventilation (air flow) and perfusion (blood flow) affects the efficiency of the gas exchange. Normally there is a balance between ventilation and perfusion; however, certain conditions can offset this balance, resulting in impaired gas exchange. Altered blood flow from a pulmonary embolus, or decreased cardiac output or shock can cause ventilation without perfusion. Conditions that cause changes or collapse of the alveoli (e.g., atelectasis, pneumonia, pulmonary edema, and adult respiratory distress syndrome) impair ventilation. Other factors affecting gas exchange include high altitudes, hypoventilation, and altered oxygen-carrying capacity of the blood from reduced hemoglobin. Older patients have a decrease in pulmonary blood flow and diffusion as well as reduced ventilation in the dependent regions of the lung where perfusion is greatest. Chronic conditions such as chronic obstructive pulmonary disease (COPD) put these patients at greater risk for hypoxia. Other patients at risk for impaired gas exchange include those with a history of smoking or pulmonary problems, obesity, prolonged periods of immobility, and chest or upper abdominal incisions.

Common Related Factors

Alveolar-capillary membrane changes
Ventilation-perfusion imbalance
Altered oxygen supply
Altered oxygen-carrying capacity of blood

Defining Characteristics

Confusion
Somnolence
Restlessness
Irritability

Inability to move secretions
Hypoxia/hypoxemia
Dyspnea
Abnormal arterial blood gases
Abnormal breathing (rate, depth, rhythm)
Tachycardia
Abnormal skin color (pale, dusky)

Common Expected Outcome

Patient maintains optimal gas exchange as evidenced by arterial blood gases (ABGs) within the patient's usual range, alert responsive mentation or no further reduction in level of consciousness, relaxed breathing, and baseline heart rate for patient.

NOC Outcome
Respiratory Status: Gas Exchange
NIC Interventions
Respiratory Monitoring; Oxygen Therapy; Airway Management

Ongoing Assessment

Actions/Interventions	Rationales
■ Assess respirations, noting quality, rate, rhythm, depth, and breathing effort.	Patients will adapt their breathing patterns over time to facilitate gas exchange. Both rapid, shallow breathing patterns and hypoventilation affect gas exchange. Shallow, "sighless" breathing patterns after surgery (as a result of the effect of anesthesia, pain, and immobility) reduce lung volume and decrease ventilation. Hypoxia is associated with signs of increased breathing effort.
■ Assess lung sounds, noting areas of decreased ventilation and the presence of adventitious sounds.	Changes in lung sounds may reveal the etiology of impaired gas exchange.
■ Assess for tachycardia, restlessness, irritability, diaphoresis, headache, visual disturbances, and confusion.	These are early nonpulmonary signs of hypoxia; lethargy and somnolence are late signs. Cognitive changes may occur with chronic hypoxia.
■ Assess for signs and symptoms of atelectasis: diminished chest excursion, limited diaphragm excursion, bronchial or tubular breath sounds, crackles, tracheal shift to affected side.	Collapse of alveoli increases shunting (perfusion without ventilation), resulting in hypoxemia.
■ Assess for signs and symptoms of pulmonary infarction: cough, hemoptysis, pleuritic pain, consolidation, pleural effusion, bronchial breath sounds, pleural friction rub, fever.	Hypoxia results from increased dead space ventilation (ventilation without perfusion) and reflex bronchoconstriction in areas adjacent to the infarct.
■ Monitor vital signs.	With initial hypoxia and hypercapnia, blood pressure (BP), heart rate, and respiratory rate all increase. As the hypoxia and/or hypercapnia becomes severe, BP and heart rate decrease, and dysrhythmias may occur. Respiratory failure may ensue when the patient is unable to maintain the rapid respiratory rate.
■ Assess for headache, dizziness, lethargy, reduced ability to follow instructions, disorientation, coma.	These are signs of hypercapnia.
▲ Monitor ABGs, and note changes.	Increasing $Paco_2$ and decreasing Pao_2 are signs of hypoxemia and respiratory acidosis. As the patient's condition deteriorates, the respiratory rate will decrease and $Paco_2$ will begin to increase. Some patients, such as those with COPD, have a significant decrease in pulmonary reserves, and additional physiological stress may result in acute respiratory failure.

■ = Independent   ▲ = Collaborative

Actions/Interventions	Rationales
▲ Use pulse oximetry to monitor oxygen saturation.	Pulse oximetry is a useful tool to detect changes in oxygenation. Oxygen saturation should be maintained at 90% or greater.
■ Assess nutritional status.	Obesity may restrict downward movement of the diaphragm, increasing the risk for atelectasis, hypoventilation, and respiratory infections. Work of breathing is increased in severe obesity due to the excessive weight of the chest wall. Hypercapnia and hypoxia result. Malnutrition may reduce respiratory mass and strength, affecting muscle function.
▲ Monitor hemoglobin levels.	Low levels reduce the uptake of oxygen at the alveolar-capillary membrane and oxygen delivery to the tissues.
■ Assess skin, nail beds, and mucous membranes for pallor or cyanosis.	Cool, pale skin may be secondary to a compensatory vasoconstrictive response to hypoxemia. As oxygenation and perfusion become impaired, peripheral tissues become cyanotic. For cyanosis to be present, 5 g of hemoglobin must be desaturated.
■ Monitor chest x-ray reports.	Chest x-ray studies reveal the etiological factors of the impaired gas exchange. Keep in mind that radiographic studies of lung water lag behind clinical presentation by 24 hours.
■ Monitor effects of position changes on oxygenation (ABGs, Svo_2, and pulse oximetry).	Putting the most compromised lung areas in the dependent position (where perfusion is greatest) potentiates ventilation and perfusion imbalances.
■ Assess the patient's ability to cough effectively to clear secretions. Note quantity, color, and consistency of sputum.	Retained secretions impair gas exchange.
■ Evaluate hydration status.	Gas exchange may be impaired by overhydration (in conditions such as heart failure). In conditions associated with increased sputum production (e.g., pneumonia, COPD), insufficient hydration may reduce the ability to clear secretions.
■ Assess use of herbal remedies (e.g., licorice and hyssop to promote expectoration, goldenseal for pneumonia, hawthorn for heart failure).	Drug interactions with prescribed drugs and contraindications need to be evaluated (e.g., licorice should not be used by patients on digitalis preparations and those with hypertension; sodium loss and retention of water and potassium may occur with long-term use of high doses).

Therapeutic Interventions

Actions/Interventions	Rationales
■ Position the patient with proper body alignment for optimal respiratory excursion (if tolerated, head of bed at 45 degrees when supine).	Upright position allows for increased thoracic capacity and full descent of diaphragm, preventing the abdominal contents from crowding the lungs and preventing their full expansion.
■ Routinely check the patient's position so that he or she does not slump down in bed.	Slumped positioning causes the abdomen to compress the diaphragm and limits full lung expansion.
■ Position the patient to facilitate ventilation-perfusion matching when a side-lying position is used.	When the patient is positioned on the side, the good side should be down (e.g., lung with pulmonary embolus or atelectasis should be up). When lung hemorrhage or abscess is present, the affected lung should be placed downward to avoid drainage to the healthy lung.
■ Change the patient's position every 2 hours.	Repositioning facilitates secretion movement and drainage and decreases atelectasis.
■ Encourage or assist with ambulation as indicated.	Ambulation promotes lung expansion, facilitates secretion clearance, and stimulates deep breathing.

Nursing Diagnosis Care Plans

Actions/Interventions	Rationales
▲ Maintain oxygen administration device as ordered, attempting to maintain oxygen saturation at 90% or greater.	Supplemental oxygen may be required to maintain Po$_2$ at an acceptable level.
• Avoid high concentration of oxygen in patients with COPD unless ordered.	Hypoxia stimulates the drive to breathe in the chronic CO$_2$ retainer patient. When applying oxygen, close monitoring is imperative to prevent unsafe increases in the patient's PaO$_2$, which could result in apnea.
• If the patient is allowed to eat, give oxygen to the patient but in a different manner (e.g., changing from mask to a nasal cannula).	Eating is an activity, and more oxygen will be consumed than when the patient is at rest. Immediately after the meal, the original oxygen delivery system should be returned.
▲ For patients who should be ambulatory, provide extension tubing or portable oxygen apparatus.	These measures may improve exercise tolerance by maintaining adequate oxygen levels during activity.
■ Encourage slow deep breathing, using incentive spirometer as indicated.	This therapy reduces tachypnea and alveolar collapse.
■ For postoperative patients, assist with splinting the chest.	Splinting optimizes deep breathing and coughing efforts.
■ Assist with coughing or suction as needed.	Excessive suctioning can interfere with gas exchange in the bronchopulmonary tree. Suctioning removes secretions to maintain a patent airway, thereby enhancing oxygenation.
■ Provide reassurance, and allay anxiety.	Anxiety increases dyspnea, respiratory rate, and work of breathing.
■ Pace activities and schedule rest periods to prevent fatigue. Assist with activities of daily living.	Activities will increase oxygen consumption and should be planned so the patient does not become hypoxic.
▲ Administer medications as prescribed.	The type depends on the etiological factors of the problem (e.g., antibiotics for pneumonia, bronchodilators for COPD, anticoagulants and thrombolytics for pulmonary embolus, analgesics for thoracic pain).
■ Anticipate need for intubation and mechanical ventilation.	Early intubation and mechanical ventilation are recommended to prevent full decompensation of the patient. Mechanical ventilation provides supportive care to maintain adequate oxygenation and ventilation to the patient.

Education/Continuity of Care

Actions/Interventions	Rationales
■ Explain the need to restrict and pace activities to decrease oxygen consumption during the acute episode.	Energy conservation reduces fatigue and dyspnea.
■ Teach the patient appropriate breathing and coughing techniques.	These techniques facilitate adequate air exchange and secretion clearance.
■ Instruct about medications: indications, dosage, frequency, side effects, and administration requirements. Include review of metered-dose inhalers if applicable.	Knowledge promotes safe and effective medication administration.
■ Explain the type of oxygen therapy being used and why its maintenance is important.	Issues related to home oxygen use, storage, or precautions need to be addressed for safe and effective treatment.
■ Teach the patient or caregivers the signs of early respiratory compromise and their appropriate management.	Early detection and treatment may reduce emergency department visits, hospitalizations, and mortality. Such instruction prevents delays in seeking help in life-threatening situations.
▲ Refer to home health services for nursing care or oxygen management as appropriate.	Referral facilitates continuation of needed services.
▲ For chronic respiratory disorders, refer for pulmonary rehabilitation.	Rehabilitation training decreases dyspnea and fatigue, and it increases exercise capacity and perception of control over condition.

■ = Independent   ▲ = Collaborative

NANDA-I NDx Grieving

Definition: A normal complex process that includes emotional, physical, spiritual, social, and intellectual responses and behaviors by which individuals, families, and communities incorporate an actual, anticipated, or perceived loss into their daily lives

Grieving is a state of an individual's emotional response to the event of a perceived or actual loss. It may apply to individuals who have had a perinatal loss or loss of a body part or to patients who have received a terminal diagnosis for themselves or a loved one. Intense mental anguish or a sense of deep sadness may be experienced by patients and their families as they face long-term illness or disability. Grief is an aspect of the human condition that touches every individual, but how an individual or a family system responds to loss and how grief is expressed varies widely. That process is strongly influenced by factors such as age, gender, and culture, as well as personal and intrafamilial reserves and strengths. The nurse will encounter the patient and family experiencing grief in the hospital setting, but increasingly, with more hospice services provided in the community, the nurse will find patients struggling with these issues in their own homes, where professional help may be limited or fragmented. This care plan discusses measures the nurse can use to help the patient and family members begin the process of grieving.

Common Related Factors

Anticipatory loss of significant object (e.g., possession, job, status, home, parts and processes of body)
Anticipatory loss of significant other
Death of a significant other
Loss of significant object (e.g., possession, job, status, home, parts and processes of body)

Defining Characteristics

Alteration in activity level
Alterations in immune function
Alterations in neuroendocrine function
Alterations in sleep patterns
Alterations in dream patterns
Anger
Blame
Detachment
Despair
Disorganization
Experiencing relief
Maintaining the connection to the deceased
Making meaning of the loss
Pain
Panic behavior
Personal growth
Psychological distress
Suffering

Common Expected Outcome

Patient or family verbalizes feelings and establishes and maintains functional support systems.

NOC Outcomes

Caregiver Emotional Health; Family Coping; Grief Resolution

NIC Interventions

Grief Work Facilitation; Presence; Emotional Support

Ongoing Assessment

Actions/Interventions

■ Identify behaviors suggestive of the grieving process.

■ Assess the phase of grieving being experienced by the patient and significant others. Many theories exist in defining the phases of grief, with the commonalities being the following:
• Notification and shock
• Experience of the loss emotionally and cognitively
• Reintegration

■ Assess the influence of the following factors on coping: past problem-solving abilities, socioeconomic background, educational preparation, cultural beliefs, and spiritual beliefs.

■ Assess whether the patient and significant others differ in their stages of grieving.

■ Identify available support systems, such as the following: family, friends, primary physician, consulting physician, nursing staff, clergy, therapist or counselor, and professional or lay support group.

■ Identify potential for a complicated grieving response.

■ Evaluate need for referral to social services, legal consultants, or support groups.

■ Observe nonverbal communication.

Rationales

Manifestations of grief are strongly influenced by factors such as age, gender, and culture. What the health care provider observes is a product of these feelings after they have been modified through these layers. The health care provider can enter dangerous territory when he or she attempts to categorize grief as appropriate, excessive, or inappropriate. Grief simply is. If its expression is not dangerous to anyone, then it is normal and appropriate.

Initially, the person may express surprise and disbelief with awareness of a loss. Sadness, despair, and other manifestations of emotional pain may develop as the person experiences loss. The person may take several months to adjust to the loss and return to normal daily functioning. The patient may move from stage to stage and back again before reintegration of the loss occurs.

These factors play a role in how grief will manifest in a particular patient or family. The nurse needs to restrain any notion that individuals of a given culture or age will always manifest predictable grief behaviors. Grief is an individual and exquisitely personal experience.

People within the same family system may become impatient when others do not reconcile their feelings as quickly as they do. Older adults may take longer to reintegrate the loss and reconcile their grief.

If the patient's main support is the object of perceived loss, the patient's need for help in identifying support is accentuated.

Anticipation of grief is helpful in preparing an individual to do actual grief work. Those who do not grieve in anticipation of a loss may be at higher risk for complicated grief.

It may be helpful to have patients and family members associated with these supports as early as possible so that financial considerations and other special needs are taken care of before the anticipated loss occurs.

Body language may communicate a great deal of information, especially if the patient and his or her family are unable to vocalize their concerns.

Therapeutic Interventions

Actions/Interventions

■ Establish rapport with the patient and significant others; try to maintain continuity in care providers. Listen and encourage the patient or significant others to verbalize feelings.

■ Provide a safe environment for expression of grief. Provide the mourners with a quiet, private environment with no interruptions.

Rationales

Open lines of communication will facilitate eventual resolution of grief. Providing emotional support for a child's grief before death may help validate the child's concerns of anticipatory grief and his or her desire to help at some level.

The environment needs to support the patient's expressions of grief (e.g., the ability to see a man cry, to see mourners make wide gestures with their hands and bodies, to listen to loud vocalizations and crying). Expression of feelings is more likely to occur in a private setting.

■ = Independent ▲ = Collaborative

Actions/Interventions	Rationales
■ Remain with the patient throughout difficult times. This may require the presence of the care provider during procedures, difficult discussions, and conferences with other family members or other members of the health care team.	The patient or family may need a trusted person present to represent their interest or feelings if they feel unable to express them. They may require someone to "witness" with them.
■ Accept the patient's or family's need to deny loss as part of the normal grief process. Recognize the patient's or family's need to maintain hope for the future.	The nurse needs to see these events as a time during which the individual or family member consolidates his or her strength to go on to the next stage of grief. Grief remains a highly dynamic and individualized process. They may continue to deny the inevitability of the loss as a means of maintaining some degree of hope. As the loss begins to manifest, the mourners start accepting aspects of the loss, piece by piece, until the whole is actually grasped.
■ Anticipate increased affective behavior. Recognize that regression may be an adaptive mechanism.	All affective behavior may seem increased or exaggerated during this time. Older adults may exhibit a preoccupation with thoughts of the impending death and confusion, especially if multiple losses are anticipated. Defense mechanisms support coping until the person is ready to acknowledge the pain of the loss. Displaced anger and hostility may occur when the loss does not occur as anticipated by those grieving.
■ Show support and positively reinforce the patient's efforts to go on with his or her life and normal activities of daily living (ADLs), stressing the strength and the reserves that must be present for the patient and family to feel enabled to do this.	This behavior is the same strength and reserve each of them will use to reconstitute their lives after the loss.
■ Offer encouragement; point out strengths and progress to date.	Patients often lose sight of their achievements while engaged in grief. When seen as a whole, the process of reorganization after a loss seems enormous, but reviewing the patient's progress toward that end is very helpful and provides perspective on the whole process.
■ Discuss the possible need for outside support systems (e.g., peer support, groups, clergy).	Support in the grieving process will come in many forms. Patients and family members often find the support of others encountering the same experiences helpful.
■ Recognize the patient's need to review (relive) the illness experience.	Telling the event allows them an opportunity to hear it described and gain some perspective on the event. This is one way in which the patient or the family integrates the event into their experience.
■ Do not force the patient to make decisions.	Grief may limit cognitive skills needed for problem solving and decision making.
■ Provide the patient with ongoing information about diagnosis, prognosis, progress, and plan of care. Involve the patient and family in decision making in all issues surrounding care.	Providing the patient and family with information acknowledges their right and responsibility for self-direction and autonomy.
■ Encourage significant others to assist with the patient's physical care.	The desire to provide care to and for each other does not disappear with illness; involving the family in care is affirming to the relationship the patient has with his or her family.
■ When the patient is hospitalized or housed away from home, facilitate flexible visiting hours and include younger children and extended family.	No individual should be excluded from being with the patient unless that is the wish of the patient. Restricted hospital guidelines for visiting serve staff members who organize care more than they serve patients.

Actions/Interventions	Rationales
■ Help the patient and significant others share mutual fears, concerns, plans, and hopes for each other, including the patient.	Secrets are rarely helpful during these times of crisis. An open sharing and exchange of information makes it easier to address important issues and facilitates effective family process. These times of stress can be used to facilitate growth and family development. They can be important and sometimes final opportunities for resolving conflict and issues. They can also be used as times for potential personal and intrafamilial growth.
■ Encourage significant others to maintain their own self-care needs for rest, sleep, nutrition, leisure activities, and time away from the patient.	Somatic complaints often accompany mourning; changes in sleep and eating patterns and interruption of normal routines are a usual occurrence. Care should be taken to treat these symptoms so that emotional reconstitution is not complicated by illness.
If the patient's death is expected:	
■ Facilitate discussion with the patient and significant others on "final arrangements"; when possible, discuss burial, autopsy, organ donation, funeral, durable power of attorney, and a living will.	The patient and family members can benefit from open communication about these topics. The family may be able to gain confidence about carrying out the patient's wishes.
■ Promote discussion on what to expect when death occurs.	Knowledge of the dying process can help the family cope with end of life.
■ Encourage significant others and the patient to share their wishes about which family members should be present at the time of death. Help significant others to accept that not being present at the time of death does not indicate a lack of love or caring.	These discussions help family members make decisions about being present and fulfilling other responsibilities.
■ When the patient is hospitalized, use a visual method to identify the patient's critical status (e.g., color-coded door marker).	This will inform all personnel of the patient's status in an effort to ensure that staff do not act or respond inappropriately to a crisis situation.
■ Initiate a process that provides additional support and resources such as clergy.	The patient and family may benefit from spiritual support resources.

Education/Continuity of Care

Actions/Interventions	Rationales
■ Involve significant others in discussions.	Involvement of others helps reinforce understanding of all individuals involved.
▲ Refer to other resources (e.g., counseling, pastoral support, or group therapy).	The patient or significant others may need additional help to deal with individual concerns.

Related Care Plan

Death and dying: End-of-life issues, p. 969

■ = Independent   ▲ = Collaborative

NANDA-I NDx Complicated Grieving

Definition: A disorder that occurs after the death of a significant other, in which the experience of distress accompanying bereavement fails to follow normative expectations and manifests in functional impairment

Complicated grieving is a state in which an individual is unable or unwilling to acknowledge or mourn an actual or perceived loss. This may subsequently impair further growth, development, or functioning. Complicated grief may be marked by a broad range of behaviors that may include pervasive denial or a refusal to partake in self-care measures or the activities of daily living. It may be marked by excessive use of alcohol or drugs or the inability to maintain one's business or home life. Because all of these behaviors can be seen at one time or another as an emotional response in individuals who are mourning a loss, a distinction must be made between the transient use of these normal adaptive responses and their sustained use, which impedes normal daily functioning and paralyzes one's ability to grow and develop as an individual. Because there is no temporal restriction on the time it takes to mourn a loss, the most reliable indicator may be the mourner himself or herself. When an individual reaches a point when he or she is discomforted by the inability to go on with his or her life, then the issue bears exploration. The nurse may encounter patients experiencing complicated grief in the outpatient setting or in the hospital. They may have physical symptoms reflective of their inability to monitor or care for their own health, or they may have symptoms reflective of chronic emotional or physical illness. Complicated grief may be the outcome of an individual's experience of being at odds with gender, cultural, or their own behavioral norms, which prohibit them from grieving successfully. The nurse may be in a position to help individuals recognize the role that complicated grief has played in their current impasse, and the nurse may be able to help the patient create a framework and environment in which it is safe to begin to mourn. Current literature may categorize complicated grieving as "dysfunctional" or "disenfranchised."

Common Related Factors

Death of a significant other
Emotional instability
Lack of social support
Sudden death of significant other

Defining Characteristics

Decreased functioning in life roles
Decreased sense of well-being
Depression
Experiencing somatic symptoms of the deceased
Fatigue
Grief avoidance
Longing for the deceased
Low levels of intimacy
Persistent emotional distress
Preoccupation with thoughts of the deceased
Rumination
Searching for the deceased
Self-blame
Separation distress
Traumatic distress
Verbalizes anxiety and distressful feelings about deceased
Verbalizes feeling dazed, empty, in shock, stunned, angry
Verbalizes feelings of detachment from others and disbelief
Verbalizes feelings of mistrust and lack of acceptance of the death
Verbalizes persistent painful memories and self-blame
Yearning

Common Expected Outcomes

Patient begins to see the role that complicated grief has played in current impasse.

Patient begins process of grieving, as evidenced by ability to discuss loss.

Symptoms of grief may be reduced or become absent.

NOC Outcomes
Coping; Family Coping; Mood Equilibrium; Psychosocial Adjustment: Life Change

NIC Interventions
Grief Work Facilitation; Family Support; Presence

Ongoing Assessment

Actions/Interventions	Rationales
■ Identify actual or potential losses.	A single loss may have resulted in a cascade of events, each of which may be perceived as a loss (e.g., the loss of a limb may have resulted in the loss of a valued job, relationship, or self-concept).
■ Explore the nature of the individual's past attitudes or relationship with lost object or person.	The degree of the patient's avoidance in dealing with his or her grief may be an indicator as to the importance of the lost object in the patient's life. Ambivalence toward the lost object or person may contribute to complicated grief. Do not assume that patients need only to free themselves from their expressive restraints to cure their complicated grief. The factors involved in obstructed grief may be quite complicated.
■ Assess the patient's past coping style and mechanisms used in stressful situations.	Avoidance may be the patient's normative style in confronting emotional conflict or pain.
■ Assess current affective state. Observe for the presence or absence of emotional distress.	Factors such as gender or cultural norms may prohibit the free expression of or filter the patient's expressions of grief.
■ Observe quality or quantity of communication; observe verbal and nonverbal cues.	These cues may be an important indicator of the patient's true affective status, especially if the patient's own normative preconceptions about himself or herself, culture, or gender prohibit the free expression of feelings.
■ Assess the degree of relatedness to others.	A patient with a limited social support network may have difficulty adjusting to a significant loss.
■ Assess satisfaction with the ability to cope and implement appropriate safety measures.	The loss may trigger feelings of powerlessness and hopelessness that are unresolved and may be accompanied by guilt and suicide ideation.
■ Determine degree of insight in the present situation.	Many patients are able to express sadness but are frozen at this point in their grief. Many patients are able to name or describe what is immobilizing them and inhibiting them from grieving effectively.
▲ Identify disturbing topics of conversation or experiences. Consider, however, that individuals may not feel comfortable discussing their issues with you or within the context that you have chosen. Provide patients with options if they seem uninterested in exploring feelings with others.	Actively listening to the patient and/or family without judgment or interruption is important to the grieving process. Repetition of their stories facilitates healing after the death of a loved one. Team member counseling may prove helpful here.
■ Estimate the degree of stress currently experienced.	Patients may feel unable to take on the resolution of complicated emotional issues in times of extreme stress; at the very least, these factors will need to be factored into an understanding of how to progress in the therapeutic approach to be used with the patient.

■ = Independent ▲ = Collaborative

Therapeutic Interventions

Actions/Interventions	Rationales
■ Communicate comfort in the patient's discussion of loss and grief.	Patients may be quite sensitive to emotional nuances communicated by the nurse. The nurse should not take on these issues with the patient if he or she is uncomfortable with certain expressions of grief or if grief carries unresolved issues for the nurse. The nurse must assume responsibility for communicating his or her own thoughts and feelings effectively. Dialogue involves mutual honesty, clarification of erroneous messages, and sensitivity to one's self and others.
■ Offer feedback regarding the patient's expressed feelings.	Dialogue necessitates this kind of reciprocity and promotes understanding of behavior during grief work.
■ Encourage or facilitate expressions of acceptance or offers of emotional support by significant others to the patient.	This type of communication is extremely helpful and healing, and it provides the patient with varied sources of support and help.
■ Recognize variation and need for individual adjustment to loss and change.	There is no one norm to conform to; the experience of the patient is perhaps the most important indicator of progress or improvement.
■ Promote culturally and spiritually competent care while respecting the patient's and family's diversity in the realm of gender, socioeconomic status, and sexual orientation.	An individual's background influences how grief is expressed. Nursing responses to support grief are based on how each patient and family interprets their own cultural, religious and ethnic traditions. The more inclusive the information gained, the more therapeutic the intervention will likely be.
■ Provide quiet and privacy when needed or requested.	Privacy allows for contemplation and reflection as part of grief work.
■ Recognize the need for the use of defense mechanisms. Do not personalize negative expression of affect or unduly challenge some use of denial. Patients will have to proceed at their own pace.	The use of defense mechanisms will support coping until the person is ready to integrate the loss.
■ Reassure the patient and significant others that some negative thoughts and feelings are normal.	Concern about how others may view one's full range of feelings may lead to further impediments in the grieving process and increase a sense of isolation and loss.
■ Support the use of adaptive coping mechanisms.	The adaptive coping mechanisms may provide respite for overwhelming pain or grief.
■ Discuss the actual loss with patient:	
• Support a realistic assessment of the event or situation.	False reassurances are never helpful and only relieve the discomfort of the care provider.
• Explore with the patient individual strengths and available resources.	Ultimately, the decision to take on the job of resolving the emotional impasse that the patient has reached is the decision of the patient. This job is certainly difficult and inevitably painful. It may be helpful to recognize that the patient has the skills and reserves of strength necessary to do the emotional work ahead.
• Explore reasons for avoidance of feeling or acknowledging loss.	These may continue to obstruct progress despite the patient's willingness to proceed. They should be factored into any care plan.
• Review common changes in behavior associated with normal grieving (e.g., change in appetite and sleep patterns) with the patient and significant others. Explain that although intensity and frequency of behaviors decrease with time, the mourning period may continue for a long time.	Understanding the range of normal behaviors associated with grieving can enhance family coping with the loss.

Actions/Interventions	Rationales
• Discuss normal coping behavior in grief recovery (e.g., the need for contact with others or the need to alternate periods of distraction with quiet time to reflect).	This places these needs within the realm of what is needed by all and may sanction the patient's need for the same considerations.
■ Encourage sharing of common problems with others.	Grief is a universal experience; people who have undergone grief over a loss can be enormously helpful to others undergoing the same feelings.

Education/Continuity of Care

Actions/Interventions	Rationales
■ Explain that emotional response to loss is appropriate and commonly experienced: • Describe the "normal" stages of grief and mourning. • Offer hope that emotional pain will decrease with time.	Many view the overt expression of feelings as a "weakness" or fear that they may lose control if they begin to acknowledge the depth of their emotions.
■ Reassure families that children should be included in grieving as much as the child or teen wants. Take your clues from the patient and family, especially in times of complicated grief.	In times of complicated grieving, children especially need to feel cared for and safe.
▲ Initiate referrals to other professional and community resources as appropriate.	It is helpful for patients to have more than one resource for helping them in this process.

Related Care Plan

Death and dying: End-of-issues, p. 969

Health-Seeking Behaviors

Definition: Active seeking (by a person in stable health) of ways to alter personal health habits and/or the environment in order to move toward a higher level of health

Health promotion activities include a wide range of topics, such as smoking cessation; stress management; weight loss; proper diet for prevention of coronary artery disease, cancer, osteoporosis, and others; exercise promotion; prenatal instruction; safe sex practices to prevent sexually transmitted diseases; protective helmets to prevent head trauma; and other practices to reduce risks for diabetes, stroke, and others.

Patients of all ages may be involved in improving health habits. Social cognitive theory identifies factors (e.g., behavior, cognition and other personal factors, and the environment) that influence how and to what extent people are able to change old behaviors and adopt new ones. Psychosocial factors such as stress and anxiety regarding perceived risk for disease, along with social support for engaging in the health-promoting behaviors, must be considered. The action plan must be tailored to fit with the patient's values and belief systems. Opportunities for self-monitoring and receiving feedback enhance the behavior change process.

The setting in which health promotion activities occur may range from the privacy of one's home, group activities such as weight maintenance groups or health clubs, or even the work setting (especially targeted programs for hypertension management and weight reduction). This care plan gives a general overview of health-seeking behaviors.

■ = Independent ▲ = Collaborative

Common Related Factors

New condition, altered health status
Lack of awareness about environmental hazards affecting personal health
Absence of interpersonal support
Limited availability of health care resources
Unfamiliarity with community wellness resources
Lack of knowledge about health promotion behaviors

Defining Characteristics

Perceives optimum health as a primary life purpose
Expresses desire to seek higher level of wellness
Expresses concern about current health status
Demonstrated or observed lack of knowledge of health promotion behaviors
Actively seeks resources to expand wellness knowledge
Expresses sense of self-confidence and personal efficacy toward health promotion
Verbalizes desire for increased control of health
Anticipates internal and external threats to health status and desires to take preventive action

Common Expected Outcomes

Patient verbalizes accurate information and necessary environmental changes to promote a healthier lifestyle.
Patient engages in desired behaviors to promote a healthier lifestyle.

NOC Outcomes

Health-Promoting Behavior; Health-Seeking Behavior; Knowledge: Health Resources

NIC Interventions

Self-Modification Assistance; Health Education; Patient Contracting

Ongoing Assessment

Actions/Interventions	Rationales
■ Assess the patient's individual perceptions of health problems.	According to models such as the Health Belief Model, the patient's perceived susceptibility to and perceived seriousness and threat of disease affect health-seeking behaviors. In addition, factors such as cultural phenomena and heritage can affect how people view their health.
■ Question the patient regarding previous experiences and health teaching.	Adults bring many life experiences to learning sessions. Often patients have previously tried unsuccessfully to engage in a specific health practice. Reasons for difficulties need to be explored.
■ Determine at what stage of change the patient is currently.	The Transtheoretical Model emphasizes that interventions for change should be matched with the stage of change at which patients are situated. For example, if the patient is only "contemplating" starting an exercise program, efforts may be directed toward emphasizing the positive aspects of exercise and reducing barriers; whereas if the patient is in the "preparation" or "action" stages, more specific directions regarding exercise (e.g., places to exercise, equipment, target heart rate, warm-up activities) can be addressed.
■ Identify priority of learning needs within the overall care plan.	Patients learn material most important to them.
■ Identify any misconceptions regarding material to be taught.	Patients must have accurate information to make appropriate behavior changes.
■ Assess the patient's confidence in his or her ability to perform desired behavior.	According to the self-efficacy theory, positive conviction that one can successfully execute a behavior is correlated with performance and successful outcome.
■ Identify the patient's specific strengths and competencies.	Every patient brings unique strengths to the health-planning task (e.g., motivation, knowledge, social support).
■ Identify health goals and areas for improvement.	Systematically reviewing areas for potential change can assist patients in making informed choices.

Actions/Interventions

- Identify possible barriers to change (e.g., lack of motivation, interpersonal support, skills, knowledge, or resources).

- Determine cultural influences on health teaching.

Rationales

If the patient is aware of possible barriers and has formulated plans for dealing with them, then successful behavioral change is more likely to occur. For example, if trying to engage in more exercise, walking in shopping malls can be substituted for outdoor activity during periods of inclement weather.

Certain ethnic and religious groups hold unique beliefs and health practices that must be considered when designing educational plans.

Therapeutic Interventions

Actions/Interventions

- Clearly define the specific behavior to be changed.

- Guide the patient in setting realistic goals.

- Promote positive expectations for success.

- Assist the patient in developing a self-contract.

- Assist in developing a time frame for implementation.

- Develop a system for the patient to monitor own progress.

- Allow periodic evaluation, feedback, and revision of the health plan as necessary.

- Reward positive efforts and achievement.

- Implement the use of modeling to assist patients.

- Provide a comprehensive approach to health promotion by giving attention to environmental, social, and cultural constraints.

- Prepare for lapses and relapses.

Rationales

The more precisely defined the behavior is, the greater the chance of success.

Goals that are too global, such as "lose 30 pounds," are difficult to achieve and can foster feelings of failure. Shorter-range goals, such as "lose 5 pounds in a month," may be more achievable and therefore reinforcing.

Patients with stronger self-efficacy to perform a behavior are much more likely to engage in it.

Contracts help clarify the goal and enhance the patient's control over the behavior, creating a sense of independence, competence, and autonomy.

Changes need to be made over a period of time to allow new behaviors to be learned well, integrated into one's lifestyle, and stabilized.

Self-management is a key component of a successful change in behavior.

This method provides a systematic approach for movement of the patient toward higher levels of health and promotes adherence to the plan. Appropriately timed feedback is critical to successful behavior change. Telephone or Internet feedback can be a convenient source.

Positive rewards, especially those inherent in the activity, such as the enjoyment of outside walking with a partner, should be encouraged because they continue to reinforce the behavior. Other rewards may consist of verbal praise, monetary rewards, special privileges (e.g., earlier office appointment, free parking), or telephone calls from the health care provider.

Observing the behavior of others who have successfully achieved similar goals helps exemplify the exact behaviors that should be developed to reach the goal. The use of videotapes with people performing the desired behavior has been quite effective.

The various health promotion models emphasize that focusing only on behavior change is doomed to failure without simultaneous efforts to alter the environment and collective behavior.

Relapse prevention needs to be addressed early in the treatment plan. Identifying high-risk situations likely to cause relapse aids problem solving. The maintenance phase of change is the longest and most challenging to sustain.

■ = Independent ▲ = Collaborative

Nursing Diagnosis Care Plans

Education/Continuity of Care

Actions/Interventions	Rationales
■ Provide instruction for specific topics/behaviors (e.g., smoking cessation, weight loss).	Correct information is needed for positive outcomes.
■ Use a variety of teaching methods to match the patient's preferred learning style.	Different people learn in different ways, so using the most effective learning style promotes success. Learning is enhanced when various approaches reinforce the material that is being taught.
■ Inform the patient regarding community resources and self-help groups as appropriate.	Self-help and support groups provide unique perspectives on "being there" and may be effective in providing alternative treatment modalities.
■ Encourage participation of family or significant others in proposed changes.	One's significant others can play an important role in providing support over the long term that may enhance overall adaptation to change.

Ineffective Health Maintenance

Definition: Inability to identify, manage, and/or seek help to maintain health

Ineffective health maintenance reflects a change in an individual's ability to perform the functions necessary to maintain health or wellness. That individual may already manifest symptoms of existing or impending physical ailment or display behaviors that are strongly or certainly linked to disease. The nurse's role is to identify factors that contribute to an individual's inability to maintain healthy behavior and implement measures that will result in improved health maintenance activities. The nurse may encounter these patients either in the hospital or in the community; the increased presence of the nurse in the community and home health settings improves the ability to assess patients in their own environment. Patients most likely to experience more than transient alterations in their ability to maintain their health are those whose age or infirmity (either physical or emotional) absorb much of their resources or those for whom the economic challenges of daily life negate an interest in personal health. The task before the nurse is to identify measures that will be successful in empowering patients to maintain their own health within the limits of their ability.

Common Related Factors

Perceptual/cognitive impairment
Presence of physical disabilities or challenges
Presence of adverse personal habits:
- Smoking
- Poor diet selection
- Morbid obesity
- Alcohol abuse
- Drug abuse
- Poor hygiene
- Lack of exercise

Low income/lack of material resources
Lack of access to care
Lack of knowledge
Poor housing conditions
Ineffective coping

Risk-taking behaviors

Inability to communicate needs adequately (e.g., deafness, speech impediment)

Dramatic change in health status

Lack of support systems

Denial of need to change current habits

Defining Characteristics

Behavioral characteristics:
- Demonstrated lack of knowledge
- Failure to keep appointments
- Expressed interest in improving behaviors
- Failure to recognize or respond to important symptoms reflective of changing health state
- Inability to follow instructions or programs for health maintenance

Physical characteristics:
- Body or mouth odor
- Unusual skin color, pallor
- Poor hygiene
- Soiled clothing
- Frequent infections (e.g., upper respiratory infection, urinary tract infection)
- Frequent toothaches
- Obesity or anorexia
- Anemia
- Chronic fatigue
- Apathetic attitude
- Substance abuse

Common Expected Outcomes

Patient demonstrates positive health maintenance behaviors as evidenced by keeping scheduled appointments, participating in smoking and substance abuse programs, making diet and exercise changes, improving home environment, and following treatment regimen.

Patient identifies available resources.

Patient uses available resources.

NOC Outcomes
Health-Promoting Behavior; Self-Direction of Care; Health-Seeking Behavior; Social Support

NIC Interventions
Health System Guidance; Support System Enhancement; Discharge Planning; Health Screening; Risk Identification

Ongoing Assessment

Actions/Interventions

■ Assess for defining characteristics, such as poor hygiene, frequent infections, and failure to keep appointments.

■ Assess the patient's knowledge of health maintenance behaviors.

■ Assess health history over past 5 years.

■ Assess to what degree environmental, social, intrafamilial disruptions, or changes have correlated with poor health behaviors.

■ Determine the patient's specific questions related to health maintenance.

Rationales

Changing ability or interest in performing the normal activities of daily living may be an indicator that commitment to health and well-being is waning.

The health care provider needs to ensure that the patient has all of the information needed to make good lifestyle choices. Some patients may know that certain unhealthy behaviors can result in poor health outcomes but continue the behavior despite this knowledge.

Assessment may give some perspective on whether poor health habits are recent or chronic in nature. History may also reflect multiple risk factors for health problems.

These changes may be precipitating factors or may be early fallout from a generalized condition reflecting decline.

Patients may have health education needs; meeting these needs may be helpful in mobilizing the patient.

■ = Independent   ▲ = Collaborative

Actions/Interventions	Rationales
■ Determine patient's motives for failing to report symptoms reflecting changes in health status.	The patient may not want to "bother" the provider, may minimize the importance of the symptoms, or may fear what may be discovered. Language barriers and poor access to care are other common reasons.
■ Discuss noncompliance with instructions or programs with the patient to determine rationale for failure.	The patient may be experiencing obstacles in compliance that can be resolved.
■ Assess the patient's educational preparation and ability to integrate and relate to information.	Patients may not have understood information because of a sensory impairment or the inability to read or understand information. Culture, literacy, language barriers, or age may impair a patient's ability to comply with the established treatment plan. Health literacy has become a patient safety issue.
■ Assess history of other adverse personal habits, including smoking, obesity, lack of exercise, and alcohol or substance abuse.	Long-standing habits may be difficult to break; once established, patients may feel that nothing positive can come from a change in behavior.
■ Determine whether the patient's manual dexterity or lack of mobility is a factor in the patient's altered capacity for health maintenance.	Patients may need assistive devices for ambulation or to complete tasks of daily living.
■ Determine to what degree the patient's cultural beliefs and personality contribute to altered health habits.	Health teaching may need to be modified to be consistent with cultural or religious beliefs.
■ Determine whether the required health maintenance facilities/equipment (e.g., access ramps, motor vehicle modifications, shower bar or chair) are available to the patient.	With adequate assistive devices, the patient may be able to effect enormous changes in maintaining his or her personal health.
■ Assess whether economic problems present a barrier to maintaining health behaviors.	Patients may be unaware of, or too proud to ask for assistance from, financial reimbursement sources such as Social Security, Medicare, or insurance benefits could be helpful to them. The growing number of uninsured and underinsured Americans is compounding this problem.
■ Assess hearing, and orientation to time, place, and person to determine the patient's perceptual abilities.	Perceptual handicaps may impair an individual's ability to maintain healthy behaviors.
■ Make a home visit to determine safety, accessibility, and quality of living conditions.	Home visits can help identify and solve problems that complicate health maintenance.
■ Assess the patient's experience of stress and disruptors as they relate to health habits.	If stressors can be relieved, patients may again be able to resume their self-care activities.

Therapeutic Interventions

Actions/Interventions	Rationales
■ Assist the patient with problem solving specific related factors as able.	Health maintenance is complicated because of the complexities of each individual's circumstance. A "one size fits all" approach will not work.
■ Define your role as patient advocate.	The nurse is in an ideal position to guide the patient through the health care system.
■ Provide the patient with a means of contacting health care providers.	Guidance will add available resources for questions or problem resolution. An ongoing relationship can establish trust and facilitate change.
■ Involve family and friends in health-planning conferences.	Family members need to understand that care is planned to focus on what is most important to the patient. This enables the patient to maintain a sense of autonomy.
■ Compliment the patient on positive accomplishments.	Positive reinforcement enhances behavior change. Patients with stronger self-efficacy are more likely to engage in positive behaviors.

Education/Continuity of Care

Actions/Interventions	Rationales
■ Provide the patient with rationale for importance of behaviors such as the following:	
• Proper nutrition	The Food and Drug Administration provides a variety of tools (e.g., MyPyramid) on recommended food groups across a variety of populations. Cardiovascular disease, cancer, type 2 diabetes, and osteoporosis are but a few of the many medical diseases related to nutrition.
• Regular exercise	Exercise promotes weight loss and increases agility and stamina. The Surgeon General recommends at least 150 minutes of moderate exercise each week.
• Proper hygiene	Hygiene decreases risk for infection and promotes maintenance and integrity of skin and teeth.
• Smoking cessation	Smoking has been directly linked to cancer, heart disease, and respiratory disease.
• Cessation of alcohol and drug abuse	In addition to physical addictions and the social consequences, the physical consequences of substance abuse mitigate against it.
• Stress management	Stress management can be considered a cornerstone to a healthy lifestyle.
• Regular physical and dental checkups and screenings	Checkups identify and treat problems early. Screening procedures are based on age and prior history (e.g., Papanicolaou, cholesterol, mammogram, blood pressure, prostate, colonoscopy).
• Regular inoculations and immunizations	These include immunizations for tetanus, diphtheria, hepatitis B (as appropriate), pneumonia, and influenza, among others.
• Early and regular prenatal care	
• Reporting of unusual symptoms to a health professional	Early contact facilitates early treatment.
▲ Ensure that other agencies (e.g., Department of Children and Family Services, Social Services, Visiting Nurse Association, Meals On Wheels) are following through with plans.	These services may be necessary to provide care. Coordinated efforts are more meaningful and effective.

NANDA-I
NDx

Impaired Home Maintenance

Definition: Inability to independently maintain a safe growth-promoting immediate environment

Individuals within a home establish a normative pattern of operation. A vast number of factors can negatively affect that operational baseline. When this happens, an individual or an entire family may experience a disruption that is significant enough to impair the management of the home environment. Health or safety may be threatened, and there may be a threat to relationships or to the physical well-being of the people living in the home. An inability to perform the activities necessary to maintain a home may be the result of the development of chronic mental or physical disabilities, or acute conditions or circumstances that severely affect the vulnerable members of the household. As a result of early hospital discharges, nurses are coordinating complicated recovery regimens in the homes of patients. The patient's home must be safe and suited to the recovery needs of the individual. Patients must have the resources needed to provide for themselves and their families during recovery or following a debilitating illness. Because there is considerable room for cultural and intrafamilial variations in the maintenance of a home, the nurse should be guided by principles of safety when evaluating a home environment.

■ = Independent   ▲ = Collaborative

Common Related Factors

Cognitive, perceptual, or emotional disturbance
Poor planning and organization
Low income
Inadequate or absent support systems
Lack of knowledge
Illness or injury of the patient or a family member
Death of a significant other
Prolonged recuperation following illness
Substance abuse

Defining Characteristics

Patient or family expresses difficulty or lack of knowledge in
maintaining home environment
Lack of preventive care such as immunizations
Poor personal habits:
  • Soiled clothing
  • Frequent illness
  • Weight loss
  • Body odor
  • Substance abuse
  • Depressed affect
Poor fiscal management
Risk-taking behaviors
Vulnerable individuals (e.g., infants, children, older adults,
infirm) in the home are neglected or often ill
Home visits reveal unsafe home environment or lack of basic
hygiene measures (e.g., presence of vermin in the home,
accumulation of waste, home in poor repair, improper
temperature regulation)

Common Expected Outcomes

Patient maintains a safe home environment.
Patient identifies available resources.
Patient uses available resources.

NOC Outcomes
Family Functioning; Safety Behavior: Home
Physical Environment; Social Support

NIC Interventions
Home Maintenance Assistance; Sustenance
Support; Discharge Planning

Ongoing Assessment

Actions/Interventions	Rationales
■ Assess financial resources for maintaining the home environment.	Families may not have sufficient money to pay rent or mortgage, utilities, and basic home maintenance or repair. Grants or special funds can sometimes be used to modify the home to suit the needs of a physically challenged patient. Other supports and services are available to reduce financial stress.
■ Assess history of substance abuse, and determine its impact on the patient's ability to maintain the home.	The financial drain of a substance abuse problem can siphon money from every available resource.
■ Perform a home assessment. Assess for basic utilities, such as electricity, running water, and heat. Evaluate for accessibility and physical barriers. Assess bathing facilities, temperature regulation, whether windows close and doors lock, presence of screens, trash disposal.	These are basic necessities for a safe environment. Beyond this, evaluate the home to determine if the special needs of the patient can be accommodated. Social service agencies can provide help in determining whether patients can live in their home safely.
■ Evaluate each member of the family to determine whether basic physical and emotional needs are being met.	A distinction must be made between optimal living conditions and a safe home environment.
■ Assess the patient's knowledge of the rationale for personal and environmental hygiene and safety.	Although this is an important starting point, knowledge deficit is unlikely to be responsible for poor home maintenance in all cases. The patient's personal priorities, culture, and age may play a role in determining individual preferences.

Actions/Interventions	**Rationales**
■ Assess the patient's physical ability to perform home maintenance.	Accurate assessment guides intervention. For example, patients may not do laundry because they are unable to carry large boxes of detergent from the store, or they may be unable to carry rubbish to the collection site because sidewalks are icy.
■ Assess whether the patient has all assistive devices necessary to perform home maintenance.	Equipment may be required to accommodate the patient's needs (e.g., bedside commode). If unavailable, other options may need to be explored (e.g., a homemaker, family assistance).
■ Assess the impact of the death of a relative who may have been a significant provider of care.	Aspects of home maintenance may have been performed by the deceased, and a new plan to meet these needs may need to be developed.
■ Assess the patient's emotional and intellectual preparedness to maintain a home.	Impaired judgment can limit the patient's ability to care for self. Some patients who are mentally challenged are capable of living alone if provided with the appropriate supports, whereas the patient with a disease such as Alzheimer's may be unable to care for himself or herself.
▲ Enlist assistance from a social worker or community resources that may be helpful to the family or patient.	Patients may be unaware of the services to which they are entitled.

Therapeutic Interventions

Actions/Interventions	**Rationales**
■ Begin discharge planning immediately after hospital admission.	Shortened hospital stays and early discharges require an organized approach to meet individual needs of the family. Patients and their families may be managing more complicated recoveries in the home than were previously encountered.
■ Integrate the family/significant other and patient into the discharge planning process.	A network of family members, friends, and community resources can facilitate safe home patient care.
■ Plan a home visit to test the efficacy of discharge plans.	The nurse may visit the home to determine its readiness to accommodate the patient, or the patient may go home briefly to help identify potential problems. A home visit can help identify and solve problems that complicate home maintenance.
▲ Arrange for ongoing home therapy. Arrange for physical therapy, dietitian, and occupational therapy consultations in the home, as needed.	Complicated recovery necessitates that services be brought to the patient. Continuity of care is facilitated through the use of community resources.
■ Assist the family in arranging for redistribution of the workload. Build in relief for caregivers.	Coordination prevents fatigue during performance of physically or emotionally exhausting tasks.

Education/Continuity of Care

Actions/Interventions	**Rationales**
■ Begin care instruction or demonstrations early in the hospital stay.	Correct techniques need to be reinforced.
■ Teach care measures to as many family members as possible.	The patient's home health needs are more likely to be met if there are multiple competent providers and intrafamilial support.
■ Ensure that the family, patient, or caregiver has been instructed in the use of all assistive devices.	During the acute period, the family and significant others may require the most teaching in preparation for discharge.
▲ Arrange for alternate placement when the family is unable to provide care.	The need for placement may be temporary or extended; the patient's status will determine needs.

■ = Independent   ▲ = Collaborative

Actions/Interventions

■ Provide telephone support or support in the form of home visits.

▲ Refer to social services for financial and homemaking concerns. Inform of community resources as appropriate (e.g., drug abuse clinic).

Rationales

A variety of methods can be used to monitor the status of the patient and the well-being of others in the home.

Specialized services may be required to meet specific needs.

NANDA-I NDx   Hopelessness

Definition: Subjective state in which an individual sees limited or no alternatives or personal choices available and is unable to mobilize energy on own behalf

Hopelessness may be expressed anywhere along the illness trajectory. It may occur secondary to an acute event, such as spinal cord injury that leaves the patient permanently paralyzed, or it may be the result of a lifetime of multiple stresses for which the patient is no longer able to mobilize the energy needed to act in his or her own behalf. It is evident in patients living in social isolation, who are lonely and have no social support system or resources. Patients living in poverty, the homeless, and those with limited access to health care all may feel hopeless about changing their health care status and being able to cope with life. Loss of belief in God's care or loss of trust in prior spiritual beliefs may foster a sense of hopelessness.

Common Related Factors

Chronic and/or terminal illness
Prolonged restricted activity
Prolonged isolation
Loss of social support
Lost belief in transcendent values or God
Prolonged discomfort
Impaired functional abilities
Prolonged treatments or diagnostic studies with no positive results
Prolonged dependence on equipment
Long-term stress

Defining Characteristics

Passivity
Decreased affect
Decreased verbalization
Lack of initiative
Decreased response to stimuli
Apathy
Verbalizes that life has no meaning
Feels "empty"
Poor problem solving and decision making
Inability to set goals
Sleep, appetite disturbances
Socially withdrawn
Suicidal thoughts

Common Expected Outcomes

Patient expresses positive expectations about the future.
Patient mobilizes energy in own behalf (e.g., making decisions).
Patient sets goals consistent with optimism, meaning in life, and belief in self and others.

NOC Outcomes

Hope; Coping; Decision Making

NIC Interventions

Hope Installation; Coping Enhancement

Ongoing Assessment

Actions/Interventions

■ Assess the role that illness plays in the patient's hopelessness.

Rationales

Level of physical functioning, endurance for activities, duration and course of illness, prognosis, and treatments involved can contribute to hopelessness.

Actions/Interventions	**Rationales**
■ Assess physical appearance (e.g., grooming, posture, hygiene).	Hopeless patients may not have the energy or interest to engage in self-care activities.
■ Assess appetite, exercise, and sleep patterns.	Deviations from normal patterns are evident during periods of hopelessness.
■ Evaluate the patient's ability to set goals, make decisions, and solve problems.	A patient who feels hopeless will feel that goal setting is futile and that goals cannot be met. They may be unable to make decisions or solve problems.
■ Note whether the patient perceives unachieved outcomes as failures or emphasizes failures instead of accomplishments.	Repeated perceptions of failure will reinforce the patient's feelings of hopelessness. The patient may express loss of level of control or an inability to change the situation.
■ Assess for feelings of hopelessness, lack of self-worth, giving up, suicidal ideas.	Hopelessness is associated with dysfunctional personality characteristics as well as suicidal ideation and behaviors.
■ Assess for potential source of hope (e.g., self, significant others, religion).	Entrusted others (e.g., clergy, family, health team) can support the patient's basic belief system that enhances hope.
■ Assess the person's expectations for the future. Clarify when the situation is only temporary.	Uncertainty about events, duration and course of illness, prognosis, and dependence on others for help and treatments involved can contribute to a feeling of hopelessness.
■ Assess the person's social support network.	Patients in social isolation find it difficult to change their condition. Evaluation of supportive persons from the past may provide the assistance the patient requires at this time. Community groups, church groups, and self-help groups may also be available for assistance.
■ Assess meaning of the illness and treatments to the individual and family.	Certain misconceptions (e.g., patients with cancer always die) may be corrected and hope restored.
■ Assess previous coping strategies used and their effectiveness. Identify patterns of coping related to illness that enhance problem-solving skills and enable the patient to achieve goals.	Successful coping is influenced by past experiences. Patients with a history of maladaptive coping may require additional resources. Past strategies may not be sufficient in the present situation.
■ Assess patient's belief in self and own abilities. Identify patient's values and satisfaction with his or her role or purpose in life.	Patients may feel that the threat is greater than their resources to handle it, and feel a loss of control over solving the threat or problem.

Therapeutic Interventions

Actions/Interventions	**Rationales**
■ Provide opportunities for the patient to express feelings of pessimism.	The nurse creates a supportive environment by listening to the patient in a nonjudgemental manner.
■ Establish a working relationship with the patient through continuity of care.	An ongoing relationship establishes trust, reduces the feeling of isolation, and may facilitate coping.
■ Encourage the patient to identify his or her own strengths and abilities.	During a crisis, patients may not be able to recognize their strengths. Fostering awareness can expedite use of these strengths.
■ Provide the physical care that the patient is unable to provide for self in a manner that communicates warmth, respect, and acceptance of the patient's abilities.	This approach reduces guilt and other negative feelings the person may experience when unable to care for self.
■ Assist the patient in developing a realistic appraisal of the situation.	Patients may not be aware of all the support services available to them that can help them move through this stressful situation (e.g., home care aides, financial assistance, free medications, community counseling programs, legal services, companion services).

■ = Independent   ▲ = Collaborative

Actions/Interventions	Rationales
■ Help the patient set realistic goals by identifying short-term goals and revising them as needed.	Patients may feel overwhelmed when viewing the situation from a "big picture" perspective. Guiding the patient to view the situation in smaller parts may make the problem more manageable. It is important that the patient set truly realistic goals so as not to be frustrated with the inability to accomplish them.
■ Encourage an attitude of realistic hope.	Emphasizing the patient's intrinsic worth and viewing the immediate problem as manageable in time may provide support. Fostering unrealistic hope is not helpful and may significantly worsen the trust the patient places in the health care provider. Belief in the nurse-patient relationship as a partnership in the journey toward hope is key to fostering hope.
■ Assure the patient and family that they will not be abandoned and that every effort will be made to optimize the highest quality of care.	Compassionate assurance gives patients and families an increased sense of feeling cared for and understood.
■ Support the patient's relationships with significant others; involve them in the patient's care as appropriate.	Interest in others may help change the patient's focus from self. Enhancing a sense of connectedness to a caring environment fosters hope.
■ Provide opportunities for the patient to control environment.	Hopeless patients may feel they have no control. Yet when given opportunities to make choices, their perception of hopelessness may be reduced.
■ Promote ego integrity by the following: • Encouraging the patient to reminisce about past life (self-validation). • Showing the patient that he or she gives something to you as a clinician.	Older patients especially find value in reviewing life's events and accomplishments.
■ Facilitate problem solving by identifying the problem and appropriate steps.	Small steps that are successful will foster confidence in oneself and may promote a more hopeful outlook. They encourage gradual mastery of the situation.
■ Expand the patient's repertoire of coping skills.	Specialized techniques may be required to help the patient gain control.
■ Encourage the use of spiritual resources as desired.	Religious practices may provide strength and inspiration.

Education/Continuity of Care

Actions/Interventions	Rationales
■ Provide accurate and ongoing information about illness, treatment effects, and care needed.	Misconceptions about diagnosis and prognosis may be contributing to hopelessness.
■ Let the patient or family know when situations are temporary.	The outlook may appear less hopeless when time is limited.
■ Educate the patient or family on using a combination of problem solving and emotive coping.	These skills can enhance the coping ability of the patient and family members.
■ Ensure that strategies to maintain hope within the patient are also used to support family caregivers.	Family caregivers are an integral component to instilling and supporting a sense of hope in their loved one.

Hyperthermia

Definition: Body temperature elevated above normal range

Hyperthermia is a sustained temperature above the normal variance, usually greater than 39° C (102.2° F) (core temperature). Adults may experience nerve damage and seizures when core body temperature is 41° C (105.8° F). Temperatures of 43° C (109.4° F) or higher are incompatible with life. Hyperthermia differs from fever in that the hypothalamic set point is not reset at a higher level. Also, hyperthermia is not stimulated by pyrogens, such as occurs with infection. Many cases of hyperthermia result from activity and from salt and water deprivation in a hot environment, such as when athletes perform in extremely hot weather or when older adults avoid the use of air conditioning because of expense. Hyperthermia may occur more readily in persons who have endocrine disorders; use alcohol; or take diuretics, anticholinergics, or phototoxic agents. Forms of accidental hyperthermia include heat cramps, heat exhaustion, and heat stroke. Malignant hyperthermia is a life-threatening response to various anesthetic agents. This inherited disorder affects calcium metabolism in muscle cells, causing fever, muscle rigidity, metabolic acidosis, dysrhythmic tachycardia, hypertension, and hypoxia. Careful evaluation of preoperative patients is essential for prevention.

Common Related Factors

Exposure to hot environment
Vigorous activity
Medications
Anesthesia
Increased metabolic rate
Illness or trauma
Dehydration
Inability to perspire

Defining Characteristics

Body temperature above the normal range
Hot, flushed skin
Increased heart rate
Increased respiratory rate
Convulsions

Common Expected Outcomes

Patient maintains body temperature below 39° C (102.2° F).
Patient maintains blood pressure, respiratory rate, and heart rate within normal limits.

NOC Outcomes
Thermoregulation; Vital Signs
NIC Interventions
Temperature Regulation; Fever Treatment;
    Malignant Hyperthermia Precautions

Ongoing Assessment

Actions/Interventions	Rationales
■ Determine precipitating factors.	Identification and management of underlying cause are essential to recovery.
■ Assess HR, BP, especially tympanic or rectal temperature.	HR and BP increase as hyperthermia progresses. Tempanic or rectal temperatures provide a more accurate indication of core temperature.
■ Obtain age and weight.	Extremes of age or weight increase the risk for inability to control body temperature.
■ Measure input and output. If patient is unconscious, central venous pressure or pulmonary artery pressure should be measured to monitor fluid status.	Fluid resuscitation may be necessary to correct dehydration. The patient who is significantly dehydrated is no longer able to sweat, which is necessary for evaporative cooling.
▲ Monitor serum electrolytes, especially serum sodium.	Sodium losses occur with profuse sweating and accidental hyperthermia.

■ = Independent   ▲ = Collaborative

Therapeutic Interventions

Actions/Interventions

- Control environmental temperature. Move heat victim to cooler area, out of direct sunlight. Transport victims with altered consciousness to a health care facility.
- Remove excess clothing and covers.

▲ Provide antipyretic medications as ordered.

▲ Provide oxygen therapy in extreme cases.
▲ Control excessive shivering with medications such as chlorpromazine (Thorazine) and diazepam (Valium), if necessary.
▲ Provide ample fluids by mouth or intravenously.

▲ Provide additional cooling mechanisms commensurate with significance of fever and related manifestations:
  - Noninvasive: cooling mattress, cold packs applied to major blood vessels
  - Evaporative cooling: cool with tepid bath; do not use alcohol
  - Invasive: gastric lavage, peritoneal lavage, cardiopulmonary bypass in an emergency

- Adjust cooling measures on the basis of physical response.

Rationales

Removing sources of heat can begin the cooling process and reduce core temperature.

Exposing skin to room air decreases warmth and increases evaporative cooling.
Temperatures above 40° C (104° F) for extended periods can cause cellular damage, delirium, and seizures.
Hyperthermia increases metabolic demand for oxygen.
Shivering increases metabolic rate and body temperature.

If patient is dehydrated or diaphoretic, fluid loss contributes to fever.

These measures help promote cooling and lower core temperature.
Alcohol cools the skin too rapidly, causing shivering.

These invasive procedures are used to quickly cool core temperature. These patients require cardiopulmonary monitoring.
Cooling too quickly may cause shivering, which increases use of energy calories and increases metabolic rate in order to produce heat.

Education/Continuity of Care

Actions/Interventions

- Explain temperature measurement and all treatments.

- Provide information regarding normal temperature and control.

- Discuss precipitating factors and preventive measures, including maintenance of adequate fluid intake, protective skin products, change in environment, taking medications as prescribed (antipyretics, antibiotics).
- Teach the patient and family to recognize early signs of hyperthermia. These signs include abdominal cramps, muscle cramps in extremities, weakness, dizziness, and nausea.
- Refer at-risk individuals to the Malignant Hyperthermia Association of the United States.
- Discuss importance of informing future health care providers of malignant hyperthermia risk; suggest a medical alert bracelet or similar identification.

Rationales

Patients may be initially disoriented, requiring repeated explanations.
This information is especially necessary for patients with conditions or in situations putting them at risk for hyperthermia (e.g., those with infection, those subject to extremely hot weather, athletes).
Patients and families need to learn how to prevent future episodes of hyperthermia. Acclimation to work or exercise in hot weather helps to reduce the risk for hyperthermia.

Early identification of signs of heat cramps allows for prompt intervention to prevent progression to heat exhaustion and heat stroke.

This organization provides information and additional resources.
Alternative anesthetic drugs or methods can be used for these patients. Patient safety is a priority.

NANDA-I NDx Hypothermia

Definition: Body temperature below normal range

Hypothermia is a temperature at a significantly lower level than normal; usually lower than 35° C (95° F) measured by the tympanic/rectal routes. Hypothermia results when the body cannot produce heat at a rate equal to that lost to the environment through conduction, convection, radiation, or evaporation. Core temperature below 32° C (89.6° F) is severe and life threatening. Hypothermia can be classified as inadvertent (seen postoperatively), intentional (for medical purposes), or accidental (exposure related). Older adults are especially vulnerable to accidental hypothermia because of age-related alterations in normal thermoregulation.

Common Related Factors

Exposure to cold environment
Illness or trauma
Inability to shiver
Poor nutrition
Inadequate clothing
Alcohol consumption
Medications
Excessive evaporative heat loss from skin
Decreased metabolic rate

Defining Characteristics

Body temperature below normal range
Shivering
Piloerection
Cool, pale skin
Slow capillary refill
Hypertension
Increased heart rate

Common Expected Outcomes

Patient maintains a body temperature above 35° C (95° F) (core).
Patient maintains HR and BP within normal limits; skin is warm.

NOC Outcomes
Thermoregulation; Vital Sign Status
NIC Interventions
Temperature Regulation; Hypothermia Treatment

Ongoing Assessment

Actions/Interventions	Rationales
■ Determine precipitating event and risk factors.	Causative factors guide appropriate treatment. Older patients have a decreased metabolic rate and reduced shivering response; therefore effects of cold may not be immediately apparent.
■ Monitor temperature.	For alert patients, oral temperature is considered more accurate than tympanic or axillary. For more hypothermic patients, core temperature can be monitored using a temperature-sensitive pulmonary artery catheter or bladder catheter.
■ Assess heart rate, rhythm, and blood pressure.	Heart rate and blood pressure decrease as hypothermia progresses. Moderate to severe hypothermia increases risk for ventricular fibrillation, along with other arrhythmias.
■ Evaluate for drug use, including psychotherapeutics, narcotics, and alcohol.	These agents cause vasodilation and heat loss.

■ = Independent   ▲ = Collaborative

Actions/Interventions

- Evaluate peripheral perfusion at frequent intervals.

- Assess nutrition and weight.

- Monitor intake and output (and/or central venous pressure).

- ▲ Monitor electrolytes, arterial blood gases, and oximetry.
- Evaluate for presence of frostbite, if applicable.

Rationales

Hypothermia initially precipitates peripheral vascular constriction as a compensatory mechanism to minimize heat loss from the extremities. As hypothermia progresses, vasodilation occurs, furthering heat loss.

Poor nutrition contributes to decreased energy reserves and limits the body's ability to produce heat by caloric consumption.

Decreased output may indicate dehydration or poor renal perfusion. Avoid fluid overload to prevent pulmonary edema, pneumonia, and taxing an already compromised cardiac and renal status.

Acidosis may result from hypoventilation and hypoxia.

Severe hypothermia causes ice crystals to form inside cells. The cells then rupture and die.

Therapeutic Interventions

Actions/Interventions

- Control environmental temperature or move patient to warmer environment. Keep patient and linen dry.

- Provide extra covering (passive warming), such as clothing and blankets; cover postoperative patients with heat-retaining blankets.
- Provide heated oral fluids for alert patients.
- ▲ Provide extra heat source:
  - Heat lamp, radiant warmer
  - Warming mattress, pads, or blankets
  - Submersion in warm bath
  - Heated, moisturized oxygen
  - Warmed intravenous fluids or lavage fluids
- Regulate heat source according to physical response.

- Avoid trauma to areas of frostbite.

Rationales

These techniques provide for a more gradual warming of the body. Rapid warming can induce ventricular fibrillation. Moisture facilitates evaporative heat loss.

Warm blankets provide a passive method for rewarming.

Warm fluids provide a heat source.

These measures raise core temperature and improve circulation. Core rewarming is indicated when body temperature is below 30° C (86° F).

Body temperature should be raised no more than a few degrees per hour. Complications of rewarming including metabolic acidosis, hypotension, and dysrhythmias.

Rubbing can further damage frozen tissue.

Education/Continuity of Care

Actions/Interventions

- Explain all procedures and treatments.

- Provide information regarding normal temperature and prevention of hypothermia, once the patient's condition is stable.
- Enlist support services as appropriate.

Rationales

Keep in mind that the patient is confused from hypothermia and decreased oxygenation; repeated explanations may be necessary.

Patients and family members need information about how to prevent hypothermia.

Social, mental, or economic problems precipitate many situations where hypothermia occurs, especially when patients are older, poor, or homeless.

Readiness for Enhanced Immunization Status

Definition: A pattern of conforming to local, national, and/or international standards of immunization to prevent infectious disease(s) that is sufficient to protect a person, family, or community and can be strengthened

Every year approximately 50,000 adults in the United States die from diseases that could be prevented by vaccines. Influenza and pneumonia are the fifth leading cause of death in older adults in the United States. Immunizations are one of the safest, most cost-effective public health measures available to patients to preserve their health. Although many adults do support immunization programs for their children, they are often less informed about the many health benefits of vaccines as adults. The Centers for Disease Control and Prevention (CDC) recommendations clearly identify who is at risk for various diseases and who should be immunized to protect against them.

Common Related Factors

Exposure to individuals with communicable disease
Interest in traveling abroad

Defining Characteristics

Expresses desire to enhance behavior to prevent infectious disease
Expresses desire to enhance identification of possible problems associated with immunizations
Expresses desire to enhance identification of providers of immunizations
Expresses desire to enhance immunization status
Expresses desire to enhance knowledge of immunization standards
Expresses desire to enhance record keeping of immunizations

Common Expected Outcomes

Patient acknowledges disease risk without immunization.
Patient obtains adult immunizations recommended by the CDC or U.S. Public Health Service.
Patient identifies community resources for immunization.
Patient develops and maintains a systematic record-keeping plan for monitoring immunization status.

NOC Outcome
Immunization Behavior
NIC Intervention
Immunization/Vaccination Management

Ongoing Assessment

Actions/Interventions

- Assess patient's prior history of immunizations as child and adult.

- Assess knowledge of latest CDC recommendations regarding immunization use.

- Assess patient's interest in travel abroad.

- Determine immunization status at every health care visit, especially emergency department visits.

Rationales

Information provides baseline to determine personal protection and adherence to immunization recommendations.

Patients may have basic knowledge about common adult illnesses like influenza and pneumococcal diseases, but they may have misinformation about vaccinations against less-common diseases, such as measles, mumps, and varicella, that may be needed by adults.

Immunizations may be required depending on country being visited, age and medical status of patient, and length of stay.

A systematic assessment program can facilitate increased awareness by both health care professionals and patients of immunization need.

■ = Independent   ▲ = Collaborative

Actions/Interventions

■ Identify any contraindications to receiving immunizations.

Rationales

Vaccines are considered to be quite safe for the general public. However, patients may have had prior anaphylaxis to a vaccine or have a moderate to severe acute illness, putting them at increased risk. Pregnant women need to discuss immunizations with their physician. All potential risks need to be weighed against benefits.

Therapeutic Interventions

Actions/Interventions

■ Review information regarding the latest CDC recommendations for prevention of common diseases. Some of these include the following:

- *Influenza:* The trivalent inactivated influenza vaccine (TIV) is recommended for persons 50 years and older, those with medical problems including compromised immune systems, those with compromised respiratory status, those living in chronic care facilities, those living with/working (including health care providers) with high-risk people, women who are or will be pregnant, and persons in institutional settings.
- *Pneumonia:* The pneumococcal polysaccharide vaccine (PPSV) does not necessarily reduce risk for getting pneumonia, but can reduce associated complications. Recommended for adults 65 years and older, those with chronic illness, younger adults without a spleen or with a damaged spleen, and immunocompromised persons.
- *Shingles (herpes zoster):* Zostavax is recommended for persons 60 years and older whether or not they have had shingles before.
- *Hepatitis B:* Hepatitis B vaccine is indicated for all persons age 18 and older, especially those whose lifestyle (e.g., intravenous [IV] drug users, those with human immunodeficiency virus [HIV], men who have sex with men, persons in a nonmonogamous relationship), travel (some international sites), occupation (e.g., health care personnel, public safety personnel, prison staff and inmates), and health conditions (chronic liver disease, renal disease, dialysis) increase their exposure to hepatitis B.
- *Hepatitis A:* Hepatitis A vaccine is indicated for adults with chronic liver disease, clotting factor disorders, IV drug users, men having sex with men, and persons traveling to certain foreign countries such as those in Central and South America.
- *Tetanus, diphtheria, pertussis:* The combined Tdap vaccine protects against all three diseases and is indicated as a booster for adults younger than 65 years. All adults need tetanus and diphtheria boosters every 10 years throughout life, especially adults in contact with younger infants and health care personnel having direct patient contact.

Rationales

The CDC provides extensive information regarding the many adult vaccines available, for whom the vaccine is recommended, the schedule for the vaccine, and any contraindications and precautions. Health care providers and patients alike need to remain current.

Actions/Interventions

- *Polio:* Routine immunization is not recommended for U.S. adult residents unless they are traveling to high-risk countries.
- *Varicella (chickenpox):* Varivax is indicated for adults not already immune to the chickenpox virus.
- *Meningitis:* Meningococcal vaccine is recommended for persons at risk during an outbreak of the disease, students living in a college dormitory, persons with spleen damage, or persons traveling to countries in which meningitis is common.
- *Measles, mumps, rubella:* Vaccine is recommended for adults born in 1957 or later if there is no evidence of immunity; high-risk persons such as health care providers, college students, travelers; and women of childbearing age.
- *Human papillomavirus (HPV):* Recommended for women through age 26 years to prevent cervical cancer.

■ Assist patient in locating potential sites for obtaining various immunizations.

■ Schedule immunizations at appropriate time intervals.

Rationales

Providing a listing of sources for vaccinations can facilitate compliance with recommendations. These sources can include family physicians, city or county health departments, local hospitals, pharmacies, or even clinics available in shopping malls, senior centers, and community centers.

Specific guidelines are offered to insure optimal protection, ranging from one-time only immunizations to 5- to 10-year boosters, to annual flu shots.

Education/Continuity of Care

Actions/Interventions

■ Teach patient about vaccinations appropriate for international travel to certain countries, referring patient to a travel clinic, local health department, or the CDC website.

■ Teach patient about resources for paying for immunizations (e.g., public health department, insurance coverage).

■ Teach patient about immunizations available for special incidence or outbreaks (e.g., cholera, tuberculosis).

■ Instruct patient in tools for maintaining personal immunization records.

Rationales

Where one travels determines disease risk, though other factors such as age, medical status, length of time in the country, type of travel (rural areas/backpacking) are also important factors. Exposure to serious disease such as malaria, yellow fever, and hepatitis is higher in developing countries with poor sanitation such as most parts of Africa and Asia and some parts of South and Central America.

Out-of-pocket expenses for immunizations vary depending on insurance coverage. Patients may need to check into own health insurance coverage plans regarding their personal benefits. Medicare pays for one influenza immunization each year, one pneumococcal vaccination (along with booster vaccine after 5 years if needed), and hepatitis B vaccination for intermediate- or high-risk individuals.

The CDC provides extensive information regarding the many adult vaccines available, for whom the vaccine is recommended, the schedule for the vaccine, and any contraindications and precautions. Health care providers and patients alike need to remain current.

Accurate record keeping helps to ensure that adults are fully protected from vaccine-preventable diseases. Such a mechanism will help prevent gaps in protection, especially when changing health care providers. It also prevents inappropriate revaccination that can occur during a health emergency.

■ = Independent   ▲ = Collaborative

Nursing Diagnosis Care Plans

Functional Urinary Incontinence

Definition: Inability of usually continent person to reach toilet in time to avoid unintentional loss of urine

The person with functional urinary incontinence has normal function of the neurological control mechanisms for urination. The bladder is able to fill and store urine appropriately. The person is able to recognize the urge to void. The most common problem is environmental barriers that make it difficult for the person to reach an appropriate receptacle for voiding. This type of incontinence occurs more often in older adults who have mobility limitations. People with arthritis of the hands may have difficulty undoing clothing buttons or zippers to prepare for voiding. The patient with limited mobility may be dependent on others for help transferring to a bedside commode or ambulating to the bathroom. If mobility assistance is not readily available, the person is not able to suppress the urge to void and becomes incontinent. Wet clothing, urine odor, and the loss of independence for toileting contribute to the person's feelings of embarrassment in this situation. Over time the person may have changes in body image and self-concept.

Common Related Factors

Altered environmental factors
Limited physical mobility

Defining Characteristics

Recognizes need to urinate but is unable to access toileting facility in a timely manner
May be incontinent only in morning upon awakening

Common Expected Outcomes

Patient receives assistance for toileting in a timely manner.
Patient has no episodes of incontinence.

NOC Outcomes

Urinary Continence; Urinary Elimination; Self-Care: Toileting

NIC Interventions

Urinary Habit Training; Urinary Incontinence Care

Ongoing Assessment

Actions/Interventions	**Rationales**
■ Assess the patient's recognition of the need to urinate.	Patients with functional incontinence are incontinent because they cannot get to an appropriate place to void. Institutionalized patients are often labeled "incontinent" because their requests for toileting are unmet. Older patients with cognitive impairment may recognize the need to void but may be unable to express the need.
■ Assess the availability of functional toileting facilities (working toilet, bedside commode).	Patients may need a bedside commode if mobility limitations interfere with getting to the bathroom.
■ Assess the patient's ability to reach a toileting facility, both independently and with help.	This information allows the nurse to plan for assistance with transfer to a toilet or bedside commode. Functional continence requires that the person be able to get to a toilet either independently or with assistance.
■ Assess frequency of the patient's need to urinate.	This information is the basis for an individualized toileting program. Many patients are incontinent in the early morning when the bladder has stored a large urine volume during sleep.

Therapeutic Interventions

Actions/Interventions

■ Establish a toileting schedule.

■ Place a bedside commode near the patient's bed.

■ Encourage use of clothing that can be easily and quickly removed.

■ Treat any existing perineal skin excoriation with a vitamin-enriched cream, followed by a moisture barrier.

Rationales

A toileting schedule assures the patient of a specified time for voiding and reduces episodes of functional incontinence.

The person needs to accept this alternative toileting facility. Some people may be embarrassed when using a toilet in a more open area.

Clothing can be a barrier to functional continence if it takes time to remove before voiding.

Moisture-barrier ointments are useful in protecting perineal skin from urine.

Education/Continuity of Care

Actions/Interventions

■ Teach the patient or caregiver the rationale behind and implementation of a toileting program.

Rationales

Successful functional continence requires consistency in use of a toileting program.

NANDA-I NDx

Reflex Urinary Incontinence

Definition: Involuntary loss of urine at somewhat predictable intervals when a specific bladder volume is reached

Reflex urinary incontinence represents dysfunction of the normal neurological control mechanisms for coordination of detrusor contraction and sphincter relaxation. Neurological disorders in the detrusor motor area of the brain result in detrusor hyperreflexia. Examples of such disorders include strokes, traumatic brain injury, hydrocephalus, tumors, Alzheimer's disease, and multiple sclerosis. Cervical and thoracic spinal cord injuries and Guillain-Barré syndrome may cause detrusor hyperreflexia with sphincter dyssynergia. The patient with reflex incontinence experiences periodic urination without an awareness of needing to void. Urination is frequent throughout the day and night. Urine volume is consistent with each voiding. Residual urine volumes are usually less than 50 mL. Urodynamic studies will indicate detrusor contraction when bladder volume reaches a specific amount.

Common Related Factors

Radiation cystitis
Radical pelvic surgery
Spinal cord lesions above S2 level
Brain injury above level of pontine micturition center

Defining Characteristics

No sensation of bladder fullness
No sensation of urge to void
Inability to initiate or inhibit voiding
Predictable pattern of voiding

Common Expected Outcomes

Patient establishes a regular voiding pattern.
Patient has no episodes of incontinence.

NOC Outcomes

Urinary Continence; Urinary Elimination;
Self-Care: Toileting

NIC Interventions

Urinary Catheterization; Urinary Catheterization:
Intermittent; Urinary Habit Training; Urinary
Incontinence Care

■ = Independent   ▲ = Collaborative

Nursing Diagnosis Care Plans

Ongoing Assessment

Actions/Interventions	Rationales
■ Assess the patient's recognition of the need to void.	Patients with neurological disorders may have damaged sensory fibers, and may not have the sensation of the need to void.
■ Measure urine volume with each voiding.	Urine volumes are usually consistent with reflex incontinence.
■ Encourage the patient to maintain a "bladder diary."	Information about fluid intake and voiding patterns provides a basis for planning bladder management techniques.
▲ Monitor the results of urodynamic studies.	A cystometrogram will measure bladder pressures and fluid volumes during filling, storage and urination. Electromyography will record detrusor activity during voiding. Test results will indicate coordination of detrusor and sphincter activity.

Therapeutic Interventions

Actions/Interventions	Rationales
■ Encourage voiding at scheduled intervals before predictable voiding.	Voiding at regular intervals, based on knowledge of the patient's voiding pattern, decreases the chance of uncontrolled incontinence.
■ Encourage the patient to limit fluid intake 2 to 3 hours before bedtime.	Limiting fluid intake reduces the need to disrupt sleep for voiding.
■ Consider use of an external catheter for the male patient.	An external catheter connected to a gravity drainage device allows the patient to remain dry.
▲ Catheterize the patient at regular intervals if spontaneous voiding is not possible. Use an indwelling catheter as a last resort.	Emptying the bladder at regular intervals will reduce incontinence episodes. The risk for infection is considerable with indwelling catheters.

Education/Continuity of Care

Actions/Interventions	Rationales
■ Teach the patient or caregiver (or perform for patient) intermittent (self-) catheterization.	This technique empties the bladder at specified intervals.
■ Discuss the use of absorbent pads in social situations.	Absorbent pads will protect clothing when the patient is in public. The patient needs to understand about changing the pads at regular intervals to prevent skin irritation from exposure to urine and moisture.

NANDA-I NDx **Stress Urinary Incontinence**

Definition: Sudden leakage of urine with activities that increase intraabdominal pressure

Stress incontinence occurs more often in women than men. The predisposing factors for women include pregnancy, obesity, decreased estrogen levels associated with menopause, and surgery involving the lower abdominal area. Men may develop stress incontinence following surgical treatment for benign prostatic hyperplasia or prostate cancer. These factors contribute to a decrease in muscle tone at the urethrovesical junction. When the muscles of the abdomen and pelvic floor are weak, they no longer provide support for the urinary sphincter. The urinary sphincter cannot remain constricted with increasing abdominal pressure. Straining with defecation, laughing, sneezing, coughing, heavy lifting, jumping, or running are examples of activities that increase intraabdominal pressure and lead to stress incontinence. The amount of urine lost may vary from a few drops to 100 mL or more. Regardless of the amount of urine lost during a stress incontinence episode, the person may experience embarrassment and changes in body image and self-concept. As a result, the person may decrease social interactions and physical activities to minimize the risks of incontinence occurring in public situations.

Common Related Factors

Multiple vaginal deliveries
Pelvic surgery
Hypoestrogenism (aging, menopause)
Diabetic neuropathy
Trauma to pelvic area
Obesity
Radial prostatectomy

Common Expected Outcomes

Patient has not episodes of incontinence.
Patient implements activities to increase abdominal and pelvic floor muscle tone.

Defining Characteristics

Observed or patient reports of involuntary leakage of small amounts of urine with activities associated with exertion and/or increased intraabdominal pressure
Observed or patient reports of involuntary leakage of small amounts of urine in the absence of detrusor contraction or an overdistended bladder

NOC Outcomes
Urinary Continence; Urinary Elimination; Self-Care: Toileting
NIC Interventions
Urinary Habit Training; Urinary Incontinence Care

Ongoing Assessment

Actions/Interventions	Rationales
■ Ask whether urine is lost involuntarily during coughing, laughing, sneezing, lifting, or exercising.	Whenever intraabdominal pressure increases, a weak sphincter and/or relaxed pelvic floor muscles allow urine to escape involuntarily.
■ Examine the perineal area for evidence of pelvic relaxation: • Cystourethrocele (sagging bladder or urethra) • Rectocele (relaxed, sagging rectal mucosa) • Uterine prolapse (relaxed uterus)	The presence of these conditions can lead to incontinence because of poor muscular control.
■ Determine parity.	Childbirth trauma weakens pelvic muscles.
■ Explore menstrual history.	Postmenopausal hypoestrogenism causes relaxation of the urethra.
■ Ask about previous surgical procedures.	In men, transurethral resection of the prostate gland can result in urinary incontinence.

Therapeutic Interventions

Actions/Interventions	Rationales
■ Encourage weight loss if obese.	Obesity is associated with increased intraabdominal pressure on the urinary bladder.
■ Encourage the patient to maintain adequate fluid intake.	Patients often restrict fluid intake to reduce incontinence episodes.
▲ Administer or encourage use of medication as ordered: • Pseudoephedrine • Vaginal estrogen	These medications increase sphincter tone and improve muscle tone.
■ Prepare the patient for surgery (Marshall-Marchetti-Krantz, Burch's colposuspension, and sling procedures) as indicated.	Many types of procedures are used to control stress incontinence. These procedures provide support to the bladder and urinary sphincter.

■ = Independent   ▲ = Collaborative

Nursing Diagnosis Care Plan

Education/Continuity of Care

Actions/Interventions	Rationales
■ Teach the patient to perform Kegel exercises.	Kegel exercises are used to strengthen the muscles of the pelvic floor and can be practiced with a minimum of exertion. The repetitious tightening and relaxation of these muscles (10 repetitions four or five times per day) helps some patients regain continence. Kegel exercises may be used in combination with biofeedback to enhance outcome.
■ Teach the patient about appropriate use of absorption pads.	Disposable pads or briefs may be worn to absorb urine and increase the person's social activities. The person needs to change the pads at regular intervals to prevent skin irritation from contact with urine and moisture.
■ Teach the patient to use transcutaneous electrical nerve stimulation (TENS), as indicated.	This device improves pelvic floor tone and inhibits the micturition reflex.
■ Teach women patients the use of a vaginal pessary (a device reserved for nonsurgical candidates).	A pessary works by elevating the bladder neck, thereby increasing urethral resistance.
▲ Refer the patient for biofeedback training.	Biofeedback techniques combined with electromyography or pressure manometry help the person learn to contract pelvic floor muscles and control incontinence.
■ Refer to stress urinary incontinence website www.nafc.org (National Association for Continence).	The site provides additional resources, support, and information.

NANDA-I NDx Urge Urinary Incontinence

Definition: Involuntary passage of urine occurring soon after a strong sense of urgency to void

Urge urinary incontinence is associated with overactivity or uncontrolled contraction of the detrusor muscle. The person has uncontrolled passage of urine within a few seconds to a few minutes after feeling a strong sense of urgency to void. The person is unable to voluntarily suppress voiding once the urge is felt. Urge incontinence may develop as a result of spinal cord lesions or following pelvic surgery. Central nervous system disorders such as Alzheimer's disease, multiple sclerosis, and Parkinson's disease may contribute to urge incontinence. Overactivity of the detrusor may be the result of interstitial cystitis or pelvic radiation. As with other types of urinary incontinence, the person with urge incontinence may experience embarrassment with loss of control of urinary elimination. The person begins to plan activities to be close to a toilet at all times. This change in behavior may affect the person's social interaction and work performance.

Common Related Factors

Alcohol intake
Caffeine intake
Diuretic use
Stroke
Spinal cord injury
Parkinson's disease
Multiple sclerosis
Infections

Defining Characteristics

Observed or reported inability to reach toilet in time to avoid urine loss
Reports of urine loss with bladder spasms
Urinary urgency

Common Expected Outcomes

Patient maintains a pattern of predictable voiding.
Patient has no periods of incontinence.

NOC Outcomes
Urinary Continence; Urinary Elimination;
   Self-Care: Toileting

NIC Interventions
Urinary Habit Training; Urinary Incontinence Care

Ongoing Assessment

Actions/Interventions

- Ask patient to describe episodes of incontinence; note descriptions of feeling the need suddenly to urinate but being unable to get to the bathroom in time.
- Instruct the patient to keep a daily bladder diary indicating voiding frequency and patterns.

▲ Culture urine.

▲ Monitor results of cystometry.

Rationales

Urge incontinence occurs when the bladder muscle suddenly contracts.

This allows the nurse to identify patterns in voiding. This information will allow for an individualized treatment plan. The patient may be voiding as often as every 2 hours.

Bladder infection can result in a strong urge to urinate; successful management of a urinary tract infection may eliminate or improve incontinence.

Diagnostic testing is used to measure bladder pressures and fluid volume during filling, storage, and urination.

Therapeutic Interventions

Actions/Interventions

- Facilitate access to toileting facilities, and teach the patient to make scheduled trips to the bathroom.
▲ Administer or encourage use of medications as ordered:
  • Anticholinergics
  • Tricyclic antidepressants

Rationales

Scheduled voiding allows for frequent bladder emptying.

Anticholinergics reduce or block detrusor contractions, thereby reducing episodes of incontinence. The tricyclics increase serotonin or norepinephrine, which results in relaxation of the bladder wall and greater bladder capacity.

Education/Continuity of Care

Actions/Interventions

- Teach the patient to limit intake of alcohol and caffeine.

- Assist the patient with developing a bladder training program.

- Teach the patient to void at scheduled intervals, gradually increasing the time between voidings.

- Teach Kegel exercises.

Rationales

These chemicals are known to be bladder irritants. They can increase detrusor overactivity.

A bladder training program helps increase bladder capacity through regulation of fluid intake, pelvic exercises, and scheduled voiding.

This behavior modification technique helps decrease detrusor overactivity and increase bladder fluid volume capacity.

These exercises improve pelvic floor muscle tone and urethrovesical junction sphincter tone.

■ = Independent   ▲ = Collaborative

Nursing Diagnosis Care Plans

Risk for Infection

Definition: At increased risk for being invaded by pathogenic organisms

Persons at risk for infection are those whose natural defense mechanisms are inadequate to protect them from the inevitable injuries and exposures that occur throughout the course of living. Infections occur when an organism (e.g., bacterium, virus, fungus, or other parasite) invades a susceptible host. Breaks in the integument, the body's first line of defense, and/or the mucous membranes allow invasion by pathogens. If the patient's immune system cannot combat the invading organism adequately, an infection occurs. Open wounds, traumatic or surgical, can be sites for infection; soft tissues (cells, fat, muscle) and organs (kidneys, lungs) can also be sites for infection either after trauma, invasive procedures, or by invasion of pathogens carried through the bloodstream or lymphatic system. Infections can be transmitted, either by contact or through airborne transmission, sexual contact, or sharing of intravenous (IV) drug paraphernalia. Being malnourished, having inadequate resources for sanitary living conditions, and lacking knowledge about disease transmission place individuals at risk for infection. Health care workers, to protect themselves and others from disease transmission, must understand how to take precautions to prevent transmission. Because identification of infected individuals is not always apparent, standard precautions recommended by the Centers for Disease Control and Prevention are widely practiced. The Agency for Healthcare Research and Quality published important guidelines and recommendations in this resource: *Patient Safety and Quality: An Evidence-Based Handbook for Nurses.* In addition, the Occupational Safety and Health Administration has set forth the Bloodborne Pathogens Standard, developed to protect workers and the public from infection. Ease of and increase in world travel have also increased opportunities for transmission of disease from abroad. Infections prolong healing and can result in death if untreated. Antimicrobials are used to treat infections when susceptibility is present. Organisms may become resistant to antimicrobials, requiring multiple antimicrobial therapy. There are organisms for which no antimicrobial is effective, such as the human immunodeficiency virus.

Common Risk Factors

Inadequate primary defenses: broken skin, injured tissue, body fluid stasis
Inadequate secondary defenses: immunosuppression, leukopenia
Malnutrition
Intubation
Indwelling catheters, drains
IV devices
Invasive procedures
Rupture of amniotic membranes
Chronic disease
Failure to avoid pathogens (exposure)
Inadequate acquired immunity

Common Expected Outcomes

Patient remains free of infection, as evidenced by normal vital signs and absence of purulent drainage from wounds, incisions, and tubes.
Infection is recognized early to allow for prompt treatment.

NOC Outcomes
Immune Status; Knowledge: Infection Control
NIC Interventions
Infection Control; Infection Protection

Ongoing Assessment

Actions/Interventions	Rationales
■ Assess for presence, existence of, and history of risk factors such as open wounds and abrasions; indwelling catheters (Foley, peritoneal); wound drainage tubes (T-tubes, Penrose, Jackson-Pratt); endotracheal or tracheostomy tubes; venous or arterial access devices; and orthopedic fixator pins.	Each of these examples represents a break in the body's normal first line of defense.
▲ Monitor white blood cell (WBC) count.	An increasing WBC count indicates the body's efforts to combat pathogens. Normal values are 4000 to 11,000/mm^3. Very low WBC count (less than 1000/mm^3) indicates severe risk for infection because the patient does not have sufficient WBCs to fight infection. NOTE: In older patients, infection may be present without an increased WBC count.
■ Monitor the following for signs of infection:	
• Redness, swelling; increased pain; purulent drainage from incisions, injury, and exit sites of tubes, drains, or catheters	Any suspicious drainage should be cultured; antibiotic therapy is determined by pathogens identified at culture.
• Elevated temperature	Temperature of up to 38° C (100.4° F) for 48 hours after surgery is related to surgical stress; after 48 hours, temperature greater than 37.7° C (99.8° F) suggests infection; fever spikes that occur and subside are indicative of wound infection; very high temperature accompanied by sweating and chills may indicate septicemia.
• Color of respiratory secretions	Yellow or yellow-green sputum is indicative of respiratory infection.
• Appearance of urine	Cloudy, foul-smelling urine with visible sediment is indicative of urinary tract or bladder infection.
■ Assess nutritional status, including weight, history of weight loss, and serum albumin.	Patients with poor nutritional status may be anergic or unable to muster a cellular immune response to pathogens and are therefore more susceptible to infection.
■ In pregnant patients, assess intactness of amniotic membranes.	Prolonged rupture of amniotic membranes before delivery places the mother and infant at increased risk for infection.
■ Assess for exposure to individuals with active infections.	This information provides warning for potential infection.
■ Assess for use of medications or treatment modalities that may cause immunosuppression.	Antineoplastic agents and corticosteroids reduce immunocompetence.
■ Assess immunization status.	Older patients and those not raised in the United States may not have completed immunizations and therefore may not have sufficient acquired active immunity.

Therapeutic Interventions

Actions/Interventions	Rationales
■ Maintain or teach asepsis for dressing changes and wound care, catheter care and handling, and peripheral IV and central venous access management.	Use of aseptic technique decreases the chances of transmitting or spreading pathogens to the patient. The CDC offers many guidelines for protecting patients from infections related to use of catheters.
■ Wash hands and teach other caregivers to wash hands before contact with patients and between procedures with the patient.	Friction and running water effectively remove microorganisms from hands. Washing between procedures reduces the risk of transmitting pathogens from one area of the body to another (e.g., perineal care or central line care). Alcohol-based hand sanitizers can be used between handwashing episodes if the hands are not visibly soiled. Use of disposable gloves does not reduce the need for hand washing. The CDC provides guidelines for hand hygiene in health care settings.

■ = Independent ▲ = Collaborative

Actions/Interventions	Rationales
■ Limit visitors.	Restricting visitation by individuals with any type of infection reduces the transmission of pathogens to the patient at risk for infection. The most common modes of transmission are by direct contact (touching) and by droplet (airborne).
■ Encourage intake of protein- and calorie-rich foods.	Optimal nutritional status supports immune system responsiveness.
■ Encourage fluid intake of 2000 to 3000 mL of water per day (unless contraindicated).	Fluids promote diluted urine and frequent emptying of bladder; reducing stasis of urine, in turn, reduces risk for bladder infection or urinary tract infection.
■ Encourage coughing and deep breathing; consider use of incentive spirometer.	These measures reduce stasis of secretions in the lungs and bronchial tree. When stasis occurs, pathogens can cause upper respiratory infections, including pneumonia.
▲ Administer or teach use of antimicrobial (antibiotic) drugs as ordered.	Antimicrobial drugs include antibacterial, antifungal, antiparasitic, and antiviral agents. All of these agents are either toxic to the pathogen or retard the pathogen's growth. Ideally, the selection of the drug is based on cultures from the infected area; this is often impossible or impractical, and in these cases, empirical management usually is undertaken with a broad-spectrum drug.
▲ Place the patient in protective isolation if he or she is at very high risk.	Protective isolation is established when WBC counts indicate neutropenia (less than 500 to 1000/mm³). Institutional protocols may vary. National guidelines, such as those published by the CDC, provide general recommendations.
■ Recommend the use of soft-bristled toothbrushes and stool softeners to protect mucous membranes.	Hard-bristled toothbrushes and constipation may compromise the integrity of the mucous membranes and provide a port of entry for pathogens.

Education/Continuity of Care

Actions/Interventions	Rationales
■ Teach the patient or caregiver to wash hands often, especially after toileting, before meals, and before and after administering self-care.	Patients and caregivers can spread infection from one part of the body to another, as well as pick up surface pathogens; hand washing reduces these risks.
■ Teach the patient the importance of avoiding contact with those who have infections or colds. Teach family members and caregivers about protecting susceptible patients from themselves and others with infections or colds.	Family members or others can spread infections or colds to a susceptible patient through direct contact, contaminated inanimate objects, or through air currents.
■ Teach the patient, family, and caregivers the purpose and proper technique for maintaining isolation.	Knowledge about isolation can help patients and family members cooperate with specific precautions.
■ Teach the patient to take antibiotics as prescribed.	Most antibiotics work best when a constant blood level is maintained; a constant blood level is maintained when medications are taken as prescribed. The absorption of some antibiotics is hindered by certain foods; patients should be instructed accordingly.
■ Instruct the patient to take the full course of antibiotics even if symptoms improve or disappear.	Not completing the entire course of the prescribed antibiotic regimen can lead to drug resistance in the pathogens and reactivation of symptoms.
■ Teach the patient and caregiver the signs and symptoms of infection, and when to report these to the physician or nurse.	Patients need to be able to recognize important signs and changes in their condition so early treatment can be initiated.

Actions/Interventions

- Demonstrate and allow return demonstration of all high-risk procedures that the patient or caregiver will do after discharge, such as dressing changes, peripheral or central IV site care, peritoneal dialysis, and self-catheterization (may use clean technique).

Rationales

Patient and caregivers need opportunities to master new skills to reduce risk for infection.

 Insomnia

Definition: A disruption in amount and quality of sleep that impairs functioning

Sleep is required to provide energy for physical and mental activities. The sleep-wake cycle is complex, consisting of different stages of consciousness: rapid eye movement (REM) sleep, non-REM sleep, and wakefulness. As persons age, the amount of time spent in REM sleep diminishes. The amount of sleep that individuals require varies with age and personal characteristics. Older patients sleep less during the night but may take more naps during the day to feel rested. Disruption in the individual's usual diurnal pattern of sleep and wakefulness may be temporary or chronic. Short-term insomnia may occur in response to changes in work schedules, temporary stressors, or travel across several time zones. Long-term insomnia is associated with alcohol and drug abuse, chronic pain, chronic depression, obesity, and aging. Such disruptions may result in both subjective distress and apparent impairment in functional abilities. Sleep patterns can be affected by environment, especially in hospital critical care units. These patients experience insomnia secondary to the noisy, bright environment and frequent monitoring and treatments. Such sleep disturbance is a significant stressor in the intensive care unit and can affect recovery.

Common Related Factors

Pain/discomfort
Environmental changes
Anxiety/fear
Depression
Medications
Excessive or inadequate stimulation
Abnormal physiological status or symptoms (e.g., dyspnea, hypoxia, or neurological dysfunction)
Normal changes associated with aging
Use of alcohol or stimulants

Defining Characteristics

Verbal complaints of difficulty falling asleep
Awakening earlier or later than desired
Interrupted sleep
Verbal complaints of not feeling rested
Lack of energy
Increased absenteeism from work or school
Decreased health status and quality of life
Difficulty concentrating
Dissatisfaction with sleep pattern

Common Expected Outcome

Patient achieves optimal amounts of sleep as evidenced by rested appearance, verbalization of feeling rested, and improvement in sleep pattern.

NOC Outcomes
Anxiety Self-Control; Sleep
NIC Intervention
Sleep Enhancement

■ = Independent   ▲ = Collaborative

Ongoing Assessment

Actions/Interventions	Rationales
■ Assess past patterns of sleep in normal environment: amount, bedtime rituals, depth, length, positions, aids, and interfering agents.	Sleep patterns are unique to each individual.
■ Assess the patient's perception of cause of sleep difficulty and possible relief measures to facilitate treatment.	For short-term problems, patients may have insight into the etiological factors of the problem (e.g., fear over results of a diagnostic test, concern over a daughter getting divorced, depression over the loss of a loved one). Knowing the specific etiological factor will guide appropriate therapy.
■ Document nursing or caregiver observations of sleeping and wakeful behaviors. Record number of sleep hours. Note physical (e.g., noise, pain or discomfort, urinary frequency) and/or psychological (e.g., fear, anxiety) circumstances that interrupt sleep.	Often the patient's perception of the problem may differ from objective evaluation.
■ Evaluate timing or effects of medications that can disrupt sleep.	In both the hospital and home care settings, patients may be following medication schedules that require awakening in the early morning hours. Attention to changes in the schedule or changes to once-a-day medication may solve the problem.

Therapeutic Interventions

Actions/Interventions	Rationales
■ Instruct the patient to follow as consistent a daily schedule for retiring and arising as possible.	Consistent schedules promote regulation of the circadian rhythm and reduce the energy required for adaptation to changes.
■ Instruct the patient to avoid heavy meals, alcohol, caffeine, or smoking before retiring.	Although hunger can also keep one awake, gastric digestion and stimulation from caffeine and nicotine can disturb sleep.
■ Instruct the patient to avoid large fluid intake before bedtime.	Evening fluid restriction helps the patient who otherwise may need to void during the night.
■ Increase daytime physical activities as indicated, but instruct the patient to avoid strenuous activity before bedtime.	Activity reduces stress and promotes sleep. However, overfatigue may cause insomnia.
■ Discourage pattern of daytime naps unless deemed necessary to meet sleep requirements or if part of one's usual pattern.	Napping can disrupt normal sleep patterns; however, older patients do better with frequent naps during the day to counter their shorter nighttime sleep schedules.
■ Suggest use of soporifics such as milk.	Milk contains L-tryptophan, which facilitates sleep.
■ Recommend an environment conducive to sleep or rest (e.g., quiet, comfortable temperature, ventilation, darkness, closed door). Suggest use of earplugs or eye shades as appropriate.	Many people sleep better in cool, dark, quiet environments.
■ Suggest engaging in a relaxing activity before retiring (e.g., warm bath, calm music, reading an enjoyable book, relaxation exercises).	These activities provide relaxation and distraction to prepare the body and mind for sleep.
■ Explain the need to avoid concentrating on the next day's activities or on one's problems at bedtime.	Planning a designated time during the next day to address these concerns may provide permission to "let go" of the worries at bedtime.
■ Encourage patients to journal or write down their problems or activities before going to sleep.	Journaling allows the patient to "put aside" the mental activities until the morning.
▲ Suggest using hypnotics or sedatives as ordered; evaluate effectiveness.	Because of their potential for cumulative effects and generally limited period of benefit, use of hypnotic medications should be thoughtfully considered and avoided if less aggressive means are effective. Different drugs are prescribed depending on whether the patient has trouble falling asleep or staying asleep. Medications that suppress REM sleep should be avoided.

Actions/Interventions	Rationales
■ If unable to fall asleep after about 30 to 45 minutes, suggest getting out of bed and engaging in a relaxing activity.	The bed should not be associated with wakefulness, TV watching, or work.
For patients who are hospitalized:	
■ Provide nursing aids (e.g., back rub, bedtime care, pain relief, comfortable position, relaxation techniques).	These aids promote rest.
■ Eliminate nonessential nursing activities.	This approach promotes minimal interruption in sleep or rest.
■ Attempt to allow for sleep cycles of at least 90 minutes.	Research studies indicate that 60 to 90 minutes are needed to complete one sleep cycle and that the completion of an entire cycle is necessary to benefit from sleep.
■ Move the patient to a room farther from the nursing station if noise is a contributing factor.	The nursing station is often the center of noise and activity.
■ Post a "Do not disturb" sign on the door.	It is important to alert people to avoid entering the room and interrupting sleep.

Education/Continuity of Care

Actions/Interventions	Rationales
■ Teach about possible causes of sleeping difficulties and optimal ways to treat them.	Considerable confusion and myths about sleep exist. Knowledge of its role in health and wellness and the wide variation among individuals may allay anxiety, thereby promoting rest and sleep.
■ Instruct in nonpharmacological sleep-enhancement techniques.	Nonpharmacological sleep-enhancement techniques can be used throughout a lifetime. Pharmacological sleep agents should only be used for a limited time.

Decreased Intracranial Adaptive Capacity

Definition: Intracranial fluid dynamic mechanisms that normally compensate for increases in intracranial volumes are compromised, resulting in repeated disproportionate increases in intracranial pressure in response to a variety of noxious and non-noxious stimuli

Intracranial pressure (ICP) reflects the pressure exerted by the intracranial components of blood, brain, and cerebrospinal fluid (CSF), each ordinarily remaining at a constant volume within the rigid skull structure. Any additional fluid or mass (e.g., subdural hematoma, tumor, or abscess) increases the pressure within the cranial vault. Because the total volume cannot change (Monro-Kellie doctrine), blood, CSF, and ultimately brain tissue are forced out of the vault. The normal range of ICP is up to 15 mm Hg; elevations above that level occur normally but readily return to baseline parameters as a result of the adaptive capacity or compensatory mechanisms of the brain and body, such as vasoconstriction and increased venous outflow. In the event of disease, trauma, or a pathological condition, a disturbance in autoregulation occurs, and ICP is increased and sustained. Exceptions include persons with unfused skull fractures (the skull is no longer rigid at the fracture site), infants whose suture lines are not yet fused (this is normal to accommodate growth), and older patients whose brain tissues have shrunk, taking up less volume in the skull (allowing for abnormal tissue growth or intracranial bleeding to occur for a longer period before symptoms appear).

■ = Independent   ▲ = Collaborative

Common Related Factors

Hydrocephalus
Increased cerebral blood flow (CBF), hypercapnia, hyperemia
Injury with cerebral edema
Intracranial mass
Systemic hypotension

Common Expected Outcome

Patient maintains optimal cerebral tissue perfusion, as evidenced by ICP less than 10 mm Hg, GCS greater than 13, and cerebral perfusion pressure (CPP) from 60 to 90 mm Hg.

Defining Characteristics

Repeated increases in ICP greater than 10 mm Hg for more than 5 minutes
Elevated ICP waveforms
Baseline ICP greater than 10 mm Hg
Wide amplitude ICP waveform
Volume pressure response test variation

NOC Outcomes

Neurological Status: Consciousness; Medication Response; Knowledge: Disease Process; Fluid Balance

NIC Interventions

ICP Monitoring; Neurological Monitoring; Cerebral Edema Management; Teaching: Disease Process; Medication Administration: Parenteral

Ongoing Assessment

Actions/Interventions	Rationales
■ Assess neurological status as follows: level of consciousness (LOC) according to Glasgow Coma Scale (GCS)—pupil size, symmetry, and reaction to light; extraocular movement; gaze preference; speech and thought processes; memory; motor sensory signs and drift; increased tone; increased reflexes; Babinski reflex.	Deteriorating neurological signs indicate increased cerebral ischemia. A decreased LOC is the first sign of increased ICP.
■ Evaluate presence or absence of protective reflexes (e.g., swallowing, gagging, blinking, and coughing).	Loss of protective reflexes increases the person's risk for injuries such as aspiration or corneal abrasions.
■ Monitor vital signs.	Continually increasing ICP results in life-threatening hemodynamic changes; early recognition is essential to survival.
▲ Monitor arterial blood gases and/or pulse oximetry (recommended parameters: Pao_2 greater than 80 mm Hg and $Paco_2$ less than 35 mm Hg with normal ICP). If the patient's lungs are being hyperventilated to decrease ICP, $Paco_2$ should be between 25 and 30 mm Hg.	A $Paco_2$ less than 20 mm Hg may decrease CBF because of profound vasoconstriction that produces hypoxia. $Paco_2$ greater than 45 mm Hg induces vasodilation with increase in CBF, which may trigger increase in ICP.
■ Monitor input and output with urine-specific gravity. Report urine-specific gravity greater than 1.025 or urine output less than 30 mL/hr.	Monitoring may indicate decreased renal perfusion and possible associated decrease in CPP.
■ Calculate CPP by subtracting ICP from the mean arterial pressure (MAP): $$CPP = MAP - ICP$$ Determine MAP using the following formula: $$\frac{Systolic\ BP - Diastolic\ BP}{3} + Diastolic\ BP$$	Pressure should be approximately 90 to 100 mm Hg and not less than 50 mm Hg to ensure blood flow to brain.
▲ Monitor serum electrolytes, blood urea nitrogen, creatinine, glucose, osmolality, hemoglobin, and hematocrit, as indicated.	These detect treatment complications such as hypovolemia.
▲ Monitor ICP closely when treatment is being tapered.	ICP may increase as treatment is tapered.

Actions/Interventions

▲ Monitor ICP if measurement device is in place. Report ICP greater than 15 mm Hg for 5 minutes. Serially monitor ICP pressure and waveforms. Types of ICP waveforms include the following:

- Lundberg A waves (plateau waves) are increased ICP greater than 50 mm Hg sustained for more than 5 minutes.
- B waves are increased ICP, usually 20 to 40 mm Hg, and may precede an A wave.
- C waves are nonpathological and often correlate with heart rate and respiratory rate.

Rationales

Sustained ICP greater than 15 mm Hg causes transtentorial herniation and brain stem compression/herniation with resultant compression of the respiratory center, apnea, and cardiac arrest. Presence of A and B waves indicates neurological deterioration; the physician should be immediately informed.

These waves indicate a neurological emergency necessitating immediate intervention to avoid brain damage.

These waves can be seen with changes in respiratory pattern and must be watched as a possible prelude to A waves.

These waves are typically less than 20 mm Hg and occur every 4 to 8 minutes.

Therapeutic Interventions

Actions/Interventions

■ Elevate head of bed 30 degrees, and keep head in neutral alignment.

■ Avoid Valsalva maneuver.

■ If ICP is elevated to 12 to 15 mm Hg, reduce nursing and medical procedures to those absolutely necessary.

▲ Maintain normothermia with antipyretics, antibiotics, and cooling blanket.

▲ If ICP increases and fails to respond to repositioning of head in neutral alignment and head elevation, recheck equipment. If ICP is increased, one or more of the following may be prescribed by the physician:
- Hyperventilate the patient.

- Administer mannitol over 30 to 60 minutes.

- Administer barbiturates as needed.

- If the patient is intubated, administer a neuromuscular blocking agent.

- Administer a short-acting pain reliever (e.g., morphine, meperidine [Demerol], or midazolam [Versed]) before painful stimulation or stress-related care such as suctioning or IV line changes.

Rationales

Elevation promotes venous outflow. Exceptions include shock and cervical spine injuries. A neutral head position prevents venous obstruction.

Valsalva increases intrathoracic pressure and CBF, thereby increasing ICP.

Both prescribed and unnecessary procedures can serve as a noxious stimulus that can further increase ICP.

Fever increases cerebral metabolic demand; fever may increase CBF and ICP.

Hyperventilation can decrease $Paco_2$ to between 25 and 30 mm Hg and induce vasoconstriction and a decrease in CBF and ICP. Hyperventilation is often reserved for brain-injured patients exhibiting signs of herniation.

Mannitol is a hyperosmotic agent that should be used carefully because it can induce cerebral ischemia. It is contraindicated with hypovolemic symptoms. A diuretic response can be anticipated within 30 to 60 minutes. A Foley catheter should be in place. An intravenous (IV) filter should be used when mannitol is infused. Electrolytes, osmolality, and serum glucose must be monitored during mannitol infusion.

Barbiturates reduce cerebral metabolism and reduce cerebral oxygen demand and lower ICP.

Neuromuscular blockers reduce shivering, coughing, bucking, and Valsalva maneuver. However, neuromuscular blocking agents have no effect on cerebration; therefore the patient should receive short-acting sedation before noxious stimulation.

Pain and agitated body movements cause further increases in ICP.

■ = Independent   ▲ = Collaborative

Actions/Interventions

▲ Drain CSF at ordered rate and amount.

Rationales

Removal of a small amount of CSF can significantly lower ICP. This can be accomplished intermittently or, as in patients with hydrocephalus, continuously.

Education/Continuity of Care

Actions/Interventions

- Teach patient and family about causes, treatment, and expected outcome.
- Reinforce discussions related to treatment (e.g., head of bed elevated, medication).
- Offer the family frequent feedback regarding the patient's status.
- Encourage family presence and participation in comfort measures.
- Provide social service, community, and/or support group information as appropriate to the primary diagnosis.

Rationales

Knowledge about increased ICP can calm anxieties about this condition.

Patient and family will be able to cooperate with care when they understand the purpose of specific interventions.

This approach will ease anxiety of family members.

This occasionally calms the patient and decreases ICP.

The primary diagnosis (e.g., a resolving head trauma versus repeated stroke) necessitates different levels of postdischarge care needs.

Deficient Knowledge

Definition: Absence or deficiency of cognitive information related to specific topic

Knowledge deficit is a lack of cognitive information or psychomotor skills required for health recovery, maintenance, or health promotion. Teaching may take place in a hospital, ambulatory care, or home setting. The learner may be the patient, a family member, a significant other, or a caregiver unrelated to the patient. Learning may involve any of the three domains: cognitive domain (intellectual activities, problem solving, and others); affective domain (feelings, attitudes, belief); and psychomotor domain (physical skills or procedures). The nurse must decide with the learner what to teach, when to teach, and how to teach the mutually agreed-upon content. Adult learning principles guide the teaching-learning process. Information should be made available when the patient wants and needs it, at the pace the patient determines, and using the teaching strategy the patient deems most effective. Many factors influence patient education, including age, cognitive level, developmental stage, physical limitations (e.g., visual, hearing, balance, hand coordination, strength), the primary disease process and comorbidities, and sociocultural factors. Older patients need more time for teaching and may have sensory-perceptual deficits and/or cognitive changes that may require a modification in teaching techniques. Certain ethnic and religious groups hold unique beliefs and health practices that must be considered when designing a teaching plan. These practices may vary from home remedies (e.g., special soups, poultices) and alternative therapies (e.g., massage, biofeedback, energy healing, macrobiotics, or megavitamins in place of prescribed medications) to reliance on an elder in the family to coordinate the care plan. Patients with low literacy skills will require educational programs that include more simplified treatment regimens, simplified teaching tools (e.g., cartoons, lower readability levels), a slower presentation pace, and techniques for cueing patients to initiate certain behaviors (e.g., pill schedule posted on refrigerator, timer for taking medications). The National Patient Safety Foundation has identified the pervasivenes of low health literacy and its implications for poorer health outcomes. It has launched the *Ask Me 3* initiative to improve health communication between patients and providers.

Although the acute hospital setting provides challenges for patient education because of the high acuity and emotional stress inherent in this environment, the home setting can be similarly challenging because of the high expectations for patients or caregivers to self-manage complex procedures such as intravenous therapy, dialysis, or even ventilator care in the home. Caregivers are often overwhelmed by the responsibility delegated to them by the health care professionals. Many have their own health problems and may be unable to perform all the behaviors assigned to them because of visual limitations, generalized weakness, or feelings of inadequacy or exhaustion.

This care plan describes adult learning principles that can be incorporated into a teaching plan for use in any health care setting.

Common Related Factors

New condition, procedure, treatment
Complexity of treatment
Cognitive/physical limitation
Misinterpretation of information
Decreased motivation to learn
Emotional state affecting learning (anxiety, denial, or depression)
Unfamiliarity with information resources
Lack of recall

Defining Characteristics

Verbalizing inaccurate information
Inaccurate follow-through of instruction
Questioning members of health care team
Incorrect task performance
Expressing frustration or confusion when performing task

Common Expected Outcomes

Patient demonstrates motivation to learn.
Patient identifies perceived learning needs.
Patient verbalizes understanding of desired content and/or performs desired skill.

NOC Outcomes
Knowledge (Specify Type); Information Processing
NIC Interventions
Learning Facilitation; Teaching: Individual

Ongoing Assessment

Actions/Interventions	**Rationales**
■ Determine who will be the learner: the patient, family, significant other, or caregiver.	Many older or terminal patients may view themselves as dependent on their caregiver and therefore will not want to be part of the educational process.
■ Assess motivation and willingness of the patient and caregivers to learn.	Adults must see a need or purpose for learning. Some patients are ready to learn soon after they are diagnosed; others cope better by denying or delaying the need for instruction. Learning also requires energy, which patients may not be ready to use. Patients also have a right to refuse educational services.
■ Assess ability to learn, remember, or perform desired health-related care.	Cognitive impairments need to be identified so an appropriate teaching plan can be designed. For example, the Mini-Mental State Examination can be used to identify memory problems that would interfere with learning. Physical limitations such as impaired hearing or vision, or poor hand coordination can likewise compromise learning and must be considered when designing the educational approach. Patients with decreased lens accommodation may require bolder, larger fonts or magnifying lenses for written material.

■ = Independent   ▲ = Collaborative

Nursing Diagnosis Care Plans

Actions/Interventions

- Identify priority of learning needs within the overall care plan.

- Question the patient regarding previous experience and health teaching.

- Identify any existing misconceptions regarding material to be taught.
- Determine cultural influences on health teaching.

- Determine the patient's learning style, especially if the patient has learned and retained new information in the past.

- Determine the patient's or caregiver's self-efficacy to learn and apply new knowledge.

Rationales

This information provides the starting base for educational sessions. Teaching standardized content that the patient already knows wastes valuable time and hinders critical learning. Adults learn material that is important to them. During the acute stages, the family or significant others may require the most teaching.

Adults bring many life experiences to each learning session. Adults learn best when teaching builds on previous knowledge or experience. This experience is the foundation for an individualized teaching plan.

Assessment provides an important starting point in education. Knowledge serves to correct faulty ideas.

To be effective, interventions need to be specific to the patient and address individual differences. Providing a climate of acceptance allows patients to be themselves and to hold their own beliefs as appropriate. Language problems can pose significant barriers to learning.

Each patient has his or her own learning style, which must be considered when designing a teaching program. Some persons may prefer written over visual materials, or they may prefer group versus individual instruction. Matching the learner's preferred style with the educational method will facilitate success in mastery of knowledge.

Self-efficacy refers to a person's confidence in his or her ability to perform a behavior. A first step in teaching may be to foster increased self-efficacy in the learner's ability to learn the desired information or skills. Some lifestyle changes can be difficult to make.

Therapeutic Interventions

Actions/Interventions

- Provide physical comfort for the learner.

- Provide a quiet atmosphere without interruption.

- Provide an atmosphere of respect, openness, trust, and collaboration.

- Involve the patient in developing the teaching plan, beginning with establishing objectives and goals for learning at the beginning of the session.
- Allow the learner to identify what is most important to him or her.

Rationales

According to Maslow's theory, basic physiological needs must be addressed before patient education. Ensuring physical comfort allows the patient to concentrate on what is being discussed or demonstrated.

A calm quiet environment assists the patient with concentrating more completely.

Conveying respect is especially important when providing education to patients with different values and beliefs about health and illness.

Goal setting allows the learner to know what will be discussed and expected during the session. Adults tend to focus on here-and-now, problem-centered education.

Adult learning is problem oriented. Priority setting is key. Allowing the patient to determine the most significant content to be presented first is most effective (i.e., what the patient needs to know now versus later). Patients may want to focus only on self-care techniques that facilitate discharge from the hospital or enhance survival at home (e.g., how to take medications, emergency side effects, suctioning a tracheal tube) and are less interested in specifics of the disease process. The *Ask Me 3* program for health literacy stresses the importance of focusing on three questions: What is my main problem? What do I need to do? Why is it important for me to do this?

Actions/Interventions	**Rationales**
■ Explore attitudes and feelings about changes.	Assessment assists the nurse in understanding how the learner may respond to the information and possibly how successful the patient may be with the expected changes.
■ Allow for and support self-directed, self-designed learning.	Adults learn when they feel they are personally involved in the learning process. Patients know what difficulties will be encountered in their own environments, and they must be encouraged to approach learning activities from their priority needs.
■ Assist the learner in integrating information into daily life.	This technique helps the learner make adjustments in daily life that will result in the desired change in behavior (or learning).
■ Allow adequate time for integration that is in direct conflict with existing values or beliefs.	Information that is in direct conflict with what is already held to be true forces a reevaluation of the old material and is thus integrated more slowly.
■ Give clear, thorough explanations and demonstrations.	Patients are better able to ask questions when they have basic information about what to expect. Accurate, clear information provides rationale for treatment and aids the patient in assuming responsibility for care at a later time.
■ Provide information using various media (e.g., explanations, discussions, demonstrations, pictures, written instructions, computer-assisted programs, and videotapes).	Different people take in information in different ways. Match the learning style with the educational approach.
■ Ensure that required supplies and equipment are available so that the environment is conducive to learning.	Adequate preparation is especially important when teaching in the home setting.
■ When presenting material, move from familiar, simple, and concrete information to less familiar, complex, or more abstract concepts.	This technique provides the patient with the opportunity to understand new material in relation to familiar material.
■ Focus teaching sessions on a single concept or idea.	Clearly focused teaching allows the learner to concentrate more completely on material being discussed. Highly anxious and older patients have reduced short-term memory and benefit from mastery of one concept at a time.
■ Pace the instruction and keep sessions short.	Learning requires energy, so shorter, well-paced sessions reduce fatigue.
■ Encourage questions.	Questions facilitate open communication between patient and health care professionals, and allow verification of understanding of given information and the opportunity to correct misconceptions. Learners often feel shy or embarrassed about asking questions and often want permission to ask them. Patients must have correct information to make valid choices.
■ Allow learner to practice new skills; provide immediate feedback on performance.	Assisting allows the patient to use new information immediately and enhances retention. Immediate feedback allows the learner to make corrections rather than practicing the skill incorrectly.
■ Encourage repetition of information or new skill.	Repeated practice by the patient will help him or her gain confidence in self-care ability.
■ Provide positive, constructive reinforcement of learning. Incorporate rewards into the learning process.	A positive approach allows the learner to feel good about learning accomplishments, gain confidence, and maintain self-esteem while correcting mistakes. Rewards help to make learning fun.
■ Document progress of teaching and learning.	Documentation allows additional teaching to be based on what the learner has completed, thus enhancing the learner's self-efficacy and encouraging the most cost-effective teaching.

■ = Independent ▲ = Collaborative

Education/Continuity of Care

Actions/Interventions	Rationales
■ Provide instruction for specific topics.	Patients must have correct information to make informed choices in their treatment, to identify when therapy adjustments are needed, and to recognize important changes in their condition that could lead to serious outcomes. Long-term care will be the patient's responsibility.
▲ Refer the patient to community resources or support groups, as needed.	Patients may be unaware of services available for questions or problem solving. These resources allow the patient to interact with others who have similar problems, learning needs, or specialty resources.
■ Include significant others whenever possible.	One's partner usually assumes a crucial supportive role when the patient is gathering information and initiating new treatments.

NANDA-I NDx Sedentary Lifestyle

Definition: Reports a habit of life that is characterized by a low physical activity level

Today's social changes have shifted lifestyles of once high physical effort to more sedentary ways of life, making physical inactivity a national problem. Unfortunately, many individuals do not actively seek out regular exercise routines, with more than 60% of Americans not exercising on a regular basis and 25% not exercising at all. The following table uses number of steps walked per day as a way to quantify levels of physical activity.

Sedentary lifestyle	<5000 steps per day
Low active	5000-7499 steps per day
Somewhat active	7500-9999 steps per day
Active	10,000-12,500 steps per day
Highly active	>12,500 steps per day

From Tudor-Locke C, Bassett DR: How many steps/day are enough? Preliminary pedometer indices for public health, *Sports Med* 34(1):1, 2004.

Lack of physical activity can lead to many chronic conditions, including diabetes, heart disease, obesity, and various cancers. The *2008 Physical Activity Guidelines for Americans* provides a science-based prescription for assisting individuals with improving their health through regular physical activity. Based on the Aerobics Center Longitudinal Study, recommendations include both aerobic and muscle-strengthening activities in the following doses: at least 150 minutes a week of moderate aerobic physical activity to obtain general health benefits and muscle-strengthening activities using major muscle groups on 2 or more days of the week. Additional health benefits can be achieved in a dose-response fashion, either by increasing the intensity to vigorous activity or by increasing the duration of moderate activity to 300 min/wk. Health benefits can be achieved in intermittent episodes of even 10 minutes of moderate physical activity. Health benefits are attainable by individuals of all ages and even those with chronic medical problems. Stressful and busy lifestyles, socioeconomic factors, physical constraints, and lack of motivation are all barriers that can contribute to low physical activity. Nursing objectives are to educate patients on the importance of adopting an active lifestyle and to assist patients in finding ways to personalize the recommended exercise prescription.

Common Related Factors

Deficient knowledge of health benefits of physical exercise
Lack of interest
Lack of motivation
Lack of resources (time, money, companionship, facilities)
Lack of training for accomplishment of physical exercise

Common Expected Outcomes

Patient verbalizes accurate information about benefits of increasing physical activity and strategies to develop a personal program of increased lifestyle activity.
Patient engages in a tailored aerobic physical activity routine that includes at least 150 minutes of moderate-intensity exercise per week.
Patient performs muscle-strengthening exercise on at least 2 days a week.

Defining Characteristics

Chooses a daily routine lacking physical exercise
Demonstrates physical deconditioning
Verbalizes preference for activities low in physical activity

NOC Outcomes
Knowledge: Prescribed activity; Physical fitness
NIC Interventions
Exercise Promotion; Exercise Promotion: Strength Training; Teaching: Prescribed Activity/Exercise

Ongoing Assessment

Actions/Interventions

■ Assess patient's current level of physical activity, including both lifestyle activity and structured exercise.
■ Assess the patient's past experiences with structured physical activity.

■ Assess patient's views on physical activity by asking questions, including the following: How do you feel about physical activity or exercise? Do you find exercise important to your health?
■ Assess patient's readiness to initiate a physical activity regimen by asking questions such as the following: How do you feel about starting an exercise routine? Are you ready to choose a time to start being more active?

■ Assess patient's confidence in his or her ability to increase physical activity using a scale of 0 to 10.

■ Assess the patient's level of mobility and physical status before prescribing an activity plan.

Rationales

This assessment provides a basis for increasing activity. Some physical activity is always better than none.
Adults bring many life experiences to learning sessions. Many patients have had positive experiences in the past that can serve as a base to build on. Similarly, often patients have previously tried unsuccessfully to become more active. Reasons for difficulties need to be explored.
Insight into the patient's priorities and values regarding physical activity will provide a basis for developing a physical activity program. Patients learn material and engage in activities most important to them.
The Transtheoretical Model emphasizes that interventions for change should be matched with the stage of change at which patients are situated. For example, if the patient is only contemplating starting an exercise program, efforts may be directed toward emphasizing the health benefits of exercise, whereas if the patient is in the preparation or action stages, more specific directions regarding exercise (e.g., walking is a great way to start, moderate versus vigorous activity, places to exercise) can be addressed.
If patients have strong self-efficacy, they are more likely to welcome the challenge and begin to initiate an exercise program, whereas patients with low self-efficacy tend to shy away from the challenges of making a change.
Many sedentary patients will have evidence of deconditioning. A baseline assessment of physical status will allow the nurse to safely initiate an exercise regimen specific to patient needs and abilities. Screening tools such as the Physical Activity Readiness Questionnaire (PAR-Q) provide guidance as to when a medical examination may be required before initiating a program. Older adults with chronic conditions may need personalized assessments.

■ = Independent　▲ = Collaborative

Actions/Interventions

■ Assess possible barriers to increasing physical activity, such as lack of motivation, interpersonal support, skills, knowledge, or resources.

■ Monitor patient's responses to new exercise routine, such as frequency of participation, length of each session, and any pain or discomfort experienced afterward.

Rationales

If the patient is aware of possible barriers and has formulated plans for dealing with them, then successful change is more likely to occur. For example, when trying to engage in a walking program, walking in a shopping mall can be substituted for outdoor activity during periods of inclement weather.

This will provide information on patient's progress and identify emotional or physical successes or setbacks.

Therapeutic Interventions

Actions/Interventions

■ Guide the patient in setting realistic short- and long-term goals for increasing physical activity.

■ Discuss ways to incorporate exercise into one's daily life by suggesting parking further away from the store, taking the stairs not the elevator, and taking walks during lunch breaks.

■ Explain to the patient how to make sedentary activities more active (e.g., pacing or walking while on the telephone, stretching while watching television, dancing while listening to favorite music).

■ Suggest purposeful physical activities.

■ For patients with decreased mobility or chronic conditions such as arthritis and chronic obstructive pulmonary disease, stress the importance of starting slow and gradually increasing activity.

■ Introduce the use of a pedometer/step counter to track steps per day. Determine the number of steps needed to accomplish at least a 10-minute walk.

Rationales

Adults have many options for increasing their current level of activity. Setting realistic achievable goals helps to maintain motivation and eventual success of the exercise regimen. Walking is a great way to get physically active. Some patients may start with simply walking for 10 minutes a day, whereas others may be ready to commit to 30 minutes. Patients may need assistance in selecting safer activities that are appropriate to their current fitness level.

Lifestyle activities are an easy starting point. Even brief episodes of activity, as little as 10 minutes each, can add up to the 150 minutes of recommended exercise per week.

Exercise can easily be incorporated into many sedentary activities and may get patients in the habit of choosing active behaviors. Some activity is always better than none.

Patients are more likely to begin and maintain activities when they perceive that the activity is beneficial and has a purpose. For example, patients may select an exercise class for the socialization, not just for the exercise, or they may focus more on lifestyle activities carried out during the course of a day, such as walking the dog, using a bathroom on another floor, or getting off a bus one stop earlier. The best activity is the one that the patient enjoys and will continue to do.

Too much exercise initially can cause injury or exacerbation of symptoms and discourage patients from continuing the exercise routine. Patients with chronic medical conditions should increase their physical activity under the supervision of their health care professional.

Pedometers can be a useful tool to quantify activity level as well as provide tangible goals. A key to successful use is to focus on number of steps walked per 10 minutes, with the idea of moving toward the 150 min/wk goal. Persons with low fitness levels tend to walk slower, so they will complete fewer steps in 10 minutes than someone with a higher fitness level. However, each person will have his or her own goal to work toward.

Actions/Interventions

■ Clarify for the patient the *2008 Physical Activity Guidelines for Americans* (adults and older adults), including aerobic and muscle-strengthening activities, and their associated health benefits:

- Adults should do 2 hours and 30 minutes (150 minutes) a week of moderate-intensity, or 1 hour and 15 minutes (75 minutes) a week of vigorous-intensity aerobic physical activity, or an equivalent combination of moderate and vigorous physical activity. Greater health benefits are derived from greater amounts of exercise.
- Examples of moderate intensity exercises include walking briskly at 3 to 4 mph, bicycling slower than 10 mph, doubles tennis, ballroom dancing.
- Examples of vigorous intensity exercises include jogging, race-walking, running, singles tennis, lap swimming, aerobic dancing, jumping rope.
- Aerobic activities should be completed in increments of at least 10 minutes, spread throughout the week.
- Adults should also engage in muscle-strengthening exercises involving major muscle groups on at least 2 days a week for additional health benefits.
- Examples of muscle-strengthening exercises include resistance training, lifting weights, using resistance bands, doing push-ups, pull-ups, sit-ups, heavy gardening, and carrying heavy loads.

■ Introduce an activity calendar, so patients can monitor their physical activity on a daily basis.

■ Suggest the patient find an activity/exercise partner.

■ Provide emotional support while increasing activity.

■ Assist in developing a time frame for achievement of the goals.

Rationales

Adults have many ways to reach their activity goals. Beyond simply increasing lifestyle activity, patients can work toward the goal of meeting the national guidelines that include both aerobic (endurance) and muscle-strengthening (resistance) exercises which convey health benefits. Patients need to have accurate information and guidance on how to achieve these goals (if feasible).

Such tracking devices serve as a visual reminder of exercise achievement as well as a self-monitoring technique.

Recruiting a support person to share in the activity can increase motivation and compliance with the regimen.

Patients may be fearful of starting an exercise regimen. Ongoing support and coaching can encourage compliance and enjoyment of physical activity.

Depending on ones' starting point, previously inactive people need to "start low and go slow" by gradually increasing the amount of activity they do. Maintaining an active lifestyle is a lifetime goal, thus starting too fast may not result in the best outcome.

Education/Continuity of Care

Actions/Interventions

■ Provide ongoing education about the benefits of physical activity to both patient and significant others.

■ Instruct patients in ways to avoid injury with exercise (e.g., starting out slowly if previously inactive, selecting the types and amount of exercise appropriate for their fitness and health status, increasing duration before intensity of activity, choosing a safe place to do the activity, and reporting any signs of overexertion or health problems to their health care professional).

■ Provide education on the use of technology to promote exercise goals, such as Internet sites for monitoring of physical activity or chat rooms to discuss exercise efforts.

Rationales

Patients and families need information on the many health benefits of exercise and the potential health risks of being sedentary. This will need to be reinforced over time.

Initiating a moderate-level of physical activity is safe for most people. However, for anyone not previously active, activity-induced injuries are possible and the patient should be informed about how best to avoid such problems.

Many Internet-based services are available to disseminate information about safe and appropriate activities and to provide a way to correspond with other patients or with the nurse about the person's progress or setbacks.

■ = Independent ▲ = Collaborative

Actions/Interventions

- Refer patients to community resources such as the YMCA, park districts, or other community activity centers.
- Teach patients to reward themselves for accomplishment of short-term and long-term goals.
- Prepare patients to anticipate setbacks in their exercise regimen.

Rationales

Patients may not be aware of resources that can be a basis of support and success.

Rewards are motivational and can give a sense of satisfaction for a job well done.

A lifetime of physical activity is difficult to maintain. Preparing and planning for setbacks will equip patients to positively cope with each challenging situation.

Related Care Plan

Activity intolerance, p. 8

NANDA-I NDx Impaired Memory

Definition: Inability to remember or recall bits of information or behavioral skills

Memory is the result of a complicated cognitive process used by an individual for learning, storing, and retrieving information. Cognitive abilities for reasoning, problem solving, interpreting information, and communication are dependent on the diverse and complex neural network that supports information processing. Structurally, memories are formed by the complex interactions of the hippocampus, thalamus, hypothalamus, and temporal lobes. Any change that disrupts these neural networks may result in problems with transferring information between immediate, short-term, and long-term memory. Amnesia is the complete loss of memory ability. This type of memory impairment represents an inability to recall previously learned information and an inability to learn new information. Memory impairment may be temporary or permanent. Situations that are associated with impaired memory include seizures, head trauma, strokes, cerebral infections, brain tumors, vitamin B1 deficiency with alcohol abuse, personality disorders, and progressive degenerative dementias. Changes in recent memory often occur with organic disorders such as delirium, dementia, or chronic alcohol abuse. Diminished long-term or remote memory is associated with damage to the area of the cerebral cortex used for storage of that memory. This type of memory loss is seen in Alzheimer's disease. Posttraumatic amnesia is an indicator of the severity of a closed head injury. Slowing of information processing and impaired episodic memory are common problems with head trauma.

Common Related Factors

Fluid and electrolyte imbalance
Neurological disturbances
Excessive environmental disturbances
Anemia
Acute or chronic hypoxia
Decreased cardiac output
Medications

Defining Characteristics

Inability to recall factual information
Inability to recall recent or past events
Inability to perform a previously learned skill
Inability to learn or retain new skills or information
Inability to determine if a behavior was performed
Observed or reported experience of forgetting
Forgets to perform a behavior at a scheduled time

Common Expected Outcomes

Patient is able to recall immediate, recent, and remote information accurately within limits of disease.

Patient is able to maintain attention and respond appropriately to environmental cues within limits of disease.

Patient is oriented to time, person, place, and self within limits of disease.

Patient uses techniques to promote retention and recall of information.

NOC Outcomes
Memory; Cognitive Orientation; Concentration

NIC Interventions
Memory Training; Reality Orientation

Ongoing Assessment

Actions/Interventions	Rationales

■ Assess neurological function with special attention to the mental status portion of the examination (e.g., Mini-Mental State Examination [MMSE])
  • Orientation to time. What is the year, season, month, day, and date?
  • Orientation to place. Where are we now (state, city, and building)?
  • Registration and recall of three words
  • Serial 7's subtraction
  • Naming familiar objects
  • Repetition of a phrase
  • Following a two-step direction
  • Reading
  • Writing a sentence
  • Copying a figure
	Memory is associated with cognitive information processing. Changes in memory will be most evident during the mental status examination of the patient.
	The MMSE is a simplified scoring tool for assessing changes in cognitive function. The tool will provide information about immediate, recent, and long-term memory function. The MMSE can help differentiate memory loss as an isolated problem from delirium or dementia. Modifications in the MMSE may be made based on the patient's heritage.

■ Assess the patient's use of alcohol.	Excessive and long-term alcohol use is associated with development of Korsakoff's syndrome and memory loss.
■ Assess the patient's use of prescription medications, over-the-counter medications, and herbal supplements. Ask about use of illegal drugs.	Memory loss may be a drug side effect or a sign of drug interactions. Benzodiazepines, H_2- histamine antagonists, β-blockers, digoxin, and glucocorticosteroids may contribute to decreases in both short-term and long-term memory function. Illegal drugs, such as marijuana, cocaine, and ecstasy, produce impaired memory as a side effect.
■ Assess the patient's nutritional status and dietary intake.	A persistent elevation of blood glucose is associated with decline in memory. Long-term nutritional deficiencies, especially vitamin deficiencies, contribute to memory loss.
■ Assess for behavioral changes such as anxiety, combativeness, or withdrawal.	The patient with memory loss and diminished orientation may exhibit restlessness, anxiety, agitation, aggressiveness, and combativeness. Depression may contribute to impaired memory, especially in the older adult.
■ Include family members and caregivers in the assessment of the patient.	Patients with impaired memory may not be able to provide detailed information about their past history or health status.
■ Assess the impact of memory loss on the patient and family members. Give special attention to assessing safety issues in the patient's living situation.	Memory loss can limit the patient's day-to-day functioning. The patient may be unable to effectively manage family and occupational responsibilities. The patient's safety may be impaired because memory loss interferes with other cognitive abilities to problem solve and make judgments. Patients may forget to turn off stoves or water faucets. Family members may experience increased frustration and stress as they cope with the patient's memory loss and safety concerns.

■ = Independent　▲ = Collaborative

Actions/Interventions	Rationales
■ Assess quality of sleep.	Normal sleep plays a role in the consolidation of memories. Inadequate sleep can limit cognitive functions such as formation of memories and new learning.
▲ Refer the patient for diagnostic testing.	Neurological and laboratory testing are indicated to rule out problems that may account for memory loss. Blood tests provide information on electrolyte imbalances or anemia. Hemodynamic assessments provide information on oxygen saturation and cardiac output. Diagnostic testing may include computed tomography scan, magnetic resonance imaging, lumbar puncture, and electroencephalogram. Psychoneurological evaluation by a trained specialist is important to arrive at a diagnosis of conditions such as Alzheimer's disease.

Therapeutic Interventions

Actions/Interventions	Rationales
■ Provide reality orientation for the patient at every contact. For example, address the patient by name, introduce yourself, and review the day, time, location, and activity being completed.	The patient with impaired memory will have difficulty maintaining orientation to the immediate environment. Reality orientation helps the patient remain mentally integrated with the immediate environment. Misinterpretations by the patient can be clarified immediately.
■ Provide a low-stimulation environment.	Excessive auditory and visual stimulation can add to disorientation and confusion. The patient needs a setting with limited distractions to enhance accurate information processing.
■ Ask the patient about recent events.	Review of events in response to questions assists the patient in encoding information for retrieval at a later time.
■ Encourage the patient to reminisce about past experiences.	The mental stimulation that occurs with recall and review of life events can enhance information retrieval from remote memory.
■ Provide opportunities for repeated practice of new information using an errorless learning approach.	An errorless learning approach provides the person with the correct information each time it is needed. The person then records the information in a memory aid such as a notebook or computer. When errors occur in learning new information, it impedes memory development of correct information.
■ Encourage use of games and puzzles as appropriate.	Games such as crossword puzzles, jigsaw puzzles, or chess have been shown to aid in stimulating important neural centers that enhance memory function.
▲ Refer the patient to a professional counselor, as needed.	The patient with memory loss associated with psychogenic problems may benefit from talk therapy.
▲ Administer medications as prescribed.	Thiamine may be given to patients with memory loss associated with Wernicke encephalopathy from alcohol abuse. Improvement in memory has been seen in patients treated with clonidine and vasopressin. Patients with Alzheimer's disease may receive medications that slow the progression of the disorder and preserve memory function for a short period of time. Acetylcholinesterase (AChE) inhibitors such as tacrine (Cognex), donepezil (Aricept), and rivastigmine (Exelon) increase acetylcholine at neuron receptors. This action improves cholinergic transmission and slows decline in memory and cognitive function.

Education/Continuity of Care

Actions/Interventions	Rationales
■ Educate the patient and family about using memory techniques.	Learning to use memory aids is a memory task itself. The patient may need extended time and reinforcement to become successful in using these techniques.
• Mnemonic devices	This internal approach to memory rehabilitation uses a variety of verbal and/or visual techniques to facilitate the encoding and retrieval of information.
• Imagery	Visual imagery techniques can be used to assist the patient in organizing and retrieving information.
• External memory aids such as calendars, alarms, timers, posted notes, lists, computers, and memory notebooks	These external strategies rely on environmental approaches to assist the patient in developing behavioral consistency to compensate for memory loss. Research indicates that external memory aids have more value than internal techniques. Learning to use them can be challenging for the patient.
■ Provide family members and caregivers with information about impaired memory and the patient's behavior.	Knowledge about impaired memory may help family members and caregivers understand the meaning of a patient's behavior. This information may help the family support the patient and provide a safer environment.
■ Allow family members and caregivers to express feelings about the patient's impaired memory and behavior.	The demands of caring for the patient with impaired memory may have a significant impact on the family's lifestyle and interactions. Unresolved stress and frustration may lead to angry verbal or physical outbursts directed toward the patient.
▲ Refer the patient and family to community resources to assist in creating safe living environments.	Patients with impaired memory may no longer be able to live alone or with family members because of safety issues. The family may need help in finding alternative living arrangements for the patient such as supervised group homes or assisted living.

Related Care Plans

Alzheimer's disease/Dementia, p. 475
Chronic confusion, p. 43

Impaired Physical Mobility

Definition: Limitation in independent, purposeful physical movement of the body or of one or more extremities

Alteration in mobility may be a temporary or more permanent problem. Most disease and rehabilitative states involve some degree of immobility (e.g., as seen in strokes, leg fracture, trauma, morbid obesity, and multiple sclerosis). With the longer life expectancy for most Americans, the incidence of disease and disability continues to grow. And with shorter hospital stays, patients are being transferred to rehabilitation facilities or sent home for physical therapy in the home environment.

Mobility is also related to body changes from aging. Loss of muscle mass, reduction in muscle strength and function, stiffer and less mobile joints, and gait changes affecting balance can significantly compromise the mobility of older patients. Mobility is paramount if older patients are to maintain any independent living. Restricted movement affects the performance of most activities of daily living (ADLs). Older patients are also at increased risk for the complications of immobility. Nursing goals are to maintain functional ability, prevent additional impairment of physical activity, and ensure a safe environment.

■ = Independent ▲ = Collaborative

Common Related Factors

Activity intolerance
Perceptual or cognitive impairment
Musculoskeletal impairment
Neuromuscular impairment
Decreased muscle endurance, strength, control, or mass
Imposed restrictions of movement, including mechanical and medical protocol
Prolonged bed rest
Sedentary lifestyle
Pain or discomfort
Depression or severe anxiety
Deconditioning/decreased endurance

Defining Characteristics

Inability to move purposefully within physical environment, including bed mobility, transfers, and ambulation
Reluctance to attempt movement
Limited range of motion (ROM)
Inability to perform action as instructed

Common Expected Outcomes

Patient performs physical activity independently or within limits of disease.
Patient demonstrates use of adaptive techniques that promote ambulation and transferring.
Patient is free of complications of immobility, as evidenced by intact skin, absence of thrombophlebitis, normal bowel pattern, and clear breath sounds.

NOC Outcomes
Ambulation: Walking; Joint Movement: Active; Mobility Level
NIC Interventions
Exercise Therapy: Ambulation; Joint Mobility; Fall Precautions; Positioning; Bed Rest Care

Ongoing Assessment

Actions/Interventions	Rationales
■ Assess for impediments to mobility.	Identifying barriers to mobility (e.g., chronic arthritis versus stroke versus pain) guides design of an optimal treatment plan.
■ Assess the patient's ability to perform ADLs effectively and safely on a daily basis using an appropriate assessment tool, such as the functional independence measures (FIM).	Restricted movement affects the ability to perform most ADLs. A variety of assessment tools are available, depending on the clinical setting. Such tools provide objective data for baselines. For example, the FIM measures 18 self-care items related to eating, bathing grooming, dressing, toileting, bladder and bowel management, transfer, ambulation, and stair climbing.
■ Assess ability to perform ROM to all joints.	This assessment provides data on extent of any physical problems and guides therapy. Testing by a physical therapist may be needed.
■ Evaluate the need for assistive devices.	Proper use of wheelchairs, canes, transfer bars, and other assistance can promote activity and reduce danger of falls.
■ Evaluate the safety of the immediate environment.	Obstacles such as throw rugs, children's toys, and pets can further impede one's ability to ambulate safely.
■ Assess emotional response to disability or limitation.	Acceptance of temporary or more permanent limitations can vary widely among individuals. Each person has his or her own definition of acceptable quality of life.
■ Monitor nutritional status.	Proper nutrition provides needed energy for ambulation, transfer techniques, and participating in an exercise or rehabilitative program. Moreover, pressure ulcers develop more quickly in patients with a nutritional deficit.
■ Evaluate need for home assistance (e.g., physical therapy, visiting nurse).	Obtaining appropriate assistance for the patient can ensure safe and proper progression of activity.

Actions/Interventions	**Rationales**
■ Assess the patient's or caregiver's knowledge of immobility and its implications.	Even patients who are temporarily immobile are at risk for effects of immobility such as skin breakdown, muscle weakness, thrombophlebitis, constipation, pneumonia, and depression.
■ Assess for developing thrombophlebitis (e.g., calf pain, Homans' sign, redness, localized swelling, and rise in temperature).	Reduced activity or immobility affects peripheral circulation and can promote clot formation.
■ Assess skin integrity for signs of redness and tissue ischemia (especially over ears, shoulders, elbows, sacrum, hips, heels, ankles, and toes).	Regular examination of the skin (especially over bony prominences) will allow for prevention or early recognition and treatment of pressure ulcers.
■ Assess elimination status (e.g., usual pattern, present patterns, signs of constipation).	Reduced activity and immobility decrease gastrointestinal motility.

Therapeutic Interventions

Actions/Interventions	**Rationales**
■ Encourage and facilitate early ambulation when possible. Assist with each initial change: dangling legs, sitting in chair, ambulation.	These activities keep the patient as functionally active as possible. Early mobility promotes confidence about regaining independence and reduces the chance that debilitation will occur.
■ Encourage appropriate use of assistive devices.	Crutches, canes, or walkers may be provided to assist the patient with mobility until activity restrictions are no longer needed. However, some patients may refuse to use assistance devices because they attract attention to a disability. Additional home environment evaluation may be needed.
■ Administer medications as appropriate.	Antispasmodic medications may reduce muscle spasms or spasticity that interferes with mobility; analgesics may reduce pain that impedes movement.
■ Facilitate transfer training by teaching or using appropriate techniques or devices when transferring patients to bed, chair, or stretcher.	Learning the correct way to transfer is important for maintaining optimal mobility and patient safety.
■ Allow the patient to perform tasks at his or her own rate. Do not rush the patient. Encourage independent activity as able and safe.	Hospital workers and family caregivers are often in a hurry and do more for patients than needed, thereby slowing the patient's recovery and reducing his or her self-esteem.
■ Encourage the patient to rest between activities that are tiring. Teach energy-saving techniques.	Rest periods are necessary to conserve energy. The patient must learn to respect the limitations of his or her restrictions.
■ Provide positive reinforcement during activity.	Patients may be reluctant to move or initiate new activity due to a fear of falling. A positive approach allows the learner to feel good about learning accomplishments.
■ Assist the patient in accepting limitations. Emphasize abilities.	Quality of life is influenced by a variety of factors that can extend beyond only physical function. Help may be required for safety and comfort, but assistance needs to be balanced to avoid making the patient unnecessarily dependent.
■ Provide a safe environment: bed rails up, bed in down position, necessary items close by.	These measures promote a safe secure environment and may reduce risk for falls.
■ Perform passive or active assistive ROM exercises to all extremities.	Exercise promotes increased venous return, prevents stiffness, and maintains muscle strength and endurance. To be most effective, all joints should be exercised to prevent contractures.
■ Encourage resistance-training exercises using light weights when appropriate.	Research supports that strength training and other forms of exercise in older adults can preserve the ability to maintain independent living status and reduce risk for falling.

■ = Independent ▲ = Collaborative

Actions/Interventions

- Institute measures to prevent skin breakdown and thrombophlebitis from prolonged immobility:
  - Clean, dry, and moisturize skin as needed.
  - Use antiembolic stockings or sequential compression devices if appropriate.
  - Use pressure-relieving devices as indicated (gel mattress).
- Turn and position the patient every 2 hours or as needed. Maintain limbs in functional alignment (e.g., with pillows, sandbags, wedges, or prefabricated splints). Support feet in dorsiflexed position. Use bed cradle.

- ▲ Encourage liquid intake of 2000 to 3000 mL/day unless contraindicated.
- Provide recommendations for nutritional intake for adequate energy resources and metabolic requirements.

- ▲ Set up a bowel program (e.g., adequate fluid, foods high in bulk, physical activity, stool softeners, laxatives) as needed. Record bowel activity level.
- Encourage coughing and deep-breathing exercises. Use suction as needed. Use incentive spirometer.

Rationales

These measures reduce skin breakdown, and the compression devices promote increased venous return to prevent venous stasis and possible thrombophlebitis in the legs.

Position changes optimize circulation to all tissues and relieve pressure. Maintaining correct alignment of extremities reduces strain in joints and prevents contractures. Supporting heavy bed linens can reduce improper alignment of feet.

Liquids optimize hydration status and prevent hardening of stool.

The patient will need adequate, properly balanced intake of carbohydrate, fats, protein, vitamins, and minerals to provide energy resources.

Prolonged bed rest, lack of exercise, and physical inactivity contribute to constipation. A variety of interventions will promote normal elimination.

Decreased chest excursions and stasis of secretions are associated with immobility. Coughing and deep breathing prevent buildup of secretions. Incentive spirometry increases lung expansion.

Education/Continuity of Care

Actions/Interventions

- Explain progressive activity to the patient. Help the patient or caregivers establish reasonable and obtainable goals.

- Instruct the patient or caregivers regarding hazards of immobility. Emphasize importance of measures such as position change, ROM, coughing, and exercises.
- Reinforce principles of progressive exercise, emphasizing that joints are to be exercised to the point of pain, not beyond.

- Instruct the patient and family regarding the need to make the home environment safe.
- ▲ Refer the patient to the multidisciplinary health team as appropriate.

Rationales

Information promotes awareness of the treatment plan. Setting small, attainable goals helps increase self-confidence and reduces frustration.

Information enables the patient to assume some control over the rehabilitative process.

"No pain, no gain" is not always true! Pain occurs as a result of joint or muscle injury. Continued stress on joints or muscles may lead to more serious damage and limit ability to move.

A safe environment will help prevent injury related to falls.

Physical and occupational therapists can provide specialized services to promote effective mobility.

Related Care Plan

Risk for falls, p. 60

NANDA-I
NDx **Nausea**

Definition: An unpleasant, wavelike sensation in the back of the throat, epigastrium, or throughout the abdomen that may or may not lead to vomiting

Nausea is a common and distressing symptom with a myriad of causes, including intracranial or labyrinthine lesions, chemical stimulation of the vomiting center by most medications, ingestion of toxins (chemotherapy), microorganisms in the gastrointestinal tract, gastrointestinal obstruction, or mucosal diseases. Decreased motility and delayed emptying of the stomach are the underlying physiological factors for most causes of nausea. Decreased peristalsis in the intestines may also contribute to nausea. Nausea may have psychogenic origins, which should be considered in cases of chronic nausea or gastroparesis. Nausea can also be associated with severe pain or aberrant motion such as in carsickness or seasickness. During the first trimester of pregnancy, nausea is common and may be related to excessive hormone production. For most women, this subsides by their second trimester; for other women, mild nausea may persist throughout the pregnancy.

Common Related Factors

Treatment related:
- Gastric irritation (drugs, alcohol, iron, blood)
- Gastric distention
- Pharmaceuticals (e.g., analgesics, medications for human immunodeficiency virus, aspirin, opioids, chemotherapy agents)

Biophysical:
- Biochemical disorders (e.g., uremia, pregnancy)
- Cardiac pain
- Cancer of stomach or colon
- Gastrointestinal diseases
- Tumors
- Motion sickness
- Physical factors (e.g., increased intracranial pressure)
- Toxins

Situational:
- Psychological factors (e.g., fear, pain, noxious stimuli)

Defining Characteristics

Reports "nausea" or "sick to stomach"
Increased salivation
Increased swallowing
Gagging sensation
Sour taste in mouth
Aversion to food

Common Expected Outcome

Patient reports diminished severity or elimination of nausea.

NOC Outcomes
Comfort Level; Symptom Severity; Hydration; Nutritional Status: Food and Fluid Intake

NIC Interventions
Nausea Management; Medication Management; Fluid Monitoring

Ongoing Assessment

Actions/Interventions

■ Assess for cause of nausea.

Rationales

Determining the cause of the nausea will guide the choice of interventions to be used. Sometimes removing the stimulus will resolve the nausea without additional treatment. Surgery may even be required to treat some etiologies.

■ = Independent   ▲ = Collaborative

Actions/Interventions	Rationales
■ Assess nausea characteristics: • History • Duration • Frequency • Severity • Precipitating factors • Medications • Measures used to alleviate the problem	A comprehensive assessment of the nausea can help determine interventions to minimize or alleviate the problem.
■ Assess hydration status such as measuring daily weights, blood pressure, intake and output, and assessing skin turgor.	Nausea is often associated with vomiting that can alter a patient's hydration status because of fluid loss.

Therapeutic Interventions

Actions/Interventions	Rationales
■ Assist the patient in preparation for diagnostic testing as ordered.	A variety of tests may be used to determine the etiology of the nausea (e.g., upper gastrointestinal study, abdominal computed tomography scan, ultrasonography).
■ Keep emesis basin within easy reach of the patient.	Nausea is often associated with vomiting. Keep emesis basin out of sight but in easy reach if nausea has a psychogenic component.
■ Offer and/or assist with oral hygiene every 2 to 4 hours if tolerated.	Nausea is often associated with anorexia and increased salivation. Oral hygiene will help promote comfort.
■ Remove noxious odors from the room (e.g., perfumes, dressings, emesis).	Strong or noxious odors can contribute to nausea.
■ Offer cold water, ice chips, ginger products, and room-temperature broth or bouillon if tolerated and appropriate to diet.	These fluids help with hydration. For some patients, ginger helps relieve nausea whether in ginger ale, ginger tea, or chewed as crystallized ginger. Fluids with extreme temperatures may be difficult to tolerate.
■ Offer frequent, small amounts of foods that appeal to the patient:	This approach will help maintain nutritional status; for some patients, an empty stomach exacerbates the nausea.
• Dry foods like toast or crackers	Dry toast or crackers before rising are especially known to be effective for pregnancy-related nausea.
• Bland, simple foods like broth, rice, bananas, or Jell-O	Patients may tolerate these types of foods. They should try to eat more when nausea is absent.
• Avoid greasy or fried foods	Fats are difficult to digest and may exacerbate the nausea.
■ Encourage the patient to use nonpharmacological nausea control techniques such as relaxation, guided imagery, music therapy, distraction, or deep breathing.	These techniques have helped patients manage their nausea, but they need to be used before nausea occurs or increases, as well as with other nausea control measures.
▲ Administer antiemetics as ordered.	Most antiemetics act by raising the threshold of the chemoreceptor trigger zone to stimulation. Other drugs that may be used to treat nausea include antihistamines, anticholinergics, dopamine antagonists, and benzodiazepines. A variety of newer antiemetic drugs are available and effective to treat chemotherapy-induced nausea and vomiting.
▲ Apply acustimulation bands as ordered, or apply acupressure.	Stimulation of the Neiguan P6 acupuncture point on the ventral surface of the wrist has been found to control nausea in some patients. This technique has been found to be especially helpful for patients who experience motion-related nausea.

Education/Continuity of Care

Actions/Interventions	Rationales
■ Teach the patient to change positions slowly.	Sudden or gross movement may increase nausea.
■ Teach the patient or caregiver about appropriate fluid and dietary choices for nausea.	Patients and caregivers can promote adequate hydration and nutritional status by knowing dietary considerations to follow when nauseated.

Actions/Interventions

- Teach the patient or caregiver nonpharmacological nausea control techniques such as relaxation, guided imagery, music therapy, distraction, or deep breathing.
- Teach the patient to take prescribed medications as ordered.
- Evaluate the patient's response to antiemetics or interventions to alleviate nausea.

- Teach the patient or caregiver how to apply acustimulation bands or acupressure.
- Teach the patient or caregiver to seek medical care if vomiting develops or persists longer than 24 hours.

Rationales

Teaching the patient and caregiver methods to control nausea increases the sense of personal efficacy in managing the nausea.

Appropriate timing for medications reduces episodes of nausea.

It is important to evaluate the interventions used to determine their effectiveness or to find other interventions that may be more effective for the patient.

Patients and caregivers may want to continue with this intervention if it was found effective in controlling nausea.

Persistent vomiting can lead to dehydration, electrolyte imbalance, and nutritional deficiencies.

Noncompliance

Definition: Behavior of person and/or caregiver that fails to coincide with a health-promoting or therapeutic plan agreed on by the person (and/or family and/or community) and health care professional. In the presence of an agreed-on health-promoting or therapeutic plan, person's or caregiver's behavior is fully or partially nonadherent and may lead to clinically ineffective or partially ineffective outcomes

The fact that a patient has attained knowledge regarding the treatment plan does not guarantee compliance. Failure to follow the prescribed plan may be related to a number of factors. Much research has been conducted in this area to identify key predictive factors. Several theoretical models, such as the Health Belief Model, Theory of Reasoned Decision Making, and Theory of Planned Behavior, serve to explain those factors that influence patient compliance. Patients are more likely to comply when they believe that they are susceptible to an illness or disease that could seriously affect their health, that certain behaviors will reduce the likelihood of contracting the disease, that the prescribed actions are less threatening than the disease itself, and when normative groups support the change. Factors that may predict noncompliance include past history of noncompliance, stressful lifestyles, contrary cultural or religious beliefs and values, lack of social support, lack of financial resources, and compromised emotional state. People living in adverse social situations (e.g., battered women, homeless individuals, those living amid street violence, the unemployed, or those in poverty) may purposefully defer following medical recommendations until their acute socioeconomic situation is improved. The rising costs of health care and the growing number of uninsured and underinsured patients often force patients with limited incomes to choose between food and medications. The problem is especially complex for older patients living on fixed incomes but requiring complex and costly medical therapies.

Common Related Factors

Conflicting health values
Health beliefs
Cultural beliefs/influences
Spiritual values
Patient-provider relationships
Health care system barriers
Complexity of therapeutic regimen

Defining Characteristics

Behavior indicative of failure to adhere to a therapeutic recommendation
Objective tests: improper pill counts or missed prescription refills; body fluid analysis inconsistent with compliance
Evidence of development of complications
Evidence of exacerbation of symptoms
"Revolving-door" hospital admissions
Missed appointments
Therapeutic effect not achieved or maintained

■ = Independent   ▲ = Collaborative

Common Expected Outcomes

Patient and/or significant other reports compliance with therapeutic plan.

Patient complies with therapeutic plan, as evidenced by appropriate pill count, appropriate amount of drug in blood or urine, evidence of therapeutic effect, maintained appointments, and/or fewer hospital admissions.

NOC Outcomes

Adherence Behavior; Compliance Behavior; Knowledge: Treatment Regimen; Participation: Health Care Decisions

NIC Interventions

Behavior Modification; Decision-Making Support; Patient Contracting; Health Education

Ongoing Assessment

Actions/Interventions	Rationales
■ Assess the patient's individual perceptions of health problems.	According to the Health Belief Model, a patient's perceived susceptibility to and perceived seriousness and threat of disease, along with perceived benefits from adhering to treatment plan, affect compliance. Some patients may not understand the chronicity of their disease or their ability to manage some of the ongoing symptoms.
■ Assess beliefs about current illness.	Determining what the patient thinks is causing his or her symptoms or disease, how likely it is that the symptoms may return, and any concerns about the diagnosis or symptoms will provide a basis for planning future care. Persons of other cultures and religious heritages may hold differing views regarding health and illness. For some cultures the causative agent may be a person, not a microbe.
■ Assess religious beliefs or practices that affect health.	Many people view illness as a punishment from God that must be treated through spiritual healing practices (e.g., prayer, pilgrimage), not medications.
■ Assess beliefs about the treatment plan.	Understanding any worries or misconceptions that the patient may have about the plan or side effects will guide future interventions.
■ Assess factors the patient feels interfere with compliance.	Identifying barriers unique to each patient allows for individualizing the corrective plan. Such barriers may include cognitive impairment, fear of actually experiencing medication side effects, failure to understand instructions regarding the plan (e.g., difficulty understanding a low-sodium diet), impaired manual dexterity (e.g., pill container is too difficult to open), sensory deficit (e.g., unable to read written instructions), and regard for nontraditional treatments (e.g., herbs, liniments, prayer, acupuncture).
■ Determine cultural or spiritual influences on importance of health care.	Not all persons view maintenance of health the same. For example, some may place trust in God for treatment and refuse pills, blood transfusions, or surgery. Others may only want to follow a "natural" or "health food" regimen.
■ Compare actual therapeutic effect with expected effect.	These data provide information on compliance; however, if therapy is ineffective or based on a faulty diagnosis, even perfect compliance will not result in the expected therapeutic effect.
■ Plot pattern of hospitalizations and clinic appointments.	These data provide objective information regarding follow-up, but do not necessarily mean that the patient is not complying with other prescribed therapies.

Actions/Interventions

■ Ask the patient to bring prescription drugs to appointments; count remaining pills.

▲ Assess serum or urine drug level.

Rationales

This technique provides some objective evidence of compliance. It is commonly used in drug research protocols.

Therapeutic blood levels will not be achieved without consistent ingestion of medication; overdosage or overtreatment can likewise be assessed.

Therapeutic Interventions

Actions/Interventions

■ Develop a therapeutic relationship with the patient and family.

■ Include patient in planning the treatment regimen.

■ Remove disincentives to compliance.

▲ Simplify therapy. Suggest long-acting forms of medications, and eliminate unnecessary medication. Eliminate unnecessary clinic visits.

■ Tailor the therapy to the patient's lifestyle (e.g., diuretics may be taken with the evening meal for patients who work outside the home) and culture (incorporate herbal medicinal massage or prayer, as appropriate).

■ If negative side effects of prescribed treatment are a problem, explain that many side effects can be controlled or eliminated.

■ Increase the amount of supervision provided; as compliance improves, gradually reduce the amount of professional supervision and reinforcement.

■ Develop a behavioral contract.

■ Develop with the patient a system of rewards that follow successful compliance.

Rationales

Compliance increases when there is a trusting relationship and a consistent caregiver. Use of a skilled interpreter is necessary for patients who do not speak the dominant language.

Patients who become comanagers of their care have a greater stake in achieving a positive outcome. They know best their personal and environmental barriers to success.

Actions such as decreasing waiting time in the clinic, recommending lower levels of activity, or suggesting medications that do not cause side effects that are unacceptable to the patient can improve compliance.

Compliance increases when therapy is short and includes as few treatments as possible. The physical demands and financial burdens of traveling must be considered. Polypharmacy is a significant problem with older patients.

Individualization will ensure a patient-centered focus and promote compliance. A "one size fits all" approach is usually ineffective.

Nonadherence because of medication side effects is a commonly reported problem. Health care providers need to determine actual etiological factors for side effects and possible interplay with over-the-counter medications. Similarly, patients may report fatigue or muscle cramps with exercise. If so, the exercise prescription may need to be revised.

Home health nurses, telephone monitoring, and frequent return visits or appointments can provide increased supervision as needed that can be tapered as appropriate.

A contract helps the patient understand and accept his or her role in the care plan and clarifies what the patient can expect from the health care worker or system.

Rewards provide positive reinforcement for compliant behavior. They may consist of verbal praise, monetary rewards, special privileges, or telephone calls by health care providers.

Education/Continuity of Care

Actions/Interventions

■ Provide specific instruction as indicated.

■ Tailor the information in terms of what the patient feels is the cause of his or her health problem and his or her concerns about therapy.

Rationales

Information enables the patient to better take control in selecting and implementing required changes in behavior.

Adult learning is problem oriented. Focus should be on strategies that reduce barriers to treatment and enhance desired outcome.

■ = Independent ▲ = Collaborative

Actions/Interventions

- Instruct the patient in the importance of reordering medications 2 to 3 days before running out.

- Teach significant others to eliminate disincentives and/or increase rewards to the patient for compliance.
- Provide social support through the patient's family and self-help groups.
- Explore community resources.

Rationales

Although many cultures in the United States are future oriented and concerned with measures to prevent illness, other cultures are more oriented to the present. This difference in time orientation needs to be addressed.

Nagging is never effective in promoting change. Incorporating rewards for positive accomplishments is more effective.

Such groups may assist the patient in gaining greater understanding of the benefits of treatment.

Churches, social clubs, and community groups can play a dominant role in some cultures. Outreach workers from a given community may effectively serve as a bridge to the health care provider.

Imbalanced Nutrition: Less Than Body Requirements

Definition: Intake of nutrients insufficient to meet metabolic needs

Adequate nutrition is necessary to meet the body's demands. Nutritional status can be affected by disease or injury states (e.g., gastrointestinal malabsorption, cancer, burns); physical factors (e.g., muscle weakness, poor dentition, activity intolerance, pain, substance abuse); social factors (e.g., lack of financial resources to obtain nutritious foods); or psychological factors (e.g., depression, boredom, dementia). During times of illness (e.g., trauma, surgery, sepsis, burns), adequate nutrition plays an important role in healing and recovery. Cultural and religious factors strongly affect the food habits of patients. Women exhibit a higher incidence of voluntary restriction of food intake secondary to anorexia, bulimia, and self-constructed fad dieting. Patients who are older experience problems in nutrition related to lack of financial resources, cognitive impairments causing them to forget to eat, physical limitations that interfere with preparing food, deterioration of their sense of taste and smell, reduction of gastric secretion that accompanies aging and interferes with digestion, and social isolation and boredom that cause a lack of interest in eating. This care plan addresses general concerns related to nutritional deficits for the hospital or home setting.

Common Related Factors

Inability to ingest foods
Inability to digest foods
Inability to absorb or metabolize foods
Inability to procure adequate amounts of food
Knowledge deficit
Unwillingness to eat
Increased metabolic needs caused by disease process or therapy

Defining Characteristics

Loss of weight with or without adequate caloric intake
10% to 20% below ideal body weight
Documented inadequate caloric intake

Common Expected Outcomes

Patient or caregiver verbalizes and demonstrates selection of foods or meals that will achieve a cessation of weight loss.
Patient weighs within 10% of ideal body weight.

NOC Outcomes
Nutritional Status: Food and Fluid Intake; Nutritional Status: Nutrient Intake

NIC Interventions
Nutrition Monitoring; Nutrition Therapy; Nutrition Management

Nursing Diagnosis Care Plans

Ongoing Assessment

Actions/Interventions	Rationales
■ Document actual weight and height; do not estimate.	Patients may be unaware of their actual weight and height or weight loss due to estimating weight.
■ Obtain nutritional history; include family, significant others, or caregiver in assessment.	The patient's perception of actual intake may differ.
■ Determine etiological factors for reduced nutritional intake.	Proper assessment guides intervention. For example, patients with dentition problems require referral to a dentist, whereas patients with memory losses may require services such as Meals On Wheels.
■ Monitor or explore attitudes toward eating and food.	Many psychological, psychosocial, and cultural factors determine the type, amount, and appropriateness of food consumed.
■ Monitor the environment in which eating occurs.	Fewer families today have a general meal together. Many adults find themselves "eating on the run" (e.g., at their desk, in the car) or relying heavily on fast foods with reduced nutritional components.
■ Encourage patient participation in recording food intake using a daily log.	Determination of type, amount, and pattern of food or fluid intake is facilitated by accurate documentation by the patient or caregiver as the intake occurs; memory is insufficient.
▲ Monitor laboratory values that indicate nutritional well-being or deterioration:	
• Serum albumin	This test indicates degree of protein depletion (2.5 g/dL indicates severe depletion; 3.8 to 4.5 g/dL is normal).
• Transferrin	Transferrin is important for iron transfer and typically decreases as serum protein decreases.
• Red blood cell and white blood cell counts	Anemia and leukopenia occur in malnutrition, leading to weakness and are usually decreased in malnutrition, indicating anemia and decreased resistance to infection.
• Serum electrolyte values	Potassium is typically increased and sodium is typically decreased in malnutrition.
■ Weigh patient weekly.	During aggressive nutritional support, patient can gain up to 0.5 pound per day.

Therapeutic Interventions

Actions/Interventions	Rationales
▲ Consult dietitian for further assessment and recommendations regarding food preferences and nutritional support.	Dietitians have a greater understanding of the nutritional value of foods and may be helpful in assessing specific ethnic or cultural foods (e.g., "soul foods," Hispanic dishes, kosher foods).
■ Establish appropriate short- and long-range goals.	Depending on the etiological factors of the problem, improvement in nutritional status may take a long time. Without realistic short-term goals to provide tangible rewards, patients may lose interest in addressing this problem.
■ Suggest ways to assist the patient with meals, as needed. Ensure a pleasant environment, facilitate proper position, and provide good oral hygiene and dentition.	Elevating the head of bed 30 degrees aids in swallowing and reduces risk for aspiration.
■ Provide companionship during mealtime.	Attention to the social aspects of eating is important in both the hospital and home settings.
■ For patients with changes in sense of taste, encourage use of seasoning.	Seasoning may enhance the flavor of foods and entice eating.
▲ For patients with physical impairments, refer to occupational therapist for adaptive devices.	The occupational therapist can offer devices such as plate guards and strap-on utensils that can help patients feed themselves.

■ = Independent   ▲ = Collaborative

Nursing Diagnosis Care Plans

Actions/Interventions

- For hospitalized patients, encourage the family to bring food from home as appropriate.
- Suggest liquid drinks for supplemental nutrition.

- Discourage beverages that are caffeinated or carbonated.
- Involve patients in all aspects of their nutritional care.

- Discuss possible need for enteral or parenteral nutritional support with patient, family, and caregiver, as appropriate.

- Encourage exercise.

Rationales

Patients with specific ethnic or religious preferences or restrictions may not be able to eat hospital foods.

Such supplements can be used to increase calories and protein without interfering with voluntary food intake.

These beverages may decrease appetite and lead to early satiety.

Involving patients in their own nutritional care has been found to raise their intake of protein and energy levels

Enteral tube feedings are preferred for patients with a functioning gastrointestinal tract. Feedings may be continuous or intermittent (bolus). Parenteral nutrition may be indicated for patients who cannot tolerate enteral feedings. Either solution can be modified to provide required glucose, protein, electrolytes, vitamins, minerals, and trace elements. Fat and fat-soluble vitamins can also be administered two or three times per week. These feedings may be used with in-hospital, long-term care, and subacute care settings, as well as in the home.

Metabolism and utilization of nutrients are enhanced by activity.

Education/Continuity of Care

Actions/Interventions

- Review and reinforce the following to the patient or caregivers:
  - The basic four food groups, MyPyramid food guide, and the need for specific minerals or vitamins
  - Importance of maintaining adequate caloric intake; an average adult (70 kg) needs 1800 to 2200 kcal/ day; patients with burns, severe infections, or draining wounds may require 3000 to 4000 kcal/day
  - Foods high in calories and protein that will promote weight gain and nitrogen balance (e.g., small frequent meals of foods high in calories and protein)
- Provide referral to community nutritional resources such as Meals On Wheels or hot lunch programs for seniors as indicated.

Rationales

Patients may not understand what is involved in a balanced diet. They are better able to ask questions and seek assistance when they know basic information.

Many seniors (especially those living alone) do not take the time or effort to cook for themselves.

NANDA-I
NDx

Imbalanced Nutrition: More Than Body Requirements

Definition: Intake of nutrients that exceeds metabolic needs

Obesity is a growing problem in the United States and is now reaching pandemic proportions, accounting for significant other health problems, including cardiovascular disease, type 2 diabetes mellitus, sleep disorders, infertility in women, aggravated musculoskeletal problems, and shortened life expectancy. Women are more likely to be overweight than men. African Americans and Hispanic individuals are more likely to be overweight than whites. Factors that affect weight gain include genetics, sedentary lifestyle, emotional factors associated with dysfunctional eating, disease states such as diabetes mellitus and Cushing's syndrome, and cultural or ethnic influences on eating. Overall nutritional requirements of older patients are similar to those of younger individuals, except calories should be reduced because of their leaner body mass.

Common Related Factors

Excessive intake in relation to metabolic need
Lack of knowledge of nutritional needs, food intake, and/or appropriate food preparation
Poor dietary habits
Use of food as coping mechanism
Metabolic disorders
Sedentary activity level

Defining Characteristics

Weight 20% over ideal for height and frame
Triceps skinfold greater than 15 mm in men, 25 mm in women
Reported or observed dysfunctional eating patterns
Eating in response to internal cues other than hunger
Eating in response to external cues such as time of day or social situation

Common Expected Outcomes

Patient verbalizes measures necessary to achieve weight reduction.
Patient demonstrates appropriate selection of meals or menu planning toward the goal of weight reduction.
Patient begins an appropriate program of exercise.

NOC Outcomes
Nutritional Status: Food and Fluid Intake; Weight Control

NIC Interventions
Nutritional Monitoring; Nutrition Counseling; Weight Reduction Assistance

Ongoing Assessment

Actions/Interventions	Rationales
■ Document weight and height; do not estimate.	Patients may be unaware of their actual weight and height.
■ Determine weight distribution by measuring waist with a tape measure.	Men with waist circumference greater than 40 inches or women with greater than 35 inches are at higher risk for obesity-related comorbidities.
■ Calculate body mass index (BMI) as a ratio of height and weight.	BMI describes relative weight for height and is significantly correlated with total body fat content. BMI is the person's weight in kilograms divided by the square of his or her height in meters. A BMI between 20 and 24 is associated with healthier outcomes. BMIs greater than 25 are associated with increased morbidity and mortality.
■ Perform a nutritional assessment to include: • Daily food intake—type and amount of food • Approximate caloric intake • Activity at time of eating • Feelings at time of eating • Where patient is when eating • Problematic eating behaviors	Environmental factors contribute to obesity more than genetics or biological vulnerability.
■ Perform behavioral assessment to include: • Importance and meaning of food • Behavioral factors that contribute to the obesity • Psychosocial consequences of being overweight • Patient's goals and expectation for weight reduction • Patient's level of motivation to lose weight • Previous attempts at weight loss	Overeating may be triggered by environmental cues and behavioral factors unrelated to physiological hunger sensations. Being overweight can negatively affect one's self-image and social interactions. Realistic goal setting is key, because patients are easily discouraged when they cannot meet unrealistic goals. This sense of failure can lead to overeating.
■ Assess knowledge regarding nutritional needs for height and level of activity or other factors (e.g., pregnancy).	A person's height, activity level, or other factors can influence his or her caloric needs.
■ Assess ability to read food labels.	Food labels contain information necessary in making appropriate selections, but can be misleading. Patients need to understand that "low-fat" or "fat-free" does not mean that a food item is calorie-free. In addition, attention should be paid to serving size and the number of servings in the food item.
■ Assess ability to plan a menu, making appropriate food selections.	Cultural or ethnic influences need to be identified and addressed.

■ = Independent ▲ = Collaborative

Actions/Interventions

■ Assess ability to accurately identify appropriate food portions.
■ Assess effects or complications of being overweight.

■ Assess usual level of activity.

Rationales

Serving sizes must be understood to limit intake according to a planned diet.
Medical complications include cardiovascular and respiratory dysfunction, higher incidence of diabetes mellitus, and aggravation of musculoskeletal disorders. Social complications and poor self-esteem may also result from obesity.
Patients may confuse routine activity with exercise necessary to enhance and maintain weight loss.

Therapeutic Interventions

Actions/Interventions

▲ Consult dietitian for further assessment and recommendations regarding a weight loss program.

■ Establish appropriate short- and long-range goals.

■ Encourage food selections that provide a caloric intake appropriate for achieving weight-loss goals.

■ Encourage the patient to keep a daily log of food or liquid ingestion and caloric intake.

■ Encourage water intake.

■ Encourage the patient to be more aware of nutritional habits that may contribute to or prevent overeating, such as the following:
• Realize the time needed for eating.

• Focus on eating, and avoid other diversional activities (e.g., reading, television viewing, or telephoning).
• Observe for cues that lead to eating (e.g., odor, time, depression, or boredom).

• Eat in a designated place (e.g., at the table rather than in front of the television).
• Recognize actual hunger versus desire to eat.

■ Encourage exercise.

■ Provide positive reinforcement as indicated. Encourage successes; assist the patient in coping with setbacks.

Rationales

Changes in eating patterns are required for weight loss. The type of program may vary (e.g., three balanced meals a day, avoidance of certain high-fat foods). Dietitians have a greater understanding of the nutritional value of foods and may be helpful in assessing or substituting specific high-fat cultural or ethnic foods.
Depending on the etiological factors of the problem, improvement in nutritional status may take a long time. Without realistic short-term goals to provide tangible rewards, patients may lose interest in addressing this problem.
One pound of adipose tissue contains 3500 kcal. Therefore to lose 1 pound per week, the patient must have a calorie deficit of 500 kcal/day.
Memory is inadequate for quantification of intake, and a visual record may also help the patient make more appropriate food choices and serving sizes.
Water assists in the excretion of by-products of fat breakdown and helps prevent ketosis.

Hurried eating may result in overeating because satiety is not realized until 15 to 20 minutes after ingestion of food.
Doing several activities at once usually results in less attention being devoted to amount of food eaten.
Identifying triggers or situations that prompt eating behaviors is the first step toward developing alternative coping strategies.
Controlling environmental stimuli can reduce impulse eating.
Eating when not hungry is a commonly recognized symptom among overeaters.
Exercise is an integral part of weight reduction programs. The combination of diet and exercise promotes loss of adipose tissue rather than lean tissue.
Positive reinforcement encourages a desired behavior. Patients need to have setbacks reframed as learning opportunities and as a normal step in making lifestyle changes.

Education/Continuity of Care

Actions/Interventions	Rationales
■ Review and reinforce teaching regarding the following:	
• Four food groups or the food pyramid (MyPyramid)	The key principle of weight loss therapy is to eat fewer calories than are expended in order to consume fat stores as fuel. Patients need to learn to eat a variety of foods in appropriate portion sizes when changing their eating pattern to ensure lifelong success at weight maintenance.
• Proper serving size	Portion distortion is a growing problem in society; consumers often perceive larger portions as more value for their money, further complicating the problem.
• Caloric content of food	Many patients are unaware of the calories present in low-fat foods.
• Methods of preparation, such as substituting baking and grilling for frying foods	These methods of food preparation decrease the fat content of food.
■ Teach and/or encourage strategies to modify patient behavior such as:	Education as the sole intervention is unlikely to achieve and maintain weight loss. Multifactorial programs that include behavioral interventions and counseling are more successful than education alone. Behavioral therapies used in conjunction with diet and exercise have been shown to be effective for long-term weight reduction.
• Stress management (e.g., meditation or relaxation techniques)	
• Stimulus control—keeping problematic foods out of house or limiting time and place of eating	
• Problem-solving strategies	
• Contingency management—rewarding changes in behavior	
• Cognitive restructuring—changing negative thoughts	
• Building social support	
• How to deal with relapses	
■ Include family, caregiver, or food preparer in nutrition counseling.	Success rates are higher when the family incorporates a healthy eating plan.
▲ Inform the patient about pharmacological agents such as appetite suppressants that can aid in weight loss.	These drugs act by chemically altering the patient's desire to eat.
■ Encourage diabetic patients to attend diabetic classes. Review and reinforce principles of dietary management of diabetes.	Obesity and diabetes are risk factors for coronary artery disease.
■ Review complications associated with obesity.	Patients need to be aware of long-term health problems as stimulus for change.
▲ Refer the patient to commercial weight-loss program as appropriate.	Some individuals require the regimented approach or ongoing support during weight loss, whereas others are able (and may prefer) to manage a weight-loss program independently.
■ Remind the patient that significant weight loss requires a long period.	Some patients are easily frustrated with the amount of time it takes to lose weight. This frustration can lead to weight loss failure. Remind patients that slow weight loss is associated with permanent weight loss.
■ Refer to community support groups as indicated.	Social support is associated with successful weight loss and weight maintenance.

■ = Independent   ▲ = Collaborative

Impaired Oral Mucous Membrane

Definition: Disruption of the lips and/or soft tissue of the oral cavity

Minor irritations of the oral mucous membrane occur occasionally in all persons and are usually viral-related, self-limiting, and easily treated. Patients who have severe stomatitis often have an underlying illness. Patients who are immunocompromised, such as the oncology patient receiving chemotherapy, are often affected with severe tissue disruption and pain. Infections such as candidiasis, if left untreated, can spread through the entire gastrointestinal tract, causing further complications and sometimes perineal pain. Oral mucous membrane problems can be encountered in any setting, especially in home care and hospice settings.

Common Related Factors

Dehydration
Nothing by mouth for more than 24 hours
Mouth breathing
Lack of or decreased salivation
Deficient knowledge of appropriate oral hygiene
Ineffective oral hygiene
Infection
Malnutrition
Medication side effects
Trauma: chemical irritants (e.g., acidic foods, drugs, noxious agents, alcohol); mechanical factors (e.g., ill-fitting dentures, braces, tubes [endotracheal or nasogastric]); surgery in oral cavity
Chemotherapy
Radiation to head or neck

Defining Characteristics

Oral pain or discomfort
Xerostomia (dry mouth)
Coated tongue
Stomatitis
Oral lesions or ulcers
Leukoplakia
Hyperemia
Oral plaque
Desquamation
Vesicles
Edema
Gingival recession
Hemorrhagic gingivitis
Halitosis

Common Expected Outcomes

Patient has healthy oral cavity as evidenced by intact, pink, moist mucous membranes.
Patient demonstrates appropriate oral hygiene practices.
Patient verbalizes absence of discomfort or inflammation of oral mucous membranes.

NOC Outcomes
Oral Health; Tissue Integrity: Skin and Mucous Membranes; Self-Care: Oral Hygiene
NIC Interventions
Oral Health Restoration; Oral Health Maintenance

Ongoing Assessment

Actions/Interventions	Rationales
■ Assess oral hygiene practices.	Information provides direction on possible causative factors and guidance for subsequent education.
■ Assess status of oral mucosa; include tongue, lips, mucous membranes, gums, saliva, and teeth. Use adequate light. Examine after removal of dental appliances. Use a moist, padded tongue blade to gently pull back the cheeks and tongue.	A systematic inspection should be performed for listed sites using a tongue blade to expose areas of the oral cavity. Denture removal is important because lesions may be underlying and further irritated by the appliance. Caregivers also need to be informed of the importance of these assessments.
■ Assess for extensiveness of ulcerations involving the intraoral soft tissues, including palate, tongue, gums, and lips.	Sloughing of mucosal membrane can progress to ulceration.

Actions/Interventions	Rationales
▲ Observe for evidence of infection, and culture lesions as needed. Report to physician or home health nurse. Severe mucositis may manifest as any of the following: • Candidiasis: cottage cheese–like white or pale yellowish patches on tongue, buccal mucosa, and palate • Herpes simplex: painful itching vesicle (typically on upper lips) that ruptures within 12 hours and becomes encrusted with a dried exudate • Gram-positive bacterial infection, specifically staphylococcal and streptococcal infections: dry, raised wartlike yellowish-brown, round plaques on buccal mucosa • Gram-negative bacterial infections: creamy to yellow-white, shiny, nonpurulent patches often seated on painful, red, superficial mucosal ulcers and erosions • Fevers, chills, rigors	Early assessment facilitates prompt treatment. Specific manifestations guide accurate treatment.
■ Assess nutrition status.	Malnutrition can be a contributing cause. Oral fluids are needed for moisture to membranes.
■ Assess for ability to eat and drink.	Inability to chew and swallow may occur secondary to pain of inflamed or ulcerated oral and/or oropharyngeal mucous membranes.

Therapeutic Interventions

Actions/Interventions	Rationales
For hospitalized or home care patients: ■ Implement meticulous mouth care regimen after each meal and every 4 hours while awake. Caregivers need to be taught these procedures. (See Education/Continuity of Care section for description of oral care.)	Mouth care prevents buildup of oral plaque and bacteria. Patients with oral catheters and oxygen may require additional care.
▲ If signs of mild stomatitis occur (sensation of dryness and burning; mild erythema and edema along the mucocutaneous junction): • Increase frequency of oral hygiene by rinsing with one of the suggested solutions between brushings and once during the night. • Discontinue flossing if it causes pain. • Provide systemic or topical analgesics as ordered.	These safety measures reduce further damage and may promote comfort. Increased sensitivity to pain is a result of thinning of oral mucosal lining and may require analgesia.
■ Instruct patient that topical analgesics can be administered as "swish and swallow" or "swish and spit" 15 to 20 minutes before meals, or painted on each lesion immediately before mealtime.	A variety of options are available to patients, such as viscous lidocaine gel (2%). Each must be performed as prescribed for optimal results. These topical analgesics provide a "numbing" feeling to ease discomfort. They may be used alone or combined with a liquid antacid or antihistamine for greater comfort.
• Instruct the patient to hold solution for several minutes before expectorating, and not to use solution if mucosa is severely ulcerated or if drug sensitivity exists.	This technique enhances full therapeutic effect.
• Explain use of topical protective agents:	A variety of more protective topical agents are available to coat the lesions and promote healing as prescribed.
• Zilactin or Zilactin-B	This medicated gel contains benzocaine for pain and is painted on the lesion and allowed to dry to form a protective seal and promote healing of mouth sores.
• Gelclair	This is a bioadherent oral gel that coats the oral cavity and forms a protective barrier to soothe pain.

■ = Independent   ▲ = Collaborative

Actions/Interventions

- Substrate of an antacid and kaolin preparation

- Palifermin

▲ For severe mucositis infection:
  - Administer local antimicrobial agents as ordered.

  - Discontinue use of toothbrush and flossing.

■ Continue use of lubricating ointment on the lips.
■ For eating problems:
  - Encourage diet high in protein and vitamins.
  - Serve foods and fluids lukewarm or cold.
  - Serve frequent small meals or snacks spaced throughout the day.
  - Encourage soft foods (e.g., mashed potatoes, puddings, custards, creamy cereals).
  - Encourage use of a straw.
  - Encourage peach, pear, or apricot nectars and fruit drinks instead of citrus juices.
▲ Refer the patient to the dietitian for instructions on maintenance of a well-balanced diet.

Rationales

This substance is prepared by allowing antacid to settle. The pasty residue is swabbed onto the inflamed areas and, after 15 to 20 minutes, rinsed with saline or water. The residue remains as a protectant on the lesion.

This agent decreases the incidence and duration of severe oral mucositis in patients with hematological cancers undergoing high-dose chemotherapy followed by bone marrow transplantation.

Mycostatin, nystatin, and Mycelex Troche are commonly prescribed.

Brushing could increase damage to ulcerated tissues. A disposable foam stick (Toothette) or sterile cotton swab is a way to gently apply cleansing solutions.

Lubrication prevents drying and cracking.

Dietary modifications may be necessary to promote healing and tissue integrity. The patient may need to select food and fluids that are less irritating to oral tissues. Soft, bland foods served at lukewarm or cool temperatures may feel soothing on oral tissues.

Nutritional expertise may be required to optimize the therapeutic diet needed to promote healing.

Education/Continuity of Care

Actions/Interventions

Instruct the patient or caregiver to perform the following:
■ Gently brush all surfaces of teeth, gums, and tongue with a soft-bristled nylon or foam brush. Floss gently.

■ Brush with a nonabrasive dentifrice such as baking soda.
■ Remove and brush dentures thoroughly during and after meals and as needed.
■ Have loose-fitting dentures adjusted.

■ Rinse the mouth thoroughly during and after brushing.

■ Avoid alcohol-containing mouthwashes and lemon/glycerin type of swabs.

■ Use the following recommended mouth rinses:
  - Baking soda and water (1 teaspoon in 8 ounces)
  - Salt (½ teaspoon), baking soda (1 teaspoon), and water (8 oz)
■ Keep lips moist. Use a lip product or a water-soluble lubricant (e.g., K-Y jelly, Aquaphor Cream).

■ Encourage use of commercial saliva products as indicated.

Rationales

Careful mechanical cleansing and flossing loosens debris, stimulates circulation, and reduces risk for infection. Toothbrushes should be replaced every few months.

Baking soda promotes further cleaning of teeth.

Dental care is key to reducing risk for infection and improving appetite.

Rubbing and irritation from ill-fitting dentures promotes disruption of the oral mucous membrane.

Removing food particles decreases risk for infection related to trapped decaying food.

Alcohol and lemon/glycerin actually dry oral mucous membranes, increasing risk for disruption of mucous membrane.

Commercial mouthwashes can be irritating; special formulas are better tolerated and may reduce irritation and promote healing. Antiplaque mouthwashes are indicated for preventive care.

Lubrication prevents drying and cracking of lips. These products minimize risk for aspirating a non–water-soluble agent.

A variety of synthetic saliva-producing products are available to treat dry mouth.

Actions/Interventions	Rationales
■ Include food items with each meal that require chewing.	Chewing stimulates gingival tissue and promotes circulation.
■ Avoid use of tobacco and alcohol, extremely hot or cold foods, and acidic or highly spiced foods.	These products are irritating and drying to the mucosa, and can aggravate xerostomia.

NANDA-I NDx Acute Pain

Definition: Unpleasant sensory and emotional experience arising from actual or potential tissue damage or described in terms of such damage (International Association for the Study of Pain); sudden or slow onset of any intensity from mild to severe with an anticipated or predictable end and a duration of less than 6 months

Pain is a highly subjective state in which a variety of unpleasant sensations and a wide range of distressing factors may be experienced by the sufferer. Pain may be a symptom of injury or illness. Pain may also arise from emotional, psychological, cultural, or spiritual distress. Pain can be very difficult to explain, because it is unique to the individual. Pain should be accepted as described by the sufferer. Pain assessment can be challenging, especially in older patients, in whom cognitive impairment and sensory-perceptual deficits are more common.

Common Related Factors

Pain resulting from medical problems
Pain resulting from diagnostic procedures or medical treatments
Pain resulting from trauma
Pain resulting from emotional, psychological, spiritual, or cultural distress

Defining Characteristics

Patient reports pain
Guarding behavior, protecting body part
Self-focused
Narrowed focus (e.g., altered time perception, withdrawal from social or physical contact)
Relief or distraction behavior (e.g., moaning, crying, pacing, seeking out other people or activities, restlessness)
Facial mask of pain
Alteration in muscle tone: listlessness or flaccidness; rigidity or tension
Autonomic responses (e.g., diaphoresis; change in blood pressure [BP], pulse rate; pupillary dilation; change in respiratory rate; pallor; nausea)

Common Expected Outcomes

Patient reports satisfactory pain control at a level less than 3 to 4 on a 0 to 10 rating scale.
Patient uses pharmacological and nonpharmacological pain-relief strategies.
Patient exhibits increased comfort such as baseline levels for pulse, blood pressure, respirations, and relaxed muscle tone or body posture.

NOC Outcomes
Comfort Status; Medication Response; Pain Control

NIC Interventions
Analgesic Administration; Conscious Sedation; Pain Management; Patient-Controlled Analgesia Assistance

■ = Independent   ▲ = Collaborative

Ongoing Assessment

Actions/Interventions	Rationales
■ Assess pain characteristics.	Assessment of the pain experience is the first step in planning pain management strategies. The patient is the most reliable source of information about his or her pain.
• Quality (e.g., sharp, burning, shooting) • Severity (scale of 0 [meaning no pain] to 10, with 10 being the most severe) • Location (anatomical description) • Onset (gradual or sudden) • Duration (how long; intermittent or continuous) • Precipitating or relieving factors	Other methods such as a visual analog scale or descriptive scales can be used to identify extent of pain.
■ Observe or monitor signs and symptoms associated with pain, such as BP, heart rate, temperature, color and moisture of skin, restlessness, and ability to focus.	Some people deny the experience of pain when it is present. Attention to associated signs may help the nurse in evaluating pain.
■ Assess for probable cause of pain.	Different etiological factors respond better to different therapies.
■ Assess patient's knowledge of or preference for the array of pain relief strategies available.	Some patients may be unaware of the effectiveness of non-pharmacological methods and may be willing to try them, either with or instead of traditional analgesic medications. Often a combination of therapies (e.g., mild analgesics with distraction or heat) may be more effective.
■ Evaluate the patient's response to pain and medications or therapeutics aimed at abolishing or relieving pain.	It is important to help patients express as factually as possible (i.e., without the effect of mood, emotion, or anxiety) the effect of pain relief measures. Discrepancies between behavior or appearance and what the patient says about pain relief (or lack of it) may be more a reflection of other methods that the patient is using to cope with than pain relief itself.
■ Assess to what degree cultural, environmental, intrapersonal, and intrapsychic factors may contribute to pain or pain relief.	These variables may modify the patient's expression of his or her experience. For example, some cultures openly express feelings, whereas others restrain such expression. However, health care providers should not stereotype any patient response but rather evaluate the unique response of each patient.
■ Evaluate what the pain means to the individual.	The meaning of the pain will directly influence the patient's response. Some patients, especially the dying, may feel that the "act of suffering" meets a spiritual need.
■ Assess the patient's expectations for pain relief.	Some patients may be content to have pain decreased; others will expect complete elimination of pain. This affects their perceptions of the effectiveness of the treatment modality and their willingness to participate in additional treatments.
■ Assess the patient's willingness or ability to explore a range of techniques aimed at controlling pain.	Some patients will feel uncomfortable exploring alternative methods of pain relief. However, patients need to be informed that there are multiple ways to manage pain.
■ Assess appropriateness of the patient as a patient-controlled analgesia (PCA) candidate: no history of substance abuse; no allergy to narcotic analgesics; clear sensorium; cooperative and motivated about use; no history of renal, hepatic, or respiratory disease; manual dexterity; and no history of major psychiatric disorder.	PCA is the IV infusion of a narcotic (usually morphine or Demerol) through an infusion pump that is controlled by the patient. This allows the patient to manage pain relief within prescribed limits. In the hospice or home setting, a nurse or caregiver may be needed to assist the patient in managing the infusion.
■ *If the patient is on PCA, assess the following:* • Pain relief	The basal or lockout dose may need to be increased to cover the patient's pain.

Actions/Interventions

- Intactness of intravenous (IV) line

- Amount of pain medication the patient is requesting

- Possible PCA complications such as excessive sedation, respiratory distress, urinary retention, nausea and vomiting, constipation, and IV site pain, redness, or swelling
- ■ *If the patient is receiving epidural analgesia, assess the following:*
  - Pain relief

  - Numbness, tingling in extremities, a metallic taste in the mouth
  - Possible epidural analgesia complications such as excessive sedation, respiratory distress, urinary retention, or catheter migration

Rationales

If the IV is not patent, the patient will not receive pain medication.

If demands for medication are quite frequent, the patient's dosage may need to be increased. If demands are very low, the patient may require further instruction to properly use PCA.

Early assessment of complications is necessary to prevent serious adverse reactions to opioid analgesics.

Intermittent epidurals require redosing at intervals. Variations in anatomy may result in a "patch effect."

These symptoms may be indicators of an allergic response to the anesthesia agent or of improper catheter placement.

Respiratory depression and intravascular infusion of anesthesia (resulting from catheter migration) can be potentially life threatening.

Therapeutic Interventions

Actions/Interventions

- ■ Anticipate need for pain relief.

- ■ Respond immediately to complaint of pain.

- ■ Eliminate additional stressors or sources of discomfort whenever possible.

- ■ Provide rest periods to facilitate comfort, sleep, and relaxation.

- ▲ Determine the appropriate pain relief method.

Pharmacological methods include the following:
- Nonopioids (acetaminophen), a nonselective nonsteroidal antiinflammatory drug (NSAID), or a selective NSAID (e.g., COX-2 inhibitor)
- Opioid analgesics

- Local anesthetic agents

Rationales

One can most effectively deal with pain by preventing it. Early intervention may decrease the total amount of analgesic required.

In the midst of painful experiences, a patient's perception of time may become distorted. Anxiety and fear about delayed pain relief can exacerbate the pain experience. Prompt responses to complaints may result in decreased anxiety in the patient. Demonstrated concern for the patient's welfare and comfort fosters the development of a trusting relationship.

Patients may experience an exaggeration in pain or a decreased ability to tolerate painful stimuli if environmental, intrapersonal, or intrapsychic factors are further stressing them.

The patient's experiences of pain may become exaggerated as the result of fatigue. In a cyclic fashion, pain may result in fatigue, which may result in exaggerated pain and exhaustion. A quiet environment, a darkened room, and a disconnected phone are all measures geared toward facilitating rest.

Unless contraindicated, all patients with acute pain should receive a nonopioid analgesic around-the-clock.

NSAIDs work in peripheral tissues. Some block synthesis of prostaglandins, which stimulate nociceptors. They are effective in managing mild to moderate pain.

Opioids may be administered orally, intravenously, systemically by PCA systems, or epidurally (either by bolus or continuous infusion). Intramuscular injections are not reliably absorbed. Opioids are indicated for severe pain, especially in the hospice or home setting.

Local anesthetics block pain transmission and are used for pain in specific areas of nerve distribution.

■ = Independent   ▲ = Collaborative

Actions/Interventions	Rationales
Nonpharmacological methods include the following:	
Cognitive-behavioral strategies as follows:	
• Imagery	The use of a mental picture or an imagined event involves use of the five senses to distract oneself from painful stimuli.
• Distraction techniques	These techniques heighten one's concentration upon non-painful stimuli to decrease one's awareness and experience of pain. Some methods are breathing modifications and nerve stimulation.
• Relaxation exercises, biofeedback, breathing exercises, music therapy	Techniques are used to bring about a state of physical and mental awareness and tranquility. The goal of these techniques is to reduce tension, subsequently reducing pain.
Cutaneous stimulation as follows:	
• Massage of affected area when appropriate	Massage interrupts pain transmission, increases endorphin levels, and decreases tissue edema. This intervention may require another person to provide the massage.
• Transcutaneous electrical nerve stimulation (TENS) units	TENS requires the application of two to four skin electrodes. Pain reduction occurs through a mild electrical current. The patient is able to regulate the intensity and frequency of the electrical stimulation.
• Hot or cold compress	Heat reduces pain through improved blood flow to the area and through reduction of pain reflexes. Cold reduces pain, inflammation, and muscle spasticity by decreasing the release of pain-inducing chemicals and slowing the conduction of pain impulses.
▲ Give analgesics as ordered, evaluating effectiveness and observing for any signs and symptoms of untoward effects.	Pain medications are absorbed and metabolized differently by patients, so their effectiveness must be evaluated individually by the patient. Analgesics may cause side effects that range from mild to life threatening.
■ Notify the physician if interventions are unsuccessful or if the current complaint is a significant change from the patient's past experience of pain.	Patients who request pain medications at more frequent intervals than prescribed may actually require higher doses or more potent analgesics.
■ Whenever possible, reassure the patient that pain is time limited and that there is more than one approach to easing pain.	When pain is perceived as everlasting and unresolvable, the patient may give up trying to cope with it or experience a sense of hopelessness and loss of control.
If the patient is on PCA:	
▲ Dedicate use of an IV line for PCA only; consult a pharmacist before mixing drug with narcotic being infused.	IV incompatibilities are possible.
If the patient is receiving epidural analgesia:	
■ Label all tubing (e.g., epidural catheter, IV tubing to epidural catheter) clearly to prevent inadvertent administration of inappropriate fluids or drugs into epidural space.	Inappropriate use of an epidural catheter can cause neurological injury or infection.
For the patient with PCA or epidural analgesia:	
■ Keep Narcan or other narcotic-reversing agent readily available.	In case of respiratory depression, these drugs reverse the narcotic effect.
■ Post "No additional analgesia" sign over bed.	This signage prevents inadvertent analgesic overdosing.

Education/Continuity of Care

Actions/Interventions	Rationales
■ Provide anticipatory instruction on pain causes, appropriate prevention, and relief measures.	Knowledge about what to expect can help the patient develop effective coping strategies for pain management.
■ Instruct the patient to report pain.	Relief measures may be instituted.
■ Instruct the patient to evaluate and report effectiveness of measures used.	Pain relief strategies can be modified to promote more satisfactory comfort levels.

Nursing Diagnosis Care Plans

Actions/Interventions

- Teach the patient effective timing of the medication dose in relation to potentially uncomfortable activities and prevention of peak pain periods.

For patients on PCA or those receiving epidural analgesia:

- Teach the patient preoperatively. Teach the patient the purpose, benefits, techniques of use and action, need for IV line (PCA only), other alternatives for pain control, and the need to notify the nurse of machine alarm and occurrence of untoward effects.

Rationales

Patients need to learn to use pain relief strategies to minimize the pain experience.

Effective pain management with PCA requires patient knowledge of how to use the equipment. Anesthesia effects should not obscure teaching.

NANDA-I NDx **Chronic Pain**

Definition: Unpleasant sensory and emotional experience arising from actual or potential tissue damage or described in terms of such damage (International Association for the Study of Pain); sudden or slow onset of any intensity from mild to severe, constant or recurring without an anticipated or predictable end and a duration of greater than 6 months

Chronic pain may be classified as chronic malignant pain or chronic nonmalignant pain. In the former, the pain is associated with a specific cause such as cancer. With chronic nonmalignant pain, the original tissue injury is not progressive or has been healed. Identifying an organic cause for this type of chronic pain is more difficult.

Chronic pain differs from acute pain in that it is harder for the patient to provide specific information about the location and the intensity of the pain. Over time it becomes more difficult for the patient to differentiate the exact location of the pain and clearly identify the intensity of the pain. The patient with chronic pain often does not present with behaviors and physiological changes associated with acute pain. Family members, friends, co-workers, employers, and health care providers question the legitimacy of the patient's pain complaints because the patient may not look like someone in pain. The patient may be accused of using pain to gain attention or to avoid work and family responsibilities. With chronic pain, the patient's level of suffering usually increases over time. Chronic pain can have a profound impact on the patient's activities of daily living, mobility, activity tolerance, ability to work, role performance, financial status, mood, emotional status, spirituality, family interactions, and social interactions.

Common Related Factor	**Defining Characteristics**
Chronic physical or psychosocial disability	Patient reports pain
	Guarding behavior protecting body part
	Self-focused
	Irritability, restlessness
	Weight changes
	Anorexia
	Changes in sleep pattern
	Fatigue
	Fear of reinjury
	Reduced interaction with people
	Depression
	Altered ability to continue previous activities
	Atrophy of involved muscle group
	Sympathetic mediated responses (e.g., temperature, cold, changes of body position, hypersensitivity)

■ = Independent   ▲ = Collaborative

Nursing Diagnosis Care Plans

Common Expected Outcomes

Patient reports pain at a level less than 3 to 4 on a 0 to 10 rating scale.

Patient uses pharmacological and nonpharmacological pain relief strategies.

Patient engages in desired activities without an increase in pain level.

NOC Outcomes
Pain Control; Quality of Life; Family Coping

NIC Interventions
Pain Management; Medication Management; Acupressure; Heat/Cold Application; Progressive Muscle Relaxation; Transcutaneous Electrical Nerve Stimulation (TENS); Simple Massage

Ongoing Assessment

Actions/Interventions	Rationales
■ Assess pain characteristics: • Quality (e.g., sharp, burning) • Severity (scale of 0 [meaning no pain] to 10 [the most severe pain]) • Location (anatomical description) • Onset (gradual or sudden) • Duration (e.g., continuous, intermittent) • Precipitating factors • Relieving factors	The most reliable source of information about the chronic pain experience is the patient's self-report. Systematic assessment and documentation of the chronic pain experience provides direction for a pain management plan.
■ Assess for signs and symptoms associated with chronic pain such as fatigue, decreased appetite, weight loss, changes in body posture, sleep pattern disturbance, anxiety, irritability, restlessness, or depression.	Patients with chronic pain may not exhibit the physiological changes and behaviors associated with acute pain. Pulse and blood pressure are usually within normal ranges. The guarding behavior of acute pain may become a persistent change in body posture for the patient with chronic pain. Coping with chronic pain can deplete the patient's energy for other activities. The patient often looks tired with a drawn facial expression that lacks animation.
■ Assess the patient's perception of the effectiveness of methods used for pain relief in the past.	Patients with chronic pain have a long history of using many pharmacological and nonpharmacological methods to control their pain. An effective pain management plan will be based on the patient's previous experience with pain relief measures.
■ Evaluate gender, cultural, societal, and religious factors that may influence the patient's pain experience and response to pain relief.	Understanding the variables that affect the patient's pain experience can be useful in developing a care plan that is acceptable to the patient. The patient's heritage will influence the meaning of pain, expressions of suffering associated with pain, and selection of pain management strategies.
■ Assess the patient's expectations about pain relief.	The patient with chronic pain may not expect complete absence of pain but may be satisfied with decreasing the severity of the pain and increasing activity level.
■ Assess the patient's attitudes toward pharmacological and nonpharmacological methods of pain management.	Patients may question the effectiveness of nonpharmacological interventions and see medications as the only treatment for pain. Patients may have misconceptions regarding alternative and complementary therapies for pain relief.
■ For patients taking opioid analgesics, assess for side effects, dependency, and tolerance.	Drug dependence and tolerance to opioid analgesics are concerns in the long-term management of chronic pain. The patient and family may have misconceptions and fears about drug tolerance, dependence, and addiction.

Actions/Interventions

■ Assess the patient's ability to accomplish activities of daily living, instrumental activities of daily living, and demands of daily living.

Rationales

Fatigue, anxiety, and depression associated with chronic pain can limit the person's ability to complete self-care activities and fulfill role responsibilities.

Therapeutic Interventions

Actions/Interventions

■ Encourage the patient to keep a pain diary to help in identifying aggravating and relieving factors of chronic pain.

■ Acknowledge and convey acceptance of the patient's pain experience.

■ Provide the patient and family with information about chronic pain and options available for pain management.

■ Assist the patient in making decisions about selecting a particular pain management strategy.

▲ Refer the patient to a physical therapist for evaluation.

Rationales

Knowledge about factors that influence the pain experience can guide the patient in making decisions about lifestyle modifications that promote more effective pain management.

The patient may have had negative experiences in the past with attitudes of health care providers toward the patient's pain experience. Conveying acceptance of the patient's pain promotes a more cooperative nurse-patient relationship.

Lack of knowledge about the characteristics of chronic pain and pain management strategies can add to the burden of pain in the patient's life.

Guidance and support from the nurse can increase the patient's willingness to choose new interventions to promote pain relief. A combination of nonpharmacological therapies and analgesic medications may be most effective. Nonopioid medications are preferred medications because of their low side-effect profile, especially among older patients. Medications should be given around-the-clock to achieve a consistent level of pain relief and comfort. The oral route is preferred.

The physical therapist can help the patient with exercises to promote muscle strength and joint mobility and therapies to promote relaxation of tense muscles. These interventions can contribute to effective pain management.

Education/Continuity of Care

Actions/Interventions

■ Teach the patient and family about using nonpharmacological pain management strategies.

• Cold applications

• Heat applications

• Massage of the painful area

Rationales

Knowledge about how to implement nonpharmacological pain management strategies can help the patient and family gain maximum benefit from these interventions.

Cold reduces pain, inflammation, and muscle spasticity by decreasing the release of pain-inducing chemicals and slowing the conduction of pain impulses. This intervention requires no special equipment and can be cost-effective. Cold applications should last about 20 to 30 min/hr.

Heat reduces pain through improved blood flow to the area and through reduction of pain reflexes. This is a cost-effective intervention that requires no special equipment. Heat applications should last no more than 20 min/hr. Special attention needs to be given to preventing burns with this intervention.

Massage interrupts pain transmission, increases endorphin levels, and decreases tissue edema. This intervention may require another person to provide the massage. Many health insurance programs will not reimburse for the cost of therapeutic massage.

■ = Independent   ▲ = Collaborative

Actions/Interventions	Rationales
• Progressive relaxation, imagery, and music	These centrally acting techniques for pain management work through reducing muscle tension and stress. The patient may feel an increased sense of control over his or her pain. Guided imagery can help the patient explore images about pain, pain relief, and healing. These techniques require practice to be effective.
• Distraction	Distraction is a temporary pain management strategy that works by increasing the pain threshold. It should be used for a short duration, usually less than 2 hours at a time. Prolonged use can add to fatigue and increased pain when the distraction is no longer present.
• Acupressure	Acupressure involves finger pressure applied to acupressure points on the body. Using the gate control theory, the technique works to interrupt pain transmission by "closing the gate." This approach requires training and practice.
• Transcutaneous electrical nerve stimulation (TENS)	TENS requires the application of two to four skin electrodes. Pain reduction occurs through a mild electrical current. The patient is able to regulate the intensity and frequency of the electrical stimulation.
■ Teach the patient and family about the use of pharmacological interventions for pain management:	
• Nonopioids (acetaminophen; nonselective, nonsteroidal antiinflammatory drugs [NSAIDs]; and selective NSAIDs [COX-2 inhibitors])	These drugs are the first step in an analgesic ladder. They work in peripheral tissues by inhibiting the synthesis of prostaglandins that cause pain, inflammation, and edema. The advantages of these drugs are that they can be taken orally and are not associated with dependency and addiction. They should be given around-the-clock to provide a consistent level of pain relief.
• Opioid analgesics (narcotics)	These drugs act on the central nervous system to reduce pain by binding with opiate receptors throughout the body. The side effects associated with this group of drugs tend to be more significant than those with the NSAIDs. Nausea, vomiting, constipation, sedation, respiratory depression, tolerance, and dependency are of concern in patients using these drugs for chronic pain management.
• Antidepressants • Anticonvulsants	Antidepressants and anticonvulsants may be useful adjuncts in a total program of pain management, especially for those with chronic neuropathic pain. In addition to their effects on the patient's mood, the antidepressants may have analgesic properties apart from their antidepressant actions.
■ Assist the patient and family in identifying lifestyle modifications that may contribute to effective pain management. Guide the patient to plan activities during periods of greatest relief from pain.	Changes in work routines, household responsibilities, and the home physical environment may be needed to promote more effective pain management. Providing the patient and family with ongoing support and guidance will increase the success of these strategies.
■ Refer the patient and family to community support groups and self-help groups for people coping with chronic pain.	Adding to the patient's network of social support can reduce the burden of suffering associated with chronic pain and provide additional resources.

Related Care Plans

Acute pain, p. 151
Fatigue, p. 66

NANDA-I NDx Post-Trauma Syndrome

Definition: Sustained maladaptive response to a traumatic, overwhelming event

Post-trauma syndrome, also called post-traumatic stress disorder (PTSD), occurs in individuals who have experienced, witnessed, or been confronted by an event or events that have involved actual or threatened death or serious injury or a threat to the physical integrity of self or others. The individual's response involves intense fear, helplessness, or horror. Typically the maladaptive response(s) continue beyond 1 month, causing significant distress or impairment in social, occupational, physical, spiritual or psychological functioning. These maladaptive responses may be acute or chronic.

Common Related Factors

Abuse (physical and psychosocial)
Being held prisoner of war
Criminal victimization
Events outside the range of usual human experience such as disasters, epidemics, and wars
Sudden destruction of one's home or community
Serious injury, accidents, or threat to self or loved one
Torture
Tragic occurrence involving multiple deaths
Witnessing mutilation or violent death

Defining Characteristics

Aggression, anger
Alienation, avoidance, detachment
Anxiety
Compulsive behavior
Denial
Depression
Difficulty concentrating, inability to make decisions
Exaggerated startle response, hypervigilance
Fear
Flashbacks, intrusive thoughts and dreams, nightmares
Gastric and neurosensory irritability
Guilt, shame
Headaches
Panic attacks
Psychogenic amnesia
Rage
Reports feeling numb
Self-injury
Sleep disturbance
Substance abuse
Suicidal thoughts/attempts

Common Expected Outcomes

Patient experiences fewer flashbacks, intrusive recollections, and nightmares.
Patient demonstrates increased concentration.
Patient contacts nurse/therapist/physician for appointment when symptoms reappear or increase.
Patient verbalizes reduction of depressed mood, anxiety, sleep disturbance, and physical symptoms.
Patient verbalizes absence of physical aggression and suicidal ideation.
Patient verbalizes hopefulness and empowerment.

NOC Outcomes
Aggression Self-Control; Coping; Hope; Mood Equilibrium; Personal Resiliency; Suicide Self-Restraint

NIC Interventions
Active Listening; Anger Control Assistance; Emotional Support; Guilt Work Facilitation; Hope Instillation; Mood Management; Support Group

■ = Independent ▲ = Collaborative

Ongoing Assessments

Actions/Interventions	Rationales
■ Identify the person's history for traumatic events.	PTSD may develop months or years following a traumatic event. Childhood losses, exposure to violence, or trauma may manifest as PTSD in adulthood. People who faced combat in wars are more likely to have delayed onset and prolonged duration of PTSD.
■ Assess the presence and degree of depression and anxiety.	A thorough assessment results in early identification and intervention to prevent escalation of symptoms. The person with PTSD may withdraw from interactions with family, friends, and co-workers.
■ Assess for statements of guilt or self-blame for the traumatic event or own survival.	The person may feel responsible for event or the deaths of others. The person's religious or cultural heritage may support feelings of guilt or shame related to behavior during the traumatic event. The person may make statements about not having done enough in the event or not deserving to survive the event.
■ Identify fearful reactions or hypervigilance to ordinary objects or situations.	Ordinary objects and situations (e.g. walking in crowded areas, sudden loud noises, driving in heavy traffic, approaching strangers) may cause the person to experience feelings from the original traumatic event. The person may startle easily or respond aggressively in response to these situations.
■ Assess the presence and degree of suicidal ideation, including a plan, means, past attempts, family history, and ability to agree to a contract for safety.	Feelings of guilt, low self-worth as a survivor, or depression may lead to thoughts of suicide. A thorough assessment results in early identification and intervention to prevent self-harm.
■ Assess the presence and degree of homicidal ideation, including a plan, identified target/person, history of violence towards others, intended means, and availability of means.	Disorganized thinking and increasing anxiety may lead to aggression and violence directed toward others. Domestic violence may develop as part of PTSD. A thorough assessment results in early identification and intervention to prevent other-directed violence.
■ Assess effectiveness of relationships with family, friends, and co-workers.	The person experiencing PTSD is more likely to react aggressively with family members, leading to domestic violence. Family members, friends, and co-workers may not know how to effectively provide support. Family and friends may be overly attentive or withdrawn. Either type of reaction is not supportive to the person with PTSD. Inability to function in the workplace may lead to being fired and unemployment.
■ Assess for adherence to prescribed medication regimen.	Adherence to drug therapy can lessen the symptoms or prevent relapse. Antidepressants (e.g., selective serotonin reuptake inhibitors [SSRIs]) have been used effectively in the management of PTSD.
■ Assess for active substance abuse.	The person may abuse alcohol or drugs to blunt the painful feelings associated with the trauma. These behaviors will interfere with and delay the recovery process.
■ Monitor sleep patterns and vital signs routinely.	Sleep disturbance is a common manifestation of PTSD. Increased temperature, heart rate, respirations and blood pressure can indicate increase in feelings of anxiety.

Therapeutic Interventions

Actions/Interventions	Rationales
■ Establish trust by being nonjudgmental and honest; offer empathy and support; allow the person to feel a sense of control.	Developing trust following trauma may be difficult for patients.

Actions/Interventions	Rationales
■ Assure patient that his or her feelings and behaviors are typical following a traumatic event.	Patients often believe they are guilty for the event and that they are going crazy. The person needs to understand that his or her feelings are a normal response to an extraordinary event.
■ Maintain safety for the patient and his or her environment.	A patient's anxiety can escalate to panic, and he or she may become suicidal or outwardly violent.
■ Provide the person with safe means for expressing feelings, especially those of anger and aggression.	Physical activities, journaling, or drawing give the person an outlet for intense emotions. These activities provide opportunities to dissipate the energy associated with these emotions. The energy is directed to the activity rather than toward self or others. Creative expression of emotions may facilitate coping with the traumatic event.
■ Assist in recognizing the connection between the trauma experience and their current feelings.	Patients are often unaware of this connection.
■ Assist in evaluating past behaviors in the context of the traumatic event, not in the context of current values.	Patients are often guilty about past behaviors and judgmental toward themselves.
■ Encourage adaptive coping behaviors based on past successes.	Patient might be using maladaptive or dysfunctional coping to avoid dealing with feelings and issues.
■ Encourage the establishment or reestablishment of healthy relationships.	Relationships may have been negatively affected by patient's feelings of detachment.
■ Monitor adherence to prescribed medication regimen.	Adherence to prescribed medication regimen can prevent or lessen exacerbation of symptoms.
■ Follow hospital/agency policy regarding legal/ethical responsibilities for reporting to authorities.	Health care professionals are mandatory reporters and are obliged to report suspected/actual abuse to safeguard protected populations.

Education/Continuity of Care

Actions/Interventions	Rationales
■ Teach distinction of anxiety that is connected to identifiable sources/objects and anxiety for which there is no identifiable object or source.	Knowledge of anxiety and its related components increases the person's feelings of control.
■ Teach anxiety-reducing strategies: • Progressive relaxation • Mindful meditation • Slow deep-breathing exercises • Focusing on single object in the room • Listening to soothing music or relaxation tapes • Visual imagery	These activities assist in lessening anxiety and its related components. Knowledge and use of them increases the patient's control over the disorder.
■ Encourage the patient to seek support persons/groups to assist with performing personal tasks and activities that are currently difficult to perform.	A strong support system will assist the patient in avoiding anxiety-provoking situations/activities.
■ Educate the patient on the actions, benefits, and side effects of prescribed medications.	Knowledge can lessen the seriousness of potential side effects and increase the likelihood of patient adherence to prescribed regimen.
■ Educate the patient on the importance of limiting caffeine, nicotine, and other central nervous system stimulants.	Limiting these substances prevents/minimizes the physical symptoms of anxiety.
■ Teach family members about post-trauma syndrome and methods to provide helpful support.	Family members who did not experience the traumatic event may have unrealistic expectations about the patient's response to and recovery from the trauma. When family members can provide effective support, they may feel less helpless.

■ = Independent ▲ = Collaborative

Powerlessness

Definition: Perception that one's own action will not significantly affect an outcome; a perceived lack of control over a current situation or immediate happening

Powerlessness may be expressed at any time during a patient's illness. During an acute episode, people used to being in control may temporarily find themselves unable to navigate the health care system and environment. The medical jargon, the swiftness with which decisions are expected to be made, and the vast array of health care providers to which the patient has to relate can all cause a feeling of powerlessness. This response is compounded by patients of cultural, religious, or ethnic backgrounds that differ from those of the dominant health care providers. Patients with chronic, debilitating, or terminal illnesses may have long-term feelings of powerlessness because they are unable to change their inevitable outcomes. Older patients are especially susceptible to the threat of loss of control and independence that comes with aging, as well as the consequences of illness and disease. Patients suffering from feelings of powerlessness may be seen in the hospital, ambulatory care, rehabilitation, or home care environment.

Common Related Factors

Health care environment
Illness-related regimen
Acute or chronic illness
Inability to communicate effectively
Dependence on others for activities of daily living
Inability to perform role responsibilities
Progressive debilitating disease
Terminal prognosis
Loss of control over life decisions
Lack of knowledge

Defining Characteristics

Expression of having no control or influence over situation or outcome
Nonparticipation in care or decision making when opportunities are provided
Reluctance to express true feelings
Diminished patient-initiated interaction
Passivity, submissiveness, apathy
Withdrawal, depression
Aggressive, acting out, and/or violent behavior
Feeling of hopelessness
Decreased participation in activities of daily living

Common Expected Outcomes

Patient begins to identify ways to achieve control over personal situation.
Patient expresses sense of personal control.
Patient makes decisions free from undue pressure from others.
Patient expresses satisfaction with life choices.

NOC Outcomes
Health Beliefs: Perceived Control; Participation: Health Care Decisions
NIC Interventions
Self-Responsibility Facilitation; Self-Esteem Enhancement

Ongoing Assessment

Actions/Interventions	Rationales
■ Assess the patient's power needs or needs for control.	Patients are usually able to identify those aspects of self-governance that they miss most and that are most important to them.
■ Assess for feelings of hopelessness, depression, and apathy.	These feelings may be a component of powerlessness.
■ Identify the patient's locus of control.	The degree to which people attribute responsibility to themselves (internal control) versus other forces (external control) determines locus of control.

Actions/Interventions

- Identify situations and/or interactions that may add to the patient's sense of powerlessness.

- Assess the patient's decision-making ability.

- Assess the role the illness plays in the patient's sense of powerlessness.

- Assess the impact of powerlessness on the patient's physical condition (e.g., appearance, oral intake, hygiene, sleep habits).

- Note whether the patient demonstrates a need for information about illness, treatment plan, and procedures.
- Evaluate the effects of the information provided on the patient's behavior and feelings.

- Assess whether the patient has an advance directive, a durable power of attorney for health care, or a living will.

- Assess the patient's desires or abilities to be an active participant in self-care.

Rationales

Many medical routines are superimposed on patients without ever receiving their permission, fostering a sense of powerlessness. It is important for health care providers to recognize the patient's right to refuse procedures such as feeding tubes and intubation.

Powerlessness is not the same as the inability to make a decision. It is the feeling that one has lost the implicit power for self-governance.

Uncertainty about events, duration and course of illness, prognosis, and dependence on others for help and treatments involved can contribute to powerlessness.

Individuals may feel as though they are unable to control very basic aspects of life. Patients most vulnerable to powerlessness are those who are increasingly susceptible to stressful events (e.g., illness with impaired mobility; older age).

This information will differentiate powerlessness from knowledge deficit.

A patient experiencing powerlessness may ignore information. A patient simply experiencing a knowledge deficit may be mobilized to act in his or her own best interest after information is given and options are explored. The act of providing information may heighten a patient's sense of autonomy.

These legal documents express the patient's desires for health care treatment and designate another person to act on his or her behalf.

Facilitating knowledge needed to improve self-care will make a difference in future health care decision making, especially in older patients. Praise and positive reinforcement for self-care are profound motivators for enhancing self-esteem.

Therapeutic Interventions

Actions/Interventions

- Encourage verbalization of feelings, perceptions, and fears about making decisions.
- Consult the patient regarding his or her care (e.g., treatment options, convenience of visits, or time of activities of daily living).
- Acknowledge the patient's knowledge of self and personal situation.
- Enhance the patient's sense of autonomy. Do this by involving the patient in decision making, by giving information, and by enabling the patient to control the environment as appropriate.

- Encourage the patient to identify strengths.

- Assist the patient in reexamining negative perceptions of the situation.

Rationales

This approach creates a supportive climate and sends a message of caring.

This approach by the nurse promotes self-control and ownership by respecting and encouraging patient involvement in decision making.

A patient's perception of powerlessness can make a profound alteration in his or her thought processes.

Patients become dependent in the "high-tech" medical environment and may relegate decision making to the health care providers. This may be especially evident in patients of cultures or ethnic heritages different from the dominant health care providers.

Review of past coping experiences and prior decision-making skills may assist the patient in recognizing inner strengths. Self-confidence and security come with a sense of control.

The patient may have misconceptions or unrealistic expectations for the situation.

■ = Independent   ▲ = Collaborative

Actions/Interventions	Rationales
■ Eliminate unpredictability of events by allowing adequate preparation for tests or procedures.	Information can provide a sense of control.
■ Encourage increased responsibility for self.	The perception of powerlessness may negate the patient's attention to areas where self-care is attainable; however, the patient may require significant support systems and resources to accomplish goals.
■ Implement individualized strategies to provide hygiene, diet, and sleep.	Allowing or helping the patient to decide when and how these things are to be accomplished will increase the patient's sense of autonomy.
■ Give the patient control over his or her environment. Encourage the patient to furnish the environment with those things that he or she finds comforting.	This technique enhances the patient's sense of autonomy and acknowledges his or her right to have dominion over controllable aspects of life. It applies to the hospital as well as the extended care or home care environment.
■ Assist with creating a timetable to guide increased responsibility in the future.	With short hospital stays, patients may find themselves helpless and dependent on discharge, and they may unrealistically perceive their situation as unchangeable. Use of realistic short-term goals for resuming aspects of self-care may foster confidence in one's abilities.
■ Provide positive feedback for making decisions and participating in self-care.	Success fosters confidence in abilities and a sense of control.
■ Assist the patient in identifying the significance of culture, religion, race, gender, and age on his or her sense of powerlessness.	Especially in the hospital environment when the patient does not speak the dominant language, food is different, and customs such as bathing, personal space, and privacy differ, patients may retreat and develop a sense of powerlessness. Use of patient advocates and outreach workers from a given ethnic community may provide a bridge to the health care providers.
■ Avoid using coercive power when approaching patient.	This approach may intensify the patient's feelings of powerlessness and result in decreased self-esteem.
■ Assist the patient in developing advance directives.	Allowing or helping the patient to decide when and how things are to be accomplished will increase his or her sense of autonomy.

Education/Continuity of Care

Actions/Interventions	Rationales
■ Assist family members or caregivers in allowing independent activities within abilities.	Caregivers may foster a sense of dependence in their efforts to be helpful and caring.
■ Refer to support groups or self-help groups and community resources as appropriate.	Persons who have "been there" may be most helpful in providing the supportive empathy necessary to move the patient to the next level of independence and control.
▲ Suggest consultation with other health care team members to ensure best practices are provided.	Access to needed health professionals ensures the provision of quality care.

Rape-Trauma Syndrome

Definition: Sustained maladaptive response to a forced, violent sexual penetration against the victim's will and consent

Rape-trauma syndrome refers to the immediate period of psychological disorganization and the long-term process of reorganization that occur as a result of attempted or actual sexual assault. Every survivor of sexual assault will express unique emotional needs and may respond differently to rape. However, almost all survivors, male and female, experience elements of the syndrome as a response to the extreme stress, profound fear of death, and sense of violation and vulnerability. Sexual assault survivors may suffer various effects of this violent crime for the remainder of their lives. Recovery from the physical trauma associated with the rape may prolong and complicate the survivor's response to and recovery from the psychological trauma. Cultural bias, social attitudes, and preconceived ideas about rape victims may make it difficult for victims to report the crime. These biases and attitudes also make effective recovery more difficult for survivors. Improved education about the impact of rape on survivors has lead to more supportive responses by law enforcement officers, emergency care first responders, and emergency department care providers.

Common Related Factors

Rape
Sexual assault trauma

Defining Characteristics

Aggression and anger
Agitation, anxiety, hyperalertness
Change in relationships
Confusion
Denial
Disorganization
Embarrassment, guilt, humiliation, self-blame, shame
Fear, paranoia, phobias
Impaired decision making, helplessness, powerlessness
Mood swings
Muscles spasms and tension
Sleep disturbances
Suicide attempts
Vulnerability

Common Expected Outcomes

Patient verbalizes relief or reduction of discomfort from physical injuries.
Patient adopts healthy coping behaviors.
Patient uses community resources to support ongoing adjustment.
Patient refers to self as a victim or survivor not as being responsible for the rape.

NOC Outcomes

Abuse Recovery: Emotional; Abuse Recovery: Sexual; Coping; Sexual Functioning; Stress Level

NIC Interventions

Rape-Trauma Treatment; Counseling; Crisis Intervention

Ongoing Assessment

Actions/Interventions

■ Assess the degree of injury sustained during the assault: bruises; lacerations; abrasions; scratches; vaginal, oral, and rectal trauma; knife wounds; gunshot wounds; strangulation marks.

Rationales

Injuries range from minor to disabling and life threatening. Serious genital injury is a common component of sexual assault. All injuries, regardless of the extent, may have a strong emotional impact on the victim. The patient may have been unconscious or psychologically guarded during the assault and may not remember details to be able to report injuries.

■ = Independent ▲ = Collaborative

Nursing Diagnosis Care Plans

Actions/Interventions

■ Assess for emotional and behavioral responses.

■ Identify the patient's previous coping mechanisms, including cultural, religious, and personal beliefs about assault.

■ Assess the survivor's readiness for a physical, genital, and/or pelvic examination.

■ Listen for the language the patient uses to describe himself or herself and his or her feelings about the assault.

■ Assess the response of family members and significant others toward the patient: blaming the victim for the rape; inability to talk about the incident; expressions of guilt, anger, embarrassment, or humiliation.

Rationales

Defensive coping behaviors that seem normal after sexual assault may become ineffective if they persist and interfere with recovery.

In a crisis, individuals fall back on old coping mechanisms that may or may not be effective in the present situation. Beliefs about sexual assault will influence the patient's ability to come to terms with the event, and whether family and friends will be effective support systems.

The patient may respond to the intrusiveness of the examination as a continuation of the sexual assault. The patient may not understand the need to determine the extent of physical trauma and collect forensic evidence.

It is considered a normal initial response for survivors to express feelings of shame or guilt about the assault. The patient may describe himself or herself as dirty and unclean. The patient may need anticipatory guidance to reframe these feelings and view himself or herself as a victim and survivor of the assault. When extremely negative feelings persist for a prolonged period of time, they pose a substantial threat to the recovery of the survivor.

Family members and significant others may struggle with their own feelings about the patient and the rape. They may experience feelings and reactions similar to the patient. They may blame the victim based on cultural, religious, or personal beliefs about rape. Their responses may interfere with the survivor's recovery.

Therapeutic Interventions

Actions/Interventions

■ Assure the survivor of immediate safety.

▲ Provide access to sexual assault advocate, crisis intervention specialist, or social services counselor.

■ Assist the survivor in identifying and contacting family or significant others.

■ Facilitate the survivor's expression of feelings and need to talk about the sexual assault. Show interest, respect, and caring without judgment. Avoid statements and questions that may be interpreted as accusing or blaming the survivor.

　• Acknowledge the survivor's mixed feelings about the assault.

　• Encourage the survivor to direct anger and hostility toward the assailant not himself or herself.

■ Prepare the patient for the physical, genital, and/or pelvic examination.

Rationales

Predominant emotions experienced by the survivor include horror, terror, fear of death, humiliation, and anger. They may feel vulnerable and threatened in unfamiliar surroundings. Survivors need to know that they are in a safe place and protected from further harm.

Specially trained sexual assault response teams provide effective support and immediate crisis intervention to survivors.

The survivor may need help identifying the person who is likely to be the most supportive at this time.

The patient may be experiencing a state of emotional or psychological shock and require time to process reactions to the sexual assault. Survivors need help understanding that they did what was necessary to survive the assault, regardless of how others may interpret their behavior during the assault.

The survivor may be feeling guilt and shame, as well as anger, aggression, and hostility.

Feelings of anger toward the offender need to be expressed to promote effective coping.

Actions/Interventions

- Obtain written consent.
- Explain each step of the procedure in advance, and ask permission.

- Collect and prepare evidence in accordance with procedures required by law

▲ Provide appropriate care for wounds and physical symptoms.
  - Administer tetanus toxoid.
  - Provide wound care.
  - Administer medications for pain, nausea, muscle tension.
  - Administer medications to prevent sexually transmitted infections.
  - Offer the survivor medication to prevent pregnancy.

■ Make sure the survivor does not go home alone upon discharge. If no family or significant other is available, the sexual assault response team may arrange for someone to accompany the patient home.

Rationales

Survivors may experience a profound loss of control over their bodies. Obtaining consent and asking permission during the examination helps the survivor regain a sense of control. The survivor needs to understand that some specimens collected during the examination will be sent to the hospital laboratory for analysis. Other specimens will be sent to a forensic laboratory and considered evidence if the offender is caught and faces criminal charges.

Evidence must be collected and protected until it can be given to the proper law enforcement officials. Deviation from procedures may result in evidence being disallowed in future court proceedings.

The extent of physical injury sustained during the assault will determine priorities for physical care. Tetanus toxoid is given as prophylaxis if the patient has not had a booster immunization in the previous 10 years. The patient needs to know that medication is available to prevent pregnancy that might occur from the rape. The survivor's cultural and religious beliefs may influence a decision to accept this type of medication.

The patient needs to feel safe and protected during the transition from hospital to home. Feelings of vulnerability and fear of strangers may continue for an extended period of time.

Education/Continuity of Care

Actions/Interventions

▲ Refer the survivor, family and significant others for individual and/or family counseling to begin within 1 to 2 days of the assault.

■ Educate the survivor, family, and significant others about the potential long-term effects of rape-trauma syndrome:
  - Mood swings
  - Sleep disorders
  - Difficulty resuming sexual activity

■ Discuss with family and significant others ways to provide support for the survivor: encouraging verbalization of feelings, help resuming usual activities, avoiding overprotecting the survivor, directing feelings of anger toward the assailant, holding and touching the survivor so as not to reinforce feelings of shame and being unclean, being nonjudgmental.

■ Refer the survivor for follow-up care to assess for complications from the physical trauma of the assault.

Rationales

Professional counseling provides the survivor and family members with a mechanism of support during this phase of crisis recovery.

The survivor needs to understand that anger, fear, sadness, hyperalertness, insomnia, depression, and nightmares are some of the symptoms that may be experienced for months and years after the assault. The survivor may be hesitant or fearful to resume intimate relationships and sexual activity. These symptoms may be triggered by new situational crises later in life. Many long-term symptoms reflect the survivor's struggle to reorganize his or her life.

The type of support and caring relationships the survivor experiences during crisis recovery will have a direct effect on long-term efforts to reorganize his or her life.

The survivor may need assessment for sexually transmitted infections, pregnancy, and human immunodeficiency virus (HIV) at appropriate intervals following the assault.

■ = Independent   ▲ = Collaborative

NANDA-I NDx **Relocation Stress Syndrome**

Definition: Physiological and/or psychological disturbance following transfer from one environment to another

The physiological and psychological stress associated with relocation is now recognized as so extreme that it is associated with the stress of divorce or the death of a loved one. Adjustment to moving from what was once familiar to what is a new environment can last for several months to several years and longer. It is suggested that, in older adults in particular, recovery from such a significant move leads to significant decline and many times leads to death. The degree of severity depends on many variables such as age, stage of life, personality, number of concurrent losses, amount of preparation, and the degree and type of support before, during, and after the move. This syndrome may also be seen in the hospitalized patient who experiences several hospital locations within one hospital stay.

Common Related Factors

Decreased health status
Feelings of powerlessness
Impaired psychosocial health
Isolation
Lack of adequate support systems
Lack of predeparture counseling
Language barrier
Move from one environment to another
Passive coping
Past, concurrent, and recent losses
Unpredictability of the experience

Defining Characteristics

Alienation
Aloneness; loneliness
Anger
Anxiety
Concern over relocation
Depression
Dependency
Fear
Frustration
Loss of identity, self-worth, or self-esteem
Increased physical symptoms or illness
Increased verbalization of needs
Insecurity
Pessimism
Sleep disturbances
Verbalizes unwillingness to move
Withdrawal
Worry

Common Expected Outcomes

The patient maintains orientation and safety in new environment.
The patient verbalizes acceptance of recent relocation.
The patient expresses satisfaction with new living arrangements.

NOC Outcomes

Anxiety Level; Coping; Personal Resiliency; Psychosocial Adjustment: Life Change

NIC Intervention

Relocation Stress Reduction

Ongoing Assessments

Actions/Interventions

■ Determine the reason for the relocation and the patient's degree of participation in the relocation decision.

■ Assess patient's orientation.

Rationales

An anticipated and planned move is often less stressful for the person than a move that is forced upon the person. This option is not usually available in acute care settings.

Loss of familiar surroundings and changes in daily routines may lead to disorientation and acute confusion, especially in the older adult.

Actions/Interventions	Rationales
■ Assess the presence and degree of anxiety.	A thorough assessment results in early identification and intervention to prevent escalation of symptoms.
■ Obtain a history of recent losses and life changes.	A person's ability to adjust to a move may be compromised when he or she is coping with other losses and significant life changes. Grief is a common reaction to the loss of familiar surroundings. Other life changes such as decreased health status and loss of independence contribute to the stress of relocation.
■ Assess the patient's physiological status and level of functioning.	The stress associated with relocation may contribute to an exacerbation of physiological symptoms and a decline in the person's level of function.
■ Explore what is most important to the person.	The impact of relocation on the person is related to the loss of things the person values, such as closeness to family and friends or loss of personal belongings.
■ Determine previous coping strategies.	Previous coping strategies may not support adjust to the current move.
■ Assess the person's level of social support.	The person's adjustment to the move may be compromised if he or she is unable to maintain desired contact with family and friends.

Therapeutic Interventions

Actions/Interventions	Rationales
■ Include the person in making decisions about the move, when possible.	The person's adjustment to the move will be less stressful when he or she participates in planning the change.
■ Include significant others in discussions and decisions as appropriate.	Decisions following acute stress can be detrimental for the person. Significant others are trusted individuals with whom the patient is familiar.
■ Avoid unplanned or abrupt transfers, especially at night or change of shift.	Unplanned or abrupt moves disrupt feelings of safety and increase the risk for acute confusion in the institutionalized patient.
■ Allow personal belongings to be arranged in the room before the person arrives.	Seeing familiar and valued objects can help the person feel less disoriented in the new surroundings.
■ Assign a current resident to be a "buddy" to the person.	The use of a buddy may reduce the person's anxiety level by providing orientation to the new surroundings. This relationship helps the person establish interpersonal relationships and a support system in the new location.
■ Arrange for maintenance of familiar routines and consistency in contact with care providers.	Maintaining familiar daily routines provides the person with a sense of normalcy. Interactions with the same people each day builds a sense of safety in the new location. Frequent changes in routines and care providers may contribute to anxiety and disorientation.
■ Encourage expression of feelings.	Exploration of feelings assists in perceiving the situation more realistically and assists with adaptability. Active listening can facilitate grief work related to losses of home, friends, and independence.
■ Reorient the person to new environment as often as needed.	Knowing where a person is, how he or she came to be here, and why he or she is here assists in the patient feeling safe. This needs to be repeated frequently for acutely ill patients in intensive care settings where environmental stimuli can overtax their coping abilities.
■ Use calm, reassuring approach.	Anxiety may be reduced in a calm environment.
■ Seek to understand the patient's perspective of the event.	Demonstration of understanding is part of building trusting relationships in the new location.
■ Arrange situations to encourage the patient's autonomy.	Autonomy reinforces self-worth and feelings of value.

■ = Independent ▲ = Collaborative

Actions/Interventions

- Provide the opportunity to actively participate in own care.
- Encourage participation in social activities.

Rationales

Taking responsibility for making choices will increase feelings of control and decrease feelings of powerlessness.

The person may need help establishing friendships in the new location.

Education/Continuity of Care

Actions/Interventions

- Allow family members to discuss their concerns and feelings related to the move.

- Teach the person the characteristics of normal grief.

- Discuss with the person and significant others the differences in patterns of adjustment.

- ▲ Refer family members to counseling and social services, as appropriate.

Rationales

Family members may feel a mixture of relief and guilt related to the move of the patient. They may have unresolved issues with the patient that come to the surface as a result of the move.

Knowing what is normal can provide reassurance and decrease anxiety. The person needs to understand that grief is part of any loss or significant life change. Many people limit their understanding of grief to death.

The person and family members need to understand that people adjust to change in different ways. Identification of differences assists in normalizing the patient's feelings.

Family members may benefit from professional support services to facilitate the relocation of the patient. The family may need help adjusting to changes in responsibilities and roles as a result of the relocation.

NANDA-I
NDx

Self-Care Deficit

Definition: Impaired ability to perform or complete activities of daily living for oneself, such as feeding, dressing, bathing, toileting

The nurse may encounter the patient with a self-care deficit in the hospital or in the community. The deficit may be the result of transient limitations, such as those one might experience while recuperating from surgery, or the result of progressive deterioration that erodes the individual's ability or willingness to perform the activities required to care for himself or herself. Careful examination of the patient's deficit is required in order to be certain that the patient is not failing at self-care because of a lack of material resources or a problem with arranging the environment to suit the patient's physical limitations. The nurse coordinates services to maximize the independence of the patient and to ensure that the environment the patient lives in is safe and supportive of his or her special needs. This care plan combines a variety of self-care deficits into one comprehensive plan.

Common Related Factors

Neuromuscular impairment
Musculoskeletal impairment
Impaired mobility or transfer ability
Cognitive impairment
Perceptual impairment
Fatigue, weakness
Pain
Severe anxiety
Decreased motivation
Environmental barriers

Defining Characteristics

Inability to feed self independently
Inability to dress self independently
Inability to bathe and groom self independently
Inability to perform toileting tasks independently
Inability to transfer from bed to wheelchair
Inability to ambulate independently
Inability to perform miscellaneous common tasks such as telephoning and writing

Common Expected Outcomes

Patient safely performs (to maximum ability) self-care activities.

Patient identifies resources that are useful in optimizing one's autonomy and independence.

NOC Outcomes
Self-Care: Eating; Self-Care: Bathing; Self-Care: Dressing; Self-Care: Grooming; Self-Care: Hygiene; Self-Care: Toileting

NIC Interventions
Self-Care Assistance: Bathing/Hygiene; Self-Care Assistance: Dressing/Grooming; Self-Care Assistance: Feeding; Self-Care Assistance: Toileting; Environment Management

Ongoing Assessment

Actions/Interventions	Rationales
■ Assess the patient's ability to perform activities of daily living (ADLs) effectively and safely on a daily basis using an appropriate assessment tool, such as the Functional Independence Measures (FIM).	The patient may only require assistance with some self-care measures. A variety of tools are available, depending on the clinical setting. Such tools provide objective data for baselines. For example, the FIM measures 18 self-care items related to eating, bathing, grooming, dressing, toileting, bladder and bowel management, transfer, ambulation, and stair climbing.
■ Assess the specific cause of each deficit (e.g., weakness, visual problems, cognitive impairment).	Different etiological factors may require more specific interventions to enable self-care.
■ Assess the patient's need for assistive devices. Assess the need for home health care after discharge.	Assistive devices increase independence in performance of ADLs. Shortened hospital stays have resulted in patients being more debilitated on discharge and therefore requiring more assistance at home. Occupational therapists have access to a wide range of self-help devices.
■ Identify preference for food, personal care items, and other things.	The patient is more likely to participate in self-care that supports his or her individual and personal preferences.
■ If indicated, assess for gag reflex or need for swallowing evaluation by speech therapist before initial oral feeding.	Absence of gag reflex or inability to chew or swallow properly may lead to choking or aspiration.

Therapeutic Interventions

Actions/Interventions	Rationales
■ Assist the patient in accepting necessary amount of dependence.	If disease, injury, or illness resulting in self-care deficit is recent, the patient may need to grieve before accepting that dependence is necessary. Patients may need help in determining the safe limits of trying to be independent versus asking for help when needed.
■ Set short-range goals with the patient.	Assisting the patient with setting realistic goals will decrease frustration.
■ Implement measures to facilitate independence, but intervene when the patient cannot perform.	An appropriate level of assistive care can prevent injury from activities without causing frustration. Nurses can be key in helping patients accept both temporary and permanent dependence.
■ Use consistent routines, and allow adequate time for the patient to complete tasks.	An established routine becomes rote and requires less effort. This helps the patient organize and carry out self-care skills.
■ Provide positive reinforcement for all activities attempted; note partial achievements.	External sources of positive reinforcement may promote ongoing efforts.
Feeding:	
■ Place the patient in optimal position for feeding, preferably sitting up in a chair; support arms, elbows, and wrists, as needed.	Proper positioning can make the task easier while also reducing risk for aspiration.

■ = Independent   ▲ = Collaborative

Actions/Interventions	Rationales
■ Encourage the patient to feed self as soon as possible (using unaffected hand, if appropriate). Assist with setup as needed.	It is probable that the dominant hand will also be the affected hand if there is upper extremity involvement.
■ Ensure that the patient wears dentures and eyeglasses if needed.	Deficits may be exaggerated if other senses or strengths are not functioning optimally.
▲ Ensure that consistency of diet is appropriate for the patient's ability to chew and swallow, as assessed by the speech therapist.	Thickened semisolid foods like pudding and hot cereal are most easily swallowed and less likely to be aspirated.
■ Provide the patient with appropriate utensils (e.g., drinking straw, plate guard, rocking knife, wide-grip utensils, nonskid placemat) to aid in self-feeding.	These items increase opportunities for success.
■ Consider appropriate setting for feeding where the patient has supportive assistance yet is not embarrassed.	Embarrassment or fear of spilling food on self may hinder the patient's attempts to feed self.
■ If the patient has visual problems, advise the patient of the placement of food on the plate.	Following cerebrovascular accident (CVA), patients may have unilateral neglect and may ignore half the plate.

Dressing/grooming:

Actions/Interventions	Rationales
■ Provide privacy during dressing.	Patients may take longer to dress and may be fearful of breaches in privacy.
■ Provide frequent encouragement and assistance with dressing as needed.	Assistance can reduce energy expenditure and frustration. However, care needs to be taken so the care provider does not rush through tasks, negating the patient's attempts.
■ Plan daily activities so the patient is rested before activity.	A plan that balances periods of activity with periods of rest can help the patient complete the desired activity without undue fatigue and frustration.
▲ Provide appropriate assistive devices for dressing as assessed by the nurse and occupational therapist.	The use of a buttonhook or of loop-and-pile closures on clothes may make it possible for a patient to continue independence in this self-care activity.
■ Place the patient in wheelchair or stationary chair.	Dressing can be fatiguing. A chair that provides more support for the body than sitting on the side of the bed conserves energy when dressing.
■ Encourage the use of clothing one size larger.	A larger size ensures easier dressing and comfort.
■ Suggest front-opening brassiere and half-slips.	Clothing that is easier to put on and remove enhances self-care with dressing.
■ Suggest elastic shoelaces or Velcro closures on shoes.	These closures eliminate tying, which can add to frustration.
■ Provide makeup and mirror; assist as needed.	Fine motor activities may take more coordinated actions and may be beyond the abilities of the patient.

Bathing/hygiene:

Actions/Interventions	Rationales
■ Maintain privacy during bathing as appropriate.	The need for privacy is fundamental for most patients.
■ Ensure that needed utensils are close by.	Nearby placement of items such as washcloth, soap, and towel conserves energy and optimizes safety.
■ Instruct the patient to select bath time when he or she is rested and unhurried.	Hurrying may result in accidents, and the energy required for these activities may be substantial.
■ Provide the patient with appropriate assistive devices (e.g., long-handled bath sponge, shower chair, safety mats for floor, grab bars for bath or shower).	Assistive devices aid in the ability to bathe self and increase safety.
■ Encourage the patient to bathe self as much as he or she is capable of. Assist with completion of bath, brushing teeth, shaving, and so on, only as needed.	Hospital workers and family caregivers are often in a hurry and do more for patients than needed, thereby slowing the patient's efforts at regaining independence.
■ Encourage the patient to comb own hair (a one-handed task). Suggest hairstyles that are low maintenance.	Simplified hairstyles enable the patient to maintain autonomy for as long as possible.
■ Assist the patient with care of fingernails and toenails as required.	Patients may require podiatric care to prevent injury to feet during nail trimming or because special implements are required to cut nails.
■ Offer frequent encouragement.	Patients often have difficulty seeing progress.

Actions/Interventions

Toileting:

- Evaluate or document previous and current patterns for toileting; institute a toileting schedule that factors these habits into the program.
- Provide privacy while the patient is toileting.

- Keep the call light within reach, and instruct the patient to call as early as possible.
- Assist the patient in removing or replacing necessary clothing.
- Encourage use of commode or toilet as soon as possible.

- Provide appropriate assistance devices (e.g., raised toilet seat and grab bar near toilet).
- Offer bedpan, or place patient on toilet every 1 to 1½ hours during the day and three times during the night.

- Closely monitor the patient for loss of balance or falls. Keep commode and toilet tissue near the bedside for nighttime use.

Transferring/ambulation:

- Plan teaching session for transferring/walking when the patient is rested.
- Assist with bed mobility by doing the following:

  - Allow the patient to work at own rate of speed.

  - Encourage the patient to use the stronger side (if appropriate) as much as possible.

- When transferring to wheelchair, always place the chair on the patient's stronger side at a slight angle to the bed and lock the brakes.
- When minimal assistance is needed, stand on the patient's weak side and place a hand under the patient's weak arm. Keep feet well apart; lift with legs, not the back, to prevent back strain.
- For moderate assistance, the caregiver places arms under both the patient's armpits with the caregiver's hands on the patient's back.
- For patients requiring maximal assistance, use a gait belt.
  - Raise the bed to tallest height that still allows patient's feet to be flat on floor.
  - Grasp gait belt with both arms, and pull patient forward.
  - Place a knee against the patient's weak knee (if applicable), and encourage the patient to put weight on the strong side during transfer.
  - Encourage the patient to use his or her arms to assist, as able, and to place them on the caregiver's forearms.

Rationales

The effectiveness of the bowel or bladder program will be enhanced if the natural and personal patterns of the patient are respected.

Lack of privacy may inhibit the patient's ability to evacuate bowel and bladder.

Staff members need time to reach patient's room to assist with transfer to commode or toilet.

Clothing that is difficult to get into and out of may compromise a patient's ability to be continent.

Patients are more effective in evacuating bowel and bladder when sitting on a commode. Some patients find it impossible to toilet on a bedpan.

These devices facilitate ease in sitting down and getting up.

This schedule eliminates incontinence. Time intervals can be lengthened as the patient begins to express the need to toilet on demand.

Patients may rush readiness to ambulate to the toilet or commode during the night because of fear of soiling themselves, and they may fall in the process.

Tasks require energy. Fatigued patients may have more difficulty and may become unnecessarily frustrated.

Bed mobility prevents disabling contractures, pressure ulcers, and muscle weakness from disuse.

Many factors may influence a patient's ability to move freely, and each of these factors must be considered when developing or teaching a patient a new system for self-care.

If stroke patients experience weakness in their dominant side, it will be necessary for them to develop muscle strength and coordination on the nondominant side.

The patient will bear weight on the stronger side. Physical or occupational therapists can provide additional guidelines.

Proper technique prevents injury to the care provider.

This technique forces the patient to keep his or her weight forward.

This technique maximizes patient support while protecting the care provider from injury.

■ = Independent   ▲ = Collaborative

Actions/Interventions

- Assist with ambulation; teach the use of ambulation devices such as canes, walkers, and crutches:
  - Stand on the patient's weak side.
  - If using a cane, place the cane in the patient's strong hand and ensure proper foot-cane sequence.

Miscellaneous skills:

- Telephone: Evaluate need for adaptive equipment through therapy department (e.g., pushbutton phone, larger numbers, increased volume).
- Writing: Supply patient with felt-tip pens. Evaluate need for splint on writing hand.
- Provide supervision for each activity until the patient performs the skill competently and is safe in independent care; reevaluate regularly to be certain that the patient is maintaining the skill level and remains safe in environment.
- Encourage maximum independence.

Rationales

These techniques enhance patient safety and assist with balance and support.

Patients will require an effective tool for communicating needs from home.

These pens mark with little pressure and are easier to use. Splints assist in holding the writing device.

The patient's ability to perform self-care measures may change often over time and will need to be assessed regularly.

The goal of rehabilitation is one of achieving the highest level of independence as possible.

Education/Continuity of Care

Actions/Interventions

- Plan teaching sessions so the patient has time to practice tasks.
- Instruct the patient in use of assistive devices as appropriate.
- Teach family and caregivers to foster independence and to intervene if the patient becomes fatigued, is unable to perform tasks, or becomes excessively frustrated.

Rationales

This allows the patient to use new information immediately, thus enhancing retention.
Information enables the patient to take some control.

This demonstrates caring and concern but does not interfere with the patient's efforts to achieve independence.

Situational Low Self-Esteem

Definition: Development of a negative perception of self-worth in response to current situation (specify)

Self-esteem is a component of an individual's self-concept. Positive self-esteem is based on the person's feeling worthwhile and capable of responding to challenges and stressors. Low self-esteem represents a mild to marked alteration in an individual's view of himself or herself, including negative self-evaluation or feelings about self or capabilities. This change in self-esteem is a temporary state in response to feeling unable to manage the current situation. One's self-esteem is affected by (and may also affect) ability to function in the larger world and relate to others within it. Self-esteem disturbance may be expressed directly or indirectly. Cultural norms, gender, and age are variables that influence how an individual perceives himself or herself. The emotional work that patients do to enhance self-esteem takes weeks, months, or even years and may require professional help beyond the scope of the bedside or community nurse. A caring individual, who is able to identify the special needs of the patient struggling with self-esteem issues, is in a unique position to provide support and compassion, enhancing the work the patient must do.

Common Related Factors

Disturbed body image
Actual or anticipated loss
Change in social roles (e.g., hospitalization, assumption of the "sick role")
Behavior inconsistent with personal values
Functional impairment
Lack of recognition
Rejections

Common Expected Outcomes

Patient verbalizes positive self-acceptance.
Patient describes successes in current situations.

Defining Characteristics

Verbally reports current situational challenge to self-worth
Self-negating statements
Indecisive, nonassertive behavior
Verbally reports feeling unable to deal with situation
Expressions of helplessness or uselessness

NOC Outcome
Self-Esteem
NIC Interventions
Self-Esteem Enhancement; Body Image Enhancement; Presence

Ongoing Assessment

Actions/Interventions	Rationales
■ Encourage patient to list past and current accomplishments: emotional, social, interpersonal, intellectual, vocational, and physical.	This exercise is sometimes helpful in providing the patient with a more realistic perspective on his or her capabilities.
■ Listen to or document how the patient describes self and the things he or she says about self.	Low self-esteem is often expressed as feeling unloved, unworthy, or incompetent. The person may be self-critical.
■ Take seriously the patient's reports of changes in self-esteem. Determine if the patient is able to relate these changes to a specific event.	The patient may be aware of the events that negatively affect his or her self-concept.
■ Determine if these feelings have resulted in a change in patient's behavior.	Patients may be able to compensate for low self-esteem through extraordinary performance in work or areas of special interest while still having problems with how he or she envisions self. Fundamentally low self-esteem will not be resolved without factoring these issues into the care plan.
■ Assess the degree to which the patient feels "in control" of his or her own behavior.	Patients may be caught in a vicious cycle of behaviors designed to camouflage the primary self-esteem problem. The acting-out feeds a sense of unworthiness and sabotages attempts at esteem building.
■ Assess the degree to which the patient feels loved and respected by others.	Rejection by others or lack of recognition of accomplishments may contribute to feelings of unworthiness. The patient's ability to establish and maintain meaningful relationships is a positive indicator for developing self-esteem. The care and support of others will be helpful in building the patient's self-esteem.
■ Assess whether the patient feels satisfied with his or her own behavior.	Patients with self-esteem disturbance may feel as though their behaviors are not in keeping with their own personal, moral, or ethical values; they may also deny these behaviors, project blame, and rationalize personal failures.
■ Assess how competent patients feel about their ability to perform and/or carry out their own and others' expectations.	The patient may have developed the ability to carry out personal responsibilities despite low self-esteem. This may be a positive indicator of the patient's potential for successful enhancement of self-esteem.
■ Assess for unresolved grief.	Unresolved grief may inhibit patients' ability to move beyond the loss or disability and to accept themselves as they are now.

■ = Independent   ▲ = Collaborative

Nursing Diagnosis Care Plans

Therapeutic Interventions

Actions/Interventions	Rationales
■ Provide environment conducive to the expression of feelings:	
• Spend time with the patient; set aside sufficient time so that the encounter is unhurried.	The patient needs time to express concerns. Spending time with the patient expresses the nurse's interest in and acceptance of the patient's feelings.
• Avoid excessive focus on physical tasks.	Successful resolution of these issues will take considerable time and energy. These issues are deserving of the patient and the nurse's complete attention.
• Use active listening and open-ended questions.	These communication techniques allow the patient to express concerns, fears, and ideas without interruption.
• Provide privacy.	Sensitive discussions need to take place in a setting where the patient is free to express self without being overheard.
■ Convey a sense of respect for the patient's abilities and strengths in addition to recognizing problems and concerns.	Assistance with problem solving and reality testing is best provided within the context of a trusting relationship.
■ Serve as role model for the patient or significant others in healthy expression of feelings or concerns. Assume responsibility for own thoughts and actions by using "I think" language in discussions.	Patients may need an example of positive ways to express feelings. Self-awareness allows the nurse to demonstrate authentic behavior.
■ Discuss "normal" impact of alteration in health status (temporary or permanent) on self-esteem. Reassure the patient that such changes often result in a variety of emotional or behavioral responses.	Disturbances in self-esteem are natural responses to significant changes. Reconstitution of the individual's self-esteem occurs after grieving has taken place and acceptance has followed.
■ Provide anticipatory guidance to minimize anxiety and fear if disturbances in self-esteem are an expected part of the rehabilitation process.	The patient needs a perspective that places the shift in self-esteem within the context of the normal recuperative process.
■ Assist the patient in his or her efforts to obtain understanding and mastery of new experiences:	If patients are unable to participate in decisions as they relate to their own care, their self-esteem may be further eroded. Significant others serve as an advocate.
• Support efforts to maintain independence, reality, positive self-esteem, sense of capability, and problem solving.	The patient needs ongoing positive feedback and reinforcement to maintain behaviors to promote self-esteem. Clearly defined goals will help the person see progress. Professional and community sources of support provide the patient with more resources to continue the work of restoring positive self-esteem.
• Provide realistic appraisal of progress.	
• Reinforce efforts at constructive change.	
• Use referral sources such as other professional or community support groups as appropriate.	

Education/Continuity of Care

Actions/Interventions	Rationales
■ Teach the patient to seek and/or plan activities likely to result in a healthy self-esteem.	The patient needs to explore alternatives to promote self-esteem.
■ Teach the patient necessary self-care measures related to primary disease.	Each success will reinforce positive self-esteem.
■ Teach the patient the harmful effects of self-negating talk.	Awareness of destructive thoughts can help the patient develop new approaches to coping.

Disturbed Sensory Perception: Auditory

Definition: Change in the amount or patterning of incoming stimuli accompanied by a diminished, exaggerated, distorted, or impaired response to such stimuli

Hearing loss is common among older adults but may also occur as the result of congenital exposure to virus; during childhood after frequent ear infections or trauma; and during adulthood as the result of trauma, infection, or exposure to occupational and/or environmental noise. Conductive hearing loss is associated with problems affecting the outer ear and middle ear. These problems include impacted cerumen and infection. Sensorineural hearing loss occurs with inner ear disorders or impaired function of cranial nerve VIII. Aging, noise exposure, and ototoxicity from some drugs contribute to this type of hearing loss. When hearing loss is profound and precedes language development, the ability to learn speech and interact with hearing peers can be severely impaired. When hearing is impaired or lost later in life, serious emotional and social consequences can occur, including depression and isolation. Some causes of hearing loss are surgically correctable. Many hearing assistive devices and services are available to help hearing-impaired individuals. Nursing interventions with the hearing impaired are aimed at assisting the individual in effective communication despite the loss of normal hearing.

Common Related Factors

Middle ear injuries secondary to penetration of eardrum
History of head trauma, especially direct blow to ear
Prolonged or cumulative exposure to environmental noise greater than 85 dB
Otosclerosis
Ménière's disease
Presbycusis (loss of hearing associated with aging)
Acoustic neuroma
Congenital rubella exposure
Ototoxic drug use
Chronic or recurring otitis media
Inoperative or poorly fitted hearing aids
Accumulated earwax (impacted cerumen)

Defining Characteristics

Asking others to repeat spoken messages
Inappropriate response to questions
Head tilting
Cupping hands around ears
Social avoidance or withdrawal
Irritability
Difficulty learning or following directions
Dizziness
Ear pain

Common Expected Outcome

Patient achieves optimal functioning within limits of hearing impairment as evidenced by ability to communicate effectively and to engage in meaningful activities.

NOC Outcomes
Hearing Compensation Behavior; Risk Control: Hearing Impairment
NIC Interventions
Communication Enhancement: Hearing Deficit; Ear Care

Ongoing Assessment

Actions/Interventions

■ Assess the patient's ability to hear by performing the following:
  • At screening, note the patient's ability to hear and appropriately respond to normal conversational voice; do this within the patient's sight, then again from out of the patient's sight.

Rationales

Difficulty responding to normal conversation may be the first indication of impaired hearing. Patients may rely on lip-reading to a greater extent than they are aware.
Sensory nerve hearing loss affects many older individuals; inability to hear high-pitched sounds or comprehend some consonants are the earliest effects.

■ = Independent   ▲ = Collaborative

Nursing Diagnosis Care Plans

Actions/Interventions

- Ask the family or caregivers about their perception of the patient's hearing impairment.

- Review audiogram, if available.

■ Assess whether hearing loss is recent, progressive, or present since childhood.

■ Review medical history.

■ Review exposure to environmental noise, either as the result of occupation, recreation, or accident.

■ Review recent use of drugs that are ototoxic.

■ Check ears for earwax.

■ Investigate and note social and emotional impact of hearing loss.

■ For patients with hearing aids:
  - Note condition and age of hearing aid.
  - Note frequency with which patient wears hearing aid.
  - Check hearing aid for fresh, functional batteries.
  - Check hearing aid for wax impaction.
■ Assess for drainage from ear canal.

▲ Culture any drainage from the ear canal.

■ Ask the patient whether the ear is painful.

■ Assess for dizziness, dysequilibrium.

■ Assess the patient's ability to effectively administer ear drops.

Rationales

Patients may be unaware of progressive hearing loss; family, friends, and caregivers often first notice requests for verbal repetition, lack of response to verbalizations, and incorrectly answered questions.

This diagnostic study indicates both type and amount of hearing loss.

Adults with new or progressive hearing loss require attention to the emotional and social implications of impaired communication, whereas those who have had hearing loss since birth or childhood probably have the skills, tools, and resources available to cope with hearing impairment.

History of head or ear trauma and frequent bouts with ear infections are often associated with hearing loss.

The Occupational Safety and Health Act requires hearing protection in workplaces with noise levels exceeding 90 dB. Young persons who frequent rock concerts or listen to very loud music place themselves at risk for hearing loss. Hearing loss that results from noise may not be reversible.

Aspirin, quinidine, some chemotherapeutic agents, and the aminoglycosides are known ototoxic agents. Withdrawal of these drugs when hearing impairment occurs often allows for full return of hearing.

Excessive wax may become impacted against tympanic membrane and prevent sound transmission.

Loss of hearing may lead to reclusiveness, isolation, depression, and withdrawal from usual activities. The decision to wear a hearing aid is often resisted because of the social stigma perceived in conjunction with aging and loss of abilities.

A hearing aid that is not functioning correctly may be the cause of decreased hearing acuity. The patient may not wear the hearing aid as needed. Wax may clog hearing aids. The patient may have trouble replacing dead batteries.

Purulent, foul-smelling drainage indicates an infection; serous, mucoid, or bloody drainage may indicate effusion of the middle ear after an upper respiratory or sinus infection.

Identification of infectious pathogens guides selection of antibiotic therapy.

Pain is a symptom of increased pressure behind the eardrum, usually a result of infection.

Disorders of the ear (e.g., Ménière's disease) may be accompanied by dizziness because of the inner ear's role in maintenance of equilibrium.

Problems with medication administration may limit effectiveness of the drug.

Therapeutic Interventions

Actions/Interventions

■ Use touch and eye contact.

Rationales

Behavioral communication techniques can support effective interactions with the patient.

Actions/Interventions	Rationales
■ When speaking, do the following: • Reduce or minimize environmental noise.	The person with a hearing impairment may have difficulty filtering background noises in order to hear the speaker.
• Face the patient in good light, and keep hands away from mouth.	This approach enhances the patient's use of lip-reading, facial expressions, and gesturing.
• Speak close to the patient's "better" ear, as appropriate. • Avoid shouting or yelling.	Loud noise may limit the patient's ability to hear. Drawing attention to the patient's hearing loss may decrease his or her willingness to communicate with others.
• Use simple language and short sentences. • Speak slowly.	The patient needs additional time to process auditory stimuli.
■ Use grease boards, computers, or other writing tools.	These tools help communicate with profoundly hearing-impaired individuals.
■ For patients with hearing aids, ensure that hearing aid is in place, clean, and working.	Patients with new hearing aids need time to adjust to the sound produced. Encouragement is often needed, especially among older patients who may decide that the hearing aid is not worth the effort.
■ Provide encouragement to use hearing aid.	Patients may stop using a hearing aid if they think it draws attention to the problem and distorts their body image. Patients may be unaware of miniature models that are now available.
■ Prepare patient for ear surgery.	Tympanoplasty (removal of dead tissue, restoration of bones with prostheses) and mastoidectomy (removal of all or portions of the middle ear structures) are common surgical treatments for hearing loss.

Education/Continuity of Care

Actions/Interventions	Rationales
■ Teach the patient or caregiver to administer ear medications.	Drops should be administered at room temperature to avoid pain and dizziness; tip of applicator or dropper should not be allowed to come into contact with anything. Head should be positioned to allow medication to flow into ear canal; this position should be maintained for 1 to 2 minutes.
■ Instruct the patient or caregiver in safe techniques for cleaning ears.	Thin washcloths and fingers are best for cleaning ears. Cotton-tipped applicators should be avoided to prevent inadvertent injury to the eardrum or pushing cerumen farther into the ear canal.
■ Teach the patient or caregiver use and care of hearing aids and/or other assistive hearing devices.	The patient and caregiver need to be able to care for and maintain the hearing aid in proper working order.
■ Explore technology such as amplifiers, modifiers for telephones, and services for the hearing impaired (e.g., closed-captioned TV, telephone hearing-impaired assistance).	These devices may assist the hearing-impaired person with functioning and participating in meaningful activities.
■ Instruct the patient in the importance of routine examination by an audiologist.	Examinations detect changes in hearing or need for change in hearing aids.

■ = Independent   ▲ = Collaborative

NANDA-I NDx Disturbed Sensory Perception: Visual

Definition: Change in the amount or patterning of incoming stimuli accompanied by a diminished, exaggerated, distorted, or impaired response to such stimuli

Visual impairment affects a significant number of people across the life span. Refractive errors are the most common form of visual problem. These correctable visual impairments include myopia, hyperopia, presbyopia, and astigmatism. Correction occurs with glasses, contact lenses, or surgery. Chronic diseases such as diabetes mellitus, glaucoma, and macular degeneration cause visual impairment that is not correctable and may lead to blindness. Cataracts contribute to visual impairment that may be corrected through surgery and lens replacement. Infections, trauma, drugs, and diseases of the brain may also cause visual impairment. Changes in visual acuity may interfere with the person's activities of daily living and productivity at work, school, or home. Loss of vision threatens the safety of the individual and puts the person at risk for falls and other injuries. Visual impairment may affect the person's psychological, emotional, and social well-being as he or she copes with adapting to the loss while attempting to remain independent. Dependence on devices to correct or adapt to visual impairment may affect the person's body image and self-concept.

Common Related Factors

Diabetes mellitus
Glaucoma
Cataracts
Refractive disorders (myopia, hyperopia, astigmatism, presbyopia)
Macular degeneration
Ocular trauma
Ocular infection
Retinal detachment
Disease or trauma to visual pathways or cranial nerves II, III, IV, and VI, secondary to stroke, intracranial aneurysms, brain tumor, trauma, myasthenia gravis, or multiple sclerosis
Advanced age

Defining Characteristics

Reported or measured changes in visual acuity
Change in usual response to visual stimuli
Failure to locate distant objects
Squinting, frequent blinking
Closing of one eye to see
Frequent rubbing of eye
Head tilting
Visual distortions
Lack of eye-to-eye contact
Abnormal eye movement
Deviation of eye
Gray opacities in eyes
Bumping into things
Clumsy behavior
Incoordination
History of falls, accidents
Disorientation
Anxiety
Anger

Common Expected Outcome

Patient achieves optimal functioning within limits of visual impairment as evidenced by ability to care for self, to navigate environment safely, and to engage in meaningful activities.

NOC Outcomes

Visual Compensation Behavior; Risk Control: Visual Impairment

NIC Interventions

Communication Enhancement: Visual Deficit; Environmental Management; Self-Esteem Enhancement

Ongoing Assessment

Actions/Interventions	Rationales
■ Determine nature of visual symptoms, onset, and degree of visual loss. Inquire about history of visual complaints, eye trauma, or ocular pain.	Recent loss, loss over a long period, and long-standing loss have different implications for nursing intervention and the patient's level of adaptation or resource use. Because visual loss may occur gradually, quantification of loss may be difficult for the patient to articulate. The incidence of macular degeneration, cataracts, retinal detachments, diabetic retinopathy, and glaucoma increases with aging.
■ Review medical history. Inquire about patient or family history of systemic or central nervous system disease.	Family or patient history of atherosclerosis, diabetes, thyroid disease, or hypertension should be investigated as possible cause for visual loss.
■ Ask patient about specifics such as ability to read, see television, history of falls, or ability to self-medicate.	Visual impairment can contribute to problems in daily activities. The risk for falls and medication errors increases if the person has diminished visual acuity.
■ Assess central vision with each eye, individually and together.	Vision loss may be unilateral, bilateral, central, and/or peripheral and may not affect both eyes to the same extent.
■ Assess peripheral field of vision and visual acuity.	Glaucoma affects peripheral vision; its onset is insidious and has no associated symptoms. Macular degeneration affects central vision, is more common among cigarette smokers, and is irreversible.
■ Assess eye and lid for inflammation, edema, positional defects, and deviation.	These findings may suggest correctable problems that can negatively affect vision.
■ Assess factors or aids that improve vision, such as glasses, contact lenses, or bright and/or natural light.	Nursing interventions should include strategies that enhance the patient's adaptive abilities.
■ Evaluate the patient's ability to function within limits of visual impairment.	Personal appearance and condition of clothing and surroundings are good indicators of the patient's adaptation to visual loss.
■ Evaluate psychological response to visual loss.	Anger, depression, and withdrawal are common responses. Self-esteem is often negatively affected.

Therapeutic Interventions

Actions/Interventions	Rationales
■ Introduce self to patient, and acknowledge visual impairment. Communicate type and degree of impairment to all involved in the patient's care.	Continuity of care is enhanced when all providers have the same information about the patient's level of functioning.
■ Orient the patient to the environment. Remove environmental barriers to ensure safety. Avoid leaving doors partially open. Do not make unnecessary changes in the environment.	Orientation reduces fear related to an unfamiliar environment. Fully open or closed doors reduce the risk for injury among the vision impaired. Providing consistency in the patient's environment ensures safety and maintains what the patient has learned. If furniture or wastebaskets are moved, notify patient of changes.
■ Provide adequate lighting.	The use of natural or halogen lighting is preferred to improve vision for patients with diminished vision.
■ Place meal tray, tissues, water, and call light within the patient's range of vision or reach. Place food on tray and plate in the same place each meal, and explain arrangement of food on tray and plate, using clockwise sequence.	This approach promotes the patient's independence, especially with self-care for feeding.
■ Recommend use of visual aids when appropriate.	Visual aids such as a magnifying glass or large-type printed books and magazines encourage reading.
■ Encourage use of sense of touch.	Touch encourages the patient to become familiar with unfamiliar objects.
■ Explain sounds or other unusual stimuli in the environment.	Explanations reduce fear.

■ = Independent   ▲ = Collaborative

Actions/Interventions	Rationales
■ Encourage use of radios, tapes, and talking books.	Diversional activities should be encouraged. Radio and television increase awareness of day and time.
■ Maintain bed in low position with side rails up, if appropriate. Keep bed in the locked position.	Side rails help remind the patient not to get up without help when needed.
■ Guide the patient when ambulating, if appropriate. Describe where you are walking; identify obstacles.	This approach helps maintain reality orientation to the environment.
■ Instruct the patient to hold both arms of the chair before sitting and to feel for the seat on chairs or sofas without arms.	These actions reduce the risk for falls.
▲ Consult the occupational therapy staff for assistive devices and training in their use.	Adaptive devices such as magnifiers for reading medication vials or syringes used for injections can increase the patient's self-care independence.
■ Supervise the patient when he or she is smoking.	Supervision prevents accidental fires.

Education/Continuity of Care

Actions/Interventions	Rationales
■ Reinforce the physician's explanation of medical management and surgical procedures, if any.	Patients and their caregivers may need periodic repetition of information to make informed decisions about treatment and procedures.
■ Teach general eye care:	
• Maintain sterility of all eyedroppers, tubes of medications, and other items.	These strategies reduce the risk for eye infection or injury.
• Care for contact lenses or eyeglasses as recommended by manufacturer.	Care and maintenance of corrective lenses enhances the effectiveness of their use to improve vision.
■ Demonstrate the proper administration of eyedrops or ointments; allow for return demonstration by the patient and/or caregiver.	Repetition of skills after demonstration promotes the patient's level of confidence in administration of eye medications.
■ Instruct the patient in use of assistive devices as appropriate.	Information allows patient to gain independence.
■ Help the family or caregiver identify the need to make modification in the home environment.	Family members may need help to provide for the patient's safety and sense of independence, as indicated.
▲ Make appropriate referrals to a home health agency for nursing and social services follow-up.	Evaluation of the home environment can identify the need for additional resources to support the patient's adaptation to visual impairment.
■ Reinforce the need to use community agencies, if indicated.	These agencies are a source of additional information and resources to support the patient's adaptation to visual impairment.

NANDA-I
NDx Ineffective Sexuality Patterns

Definition: Expressions of concern regarding own sexuality

A patient or significant other may express concern regarding the means or manner of sexual expression or physical intimacy within their relationship. Alterations in human sexual response may be related to genetic, physiological, emotional, cognitive, religious, and/or sociocultural factors or to a combination of these factors. All of these factors play a role in determining what is normative for each individual within a relationship. The problem of altered patterns of sexuality is not limited to a single gender, age, or cultural group; it is a potential problem for all patients, whether the nurse encounters them in the hospital or in the community. It is probable that most couples encounter some point in their relationship where patterns of sexual expression become altered to the dissatisfaction of one or both members. The ability to communicate effectively, to seek professional help whenever necessary, and to modify existing patterns to the mutual satisfaction of both members are skills that enable the couple to grow and evolve in this aspect of their relationship. The nurse is in a unique position to provide anticipatory guidance relative to altered patterns of sexual function when the problem is an inevitable or probable result of illness or disability. The ability to discuss these issues openly when the patient raises concerns about sexual expression highlights the legitimacy of the couple's feelings and the normalcy of sexual expression as a part of intimacy, as well as emotional and physical well-being.

Common Related Factors

Absent or ineffective role model
Conflicts with sexual orientation or variant preferences
Fear of sexually transmitted infections (STIs)
Fear of pregnancy
Impaired relationship with significant other
Lack of knowledge about alternative responses to changes in sexual response related to illness or medical treatment
Lack of privacy
Loss of significant other

Defining Characteristics

Alterations in achieving perceived sexual role
Alteration in relationship with significant other
Values conflicts
Reported changes in sexual activities or behaviors
Reported difficulties in sexual activities or behaviors
Reported limitations in sexual activities or behaviors

Common Expected Outcomes

Patient or couple verbalizes satisfaction with the way they express physical intimacy.
Both members of the couple exhibit behavior that is acceptable to his or her partner.

NOC Outcomes
Abuse Recovery: Sexual; Body Image; Sexual
    Identity: Acceptance
NIC Interventions
Sexual Counseling; Anticipatory Guidance;
    Teaching: Sexuality

Ongoing Assessment

Actions/Interventions	Rationales
■ Identify level of comfort in discussion for patient and/or significant other.	It is important for the nurse to create an environment where the couple or patient feels safe and comfortable in discussing feelings.
■ Assess level of understanding regarding human sexuality and functioning.	Many persons have misconceptions about sexual intimacy.
■ Explore current and past sexual patterns, practices, and degree of satisfaction.	This information determines a realistic approach to care planning.
■ Solicit information from the patient about the nature, onset, duration, and course of sexual difficulty.	Problems with sexuality may be long-standing or of short duration.
■ Identify potential or actual factors that may contribute to current alteration in sexual functioning.	The care plan will be developed in the context of the patient's overall health status. Different interventions will address specific contributing factors.

Therapeutic Interventions

Actions/Interventions	Rationales
■ Use a relaxed, accepting manner in discussing sexual issues. Convey acceptance and respect for patient concerns.	Patients are often hesitant to report such concerns and/or difficulties because sexuality remains a private matter within many cultures, and it is uncomfortable to discuss.
■ Provide privacy and adequate time to discuss sexuality.	Respecting the individual and treating his or her concerns and questions as normal and important may foster greater self-acceptance and decrease anxiety.

■ = Independent ▲ = Collaborative

Actions/Interventions

■ Encourage sharing of concerns, feelings, and information between patient and current or future partner. Whenever possible, involve both in sexual health education and counseling efforts.

■ Discuss the multiplicity of influences on sexual functioning (both physiological and emotional). Offer opportunities to ask questions and express feelings.

■ Explore awareness of and comfort with a range of sexual expression and activities (not just sexual intercourse).

■ Assist the patient and significant other in identifying possible options to overcome situational, temporary, or long-term influences on sexual functioning.

■ Encourage patient and significant other to locate and read relevant educational materials regarding sexuality.

Rationales

For some sexual problems, it is the couple's relationship that provides the focus for intervention.

Patients and couples may have limited knowledge of sexual function and factors that influence sexuality. Open discussion can relieve feelings of guilt or shame.

Patients and couples may have limited knowledge of ways to express their sexuality. They may be uncomfortable with some types of sexual expression based on cultural, social, or religious beliefs.

The nurse can facilitate open discussion by the couple of possible ways to adapt to changes in sexual function. The couple needs to share responsibility for exploring options.

Many excellent books are available that undo myths and errors and promote increased knowledge and communication about sexual concerns.

Education/Continuity of Care

Actions/Interventions

■ Provide accurate and timely health teaching regarding the "normal" range of sexual expression and sexual practices throughout the life cycle.

■ Discuss range of possibilities and consequences (both positive and negative) associated with sexual expression of all types (e.g., change in relationship, impact on physical and/or emotional health, possibility of pregnancy, STIs).

■ Offer information regarding birth control methods and "safe sex" practices.

■ Be specific in providing instruction to the patient and significant other regarding any limitations on sexual activity resulting from illness, surgery, medications, or other events.

■ Explain alternative means or forms of expressing intimacy and/or sexual expression (e.g., alternative positions for intercourse) that decrease discomfort or degree of physical exertion for those with impaired mobility or cardiopulmonary disease. Consider concerns imposed by the patient's or significant other's health status, illness, or other situation.

▲ Consider referral for further workup and/or treatment (e.g., primary health care provider, specialized physician or mental health consultant, substance abuse treatment program, or sexual dysfunction clinic).

■ Consider referral to self-help and/or support groups (e.g., Reach for Recovery, ostomy association, Mended Hearts, Huff and Puff, Sexual Impotence Resolved, Us TOO, HIV support groups, Breast Cancer Network of Strength, Survivors of Abuse, or Resolve).

Rationales

Satisfying sexual functioning and practice are not automatic and need to be learned.

Information is necessary to support the couple or the individual patient making decisions about sexual activity.

The patient and significant other need accurate information about preventing unintended pregnancy or transmission of infections through sexual contact.

The patient needs to understand the relationship between illness, treatment methods, and sexuality.

The amount and type of information provided should match the patient's or couple's level of interest and comfort. Alternative ways of sexual expression should be mutually pleasing and acceptable to the patient and the significant other.

The counseling needs of the couple or patient may be beyond the skill or training of the nurse.

Self-help support groups are unique sources of empathy, information, and successful role models. These organizations can provide information about sexuality and specific health problems.

Risk for Impaired Skin Integrity

Definition: At risk for skin being adversely altered

Maintenance of skin integrity and prevention of pressure ulcers is identified as a key marker of quality care. The Centers for Medicare and Medicaid Services (CMS) and The Joint Commission (TJC) have identified pressure ulcer prevention as one of the first major nursing-sensitive outcomes. Although the literature suggests that not all pressure ulcers can be prevented, the nurse is in a key role to implement comprehensive guidelines to aid in the prevention and early detection of impaired skin integrity. Nurses must be aware of the myriad factors that place patients at risk for skin breakdown. The literature reports that pressure ulcers can develop in 2 to 6 hours; thus identifying at-risk individuals is key.

Immobility, which leads to pressure, shear, and friction, is the factor most likely to put an individual at risk for altered skin integrity. Advanced age, the normal loss of elasticity, inadequate nutrition, environmental moisture (especially from incontinence), and vascular insufficiency potentiate the effects of pressure and hasten the development of skin breakdown. Groups of persons with the highest risk for altered skin integrity are those with spinal injuries, those who are confined to bed or wheelchair for prolonged periods of time, those with edema, and those who have altered sensation that triggers the normal protective weight shifting. Pressure relief and pressure redistribution devices for the prevention of skin breakdown include a wide range of surfaces, specialty beds and mattresses, and other devices. Preventive measures are usually not reimbursable, even though costs related to treatment once breakdown occurs are greater.

Evidence is accumulating to support the significant reductions in the prevalence of pressure ulcers when a standardized program for prevention is implemented. Several guidelines can be found in the literature. This care plan is based on recommendations from the National Pressure Ulcer Advisory Panel (NPUAC), the National Guideline Clearinghouse, and the Agency for Healthcare Research and Quality (AHRQ).

Common Risk Factors

Extremes of age
Immobility
Imbalanced nutritional state
Mechanical factors (e.g., pressure, shear, friction)
Pronounced bony prominences
Impaired circulation
Impaired sensation
Incontinence
Edema
Moisture
History of radiation
Hyperthermia or hypothermia
Immunological deficit
Impaired cognition
Dermatitis
Mechanical trauma (e.g., scratches, skin tear, surgical
    incision)
Chemical skin irritants (e.g., formaldehyde, hair dyes, epoxy,
    soaps, adhesives)
Pruritus or itching (e.g., dry skin, allergic reactions)
Long-term steroid use
NOTE: Risk should be determined by the use of a risk assessment tool (e.g., Braden Scale).

■ = Independent   ▲ = Collaborative

Common Expected Outcome

Patient's skin remains intact, as evidenced by no redness over bony prominences and capillary refill less than 6 seconds over areas of redness.

NOC Outcomes
Risk Control; Risk Detection; Tissue Integrity: Skin and Mucous Membranes

NIC Interventions
Pressure Ulcer Prevention; Skin Surveillance

Ongoing Assessment

Actions/Interventions	Rationales
■ Assess general condition of skin.	Healthy skin varies among individuals but should have good turgor (an indication of moisture), feel warm and dry to the touch, be free of impairment (scratches, bruises, excoriation, rashes), and have quick capillary refill (less than 6 seconds). Older patients' skin is normally less elastic and has less moisture and thinning of the epidermis, making for higher risk for skin impairment.
■ Specifically assess skin over bony prominences (e.g., sacrum, trochanters, scapulae, elbows, heels, inner and outer malleolus, inner and outer knees, back of head).	Areas where skin is stretched tautly over bony prominences are at higher risk for breakdown because the possibility of ischemia to skin is high as a result of compression of skin capillaries between a hard surface (e.g., mattress, chair, or table) and the bone. Pressure areas initially appear as persistent reddened areas in light pigmented skin. In darker skin tones, the area may appear as red, blue, or purple hue spots.
■ Assess the patient's awareness of the sensation of pressure.	Normally, individuals shift their weight off pressure areas every few minutes; this occurs more or less automatically, even during sleep. Patients with decreased sensation are unaware of unpleasant stimuli (pressure) and do not shift weight. This results in prolonged pressure on skin capillaries and ultimately in skin ischemia.
■ Use an objective tool for pressure ulcer risk assessment. • Braden Scale • Norton Scale	These are validated tools for risk assessment. The Braden Scale is the most widely used. It consists of six subscales: sensory, perception, moisture, activity and mobility, nutrition, and fraction/sheer. • Acute care: Assessment should be carried out on all patients on admission and every 24 to 48 hours or sooner if the patient's condition changes. • Long-term care: Assess on admission, weekly for 4 weeks, and then quarterly and whenever resident's condition changes. • Home care: Assess on admission and at every visit (see http://www.NPUAP.org).
■ Assess the patient's ability to move (e.g., shift weight while sitting, turn over in bed, move from bed to chair).	Immobility is the greatest risk factor in skin breakdown.
■ Assess the patient's nutritional status, including weight, weight loss, and serum albumin levels.	An albumin level less than 2.5 g/dL is a grave sign, indicating severe protein depletion. Research has shown that patients whose serum albumin level is less than 2.5 g/dL are at high risk for skin breakdown, all other factors being equal.
■ Assess for edema.	Skin stretched tautly over edematous tissue is at risk for impairment.
■ Assess for history of radiation therapy.	Radiated skin becomes thin and friable, may have less blood supply, and is at higher risk for breakdown.

Actions/Interventions	**Rationales**
■ Assess for history or presence of AIDS or other immunological problems.	Early manifestations of diseases related to human immunodeficiency virus may include skin lesions (e.g., Kaposi's sarcoma); in addition, because of their immunocompromised state, patients with AIDS often have skin breakdown.
■ Assess for fecal and/or urinary incontinence.	The urea in urine turns into ammonia within minutes and is caustic to the skin. Stool may contain enzymes that cause skin breakdown. Use of diapers and incontinence pads with plastic liners traps moisture and hastens breakdown.
■ Assess for environmental moisture (e.g., wound drainage, high humidity).	Moisture may contribute to skin maceration.
■ Assess the surface that the patient spends a majority of time on (e.g., mattress for bedridden patient, cushion for persons in wheelchairs).	Patients who spend the majority of time on one surface need a pressure reduction or pressure relief device to distribute pressure more evenly and lessen the risk for breakdown.
■ Assess amount of shear (pressure exerted laterally) and friction (rubbing) on the patient's skin.	A common cause of shear is elevating the head of the patient's bed: the body's weight is shifted downward onto the patient's sacrum. Common causes of friction include the patient rubbing heels or elbows against bed linen, and moving the patient up in bed without the use of a lift sheet.
■ Reassess skin often and whenever the patient's condition or treatment plan results in an increased number of risk factors.	The incidence and onset of skin breakdown is directly related to the number of risk factors present.
■ Assess skin for:	
• Dermatitis or exposure to chemical irritants	These conditions can cause inflammation, resulting in redness and itching, and may cause blisters.
• Pruritus or itching	Itching or mechanical traumas can result in disruptions to skin integrity and reduce its barrier function.
• Mechanical trauma	
• Long-term steroid use	Long-term steroid use may leave skin papery thin and prone to injury.

Therapeutic Interventions

Actions/Interventions	**Rationales**
■ If patient is restricted to bed, encourage implementation and posting of a turning schedule, restricting time in one position to 2 hours or less, and customizing the schedule to the patient's routine and caregiver's needs.	A schedule that does not interfere with the patient's and caregiver's activities is most likely to be followed. Use of a written schedule may be effective. Turning every 2 hours is key. The head of the bed should be kept at 30 degrees or less (or as condition allows) to avoid sliding down on bed.
■ Encourage implementation of pressure-relieving devices commensurate with degree of risk for skin impairment:	
• For low-risk patients: good-quality (dense, at least 5 inches thick) foam mattress overlay	Egg crate–type mattresses less than 4 to 5 inches thick do not relieve pressure. Because they are made of foam, moisture can be trapped. A false sense of security with the use of these mattresses can delay initiation of devices useful in relieving pressure.
• For moderate-risk patients: water mattress, static or dynamic air mattress	Dynamic devices electronically alternate inflation and deflation of the device. Static devices consist of gel, foam, water, or air that remain in a constant state of inflation. In the home, a waterbed is a good alternative.

■ = Independent ▲ = Collaborative

Actions/Interventions

- For high-risk patients or those with existing stage III or IV pressure ulcers (or with stage II pressure ulcers and multiple risk factors): low–air-loss beds (Mediscus, Flexicare, KinAir) or air-fluidized therapy (Clinitron, Skytron)

■ Encourage the patient and/or caregiver to maintain functional body alignment.

■ Change chair-bound position every hour and encourage the patient to shift weight every 15 minutes.

■ Encourage ambulation if the patient is able.

■ Increase tissue perfusion by massaging *around* affected area.

■ Clean, dry, and moisturize skin, especially over bony prominences, twice daily or as indicated by incontinence or sweating. Avoid hot water. If powder is desirable, use medical grade cornstarch; avoid talc.

▲ Encourage adequate nutrition and hydration:
- 2000 to 3000 kcal/day (more if increased metabolic demands)
- Fluid intake of 2000 mL/day unless medically restricted

■ Encourage use of lifting devices (bed linen or trapeze) to move patient in bed, and discourage patient or caregiver from elevating head of bed repeatedly.

■ Use pillows or foam wedges to keep bony prominences from direct contact with each other. Keep pillows under heels to raise off bed.

▲ Leave blisters intact by wrapping in gauze or applying a hydrocolloid or a vapor-permeable membrane dressing.

Rationales

Low–air-loss beds allow elevated head of bed and patient transfer. These should be used when pulmonary concerns necessitate elevating the head of bed or when getting the patient up is feasible. Air-fluidized therapy supports the patient's weight at well below capillary closing pressure but restricts getting the patient out of bed easily.

Misalignment can lead to discomfort and injury to joints, nerves, or limbs.

Pressure over the sacrum may exceed 100 mm Hg during sitting. The pressure necessary to close skin capillaries is around 32 mm Hg; any pressure greater than 32 mm Hg results in skin ischemia.

Ambulation reduces pressure on the skin from immobility.

Massaging the actual reddened area may damage the skin further.

Smooth, supple skin is more resistant to injury. Use a mild cleansing agent. Moisturizers or emollients should contain lipids that help to trap water and prevent evaporation away from skin. Emollients also attract water from the dermis and retain it in the epidermis. Avoid talc, which can be inhaled and cause lung injury.

Adequate hydration and nutrition help maintain skin turgor, moisture, and suppleness, which provide resilience to damage caused by pressure.

Hydrated skin is less susceptible to breakdown. Patients with limited cardiovascular reserve may not be able to tolerate this much fluid.

These measures reduce shearing forces on the skin.

Blisters are sterile natural dressings. Leaving them intact maintains the skin's natural function as a barrier to pathogens while the impaired area below the blister heals.

Education/Continuity of Care

Actions/Interventions

▲ Consult dietitian as appropriate.

■ Teach the patient and caregiver the causes of pressure ulcer development:
- Pressure on skin, especially over bony prominences
- Incontinence
- Poor nutrition
- Shearing or friction against skin

■ Reinforce the importance of mobility, turning, or ambulation in prevention of pressure ulcers.

■ Teach the patient or caregiver the proper use and maintenance of pressure-redistribution devices to be used at home.

Rationales

The dietitian can assist the patient and family in food choices to meet adequate nutritional and hydration goals.

This information can assist the patient or caregiver in finding methods to prevent skin breakdown.

Teaching the patient or caregiver methods to prevent pressure ulcers will enhance their sense of self-efficacy and can improve compliance with the prescribed interventions.

Care and maintenance of pressure-redistribution devices will promote their ongoing effectiveness.

Actions/Interventions

■ Teach patients and caregivers about proper skin care to prevent skin breakdown:

- Avoid bar soaps. Use soap substitutes such as aqueous creams.

- Moisturize skin with creams and lotions or emollients.

- Avoid soaps or lotions with perfumes/dyes or alcohol.

▲ Consult wound, ostomy and continence nurse (WOCN).

Rationales

Teaching patients and caregivers methods to maintain skin integrity enhances their sense of self-efficacy and prevents skin breakdown.

Bar soaps can strip skin of natural oils needed for elasticity and hydration. Soaps change the acidity of the skin, which can lead to breakdown.

Moisturizers rehydrate the skin and optimize skin integrity. Drier skin may need emollients (greasier moisturizers).

The perfumes or dyes may cause skin irritation, and the alcohol can lead to skin dryness.

The WOCN nurse can assist staff, patient, and family in product selection, education, and development of a prevention plan.

Related Care Plan

Pressure ulcers, p. 946

Spiritual Distress

Definition: Impaired ability to experience and integrate meaning and purpose in life through connectedness with self, others, art, music, literature, nature, and/or a power greater than oneself

Spiritual distress is an experience of profound disharmony in the person's belief or value system that threatens the meaning of his or her life. During spiritual distress the patient may lose hope, question his or her belief system, or feel separated from his or her personal source of comfort and strength. Pain, chronic or terminal illness, impending surgery, and the death or illness of a loved one are crises that may cause spiritual distress. Prescribed treatments may present conflicts with the person's values, beliefs, or faith traditions. The health care environment may limit the person's ability to engage in practices or rituals that support spiritual well-being and a sense of connectedness. Being physically separated from family and familiar culture contributes to feeling alone and abandoned. Nurses in the hospital, home care, and ambulatory settings can assist the patient in reestablishing a sense of spiritual well-being.

Common Related Factors

Active dying
Anxiety
Chronic illness
Death of a family member
Developmental or situational crises
Life changes
Self-alienation
Social alienation or isolation

Defining Characteristics

Connections to self
- Anger
- Expresses lack of acceptance, forgiveness of self, courage, or hope
- Expresses lack of meaning or purpose in life
- Expresses lack of serenity or peace

Connections with others
- Expresses alienation or separation from support system
- Refuses interactions with significant others or spiritual leaders

Connections with art, music, literature, nature
- Disinterest in engaging in connection activities
- Inability to engage in previous creative activities

■ = Independent   ▲ = Collaborative

Connections with power greater than self
- Expresses abandonment, hopelessness, suffering
- Expresses anger toward a higher power or God
- Inability to experience the transcendent or to be introspective
- Inability to participate in prayer or religious activities
- Requests to see spiritual leader
- Sudden change in spiritual practices

Common Expected Outcomes

Patient expresses hope in and value of his or her own belief system and inner resources.

Patient expresses a sense of well-being through art, music, or writing.

Patient participates in spiritual activities.

Patient expresses connectedness with self, others, or a higher power.

NOC Outcomes
Hope; Spiritual Well-Being
NIC Interventions
Spiritual Support; Coping Enhancement; Emotional Support

Ongoing Assessment

Actions/Interventions	Rationales
■ Assess history of formal religious affiliation and desire for religious contact.	Information regarding specific religion and importance of rituals or practices may improve understanding of the patient's needs.
■ Assess cultural beliefs.	All people have a spiritual dimension even if they do not express association with a specific religion or faith tradition. Individuals may have other important beliefs besides religion that provide strength and inspiration.
■ Assess spiritual meaning of illness or treatment. Questions such as the following provide a basis for future care planning: • "What is the meaning of your illness?" • "How does your illness or treatment affect your relationship with God, your beliefs, or other sources of strength?" • "Does your illness or treatment interfere with expressing your spiritual beliefs?"	Level of physical functioning, duration and course of illness, prognosis, and treatments involved can contribute to spiritual distress. Physical impairments or suffering may be seen as "punishment from God."
■ Assess hope.	Being hopeful provides a link to spiritual well-being.
■ Assess whether patient has any unfinished business.	Patients may not find peace or harmony until business is completed, such as resolving strained family relations.

Therapeutic Interventions

Actions/Interventions	Rationales
■ Encourage verbalization of feelings of anger or loneliness.	When interviewed later, after the crisis is resolved, usually patients list the nurse's listening to concerns and the nurse's technical competence as two of the most important items that helped create a sense of well-being.
■ Acknowledge understanding of the patient's spiritual beliefs and practices.	Patients have a right to their beliefs and practices, even if they conflict with the nurse's.
■ Develop an ongoing relationship with the patient.	An ongoing relationship establishes trust, reduces the feeling of isolation, and may facilitate resolution of spiritual distress.

Actions/Interventions

■ Facilitate decision making consistent with the patient's beliefs and values.

■ When requested by patient or family, arrange for visits from spiritual leaders, religious rituals, or the display of religious objects, especially when the patient is hospitalized.

■ Assist the patient with spiritual rituals. If requested, pray with the patient.

■ Acknowledge and support the patient's hopes.

■ Do not provide logical solutions for spiritual dilemmas.

■ Facilitate communication between patient and family, spiritual leaders, and other caregivers.

Rationales

The nurse may advocate and support a patient's decision to accept or refuse health care treatment consistent with his or her spiritual beliefs.

Religious rituals and objects help lessen feelings of separation and provide strength and inspiration. If the patient belongs to a highly codified or ritualized religion, such as Orthodox Judaism, spiritual leaders are important at times of passage, such as birth or death. In times of crisis the patient may not have the inner strength to call spiritual leaders without assistance.

Spiritual rituals and prayer provide a sense of connectedness to others. Prayer combined with authentic empathy from the nurse can help patients meet their spiritual needs. Some faith traditions may require the patient to face a specific direction during prayer. The patient may need assistance to change positions for prayer.

Hopes are different from denial or delusions. Supporting a hope for discharge does not mean supporting a denial of the seriousness of the patient's condition. Hope allows the patient to face the seriousness of the situation.

Spiritual beliefs are based on faith and are independent of logic.

The patient may desire privacy or rest or may not want spiritual leaders present, but may find it difficult to express.

Education/Continuity of Care

Actions/Interventions

■ Provide information in a way that does not interfere with the patient's beliefs, faith, or hopes.
■ Inform the patient and family of how to obtain religious rites or seek spiritual guidance.

Rationales

Providing information in this way demonstrates respect for the patient's individuality.

Religious rites or spiritual guidance may be essential when decisions about prolonging life, organ donation, or some medical therapy (e.g., blood transfusion) is a question in the patient's mind.

Impaired Swallowing

Definition: Abnormal functioning of the swallowing mechanism associated with deficits in oral, pharyngeal, or esophageal structure or function

Impaired swallowing can be a temporary or permanent complication that can be life threatening. Aspiration of food or fluid is the most serious complication. Impaired swallowing can be caused by a structural problem, interruption or dysfunction of neural pathways, decreased strength or excursion of muscles involved in mastication, facial paralysis, or perceptual impairment. Swallowing difficulties are a common complaint among older adults, in those individuals who have had a stroke, suffered head trauma, have head or neck cancer, or experience progressive neurological diseases like Parkinson's disease, multiple sclerosis, and amyotrophic lateral sclerosis. Dysphagia severity rating scales are available to guide extent of modification in diet plan.

■ = Independent   ▲ = Collaborative

Common Related Factors

Neuromuscular:
- Decreased or absent gag reflex
- Decreased strength or excursion of muscles involved in mastication
- Perceptual impairment
- Facial paralysis (cranial nerves VII, IX, X, XII)

Mechanical:
- Edema
- Tracheostomy tube
- Tumor

Fatigue

Limited awareness

Reddened, irritated oropharyngeal cavity (stomatitis)

Defining Characteristics

Observed evidence of difficulty in swallowing (coughing, choking, stasis of food in oral cavity)

Verbalized difficulty swallowing

Complaints of "something stuck" in throat

Abnormality in swallow study

Evidence of aspiration

Common Expected Outcomes

Patient exhibits ability to safely swallow, as evidenced by absence of aspiration, no evidence of coughing or choking during eating/drinking, no stasis of food in oral cavity after eating, and ability to ingest foods/fluid.

Patient verbalizes appropriate maneuvers to prevent choking and aspiration: positioning during eating, type of food tolerated, and safe environment.

Patient and caregiver verbalize emergency measures to be enacted should choking occur.

NOC Outcomes
Swallowing Status; Risk Control; Self-Care: Eating
NIC Interventions
Aspiration Precautions; Swallowing Therapy

Ongoing Assessment

Actions/Interventions	Rationales
■ Assess for presence of gag and cough reflexes.	The lungs are normally protected against aspiration by reflexes such as cough or gag. When reflexes are depressed, patient is at increased risk for aspiration.
■ Assess strength of facial muscles.	Cranial nerves VII, IX, X, and XII regulate motor function in the mouth and pharynx. Coordinated function of muscles innervated by these nerves is necessary to move a bolus of food from the front of the mouth to the posterior pharynx for controlled swallowing.
■ Assess coughing or choking during eating and drinking.	These signs indicate aspiration risk.
■ Assess ability to swallow small amount of water.	If aspirated, little or no harm to patient occurs.
■ Assess for residual food in mouth after eating.	Pocketed food may be easily aspirated at a later time.
■ Assess regurgitation of food or fluid through nares.	Regurgitation indicates a decreased ability to swallow food or fluids and an increased risk for aspiration.
▲ Assess results of swallowing studies as ordered.	A video-fluoroscopic swallowing study may be indicated to determine nature and extent of any oropharyngeal swallowing abnormality, which aids in designing interventions.

Therapeutic Interventions

Actions/Interventions	Rationales
For the hospitalized or home care patient:	
■ Before mealtime, provide adequate rest periods.	Fatigue can further contribute to swallowing impairment.
■ Remove or reduce environmental stimuli (e.g., television, radio).	With distractions removed, the patient can concentrate on swallowing.
■ Provide oral care before feeding. Clean and insert dentures before each meal.	Optimal oral care facilitates appetite and eating.

Actions/Interventions

▲ If swallowing study was completed, consult with speech pathologist regarding level of dysphagia severity and implications for meal planning.

■ Place suction equipment at bedside, and suction as needed.

■ If decreased salivation is a contributing factor:
  • Before feeding, give the patient a lemon wedge, pickle, or tart-flavored hard candy.
  • Use artificial saliva.
■ Maintain the patient in high-Fowler's position with head flexed slightly forward during meals.

■ Encourage intake of food that the patient can swallow; provide frequent small meals and supplements. Use thickening agents as recommended by a speech pathologist.

■ Instruct the patient to (1) hold food in mouth, (2) close lips, (3) think about swallowing, and then (4) swallow.
■ Instruct the patient not to talk while eating. Provide verbal cueing as needed.
■ Encourage the patient to chew thoroughly, eat slowly, and swallow frequently, especially if extra saliva is produced. Provide patient with direction or reinforcement until he or she has swallowed each mouthful.
■ Identify food given to the patient before each spoonful if the patient is being fed.

■ Proceed slowly, giving small amounts; whenever possible, alternate servings of liquids and solids.
■ Encourage a high-calorie diet that includes all food groups, as appropriate. Avoid milk and milk products.
■ If patients pouch food to one side of their mouth, encourage them to turn their head to the unaffected side and manipulate the tongue to paralyzed side.

■ If patient has had a stroke, place food in back of mouth, on unaffected side, and gently massage unaffected side of throat.
■ Place whole or crushed pills in custard or gelatin. (First ask a pharmacist which pills should not be crushed.) Substitute medication in elixir form as indicated.
■ Encourage the patient to feed self as soon as possible.

■ If oral intake is not possible or is inadequate, initiate alternative feedings (e.g., nasogastric feedings, gastrostomy feedings, or hyperalimentation).

Follow-up:
▲ Initiate dietary consultation for calorie count and food preferences.

Rationales

Levels on rating scales can range from minimal dysphagia, in which no change in diet is required, to mild-moderate dysphagia, in which specific swallow techniques and a modified diet may be indicated, to severe dysphagia, in which nothing by mouth is recommended.

With impaired swallowing reflexes, secretions can rapidly accumulate in the posterior pharynx and upper trachea, increasing risk for aspiration.

Moistening and use of tart flavors stimulate salivation, lubricate food, and enhance ability to swallow.

Upright position facilitates gravity flow of food or fluid through alimentary tract. Aspiration is less likely to occur with head tilted slightly forward (position narrows airway).

Thickened foods with consistency of pudding, cooked cereal, and semisolid food are easier for the patient to manage in the mouth and pharynx for controlled swallowing. Thin foods are most difficult; gravy or sauce added to dry foods facilitates swallowing.

Proper instruction and focused concentration on specific steps reduces risks.

Concentration must be focused on swallowing.

Such directions assist in keeping one's focus on the task.

Knowledge of consistency of food to expect can prepare the patient for appropriate chewing and swallowing technique.

This technique helps prevent foods from being left in the mouth.

Dairy products can lead to thickened secretions.

Foods placed in unaffected side of mouth facilitate more complete chewing and movement of food to back of mouth, where it can be swallowed. These strategies aid in cleaning out residual food.

Massage helps stimulate act of swallowing.

Mixing some pills with foods helps reduce risk for aspiration.

With self-feeding, the patient can control the volume of a food bolus and the timing of each bite to facilitate effective swallowing.

Optimal nutrition is a patient need.

Dietitians have a greater understanding of the nutritional value of foods and may be helpful in guiding treatment.

■ = Independent ▲ = Collaborative

Nursing Diagnosis Care Plans

Education/Continuity of Care

Actions/Interventions	Rationales
■ Discuss with and demonstrate the following to the patient or caregiver: • Avoidance of certain foods or fluids • Upright position during eating • Allowance of time to eat slowly and chew thoroughly • Provision of high-calorie meals • Use of fluids to help facilitate passage of solid foods • Monitoring of patient for weight loss or dehydration	Both the patient and caregiver may need to be active participants in implementing the treatment plan to optimize safe nutritional intake.
■ Teach patient/caregiver exercises to enhance muscular strength of face and tongue to enhance swallowing.	Muscle strengthening can facilitate greater chewing ability and positioning of food in mouth.
■ Facilitate home care aide or meal provision, if needed.	Homebound patients may require additional assistance to maintain adequate nutrition.
■ Demonstrate to the patient, caregiver, or family what should be done if the patient aspirates (e.g., chokes, coughs, becomes short of breath). For example, use suction, if available, and the Heimlich maneuver if the patient is unable to speak or breathe. If liquid aspiration, turn the patient three-fourths prone with head slightly lower than chest. If patient has difficulty breathing, call the Emergency Medical System (9-1-1).	Respiratory aspiration requires immediate action by the caregiver to maintain the airway and promote effective breathing and gas exchange. Being prepared for an emergency helps prevent further complications.
■ Encourage family members or caregiver to seek out cardiopulmonary resuscitation (CPR) instruction.	Mastery of emergency measures may provide confidence to both the patient and caregiver.

NANDA-I
NDx Ineffective Therapeutic Regimen Management

Definition: Pattern of regulating and integrating into daily living a program for treatment of illness and the sequelae of illness that is unsatisfactory for meeting specific health goals

With the ongoing changes in health care, patients are being expected to be comanagers of their care. They are being discharged from hospitals earlier and are faced with increasingly complex therapeutic regimens to be handled in the home environment. Likewise, patients with chronic illness often have limited access to health care providers and are expected to assume responsibility for managing the nuances of their disease (e.g., heart failure patients taking an extra furosemide [Lasix] tablet for a 2-pound weight gain).

Patients with sensory perception deficits, altered cognition, or financial limitations and those who lack support systems may find themselves overwhelmed and unable to follow the treatment plan. Older patients, who often experience most of the above problems, are especially at high risk for ineffective management of the therapeutic plan. Other vulnerable populations include patients living in adverse social conditions (e.g., poverty, unemployment, little education); patients with emotional problems (e.g., depression over the illness being treated or other life crises or problems); and patients with substance abuse problems. Culture, ethnicity, and religion may influence one's health beliefs, health practices (e.g., folk medicine, alternative therapies), access to health services, and assertiveness in pursuing specific health care services.

Common Related Factors

Complexity of health care
Complexity of therapeutic regimen
Economic difficulties
Excessive demands made on individual or family
Decisional conflicts
Family conflict
Family patterns of health care
Inadequate number and types of cues to action
Knowledge deficit of prescribed regimen
Mistrust of regimen of health care providers
Perceived seriousness
Perceived susceptibility
Perceived barriers
Social support deficits
Perceived powerlessness

Defining Characteristics

Choices of daily living ineffective for meeting the goals of treatment or prescription program
Increased illness symptoms
Verbalized desire to manage the treatment of and prevention of sequelae from illness
Verbalized difficulty with prescribed regimen
Verbalization by patient that he or she did not follow prescribed regimen

Common Expected Outcomes

Patient verbalizes intention to follow prescribed regimen.
Patient describes or demonstrates required competencies.
Patient identifies appropriate resources.
Patient demonstrates ongoing adherence to treatment plan.

NOC Outcomes

Compliance Behavior; Knowledge: Treatment Regimen

NIC Interventions

Self-Modification Assistance; Teaching: Individual; Health System Guidance

Ongoing Assessment

Actions/Interventions	Rationales
■ Assess prior efforts to follow a regimen.	This knowledge provides an important starting point in understanding any complexities in implementation of the treatment plan.
■ Assess for related factors that may negatively affect success with following the regimen.	Knowledge of causative factors provides direction for subsequent intervention. This may range from financial constraints to physical limitations.
■ Assess the patient's individual perceptions of health problems.	According to the Health Belief Model, the patient's perceived susceptibility to and perceived seriousness and threat of disease affect compliance with the treatment plan. In addition, factors such as cultural phenomena and heritage can affect how people view their health.
■ Assess the patient's confidence in his or her ability to perform desired behavior.	According to the self-efficacy theory, positive conviction that one can successfully execute a behavior is correlated with performance and successful outcome.
■ Assess the patient's ability to learn or remember the desired health-related activity.	Cognitive impairments need to be identified so an appropriate alternative plan can be devised. For example, the Mini-Mental State Examination can be used to identify memory problems that could interfere with accurate pill taking. Once these problems are identified, alternative actions, such as using egg cartons to dispense medications or receiving daily phone reminders, can be instituted.

■ = Independent   ▲ = Collaborative

Actions/Interventions

■ Assess the patient's ability to perform the desired activity.

Rationales

The patient's ability to perform the activity determines the amount and type of education that needs to be provided. For example, patients with limited financial resources may be unable to purchase special diet foods such as those low in fat or low in salt. Patients with arthritis may be unable to open childproof pill containers.

Therapeutic Interventions

Actions/Interventions

■ Include the patient in planning the treatment regimen.

■ Inform the patient of the benefits of adherence to the prescribed regimen.

■ Tailor the therapy to the patient's lifestyle (e.g., taking diuretics at dinner if working outside the home during the day).

■ Simplify the regimen. Suggest long-acting forms of medications, and eliminate unnecessary medication.

■ Eliminate unnecessary clinic visits.

■ Develop a system for the patient to monitor own progress.

■ Develop with the patient a system of rewards that follow successful follow-through.

■ Concentrate on the behaviors that will make the greatest contribution to the therapeutic effect.

■ If negative side effects of prescribed treatment are a problem, explain that many side effects can be controlled or eliminated.

■ If the patient lacks adequate support in following the prescribed treatment plan, initiate referral to a support group (e.g., AARP, American Diabetes Association, senior groups, weight loss programs, Breast Cancer Network of Strength, smoking cessation clinics, stress management classes, social services).

Rationales

Patients who become comanagers of their care have a greater stake in achieving a positive outcome. They know best their personal and environmental barriers to success.

Patients who believe in the efficacy of the recommended treatment to reduce risk or to promote health are more likely to engage in it.

Tailoring the therapy will foster a patient-centered focus and promote compliance. A "one size fits all" approach is usually ineffective.

The greater the number of times during the day that patients need to take medications, the greater the risk of not following through. Polypharmacy is a significant problem with older patients. Attempt to reduce nonessential drug usage.

The physical demands of traveling to an appointment, the financial costs incurred (loss of day's work, child care), the negative feelings of being "talked down to" by health care providers not fluent in the patient's language, as well as the commonly long waits can cause patients to avoid follow-ups when they are required. Telephone follow-up may be substituted as appropriate.

Self-monitoring is a key component of a successful change in behavior.

Rewards may consist of verbal praise, monetary rewards, special privileges (e.g., earlier office appointment, free parking), or telephone calls.

Behavior change is never easy. Efforts should be directed to activities known to result in specific benefits (e.g., smoking cessation, fluid control in heart failure patients).

Nonadherence because of medication side effects is a commonly reported problem. Health care providers need to determine actual etiological factors for side effects and possible interplay with over-the-counter medications. Similarly, patients may report fatigue or muscle cramps with exercise. If so, the exercise prescription may need to be revised.

Groups that come together for mutual support and information can be beneficial, especially to patients coping with chronic illness.

Education/Continuity of Care

Actions/Interventions	Rationales
■ Use a variety of teaching methods to match the patient's preferred learning style.	Different people learn in different ways. Match the learning style with the educational approach. For some patients this may require grocery shopping for "healthy foods" with a dietitian or a home visit by the nurse to review a psychomotor skill.
■ Introduce complicated therapy one step at a time.	This format allows the learner to concentrate more completely on one topic at a time.
■ Instruct the patient in the importance of reordering medications 2 to 3 days before running out.	Although many cultures in the United States are future oriented and are concerned with measures to prevent illness, other cultures are more oriented to the present. This difference in time orientation may need to be addressed.
■ Include significant others in explanations and teaching. Encourage their support and assistance in following plans.	Inclusion of significant others encourages support and assistance in reinforcing appropriate behaviors and facilitating lifestyle modification.
■ Allow the learner to practice new skills; provide immediate feedback on performance.	Practice allows the patient to use new information immediately, thus enhancing retention. Immediate feedback allows the learner to make corrections rather than practice the skill incorrectly.
■ Role-play scenarios when nonadherence to the plan may easily occur. Demonstrate appropriate behaviors.	Relapse prevention needs to be addressed early in the treatment plan. Helping the patient expand his or her repertoire of responses to difficult situations assists in meeting treatment goals.

NANDA-I NDx Impaired Tissue Integrity

Definition: Damage to mucous membrane, corneal, integumentary, or subcutaneous tissues

Tissue is a collection of cells with similar structure or function. The four types of tissue are epithelial, connective, muscular, and nervous. Tissue can be damaged by physical trauma, including thermal injury (e.g., frostbite); chemical insult, including reactions to drugs, especially chemotherapeutic drugs; radiation; and ischemia. Inflammation of subcutaneous tissue is called cellulitis. Some damaged tissue is able to regenerate (e.g., skin, mucous membranes) whereas other damaged tissue may be replaced by connective tissue (e.g., cardiac and smooth muscle cells). If untreated, impaired tissue is at risk for infection and/or necrosis (tissue death) and can lead to systemic infection (e.g., sepsis or septicemia). Persons at risk for impaired tissue integrity include the homeless, individuals undergoing cancer therapy, and individuals with altered sensation.

Common Related Factors	Defining Characteristics
Trauma	Affected area hot, tender to touch
Temperature extremes	Skin purplish
Infection	Swelling around initial injury
Altered circulation	Local pain
Chemical irritants	Protectiveness toward site
Fluid imbalances	
Nutritional deficits or extremes	
Radiation	

■ = Independent   ▲ = Collaborative

Common Expected Outcome

Patient's tissues return to normal structure and function.

NOC Outcome

Tissue Integrity: Skin and Mucous Membranes

NIC Interventions

Wound Care; Infection Protection; Teaching:
Prescribed Medication

Ongoing Assessment

Actions/Interventions	Rationales
■ Determine the etiology of tissue damage.	Information guides design of optimal treatment plan (e.g., infection versus burns).
■ Assess condition of tissue.	Redness, swelling, pain, burning, and itching are signs of the body's immune response to localized tissue trauma.
■ Assess characteristics of the wound, including color, size, drainage, and odor.	These data provide information on extent of damage. Color of tissue is an indication of tissue viability and oxygenation. Odor may arise from infection present in the wound; it may also arise from necrotic tissue. Wound drainage or exudate is a normal part of wound physiology and must be differentiated from pus, which is an indication of infection. Purulent drainage from the injured area is an indication of infection.
■ Assess for elevated body temperature.	Fever can be an indication of infection unless the patient is immunocompromised.
■ Assess the patient's level of discomfort.	Depth of wound may affect pain sensations.
■ Identify signs of itching and scratching.	The patient who scratches the skin in attempts to relieve intense itching may open skin lesions and increase risk for infection.

Therapeutic Interventions

Actions/Interventions	Rationales
■ Remove any embedded material (e.g., glass, metal), as needed.	Removal facilitates wound healing and prevention of infection.
■ Cleanse with normal saline or a nontoxic cleanser, as appropriate.	Cleansing removes debris and pathogens.
▲ Provide skin care as needed. For example, cover wound with wet or dry dressing, using topical creams or lubricants, using hydrocolloid dressing (e.g., DuoDerm) or vapor-permeable membrane dressing such as Tegaderm.	Each type of wound is best treated based on its etiology.
■ Maintain sterile dressing technique during wound care.	Sterile technique reduces risk for infection.
▲ Premedicate for dressing changes as needed.	Manipulation of deeper or extensive wounds may be painful.
■ Saturate dressings with sterile normal saline solution before removal.	Saturating dressings will ease dressing removal by loosening adherents and decreasing pain, especially with burns.
▲ Administer antibiotics as ordered.	Wound infections may be treated more easily with topical agents, although intravenous antibiotics may be indicated.
■ Discourage rubbing and scratching. Provide gloves or clip nails if necessary.	Rubbing and scratching can cause further injury and delay healing.
■ Encourage diet that meets nutritional needs.	A high-protein, high-calorie diet may be needed to promote healing.

Education/Continuity of Care

Actions/Interventions	Rationales
■ Teach patient or caregiver about cause of tissue integrity impairment.	Thorough understanding of specific cause is necessary for appropriate follow-through of treatment plan.
■ Instruct the patient or caregiver in proper care of wound (i.e., cleansing, dressing, and application of topical medications).	Teaching increases the patient's ability to manage therapy independently.
■ Teach the patient or caregiver signs and symptoms of infection and when to notify the physician or nurse.	The patient needs to be aware of potential complications to facilitate prompt intervention in the event of a problem.
■ Teach the patient or caregiver pain control measures (e.g., soaks, use of analgesics, and distraction).	Information allows the patient to identify when therapy adjustments need to be made.

Related Care Plans

Burns, p. 933
Risk for impaired skin integrity, p. 185
Pressure ulcers, p. 946

Ineffective Tissue Perfusion (Peripheral, Cerebral, Cardiopulmonary, Renal, Gastrointestinal)

Definition: Decrease in oxygen resulting in failure to nourish the tissues at the capillary level

Reduced arterial blood flow causes decreased nutrition and oxygenation at the cellular level. Decreased tissue perfusion can be transient with few or minimal consequences to the health of the patient, or it can be more acute or protracted with potentially devastating effects on the patient. Diminished tissue perfusion, which is chronic in nature, invariably results in tissue or organ damage or death. Management is directed at removing vasoconstricting factors, improving peripheral blood flow, and reducing metabolic demands on the body.

In practice, patients often present with a combination of causative factors. Therefore this care plan will focus on the general assessment and therapeutic interventions common to many etiologies. The reader is referred to the more specific medical disorder care plans that follow in later chapters. A list of some of these is provided toward the end of this care plan.

Common Related Factors

Impaired transport of oxygen
Interruption in blood flow
Mismatch of ventilation with blood flow
Decreased hemoglobin concentration in blood
Hypoventilation
Hypovolemia
Hypervolemia
Exchange problems
Altered affinity of hemoglobin for oxygen

Defining Characteristics—Peripheral

Weak or absent peripheral pulses
Numbness, pain, ache, claudication in extremities
Skin temperature changes/cool extremities/clammy skin
Shiny skin/loss of hair
Thickened discolored nails
Difference in blood pressure in opposite extremity
Skin color pales on elevation/dependent rubor
Prolonged capillary refill
Bruits
Delayed healing
Altered sensation

Defining Characteristics—Cerebral

Altered level of consciousness
Changes in motor response
Speech abnormalities

■ = Independent ▲ = Collaborative

Changes in pupillary reactions
Behavioral changes
Dysphagia

Defining Characteristics— Cardiopulmonary

Tachycardia
Dysrhythmias
Hypotension
Tachypnea
Dyspnea
Chest pain
Prolonged capillary refill
Abnormal arterial blood gases
Bronchospasm

Defining Characteristics—Renal

Elevation in blood urea nitrogen [BUN]/creatinine ratio
Oliguria
Anuria
Hematuria
Altered blood pressure outside of normal ranges

Defining Characteristics— Gastrointestinal

Abdominal distention
Abdominal pain or tenderness
Absent bowel sounds
Hypoactive bowel sounds
Nausea

Common Expected Outcomes

Patient maintains optimal peripheral tissue perfusion as evidenced by strong palpable peripheral pulses, reduction in or absence of pain, warm and dry extremities, adequate capillary refill (less than 2 seconds), and prevention of ulceration.

Patient maintains optimal cardiopulmonary perfusion as evidenced by cupnea, blood pressure within normal range for patient, absence of chest pain, warm and dry skin, palpable peripheral pulses, normal arterial blood gases, absence of adventitious breath sounds, and urinary output greater than or equal to 30 mL/hr.

Patient maintains optimal cerebral tissue perfusion as evidenced by alert responsive mentation, absence of neurological deficits, normoreactive pupils, normal/baseline motor function, stable blood pressure with position changes, and absence of dizziness.

Patient maintains optimal renal perfusion as evidenced by urinary output greater than or equal to 30 mL/hr, normal BUN/creatinine ratio, absence of hematuria, and acceptable blood pressure for patient.

Patient maintains optimal gastrointestinal perfusion as evidenced by absence of abdominal pain, normal bowel sounds, good appetite, and absence of nausea.

NOC Outcomes

Tissue Perfusion: Cardiopulmonary; Tissue Perfusion: Cerebral; Tissue Perfusion: Abdominal Organs; Tissue Perfusion: Peripheral; Fluid Balance; Electrolyte and Acid/Base Balance

NIC Interventions

Circulatory Care: Arterial Insufficiency; Circulatory Care: Venous Insufficiency; Cardiac Care: Acute; Cerebral Perfusion Promotion; Hypovolemia Management

Ongoing Assessment

Actions/Interventions

■ Assess for signs of decreased tissue perfusion.

■ Assess for possible causative factors of reduced tissue perfusion. Some examples include:
- *Peripheral:* Vasospasm, indwelling arterial catheters, constricting cast, compartment syndrome, embolism or thrombus, positioning
- *Cardiopulmonary:* Pulmonary embolism, low hemoglobin, myocardial ischemia, vasospasm
- *Cerebral:* Hypovolemia, positioning, increased intracranial pressure, intracranial bleeding, cerebral edema, vasoconstriction

■ Monitor blood pressure for orthostatic changes.

▲ Use pulse oximetry to monitor oxygen saturation and pulse rate.

▲ Monitor hemoglobin levels.

Rationales

Specific clusters of signs and symptoms occur with differing etiologies. Evaluation provides baseline for future comparisons.

Early detection of causes facilitates prompt, effective treatment.

Stable blood pressure is necessary to maintain adequate tissue perfusion, especially cerebral perfusion. Medication effects such as vasodilation, altered autonomic control, reduced fluid volume, and decompensated heart failure are among many factors potentially compromising optimal blood pressure.

Pulse oximetry is a useful tool to detect changes in oxygenation.

Low levels reduce the uptake of oxygen at the alveolar-capillary membrane and oxygen delivery to the tissues.

Therapeutic Interventions

Actions/Interventions

▲ Assist with diagnostic testing as indicated.

▲ Administer optimal fluid balance. For patients with decreased preload, administer intravenous fluids as ordered.

■ Assist with position changes.

■ Promote active/passive range-of-motion (ROM) exercises.

▲ If venous insufficiency is a cause, apply appropriate venous compression devices such as support hose or pneumatic compression.

▲ Maintain adequate ventilation and perfusion as in the following:
- Place patient in semi- to high-Fowler's position as tolerated
- Administer oxygen therapy as prescribed.

Rationales

A variety of tests are available depending on the etiology of the impaired tissue perfusion. These include segmental limb pressure measurement such as ankle-brachial index (ABI) for lower extremities, Doppler flow studies, vascular stress testing, and angiograms.

Volume therapy may be required to maintain adequate filling pressures and optimize cardiac output needed for tissue perfusion. Oral fluid replacement is indicated for mild fluid deficit. Older patients have a decreased sense of thirst and may need ongoing reminders to drink.

Slowly changing from supine to sitting/standing position can reduce the risk for orthostatic blood pressure changes. Older patients are more susceptible to such drops in pressure with position changes.

Exercise prevents venous stasis and further circulatory compromise.

These therapies promote increased venous return, contributing to improved cardiac output.

Upright positioning promotes improved alveolar gas exchange. Oxygen saturation needs to be greater than 90%. Increasing arterial oxygen saturation delivers more oxygen to the tissues and relieves oxygen supply and demand imbalances.

■ = Independent   ▲ = Collaborative

Nursing Diagnosis Care Plans

Actions/Interventions

▲ Administer medications as prescribed to treat underlying problem. Note response.
- Antiplatelets/anticoagulants (to reduce blood viscosity and coagulation)
- Peripheral vasodilators (to enhance arterial dilation and improve peripheral blood flow)
- Antihypertensives (to reduce systemic vascular resistance and optimize cardiac output and perfusion)
- Inotropes (to improve cardiac output)

▲ In acute situations, anticipate the need for more invasive therapies as indicated.

▲ For specific etiologies, anticipate directed interventions (e.g., fasciotomy for compartment syndrome; bivalving a constricting cast; nitroglycerine for complaints of angina; intracranial pressure catheters for some cerebral problems).

■ See also selected medical disorder care plans throughout this book that focus on specific etiologies for tissue impairment, such as chronic peripheral arterial occlusive disease, chronic venous insufficiency, transient ischemic attack, decreased intracranial adaptive capacity, stroke, angina pectoris, acute coronary syndromes, aortic aneurysm, and pulmonary embolism, to name a few.

Rationales

These medications facilitate perfusion for most etiologies of impairment.

Therapies such as percutaneous transluminal angioplasty/stenting, atherectomy, surgical revascularization, embolectomy, and thrombolytic therapy may be indicated.
Therapies help optimize tissue perfusion.

Education/Continuity of Care

Actions/Interventions

■ Provide information on normal tissue perfusion and possible causes for impairment.

■ Discuss examples of lifestyle factors that can promote improved tissue perfusion (avoiding crossed legs at the knee when sitting, changing positions at frequent intervals, rising slowly from supine/sitting to standing position, avoiding smoking, reducing risk factors for atherosclerosis [obesity, hypertension, dyslipidemia, inactivity]).

■ Explain all procedures and treatments.

■ Instruct the patient to inform the nurse immediately if symptoms of decreased tissue perfusion persist, increase, or return.

Rationales

Knowledge of causative factors provides rationale for treatments.
These measures reduce venous compression/venous stasis and arterial vasoconstriction.

Explaining expected events and sensations can help reduce anxiety associated with the unknown.
Early assessment facilitates prompt treatment.

 NANDA-I NDx **Urinary Retention**

Definition: Incomplete emptying of the bladder

Urinary retention may occur in conjunction with or independent of urinary incontinence. Urinary retention, the inability to empty the bladder even though urine is present, may occur as a side effect of certain medications, including anesthetic agents, antihypertensives, antihistamines, antispasmodics, and anticholinergics. These drugs interfere with the nerve impulses necessary to cause relaxation of the sphincters, which allow urination. Obstruction of outflow is another cause of urinary retention. Most commonly, this type of obstruction in men is the result of benign prostatic hyperplasia.

Common Related Factors

General anesthesia
Regional anesthesia
High urethral pressures caused by disease, injury, or edema
Pain, fear of pain
Infection
Inadequate intake
Urethral blockage

Defining Characteristics

Decreased (less than 30 mL/hr) or absent urinary output for 2 consecutive hours
Frequency
Sensation of bladder fullness
Bladder distention
Abdominal discomfort
Dribbling
Increased residual urine volume

Common Expected Outcome

Patient empties bladder completely as evidenced by urine volume greater than or equal to 300 mL with each voiding and residual volume less than 100 mL.

NOC Outcomes
Urinary Continence; Urinary Elimination; Infection Status
NIC Intervention
Urinary Retention Care

Ongoing Assessment

Actions/Interventions	Rationales
■ Evaluate previous patterns of voiding.	There is a wide range of "normal" voiding frequency.
■ Visually inspect and palpate lower abdomen for distention.	The bladder lies below the umbilicus. The lower abdomen becomes distended as the urine volume increases in the bladder.
■ Evaluate time intervals between voidings, and record the amount voided each time.	Keeping an hourly log for 48 hours gives a clear picture of the patient's voiding pattern and amounts and can help to establish a toileting schedule.
▲ Catheterize the patient or use a bladder scan (portable ultrasound instrument) to measure residual urine if incomplete emptying is suspected.	Retention of urine in the bladder predisposes the patient to urinary tract infection and may indicate the need for an intermittent catheterization program.
■ Assess amount, frequency, and character (e.g., color, odor, and specific gravity) of urine.	These characteristics allow for assessment of residual urine volumes and risk factors for a urinary tract infection.
■ Determine balance between intake and output.	Intake greater than output may indicate retention.
▲ Monitor urinalysis, urine culture, and sensitivity.	Urinary tract infection can cause retention, but it is more likely to cause frequency.
■ If an indwelling catheter is in place, assess for patency and kinking.	An occluded or kinked catheter may lead to urinary retention in the bladder.
▲ Monitor blood urea nitrogen and creatinine.	Elevation in these values will differentiate between urinary retention and renal failure as causes of decreased urine output.

Therapeutic Interventions

Actions/Interventions	Rationales
■ Initiate the following methods to facilitate voiding:	
• Encourage fluids unless the patient is on a fluid restriction.	Unless medically contraindicated, fluid intake should be at least 1500 mL/24 hr.
• Encourage intake of cranberry juice daily.	Cranberry juice keeps urine acidic. This helps prevent infection because cranberry juice metabolizes to hippuric acid, which maintains an acidic urine; acidic urine is less likely to become infected.
• Place bedpan, urinal, or bedside commode within reach.	

■ = Independent   ▲ = Collaborative

Actions/Interventions	Rationales
• Position patient upright if possible to facilitate successful voiding.	An upright position on a commode or in bed on a bedpan increases the patient's voiding success through force of gravity; it also decreases embarrassment of soiling self or bed linens.
• Provide privacy.	Privacy helps the patient relax urinary sphincters.
• Encourage the patient to void at least every 4 hours.	Voiding at frequent intervals empties the bladder and reduces risk for urinary retention.
• Have the patient listen to the sound of running water, or place the patient's hands in warm water and/or pour warm water over the perineum.	These actions stimulate urination.
• Offer fluids before voiding.	Sufficient urine volume is needed to stimulate the voiding reflex.
• Perform Credé's method over bladder.	Credé's method (pressing down over the bladder with the hands) increases bladder pressure, which stimulates relaxation of the sphincter to allow voiding.
▲ Encourage the patient to take bethanechol (Urecholine) as ordered.	Bethanechol stimulates the parasympathetic nervous system to release acetylcholine at nerve endings and to increase tone and amplitude of contractions of smooth muscles of the urinary bladder.
▲ Institute intermittent catheterization.	Because many causes of urinary retention are self-limited, the decision to leave an indwelling catheter in place should be avoided.
▲ Insert an indwelling (Foley) catheter as ordered: • Tape the catheter to abdomen (male) and thigh (female).	Taping catheter prevents inadvertent displacement.

Education/Continuity of Care

Actions/Interventions	Rationales
■ Educate the patient or caregiver about the importance of adequate fluid intake (e.g., 8 to 10 glasses of fluids daily) unless the patient is on a fluid restriction.	Increased fluid stimulates voiding and decreases the risk for development of urinary tract infections due to flushing of bacteria from the genitourinary tract.
■ Instruct the patient or caregiver in measures to stimulate voiding.	Knowledge of a variety of methods to enhance voiding optimizes success.
■ Instruct the patient or caregiver in signs and symptoms of overdistended bladder (e.g., decreased or absent urine, frequency, hesitancy, urgency, lower abdominal distention, or discomfort).	Knowing signs and symptoms allows for early recognition of the condition and treatment.
■ Instruct the patient or caregiver in signs and symptoms of urinary tract infection (e.g., chills and fever, frequent urination or concentrated urine, and abdominal or back pain).	Knowing signs and symptoms allows the patient or caregiver to recognize them and seek treatment.
■ Teach the patient or caregiver to perform meatal care twice daily with soap and water and to dry thoroughly.	Meatal care reduces the risk for infection.
■ Teach the patient to achieve an upright position on the toilet if possible.	An upright position is the natural position for voiding and uses the force of gravity.

Dysfunctional Ventilatory Weaning Response

Definition: Inability to adjust to lowered levels of mechanical ventilator support that interrupts and prolongs the weaning process

A patient is who is reliant on ventilatory support and unable to tolerate the weaning process is experiencing dysfunctional ventilatory weaning response (DVWR). This may result from physiological, psychological, or situational factors. Their influence should be evaluated before weaning and after each unsuccessful weaning attempt. In addition to the listed related factors, physiological factors associated with the inability to wean may include left ventricular failure, use of medications that depress the respiratory drive (e.g., sedatives, narcotics) or cause respiratory muscle weakness (neuromuscular blocking agents or aminoglycosides), alterations in metabolic status (hypophosphatemia, hypothyroidism, hypomagnesemia), acid-base imbalances (metabolic acidosis, respiratory alkalosis), respiratory tract infection, overhydration, anemia, significant alterations in vital signs, abnormal weaning parameters (negative inspiratory force, tidal volume, vital capacity, minute ventilation, rapid shallow breathing index), and an Fio_2 of greater than 0.50 on the ventilator. Additional psychological factors may include psychological ventilator dependence and agitation associated with intensive care unit psychosis, delirium, increased anxiety, and fear. Inability to wean may also be a result of lack of motivation secondary to depression, cognitive impairments, or personality disorders. Unfavorable situational factors such as an inappropriate weaning plan may also contribute to weaning failure. When abnormalities or adverse conditions are identified, the weaning plan should incorporate measures to eliminate them or minimize their effects so the risk for DVWR is reduced. Weaning may be postponed when the patient does not demonstrate readiness to wean. This reduces patient frustration and anxiety and avoids potentially life-threatening situations.

Common Related Factors

Physical:
- Ineffective airway clearance
- Sleep pattern disturbance
- Inadequate nutrition
- Uncontrolled pain or discomfort

Psychological:
- Knowledge deficit of the weaning process or patient role
- Patient-perceived inefficacy about the ability to wean
- Decreased motivation
- Decreased self-esteem
- Anxiety: moderate, severe
- Fear
- Hopelessness
- Powerlessness
- Insufficient trust in the nurse

Situational:
- Uncontrolled episodic energy demand or problems
- Inappropriate pacing of diminished ventilator support
- Inadequate social support
- Adverse environment (e.g., noisy, active environment; negative events in the room; low nurse-patient ratio; extended nurse absence from bedside; unfamiliar nursing staff)
- History of ventilator dependence greater than 1 week
- History of multiple unsuccessful weaning attempts

Defining Characteristics

Mild DVWR:
- Restlessness
- Slight increased respiratory rate (RR) from baseline
- Expressed feelings of increased need for oxygen, breathing discomfort, fatigue, and warmth

Moderate DVWR:
- Slight increase in blood pressure (BP) (less than 20 mm Hg)
- Slight increase in heart rate (HR) (less than 20 beats/min)
- Increase in RR (less than 5 breaths/min)
- Hypervigilance to activities
- Inability to respond to coaching
- Inability to cooperate
- Apprehension
- Diaphoresis
- Pale, slight cyanosis
- "Wide-eyed" look
- Decreased air entry on auscultation
- Slight respiratory accessory muscle use

Severe DVWR:
- Agitation
- Deterioration in arterial blood gases (ABGs) from current baseline
- Increase in BP (greater than 20 mm Hg)

■ = Independent   ▲ = Collaborative

- Increase in HR (greater than 20 beats/min)
- Increase in RR
- Profuse diaphoresis
- Full respiratory accessory muscle use
- Shallow, gasping breaths
- Paradoxical abdominal breathing
- Discoordinated breathing with the ventilator
- Decreased level of consciousness
- Adventitious breath sounds, audible airway secretions
- Cyanosis

Common Expected Outcome

Patient experiences a functional ventilatory weaning response as evidenced by BP, HR, and RR in normal range for patient; expressed feelings of comfort; being responsive or cooperative to coaching; ABGs within baseline range; and effective breathing pattern.

NOC Outcomes
Respiratory Status: Ventilation; Respiratory Status: Gas Exchange
NIC Interventions
Mechanical Ventilatory Weaning; Mechanical Ventilation

Ongoing Assessment

Actions/Interventions	**Rationales**
■ Assess for increasing dyspnea, restlessness, apprehension, and agitation.	These signs are associated with DVWR.
■ Monitor vital signs closely during weaning process, watching for increases in BP, HR, and RR.	Abnormal increases in these parameters indicate respiratory compromise and are signs of weaning failure.
■ Assess lungs for adventitious sounds.	When coarse crackles or sonorous wheezes are present, suctioning may be required to reduce airway resistance and the work of breathing.
■ Assess skin color and warmth. Assess for presence of cyanosis.	Cool, pale diaphoretic skin may be caused by a compensatory peripheral vasoconstrictive response to hypoxemia. Cyanosis may occur when 5 g of hemoglobin are desaturated.
■ Assess the patient's ability to cooperate and respond to coaching.	Cooperation and ability to be coached facilitate implementation of measures used to help patients control their breathing and anxiety and remain motivated to perform the work of breathing.
■ Monitor for signs of respiratory muscle fatigue (e.g., abrupt rise in $Paco_2$, rapid shallow ventilation, paradoxical abdominal wall motion) while weaning is in progress.	These signs of DVWR require resumption of preweaning level of ventilatory support.
■ Assess for presence of discoordinated breathing with the ventilator.	Discoordinated breathing increases the work of breathing, dyspnea, anxiety, and feelings of loss of control over breathing.
▲ Continuously monitor pulse oximetry for oxygen saturation. ABGs and capnography should also be evaluated when available.	These tools are used to assess the adequacy of oxygenation and ventilation during weaning and the need to resume previous level of ventilatory support.
■ For patients with chronic dyspnea, assess usual symptom management.	This information may reveal effective strategies for reducing dyspnea during weaning.
■ Before weaning and after each unsuccessful attempt, assess for physiological (e.g., lack of adequate sleep, poor nutrition), psychological (e.g., anxiety, fear), and situational (e.g., adverse environmental conditions) factors that contribute to DVWR.	Addressing these factors promotes successful weaning and reduces patient frustration and anxiety related to multiple unsuccessful weaning attempts and avoids potentially life-threatening situations.

Therapeutic Interventions

Actions/Interventions	Rationales
▲ Notify physician, and anticipate altering ventilator support depending on the degree of DVWR.	When DVWR occurs, greater ventilatory support is needed. Inappropriate settings can increase work of breathing and lead to respiratory muscle fatigue. The respiratory muscles can be rested with appropriate ventilator settings.
▲ Maintain the prescribed oxygen level and ventilatory settings.	Oxygen saturation of 90% or greater is needed to maintain adequate tissue oxygenation.
■ Suction the airway as needed to maintain patency.	Suctioning decreases airflow resistance and minimizes work of breathing.
▲ Individualize the patient's weaning program through collaboration with other health care team members. • Method of weaning (e.g., using the synchronized intermittent mandatory ventilation [SIMV] mode to slowly decrease ventilatory support versus use of continuous positive airway pressure and pressure support or short trials of oxygen alone with full suspension of ventilatory support) • Provision of adequate rest between weaning trials • Scheduled weaning for certain parts of the day	Patients respond differently to weaning efforts. Tailoring weaning strategies to the patient's needs and ensuring consistency among team members increase the potential for successful weaning.
▲ Maintain the patient's required nutrient intake. Collaborate with the dietitian to ensure that nutritional replacement is matched to metabolic needs.	Attention to required intake ensures sufficient nutrients to enable weaning. Malnutrition reduces respiratory mass and strength. Overfeeding increases metabolic production of carbon dioxide that increases respiratory drive and respiratory muscle fatigue.
▲ Administer pain medications and antianxiety medications, as required.	Pain medications are used to relieve uncontrolled pain or discomfort; however, oversedation could prevent the patient from ventilating adequately by blunting the respiratory drive.
■ Assist the patient with turning and repositioning during the weaning process. Postpone nonessential physical activities during weaning.	These measures decrease energy expenditure and reduce oxygen demand.
■ Coach the patient through ineffective breathing patterns and episodes of anxiety, assisting him or her to focus on breathing pattern. Demonstrate effective breathing techniques.	Coaching can reduce anxiety and assist in reestablishment of an effective breathing pattern.
■ Give frequent feedback to the patient regarding progress.	Feedback helps keep the patient working toward weaning.
■ Establish patient trust with the following measures: • Use a calm, empathetic approach. • Demonstrate confidence in the patient's abilities. • Explain things before doing them. • Collaborate with the patient in planning his or her care. • Provide individual attention. • Answer call light in a timely manner. • Do not minimize reports of dyspnea.	Patient trust and confidence in the nurse helps motivate the patient in the weaning process and decreases anxiety and fear. Patients who have had previous near-death experiences or feared dying during severe episodes of dyspnea may perceive subsequent occurrences as life-or-death situations. Failure to respond to patient requests/needs in an appropriate manner may result in mistrust.
■ Determine significant others' effect on the patient during the weaning process. Establish and control visiting times as appropriate.	Significant others may be a positive factor and a great support during the weaning process and should be allowed to remain at the bedside for extended periods; however, some significant others may have a negative effect, causing the patient to become restless and fight the ventilator.
■ Provide an appropriate environment for weaning: personalized space, a quiet room with a controllable temperature.	Attention to providing a comfortable environment can reduce some of the stress associated with weaning.
■ Assist the patient into a position that is comfortable for breathing (usually semi-Fowler's or Fowler's).	This position facilitates lung expansion and minimizes dyspnea.

■ = Independent   ▲ = Collaborative

Actions/Interventions

- Provide the means for communicating (e.g., alphabet board, call light).

Rationales

Frustration, anxiety, fear, panic, and anger can occur when patients cannot communicate their needs. These emotions may increase dyspnea. Communication of breathing difficulties is needed to prevent life-threatening situations.

Education/Continuity of Care

Actions/Interventions

- Discuss with the patient, significant others, or caregiver the individualized weaning plan and the importance of actively engaging in the work of weaning.
- Reassure the patient that multiple weaning trials are normal and expected.

- Discuss with the patient and significant others/caregiver the importance of setting achievable goals, and explain the probable weaning process, including the potential for setbacks.
- Give positive reinforcement for achievements.

- Avoid instructions to "control your breathing," "relax," or "calm down."

- Before weaning, explain that anxiety and dyspnea may occur during the process, and discuss the measures that may be used to decrease these symptoms (e.g., music, progressive muscle relaxation techniques, imagery, prayer, meditation).
- If the patient is to be removed from ventilator support during weaning attempts, explain that when usual support is reinitiated, there may be some temporary difficulty synchronizing his or her breathing with the ventilator.

Rationales

Increased understanding promotes cooperation with the plan.

This information helps prevent anxiety, frustration, and feelings of hopelessness. Patients may fear that they will not be able to be weaned.

Minimizing setbacks may help motivate the patient to try again.

Positive reinforcement increases the patient's sense of well-being and motivation to continue the weaning process.

These instructions increase patient frustration and feelings of helplessness because they may not be possible when the patient is dyspneic.

Management of dyspnea and anxiety can prevent premature cessation of weaning trials. Music may increase exercise tolerance in pulmonary patients, decrease heart rate and respiratory rate in ventilator patients, and reduce situational dyspnea.

Prior knowledge decreases fear and anxiety.

CHAPTER

3

Cardiac and Vascular Care Plans

Acute Coronary Syndromes/Myocardial Infarction

Unstable Angina; ST-Segment Elevation Myocardial Infarction; Non–ST-Segment Elevation Myocardial Infarction; Non–Q-Wave Myocardial Infarction; Q-Wave Myocardial Infarction

Acute coronary syndromes (ACS) represent a spectrum of clinical conditions that are associated with acute myocardial ischemia. Most patients who experience ACS have atherosclerotic changes in the coronary arteries. Chronic inflammatory processes play a key role in the pathogenesis of atherosclerosis. The presence of atherosclerotic plaques narrows the lumen of the arteries, and disruption or rupture of those plaques exposes a thrombogenic surface on which platelets aggregate, contributing to thrombus formation that diminishes blood flow to the myocardium. The resulting imbalance between myocardial oxygen demand and supply is the primary cause of the clinical manifestation in ACS. Other causes of ACS include coronary artery spasm and arterial inflammation related to infection. Noncardiac conditions that increase myocardial oxygen demand can precipitate ACS in patients with preexisting coronary artery disease (CAD). These conditions include fever, tachycardia, and hyperthyroidism. Decreased myocardial oxygen supply can occur in noncardiac conditions such as hypotensive states, hypoxemia, and anemia.

Clinical conditions included in ACS are unstable angina, variant angina, non–ST-segment elevation myocardial infarction (NSTEMI), and ST-segment elevation MI (STEMI). Evaluation of chest pain related to these disorders is a major cause of emergency department visits and hospitalizations in the United States. The term *ACS* is used prospectively to diagnose patients with chest pain or other clinical manifestations indicating the need to be triaged for treatment of unstable angina or acute MI. Although their pathogenesis and clinical presentation are similar, they differ primarily by whether ischemia is severe enough to cause sufficient myocardial damage to release detectable quantities of cardiac biomarkers (e.g., troponin, creatine kinase–myocardial bound [CK-MB], myoglobin) denoting acute MI. Early identification of ACS and intervention to improve myocardial perfusion reduces the risk for sudden cardiac death and acute MI in these patients.

Unstable angina is characterized by (1) angina that occurs when the paient is at rest; (2) angina that significantly limits the patient's activity; or (3) previously diagnosed angina that becomes more frequent, lasts longer, and increasingly limits the patient's activity. Patients typically do not have ST-segment elevation and do not release cardiac biomarkers indicating myocardial necrosis.

NSTEMI is distinguished from unstable angina by the presence of cardiac biomarkers, indicating myocardial necrosis. Most patients do not develop new Q waves on the electrocardiogram (ECG) and are diagnosed with non–Q-wave MI. STEMI is characterized by release of cardiac biomarkers and the presence of new Q waves on the ECG. This care plan focuses on the assessment of and interventions for patients with all these conditions. The American Heart Association and the American College of Cardiology have developed treatment guidelines for patients with unstable angina and NSTEMI, as well as for STEMI. Each guideline addresses initial and ongoing drug therapy, indications for fibrinolytic and percutaneous coronary interventions, and discharge considerations. For patients with MI, the therapeutic goals are to establish reperfusion, to reduce infarct size, to prevent and treat complications, and to provide emotional support and education. The Centers for Medicare and Medicaid Services (CMS) and The Joint Commission (TJC) have developed core performance measures/quality indicators for acute MI treatment. This care plan focuses on acute management of ACS. The cardiac rehabilitation care plan presented later in this chapter addresses specific learning needs.

 NANDA-I NDx **Acute Chest Pain**

Common Related Factors
Myocardial ischemia
Myocardial infarction

Defining Characteristics
Chest pain/discomfort occurring at rest or with minimal exertion
New-onset (less than 2 months) angina
Changing pattern of previously stable angina
Facial mask of pain
Shortness of breath
Pallor, weakness
Epigastric discomfort/indigestion
Palpitations
Nausea/vomiting
Diaphoresis or cold sweat
ECG changes: ST-segment depression or elevation, deep symmetrical T-wave inversion in multiple leads, or any transient ECG changes occurring during pain

Common Expected Outcomes
Patient verbalizes relief of pain to a level no higher than 3 to 4 on a scale of 0 to 10.
Patient appears comfortable.

NOC Outcomes
Pain Control; Pain Control Medication Response
NIC Interventions
Cardiac Care: Acute; Pain Management

Ongoing Assessment

Actions/Interventions

■ Assess the following pain characteristics:
  • Quality: squeezing, tightening, choking, pressure, burning, "viselike," aching
  • Location: substernal area; may radiate to arms, shoulders, neck, back, jaw
  • Severity: more intense than stable angina pectoris
  • Duration: persists longer than 20 minutes, usually several hours
  • Onset: with minimal exertion or during rest or sleep
  • Relieving factors: usually do not respond to sublingual nitroglycerin (NTG) or rest; may respond to intravenous (IV) NTG; not affected by position change or breathing

Rationales

Patients with presenting symptoms for MI can have a variety of pain characteristics, making diagnosis difficult. Older patients, women, patients with diabetes mellitus, and patients with heart failure often have atypical symptoms. Sudden shortness of breath and fatigue are more common than typical substernal chest pain. Associated diaphoresis may be present. Careful assessment facilitates early or appropriate treatment when time is critical for saving salvageable myocardium. If patients are phoning the health care provider about the pain, they should be advised to seek evaluation in a medical facility. Triage to the appropriate medical setting is a priority task. Patients with significant pain are usually admitted to rule out MI until serial laboratory data provide definitive diagnosis.

Actions/Interventions	**Rationales**
■ Assess any prior treatments for pain.	The nurse should note treatment that patient received before hospital admission. Patients may have tried several pain relief methods at home, including antacids. Some patients may have taken sublingual nitroglycerin and a single dose of aspirin before contacting emergency medical services.
■ Monitor ECG immediately during pain for evidence of myocardial ischemia or injury.	MI occurs over several hours. The time course of ST-T wave changes and development of Q waves guides diagnosis and treatment. If ECG is unchanged from prior tracings, patient is considered low risk and can be managed on an outpatient basis.
■ Note time since onset of first episode of chest pain.	If less than 6 hours since first pain occurred and patients have evidence of acute ST-segment elevation or new left bundle branch block on ECG, they may be candidates for IV thrombolytic therapy.
▲ Monitor serial cardiac biomarkers.	CK-MB, troponin, and myoglobin are released into the circulation from necrotic myocardial cells. Their serum levels rise in characteristic patterns over time after an MI. Myoglobin and CK-MB are detectable first, but troponin is more sensitive and specific for myocardial injury, in that it remains elevated for 10 to 14 days. Enzymes and proteins do not elevate with unstable angina because cellular death is not occurring.
▲ If cardiac biomarkers are negative, anticipate other diagnostic studies: • Echocardiography with or without stress testing • Exercise stress testing • Pharmacological stress testing with dipyridamole, adenosine, or dobutamine and nuclear imaging	Exercise and pharmacological stress testing and echocardiography are useful in evaluating ventricular function and myocardial perfusion in patients with ACS. Choice of test is based on resting ECG, ability to perform exercise, and technologies available. The results of these tests are used to determine the extent of CAD and patient's risk for MI. The test results can be used in making decisions about the need for coronary angiography.
■ Monitor heart rate (HR) and blood pressure (BP) during pain episodes and during medication administration.	Pain causes increased sympathetic stimulation, which increases oxygen demands on the heart. Tachycardia and increased BP are seen during pain and anxiety; hypotension is seen with nitrate and morphine administration; bradycardia is seen with morphine and β-blocker administration.
■ Continually reassess patient's chest pain and response to medication. If no relief from optimal dose of medication is achieved, report to physician for evaluation for thrombolytic treatment, angioplasty, coronary angiography, or bypass surgery revascularization.	Ongoing pain can signify prolonged myocardial ischemia that warrants immediate intervention.
■ For patients experiencing an acute STEMI, assess for absolute and relative contraindications to thrombolytic agents.	Thrombolytic agents do not distinguish a pathological occlusive coronary thrombus from a protective hemostatic clot; therefore patient selection is critical. Guidelines for absolute versus relative contraindications continue to be revised because risk/benefit assessments may change depending on availability of newer treatment modalities. Guidelines recommend that fibrinolytic agents be given within 30 minutes of hospital admission for STEMI when indicated.

Therapeutic Interventions

Actions/Interventions	**Rationales**
■ Maintain quiet environment.	Reduced stimulation decreases oxygen demands and may reduce anxiety.

■ = Independent   ▲ = Collaborative

Actions/Interventions	Rationales
■ Instruct patient to report pain as soon as it starts.	The patient needs to learn the meaning of this chest discomfort/pain as a sign of myocardiac injury, the benefits of obtaining prompt treatment, and the risks of delaying treatment of chest pain.
■ Respond immediately to complaint of pain.	Prompt treatment may decrease myocardial ischemia and prevent damage.
■ Obtain 12-lead ECG during pain episodes.	ST segment and T-wave changes help provide definitive diagnosis. Unstable angina and non–ST elevation have similar ECG changes, in contrast to those seen with STEMI.
▲ Administer oxygen as prescribed. Measure oxygen saturation.	Oxygen improves arterial saturation. When more oxygen is available to the myocardium, ischemia is reduced or reversed.
▲ Give antiischemic therapy as prescribed, evaluating effectiveness and observing signs or symptoms of untoward reactions:	Early, effective treatment aids in salvaging at-risk myocardium.
• Administer aspirin at admission and daily as ordered.	Aspirin decreases platelet aggregation and significantly improves mortality and morbidity rates when used within 24 hours of onset of chest pain. Use of aspirin is a core performance indicator. Treatment should be started at home or in the emergency department and not delayed until admission.
• Anticipate administration of anticoagulants or antiplatelet therapy for high-risk patients.	Anticoagulants reduce development or magnitude of MI when administered during the acute phases of ACS.
• Administer NTG drip. Titrate dose until relief of pain as long as BP remains stable.	NTG relaxes smooth muscles in the vascular system, causing peripheral arterial and venous vasodilation. This reduction in both preload and afterload results in lower BP, decreased venous return to the ventricle, and decreased myocardial demand. Do not give if systolic BP is less than 90 mm Hg.
• Administer morphine sulfate intravenously.	Morphine sulfate is an opioid analgesic that reduces the workload on the heart through venodilation. It reduces anxiety and decreases patient's perception of pain. Side effects include hypotension, bradycardia, decreased respirations, and nausea.
• Administer β-blockers. Anticipate IV administration; observe for side effects: hypotension, bradycardia, congestive heart failure, and bronchospasm.	Beta blockers decrease myocardial oxygen demand, the magnitude of infarction, and the incidence of associated complications. Research reports reduced mortality in acute phase of MI and at 1-year follow-up, as well as chances of reduced reinfarction. Do not give in patients with chronic obstructive pulmonary disease, heart block, bradycardia, decompensated left ventricular failure, hypotension, or cocaine toxicity.
• Administer calcium channel blockers.	Calcium channel blockers are indicated for patients with significant hypertension, cocaine toxicity, contraindications to β-blocker therapy, or refractory ischemia with coronary spasm. For contraindication to β-blocker therapy, a nonhydropyridine calcium channel blocker such as diltiazem (Cardizem) should be given in absence of left ventricular (LV) dysfunction.
• Administer ACE inhibitors or angiotensin receptor blockers (ARBs).	Research supports use after large transmural MIs, in patients with LV dysfunction, and in patients with diabetes because the risk for recurrent MI and progression to heart failure and death is reduced.

Actions/Interventions

- Administer thrombolytic agent according to unit protocol.

- Anticipate coronary angiography to diagnose and, depending on results, anticipate revascularization by percutaneous transluminal coronary angioplasty with stenting or coronary artery bypass surgery.

Rationales

Thrombolytic agents are enzymes that convert plasminogen to plasmin, which has potent fibrinolytic activity. These drugs break down fibrin clots and restore perfusion of myocardial tissue through previously blocked coronary arteries. IV therapy is preferred because it is fastest. Guidelines recommend administration within 30 minutes of hospital arrival.

Definitive diagnosis and early revascularization optimize myocardial perfusion and reduce risk for ischemia, infarction, and related complications. If indicated, percutaneous coronary intervention should be done within 120 minutes of hospital arrival.

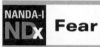 **Fear**

Common Related Factors

Recurrent anginal attacks
Incomplete relief from pain by usual means (NTG and rest)
Threat of MI
Threat of death
Threat of unknown
Unfamiliar environment
Separation from support system

Defining Characteristics

Identifies fearful feelings or object of fear
Restlessness
Increased awareness/tension
Increased questioning
Increased HR, BP, respiratory rate

Common Expected Outcomes

Patient verbalizes or manifests a reduction or absence of fear.
Patient uses effective coping mechanisms.

NOC Outcomes

Fear Self-Control; Coping

NIC Interventions

Cardiac Care; Anxiety Reduction; Coping Enhancement; Emotional Support

Ongoing Assessment

Actions/Interventions

- Assess level of fear (mild to severe).

- Assess cause of fear.

Rationales

Fear is associated with the physiological reactions (increased BP and HR) that can increase myocardial oxygen demand.

Determining specific cause guides therapy. Patient may be afraid of the pain experience itself, of interventions associated with emergency care, outcomes such as MI or dying, being separated from loved ones, or being in an unfamiliar environment.

Therapeutic Interventions

Actions/Interventions

- Acknowledge awareness of patient's fear.

- Encourage verbalization of fears and feelings.

Rationales

Acknowledgment of the patient's feelings validates the feelings and communicates acceptance of those feelings.

Verbalization provides clarity of patient's perception and enhances coping.

■ = Independent   ▲ = Collaborative

Actions/Interventions

- Maintain confident, assured manner.

- Assure patient and significant others of close, continuous monitoring that will ensure prompt intervention.
- Reduce unnecessary external stimuli.

- Explain all procedures as appropriate, using simple, concrete terms.

▲ Administer mild tranquilizer as needed.

- Establish rest periods between care and procedures.

Rationales

The staff's anxiety is easily noticed by the patient. The patient's feeling of stability increases in a calm and non-threatening atmosphere.

Continuous monitoring provides a measure of safety and security.

Anxiety may escalate with excessive conversation, noise, and equipment around the patient.

Information and open communication help allay anxiety. Patients who are anxious may not be able to comprehend anything more than simple, clear, brief instructions.

Medication may be indicated to reduce stress and anxiety that aggravate fear.

Quiet periods assist in relaxation and regaining emotional balance.

Risk for Decreased Cardiac Output

Common Risk Factors

Prolonged episodes of myocardial ischemia affecting contractility

Acute MI (especially at anterior site) affecting pumping ability of the heart

Right ventricular infarct (RVI) with reduced right ventricular (RV) pumping

Papillary muscle rupture and mitral insufficiency

Common Expected Outcome

Patient maintains adequate cardiac output, as evidenced by strong peripheral pulses, systolic blood pressure within 20 mm Hg of baseline, HR 60 to 100 beats/min with regular rhythm, urinary output ≥30 mL/hr, warm and dry skin, clear breath sounds, good capillary refill, and normal level of consciousness.

NOC Outcomes
Cardiac Pump Effectiveness; Vital Signs; Fluid Balance

NIC Interventions
Invasive Hemodynamic Monitoring; Hemodynamic Regulation; Cardiac Care: Acute

Ongoing Assessment

Actions/Interventions

- Monitor HR and BP.

- Assess skin color, temperature, and moisture.

- Assess peripheral pulses, including capillary refill.

- Assess for any changes in level of consciousness.

Rationales

Sinus tachycardia and increase in arterial BP are early signs of ventricular dysfunction and occur as compensatory responses.

Decreased cardiac output results in compensatory increase in sympathetic nervous system activity that causes cool, pale, clammy skin.

Reduced stroke volume and cardiac output cause weak peripheral pulses and slow capillary refill.

Early signs of cerebral hypoxia are restlessness, anxiety, and difficulty concentrating. Older patients are especially susceptible to reduced perfusion to vital organs.

Actions/Interventions	Rationales
■ Assess respiratory rate, rhythm, and breath sounds.	Rapid, shallow respirations and presence of crackles and wheezes are characteristic of reduced cardiac output. Crackles reflect accumulation of fluid secondary to impaired ventricular emptying.
■ Assess urine output.	The renal system compensates for low blood pressure by retaining water. Oliguria is a classic sign of inadequate renal perfusion from reduced cardiac output.
■ Auscultate for presence of S_3, S_4, or systolic murmur.	S_3 denotes LV dysfunction; S_4 is a common finding with MI, usually indicating noncompliance of the ischemic ventricle. Loud holosystolic murmur may be caused by papillary muscle rupture.
■ Use pulse oximetry to monitor oxygen saturation; assess arterial blood gases.	Pulse oximetry is a useful tool to detect changes in oxygenation. Oxygen saturation should be kept at 90% or greater. As shock increases, aerobic metabolism ceases and lactic acidosis ensues, raising level of carbon dioxide and pH.
■ If patient had an inferior MI, evaluate ECG using right precordial leads ($_RV_4 - _RV_6$). Assess for signs of RVI and RV failure.	These leads may show ECG changes indicative of RVI. RVI is seen in 30% to 50% of patients with symptoms for inferior MI. Signs of RV dysfunction include increased central venous pressure, increased jugular venous distention, absence of crackles or rales, and decreased BP.

Therapeutic Interventions

Actions/Interventions	Rationales
■ Anticipate insertion of hemodynamic monitoring catheters.	Pulmonary artery diastolic pressure and PCWP are excellent guides of filling pressures in the left ventricle; monitoring of central venous pressure and right atrial pressure guides management of RVI.
▲ Administer IV fluids to keep pulmonary capillary wedge pressure (PCWP) at 16 to 18 mm Hg for optimal filling of ventricle.	Too little fluid reduces preload or blood volume and BP; too much fluid can overload the heart and lead to pulmonary edema.
▲ If signs of LV failure occur:	
• Administer diuretic and vasodilator medications as prescribed.	These medications reduce filling pressures and workload of the infarcted heart and improve fluid balance.
• Administer IV inotropic medications.	These medications improve pumping of the heart.
• Initiate oxygen as needed.	Oxygen increases arterial saturation. When more oxygen is available to the myocardium, ischemia is reduced or reversed and ventricular pumping may be improved.
▲ If signs of RV failure occur:	
• Anticipate aggressive fluid resuscitation (3 to 6 L/24 hr).	The right ventricle is a low-pressure system that is dependent on a full venous return and strong filling in the ventricle to produce effective cardiac output. The damaged myocardium requires a greater amount of fluid to maintain adequate filling. Aggressive fluid therapy is a key therapy.
• Anticipate inotropic and peripheral vasodilator medication.	These medications improve ventricular contraction and reduce RV and LV afterload, thereby enhancing stroke volume.
▲ Avoid or carefully administer nitrates and morphine sulfate for pain.	These medications reduce preload and filling pressures, which may compromise cardiac output.
■ Anticipate intraaortic balloon pump (IABP) management if pain and ischemic changes persist despite maximal medical therapy.	IABP increases coronary blood flow during diastole while reducing work by left ventricle during systolic contraction.

■ = Independent   ▲ = Collaborative

Risk for Decreased Cardiac Output: Dysrhythmias

Common Risk Factor

Electrical instability or dysrhythmias secondary to ischemia or necrosis, sympathetic nervous system stimulation, or electrolyte imbalance (hypokalemia or hypomagnesemia)

Common Expected Outcome

Patient maintains adequate cardiac output as evidenced by strong peripheral pulses, systolic BP within 20 mm Hg of baseline, HR 60 to 100 beats/min with regular rhythm, urinary output greater than or equal to 30 mL/hr, strong peripheral pulses, warm and dry skin, clear breath sounds, good capillary refill, and normal level of consciousness.

NOC Outcomes
Cardiac Pump Effectiveness; Circulation Status
NIC Interventions
Dysrhythmia Management; Hemodynamic Regulation; Cardiac Care: Acute

---

Ongoing Assessment

Actions/Interventions	Rationales
■ Monitor patient's HR and rhythm continuously. Monitor PR, QRS, and QT intervals, and note change.	Dysrhythmias produce alterations in both heart rate and rhythm. Changes in electrical properties of myocardial cells occur with prolonged ischemia and infarction. These changes include increased automaticity of ectopic pacemakers and increased refractoriness in normal conduction pathways. Many antidysrhythmic drugs also depress the conduction of normal impulses and can cause further dysrhythmias.
■ Observe for or anticipate the following common dysrhythmias specific site of infarction: • With anterior MI: second-degree heart block, complete heart block, right bundle branch block, left anterior hemiblock, left bundle branch block, or bifascicular block • With inferior MI: sinus bradycardia, sinus pause, and first- and second-degree heart block (Wenckebach phenomenon), and third-degree heart block	Specific areas of infarction correlate with expected dysrhythmias.
■ Monitor with continuous ECG monitoring in appropriate lead. • Monitor in lead II, observing for left anterior hemiblock.	Monitoring facilitates prompt detection of conduction problem. Left anterior hemiblock is characterized by normal QRS width and left axis deviation with deep S waves in leads II, III, and aVF. By anticipating these dysrhythmias, early assessment is made and treatment is initiated.
• If anterior MI with left anterior hemiblock is already present, monitor in modified chest lead (MCL$_1$) for right bundle branch block.	Right bundle branch block is characterized by a QRS of greater than 0.12 second and an rSR′ complex in V$_1$ or V$_2$.
■ Assess for signs of decreased cardiac output that accompany dysrhythmias: hypotension, reduced urine output, weak pulses, cool skin, reduced level of consciousness.	The patient's tolerance to the dysrhythmia guides intervention. Hemodynamic status is more important than "treating the dysrhythmia" per se.
■ Assess response to antidysrhythmic treatment.	Follow-up evaluation guides ongoing treatment.

Therapeutic Interventions

Actions/Interventions	Rationales
■ Institute treatment as appropriate and according to protocol: • Potassium or magnesium supplement as guided by serum electrolyte levels • Amiodarone or procainamide (Pronestyl) for PVC and ventricular tachycardia • Atropine sulfate for symptomatic bradycardia; external pacemaker on standby • Calcium channel blockers, β-blockers, adenosine, and cardioversion for atrial tachydysrhythmias • Temporary pacemaker for Mobitz type II, new complete heart block, new bifascicular bundle branch block, or left bundle branch block with anterior wall MI • Implantable cardioverter-defibrillator for recurrent ventricular tachycardia, as indicated • Defibrillation for ventricular fibrillation • Cardiopulmonary resuscitation as appropriate	Current Advanced Cardiac Life Support guidelines provide protocols for management of dysrhythmias.

NANDA-I NDx Deficient Knowledge

Common Related Factors

Unfamiliarity with disease process, treatment, and recovery
Information misinterpretation

Defining Characteristics

Multiple or no questions
Confusion over events
Expressed need for information
Verbalized confusion

Common Expected Outcome

Patient verbalizes understanding of condition, diagnosis or treatment of ACS, and recovery process.

NOC Outcomes
Knowledge: Disease Process; Knowledge: Treatment Regimen
NIC Interventions
Teaching: Disease Process; Teaching: Prescribed Medications

Ongoing Assessment

Actions/Interventions	Rationale
■ Assess knowledge of ACS: causes, treatment, and early recovery process.	Information provides the basis for education. Many patients have been exposed to media information or family and friends experiencing cardiac events. Misconceptions may exist.

Therapeutic Interventions

Actions/Interventions	Rationales
■ Teach patient or significant others the following: • Anatomy and physiology of the coronary condition and atherosclerotic process	Information provides rationale for treatment.

■ = Independent   ▲ = Collaborative

Cardiac and Vascular Care Plans

Actions/Interventions	Rationales
• Angina versus unstable angina versus MI	Information aids the patient in assuming responsibility for care at later time. It is critical that patients are able to recognize when chest pain symptoms require immediate attention.
• Diagnostic procedures (stress test, echocardiogram, or angiogram)	Information can clarify diagnostic process and reduce anxiety. Follow-up testing is common to assess response to medical therapy and evaluate functional capacity.
• Medical therapy, as in the following:	Patients are better able to ask questions and seek assistance when they know basic information about prescribed medications. CMS and TJC have quality indicators for acute MI related to prescribing at discharge (antiplatelet medication [acetylsalicylic acid], ACE inhibitor/ARBs) for those with left ventricular dysfunction, and β-blocker medications.
• Antiplatelet medicines	Antiplatelet medications reduce the risk for thrombosis formation by inhibiting platelet aggregation.
• Use of NTG if chest pain occurs	Nitroglycerin causes vasodilation that reduces myocardial demands. Patients need clear directions on self-administration.
• Use of calcium channel blockers	Calcium channel blockers are useful if unstable angina has a spasm component or if β-blockers are contraindicated.
• Use of ACE inhibitors or ARBs; β-blockers	These medications decrease mortality and morbidity post MI.
• Indicated lifestyle changes (smoking cessation, exercise, diet, hypertension and lipid management)	Modification in risk factors can decrease risk for CAD events. Smoking cessation counseling is a CMS and TJC quality indictor for acute MI.
■ Explain that the acute phase of unstable angina is usually over in 4 to 6 weeks and return to prior lifestyle post MI is 2 to 3 months.	Recovery from unstable angina is shorter than with an MI because only ischemic, not infarcted, tissue occurs. More than 85% of patients experiencing an MI return to full activity level.
■ Inform patient that more extensive teaching sessions will be instituted when the next stage of cardiac rehabilitation is initiated.	Readiness for learning is key to effective teaching. The complexities of an acute care setting do not provide an optimal environment for learning.
■ Refer to cardiac rehabilitation program as indicated.	These programs can assist with risk factor reduction and provide education and emotional support.
■ Screen for depression.	It is reasonable to screen for depression because the disease process can alter prognosis and quality of life. Depression is linked to cardiac events.
■ Encourage flu vaccine.	Vaccine is recommended by National Clinical Practice guidelines, because the flu infection has been found to have a direct influence on the atherosclerotic plaque, potentially leading to plaque rupture and subsequent cardiac events.

Related Care Plans

Angina Pectoris, Chronic

Chest Pain

Chronic stable angina pectoris is a clinical syndrome characterized by the abrupt or gradual onset of substernal discomfort (often with radiation to the neck, jaw, shoulder, back, or arm) caused by insufficient coronary blood flow and/or inadequate oxygen supply to the myocardial muscle. The patient with chronic angina will have episodes of chest pain that are usually predictable. Chest pain will occur in response to or is aggravated by physical exertion or emotional stressors. Situations that increase myocardial oxygen demand or decrease oxygen supply include both cardiac and noncardiac causes. Chronic angina usually persists for only a few minutes and subsides with cessation of the precipitating factor, rest, or use of nitroglycerin (NTG). Patients may present in ambulatory settings or during hospitalization for other medical problems. Chronic angina usually can be controlled with medications on an outpatient basis. Chronic angina can significantly affect one's quality of life. A person may limit activities based on fear of precipitating episodes of chest pain.

 NANDA-I NDx   Acute Chest Pain

Common Related Factors

Myocardial ischemia caused by the following:
- Atherosclerosis and/or coronary spasm
- Less common causes: severe aortic stenosis, cardiomyopathy, mitral valve prolapse, hypothyroidism, hypertension, anxiety, tachydysrhythmias, hyperviscosity of blood

Common Expected Outcomes

Patient reports relief of chest discomfort.
Patient appears relaxed and comfortable.

Defining Characteristics

Chest pain or discomfort of chest pain
No change in the frequency, duration, time of appearance, or precipitating factors of chest pain during the previous 60 days

NOC Outcomes
Pain Level; Medication Response; Pain Control
NIC Interventions
Pain Management; Cardiac Care

Ongoing Assessment

Actions/Interventions

- Assess the following pain characteristics:
  - Quality: choking, strangling, pressure, burning, tightness, ache, heaviness, griplike, squeezing
  - Location: substernal area, may radiate to arms and shoulders, neck, back, jaw
  - Severity: scale 0 to 10 (usually not at top of scale)
  - Duration: typically minutes in duration
  - Onset and aggravating factors: episodic and usually precipitated by physical exertion, emotional stress, smoking, heavy meal, or exposures to extreme temperature
  - Relieving factors: rest, use of NTG, or removal of precipitating factor

Rationales

The discomfort of angina is often difficult for patients to describe, and many patients do not consider it to be "pain." Older patients, patients with diabetes, and women tend to have more fatigue or shortness of breath as anginal symptoms/angina equivalents.

■ = Independent   ▲ = Collaborative

Actions/Interventions

- Evaluate whether this is a chronic problem (stable angina) or a new presentation.

- Assess for the appropriateness of performing an electrocardiogram (ECG) to evaluate ST-segment and T-wave changes.

- Monitor vital signs during chest pain and after nitrate administration.

- Monitor effectiveness of interventions.

Rationales

New-onset angina that is less than 2 months in occurrence, severe, or frequent (more than three times per day) is considered "unstable" angina/ acute coronary syndrome until proven otherwise. It requires immediate assessment (see Acute Coronary Syndromes/Myocardial Infarction, p 209).

Differentiating between angina and myocardial infarction (MI) is important in making decisions about implementing appropriate interventions. Anginal changes are transient, occurring during the actual ischemic episode.

Blood pressure (BP) and heart rate (HR) are usually elevated secondary to sympathetic stimulation during pain; however, nitrates cause vasodilation and a resultant drop in BP. Older patients may experience more significant postural hypotension secondary to decreased responsiveness of the baroreceptors.

Chest pain unresponsive to the patient's usual use of rest or nitroglycerin requires immediate evaluation.

Therapeutic Interventions

Actions/Interventions

- At first signs of pain or discomfort, instruct patient to relax and/or rest.

- Instruct patient to take sublingual NTG. Sit or lie down when taking NTG. Put pill under tongue and let dissolve. If pain is not relieved in 5 minutes, take another. If still not relieved, take a third. If this does not relieve pain, call physician or go to emergency department.

- If pain continues after repeating sublingual dose every 5 minutes for total of three pills, seek immediate medical attention.

- If in a medical setting, administer oxygen as ordered.

- Offer assurance and emotional support by explaining all treatments and procedures and by encouraging questions.

Rationales

Decreasing myocardial oxygen demand restores the balance between oxygen supply and demand. When more oxygen is available to the myocardium, ischemia is reversed.

The patient needs to learn the meaning of chest pain as a sign of myocardial ischemia and the benefits of prompt therapy. Information allows patient to initiate effective therapy when needed. A stinging or burning in the mouth should occur if medication is effective. Many patients find NTG spray easier to use.

Patients with chronic disease need to be able to recognize important changes in their condition to avert complications. Chest pain unrelieved by NTG may represent unstable angina or MI and should be evaluated immediately.

Increasing arterial oxygen saturation delivers more oxygen to the myocardium and relieves oxygen supply and demand imbalance.

Anxiety can increase cardiac workload and myocardial oxygen demand through stimulation of the sympathetic nervous system.

NANDA-I NDx **Deficient Knowledge**

Common Related Factors

Unfamiliarity with disease process and treatment
Misinterpretation of information
Lack of recall

Defining Characteristics

Multiple questions to health care team
Inaccurate follow-through of prescribed treatment
Verbalizing inaccurate information

Common Expected Outcomes

Patient or significant others verbalize understanding of angina pectoris, its causes, and appropriate relief measures for pain.

Patient describes own cardiac risk factors and strategies to reduce them.

NOC Outcomes
Knowledge: Disease Process; Knowledge: Treatment Regimen

NIC Interventions
Teaching: Disease Process; Teaching: Medication; Cardiac Care: Rehabilitation

Ongoing Assessment

Actions/Interventions	Rationales
■ Assess knowledge regarding the causes of angina, diagnostic procedures, treatment plan, and risk factors for coronary artery disease (CAD).	Information provides starting base for educational sessions. Teaching standardized content that patient already knows wastes valuable time and hinders critical learning.
■ Evaluate compliance with any previously prescribed lifestyle modifications.	Smoking, heavy meals, and obesity can easily precipitate anginal attacks. Behavior change is never easy. This knowledge provides an important starting point in understanding any complexities in implementation of the treatment plan.

Therapeutic Interventions

Actions/Interventions	Rationales
■ Provide information regarding the following:	
• Anatomy and physiology of coronary circulation and the atherosclerotic process.	Patient understanding of the role of normal versus atherosclerotic coronary arteries in supplying oxygen to the myocardial tissue will provide a rationale for treatment.
• Diagnostic tests for evaluating CAD, such as the following:	
• ECG	Usually ST-segment depression or inverted T wave is present, indicating subendocardial ischemia.
• Exercise stress test/stress echocardiogram	ST-segment changes provide an indirect assessment of coronary artery perfusion. Significant ST depression on stress testing and reversible defects indicate the need for angiography. However, the exercise stress test is not always conclusive for CAD. Women often have false-positive results, and false-negative results can occur if only submaximal exercise is performed. Exercise echocardiograms are often used to evaluate wall motion abnormality present during myocardial ischemia.
• Pharmacological stress test with nuclear imaging	This test is indicated for subgroups of patients who are unable to exercise and have findings that are highly suggestive of CAD. Two types of agents may be used: coronary vasodilators (adenosine and dipyridamole) and those that increase HR (dobutamine). Scans of the heart identify poorly perfused areas of the myocardium.
• Coronary angiography	Angiography is the definitive test for directly identifying the extent of the CAD.
• Differentiating angina from noncardiac pain	Chest pain is very challenging to interpret, because pulmonary, GI, and musculoskeletal etiologies can mimic myocardial problems. Patients must have correct information for long-term care.
• Differentiating stable versus unstable angina versus MI	Patients need to understand the importance of reporting changes in chest pain pattern that may indicate progression of CAD.

■ = Independent   ▲ = Collaborative

Actions/Interventions

- Need to avoid angina-provoking situations (e.g., heavy meals, physical overexertion, temperature extremes, cigarette smoking, emotional stress, and stimulants such as caffeine or cocaine)
- Use of sublingual NTG to relieve attacks, as in the following. Note that nitroglycerin spray may be preferred by some patients.

  - Carry pills at all times.

  - Keep pills in dark, dry container, away from heat.
  - Replace pills every 3 to 4 months.

- Use of other medications for long-term management:
  - Long-acting nitrates

  - β-Blockers

  - Calcium channel blockers

  - Antiplatelet aggregation therapy (aspirin); Plavix if aspirin is contraindicated for high-risk patients (determined by testing)

  - Angiotensin-converting enzyme (ACE) inhibitors for those with CAD and diabetes and/or left ventricular systolic dysfunction. ARBs may be substituted for those intolerant to ACE inhibitors.
  - Ranolazine

Rationales

Long-term care is the patient's responsibility; enough information is needed for successful intervention.

NTG relaxes smooth muscles in the vascular system, causing peripheral arterial and venous vasodilation, which can lower BP and cause dizziness. Early, effective treatment aids in salvaging at-risk myocardium. The patient needs to understand the importance of obtaining prompt treatment and the risk of delaying treatment.

NTG pills (or spray) need to be taken immediately at the first sign of pain.

NTG is volatile and inactivated by heat, moisture, and light.

Once bottle is opened, NTG begins to lose its strength. Tablets that are effective should sting in the mouth.

Long-acting nitrites act by producing vasodilation, which increases coronary blood flow and reduces oxygen demands of the heart. They must be used cautiously in older patients who are more susceptible to postural hypotension secondary to reduced response of baroreceptors.

β-Blockers reduce contractility and HR, thereby decreasing myocardial oxygen demand. They must be used cautiously in older patients who have degeneration of the conduction system and who are at risk for bradycardia, conduction heart blocks, and chronic obstructive pulmonary disease (COPD). They are usually prescribed along with a nitrate.

Calcium channel blockers cause vasodilation, which increases coronary blood flow and reduces oxygen demands of the heart. They are usually prescribed along with a nitrate.

Aspirin is strongly recommended as a long-term therapy for those with coronary artery disease (angina) who can tolerate it. Aspirin chemically blocks the synthesis of prostaglandins and thromboxane A_2 in platelets. Without prostaglandins, platelets are unable to aggregate and form clots in coronary blood vessels. The effect of aspirin on platelet aggregation is irreversible for the life of the platelet, about 3 to 7 days.

These drugs decrease afterload, causing vasodilation, and prevent activation of renin-angiotensin-aldosterone system.

Ranolazine provides a new approach for treating chronic angina. It is one of a new class of drugs called partial fatty acid oxidation inhibitors. It acts by increasing efficiency of oxygen use by the heart by shifting metabolism to a fuel source that requires less oxygen (glucose) to generate the same amount of energy.

Actions/Interventions

- Need to reduce modifiable risk factors for atherosclerosis:
  - Smoking: Provide counseling, pharmacological therapy, and referral to cessation programs. The American Heart Association, the American Lung Association, and the American Cancer Society provide support groups and interventions.
  - Hypertension: Instruct in need to maintain healthy weight control, reduce salt intake, initiate an exercise program, and take antihypertensive medications as prescribed. Moderate alcohol intake, a diet high in fruits and vegetables (DASH), and low-fat dairy products are key.
  - Elevated serum lipid levels: Emphasize need to reduce intake of foods high in saturated fat, cholesterol, or both (e.g., fatty meats, organ meats, lard, butter, egg yolks, dairy products). Arrange for evaluation by dietitian as needed. Include spouse or significant others in meal planning. Treatment usually requires antihyperlipidemic medication. Consider adding plant stanols, fiber, and omega-3 fatty acids as appropriate.
  - Diabetes: Emphasize control through lifestyle and medication.

  - Obesity: Refer to weight management specialty programs as appropriate.

  - Stress: Refer to programs for stress management as appropriate.
  - Flu vaccine

  - Physical inactivity: Emphasize benefits of exercise in reducing risk for heart attack. Refer to cardiac rehabilitation program as needed. Keep exercise intensity below angina threshold.

- Therapeutic procedures to relieve angina unresponsive to medications and lifestyle changes:
  - Percutaneous coronary interventions: angioplasty, atherectomy, stent implantation, laser angioplasty

  - Coronary artery bypass graft surgery

  - Enhanced external counterpulsation

  - New therapies under study

■ Refer patient to cardiac rehabilitation services for specialized teaching and assistance with recommended lifestyle changes as appropriate.

Rationales

Smoking causes vasoconstriction and reduces myocardial oxygen supply. Risk for developing CAD is 2 to 6 times greater in cigarette smokers. Risk is proportional to number of cigarettes smoked.

The stress of constantly elevated BP can increase the rate of atherosclerosis development. The Joint National Committee on Prevention, Detection, Evaluation, and Treatment of High Blood Pressure (JNC) guidelines provide goals and treatment approaches.

There is a positive correlation between serum lipids (especially low-density lipoprotein [LDL]) and atherosclerosis. Treatment goal for patients with CAD is LDL (bad cholesterol) level less than 100 mg/dL. Newer National Cholesterol Education Program Adult Treatment Panel III guidelines suggest a goal of less than 70 mg/dL as a therapeutic option in patients at high risk for CAD.

Eighty percent of diabetic patients have cardiovascular disease. Diabetes eliminates the lower incidence of cardiovascular disease in women. Diabetes is associated with a high incidence of silent ischemia.

Obesity affects hypertension, diabetes, and lipid levels and contributes to metabolic syndrome, which is highly associated with CAD. Target body mass index (BMI) is 18.5 to 24.9.

Persistent stress causes the release of catecholamines that contribute to elevated blood pressure and CAD.

Annual flu vaccine is recommended for those with cardiovascular disease. The flu vaccine has been found to have a direct influence on the atherosclerotic plaque, potentially leading to plaque rupture and subsequent cardiac events.

Exercise increases high-density lipoprotein levels (good cholesterol), assists with weight loss, lowers hypertension, improves diabetes, and reduces the risk for clot formation (fibrinolytic activity). One hundred fifty minutes of moderate activity is recommended per week.

These interventions provide a means to nonsurgically improve coronary blood flow and revascularize the myocardium.

Surgery may be recommended for significant left main CAD, triple vessel disease, and disease unresponsive to other treatments.

Counterpulsation devices use air via cuffs attached to the lower extremities to propel blood back to the heart.

Several other therapies such as spinal cord stimulation, transcutaneous electrical nerve stimulation, and stem cell transplant are being readied for research trials.

Specialty services may be required to ensure that patients' needs are met and outcomes achieved.

■ = Independent   ▲ = Collaborative

NANDA-I NDx Activity Intolerance

Common Related Factors

Occurrence or fear of chest pain
Side effects of prescribed medications
Imbalance between oxygen supply and demand
Sedentary lifestyle

Defining Characteristics

Exertional chest pain or dyspnea
Fatigue/weakness
Abnormal HR or BP response to activity
ECG changes reflecting ischemia or dysrhythmias
Unable to complete desired activities

Common Expected Outcomes

Patient performs activity within limits of ischemic disease, as evidenced by absence of chest pain or discomfort and no ECG changes reflecting ischemia.
Patient recognizes activity and energy limitations and balances activity and rest.

NOC Outcomes

Knowledge: Prescribed Activity; Activity Tolerance; Energy Conservation

NIC Interventions

Teaching: Prescribed Activity/Exercise; Energy Management and Promotion

Ongoing Assessment

Actions/Interventions

- Assess patient's level of physical activity before experiencing angina.
- Assess BP and HR before, during, and after activity.

- Assess emotional response to limitations in physical abilities.

Rationales

Sometimes patients have significantly reduced their activity to avoid anginal symptoms.
Information provides a basis for determining activity intolerance and realistic short- and long-term goals and subsequent therapies.
Depression over inability to perform desired/required activities can be a source of stress and aggravation.

Therapeutic Interventions

Actions/Interventions

- Assist in reviewing required home, work, or leisure activities and in developing an appropriate plan for accomplishing them (e.g., what to do in morning versus afternoon or how to pace tasks throughout the week).
- Evaluate need for additional support at home (e.g., housekeeper, neighbor to shop, family assistance).
- Encourage adequate rest periods between activities.

- Remind patient not to work with arms above shoulders for long periods.
- Remind patient to continue taking medications (e.g., β-blockers), despite side effect of fatigue.
- Instruct in prophylactic use of NTG before physical exertion as needed.

- Encourage a program of progressive aerobic exercise. Refer to cardiac rehabilitation as appropriate.

Rationales

Devising plan that facilitates accomplishment of small, attainable goals can be satisfying.

Coordinated efforts are more meaningful and effective in assisting patient in conserving energy.
Rest between activities provides time for energy conservation and recovery.
Arm activity increases myocardial demands.

Often the body does adjust to the medications after several weeks.
Prophylactic NTG use is an important measure for patients with predictable angina patterns. It is an underutilized therapy.
Routine exercise can increase functional capacity, making the heart more efficient.

Related Care Plans

Anxiety, p. 18
Cardiac rehabilitation, p. 230
Health-seeking behaviors, p. 89
Ineffective coping, p. 49

Aortic Aneurysm

Dissecting Aneurysm; Thoracic Aneurysm; Abdominal Aneurysm

An aneurysm is a localized, circumscribed, blood-filled abnormal dilation of an artery caused by disease or weakening of the vessel wall. True aneurysms involve dilation of all layers of the vessel wall. The two types of true aneurysms are (1) saccular, which is characterized by a bulbous out-pouching of one side of the artery resulting in localized stretching of the artery wall, and (2) fusiform, which is characterized by a uniformly shaped dilation of the entire circumference of the artery. True aneurysms are asymptomatic and are typically diagnosed by physical examination or a diagnostic ultrasound or computed tomography (CT) scan. The natural history of an aneurysm is enlargement; as a rule, the larger it is, the greater the chance of rupture. Aneurysms are most commonly seen in the abdominal aorta. Abdominal aortic aneurysms (AAAs) account for about 75% and thoracic aneurysms for about 25% of all cases. They occur more often in men than in women. Risk factors include smoking and having a family history of aneurysms. When an aneurysm becomes big enough for risk for rupture, it can be repaired by open surgical repair or a less-invasive endograft-covered stent repair.

Dissecting aneurysms occur when the inner layer of the blood vessel wall tears and splits, creating a false channel and cavity of blood between the intimal and adventitial layers. They are typically classified according to the location. According to the Stanford Classification, type A involves the ascending aorta and its transverse arch, and type B involves the descending aorta. A dissecting AAA is the most common catastrophe involving the aorta, and it has a high mortality rate if not detected early and treated with surgery. Over 90% of patients present with sudden onset of severe pain, which is usually described as sharp, tearing, or stabbing in nature. Symptoms depend on the size and location of the dissection or rupture. Risk factors for dissection include hypertension, pregnancy, trauma, and Marfan syndrome.

NANDA-I NDx Risk for Ineffective Tissue Perfusion

Common Risk Factors

Conditions that increase stress on the arterial wall, leading
   to risk for dissection:
- Hypertension
- Pregnancy with hypervolemia
- Coarctation of the aorta

Defect in the vessel wall, leading to risk for dissection:
- Marfan syndrome
- Cystic degeneration in the media

Trauma
Iatrogenic causes

 = Independent ▲ = Collaborative

Common Expected Outcomes

Patient has reduced risk for complications from progressive dissection or rupture as a result of early detection of symptoms and appropriate intervention.

Patient maintains optimal tissue perfusion as evidenced by strong palpable peripheral pulses; warm, dry extremities; blood pressure within normal range for patient; urinary output greater than or equal to 30 mL/hr; alert, normal level of consciousness; normal bowel sounds; absence of abdominal or chest pain.

NOC Outcomes
Vital Signs; Circulation Status; Pain Level
NIC Interventions
Vital Sign Monitoring; Circulatory Precautions; Pain Management; Analgesic Administration

Ongoing Assessment

Actions/Interventions	Rationales
■ Obtain a thorough history regarding risk factors for dissection or rupture.	Most patients are asymptomatic unless their aneurysm is dissecting or ruptures. History aids in ruling out cerebrovascular, cardiac, vascular occlusive, and/or renal disease. Poorly controlled hypertension increases stress on the aortic wall and its risk for dissection or rupture.
■ Assess and monitor location and characteristics of pain. • Abdominal: pain in abdomen or back, flank, or groin caused by pressure on adjacent structures • Thoracic: pain in neck, low back pain, shoulders, or abdomen	Description of pain can help differentiate location and determine treatment. Over 90% of patients with AAA present with sudden onset of severe pain described as sharp, tearing, or stabbing in nature.
■ Monitor for signs and symptoms indicating progressive dissection.	A high index of suspicion can determine the treatment to reduce mortality. Clinical signs and symptoms indicate the site and progression of dissection. Acute aortic dissection usually occurs along the thoracic aorta. Pain is severe and may mimic the pain associated with myocardial infarction. Pain may be located both above and below the diaphragm if the dissection is extensive. Changes in level of consciousness and diminished carotid pulses are associated with dissection of the aortic arch. Dissection of the abdominal aorta can cause decreased urine output, diminished motor and sensory function in the lower extremities, abdominal pain, and bloody diarrhea.
For abdominal aneurysms: ■ Monitor urine output.	Reduction may result from compression of the renal arteries from infrarenal abdominal aneurysm, cross-clamping of the aorta during surgery, or embolization. However, most aneurysms are located below the renal artery.
■ Monitor for abnormal bowel function.	Abnormal function is caused by partial intestinal obstruction.
■ Gently palpate abdomen for midline mass or pulsations.	An enlarging AAA may present as a midline pulsatile mass in the abdomen. The pulsations may equal apical heart rate. The technique for palpation should be as gentle as possible to avoid trauma to the aneurysm.
■ Observe for abdominal distention, diarrhea, or severe abdominal pain and/or fever.	These signs rule out embolization or decreased perfusion to the mesenteric artery and rupture into the abdominal cavity.
■ Assess for gastrointestinal bleeding.	Bleeding is caused by erosion of the duodenum.
■ Assess lower extremities for signs of peripheral ischemia and insufficiency. These include pain, pallor, pulselessness, paresthesia, poikilothermia (decreased temperature, coolness), and paralysis.	Dissection can cause reduced sensory and motor function in the lower extremities.

Actions/Interventions

For thoracic aneurysms:

■ Monitor blood pressure (BP) for hypertension.

■ Auscultate for bruits over palpable pulsatile mass.

■ Monitor quality of peripheral pulses.

■ Assess for dysphagia.
■ Assess for hemoptysis.
■ Assess for respiratory compromise.

■ Observe for upper-extremity and head swelling with cyanosis.
■ Anticipate further diagnostic studies:
  • Chest x-ray (thoracic) study and abdominal or lateral x-ray study of spine (abdominal)
  • Computed tomography angiography (CTA) scan
  • Magnetic resonance imaging scans
  • Ultrasonography
  • Aortography

Rationales

Hypertension is a risk factor for rupture. Differential arm BP may be present as a result of compression of the subclavian artery.
Bruit denotes abnormal blood flow common with aneurysms.
Peripheral pulses assure distal perfusion. A suggested grading system is as follows: 0 = absent, 1+ = present, 2+ = strong.
Dysphagia may be caused by esophageal compression.
Hemoptysis results from compression of the trachea or lung.
Respiratory compromise is a result of compression of the trachea or bronchus.
These signs can be caused by superior vena cava obstruction.

Tests are required to confirm diagnosis and delineate anatomy (size, shape, and location of aneurysms).

Therapeutic Interventions

Actions/Interventions

■ Provide nonpharmacological measures to alleviate pain:
  • Position of comfort (e.g., place patients exhibiting back pain in a side-lying position)
  • Physical comfort (e.g., hand-holding; application of cold towel)
  • Relaxation techniques
▲ Administer pain medicines as prescribed.

▲ Administer medications to control blood pressure: β-blocker medication or angiotensin-converting enzyme (ACE) inhibitor medication.

■ For type A dissections (involving ascending aorta or transverse arch), anticipate surgical treatment and prepare patient.
■ For type B dissections (involving descending thoracic aorta), anticipate chronic medical treatment, which consists of the following long-term measures:
  • Decrease or eliminate identified factors that will increase BP and heart rate (HR).
  • Provide a quiet environment as much as possible.
  • Pace activities (eating, personal hygiene, visitors) appropriately.
  • Administer sedatives as prescribed.

Rationales

These measures may be tried initially, but depending on status of the aneurysm, these measures may not be effective.

Persistent acute pain suggests ongoing dissection or rupture. Surgical intervention may be required to relieve pain.
BP control is imperative for maintaining tissue perfusion. Goal is to maintain systolic BP less than 120 mm Hg. These medications reduce the stress applied to the arterial walls and may reduce risk for dissection in hypertensive patients.
The surgical procedure involves replacement of the ascending aorta to prevent aortic rupture or retrograde progression of the dissection.
The major treatment approach for type B involves a pharmacological regimen to control BP. It may require surgical treatment if hypertension is uncontrollable, persistent pain occurs, compromise to major organs occurs, or the aorta ruptures.

■ = Independent   ▲ = Collaborative

NANDA-I NDx   Risk for Decreased Cardiac Output

Common Risk Factors

Side effects of medications
Progressive dissection
Rupture of the aorta

Common Expected Outcome

Patient maintains adequate cardiac output, as evidenced by HR of 60 to 100 beats/min, palpable pulses, clear lung sounds, urine output more than 30 mL/hr, and normal level of consciousness.

NOC Outcome
Cardiac Pump Effectiveness
NIC Intervention
Hemodynamic Regulation

Ongoing Assessment

Actions/Interventions

■ Assess hemodynamic status. Monitor for signs of decreasing cardiac output, such as tachycardia, decreased urine output, and restlessness.

■ Assess for signs of myocardial ischemia: chest pain, tachycardia, or ST-segment and T-wave changes on electrocardiogram (ECG).

Rationales

A dissecting AAA is the most common catastrophe involving the aorta, and it has a high mortality rate if not detected early and treated with surgery. Patients with dissecting or rupturing aneurysm are hemodynamically compromised. Early evaluation of warning signs facilitates prompt intervention.

ECG changes help guide timing of interventions.

Therapeutic Interventions

Actions/Interventions

▲ If decreased cardiac output is drug induced, anticipate the following:
  • For β-blocker:
    • May stop the drug or reduce dose.

  • For vasodilators:
    • Stop the drug, and administer isotonic solution (0.9% normal saline solution) or plasma expanders.

▲ If decreased cardiac output is related to further dissection (severe aortic insufficiency) or ruptured aorta, anticipate emergency angiography and surgery:
  • Send blood specimen for type and crossmatch and other routine preoperative blood work.
  • Stay with patient.

  • Administer medications, intravenous fluids, and blood as ordered.
  • Prepare patient for surgical repair.

Rationales

β-Blockers have a negative inotropic effect, which can potentiate heart failure. Presence of rales and S_3 indicates heart failure.

Fluids are usually required to maintain increased intravascular volume.

Rapid, efficient intervention is critical to preserve circulation and life.

Blood replacement therapy may be required to maintain effective blood volume.

The presence of competent, calm staff may provide emotional support and reduce fear.

These maintain adequate cardiac output before surgical intervention.

Information helps to allay anxiety. Patients who are anxious may not be able to comprehend anything more than simple, brief instructions and explanations.

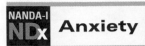

Anxiety

NANDA-I NDx

Common Related Factors

Sudden onset of illness
Impending surgery
Close monitoring by medical or nursing staff
Fear of death
Multiple tests and procedures

Defining Characteristics

Tense, anxious appearance
Request to have family at bedside all the time
Restlessness
Increased questioning
Constant demands
Glancing about or increased alertness

Common Expected Outcomes

Patient verbalizes reduced anxiety.
Patient demonstrates positive coping method.

NOC Outcome

Anxiety Self-Control

NIC Interventions

Anxiety Reduction; Teaching: Procedure/
Treatment; Calming Techniques

Cardiac and Vascular Care Plans

Ongoing Assessment

Actions/Interventions	Rationales
■ Assess anxiety level (mild, severe). Note signs and symptoms, especially nonverbal communication.	Aortic dissection/rupture can result in an acute life-threatening situation that will produce high levels of anxiety in the patient as well as in significant others.

Therapeutic Interventions

Actions/Interventions	Rationales
■ Acknowledge awareness of patient's anxiety.	Acknowledgment of the patient's feelings validates the feelings and communicates acceptance of those feelings.
■ Reduce unnecessary external stimuli.	Anxiety may escalate with excessive conversation, noise, and equipment around patient.
■ Explain all procedures as appropriate, using simple, concrete words.	Information helps allay anxiety. Patients who are anxious may not be able to comprehend anything more than simple, clear, brief instructions.
■ Provide a quiet, private place for significant others to wait.	A quiet environment can reduce anxiety.

Deficient Knowledge: Follow-Up Care

NANDA-I NDx

Common Related Factors

New medical problem
Unfamiliarity with surgical procedure and hospital care

Defining Characteristics

Expressed need for information
Multiple questions

Common Expected Outcome

Patient or family verbalizes understanding of disease process, treatment options, and goals of therapy.

NOC Outcomes

Knowledge: Disease Process; Knowledge: Treatment Regimen

NIC Interventions

Teaching: Disease Process; Teaching: Procedure/ Treatment

■ = Independent   ▲ = Collaborative

Ongoing Assessment

Actions/Interventions	Rationales
■ Assess knowledge of the disease and treatment options.	This information provides an important starting point in education.

Therapeutic Interventions

Actions/Interventions	Rationales
■ Instruct medically treated patient about the following: • Importance of follow-up CT scanning • Goals of therapy (avoidance of excess BP and strain on the diseased arterial wall) • Use of antihypertensive medications as prescribed; importance of compliance • Side effects of medicines • Signs and symptoms to report	Patients treated medically need to maintain goal BP levels and comply with scheduled CT scans to monitor size of the aneurysm. Knowledge of early warning signs facilitates rapid treatment. These may include pain in chest, abdomen, back, groin; weakness; decreased urine output; cool, pale extremities.
■ Instruct endograft patients about need for follow-up CT scans at 1 and 6 months and yearly for the rest of their lives.	The endograft may incur a leak; ongoing evaluation is needed, so appropriate treatment can be initiated.
■ Instruct surgical patients about the following: • Activity restrictions • Wound care • Avoiding activities that are isometric or abruptly raise BP (e.g., lifting and carrying of heavy objects, straining for bowel movement) • Signs and symptoms to report	Discharge instructions guide patients regarding self-care measures. Heavy lifting of more than 5 to 10 pounds is restricted for 4 to 6 weeks after surgical repair of an aortic aneurysm. These restrictions reduce strain on suture lines until they are completely healed.

Related Care Plans

Acute pain, p. 151
Deficient fluid volume, p. 72
Ineffective tissue perfusion, p. 199

Cardiac Rehabilitation

Post–Myocardial Infarction; Post–Cardiac Surgery; Post–Percutaneous Transluminal Coronary Angioplasty; Chronic Heart Failure; Chronic Angina; Activity Progression; Cardiac Education

Cardiac rehabilitation is the process of actively assisting patients with known heart disease to achieve and maintain optimal physical and emotional health and wellness. It has undergone significant evolution, redesigning itself from a primarily exercise-focused intervention into a comprehensive disease management program. Core components of these programs include the following: baseline and follow-up patient assessments; aggressive strategies for reducing modifiable risk factors for cardiovascular disease (CVD; e.g., lipids, hypertension, diabetes, obesity); counseling on heart-healthy nutrition, smoking cessation, and stress management; assistance in adhering to prescribed medications; promotion of lifestyle physical activity; exercise training; and psychosocial and vocational counseling. These integrated services are best provided by a multidisciplinary team composed of physicians, nurses, health educators, exercise physiologists, dietitians, and behavioral medicine specialists. More recently, the nurse has changed from team member to case manager. Key to providing cost-effective help is the provision of interventions based on each patient's unique needs, interests, and skills.

Cardiac rehabilitation programs typically begin in the hospital setting and progress to supervised (and often electrocardiographically monitored) outpatient programs. However, with shorter hospital stays, little time may be available for adequate instruction regarding lifestyle management and activity progression. Only 11% to 38% of eligible patients reportedly participate in any outpatient programs, usually because of lack of physician referral, lack of insurance coverage, transportation difficulties, gender-related barriers, conflicts with returning to work, and associated medical problems. Therefore newer models are being considered, such as transtelephonic electrocardiogram (ECG) monitoring at home.

Activity Intolerance

Common Related Factors

Imposed activity restrictions secondary to medical condition or high-technology therapies or procedures

Pain (ischemic, postsurgery incisional, related to other underlying conditions or health problems)

Generalized weakness or fatigue (sedentary lifestyle before event, lack of sleep, decreased caloric intake after surgery)

Reduced cardiac output (secondary to myocardial dysfunction, dysrhythmias, postural hypotension)

Fear or anxiety (of overexerting heart, of experiencing angina or incisional pain)

Defining Characteristics

Verbal report of fatigue or weakness

Verbal report of chest pain/other pain

Abnormal heart rate (HR) or blood pressure (BP) in response to activity

Exertional dyspnea

ECG changes reflecting ischemia

Dysrhythmias precipitated by activity

Common Expected Outcomes

Patient exhibits activity tolerance as evidenced by heart rate and blood pressure within prescribed ranges during activity progression, absence of activity-related chest pain or discomfort, absence of dyspnea, no occurrence of or increase in dysrhythmias during activity.

Patient reports readiness to perform activities of daily living (ADLs) and routine home activities.

NOC Outcomes

Circulation Status; Activity Tolerance; Physical Fitness

NIC Interventions

Exercise Promotion; Cardiac Care: Rehabilitation; Teaching: Prescribed Exercise/Activity

Ongoing Assessment

Actions/Interventions	Rationales
■ Assess patient's activity tolerance and exercise habits before current illness.	This information will serve as a basis for formulating short- or long-term goals. Some patients may have participated in regular exercise programs and be quite fit, whereas others may have been incapacitated by chronic angina or chronic heart failure (CHF) or have other health problems that interfere with activity.
■ Assess patient's HR, BP, and cardiac rhythm before initiating activity or exercise session.	Hospital patients with complications need close observation and may require supplemental oxygen and telemetry monitoring. Outpatients may exhibit hemodynamic changes such as orthostatic hypotension secondary to changes in prescribed medications or associated illnesses.
■ Assess patient's emotional readiness to increase activity.	Many patients with myocardial infarction (MI) may still be denying they even had a heart attack and may want to do more than prescribed; some post-MI or surgical patients or older patients with CHF can be quite fearful of overexerting their hearts or causing discomfort.

■ = Independent   ▲ = Collaborative

Cardiac and Vascular Care Plans

Actions/Interventions

- Assess motivation level and interest regarding initiation of outpatient exercise program.

- Monitor response to progressive activities. Signs of abnormal responses include:
  - Heart rate outside target range (depending on patient's baseline and stage of recovery)
  - Pulse greater than 20 beats/min over baseline, or greater than 120 beats/min (while inpatient)
  - Chest pain or discomfort; dyspnea
  - Occurrence of or increase in dysrhythmias (inappropriate bradycardia, symptomatic supraventricular tachycardia)
  - Excessive fatigue/weakness
  - Significant decrease of 15 to 20 mm Hg in systolic BP
  - Significant systolic BP of 200 mm Hg or more, or diastolic BP greater than 110 mm Hg
  - ST-segment displacement, if ECG is monitored
  - Light-headedness, dizziness
- For inpatients, monitor oxygen saturation.

- Assess patient's perception of effort required to perform each activity.

Rationales

Some patients with no prior history of exercise may benefit from more supervised sessions to facilitate adherence. However, other patients may prefer to exercise independently at home, for example, using a stationary bicycle.

Physical activities increase demands on the heart. Close monitoring of the patient's response provides guidelines for optimal activity progression.

A saturation of greater than 90% is recommended. Lower values require supplemental oxygen during activity and slower activity progression.

The Borg scale uses ratings from 6 to 20 to determine rating of perceived exertion. A rating of 11 (fairly light) to 13 (somewhat hard) is an acceptable level for most inpatients, whereas 11 to 15 may be appropriate for outpatients.

Therapeutic Interventions

Actions/Interventions

- Encourage verbalization of feelings regarding exercise or need to increase activity.
- Inform patient about health benefits and physical effects of activity or exercise.

- ▲ For inpatients, maintain progression of activities as ordered by cardiac rehabilitation team or physician, and as tolerated by patient. The following are provided as a guide.

Cardiac Rehabilitation Activity Progression:
- Self-care activities at bedside
- Selected range-of-motion (ROM) exercises in bed—progressing to chair
- Sitting up in chair for 30 to 60 minutes 3 times a day—progressing "as tolerated"
- Partial bath in chair progressing to sink
- Walking 75 to 100 feet in hall 2 to 3 times a day—progressing to "ambulate ad lib"
- Calisthenic exercises while standing
- Stair climbing

Rationales

An honest relationship facilitates problem solving and successful coping.

Activity prevents complications related to immobilization, improves feelings of well-being, and may improve mortality (with long-term exercise).

Not everyone progresses at the same rate. Some patients progress slowly because of complicated MI, lack of motivation, inadequate sleep, fear of "overexertion," related medical problems, and previous sedentary lifestyle. In contrast, others who experience small infarcts and who had high fitness and activity levels before hospitalization may progress rapidly. Activities are progressed by increasing either distance or time walked, as the patient tolerates or prefers.

Gradual resumption of activities promotes feeling of independence. ROM exercises reduce risk for thromboembolism. Early chair sitting reduces postural hypotension and promotes better lung function Repetition of exercises helps maintain muscle strength and build confidence. Increase in distance or speed is used to increase level of activity. Success in stair climbing promotes confidence before discharge.

Actions/Interventions

- Perform discharge submaximal exercise stress test as prescribed (for most post-MI patients).
▲ For patients with neurological or musculoskeletal problems, refer to physical therapy for assessment of ambulatory assistive device.
■ Encourage adequate rest periods before and after activity.

■ Assist and provide emotional support when increasing activity.

Before discharge:
■ Provide written guidelines in activity progression for home exercise programs.

■ Include metabolic equivalent task (MET) level guides for determining when to resume various ADLs.

■ Provide instructions for warm-up and cool-down exercises.

■ Provide a target HR guide (usually around 20 beats/min above standing resting HR).
■ Instruct patients regarding whom (e.g., cardiac rehabilitation nurse, physician) to call if any abnormal response to exercise is noted.
■ For older patients or patients with significant medical complications, consider referral to a home care nurse or physical therapy sessions.

Outpatient programs:
■ Assist patient with setting appropriate short- and long-term goals.

■ Determine patient's projected length of time in a supervised program.

■ Design an individualized plan, including intensity, duration, frequency, and mode of exercise.

■ Gradually adjust duration and/or intensity of exercise until target HR is reached.

Rationales

Exercise stress testing is used to risk-stratify patients.

Assistive aids help reduce energy consumption during physical activity.

Rest decreases cardiac workload and provides time for energy conservation and recovery.
Patients may be fearful of overexertion and potential damage to the heart. Appropriate supervision during early efforts can enhance confidence.

Exercise programs must be individualized, because each patient recovers at his or her own rate. Most patients are not enrolled in outpatient rehabilitation until 2 to 3 weeks after hospital discharge (if at all). Thus patients need to initiate some exercise progression on their own.
Tables have been developed that indicate the MET level for most ADLs and sports activities. For example, resting in a supine position is 1 MET. Sitting on a bedside commode is about 3 METs, as is walking at 2.5 mph. Walking briskly up stairs is about 7 METs. Shoveling snow is about 8 to 9 METs.
Warm-up exercises facilitate the heart and body's transition from rest to physical activity. Cool-down exercises facilitate hemodynamic adjustments and return of HR and BP to near-normal levels.
Having a target guide aids in monitoring intensity of exercise.

Information enables patient to take control of situation.

Some patients require more supervision or specialized therapy to regain activity tolerance.

Some patients are only interested in regaining strength after a cardiac event, whereas others are motivated to improve their functional capacities by beginning new lifelong exercise habits.
Some insurance carriers reimburse for 36 sessions and others for only 6 sessions. Some patients may prefer home exercise rather than the group environment and may attend only a few sessions to get started.
Age and fitness level must be considered in designing the exercise prescription. Although the benefits are the same as for younger patients, older patients need more warm-up and cool-down time. Intensity is usually guided by the target HR, which is about 20 beats/min above standing resting HR. For patients who had symptom-limited exercise stress tests, a more individualized and precise target HR can be calculated.
For patients less familiar with exercise or with more complications, it may take several sessions to reach target HR.

■ = Independent   ▲ = Collaborative

Actions/Interventions

- Provide instruction in appropriate warm-up and cool-down exercises.

- Instruct in self-monitoring of appropriate and abnormal responses to exercise.
- Teach patients how to self-monitor their pulse rate if appropriate.
- Reinforce positive effects of exercise in improving mortality and quality of life.

- Provide positive feedback to patients' efforts.

Rationales

Stretching exercises promote flexibility and prepare the muscles and joints for the upcoming stress from exercise. Cool-down is especially important because it helps to pump blood pooled in the primary muscle groups back to the upper part of the body. It also helps prevent muscle soreness. It is especially important for older patients to perform adequate warm-up and cool-down exercises.

Cardiac patients must be aware of warning signs that warrant cessation of exercise.

HR is a guide for monitoring intensity or duration of exercise.

Studies of cardiac rehabilitation programs have reported significant reduction in mortality in patients with coronary heart disease.

Ongoing feedback facilitates adherence to a sometimes difficult behavior change.

NANDA-I NDx Deficient Knowledge

Common Related Factor

Unfamiliarity with cardiac disease process, treatments, recovery process, follow-up care

Defining Characteristics

Questioning members of the health care team
Verbalized misconceptions/inaccurate information
Lack of questions

Common Expected Outcomes

Patient verbalizes understanding of disease state, recovery process, and follow-up care.
Patient identifies available resources for lifestyle changes.

NOC Outcomes

Knowledge: Disease Process; Knowledge: Treatment Regimen

NIC Interventions

Cardiac Care: Rehabilitative; Teaching: Disease Process; Teaching: Prescribed Medications; Teaching: Prescribed Diet; Behavior Modification

---

Ongoing Assessment

Actions/Interventions

- Assess understanding of disease process, specific cardiac event, treatments, recovery, and follow-up care.
- Identify specific learning needs and goals before discharge.

For outpatients:

- Conduct intake interviews regarding prior experiences with risk factor reduction and lifestyle changes that the patient is interested in pursuing.

Rationales

Teaching standardized content that patient already knows wastes valuable time and hinders critical learning.

Shortened hospital stays and complex risk factor reduction programs provide challenges to the nurse and patient. Priority needs must be identified and satisfied first.

Coronary atherosclerosis is a chronic disease requiring risk factor modification. Patients may have been told to change their lifestyle at an earlier time. Knowledge of prior behaviors serves to guide management plan.

Actions/Interventions

■ Assess the patient's readiness for and self-efficacy to initiate and maintain recommended behavioral changes.

Rationales

Lifestyle changes can be extremely difficult to make. Many behavior modification techniques based on social learning theory stress the importance of self-efficacy in initiating change.

Therapeutic Interventions

Actions/Interventions

■ Develop a plan for meeting individual goals. Include topics to be covered, format (individual versus group session), frequency (after each exercise session versus monthly), available audiovisual resources (video library, books, Internet, telephone), and specialty personnel (nutritionist, exercise physiologist, others).

■ Encourage meetings or conferences with family or significant others to discuss home recovery plan.

■ Provide information on the following needed topics:
- Pathophysiology of cardiac event (MI, HF, coronary artery disease, percutaneous transluminal coronary angioplasty, stent, valve disease)
- Healing process after cardiac event
- Incisional pain versus angina versus heart attack
- Resumption of ADLs, such as lifting, household chores, driving a car, climbing stairs, social activities, sexual activity, and recreational activity
- Return to work

■ Provide information regarding follow-up medications.

■ Provide referral to comprehensive risk reduction programs as indicated:
- Lipid management
- Hypertension management
- Diabetes management
- Weight management
- Counseling on heart-healthy nutrition
- Smoking cessation
- Stress management

■ Stress the importance of the patient's own role in maximizing his or her health status.

■ Provide information on available educational or support resources: American Heart Association, Mended Hearts groups, cardiac rehabilitation programs, stress management programs, smoking-cessation programs, and weight management programs.

Rationales

Each patient has his or her own learning style, which must be considered when designing a teaching program.

This approach enhances smooth transition to the home and may help guard against "overprotectedness."

Specific instructions, especially in written form, help reduce the patient's postdischarge fears and reduce risks of either overexertion or "cardiac invalidism."

Secondary prevention guidelines recommend that patients should take aspirin (to reduce platelet aggregation), β-blockers (to reduce mortality), lipid-lowering medication (to achieve a low-density lipoprotein level less than 100 mg/dL), and angiotensin-converting enzyme inhibitors (if ejection fraction is less than 40%). Antihypertensive and glucose-lowering medications are added as needed.

Staff is challenged to individualize services. Programs should focus on increasing awareness of personal risk factors and offer clear directions and strategies for risk reduction.

Patients need to understand that reduction of cardiac risk factors and health maintenance depend on them. Health professionals and family members can only provide information and support.

Lifestyle changes may require the assistance of professionals. Support groups provide contact with other individuals "who have been there" and can be beneficial in reducing anxiety and dealing with the impact of a cardiac event.

■ = Independent ▲ = Collaborative

NANDA-I NDx **Risk for Ineffective Coping**

Common Risk Factors

Recent changes in health status
Perceived change in future health status
Perceived change in social status and lifestyle
Feeling powerless to control disease progression
Unsatisfactory support systems
Inadequate psychological resources

Common Expected Outcomes

Patient implements an effective coping mechanism.
Patient identifies available resources for psychological and
    social support.

NOC Outcomes
Coping; Anxiety Self-Control
NIC Interventions
Coping Enhancement; Support System Enhance-
    ment; Anxiety Reduction; Teaching: Individual

Ongoing Assessment

Actions/Interventions	Rationales
■ Assess specific stressors.	Accurate appraisal can facilitate development of appropriate coping strategies. A patient's concerns may include fear of overexerting the heart with activity, expectation of becoming a cardiac invalid, inability to resume satisfying sexual activity, or inability to maintain recommended lifestyle changes.
■ Assess effectiveness past and present coping mechanisms.	Successful adjustment is influenced by previous coping success. Patients with a history of maladaptive coping may need additional resources.
■ Evaluate resources or support systems available to patient in hospital and at home.	Women (who manifest cardiac disease at a later age) are often widows living alone with limited support systems. Likewise, older patients with lifelong cardiac disease may have reduced contact with significant others.

Therapeutic Interventions

Actions/Interventions	Rationales
■ Encourage verbalization of concerns.	Acknowledging awareness of the challenges faced by the patient related to recovery from chronic cardiac disease can open doors for ongoing communication.
■ Encourage patient to seek information that will enhance coping skills.	Patients who are not coping well may need more guidance initially.
■ Provide information that patient wants or needs. Do not provide more than patient can handle.	With shortened exposure to cardiac rehabilitation services, patients can easily become overwhelmed by the large number of changes that are expected of them in a short time. Lifestyle changes should be considered over a lifelong period.
■ Provide reliable information about future limitations (if any) in physical activity and role performance.	At least 85% of patients can resume a normal lifestyle. Patients with more complications need guidance in understanding which limitations are temporary during recovery and which may be more permanent.

Actions/Interventions

- Provide information about the healing process so that misconceptions can be clarified. Refer to famous people (politicians, athletes, movie stars) who had similar cardiac problems or procedures and are now leading productive lives.
- Explain that patients are often "healthier" after cardiac events.

- Point out signs of positive progress or change.

- Encourage referral to a cardiac rehabilitation program and/or "coronary club."

Rationales

Examples such as Lyndon Johnson serving as President after a heart attack can provide reassurance and confidence about resuming activities.

Patients' blocked arteries may have been opened with revascularization, they are more knowledgeable about their specific risk factors and treatment plan, and they may be taking medication to improve their health.

Patients who are coping ineffectively may not be able to assess their own progress.

These programs provide opportunities to discuss fears with specialists and patients experiencing similar concerns.

Related Care Plans

Disturbed body image, p. 24
Health-seeking behaviors, p. 89
Ineffective sexuality patterns, p. 182

Coronary Bypass/Valve Surgery: Postoperative Care

Coronary Artery Bypass Grafting (CABG); Valve Replacement; Minimally Invasive Surgery; Off-Pump CABG (OPCAB)

Coronary Bypass Surgery

The surgical approach to myocardial revascularization for coronary artery disease is bypass grafting. An artery from the chest wall (internal mammary) or a vein from the leg (saphenous) is used to supply blood distal to the area of stenosis. Internal mammary arteries have a higher patency rate. Today's CABG patients are older (even octogenarians unresponsive to medical therapy or with failed coronary angioplasties or stents), have poorer left ventricular function, and may have undergone prior sternotomies. Older patients are at higher risk for complications and have a higher mortality rate. Women tend to have CABG surgery performed later in life. They have more complicated recovery courses than men because of the smaller diameter of women's vessels and their associated comorbidity. Women have also been noted to have less favorable outcomes, with more recurrent angina and less return to work. Newer techniques for revascularization are available, such as transmyocardial revascularization with laser and video-assisted thoracoscopy. These techniques use limited incision and reduce the need for cardiopulmonary bypass and related perioperative complications. Surgical procedures for CABG without cardiopulmonary bypass or cardioplegia (off-pump) hold promise for reductions in postoperative morbidity.

Valve Replacement Surgery

Rheumatic fever, infection, calcification, or degeneration can cause the valve to become stenotic (incomplete opening) or regurgitant (incomplete closure), leading to valvular heart surgery. Whenever possible, the native valve is repaired. If the valve is beyond repair, it is replaced. Replacement valves can be tissue or mechanical. Tissue valves have a short life span; mechanical valves can last a lifetime but require long-term anticoagulation. Valve surgery involves intracardiac suture lines; therefore these patients are at high risk for conduction defects and postoperative bleeding.

This care plan focuses only on acute care. See Cardiac Rehabilitation care plan presented earlier in this chapter for patient education information.

■ = Independent   ▲ = Collaborative

NANDA-I NDx ## Decreased Cardiac Output

Common Related Factor

Low cardiac output syndrome (occurs to some extent in all patients after extracorporeal circulation [ECC] secondary to reduced ventricular function)

Defining Characteristics

Left ventricular failure (LVF):
- Increased left arterial pressure (LAP), pulmonary capillary wedge pressure (PCWP), and pulmonary artery diastolic pressure (PADP)
- Tachycardia
- Decreased blood pressure (BP) and decreased cardiac output (CO)
- Slow capillary refill
- Diminished peripheral pulses
- Changes seen on chest x-ray films
- Crackles
- Decreased arterial and venous oxygen
- Acidosis
- Decreasing urine output
- Changes in level of consciousness

Right ventricular failure (RVF):
- Increased right arterial pressure (RAP), central venous pressure (CVP), and heart rate (HR)
- Decreased LAP, PCWP, and PADP (unless biventricular failure present)
- Jugular venous distention
- Decreased BP, decreased perfusion, decreased cardiac output, change in level of consciousness

Common Expected Outcome

Patient maintains adequate cardiac output, as evidenced by strong peripheral pulses, systolic BP within 20 mm Hg of baseline, HR 60 to 100 beats/min with regular rhythm, urinary output greater than 30 mL/hr, clear breath sounds, good capillary refill, warm and dry skin, and normal level of consciousness.

NOC Outcomes
Cardiac Pump Effectiveness; Circulation Status
NIC Interventions
Invasive Hemodynamic Monitoring; Hemodynamic Regulation

Ongoing Assessment

Actions/Interventions

- Document the pump time (ECC) during surgery.

- Assess HR, BP, and pulse pressure. Use direct intraarterial monitoring as ordered.

Rationales

The ECC pump, or the heart-lung machine, is used to divert blood from the heart and lungs, to oxygenate it, and to provide flow to the vital organs while the heart is stopped. For on-pump procedures, the more prolonged the pump run, the more profound the ventricular dysfunction. Newer surgical techniques are performing CABG without extracorporeal bypass (off-pump, or "surgery on the beating heart" to avoid this complication).

Sinus tachycardia and increased arterial BP are seen in early stages to maintain an adequate cardiac output; BP drops as condition deteriorates. Older patients have reduced response to catecholamines; thus their response to decreased CO may be blunted with less increase in heart rate.

Actions/Interventions	**Rationales**
■ Assess peripheral and central pulses, including capillary refill.	Pulses are weak with reduced stroke volume and cardiac output. Capillary refill is slow.
■ Assess for changes in level of consciousness.	Early signs of cerebral hypoxia are restlessness and anxiety, with confusion and loss of consciousness occurring in later stages. Older patients are especially susceptible to reduced perfusion to vital organs.
■ Assess respiratory rate and rhythm.	Rapid shallow respirations are characteristic of decreased cardiac output.
■ Assess urine output.	The renal system compensates for low blood pressure by retaining fluid and sodium. Oliguria is a classic sign of inadequate renal perfusion from reduced cardiac output.
■ Use pulse oximetry to monitor oxygen saturation; assess arterial blood gases.	Pulse oximetry is a useful tool to detect changes in oxygenation. Oxygen saturation should be kept above 90% or greater. As shock increases, aerobic metabolism ceases and lactic acidosis ensues, raising levels of carbon dioxide and pH.
■ If hemodynamic monitoring is in place, assess CVP, PADP, PCWP, cardiac output/cardiac index (CO/CI), and SVo_2 level.	CVP provides information on filling pressures of the right side of the heart; PADP and PCWP reflect left-sided fluid volumes. Cardiac output provides information on end-organ perfusion and objective numbers to guide therapy. SVo_2 provides information on tissue oxygenation at the cellular level. Change in oxygen saturation of mixed venous blood is one of the earliest indications of decreased cardiac output.
■ Auscultate breath sounds.	Crackles are evident in LVF but not in RVF.
▲ Monitor serial chest x-ray films.	X-ray studies provide information on enlarged heart, increased pulmonary vascular markings, and pulmonary edema.

Therapeutic Interventions

Actions/Interventions	**Rationales**
▲ Maintain hemodynamics within set parameters by titration of vasoactive drugs, most commonly:	
• Intravenous (IV) nitroglycerin	Nitroglycerin is a vasodilator that acts on the coronary vasculature, decreases spasm of mammary grafts, and dilates venous system.
• Sodium nitroprusside (Nipride)	Sodium nitroprusside is a vasodilator that lowers systemic vascular resistance and decreases BP. Elevated pressure on new grafts may cause bleeding.
• Dopamine	Dopamine is an inotrope and vasopressor that has varying effects at different doses. Low doses increase renal blood flow. Higher doses increase SVR and contractility.
• Dobutamine (Dobutrex)	Dobutamine is an inotrope that increases contractility with slight vasodilation.
• Milrinone	Milrinone is a cyclic AMP–specific PDE inhibitor that has inotropic and vasodilator effects.
• Norepinephrine (Levophed)	Norepinephrine is a vasopressor that increases SVR and contractility.
• Epinephrine	Epinephrine is an inotrope and vasopressor that increases SVR and contractility.
• Phenylephrine (Neo-Synephrine)	Neosynephrine is a vasopressor that increases SVR.
• Vasopressin	Vasopressin is a vasopressor that increases SVR.
• Nicardipine	Nicardipine is a calcium channel blocker that increases cardiac output and decreases peripheral vascular resistance.
▲ Maintain oxygen therapy as prescribed.	Oxygen saturation needs to be greater than 90%. When more oxygen is available to the myocardial tissues, ventricular function may improve.

■ = Independent   ▲ = Collaborative

Actions/Interventions

■ If patient is unresponsive to usual treatments, anticipate use of mechanical assistance.

Rationales

Mechanical devices such as the ventricular assist device or the intraaortic balloon pump provide temporary circulatory support to improve cardiac output. These devices can be used in cardiac surgery patients who cannot be weaned from cardiopulmonary bypass. The intraaortic balloon pump is used to increase coronary artery perfusion and decrease myocardial workload. The nurse needs to follow unit protocols for the management of the patient with a mechanical assist device.

NANDA-I
NDx **Deficient Fluid Volume**

Common Related Factors

Fluid leaks into extravascular spaces
Diuresis
Blood loss or altered coagulation factors

Defining Characteristics

Decreased filling pressures (CVP, RAP, PADP, PCWP, LAP)
Hypotension/tachycardia
Decreased cardiac output or cardiac index
Decreased urine output with increased specific gravity
If blood loss occurs:
• Decreased hemoglobin level or hematocrit
• Increased chest tube drainage

Common Expected Outcome

Patient is normovolemic, as evidenced by normal filling pressures, systolic BP greater than or equal to 90 mm Hg, HR 60 to 100 beats/min at regular rate, and urine output at 30 mL/hr or greater.

NOC Outcomes

Circulation Status; Fluid Balance

NIC Interventions

Hemodynamic Regulation; Invasive Hemodynamic Monitoring; Hypovolemia Management

---

Ongoing Assessment

Actions/Interventions

▲ Assess hemodynamic parameters.

■ Monitor fluid status: intake, output, and urine-specific gravity.

▲ Monitor coagulation factors on complete blood count.

▲ Monitor platelets for thrombocytopenia. If platelet count drops below 100,000 mm³, or if platelets drop below 50% of preoperative platelet level, check heparin-induced platelet antibody (HIPA).

▲ If HIPA result is positive, stop all heparin products and obtain a hematology consult.

Rationales

Most patients have hypotension and compensatory tachycardia in response to a low fluid volume. Invasive hemodynamic measurements (e.g., CVP, PADP) may be required to determine status and guide therapy.

During ECC, the blood is diluted to prevent sludging in the microcirculation. Total fluid volume may be normal or increased, but because of ECC, changes in membrane integrity cause fluid leaks into extravascular spaces. Concentrated urine denotes fluid deficit.

Heparin is used with ECC to prevent clots from forming. Clotting derangements and bleeding are common postoperative problems.

Increasing numbers of patients on heparin develop heparin antibodies that activate platelets, causing new or worsening thrombosis. This heparin-induced thrombocytopenia (HIT) results in a low platelet count.

No specific guidelines on positive HIPA are yet defined. Each patient must be evaluated individually. Argatroban is used for anticoagulation in heparin-induced thrombocytopenia.

Actions/Interventions	Rationales
■ Obtain report of blood loss from operating room and type and amount of fluid replacement.	These data provide key information on level of fluid balance.
■ Assess chest tube drainage.	Significant blood loss from chest tubes can contribute to decreased fluid volume.

Therapeutic Interventions

Actions/Interventions	Rationales
▲ Administer IV fluid as prescribed (e.g., lactated Ringer's solution).	A cell-saver from the ECC is used to replace blood intra-operatively. Further fluid volume replacement is initiated after surgery. These maintain adequate filling pressures.
▲ Keep cross-matched blood available.	In case major bleeding occurs, blood replacement must be immediately available.
▲ Administer coagulation drugs as prescribed: vitamin K, protamine.	Specific drugs work for different etiologies.
▲ Administer blood products (packed red blood cells, fresh frozen plasma, platelets, cryoprecipitate).	Transfusion therapy is used to correct deficiencies.

 Risk for Decreased Cardiac Output: Dysrhythmias

Common Risk Factors

Dysrhythmias resulting from the following:
- Ectopy (ischemia, electrolyte imbalance, and mechanical irritation)
- Bradydysrhythmias and heart block (edema or sutures in the area of the specialized conduction system)
- Supraventricular tachydysrhythmias (atrial stretching, mechanical irritability secondary to cannulation, or rebound from preoperative β-blockers)

Common Expected Outcome

Patient maintains optimal cardiac output as evidenced by baseline cardiac rhythm, HR between 60 and 100 beats/min, and adequate BP to meet metabolic needs.

NOC Outcomes
Vital Signs; Electrolyte and Acid-Base Balance; Cardiac Pump Effectiveness
NIC Interventions
Dysrhythmia Management; Electrolyte Monitoring; Electrolyte Management (Specify)

Ongoing Assessment

Actions/Interventions	Rationales
■ Continuously monitor cardiac rhythm.	Ability to recognize dysrhythmias is essential to early treatment. Atrial fibrillation, premature ventricular contractions, and heart blocks are the most common postoperative dysrhythmias.
▲ Monitor 12-lead electrocardiogram (ECG) as prescribed.	Besides providing information on dysrhythmias, the ECG may document intraoperative myocardial ischemia that may also affect cardiac output.

■ = Independent   ▲ = Collaborative

Actions/Interventions

▲ Monitor electrolyte levels, especially potassium, magnesium, and calcium.

Rationales

Electrolyte imbalances are common causes of dysrhythmias and guide treatment. Potassium and magnesium loss results from diuresis.

Therapeutic Interventions

Actions/Interventions

■ Maintain temporary pacemaker generator at bedside.

▲ Administer potassium as prescribed to keep serum level at 4 to 5 mEq/L.

▲ Administer magnesium as prescribed to keep level greater than 2 mEq/L.

▲ Administer calcium as prescribed to keep level at 8 to 10 mg/dL.

▲ Treat dysrhythmias according to unit protocol.

▲ If dysrhythmias are unresponsive to medical treatment, avoid precordial thump. Use countershock instead.

Rationales

Dysrhythmias are common after cardiac surgical procedures. Temporary epicardial pacing wires are often placed prophylactically during surgery for use in overdriving tachy-dysrhythmias or for backup pacing bradydysrhythmias. During the first 24 hours the wires may be connected to a pulse generator kept on standby.

Both hypokalemia and hyperkalemia can initiate cardiac dysrhythmias.

A variety of dysrhythmias can be precipitated by magnesium imbalance.

Although cardiac dysrhythmias are less common with hypocalcemia, they can be dangerous when present.

Advanced Cardiac Life Support (ACLS) and other evidence-based clinical guidelines provide direction for treatment. Amiodarone has become the drug of choice for most dysrhythmias. Pacing through epicardial pacing wires is often ordered.

Avoidance of precordial thump reduces risk for trauma to vascular suture lines.

Decreased Cardiac Output: Cardiac Tamponade

Common Related Factor

Cardiac tamponade resulting in external compression of cardiovascular structures causing reduced diastolic filling

Defining Characteristics

Decreased BP
Narrow pulse pressure
Pulsus paradoxus (systolic pressure decreases 10 mm Hg or more during inspiration)
Tachycardia
Electrical alternans (decreased QRS voltage during inspiration)
Equalization of pressures (CVP, right ventricular diastolic pressure [RVDP], PADP, PCWP)
Jugular venous distention (JVD)
Chest tubes (if present) suddenly stop draining (suspect clot)
Distant or muffled heart tones
Restlessness, confusion, and anxiety
Decrease in hemoglobin and hematocrit
Cool, clammy skin
Diminished peripheral pulses
Decreased urine output
Decreased arterial and venous oxygen saturation
Acidosis
Unwillingness to lie supine

Common Expected Outcome

Patient maintains adequate cardiac output as evidenced by the following: BP within normal limits for patient, strong regular pulses, absence of JVD, absence of pulsus paradoxus, skin warm and dry, and normal level of consciousness.

NOC Outcomes

Cardiac Pump Effectiveness; Fluid Balance; Blood Coagulation

NIC Interventions

Hemodynamic Regulation; Invasive Hemodynamic Monitoring; Fluid Resuscitation; Shock Management: Cardiac; Emergency Care

Ongoing Assessment

Actions/Interventions	Rationales
■ Assess for classic signs associated with acute cardiac tamponade:	Accumulation of blood in the mediastinum or pericardium applies pressure on the heart and causes tamponade with a resulting decrease in cardiac output. Cardiac tamponade is a life-threatening condition. Early assessment of reduced cardiac output facilitates early emergency treatment. Symptoms are related to the degree of tamponade.
• Low arterial BP with narrowed pulse pressure	An initial elevation in BP may occur with compensatory vasoconstriction; however, as venous return is compromised from the cardiac compression, a significant decrease in cardiac output occurs.
• Tachycardia	Tachycardia is related to compensatory catecholamine release.
• Distant or muffled heart sounds	These characteristic sounds are related to fluid accumulation in the pericardial sac.
• CVP	The CVP may rise to 15 to 20 cm H_2O as a result of impedance to diastolic filling by atrial compression.
• Pulsus paradoxus	Pulsus paradoxus is characterized by a drop of more than 10 mm Hg in systolic BP with inspiration.
• Dyspnea	Dyspnea is related to fluid backup in the pulmonary system.
■ Assess level of consciousness.	Symptoms may range from anxiety to altered level of consciousness in shock.
■ Monitor chest tube drainage.	A decrease in chest tube drainage occurring with decreased cardiac output may indicate cardiac tamponade.
▲ Assess 12-lead ECG.	ECG may reveal ST-segment elevation, nonspecific ST and T-wave changes, and/or electrical alternans (caused by pendulum-like movement of the heart within the pericardial effusion).
▲ Assist with performance of bedside echocardiogram if time permits.	Echocardiography evaluation provides the most helpful diagnostic information. Effusions seen with acute tamponade are usually smaller than with chronic tamponade. However, in light of circulatory collapse, treatment may be indicated before the echocardiogram can be performed.
▲ Assess hemodynamic profile using pulmonary artery catheter; assess for equalization of pressures.	The CVP, RVDP, PADP, and PCWP are all elevated in tamponade and within 2 to 3 mm Hg of each other. These pressures confirm diagnosis.
▲ Assess chest x-ray study.	X-ray study reveals a widened mediastinum with a normal cardiac silhouette, clear lung fields, and dilation of superior vena cava.

■ = Independent ▲ = Collaborative

Therapeutic Interventions

Actions/Interventions	Rationales
■ Implement unit protocols to remove clots from chest and/or mediastinal drainage tubes.	Impaired drainage can cause buildup of blood in the pericardial sac or mediastinum, resulting in tamponade.
▲ If cardiac tamponade is rapidly developing with cardiovascular decompensation and collapse:	
• Maintain aggressive fluid resuscitation.	Fluids are required to maintain adequate circulating volume as tamponade is evacuated.
• Administer vasopressor agents (dopamine, norepinephrine) as prescribed.	Vasopressor medications maximize systemic perfusion pressure to vital organs.
• Assemble open chest tray for bedside intervention; prepare patient for transport to surgery.	Acute tamponade is a life-threatening complication, but immediate prognosis is good with fast, effective treatment.

NDx Risk for Ineffective Myocardial Tissue Perfusion

Common Risk Factors

Spasm of native coronary or of internal mammary artery graft
Low flow or thrombosis of vein grafts
Coronary embolus
Perioperative ischemia
Chronic myocardial ischemia

Common Expected Outcome

Risk for perioperative ischemia and/or infarction is reduced through early assessment and treatment.

NOC Outcomes
Circulation Status; Tissue Perfusion: Cardiac
NIC Interventions
Cardiac Care: Acute; Hemodynamic Regulation

Ongoing Assessment

Actions/Interventions	Rationales
■ Continuously monitor ECG.	Cardiac rhythm changes may occur secondary to myocardial ischemia.
▲ Obtain a 12-lead ECG on admission and as needed. Compare with preoperative ECG. Note any acute changes: T-wave inversions, ST-segment elevation or depression.	Primary nurse must know which vessels were bypassed and must carefully evaluate the corresponding areas on the 12-lead ECG. Patients commonly have chronic myocardial ischemia that is further compromised during surgery, or they may have spasms in specific coronary arteries:
	• Right coronary artery (RCA): leads II, III, aVF
	• Posterior descending: R waves in V_1 and V_2
	• Left anterior descending: V_1 to V_4
	• Diagonals: V_5 to V_6
	• Circumflex, obtuse marginal: I, aVL, and V_5
▲ Monitor cardiac biomarkers (creatine kinase–myocardial bound [CK-MB] and troponin) for signs of perioperative ischemia or infarct per institutional policy.	Patients usually do not express characteristic chest pain because of the effects of general anesthesia during surgery. Laboratory data aid in diagnosis. However, many programs no longer measure these postoperatively, because there are no consistent standards to substantiate normal postoperative levels. New wall motion abnormality on echocardiogram can be used to document changes.

Therapeutic Interventions

Actions/Interventions	Rationales
▲ Maintain adequate diastolic BP with vasopressors.	Coronary artery flow occurs during diastole. Adequate pressures of at least 40 mm Hg are needed to drive coronary flow and prevent graft thrombosis.
▲ Maintain arterial saturation greater than 95%.	Adequate oxygenation is required for effective gas exchange.
▲ If signs of ischemia are noted, administer medications (IV nitroglycerin and/or calcium channel blocker).	Nitroglycerin and calcium channel blockers increase coronary perfusion and alleviate possible coronary spasm.
▲ Anticipate insertion of intraaortic balloon.	This assist device improves coronary artery blood flow during diastole.

Risk for Electrolyte Imbalance

Common Risk Factors

Fluid shifts
Diuretics

Common Expected Outcome

Patient maintains normal electrolyte balance, as evidenced by sodium level within 130 to 142 mEq/L; potassium, 4 to 5 mEq/L; chloride, 98 to 115 mEq/L; calcium, 9 to 11 mg/dL; and magnesium, 1.7 to 2.4 mEq/L.

NOC Outcomes
Electrolyte and Acid/Base Balance; Fluid Balance
NIC Intervention
Fluid/Electrolyte Management

Ongoing Assessment

Actions/Interventions	Rationales
▲ Observe and document serial laboratory data: sodium, potassium, chloride, magnesium, and calcium levels.	Hemodilution from ECC and resultant fluid shifts cause changes in fluid composition.
■ Monitor ECG for changes.	Widening QRS complex, ST segment changes, dysrhythmias, and atrioventricular blocks are seen with electrolyte imbalance.

Therapeutic Interventions

Actions/Interventions	Rationales
▲ Maintain adequate electrolyte balance by administering desired electrolytes as prescribed.	Hypertonic solutions may be used to correct sodium and chloride deficiencies. Potassium, calcium, and magnesium imbalances may be corrected by IV administration.

Risk for Impaired Gas Exchange

Common Risk Factors

Retraction and compression of lungs during surgery
Surgical incision, making coughing difficult
Secretions
Pulmonary vascular congestion

■ = Independent   ▲ = Collaborative

Common Expected Outcome

Patient maintains optimal gas exchange as evidenced by clear breath sounds, normal respiratory pattern, normal arterial blood gases (ABGs), and no further change in level of consciousness.

NOC Outcomes

Respiratory Status: Gas Exchange; Respiratory Status: Ventilation

NIC Interventions

Respiratory Monitoring; Ventilation Assistance; Airway Management; Endotracheal Extubation

Ongoing Assessment

Actions/Interventions	Rationales
■ Assess breath sounds, noting areas of decreased ventilation and presence of adventitious sounds.	Changes in breath sounds may reveal the etiology of impaired gas exchange. Diminished breath sounds are associated with poor ventilation.
▲ Monitor serial ABGs and oxygen saturation.	Low Po_2 and oxygen saturations and increasing $Paco_2$ are characteristic of hypoxemia and respiratory failure.
■ Assess for restlessness or changes in level of consciousness.	Hypoxemia results in cerebral hypoxia.
▲ Monitor serial chest x-ray films.	Chest x-ray studies can reveal the etiology of the impaired gas exchange. Pleural effusions, pulmonary edema, or infiltrates are contributing factors.
▲ Verify that ventilator settings are maintained as prescribed: • Tidal volume 10 to 15 mL/kg • Rate 10 to 14 per minute • Fio_2 to keep Po_2 greater than 80 mm Hg • Positive end-expiratory pressure (PEEP) starting at 5 cm H_2O	Safety is a priority. Ongoing titration may be required to maintain ABGs within acceptable limits.
▲ Monitor rising pulmonary artery pressures and peripheral vascular resistance.	Data provide information on pulmonary hypertension and cor pulmonale.
▲ Anticipate use of nitric oxide therapy with other ventilation therapy for patients with pulmonary hypertension.	Nitric oxide reduces the pulmonary vascular resistance for patients with persistent pulmonary hypertension.

Therapeutic Interventions

Actions/Interventions	Rationales
■ Suction as needed. Hyperventilate and hyperoxygenate during suctioning.	Suctioning removes secretions when the patient is unable to effectively clear the airway while ventilated. However, repeated and prolonged suctioning may lead to desaturation of blood and impaired gas exchange. Hyperoxygenation helps decrease hypoxia related to the suctioning procedure. Hyperventilation helps expand lungs that were deflated during surgery.
▲ Change ventilator settings as ordered.	Ongoing titration is expected to maintain ABGs within accepted limits. (Note: Patients with preexisting pulmonary dysfunction will have lower Po_2 and higher Pco_2 values.) PEEP may be increased in increments of 2.5 cm to maintain adequate oxygenation on Fio_2 of 50%. Patients can usually tolerate up to 20 cm H_2O of PEEP if they are not hypovolemic or hypotensive.
■ Initiate calming techniques if patient is "fighting" ventilator.	Patients expend energy and increase oxygen demands when their breathing is asynchronous with the ventilator. This breathing pattern may trigger high-pressure alarms on the ventilator.

Actions/Interventions	Rationales
■ Instruct patient or family of rationale and expected sensations associated with use of mechanical ventilation.	Adequate educational preparation can reduce anxiety and facilitate adjustment to mechanical ventilation process.
▲ Administer sedation as needed: • Midazolam (Versed): short-acting central nervous system depressant • Morphine sulfate • Propofol (Diprivan) drip	Sedation with midazolam and/or morphine sulphate helps decrease anxiety, which may reduce myocardial oxygen consumption. Patients are usually kept sedated for at least 4 hours to facilitate hemodynamic stability. Sedation with propofol IV infusion can be used for patients requiring longer mechanical ventilation therapy.
▲ Wean from ventilator, and extubate as soon as possible.	Initially the cardiac surgical patient requires mechanical ventilation because of use of general anesthesia. Weaning and extubation occur as soon as the anesthetic agents wear off, after 4 hours in most patients.
■ Encourage coughing and deep breathing. Use a pillow to splint the incision.	Coughing is an effective way to clear secretions. The surgical incision may cause chest discomfort and inhibit deep breathing and coughing. Splinting the chest may enhance coughing efforts.
▲ Use pain medications as needed.	Medications decrease incisional discomfort so that patient will cough and breathe deeply.
▲ Provide supplemental oxygen as indicated.	Oxygen saturation needs to be greater than 90%. Adequate oxygenation is required for effective gas exchange.
■ Instruct in need to use incentive spirometer.	Incentive spirometry increases lung volume and reduces alveolar collapse.
■ Encourage dangling of legs or progressive activity as tolerated.	Progressive activity increases lung volume and ventilation.
■ Consider chest physiotherapy.	Postural drainage and percussion techniques aid in mobilizing respiratory secretions for removal by suctioning or coughing.

NANDA-I NDx **Fear**

Common Related Factors
Intensive care unit environment
Unfamiliarity with postoperative care
Altered communication secondary to intubation
Dependence on mechanical equipment
Threat of pain related to major surgery
Threat of death

Defining Characteristics
Restlessness
Increased awareness
Glancing about
Trembling/fidgeting
Constant demands
Facial tension
Insomnia
Wide-eyed appearance

Common Expected Outcomes
Patient appears calm and trusting of medical care.
Patient verbalizes fears and concerns.

NOC Outcomes
Fear Self-Control; Coping
NIC Interventions
Anxiety Reduction; Preparatory Sensory Information; Emotional Support

■ = Independent   ▲ = Collaborative

Ongoing Assessment

Actions/Interventions	Rationales
■ Recognize patient's level of fear. Note signs and symptoms, especially nonverbal communication.	Controlling fear helps reduce physiological reactions that can aggravate condition and increase oxygen consumption.

Therapeutic Interventions

Actions/Interventions	Rationales
■ Orient to the intensive care environment.	The noise and continuous lighting in the intensive care unit environment increase the amount of sensory stimuli for the patient and add to the level of anxiety. Patient and family need to be aware of the source of noise such as normal sounds from mechanical ventilators, monitoring equipment, and mechanical ventricular assist devices. Because equipment alarms should not be silenced, nurses need to explain each alarm sound and respond to each alarm as quickly as possible to resolve the problem and restore normal function.
■ Display calm, confident manner.	This approach increases the patient's feeling of security.
■ Prepare for and explain common postoperative sensations (coldness, fatigue, discomfort, coughing, uncomfortable endotracheal tube). Clarify misconceptions.	Anticipatory preparation can help reduce anxiety associated with the unknown.
▲ Explain purpose of tubes, monitoring equipment, medication pumps, mechanical ventilators, and other equipment and devices that are part of postoperative care. Explain each procedure before doing it, even if previously described.	Misconceptions about the use of the equipment can add to patients' fear of equipment failure and feelings of dependency on machines. Information can promote trust or confidence in medical management. However, high anxiety levels can reduce attention level and retention of information.
■ Avoid unnecessary conversations between team members in front of patients.	This measure can reduce patients' misconceptions and fear or anxiety.
▲ Provide pain medication at first sign of discomfort.	Effective pain management will reduce discomfort and fear.
■ For intubated patients, provide nonverbal means of communication (slate, paper and pencil, gestures). Be patient with attempts to communicate. Know and anticipate typical patient concerns.	Patients' inability to talk can add to their anxiety.
■ Ensure continuity of staff.	Continuity facilitates communication efforts and provides stability in care.
■ Encourage visiting by family/significant others.	Visitors can promote a feeling of security; patient does not feel alone.

Related Care Plans

Cardiac rehabilitation, p. 230
Dysrhythmias, p. 249
Mechanical ventilation, p. 418

Dysrhythmias

Tachycardia; Bradycardia; Atrial Flutter; Atrial Fibrillation; Paroxysmal Supraventricular Tachycardia (PSVT); Heart Block; Pacemakers

Dysrhythmias involve any disturbance in the rhythm, rate, or conduction in the cardiac electrical system. They can occur for a variety of reasons. Dysrhythmias can develop as a result of myocardial ischemia, electrolyte imbalances, acid-base imbalances, and adverse reactions to drugs. Even the aging process causes changes in the electrical properties of myocardial cells. Changes in electrical events in the heart have a direct effect on contraction and relaxation of the myocardium. The end result is hemodynamic alterations that may lead to decreased cardiac output. The clinical significance of dysrhythmias can range from benign occurrences not requiring treatment to life-threatening situations. For some patients, syncope or even sudden cardiac death is the first occurrence of the dysrhythmia. Evaluation of the etiological factors for and the clinical significance of the dysrhythmia guide the therapeutic management. Treatment usually consists of drug therapy but may also include pacemaker support, electrical cardioversion, radiofrequency catheter ablation, an implantable defibrillator, or cardiopulmonary resuscitation (CPR). The American Heart Association Guidelines for Advanced Cardiac Life Support (ACLS) provide treatment protocols for the management of patients experiencing dysrhythmias. This care plan focuses on acute management in a medical setting.

Risk for Decreased Cardiac Output

Common Risk Factors

Rapid heart rate (HR) or rhythm secondary to the following:
- Myocardial ischemia
- Electrolyte imbalance (especially hypokalemia and hypomagnesemia)
- Anxiety or emotional factors
- Drugs (e.g., aminophylline, isoproterenol, dopamine, digoxin toxicity)
- Stimulant intake (coffee, tea, tobacco)
- Substance abuse (e.g., cocaine, alcohol)
- Physical activity
- Heart failure
- Pulmonary embolism
- Hypoxemia
- Chronic lung disease
- Edema
- Thyrotoxicosis

Slow HR or rhythm secondary to the following:
- Myocardial ischemia
- Drugs (e.g., calcium channel blockers, digoxin toxicity, β-blockers)
- Excessive parasympathetic stimulation (e.g., sensitive carotid sinus artery, inferior wall myocardial infarction)
- Diseases or degeneration of the conduction system
- Cardiomyopathy
- Hypothyroidism
- Increased intracranial pressure

■ = Independent   ▲ = Collaborative

Cardiac and Vascular Care Plans

Common Expected Outcome

Patient maintains adequate cardiac output as evidenced by strong peripheral pulses, systolic BP within 20 mm Hg of baseline, HR 60 to 100 beats/min with regular rhythm, urinary output >30 mL/hr, warm and dry skin, and normal level of consciousness.

NOC Outcomes
Vital Signs; Cardiac Pump Effectiveness
NIC Intervention
Dysrhythmia Management

Ongoing Assessment

Actions/Interventions	Rationales
■ Auscultate the heart for tachycardia (rate greater than 100 beats/min), bradycardia (rate less than 60 beats/min), and irregular rhythm.	Clinical assessment of patient is important to verify rhythm noted on monitor or the electrocardiogram (ECG).
■ Assess for signs of reduced cardiac output: rapid, slow, or weak peripheral pulses; hypotension; dizziness; syncope; shortness of breath; chest pain; fatigue; and restlessness.	The patient's tolerance of a dysrhythmia and the need for specific treatment is based on clinical manifestations of decreased cardiac output.
■ Determine acuteness or chronicity of the dysrhythmia.	The persistence of a dysrhythmia will determine the type of therapy needed to restore normal sinus rhythm or control the dysrhythmia to maintain adequate cardiac output.
■ Review history, and assess for causative factors.	Dysrhythmias are best suppressed when precipitating factors are eliminated or corrected. Some dysrhythmias such as those caused by heart failure are difficult to eradicate. Lifestyle behaviors such as smoking, caffeine intake, and emotional stress can stimulate some dysrhythmias.
■ If the patient is monitored electrocardiographically, determine specific type of dysrhythmia: sinus bradycardia, second- or third-degree heart block, atrial flutter or fibrillation with fast or slow ventricular response, junctional tachycardia, ventricular tachycardia, or paroxysmal supraventricular tachycardia (PSVT).	Ability to recognize dysrhythmias is essential to early and appropriate treatment.
■ Evaluate monitor leads that show the most prominent P waves such as lead II, V_1, or modified chest lead (MCL$_1$).	These leads aid in differentiating atrial from ventricular dysrhythmias.
■ Assess need for intravenous (IV) line.	An IV line provides immediate access in case IV medications are prescribed.
■ Carefully monitor patient's response to activity.	The patient with a dysrhythmia may have adequate CO at rest but inadequate CO to support increased activity levels.
■ Monitor for side effects of medication therapy.	Medications prescribed to "treat" dysrhythmias can themselves be proarrhythmogenic.

Therapeutic Interventions

Actions/Interventions	Rationales
■ If the patient is asymptomatic, provide reassurance if the dysrhythmia is not life threatening. Consult physician about further medical treatment.	Assessment of patient's hemodynamic status provides guidance for treatment. The patient, not the dysrhythmia, should be treated. No treatment may be indicated if patient demonstrates adequate CO.
▲ Provide oxygen therapy as ordered.	Oxygen decreases myocardial cell irritability and can relieve hypoxia-induced dysrhythmias.
▲ If the patient has acute dysrhythmia, obtain ECG immediately to document it.	ECGs provide the necessary information for diagnosing the type of dysrhythmia. An ECG should be obtained before patient reverts to baseline rhythm.

Actions/Interventions

■ Anticipate need for additional testing.

▲ Anticipate specific therapy based on identification of dysrhythmia.

For PSVT (rapid atrial tachycardia, junctional tachycardia, atrial flutter, and atrial fibrillation) with a pulse:

- Anticipate use of vagal maneuvers such as carotid sinus massage (compression), the Valsalva maneuver, or the administration of IV adenosine.

- Anticipate or prepare medications to reduce ventricular response: adenosine, calcium channel blockers, β-blockers, amiodarone.

- If the patient is unresponsive to medications, anticipate treatment with overdrive pacing, especially for atrial fibrillation and atrial flutter after cardiac surgery.

- If the ventricular rate is greater than 150 beats/min in unstable patients or if dysrhythmia is chronic and unresponsive to medical therapy, anticipate electrical cardioversion.

- For persistent, recurrent PSVT, anticipate use of radiofrequency catheter ablation.

- Instruct patient to avoid intake of stimulants as indicated: caffeine, alcohol, tobacco, and amphetamines.

For sinus bradycardia or second- or third-degree heart block with slow ventricular response:

- Instruct the patient to avoid the Valsalva maneuver (e.g., straining for stool) and vagal stimulating activities (e.g., vomiting).
- If the patient is symptomatic, administer atropine IV push, according to ACLS protocol.

- Anticipate transcutaneous pacing or temporary pacemaker insertion.

Rationales

A variety of tests are available to aid in diagnosis and to evaluate treatment (e.g., electrophysiology testing, ambulatory Holter monitoring, signal-averaged ECG, exercise stress testing).

Knowledge of specific rate or rhythm problem is necessary to accurately anticipate appropriate treatment.

These vagal maneuvers stimulate the vagus nerve, which may slow the heart. They may also be used to help diagnose the underlying dysrhythmia. (NOTE: These measures should be avoided in older patients.) Adenosine slows AV node conduction and may facilitate recognition of the origin of the dysrhythmia.

The type of medication to be given and the route of administration (by mouth or intravenously) depends on patient's hemodynamic status, underlying medical condition, acuteness or chronicity of dysrhythmia, and clinical setting. Current guidelines for ACLS provide protocols for management of dysrhythmias, including medications and electrical therapies. Using the ACLS protocols, the nurse can anticipate and prepare for the administration of appropriate medications or electrical therapies based on the progression of the dysrhythmia and the patient's response to each stage of therapeutic intervention.

Overdrive pacing involves pacing the heart for several seconds at a rate about 20% faster than the tachycardia and then stopping the pacemaker to allow the heart's natural rhythm to resume control. It is appropriate when atrial pacing leads are in place.

During cardioversion, low levels of energy are used to reset the natural cardiac cycle by electrically interfering with existing dysrhythmia. In nonemergencies, the patient should be sedated before the procedure. Anticoagulation is indicated before cardioversion to reduce the risk for embolization when normal cardiac function is restored.

Radiofrequency current is passed through an endocardial catheter positioned at the site of the dysrhythmia. Heat is created that abolishes the ectopic dysrhythmia.

Stimulants increase the automaticity of the heart, which can precipitate dysrhythmias.

Activities that increase vagal stimulation reduce HR.

Atropine decreases vagal tone and increases conduction through the atrioventricular node. Repeat doses may be indicated at 3- to 5-minute intervals.

Pacemakers supplement the body's natural pacemaker to maintain a preset HR. Transcutaneous pacemakers can be applied quickly. However, some patients may not tolerate the pacing stimulus to the skin and chest wall.

Cardiac and Vascular Care Plans

■ = Independent   ▲ = Collaborative

Actions/Interventions	**Rationales**
• If the patient is unresponsive to atropine, initiate epinephrine or dopamine, according to ACLS protocol.	These sympathetic stimulating medications increase BP and HR. NOTE: Sometimes the hypotension is not a result of the bradycardia but rather of hypovolemia or myocardial dysfunction and needs to be treated as such.
• Anticipate permanent pacemaker for chronic conditions.	Several cardiology national associations provide class I indications for permanent pacemaker implantation to improve cardiac output.
For ventricular tachycardia with a pulse:	
• Recognize that this is a potentially life-threatening dysrhythmia.	Ventricular tachycardia requires immediate attention and efficient treatment. Rapid hemodynamic collapse is possible.
• Administer medications as ordered (i.e., amiodarone [IV]), noting effectiveness. Alternative drugs include sotalol and procainamide.	For patients with wide complex tachycardias, ACLS protocols recommend amiodarone as the first-choice drug, followed by procainamide and sotalol.
• Anticipate use of elective synchronized cardioversion if unresponsive to medications.	Elective cardioversion using 200 J for biphasic cardioverter may be needed to convert rhythm before patient becomes unstable.
If patient has torsades de pointes:	This dysrhythmia is a specific type of multidirectional ventricular tachycardia that alternates in amplitude and direction of electrical activity; the dysrhythmia often requires no immediate intervention but may be life threatening.
• Evaluate QT interval on 12-lead ECG. Be especially alert for a 25% or greater increase from the normal QT adjusted for HR and gender.	Generally torsades de pointes dysrhythmia is associated with a prolonged QT interval on the ECG.
• Anticipate the need to obtain serum antidysrhythmic drug levels and/or electrolyte levels (potassium, calcium, magnesium).	Hypokalemia, hypomagnesemia, and hypocalcemia, along with elevated quinidine, procainamide, or tricyclic levels, can precipitate torsades de pointes.
• Anticipate medical therapies assistive to the treatment of torsades de pointes:	
• Amiodarone	Amiodarone may be effective for stable polymorphic VT.
• Magnesium sulfate	Hypomagnesemia is often the cause of delayed repolarization that precipitates torsades de pointes.
• Overdrive pacing	ACLS lists overdrive pacing as the treatment of choice to capture/convert the ventricular rhythm.
• Isoproterenol	This drug helps to overdrive the ventricular rate and break the dysrhythmic mechanism.
• Anticipate or prepare for emergency cardioversion or defibrillation, or CPR.	Being prepared for an emergency helps save life.
For ventricular fibrillation or pulseless ventricular tachycardia:	
• Anticipate the use of adjunct therapies, such as CPR and defibrillation by trained personnel.	A patient with a pulseless dysrhythmia should receive basic cardiac life support measures to support airway, breathing, and circulation, including automatic electrical defibrillation until personnel trained to provide ACLS are on the scene.
• Defibrillate patient.	ACLS protocols recommend beginning at 200 J for biphasic defibrillator and 360 J for monophasic defibrillator.
• Prepare for airway intubation and oxygen therapy.	Airway maintenance and supplemental oxygen therapy are needed until cardiac function is restored.
• Prepare for administration of IV medications: epinephrine, vasopressin, amiodarone, lidocaine, magnesium.	ACLS protocols provide guidelines for appropriate dosages and frequency of administration. Vasopressors are key for their vasoconstricting effects to improve cardiac output and coronary perfusion. If patient is unresponsive to defibrillation shocks, antidysrhythmic medications can be added. Magnesium is used only if the rhythm is torsades de pointes or caused by hypomagnesemia.

Deficient Knowledge: Cause and Treatment of Dysrhythmia

Common Related Factors

New condition/treatment
Complexity of treatment
Emotional state affecting learning (anxiety)

Common Expected Outcome

Patient verbalizes understanding of cause of and treatment regimen for dysrhythmia.

Defining Characteristics

Verbalized knowledge deficit
Verbalized inaccurate information
Questioning of staff about medication and/or management
Noncompliance with treatment
Inappropriate or inaccurate self-treatment

NOC Outcomes

Knowledge: Disease Process; Knowledge: Treatment Regimen

NIC Interventions

Teaching: Disease Process; Teaching: Prescribed Medications

Ongoing Assessment

Actions/Interventions	Rationales
■ Assess current knowledge of dysrhythmia, diagnostic procedures, and treatments.	Information provides basis for educational session.

Therapeutic Interventions

Actions/Interventions	Rationales
■ Instruct patient regarding cause of dysrhythmia if known.	Cause may be related to an acute event such as myocardial infarction, cardiac surgery, or electrolyte imbalance. However, it may be a chronic problem secondary to cardiomyopathy or other disorder.
■ If patient is having a procedure to diagnose or treat dysrhythmias, show patient equipment and/or procedure room beforehand.	Explanations enhance understanding and reduce anxiety.
■ Instruct patient regarding treatment versus maintenance medications: dose, method of administration.	Patients in acute setting may need explanation as to the variety of medications that may be required to successfully treat the problem. Patients with chronic conditions may require long-term self-management.
■ Instruct patient regarding adjunct therapies (cardioversion, pacemaker therapy) as appropriate.	In the acute setting, health care providers need to reserve time to explain rationale for and use of adjunct and often emergency therapies to reassure the patient that he or she is being safely cared for.
■ Instruct patient in the side effects of medications.	Most antidysrhythmics can have significant side effects. If side effects occur, patients need to report immediately so that appropriate therapy can be initiated.
■ If patient is taking a medication that requires maintenance of potassium level (e.g., digoxin), inform patient of foods high in potassium.	Foods that are sources of potassium include bananas, dried apricots, prune juice, cooked lima or pinto beans, cantaloupe, and winter squash.
■ Instruct patient and/or family members in method for checking pulse. State patient's normal rate and abnormal rate that should be reported to the physician. Explain any medications that are to be withheld or administered on the basis of pulse rate finding.	Eliciting patient as comanager of care empowers the patient and ensures more appropriate treatment.

■ = Independent ▲ = Collaborative

Actions/Interventions

- Instruct patient with tachydysrhythmias to avoid stimulant intake: caffeine, tobacco, alcohol, and amphetamines.
- ▲ By physician's order and hospital protocol, instruct patient in non medicinal methods to assist with controlling tachydysrhythmias (e.g., Valsalva maneuver, carotid sinus massage).
- Instruct patients with bradydysrhythmias to avoid straining for bowel movements. Provide information on natural laxatives as needed.
- Inform patient of proper procedure to follow in case dysrhythmia recurs (as evidenced by specific signs and symptoms).
- Instruct patient that fluid volume deficits caused by gastrointestinal influenza, diarrhea, and dehydration may lead to subsequent electrolyte imbalances and dysrhythmias.
- Instruct patient's family about sources for learning CPR.

Rationales

Stimulants increase the automaticity of the heart, which can precipitate dysrhythmias.

These procedures increase patient's sense of control and ensure prompt treatment.

Straining stimulates the vagal nerve, which can further slow the heart rate.

Developing a specific plan of care provides reassurance regarding ability of the patient to care for self at home.

Electrolyte abnormalities are major causes for dysrhythmias.

Knowledge of lifesaving skills may reduce anxiety related to "life-threatening" dysrhythmias. CPR training saves lives.

NANDA-I NDx **Risk for Ineffective Coping**

Common Risk Factors

Misinterpretation of condition or treatment
Situational crisis
Disturbances in self-concept or body image
Disturbances in lifestyle or role
Inadequate coping methods
Prolonged hospitalization
History of ineffective medical treatments
Perceived personal stress resulting from chronic condition or treatment
Lack of support system

Common Expected Outcomes

Patient verbalizes acceptance of possible chronic medical problem.
Patient describes and maintains effective coping strategist.
Patient uses available resources and support systems.

NOC Outcomes
Coping; Social Support
NIC Intervention
Coping Enhancement

Ongoing Assessment

Actions/Interventions

- Evaluate patient's emotional response to the dysrhythmia. Assess for coping difficulties.

- Assess patient's specific stressors (e.g., difficulty diagnosing cause of dysrhythmia, ineffective therapies, change in self-image related to problem).

Rationales

Palpitations or syncope occurring at home can be especially frightening. For patients in whom dysrhythmias are resistant to therapy, chronic episodes of tachycardia can lead to coping difficulties and body image disturbances. Behavioral and physiological responses to life threatening situations provide clues to level of coping difficulties.

Stressors may exhaust the patient's ability to maintain effective coping.

Actions/Interventions	Rationales
■ Evaluate patient's available resources or support systems.	Patients may have support in one setting, such as during hospitalization, yet be discharged home without sufficient support for effective coping. Resources may include significant others, health care providers such as home health nurse, community resources, and spiritual counseling.

Therapeutic Interventions

Actions/Interventions	Rationales
■ Encourage the patient and family to verbalize feelings about dysrhythmia, diagnostic procedures and treatment plan, and any lifestyle changes imposed by this medical problem.	Verbalization may help reduce anxiety and open doors for ongoing communication.
■ Explain dysrhythmias, procedures, and medications in a clear and concise manner to the patient and family.	Information provides rationale for therapy and aids the patient in understanding treatment and assuming responsibility for ongoing care. However, patients who are coping ineffectively have reduced ability to assimilate information.
■ Assist patient with evaluating situation accurately.	Patient response to acute episode is highly variable, depending on prior experiences and the like. Accurate appraisal can facilitate development of coping strategies.
■ Maintain appropriate level of intensity of action when responding to current dysrhythmia.	Overreaction or excessive response to a patient's dysrhythmia may encourage or increase feelings of anxiety.
■ As necessary, remain with the patient during episodes of dysrhythmia or during treatments.	The staff's presence is reassuring to the patient.

Heart Failure, Chronic

Congestive Heart Failure; Cardiomyopathy; Left-Sided Failure; Right-Sided Failure; Pump Failure; Systolic Dysfunction; Diastolic Dysfunction

Heart failure is described as a common clinical syndrome resulting in the inability of the heart to meet the hemodynamic and metabolic demands of the body, producing in a variety of biochemical and neurohormonal changes and manifesting in a variety of ways. With almost 5 million persons in the United States having heart failure, it is a major health problem associated with high mortality rates, major morbidity, and rehospitalization. There is an increased prevalence with age, especially with women, making this a key geriatric concern. Heart failure remains one of the most disabling conditions, carrying a high economic burden related to the frequency of hospital readmissions.

Heart failure (HF) is the final syndrome of a wide spectrum of endothelial and myocardial injuries that produce ventricular systolic dysfunction (poor pumping function) and/or diastolic dysfunction (poor relaxation and filling function). Hypertension and coronary artery disease are the most common contributing factors to heart failure, though the list of causative factors is quite extensive. These causes are often described as resulting from myocardial ischemia and chamber enlargement from a variety of causes, volume-related factors, pressure-loading etiologies, and restrictive causes. Because of the health consequences of heart failure, attention is being directed to identifying and treating earlier those at risk for heart failure. A lettered classification system has been developed with characteristics defined for stages A, B, C, and D, with A being high risk but without structural problems or HF symptoms to D being refractory heart failure requiring specialized interventions. This somewhat parallels the classic New York Heart Association functional classification system based on severity of symptoms. Class I patients have no symptoms or physical limitations. Class II patients have slight limitations in their physical activity, whereby ordinary physical activities can cause symptoms such as fatigue, palpitations, dyspnea, or angina. Class III patients have marked physical limitations, with less than ordinary level of activities causing symptoms. Class IV patients experience dyspnea even at rest; activity is severely restricted.

The goals of treatment are to prevent progression of HF, reduce exacerbations, recognize early signs of decompensation, control symptoms, assist patient in comanaging the disease, and improve quality of life. The basis of medical therapy is neurohormonal inhibition. Angiotensin-converting enzyme (ACE) inhibitors, angiotensin II receptor blockers (ARBs), β-blockers (e.g., carvedilol), and aldosterone antagonists vasodilate, prevent decompensation, and reduce mortality. These drugs are used in combination with diuretics that reduce fluid overload. Digoxin is sometimes used in appropriate patients but does not reduce mortality. As patients deteriorate and experience acute decompensation, additional therapies of intravenous (IV) vasodilators and inotropes are indicated. Additional device therapies are available for more complicated patients. These include ultrafiltration to remove excess fluids and sodium, cardiac resynchronization therapy (CRT) pacemakers to optimize cardiac output (CO), implantable defibrillators to reduce risk for sudden cardiac death, and ventricular assist devices (VADs) to extend life.

Innovative programs such as cardiac case-managed home care, community-based HF case management, telemanagement, and HF cardiac rehabilitation programs are being developed to reduce the need for acute care or hospital services for this growing population. Because the goal of therapy is to manage patients outside the hospital, this care plan focuses on treatment in an ambulatory setting for patients with HF symptoms (Stage C, Functional Class II-III).

NOTE: Several national organizations have performance outcome goals related to HF: the American Heart Association's Get With the Guidelines—HF initiative and The Joint Commission's (TJC's) National Patient Safety Goals and National Quality Improvement Goals.

 NANDA-I NDx **Decreased Cardiac Output**

Common Related Factors

Increased or decreased preload
Increased afterload
Impaired contractility
Alteration in heart rate (HR), rhythm, conduction
Impaired diastolic function
Cardiac muscle disease
Medication side effects

Defining Characteristics

Low blood pressure (BP)
Increased HR
Decreased urine output
Decreased peripheral pulses
Cold, clammy skin
Crackles/tachypnea
Dyspnea
Orthopnea or paroxysmal nocturnal dyspnea (PND)
Decreased activity tolerance or fatigue
Edema/weight gain
Restlessness
Changes in level of consciousness
Dysrhythmias
Abnormal heart sounds (S_3, S_4)

Common Expected Outcome

Patient maintains adequate cardiac output as evidenced by strong peripheral pulses, systolic BP within 20 mm Hg of baseline, HR 60 to 100 beats/min with regular rhythm, urinary output ≥30 mL/hr, warm and dry skin, normal level of consciousness, and eupnea with absence of pulmonary crackles.

NOC Outcomes

Circulation Status; Cardiac Pump Effectiveness

NIC Interventions

Hemodynamic Regulation; Dysrhythmia Management

Ongoing Assessment

Actions/Interventions	Rationales
■ Assess rate and quality of apical and peripheral pulses, including capillary refill.	Most patients have compensatory tachycardia in response to low cardiac output. If dysrhythmias are present (premature atrial contractions, premature ventricular contractions, atrial fibrillation, runs of chronic ventricular tachycardia), the pulse rhythm will be irregular. Peripheral pulses may be weak, with reduced stroke volume and CO. Capillary refill is slow, sometimes absent.
■ Assess BP, noting any orthostatic changes.	Most patients have significantly reduced BP secondary to a low cardiac output state, as well as the vasodilating effects of prescribed medications. Typically patients can have systolic BPs in the range of 80 to 100 mm Hg and still be adequately perfusing target organs. However, symptomatic hypotension, systolic BP below 80 mm Hg, or a mean arterial pressure less than 60 mm Hg needs to be reported and further evaluated.
■ Assess heart sounds for presence of S_3 and/or S_4.	S_3 denotes reduced left ventricular ejection and is a classic sign of left ventricular failure (LVF). S_4 occurs with reduced compliance of the left ventricle, which impairs diastolic filling.
■ Assess respiratory rate, rhythm, and breath sounds. Determine any recent occurrence of PND or orthopnea.	Rapid shallow respirations are characteristic of reduced cardiac output. Crackles reflect accumulation of fluid in pulmonary circulation secondary to impaired left ventricular emptying. They are more evident in the dependent areas of the lung. Orthopnea is difficulty breathing when supine. PND is difficulty breathing during the night.
■ Weigh patient, and evaluate trends in weight.	Body weight is a more sensitive indicator of fluid or sodium retention than intake and output. A 2- to 3-pound increase in weight usually indicates retention of 1 liter of fluid and a need to adjust diuretic drug therapy. Patients need to understand that the focus of daily weighing is on fluid, not changes in body fat.
■ Assess skin color, temperature, and moisture.	Cool, pale, clammy skin is secondary to compensatory increases in sympathetic nervous system stimulation, low CO, and desaturation.
■ Assess for complaints of fatigue and reduced activity tolerance. Determine at what level of activity fatigue or exertional dyspnea occurs.	Fatigue and exertional dyspnea are common problems with low cardiac output states.
■ Assess urine output. Determine how frequently the patient urinates.	Oliguria can reflect decreased renal perfusion.
■ Determine any changes in level of consciousness.	Hypoxia and reduced cerebral perfusion are reflected in restlessness, irritability, and difficulty with concentrating. Older patients are especially susceptible to reduced perfusion.
■ Assess oxygen saturation with pulse oximetry both at rest and after/during ambulation.	Changes in oxygen saturation of mixed venous blood is one of the earliest indicators of decreased CO. Hypoxemia is common, especially with activity.
▲ Monitor serum electrolytes, especially sodium and potassium.	Hypokalemia and hypomagnesemia are causative factors for dysrhythmias, which can further reduce cardiac output.
▲ Assess B type natriuretic peptide (BNP).	BNP is elevated with increased filling pressure and volume in the left ventricle and serves as a critical indicator for HF. It aids in differentiating cardiac from noncardiac causes of dyspnea.

■ = Independent   ▲ = Collaborative

Actions/Interventions

▲ Assess left ventricular function as ordered.

▲ Monitor patient for signs and symptoms of digitalis toxicity. Obtain blood specimens to measure the serum digoxin level.

Rationales

Several national guidelines recommend that LVF assessment must be completed and documented either before admission, during the admission, or plans made to assess post discharge because ejection fraction status guides treatment.

The margin between therapeutic and toxic doses of digoxin therapy is narrow. The margin is further reduced in older patients and in patients with hypokalemia and renal insufficiency. Patients with digitalis toxicity may develop cardiac dysrhythmias such as sinus bradycardia, atrioventricular blocks, and ventricular tachycardia. Serum drug levels greater than 2.5 ng/mL are associated with toxicity.

Therapeutic Interventions

Actions/Interventions

■ Administer or evaluate patient's home compliance with prescribed medications:

• ACE inhibitors (or angiotensin II receptor blockers)

• β-Blockers (e.g., carvedilol, metoprolol)

• Diuretics (loop, thiazide, K$^+$ sparing)

• Aldosterone antagonists (e.g., spironolactone)

• Vasodilators (e.g., nitrates, hydralazine)

• Positive inotropes (e.g., digoxin, dopamine, dobutamine, milrinone)

Rationales

HF therapy requires administration of several types of medications. The cornerstone of treatment is ACE inhibitors, β-blockers, and diuretics. Aldosterone antagonists, digoxin, and vasodilators are included as appropriate. Polypharmacy is an ongoing challenge for HF patients.

These medications decrease peripheral vascular resistance and venous tone and suppress aldosterone output, thus reducing BP and demands on heart. This category of drugs has been shown to increase exercise tolerance and is the only one to increase survival in HF patients. It is very important to titrate to symptoms, not BP. National guidelines (AHA, TJC) recommend that the ACE inhibitors or ARBs should be prescribed for patients with ejection fraction less than 40%. In addition, the guidelines require that the reason for contraindication or for any delayed starting needs to be documented.

β-Blockers are used to decrease neurohormonal activity. They have been shown to reduce mortality, slow disease progression, and improve quality of life. Careful titration of starting doses is required because some patients exhibit fatigue, mood disturbances, or dizziness when medication is started or titrated up. These drugs should be given with food and separated from other vasodilators to reduce side effects (e.g., carvedilol with breakfast and dinner, ACE inhibitor with lunch) if side effects are troublesome.

Diuretics reduce circulating volume, enhance sodium and water excretion, and improve symptoms. Loop diuretics are preferred. The correct dose is the dose that works. Often combination therapy is needed.

Aldosterone antagonists are not given primarily for their diuretic effect, but rather for the beneficial effects on left ventricular (LV) remodeling, reduction in sympathetic activity, and improvement in mortality. Patients need to be closely monitored for hyperkalemia.

Vasodilators reduce preload, which decreases pulmonary congestion, and reduce afterload, which enhances the pumping ability of the ventricle.

Inotropes improve myocardial contractility. In stable class III to IV patients, intravenous medications may be administered intermittently in the outpatient or home setting.

Actions/Interventions

- Antidysrhythmics (e.g., amiodarone, β-blockers, potassium and magnesium supplements)

▲ Provide oxygen as indicated by the patient's condition and saturation levels (home oxygen through cannula or partial rebreather).

▲ If increased preload is a problem, restrict fluids and sodium as ordered.

▲ If decreased preload is a problem, increase fluids and closely monitor.

■ If the condition does not respond to therapy, consider referral to an acute care setting or hospital for invasive hemodynamic monitoring, more intensive medical therapy, and mechanical assist devices such as intraaortic balloon pump (IABP) and right or left VAD.

▲ If chronic life threatening dysrhythmias are the problem, anticipate treatment with an implantable cardiac defibrillator (ICD).

▲ For patients with intraventricular conduction delay (greater than 0.13 QRS interval), anticipate possible treatment with CRT pacemakers.

Rationales

These medications correct dysrhythmias such as premature ventricular contractions, ventricular tachycardia, and atrial fibrillation. HF is one of the most arrhythmogenic disorders. Unfortunately, management of dysrhythmias in this population is usually unsuccessful or even harmful because some antidysrhythmics have a negative inotropic effect, which may exacerbate HF or actually cause additional dysrhythmias. Atrial fibrillation with its resultant loss of atrial kick can cause significant decompensation. Some dysrhythmias require treatment with pacemakers and/or ICDs.

The failing heart may not be able to respond to increased oxygen demand. Oxygen supply may be inadequate when there is fluid accumulation in the lungs. Therefore supplemental oxygen may be indicated.

Fluid restriction decreases extracellular fluid volume and reduces cardiac workload.

Fluids increase extracellular fluid volume to optimize ventricular filling.

Hemodynamic monitoring provides information on filling pressures on the right side (central venous pressure) and left side (pulmonary artery diastolic; pulmonary capillary wedge pressure) of the heart. Mechanical assist devices such as the VAD or the IABP provide temporary circulatory support for the failing ventricle. These devices can be used in a variety of patients with chronic HF, including patients waiting for heart transplants, patients with severe ventricular failure after a myocardial infarction, and cardiac surgery patients who cannot be weaned from cardiopulmonary bypass. VAD can be inserted in the right ventricle, the left ventricle, or both ventricles depending on the site of the failure. Newer technologies include portable VADs that allow the patient to ambulate. IABP is used to increase coronary artery perfusion and decrease myocardial work load.

ICDs are indicated for documented ventricular tachycardia or ventricular fibrillation that puts patients at risk for sudden death.

Research demonstrates improved LV synchrony and hemodynamics when pacemakers are implanted in both right and left ventricular areas.

NANDA-I NDx **Excess Fluid Volume**

Common Related Factors	Defining Characteristics
Decreased cardiac output causing the following: - Decreased renal perfusion, which stimulates the renin-angiotensin-aldosterone system and causes release of antidiuretic hormone - Altered renal hemodynamics (diminished medullary blood flow), which results in decreased capacity of nephron to excrete water	Weight gain Edema Intake greater than output Decreased urine output Abnormal breath sounds: crackles Shortness of breath/orthopnea/dyspnea Restlessness

■ = Independent   ▲ = Collaborative

Pulmonary congestion on x-ray study
Jugular vein distention
Elevated central venous pressure and pulmonary capillary
 wedge pressure
Ascites/hepatojugular reflux
Elevated BP
Tachycardia
Third heart sound (S_3)

Common Expected Outcome

Patient maintains optimal fluid balance, as evidenced by urine output greater than or equal to 30 mL/hr, HR less than 100 beats/min, balanced intake and output, stable weight/dry weight (or loss attributed to fluid loss), absence of or reduction in edema, absence of pulmonary congestion.

NOC Outcome
Fluid Balance
NIC Interventions
Fluid Monitoring; Fluid Management

Ongoing Assessment

Actions/Interventions	Rationales
■ Assess for a significant (greater than 2 pounds) weight change in 1 day or trend over several days. Verify that patient has weighed consistently (e.g., before breakfast, on the same scale, after voiding, in the same amount of clothing, without shoes).	Body weight is a more sensitive indicator of fluid or sodium retention than intake and output. A 2 to 3 pound increase in weight in a day normally indicates retention of about 1 liter of fluid and a need to adjust fluid or diuretic therapy.
■ Evaluate weight in relation to nutritional status.	In some HF patients, weight may be a poor indicator of fluid volume status. Poor nutrition and decreased appetite over time result in a decrease in weight, which may be accompanied by fluid retention, although the net weight remains unchanged.
■ Assess for presence of edema by palpating area over tibia, ankles, feet, and sacrum.	Edema occurs when fluid accumulates in the extravascular spaces. Symmetrical dependent edema is characteristic in HF; it is graded on a trace to 4+ scale. Pitting edema is manifested by a depression that remains after the finger is pressed over an edematous area and then removed.
■ Assess for crackles in lungs, change in respiratory pattern, shortness of breath or orthopnea.	These respiratory changes are signs of fluid accumulation in the lungs.
■ Monitor HR and BP.	Sinus tachycardia and elevated BP are seen in early stages. Older patients have a reduced response to catecholamines; thus their response to fluid overload may be blunted with less change in HR.
■ Assess for jugular vein distention, ascites, nausea, and vomiting.	Patients with hypertonic overhydration exhibit cellular swelling. Right HF causes increased venous pressure and fluid congestion in hepatic and abdominal systems.
■ If the patient is on fluid restriction, review the daily log for recorded intake.	All sources of oral fluid need to be recorded. The patient should be reminded to include items that are liquid at room temperature, such as gelatin, soup, sherbet, and frozen juice bars.
■ Evaluate urine output in response to diuretics.	Focus is on monitoring response to the diuretics, rather than actual amount voided. It is unrealistic to expect patients to measure each void. Therefore recording two voids versus six voids after a diuretic medication may provide more useful information. NOTE: Fluid volume excess in the abdomen may interfere with absorption of oral diuretic medications. Medications may need to be given intravenously by a nurse in the home or outpatient setting.

Actions/Interventions

■ Monitor for excessive response to diuretics: 2-pound weight loss in 1 day, hypotension, weakness, and blood urea nitrogen level elevated out of proportion to serum creatinine level.

▲ Monitor for potential side effects of diuretics: hypokalemia, hyponatremia, hypomagnesemia, elevated serum creatinine level, and hyperuricemia (gout).

▲ Monitor chest x-ray reports.

Rationales

Significant increased response to diuretic therapy can result in fluid volume deficit and electrolyte imbalances that can cause significant complications. Moreover, excess fluid loss can stimulate compensatory mechanisms to promote activation of renin angiotensin aldosterone system. That can begin the vicious cycle of fluid retention.

The electrolyte and other abnormalities related to diuretic therapy can cause significant problems.

As interstitial edema accumulates, the x-ray studies show cloudy white lung fields

---

Therapeutic Interventions

Actions/Interventions

■ Instruct the patient/caregiver regarding fluid restriction as appropriate.

■ Provide innovative techniques for monitoring fluid allotment at home. For example, suggest that patient measure out and pour into a large pitcher the prescribed daily fluid allowance (e.g., 1000 mL). Then, every time the patient drinks some fluid, he or she should remove that same amount from the pitcher.

▲ Administer or instruct patient to take diuretics as prescribed.

▲ Instruct patients to avoid foods and fluids that are high in sodium. Restrict sodium intake as prescribed.

■ Instruct patient to avoid medications that may cause fluid retention, such as over-the-counter nonsteroidal antiinflammatory drugs (NSAIDs) and certain vasodilators (e.g., calcium channel blockers).

■ Instruct patient to notify health care provider about any significant weight changes, leg swelling, or breathing changes.

Rationales

Restriction helps reduce extracellular volume. For patients with mild or moderate HF, it may not be necessary to restrict fluid intake. In advanced HF, fluids may be restricted to 1000 mL/day. Information is key for patients who will be comanaging fluids.

Strategies such as this provide a visual guide for how much fluid is still allowed throughout the day, enhancing compliance with the regimen.

Diuretics aid in the excretion of excess body fluids. Therapy may include several different types of diuretic agents for optimal effect, depending on the acuteness or chronicity of the problem. Compliance is often difficult for patients trying to maintain a more normal lifestyle outside the home, who find frequent urination especially troublesome. Some patients prefer taking diuretics later in the day, after their activities. Such creative schedules can increase compliance.

Restriction decreases excess fluid volume. Diets containing 2 to 3 g of sodium are usually prescribed. Patient can begin sodium restriction by eliminating the use of the salt shaker at the table, avoiding obviously salty foods, and not adding salt to food when cooking. The patient needs to learn to read package labels for sources of hidden salt and sodium often used as preservatives and flavoring agents in processed foods. Current federal guidelines require that the total milligrams of sodium be listed on food labels. Instruct that soups and many ethnic foods contain high amounts of sodium, especially if eaten in restaurants.

NSAIDs can cause renal insufficiency. COX-2 inhibitors (e.g., rofecoxib [Vioxx]) cause fluid retention. Some calcium channel blockers have significant negative inotropic effects.

Early recognition and treatment of symptoms at home can help break the cycle of frequent hospital readmission for HF. Patients need to understand their roles in symptom management. Telephone nursing can be initiated to provide for consistent monitoring between office visits.

■ = Independent   ▲ = Collaborative

Actions/Interventions	Rationales
■ Teach the patient about measures to relieve dry mouth, such as frequent oral hygiene, sucking on hard candy, or chewing gum.	Patients on fluid restrictions may experience increased thirst and dry mouth. Measures to stimulate saliva secretion will help keep oral mucous membranes moist. The patient with diabetes mellitus may need to use sugar-free gums and candy. The patient should avoid ice chips because they can add to fluid intake. An 8-ounce cup of ice chips equals approximately 4 ounces of water.
▲ For significant fluid volume excess, consider admission to an acute care setting for hemofiltration or ultrafiltration.	These therapies are very effective methods to draw off excess fluid, but patients should be reminded that compliance with medication regimens and sodium restriction will help keep their conditions stable.

NANDA-I NDx Risk for Electrolyte Imbalance

Common Risk Factors

Fluid imbalance (increased total body fluid dilutes electrolyte concentration)

Renal dysfunction (decreased renal perfusion results in greater reabsorption of sodium and potassium)

Diuretic therapy (enhances renal excretion of total body water and sodium and potassium)

Low-sodium diet

Common Expected Outcomes

Patient maintains electrolytes within normal range when therapy is stable.

Patient receives medication adjustments as needed if electrolyte imbalance is noted.

NOC Outcome
Electrolyte and Acid/Base Balance
NIC Interventions
Fluid/Electrolyte Management; Electrolyte Management (Specify)

Ongoing Assessment

Actions/Interventions	Rationales
■ Monitor for manifestations of serum electrolyte imbalances:	Monitoring is especially important for patients receiving diuretics, ACE inhibitors, and digoxin, especially in the event of large weight gain or loss or in the presence of renal insufficiency.
• Hyponatremia (sodium less than 136 mEq/liter): may be accompanied by headache, confusion, apathy, tachycardia, and generalized weakness.	In chronic HF, hyponatremia is usually dilutional; it is caused by a greater concentration of water than sodium occurring with fluid volume excess.
• Hypokalemia (potassium less than 4 mEq/liter): may cause fatigue; gastrointestinal distress; leg cramps; increased sensitivity to digoxin; atrial and ventricular dysrhythmia; ST-segment depression; broad, sometimes inverted, progressively flatter T wave; and enlarging U wave.	Patients with HF require a higher safety range for "normal" potassium level because they are already prone to ventricular irritability from their dilated hearts. Hypokalemia usually occurs as a side effect of diuretic therapy.
• Hypomagnesemia (magnesium less than 1.5 mEq/liter): may cause lethargy, mood changes, nausea, and paresthesia.	Dysrhythmias and sudden death increase with hypomagnesemia, especially in patients with HF. Hypomagnesemia is usually associated with hypokalemia.

Actions/Interventions

- Hypernatremia (sodium greater than 147 mEq/liter): may be accompanied by thirst, dry mucous membranes, fever, and neurological changes if severe.
- Hyperkalemia (potassium greater than 5.1 mEq/liter): may be accompanied by muscular weakness, diarrhea, and electrocardiogram (ECG) changes.
- ■ Monitor fluid losses and gains.
- ▲ Monitor digoxin level and effects in presence of hypokalemia.

Rationales

Hypernatremia is commonly caused by large loss of water.

Coadministration of ACE inhibitors, ARBs, or aldosterone blockers can cause significant potassium retention.

Patients with HF have a precarious fluid balance status. Hypokalemia sensitizes the myocardium to digitalis, thus predisposing the patient to digoxin toxicity.

Therapeutic Interventions

Actions/Interventions

For hyponatremia:

▲ Encourage sodium restriction as prescribed. Provide dietary instruction.

▲ Encourage fluid restriction as indicated. Teach the patient about measures to relieve dry mouth, such as frequent oral hygiene, sucking on hard candy, or chewing gum.

■ Instruct the patient to avoid salt contained in over-the-counter preparations such as antacids (e.g., Alka-Seltzer).

▲ Administer or prescribe diuretics as indicated.

For hypokalemia (commonly caused by prolonged use of thiazide or loop diuretics):

▲ Administer oral or IV potassium supplement as prescribed.

■ Encourage daily intake of potassium-rich foods (raisins, bananas, cantaloupe, dates, and potatoes).

For hypomagnesemia:

▲ Administer magnesium replacement as indicated.

For hypernatremia:

▲ Carefully replace water orally or intravenously.

■ Anticipate reduction in diuretic dosage.

For nonacute hyperkalemia:

■ Anticipate reduction in potassium supplement.

▲ Provide diet with potassium restriction as prescribed.

▲ Discontinue potassium-sparing diuretics as prescribed.

■ Instruct the patient to avoid salt substitutes containing potassium.

For acute hyperkalemia (serum potassium greater than 6 mEq/liter):

■ Place patient on ECG monitor.

Rationales

Sodium promotes water retention, which can lead to fluid overload.

Restriction of intake reduces the work of the heart and reduces the need for diuretic therapy. Patients on fluid restrictions may experience increased thirst and dry mouth. Measures to stimulate saliva secretion will help keep oral mucous membranes moist. The patient should avoid ice chips because they can add to fluid intake. An 8-ounce cup of ice chips equals approximately 4 ounces of water.

Thorough understanding of hidden salt products is necessary for appropriate self-care.

Diuretics help restore water and sodium balance. Some HF patients are given a sliding scale protocol.

Oral supplements should be given directly after meals or with food to minimize gastrointestinal irritation.

These foods will assist in correcting deficiency.

Replacement may be an oral or IV supplement.

HF patients have a precarious fluid balance status.

Diuretics are commonly the cause of the large water loss resulting in hypernatremia.

Some conditions may be easily corrected with reduced supplements.

Foods with high potassium nutrients can exacerbate the problem.

The potassium-sparing class of diuretics is often used to counteract the potassium loss associated with loop or thiazide diuretics. However, they can easily lead to hyperkalemia.

All sources of potassium need to be considered.

Common ECG changes associate with hypokalemia may include the following: tall, peaked T waves; widened QRS; prolonged PR interval; decreased amplitude and disappearance of P wave; or ventricular dysrhythmia.

■ = Independent   ▲ = Collaborative

Actions/Interventions

▲ Administer the following temporary measures as ordered:

- Regular IV insulin and hypertonic dextrose

- Sodium bicarbonate

- Cation-exchange resins

- IV calcium chloride

- Dialysis

■ Anticipate admission to an acute care setting.

Rationales

Insulin causes a shift of potassium into the cells. Onset of action is 30 minutes, and duration is several hours.

Sodium bicarbonate causes rapid movement of potassium into the cells. Onset is within 15 minutes, and duration of action is 1 to 2 hours.

These resins reduce serum potassium levels slowly but have the advantage of actually removing potassium from the body. Routes of administration include oral or rectal. They are often given with one of the other measures.

Calcium chloride immediately antagonizes the cardiac and neuromuscular toxicity of hyperkalemia. Duration of action is 1 hour.

Hemodialysis is an effective method for removing potassium but is reserved for situations in which more conservative measures fail.

Vigilant monitoring and rapid interventions reduce life-threatening consequences of hyperkalemia.

Activity Intolerance

Common Related Factors

Decreased cardiac output
Deconditioned state
Sedentary lifestyle
Imbalance between oxygen supply and demand
Insufficient sleep or rest periods
Lack of motivation or depression
Side effects of medications

Defining Characteristics

Verbal report of fatigue or weakness
Unable to endure or complete desired activities
Abnormal HR, BP, or respiratory response to activity
Exertional discomfort or dyspnea

Common Expected Outcomes

Patient exhibits activity tolerance, as evidenced by rating of perceived exertion of 3 or less (0 to 10 scale), HR within 20 beats/min of resting HR, SBP within 20 mm Hg increase over resting SBP, respiratory rate less than 20 breaths/min.

Patient reports ability to perform required activity of daily living.

Patient verbalizes and uses energy conservation techniques.

NOC Outcomes

Activity Tolerance; Energy Conservation; Self-Care: Activities

NIC Interventions

Energy Management; Exercise Therapy; Exercise Promotion

Ongoing Assessment

Actions/Interventions

■ Assess patient's current level of activity. Determine reasons for limiting activity.

Rationales

Although newer pharmacological therapies have alleviated many of the disabling symptoms experienced by patients with HF, chronic symptoms of activity intolerance and limited exercise capacity often occur. Changes in functional capacity with chronic HF have a direct impact on the patient's quality of life. The patient may have restricted activity over time to avoid symptoms. Therefore it is important to ask the patient about tolerance for specific activities, such as walking a specific distance (e.g., 100 feet) or climbing a flight of stairs.

Actions/Interventions

- Observe or document response to activity. Have the patient walk in the hall for several minutes as a nurse evaluates HR, BP, and oxygen saturation response to exertion. If the patient is able, evaluate response to stair climbing.
- Assess patient's perception of effort to perform each activity.

- Evaluate the need for oxygen during increased activity.

Rationales

HR increases of more than 20 beats/min, BP drop of more than 20 mm Hg, dyspnea, light-headedness, and fatigue signify abnormal responses to activity. Pulse oximetry provides information on hypoxemia with exertion.

The Borg Scale uses ratings from 0 to 10 to determine ratings of perceived exertion. A rating of 2 (light) to 3 (moderate) is an acceptable level for most HF patients doing daily work.

Portable pulse oximetry can be used to assess for oxygen desaturation. Supplemental oxygen may help compensate for the increased oxygen demand.

Therapeutic Interventions

Actions/Interventions

- Establish guidelines and goals of activity with the patient and significant others.

- Use slow progression of activity (e.g., walking in a room, walking short distances around the house, and then progressively increasing distances outside of the house) saving energy for return trip.
- Teach appropriate use of environmental aids (e.g., bedside commode, chair in bathroom, hall rails).
- Teach energy conservation techniques, for example:
  - Sitting to do tasks
  - Pushing rather than pulling
  - Sliding rather than lifting
  - Storing frequently used items within easy reach
  - Organizing a work-rest-work schedule
- Recommend use of light weights (1 to 2 pounds) for upper extremity strengthening.

▲ Consult cardiac rehabilitation or physical therapy departments for assistance in increasing activity tolerance.

- Instruct the patient to recognize signs of overexertion.

- Provide emotional support and encouragement while increasing activity levels.

Rationales

Motivation is enhanced if the patient participates in goal setting. Depending on the classification of HF, some class I or II patients may be able to successfully work outside the home on a part-time or full-time basis. However, other patients may be class III or IV and be relatively homebound.

Appropriate progression prevents overexerting the heart while attaining short-range goals. Duration and frequency should be increased before intensity.

Appropriate aids enable the patient to achieve optimal independence for self-care.

These techniques reduce oxygen consumption, allowing for more prolonged activity.

Strength training can enhance endurance and facilitate performance of activities of daily living; such exercises can be performed while sitting in a chair.

Specialized therapy or cardiac monitoring may be necessary when initially increasing activity. Some exercises may be provided in the home. A structured program of low-intensity exercise can improve functional capacity, increase self-confidence to exert self, improve quality of life, and provide an environment for early triage of symptoms.

Knowledge promotes awareness of when to reduce activity and provides data for activity progression.

Patients may be fearful of overexertion and potential damage to the heart. Appropriate supervision and support during activity progression can enhance confidence.

■ = Independent ▲ = Collaborative

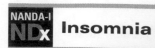 **Insomnia**

Common Related Factors
Anxiety/fear
Physical discomfort or shortness of breath
Medication schedule and effects or side effects
Sleep-disordered breathing

Defining Characteristics
Fatigue
Frequent daytime dozing
Irritability
Inability to concentrate
Complaints of difficulty falling asleep
Interrupted sleep

Common Expected Outcome
Patient achieves optimal amounts of sleep, as evidenced by rested appearance, verbalization of feeling rested, and improvement in sleep pattern.

NOC Outcome
Sleep
NIC Intervention
Sleep Enhancement

Ongoing Assessment

Actions/Interventions	Rationales
■ Assess current sleep pattern and sleep history.	Sleep patterns are unique to each individual. Some patients are unaware of their poor sleep patterns, but their significant others report sleeping problems.
■ Assess for possible deterrents to sleep: • Nocturia	Supine position during sleep promotes increased venous return and increased renal blood flow. The patient's sleep is interrupted by the need to urinate.
• Volume excess causing dyspnea, orthopnea, and PND	When patient is supine, the fluid returning to the heart from the extremities may cause pulmonary congestion.
• Fear of PND	Patients report this as a significant factor in sleeping difficulties.
• Timing of medications	Patients may be following medication schedules that require awakening in the early morning hours. Diuretics taken in the evening may increase nocturia.
■ Assess for history of signs of sleep-disordered breathing.	Sleep-disordered breathing is common with HF, with reports of occurrence in more than 50% of patients. These patients experience interrupted sleep and periods of desaturation during the nighttime. This disorder is associated with increased dysrhythmias, reduced quality of life, and increased mortality.

Therapeutic Interventions

Actions/Interventions	Rationales
■ Instruct patient to reduce daytime napping and to increase daytime activity.	Napping can disrupt normal sleep patterns. However, older patients do better with frequent naps during the day to counter the shorter nighttime sleep schedule.
■ Instruct patient to decrease fluid intake before bedtime.	Careful scheduling of evening medications reduces the need to awaken to void.
■ Plan a medication schedule so that prescribed medications, especially diuretics, are not given during the late evening or night.	Evening fluid restriction facilitates an undisturbed night.

Actions/Interventions

- Encourage patient to follow as consistent a daily schedule for retiring and arising as possible; avoid caffeine and smoking.
- Encourage patient to elevate head with two pillows or put head of bed frame on 6-inch blocks.
- Encourage verbalization of fears.

- Review measures that the patient can take to prevent or treat PND, chest pain, or palpitations.
- Review how the patient can summon help during the night.
- Provide instruction in use of continuous positive airway pressure (CPAP) device if ordered.

Rationales

A regular schedule promotes regulation of the circadian rhythm. Stimulation from caffeine and nicotine can disturb sleep.

Elevating the head of the bed can reduce pulmonary congestion and nighttime dyspnea.

Verbalization may help reduce anxiety and open doors for further problem solving and intervention.

Prevention is key and may require medication adjustments by the physician.

Information enables the patient to take control.

CPAP applied during sleep periods has been shown to improve sleep efforts and reduce episodes of hypopnea and apnea, thereby enhancing oxygen saturation.

NANDA-I NDx **Deficient Knowledge**

Common Related Factors
Unfamiliarity with pathology and treatment
Misinterpretation of information
New medications
Chronicity of disease
Ineffective teaching or learning in past
Cognitive limitation
Emotional states affecting learning (depression, denial, anxiety)

Defining Characteristics
Verbalizes incorrect or inaccurate information
Inaccurate follow-through of instructions
Questioning members of health care team
Denial of need to learn
Development of avoidable complications

Common Expected Outcome
Patient or significant others verbalize understanding of desired content.
Patient performs desired skills.

NOC Outcomes
Knowledge: Disease Process; Knowledge: Treatment Regimen

NIC Interventions
Teaching: Disease Process; Teaching: Prescribed Medications; Teaching: Prescribed Diet; Teaching: Prescribed Activity/Exercise

---

Ongoing Assessment

Actions/Interventions

- Assess knowledge of causes, treatment, and follow-up care related to HF.

- Identify existing misconceptions regarding care.

Rationales

This information provides starting base for educational sessions. Teaching standardized content that patient already knows wastes valuable time and hinders critical learning.

Understanding any misconceptions the patient may have about the treatment or side effects will guide future interventions.

■ = Independent   ▲ = Collaborative

Therapeutic Interventions

Actions/Interventions	Rationales
■ Educate patient or significant others about the following:	Patients are better able to ask questions and seek assistance when they know basic information about disease and treatment. The AHA and TJC provide excellent tools for providing education to meet national guidelines.
• Normal heart and circulation	Information helps the patient understand the disease process.
• HF disease process	Knowledge of disease and disease process will promote adherence to suggested medical therapy.
• Importance of adhering to therapy	HF is the most common reason for readmission, especially in the older population. Strict adherence to therapy aids in reducing symptoms and readmission. Therapy must be simplified as much as possible to facilitate adherence. Patients must be encouraged to follow up closely with health care providers and/or HF nurses.
• Symptoms (e.g., weight gain, edema, fatigue, dyspnea) and when to report them to health care providers	When patients can identify symptoms that require prompt medical attention, complications can be minimized or possibly prevented. Telemanagement, home care nurses, and HF case managers can aid in this education and assessment.

• Dietary modification to limit sodium ingestion, including the following:
  • Rationale for restriction
  • Alternative seasonings
  • Foods to generally avoid: canned soups and vegetables, prepared frozen dinners, and fast-food meals
  • Ways to recognize hidden sodium: preservatives, labels, and consumer information services
	Understanding the rationale behind dietary restrictions may establish motivation necessary for making this adjustment in lifestyle. Diet and fluid restriction education is part of national performance guidelines.

• Activity guidelines	Providing specific information lessens uncertainty and promotes adjustment to recommended activity levels.
• Medications: instruct in action, use, side effects, and administration	Prompt reporting of side effects can prevent drug-related complications. Compliance is improved when patients understand "why" they are expected to take so many medications. Key medications need to be prescribed and taken to meet national guidelines and reduce morbidity and mortality associated with HF.
• Psychological aspects of chronic illness	Living with a chronic illness can be depressing, especially for older patients, who may have limited support systems. Referral to support groups may be indicated.
• Smoking cessation	Anyone who has smoked cigarettes within 12 months before admission needs to receive smoking cessation counseling, not just current smokers, per national guidelines.
• Overall goals of medical therapy	Discussion of long-range goals will help clarify misconceptions and may promote compliance.
• Community resources	Referral may be helpful for financial and emotional support.

■ Provide information on ways to enhance self-management efforts:
  • Recognizing changes in one's condition and their importance
  • Decisions regarding appropriate treatment and evaluation of effectiveness
	The burden of living with chronic HF rests with patient and caregiver. Patients are at the front line in reacting to changes in symptoms and condition. They need to be able to self-treat for minor changes (e.g., increase diuretics, reduce fluids) before contacting health care providers.

Actions/Interventions

- Provide information on medical devices and therapies that may be indicated for optimal cardiac output:
  - ICD
  - CRT pacing
  - Ventricular assist device
  - Heart transplant surgery
- Encourage questions from the patient or significant others.

Rationales

A select group of HF patients, especially Class III and IV, can benefit from adjunct medical therapies.

Questions facilitate open communication between patient and health care provider and allow verification of understanding of information given and opportunity to correct misconceptions.

Related Care Plans

Cardiac rehabilitation, p. 230
Impaired gas exchange, p. 78
Ineffective therapeutic regimen management, p. 194
Sleep-disordered breathing, p. 451
Powerlessness, p. 162

Hypertension

High Blood Pressure; Isolated Systolic Hypertension

High blood pressure (BP) is classified according to the level of severity. The following table is from the Report of the Joint National Committee on Prevention, Detection, Evaluation, and Treatment of High Blood Pressure (JNC).

Classification of BP for Adults 18 Years of Age and Older			
	Systolic (mm Hg)		**Diastolic (mm Hg)**
Normal:	<120	and	<80
Prehypertension:	120 to 139	or	80 to 89
Hypertension:			
Stage 1:	140 to 159	or	90 to 99
Stage 2:	≥160	or	≥100

Epidemiological studies report that 1 in 3 U.S. adults have hypertension, with 65 million people in the United States having BPs greater than or equal to 140/90 mm Hg or taking antihypertensive medications. Age, gender, and ethnic differences are evident. African Americans in the United States develop hypertension earlier, have more significantly elevated BP, and have more target organ disease than whites. Likewise, African American women have a higher incidence of hypertension than white women.

Although hypertension can be initiated in childhood, it is most evident in middle life. As the population ages, the prevalence of hypertension will increase unless effective prevention measures are implemented. The category of prehypertension identifies a significant segment of the population who are at twice the risk for developing hypertension than people in the normal category. Preventive efforts in this population are aimed at reducing risk factors through therapeutic lifestyle changes, which are detailed in the JNC guidelines.

Blood pressure self-management is key to successful treatment. Ambulatory BP monitoring may be indicated to document changes in BP throughout the day (circadian pattern) and provide information for treating drug-resistant patients and those experiencing hypotension secondary to medication. Several classes of drugs are available for treatment. Usually two or more antihypertensive medications are needed to achieve optimal BP control.

This care plan focuses on patients with hypertension in an ambulatory care setting.

■ = Independent   ▲ = Collaborative

Deficient Knowledge: Nature of and Complications of Hypertension or Management Regimen

Common Related Factors

Lack of exposure
Cognitive limitation
Misinterpretation
Lack of recall
Complexity of treatment

Defining Characteristics

Verbalizing inaccurate information
Inaccurate follow-through of instruction
Questioning members of health care team

Common Expected Outcomes

Patient verbalizes understanding of the disease and its long-term effects on target organs.
Patient describes strategies for managing hypertension.

NOC Outcomes

Knowledge: Disease Process; Knowledge: Treatment Regimen

NIC Intervention

Teaching: Disease Process

Ongoing Assessment

Actions/Interventions	Rationales
■ Assess knowledge of disease and prescribed management.	Assessment provides an important starting point in education. Patients need to understand that hypertension is a chronic, lifelong disease in which they have a vital role in effective management.

Therapeutic Interventions

Actions/Interventions	Rationales
■ Encourage questions about hypertension and prescribed treatments.	Questions facilitate open communication between patient and health care provider and allow verification of understanding of given information and the opportunity to correct misconceptions.
■ Involve family in teaching about hypertension.	Family members play an important role in supporting the patient's efforts to adopt new health behaviors for management of hypertension. Family members may also need to be screened for hypertension because of its familial tendency. Genetic factors are strong risk factors for hypertension.
■ Instruct the patient that hypertension cannot be diagnosed with only one measurement.	There are wide variations in "normal" blood pressure over the course of a day or week because of biological and diurnal effects. Clinical practice guidelines state that a diagnosis can be established only with the average of two or more BP readings on two or more occasions.
■ Instruct the patient to self-measure BP, and suggest home monitoring equipment as appropriate.	Many patients have "white coat" hypertension, in which BP is elevated during a doctor's office visit because of apprehension or pain. Therefore at least two elevated measurements are required to diagnose hypertension. BP self-measurement can be useful in identifying true hypertension versus white coat hypertension, in documenting response to medication regimen, and in facilitating adherence to treatment. Patients should be guided to only purchase home equipment that meets established criteria for accuracy.

Actions/Interventions	**Rationales**
■ Plan teaching in stages, providing information in the following areas:	Providing information in short sessions over a longer period of time prevents information overload and promotes comprehension.
• Definition of hypertension, differentiating between systolic and diastolic pressures; prehypertension	Patients may falsely believe that only elevated diastolic blood pressure requires treatment, when elevated systolic BP is also associated with high risk. Most patients are not aware of the newest classification of "prehypertension."
• Causes of hypertension	Patients need to realize that 90% of hypertension is not related to a primary cause.
• Risk factors: family history, obesity, diet high in saturated fat and cholesterol, smoking, and stress	Implementing lifestyle changes is the cornerstone of treatment.
• Nature of disease and its effect on target organs (e.g., renal damage, visual impairment, heart disease, stroke)	There are few signs and symptoms associated with hypertension until target organ damage occurs.
• Treatment goal: "control" versus "cure"	Hypertension is a chronic, lifelong disease. It is treated with medication and lifestyle changes. Treatment should not be stopped because the patient feels better or has problems with medication side effects.
• Rationale and strategy for weight reduction (if overweight)	Of all lifestyle changes, weight reduction has most consistently demonstrated BP-lowering effects. Studies show weight reduction lowers BP at all ages and in both genders. A body mass index of 25 or higher is strongly correlated with increased BP. Weight loss of just 10 pounds can lower BP.
• Rationale and strategy for adopting the Dietary Approaches to Stop Hypertension (DASH) diet	The DASH diet is high in fruits, vegetables; low-fat dairy products; low in total and saturated fats; and rich in potassium, magnesium, protein, and fiber. The mix of potassium, magnesium, and calcium in the diet serves as a diuretic in helping the body excrete salt. This diet is especially effective in treating African American patients.
• Rationale and strategies for low-sodium diet	Dietary sodium contributes to fluid retention and elevated BP, although not all patients are "salt sensitive" who effectively lower blood pressure with sodium restriction. African American and older patients seem to be most salt sensitive.
• Common medications: thiazide diuretics, β-blockers, angiotensin II receptor blockers (ARBs), calcium channel blockers, and angiotensin-converting enzyme (ACE) inhibitors	A wide range of medications is available. They are indicated when BP remains above 140/90 mm Hg after lifestyle modification. National guidelines recommend a thiazide diuretic for initial therapy, either alone or in combination with other medications. Coexisting "compelling conditions," such as myocardial infarction, high risk coronary artery disease, heart failure, diabetes, chronic kidney disease, and risk for stroke, also guide drug selection.
• Establishment of medication routine considering daily activities and sleep habits	A consistent medication schedule will minimize the chance of error and encourage better compliance with therapy.
• Possible side effects of medications	Side effects are the most common reason for noncompliance with medications. Warning the patient of possible side effects enhances attention on what to do if they occur. Not all persons experience side effects. If they do occur and are bothersome (pedal edema, fatigue, hypokalemia, impotence), instruct patient to discuss them with the health care provider before discontinuing any medications.
• Interaction with over-the-counter drugs such as cough and cold medicines, aspirin compounds, and herbal medications	Patients should be encouraged to bring in all sources of medications (over-the-counter, complementary, and prescription) to review and rule out iatrogenic causes of hypertension.

■ = Independent ▲ = Collaborative

Actions/Interventions	Rationales
• Rationale and strategy for reduction of alcohol intake: no more than two drinks per day for men and one drink per day for women	Research indicates that alcohol intake of more than three to four standard drinks per day is associated with high BP.
• Need for potassium-rich foods (e.g., fruit juices, bananas) as appropriate	Some diuretics are potassium wasting; however, most ACE inhibitors and ARBs retain potassium.
• Smoking cessation	Smoking causes vasoconstriction and an increase in blood pressure.
• Role of physical exercise	Research supports a positive effect of aerobic exercise in independently lowering BP, as well as maintaining weight loss.
• Relaxation techniques to combat stress	The physiological response to physical and/or emotional stressors includes neuroendocrine changes associated with increased sympathetic nervous system activity and increased cortisol secretion. These changes produce vasoconstriction and increase sodium and water retention. Unrelieved persistent stress contributes to increased blood pressure. Relaxation techniques can positively influence physiological responses that reduce blood pressure.
• Signs and symptoms to report to health care provider: chest pain, shortness of breath, edema, weight gain greater than 2 pounds per day or 5 pounds per week, nosebleeds, changes in vision, headaches, and dizziness	Patients need to recognize important changes in their condition that could lead to serious outcomes.

• Important safety measures to reduce orthostatic hypotension:
  • Avoid sudden changes in position.
  • Avoid hot tubs and saunas.
  • Avoid prolonged standing; wear support stockings as needed.
	Orthostatic hypotension is a common side effect of many drugs used to manage hypertension. If the patient is taking more than one drug for hypertension, this side effect may be magnified. These measures reduce severity of orthostatic hypotension. Hypotension associated with quickly assuming an upright position is especially evident in older patients with long-standing hypertension that is reduced too rapidly. Hot tubs and saunas cause vasodilation and potential hypotension. Standing can cause venous pooling.

■ Provide information about community resources and support groups (e.g., American Heart Association, weight loss programs, smoking cessation programs).	These resources can assist and support the patient when lifestyle changes are needed.

Risk for Ineffective Therapeutic Regimen Management

Common Risk Factors

Complexity of therapeutic regimen
Financial costs
Social support deficits
Conflicting health values
Fears about treatment and possible side effects

Common Expected Outcomes

Patient describes system for taking medications.
Patient describes positive effort to lose weight and restrict sodium as appropriate.
Patient verbalizes intention to follow prescribed regimen.
Patient demonstrates ongoing adherence to treatment plan.

NOC Outcomes
Compliance Behavior; Participation: Health Care Decisions
NIC Interventions
Mutual Goal Setting; Support System Enhancement; Teaching: Individual

Ongoing Assessment

Actions/Interventions	Rationales
■ Assess patient's health values and beliefs.	Health behavior models propose that patients compare factors such as perceived susceptibility to and severity of illness or complications with perceived benefits of treatment in making decisions regarding adherence to therapies.
■ Assess previous patterns of adherence.	Past history of noncompliance is a significant risk factor for future adherence problems.
■ Assess for risk factors that may negatively affect adherence to regimen.	Knowledge of causative factors provides direction for subsequent interventions. Some factors may include contrary beliefs and values, lack of social support, lack of financial resources, and compromised emotional states.

Therapeutic Interventions

Actions/Interventions	Rationales
▲ Simplify drug regimen.	Many patients require three to four BP-lowering medications to achieve treatment goals. Simplifying the regimen can enhance compliance. Combined medications should be used as available. The more often patients have to take medicines during the day, the greater the risk for noncompliance.
■ Include patient in planning treatment regimen.	Patients who become comanagers of their care have a greater stake in achieving a positive outcome. Health care providers need to be willing to change unsuccessful regimens and search for those most likely to succeed.
■ Instruct in importance of reordering medications 2 to 3 days before running out.	Missing doses of antihypertensive medications while waiting to obtain prescription refills may contribute to rebound hypertension as an adverse reaction. This reaction is most likely to occur with ACE inhibitors, α-adrenergic blockers, β-blockers, and α-2 agonists. Attention to the best time for reordering medications ensures ongoing therapy but is not easy to accomplish because of many insurance rules.
■ Inform the patient of the benefits of adherence to the prescribed regimen.	Information provides rationale for therapy and aids the patient in assuming responsibility for care.
■ If negative side effects of prescribed treatment are a problem, explain that many side effects can be controlled or eliminated.	Patients need to be aware that adjustments and substitutions can be made to relieve side effects.
■ Instruct patient to self-monitor BP.	Self-monitoring provides the patient with immediate feedback and a sense of control.
■ Include significant others in explanations and teaching.	Including significant others encourages support and assistance in reinforcing appropriate behavior and facilitating lifestyle modification.
■ When the patient has inadequate support regarding lifestyle changes, refer him or her to appropriate support groups (e.g., American Heart Association, weight loss programs, smoking cessation programs, stress management classes, social services).	Groups that come together for mutual support can be beneficial.

■ = Independent   ▲ = Collaborative

Mitral Valve Prolapse

Barlow's Disease; Floppy Valve, Click-Murmur Syndrome

Mitral valve prolapse (MVP) is the most common abnormality of the heart valves. The mitral valve rests between the left atrium and ventricle. Prolapse of this valve refers to the upward movement of the mitral leaflets back into the left atrium during systole. Mitral valve prolapse usually results from abnormality in the connective tissue of the leaflets, annulus, or chordae tendineae and occurs in about 2% to 3% of the general population, usually in people ages 20 to 40 years. It is seen in both men and women. MVP can be inherited, especially if associated with connective tissue disorders like Marfan's syndrome. Most persons with MVP are asymptomatic and do not require treatment, except reassurance that this is a benign condition. Others may experience symptoms associated with mitral regurgitation, atypical chest pain related to tension the prolapsed valve exerts on the papillary muscle, harmless palpitations as the result of an autonomic nervous system imbalance, and fatigue. Diagnostic findings include midsystolic click, late systolic murmur, echocardiogram abnormalities, and angiographic findings. This disease is treated in an ambulatory care setting.

 NANDA-I NDx ## Deficient Knowledge

Common Related Factor

New diagnosis

Defining Characteristics

Asking multiple questions
Expressing fears
Being overly anxious
Asking no questions
Verbalizing misconceptions

Common Expected Outcome

Patient or significant others verbalize understanding of occurrence of disease, causative factors, physiology of disease, diagnostic procedure, treatment, and possible complications.

NOC Outcome
Knowledge: Disease Process
NIC Intervention
Teaching: Disease Process

Ongoing Assessment

Actions/Interventions	Rationales
■ Assess knowledge of MVP: etiological factors, treatment, and prognosis.	Assessment provides an important starting point in education. Many misconceptions may be present among the lay public.

Therapeutic Interventions

Actions/Interventions	Rationales
■ Teach patient about occurrence of disease: • Most common form of valvular heart disease • Large number of undiagnosed, asymptomatic people in general population • Common in women but also diagnosed in men	Providing the patient with accurate knowledge about MVP can reduce the anxiety and fear he or she may experience about a diagnosis of heart valve disease. Knowledge helps the patient participate in decisions about management of this disease.

Actions/Interventions

- Teach patient about the following causative factors to increase understanding of disease process:
  - Etiological factors usually unknown
  - Important to understand that serious heart disease usually is not present, symptoms are more a nuisance than significant, and prognosis is excellent
- Teach patient the physiology of the disease:
  - Leaflet enlargement causing prolapse of one or both valve leaflets into left atrium
- Inform patient of the following typical diagnostic procedures:
  - Cardiac auscultation for nonejection click and a crescendo murmur that continues to the second heart sound, heard best at the apex
  - Echocardiogram to evaluate valve motion
  - Ambulatory Holter ECG monitoring for complaint of palpitations
  - Exercise stress test for complaint of chest pain
- Teach patient the following about the treatment of the disease:
  - Usually no treatment is indicated; patients need reassurance that this is not a severe cardiac condition
  - Use of exercise to reduce anxiety over condition and increase self-esteem
  - β-Blocker (or calcium channel blocker medication if cannot tolerate β-blocker)
  - Antiplatelet therapy (aspirin)
  - Self-limitation of activities, foods or drinks, and stressors that precipitate symptoms
- Teach patient about controversial use of endocarditis prophylaxis.

- Instruct about need for follow up examination every few years.
- Teach about options for surgical treatment (valve repair or replacement).

Rationales

Thorough understanding of specific causes is necessary for appropriate follow-through of the treatment plan.

This information helps the patient understand the rationale for therapy.

Auscultation of characteristic findings may be sufficient for diagnosis. A click is associated with tightening of the prolapsed leaflets against the high pressures of the left ventricular chamber. The murmur is associated with the leakage through the prolapsed (open) valve during systole. A Doppler echocardiogram is a particularly sensitive means of detecting minor degrees of MVP (abnormal posterior systolic motion of mitral valve leaflets) in apparently healthy adults.

MVP is a harmless condition and should not interfere with a normal lifestyle. Regular aerobic exercise is encouraged for patients who are asymptomatic. β-blocker and calcium channel blocker medications are used to treat symptomatic palpitations and/or chest pain. Antiplatelet therapy may be indicated if patient has a history of focal neurological events. Reducing caffeine may be helpful if palpitations are a problem.

In 2007 the American Heart Association changed its recommendations for routine prophylactic antibiotic use to prevent endocarditis. Attention is now directed to effective oral hygiene to reduce risk. Antibiotic therapy is indicated only if the patient has associated moderate to severe symptoms of mitral insufficiency.

Ongoing evaluation promotes optimal care.

Current clinical practice guidelines recommend repair over replacement. Patient needs to know that this is indicated only for severe cases of mitral regurgitation.

Risk for Disturbed Body Image

Common Risk Factors

Concern over "cardiac" condition
Fatigue secondary to β-blocker medication or sequelae of disease

Common Expected Outcome

Patient demonstrates enhanced body image and self-esteem as evidenced by ability to talk about altered heart function.

NOC Outcomes
Body Image; Coping

NIC Interventions
Body Image Enhancement; Teaching: Disease Process

■ = Independent   ▲ = Collaborative

Ongoing Assessment

Actions/Interventions

- Assess perception of change in body function and meaning of cardiac diagnosis.

- Note verbal references to heart and related discomfort, as well as any change in lifestyle.

Rationales

A distinction should be made between patients who present without symptoms and who are unintentionally diagnosed during routine examination and patients who sought medical attention because of symptoms.

Despite being a harmless, benign condition for most, some patients may develop "cardiac neurosis" when the condition is brought to their attention.

Therapeutic Interventions

Actions/Interventions

- Encourage the patient to talk about positive and negative feelings about the diagnosis of MVP.

- Provide accurate information about causes, prognosis, and treatment of condition.
- Provide reassurance that it is possible to lead a normal life with MVP.

- Teach the patient adaptive behaviors for problems with fatigue:
  - Encourage to allow several weeks for adjustment to β-blocker side effects.
  - Encourage appropriate pacing of daily activities.
- For female patients of childbearing age, instruct that pregnancy is usually not contraindicated.
- Refer to support group as indicated.

Rationales

It is worthwhile to encourage the patient to separate feelings about changes in heart function from feelings about self-worth. Expression of feelings can enhance the person's coping strategies.

Many patients have anxiety when diagnosed with a heart disease about which they know little.

Professional caregivers represent a microcosm of society, and their actions and behaviors are scrutinized as the patient finds meaning in and adjusts to new diagnoses.

Adaptive behaviors compensate for actual or perceived changes in activity level. Information enables the patient to assume some control. Fatigue can be caused by the disorder itself, though this is not clearly understood.

Patients are encouraged to live normal lives.

Participation in a support group may allow the patient to realize that others have the same problem; they may use this as a means to help make needed lifestyle alterations.

Risk for Chest Pain

Common Risk Factor

Etiological factors of pain are unknown but may be related to excessive stretch of chordae tendineae and papillary muscles or to coronary artery spasm.

Common Expected Outcomes

Patient verbalizes reduced or relieved pain.
Patient appears relaxed and comfortable.

NOC Outcomes

Pain Level; Knowledge: Treatment Regimen

NIC Interventions

Teaching: Disease Process; Teaching: Medications Prescribed

Ongoing Assessment

Actions/Interventions

- Assess atypical chest pain:
  - May last seconds to several hours
  - Typically left precordial, sharp, stabbing
  - May be substernal or diffuse
  - Usually not specifically related to exertion or stress; may be precipitated by fatigue
  - Usually not relieved by nitroglycerin
  - May present with inverted T waves and ST depression associated with exercise
- Assess hemodynamic status during pain occurrence: heart rate, blood pressure, and skin changes.

Rationales

Patients with MVP usually experience atypical chest pain that is not characteristic of angina pectoris. MVP does not involve pathology of coronary arteries. However, some patients with MVP may also have unrelated but additional problem of coronary spasm that can cause angina.

Associated symptoms help guide treatment.

Therapeutic Interventions

Actions/Interventions

- Permit unrestricted activity if the patient is asymptomatic.

- Encourage rest if pain is exertionally induced.

- Encourage a nonstressful environment.
- Provide psychological and emotional support.
- ▲ Instruct the patient to take medications as prescribed:
  - β-Blockers
  - Calcium channel blockers (if β-blocker not tolerated)
- Suggest patient undergo exercise stress testing to rule out coronary artery disease.
- Instruct patient about positions that may reduce chest pain:
  - Lying down
  - Squatting

Rationales

Because chest pain is not related to "angina," patients are encouraged to participate in regular physical activity.
Attention to simple measures to reduce duration/intensity of pain can enhance the quality of one's life for patients experiencing this associated symptom.
Stress has been related to increased occurrence of chest pain.
Support allays fears of the seriousness of this benign disease.
These medications are usually effective in relieving chest pain and associated palpitations.

Because most atypical chest pain with MVP is not anginal in etiology, a negative stress test can be reassuring to patient.
These positions increase venous return and lessen MVP.

Related Care Plan

Disturbed body image, p. 24

Pacemaker/Cardioverter-Defibrillator

Implantable (Permanent); External Pacemaker (Temporary); Cardioverter-Defibrillator (ICD)

Cardiac rhythm management (CRM) devices is a new term to encompass the spectrum of pacemaker and defibrillation systems now available to treat symptomatic bradydysrhythmias and tachydysrhythmias, terminate lethal dysrhythmias, and improve conduction system abnormalities. An implantable, permanent pacemaker delivers an electrical stimulus to the heart muscle when needed. The types of pacemakers currently available are as follows. (1) *Bradycardia pacemaker*—its mode of response is inhibited, triggered, or asynchronous. It is indicated for chronic symptomatic bradydysrhythmias or for second- or third-degree atrioventricular (AV) block. A dual-chamber pacemaker is indicated for bradycardia with competent sinus node to provide AV synchrony and rate variability. (2) *Rate-modulated pacemaker*—this is indicated for patients who can benefit from an increase in pacing rate, either atrial or ventricular, in response to their body's metabolic (physiological) needs or to

■ = Independent　▲ = Collaborative

activity (nonphysiological) for increased cardiac output. (3) *Antitachycardia pacemaker*—this is indicated for pace-terminable conditions: recurrent supraventricular tachycardia (e.g., AV reciprocating tachydysrhythmias [as in Wolff-Parkinson-White], atrial flutter, and other AV tachydysrhythmias). (4) *Cardiac resynchronization pacemakers*—this biventricular pacing system is indicated for severe heart failure and cardiomyopathy patients with intraventricular conduction delays who can benefit from synchronized septal wall motion and improved left ventricular contraction.

An external pacemaker delivers an electrical stimulus to the heart for the acute management of bradydysrhythmias and certain types of tachydysrhythmias and for use in provocative diagnostic cardiac procedures. Transcutaneous cardiac pacing (noninvasive) is rapidly initiated by delivering an electrical current from an external power source through large electrodes applied to the patient's chest. It is an alternative method to transvenous pacing for the initial management of bradyasystolic arrest situations until definitive treatment can be instituted or to overdrive tachydysrhythmias in emergency situations. Transvenous endocardial pacing directly stimulates the myocardial tissue with electrical current pulses through an electrode catheter inserted through a vein into the right atrium or right ventricle. Cardiac resynchronization pacemakers use transvenous pacing electrodes positioned in the right ventricle and in the coronary sinus (to pace left ventricle). Epicardial pacing stimulates the myocardium through one or two pacing electrodes sutured loosely through the epicardial surface of the heart. It is most commonly used after open heart surgery for temporary relief of bradyarrhythmias or for overdrive pacing for tachyarrhythmias.

An implanted cardioverter-defibrillator (ICD) delivers one or more countershocks (depending on device model) directly to the heart after it recognizes a dysrhythmia through rate-detection criteria. It is a life-prolonging therapy for patients with serious ventricular dysrhythmias. Ongoing randomized controlled trials continue to identify patients most likely to benefit from ICD implants. Some of the national recommendations for implantation include (1) secondary prevention for those who have survived sudden cardiac death caused by the tachydysrhythmias not due to transient or reversible cause and (2) for primary prevention in patients with and without ischemic heart disease or cardiomyopathy with an ejection fraction of less than 30%, with New York Heart Association Functional Class II-III symptoms while undergoing optimal medical therapy. After a preset sensing period in which the system detects a lethal dysrhythmia, the defibrillator mechanism delivers a shock (usually 25 J) to the heart muscle. If needed, repeat shocks are delivered. The shock delivered is often described as a hard thump or as a kick to the chest. Most ICDs also contain antitachycardia (overdrive) and antibradycardia (backup pacing) pacemakers.

NANDA-I NDx Risk for Decreased Cardiac Output

Common Risk Factors

Pacemaker malfunction caused by the following:
- Electrode dislodgment
- Faulty connection between lead and pulse generator
- Faulty lead system (e.g., lead fracture, insulation break)
- Pulse generator circuitry failure
- Battery depletion
- Inadequate pacemaker parameter settings
- Inappropriate type of pacemaker
- Ventricular dysrhythmias caused by irritation from pacing electrode or asynchronous pacing resulting from malsensing problem

- Change in myocardial threshold
- Competitive rhythms

Cardioverter-defibrillator malfunction caused by the following:

- Difficulty determining defibrillation thresholds during electrophysiology study or implant procedure
- Failure to sense and/or emit charge to break tachydysrhythmias
- Failure of myocardium to respond to the charged energy delivered as a result of low-energy output
- Inappropriate sensing of atrial tachydysrhythmias
- Postoperative complications as a result of concomitant cardiac surgery (pericardial effusion, cardiac tamponade)
- Extreme bradycardia or asystole after defibrillation

Common Expected Outcome

Patient maintains adequate cardiac output as evidenced by strong peripheral pulses, systolic BP within 20 mm Hg of baseline, HR 60 to 100 beats/min with regular rhythm, urinary output ≥30 mL/hr, warm and dry skin, and normal level of consciousness.

NOC Outcomes
Circulation Status; Cardiac Pump Effectiveness
NIC Intervention
Dysrhythmia Management

Ongoing Assessment

Actions/Interventions

■ Assess apical or radial pulses and hemodynamic status.

■ If electrocardiogram (ECG) is monitored:
  • Assess for proper pacemaker function: capture, sensing, firing, and configuration of paced QRS.

  • Assess for pacemaker-induced dysrhythmias.

For Permanent Implantable Pacemaker
Immediately after pacemaker implantation:

▲ Check implant data for the following: type of pacemaker (e.g., single-chamber, dual-chamber, AV sequential, demand, programmable, rate response) and programmed parameters.

▲ Monitor chest x-ray and ECG studies after patient returns to room and as prescribed.

■ Keep ECG monitor alarms on at all times.

■ Record rhythm strips as follows:
  • Routinely according to unit policy
  • If pacemaker malfunction is suspected
  • When pacemaker parameter adjustments are made

Rationales

Electrical stimulation of the heart does not guarantee effective "pumping" of the heart; hemodynamics need to be assessed.

The nurse's role is to verify proper pacemaker function to reduce risk for malfunction and complications. Each type of pacemaker will have its own pacing configuration depending on which leads are viewed.

The challenge is to determine the relationship between isolated and pacemaker-induced dysrhythmias.

Certain types of pacemakers have variable functions, which can be difficult to interpret. If using a dual-chamber pacemaker, then preprogrammed, timed intervals and lower and upper rate limits need to be known.

It is necessary to verify correct placement of lead and pacemaker function. Ventricular lead placement is usually in the right ventricular apex; atrial lead placement is in the right atrial appendage.

Alarm signals alert the nurse to potential life-threatening dysrhythmias or pacemaker malfunction. Disabling or turning off alarms places the patient at higher risk.

Recordings provides data for serial comparison.

■ = Independent   ▲ = Collaborative

Actions/Interventions	Rationales
▲ If pacemaker malfunction is suspected, conduct the following: • Assess hemodynamic stability with spontaneous or competitive rhythm. • Obtain 12-lead ECG.	Not all malfunctions result in hemodynamic compromise. Level of compromise guides level of intervention. The ECG complex verifies function of pacemaker and lead placement. Left bundle branch block–paced QRS configuration suggests good right ventricular lead position.
If failure to sense is noted:	Failure to sense occurs when the pacemaker does not recognize spontaneous atrial or ventricular activity and it fires inappropriately.
▲ Monitor chest x-ray films.	X-ray studies are used to verify placement and status of pacemaker electrode.
■ Observe for phrenic nerve stimulation (hiccups) and intercostal or abdominal muscle twitching.	Stimulation of chest wall and diaphragm indicates possible dislodged pacemaker.
■ Observe for induced ventricular dysrhythmias caused by pacemaker competition.	Pacing stimulus may excite a repolarized cell during the relative refractory period when the heart is at risk for fibrillation; this represents an "R on T" phenomenon.
If loss of capture is noted:	Electrical stimulus from pacemaker to myocardium is insufficient to produce an atrial or ventricular beat.
■ Follow the three steps under "failure to sense" above.	
■ Assess for factors that increase myocardial threshold (e.g., ischemia, fibrosis around electrode tip, acidosis, electrolyte imbalance, antidysrhythmic drugs).	Threshold is the minimum amount of electrical energy needed to pace and capture the heart rhythm.
■ If ventricular dysrhythmias occur, assess hemodynamic status.	Level of hemodynamic compromise guides intensity of intervention.
If patient is at home:	
■ Instruct to come to ambulatory care setting.	Pacemaker function must be further evaluated.
■ For repetitive pacemaker problems, consider using transtelephonic monitoring devices.	These devices provide immediate evaluation of cardiac rhythm.
■ Consider registering patients with a 24-hour service.	Such service provides ongoing evaluation as well as a source of support and security for the patient.
For Temporary External Pacemaker ▲ Check that the prescribed pacemaker parameters are maintained (rate, pacing output in milliamperes, sensitivity).	Each patient has a different pacing threshold. Also, each type of pacemaker requires different settings (e.g., transvenous uses low milliamperes [2 to 10 mA], whereas transcutaneous may have 40 to 100 mA for capture). Patients with large hearts, large chest muscles, or pleural or pericardial effusions will require more energy.
■ Observe or monitor ECG continuously for appropriate pacemaker function: sensing, capturing, and firing (pacing spikes).	These data verify function and provide early warning for malfunction.
■ Record rhythm strips as follows: • Routinely according to unit policy • When changes in pacing parameters are made • For presence of spontaneous rhythm	Recordings provide data for serial comparison.
■ If pacemaker is on standby, evaluate pacemaker capture daily and as needed.	Capture is represented by a pacing spike followed by ventricular depolarization (QRS).
■ Assess for proper environmental and electrical safety measures.	The pacemaker lead is directly in contact with the myocardium. A small amount of current can initiate fibrillation.
■ If signs of pacemaker malfunction or dysrhythmia occur, assess hemodynamic status until stable.	Level of hemodynamic compromise guides intervention.
■ Assess for pacemaker-induced dysrhythmias.	These dysrhythmias may be caused by competitive rhythm secondary to asynchronous pacing or tissue excitability.

Actions/Interventions

Rationales

For Implanted Cardioverter-Defibrillator

■ Observe or monitor closely for the following:
  • Presence of sustained ventricular dysrhythmias

Such dysrhythmias significantly reduce cardiac output and can be life threatening.

  • Symptomatic bradycardia or atrial tachydysrhythmias

Such dysrhythmias significantly reduce cardiac output.

  • Prolongation of QT interval if patient is receiving anti-dysrhythmic therapy

Prolonged refractory period can precipitate dysrhythmias.

■ Assess for improper function of implantable defibrillator:
  • Failure to sense ventricular dysrhythmia
  • Failure to emit energy charge
  • Failure to terminate ventricular dysrhythmia
  • Improper sensing of tachydysrhythmias and inappropriate shocks

Vigilant monitoring helps reduce consequences of malfunction.

Therapeutic Interventions

Actions/Interventions

Rationales

For Permanent Implantable Pacemaker

If malfunction is suspected:

■ Turn patient on left side (for endocardial pacemaker).

This position facilitates good ventricular wall contact. Malpositioning is a common cause of malfunction, especially in the acute setting.

■ Notify physician.

Pacemaker malfunction can signify a potentially life-threatening condition and warrants immediate intervention.

▲ Call pacemaker specialist to evaluate further pacemaker function and to make changes in parameters if needed through the use of pacemaker programmer.

This is a noninvasive technique of pacemaker programming through radiofrequency signal.

▲ Prepare atropine sulfate, dopamine, epinephrine, and isoproterenol (Isuprel) for standby.

Atropine is an anticholinergic drug that increases cardiac output and heart rate (HR) by blocking vagal stimulation in the heart. Dopamine is an adrenergic stimulator and inotropic drug. Epinephrine and isoproterenol are sympathetic drugs that increase HR and cardiac output by stimulating β-receptors in the heart; these are used to stimulate the ventricles.

▲ Prepare for temporary pacemaker insertion.

Transcutaneous pacing is effective in providing adequate HR and rhythm to patients in emergency situations.

■ Initiate basic life support measures as needed.

Life-threatening situations warrant immediate attention. Basic cardiopulmonary resuscitation can maintain circulation and perfusion until rhythm is restored.

■ Anticipate need for medical correction of pacemaker in laboratory.

Depending on the source of the problem, electrode lead system may need to be replaced. For chronically used pacemakers, battery depletion may be the problem.

For Temporary External Pacemaker

■ When a transcutaneous pacemaker is used, ensure that a large R wave is obtained on the ECG monitor.

This pacing system reads the signal from the surface ECG, not intracardiac as with the transvenous and epicardial pacemakers.

If failure to sense is noted:

Pacemaker is not sensing spontaneous rhythm, which could lead to dysrhythmias. Pacing stimulus may excite a repolarized cell during a relative refractory period (R-on-T phenomenon).

■ Check that the dial is not on asynchronous pacing (fixed rate).

When the pacer is in asynchronous mode, it does not use the sensing circuit and instead paces at the preset (fixed) rate regardless of underlying cardiac rate and rhythm.

■ Check for loose connections. For transcutaneous pacing, check for adherence of ECG electrodes.

The pacemaker is not picking up cardiac signal when the line of communication is interrupted.

■ = Independent   ▲ = Collaborative

Actions/Interventions	Rationales
■ Reposition limb of body if lead insertion is through the brachial or femoral vein. If transcutaneous pacing is used, increase size of ECG pattern on monitor, or try a different lead.	Malpositioning can dislodge the pacemaker lead from the wall of the ventricle.
▲ Notify the physician of need to adjust sensitivity dial.	Increasing sensitivity increases the gain of the spontaneous cardiac rhythm signal.
▲ Check position of the endocardial lead by chest x-ray examination. If the problem is not corrected and the patient has adequate rhythm, check with the physician whether the pacemaker should be on standby.	Placing the pacemaker on standby avoids risk for pacemaker-induced dysrhythmia from competitive rhythms.
▲ If the problem is not corrected and the patient is hemodynamically compromised: with transvenous lead, anticipate use of transcutaneous external pacemaker while awaiting electrode repositioning; with epicardial pacing, anticipate removal of lead and use of transcutaneous external pacemaker or insertion of transvenous pacemaker, depending on patient's status.	Transcutaneous pacing is a rapid, efficient, noninvasive means to restore a cardiac rhythm.

If loss of capture is noted:

Actions/Interventions	Rationales
■ Check all possible connections.	The pacemaker fails to depolarize the myocardium.
■ Turn patient on left side (endocardial catheter).	An intact system is required for conducting the cardiac signal.
	This position facilitates optimal lead placement (right ventricular apex). Capture requires contact between the distal pacing lead and healthy myocardium.
▲ Increase pacing output (milliamperes), and evaluate for good capture.	The pacing threshold may have changed for a variety of reasons and needs to be increased.
■ For transcutaneous pacing, also check for adequate adherence of anterior or posterior electrodes to the patient's skin.	A posterior electrode may have slipped out of position because of diaphoresis.
■ Correct any underlying causes that may reduce myocardial response to electrical stimulation, such as hypoxia or acidosis.	Besides increasing pacing output, treating specific causes for change in threshold optimizes pacemaker function.

If loss of pacing spikes is noted:

Actions/Interventions	Rationales
■ Check that the power switch is "on."	The pacemaker fails to emit electrical stimulus.
	The first step in evaluating the loss of pacer spikes is making sure the power switch is in the "on" position.
■ Check whether the needle gauge on the external pacemaker box is fluctuating.	Flucuation verifies that the pacemaker senses intrinsic activity.
■ If the needle gauge is not fluctuating, replace batteries in the generator.	Temporary pulse generators use 9-volt batteries. The life of a battery depends on how "pacemaker-dependent" each patient is.
■ Check all possible connections.	An intact system is required for conducting the cardiac signal.
■ Check for electromagnetic interference.	Interference from equipment (e.g., radiation, from cautery, or from imaging resonance) can inhibit pacing output by temporarily turning off the pacemaker.
■ Replace generator as needed.	An effective power source is required for optimal function.

If pacemaker malfunction is noted and not easily corrected by the preceding steps:

Actions/Interventions	Rationales
■ Evaluate adequate spontaneous rhythm.	An unreliable escape rhythm will lead to hemodynamic collapse.
■ Monitor vital signs every 15 to 30 minutes.	Treat the patient according to unit protocol and Advanced Cardiac Life Support (ACLS) guidelines.
■ Prepare atropine sulfate, dopamine, epinephrine, and isoproterenol for standby.	Atropine is an anticholinergic drug that increases cardiac output and HR by blocking vagal stimulation in the heart. Dopamine is an adrenergic stimulator and inotropic drug. Epinephrine and isoproterenol are sympathetic drugs that increase cardiac output and HR by stimulating β-receptors in the ventricle.

Actions/Interventions

If pacemaker-induced dysrhythmia is noted:
- ■ Maintain proper environmental and electrical safety measures.
- ■ Ensure that all electrical equipment is properly grounded with three-prong plugs.
- ▲ Ensure that a biomedical engineer has checked room.
- ■ Ensure that exposed pacing wire terminals and generator are insulated in a rubber glove or enclosed in a plastic case.
- ■ Ensure that bed linen and gown are kept dry.

For Implanted Cardioverter-Defibrillator
- ▲ Get information from the electrophysiologist on functions of the implantable defibrillator and how it is programmed. Ask if the device is active (on) or inactive (off).
- ▲ Ensure that a special ring-type magnet is available on the nursing unit.

If ventricular tachycardia or ventricular fibrillation occurs:
- ▲ Check whether the patient received an internal shock or shocks. If the patient received an internal shock:
  - • Notify physician and electrophysiologist.
  - • Document total number of shocks that the patient received before conversion.
  - • Save rhythm strips in the chart.
  - • Check electrolyte level or other factors that predispose to ventricular arrhythmias.
- ■ If the patient did not receive an internal shock and his or her condition is decompensating:
  - • Initiate basic life support measures. Proceed with external defibrillation protocol. Do not wait for the device to emit charges.

  - • Apply defibrillation paddles 3 to 4 inches from the pulse generator.

For sustained nonsymptomatic ventricular tachycardia:

- ■ Notify physician.
- ▲ Administer antidysrhythmic drug as ordered.
- ▲ Check potassium and magnesium blood levels or other factors that predispose to ventricular dysrhythmia.
- ▲ Reevaluate the patient's hemodynamic status for ventricular tachycardia of longer duration.

If implantable defibrillator malfunction is noted:
- ▲ Notify electrophysiologist at once.
- ▲ Prepare antidysrhythmic medication.
- ■ Have emergency cart and external defibrillator ready within reach.

Rationales

Stray electrical current may enter the heart through the external lead, which can cause dysrhythmia.
Safety measures reduce complications.

Attention must be directed to ensuring a safe environment.
Insulation reduces risk for stray current to travel to heart.

Moisture conducts current and increases the risk for accidental shocks.

There are a variety of types and models of ICDs. Each can have variable functions that can be difficult to interpret.

The magnet is to be used only by qualified personnel to check for proper lead signal (synchronous pulse tone means proper R-wave sensing). Applying the magnet for 30 seconds or more will deactivate the device (constant tone).

Most ICD devices have memory and ECG storage capability so the physician or pacemaker nurse can "interrogate" the programmer to determine the sequence or outcome of events.

Prompt intervention is essential to controlling life-threatening dysrhythmias. Never assume that the internal defibrillator is functioning normally. The magnet can be used over the pulse generator to suppress function during an emergency.
This position is to prevent the occurrence of circuit failure and muscle tissue burns. If anterolateral positioning is unsuccessful, try anteroposterior.
The implantable defibrillator does not sense ventricular tachycardia with a rate slower than the programmed cutoff rate (e.g., less than 150 beats/min).
Rapid efficient intervention may be warranted.
ACLS protocols provide guidelines.
Dysrhythmias are best treated by treating the cause.

Patients may be able to sustain ventricular tachycardia only when they are of short duration. Sustained dysrhythmia may significantly compromise cardiac output.

ICD malfunction requires specialty intervention.
ACLS protocols provide guidelines.
This equipment needs to be available for emergency use in case external defibrillation is needed to stabilize the patient's rhythm and to support life.

■ = Independent ▲ = Collaborative

Actions/Interventions	Rationales
▲ If implantable defibrillator exhibits false emission of multiple shocks and is activated:	
• Deactivate the device by applying a magnet over the upper right corner of the device for 30 seconds.	Deactivation prevents inappropriate shocks that could worsen dysrhythmias and further damage the myocardium. NOTE: When the defibrillator is deactivated, a constant tone is heard instead of a pulse tone (activated).
• Anticipate return to the operating room for possible pulse generator replacement or lead reconfiguration.	
• Document implantable defibrillator malfunction.	
If symptomatic extreme bradycardia or asystole occurs after defibrillation:	
▲ Initiate routine emergency procedure.	Rapid efficient intervention is critical.
▲ Prepare for temporary pacemaker insertion.	The pacemaker will provide a new source for stimulating cardiac rhythm.
▲ Prepare atropine sulfate, dopamine, epinephrine, and isoproterenol drip. Administer as ordered.	These medications accelerate the HR and improve cardiac output.
■ Instruct outpatient to do the following:	
• Lie down when device fires.	Each patient needs to understand the plan of care if the ICD discharges inappropriately.
• Report to health care provider any physical symptoms such as chest pain, palpitation, diaphoresis, fainting, dizziness, or other symptoms before receiving shock.	These data provide information on degree of hemodynamic compromise associated with specific dysrhythmias.
• Report to staff the delivery of any internal shock or shocks and total number of shocks received.	Protocols vary as to how soon and to whom the patient should report.
• Go to the nearest hospital emergency department if multiple discharges occur in rapid succession and/or if symptomatic.	Immediate medical care is necessary in this situation to restore ICD function and maintain cardiac output.

NANDA-I NDx Acute Pain/Discomfort

Common Related Factors
Insertion of pacemaker or ICD
Lead displacement
High-pacing energy output
Self-imposed and imposed activity restriction
"Frozen" shoulder
Hiccupping (phrenic nerve stimulation); intercostal or pectoral muscle stimulation

Defining Characteristics
Restlessness, irritability
Verbalized discomfort
Splinting of wound with hands
Limited range of motion (ROM) of affected extremity

Common Expected Outcomes
Patient verbalizes relief or reduction in pain or discomfort.
Patient appears relaxed and comfortable.

NOC Outcomes
Pain Level; Pain Control
NIC Intervention
Pain Management

Ongoing Assessment

Actions/Interventions	Rationales
■ Assess pain characteristics: source, quality, location, onset, and precipitating and relieving factors.	Assessment of the pain experience is the first step to planning effective treatment strategies.

Actions/Interventions	**Rationales**
■ Assess for probable cause of pain.	Different etiological factors respond better to different therapies. For example, transcutaneous pacing can be especially uncomfortable, and diaphragmatic stimulation requires repositioning of pacemaker lead.
■ Assess for hiccups or muscle twitching.	Hiccups occur with phrenic nerve stimulation; muscle twitching occurs with high-energy output.
■ Palpate affected site for presence of permanent pulse generator pocket stimulation.	High pacing output or lead detachment from generator can cause stimulation.

Therapeutic Interventions

Actions/Interventions	**Rationales**
■ Provide comfort measures (e.g., back rubs, change in position, gentle massage of shoulder on operative side).	Nonpharmacological measures can promote comfort.
▲ Administer pain medication as prescribed.	Analgesics or sedatives may be used to reduce painful skeletal muscle contractions with transcutaneous pacing.
■ Instruct patient to report pain and effectiveness of interventions.	Patient comfort is a priority.
■ Explain reasons for any activity restriction. Emphasize that most are temporary.	Restricted activity and limited ROM can be sources of discomfort in the early postprocedure period, but they are required to ensure correct placement of the pacing lead.
▲ If hiccups, muscle twitching, or pulse generator pocket stimulation are present, do the following: • Notify physician. • Obtain chest x-ray film. • Obtain ECG. • Anticipate return to procedure room for lead repositioning.	These symptoms can indicate dislodged pacemaker.

Risk for Impaired Physical Mobility

Common Risk Factors
Imposed activity restriction with transvenous pacemaker
Reluctance to attempt movement because of pain at site of
 pulse generator/ICD or fear of lead dislodgment

Common Expected Outcomes
Patient engages in activity within prescribed restrictions.
Patient avoids any complications of immobility.

NOC Outcome
Joint Movement
NIC Interventions
Positioning; Joint Mobility

Ongoing Assessment

Actions/Interventions	**Rationales**
■ Assess whether patient with an implanted pacemaker/ ICD is restricting activity because of physician order, discomfort, or fear of malfunction.	Many patients, especially older patients, avoid moving for fear of dislodging the pacemaker/ICD.
■ Assess for potential complications related to reduced activity.	Reduced activity can affect peripheral circulation, pulmonary ventilation, ability to sleep, and the gastrointestinal system.

■ = Independent   ▲ = Collaborative

Actions/Interventions

- Assess specific activity restrictions for patients with temporary transvenous external pacemakers.

Rationales

Femoral vein site insertion of pacing leads requires complete bed rest. To prevent dislodging the pacing lead, the affected leg should not be bent. Patients with brachial or internal jugular leads may transfer to a chair with assistance.

Therapeutic Interventions

Actions/Interventions

- Explain the importance of imposed activity restriction.
- Assist in turning every 2 hours. For endocardial pacemaker, avoid turning to right side.

- Assist with active ROM exercises to the nonaffected extremities 3 times daily.
- Assist patient in using affected extremity carefully.

- Provide passive ROM exercise to the shoulder on the operative side.

Rationales

Restrictions reduce risk for electrode displacement.

The endocardial pacing lead is positioned in the right ventricular apex. Turning to the right side can cause the lead to float or move away from the apex, thereby causing pacemaker malfunction.

Exercises maintain function without compromising pacemaker positioning.

Patient may require assistance with activities of daily living so as not to compromise pacemaker function.

Careful ROM exercises serve to prevent "frozen" shoulder from disuse.

NANDA-I NDx Deficient Knowledge

Common Related Factors

Inability to comprehend
New procedure or equipment
Misinterpretation of information
Advanced age of patient

Defining Characteristics

Verbalized inaccurate information
Questioning members of health care team
Inaccurate follow-through of instruction

Common Expected Outcomes

Patient and family verbalize understanding about pacemaker or ICD.
Patient accepts activity limitation.
Patient understands role in detecting early signs of equipment malfunction or failure.

NOC Outcomes
Knowledge: Disease Process; Knowledge: Treatment Regimen

NIC Interventions
Teaching: Disease Process; Teaching: Procedure/Treatment

Ongoing Assessment

Actions/Interventions

- Assess level of understanding about pacemaker and/or ICD and reasons for insertion.
- Assess understanding of how to care for insertion site, activity prescriptions, and need for follow-up pacemaker checks.

Rationales

Evaluation provides starting point for educational session.

Thorough understanding is necessary for appropriate care and follow-up.

Therapeutic Interventions

Actions/Interventions

- Before procedure, explain the anatomy and physiology of the heart, the pacemaker or ICD function and its advantages, and the insertion procedure.

Rationales

Thorough understanding is necessary for informed consent to be given.

Actions/Interventions

Rationales

- After procedure for a permanent pacemaker insertion:
  - Stress importance of bed rest after implantation.
  - Instruct patient to avoid turning to the right side if endocardial pacemaker was inserted.
  - Explain importance of notifying the nurse of the following:
    - Any pain or drainage from the insertion site
    - Complaints of headache, dizziness, confusion, chest pain, shortness of breath, hiccups, or muscle twitching
  - Explain the need for chest x-ray evaluation and 12-lead ECG.
- Before discharge and routinely in the ambulatory care setting, teach the patient and reinforce the following for a permanent pacemaker:
  - Need for regular follow-up care

  - Signs and symptoms of infection; wound care for insertion site
  - The need to discuss with the physician the types of sports activities in which the patient can participate (avoid contact sports)
  - The need to avoid over-the-head arm motion or overstretching for 1 month

  - The need to carry a pacemaker identification card with the type of pacemaker, brand name, model number, and programmed pacing rate
  - Signs and symptoms of pacemaker malfunction

  - How to take and record pulse as needed
  - Need to notify physician or pacemaker follow-up office if pulse rate is 5 to 10 beats slower than programmed rate or to inform health care providers of any signs and symptoms of pacemaker malfunction
  - Pacemaker longevity and need for pacemaker battery replacement when elective replacement indication time has been reached
  - Avoidance of strong magnetic field (magnetic resonance, electrocautery equipment, laser, diathermy, lithotripsy, direct radiation, current industrial machinery)
  - Safety of using newer-model microwave ovens; if dizziness is felt while near the appliance being used, advise patient to move at least 5 to 10 feet away
  - Need to alert airport personnel, dentist, and others of presence of pacemaker
- Before discharge, instruct the patient or family regarding the following for an ICD:
  - Need to carry identification card at all times
  - Need to apply for medical alert identification and wear it at all times
  - Need for regular follow-up care (every 2 to 4 months until the end of life of battery)
  - Procedure for taking pulse

Bed rest prevents lead displacement.
Correct positioning ensures good ventricular wall contact.

These are symptoms that require immediate follow-up.
These complaints may suggest pacemaker malfunction.

These diagnostic measures are required to assess pacemaker function.

Follow-up may be according to routine physician appointment or follow-up at specialized pacemaker clinic or by transtelephonic methods.
Patients are better able to seek assistance when they know basic information.
Knowledge helps prevent pacemaker complications.

This restriction is necessary to prevent lead displacement because it takes about 1 month for scar tissue to form around the electrode tip.
Pacemakers are becoming more complex. Timely troubleshooting requires knowledge of the specifics of the patient's own pacemaker.
Information aids the patient in assuming responsibility for ongoing care.
Daily pulse checks aid in detecting early battery failure.
Vigilant monitoring helps reduce consequences of malfunction.

Most lithium batteries last 5 to 10 years. Pulse generator replacement (battery) using the same electrode can be done on an outpatient basis.
Magnetic fields may cause pulse generator circuitry failure or may cause certain pacemakers to go into backup mode.

Pacemaker assumes normal function without permanent effects.

Newer pacemakers rarely trigger airport screening devices.

Long-term care will be the patient's responsibility. Enough information is required for successful follow-up.

■ = Independent   ▲ = Collaborative

Cardiac and Vascular Care Plans

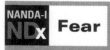

Cardiac and Vascular Care Plans

Actions/Interventions

- How patient can do cough cardiopulmonary resuscitation in case of ICD failure
- How to enroll family for cardiopulmonary resuscitation course
- Chest and abdominal wound care
- Signs and symptoms of infection
- Signs and symptoms of tachydysrhythmias and implantable defibrillator malfunction
- Anticipating shock when symptoms occur
- Tingling sensation by person who touches patient being shocked
- Avoiding strong magnetic field: diathermy, computed tomography scans, lithotripsy, electrocautery equipment, stimulator, magnetic resonance imaging, laser, and current industrial machinery (newer-model microwave ovens have no reported effect); for radiation therapy, device should be shielded
- Remembering that the device will emit a beeping noise when near magnetic field
- Immediately notifying physician or pacemaker laboratory of shocks received
- Alerting dentists or other physicians for presence of implantable defibrillator
- Alerting airport personnel regarding implantable defibrillator
- Avoiding contact sports like baseball, basketball, football, and other activities
- Magnet testing during scheduled follow-up care
- State-specific driving restriction

■ Use a variety of teaching materials, such as the following:
- Video of patients with ICD
- Demonstration model of ICD and equipment
- Handout materials

■ Review ICD manual with patient and family.

■ Refer to support group.

Rationales

Different people take in information in different ways. Match the learning style with the educational approach.

Patients are better able to ask questions and seek assistance when they know basic information about ICDs.

Support groups provide emotional support and information that may assist patients in coping with pacemaker/ICD devices.

NANDA-I NDx **Fear**

Common Related Factors

Diagnosis of inducible life-threatening dysrhythmia
History of sudden cardiac death, syncope, and multiple diagnostic studies
Anticipation of perceived threat, danger, or death
Insertion of ICD
Anticipation of how receiving a shock will feel
Potential for ICD system malfunction
Loss of independence caused by change in role functions or routines

Defining Characteristics

Report of being scared
Report of increased tension
Increased alertness
Narrowed focus on the source of fear

Common Expected Outcome

Patient verbalizes or manifests a reduction or absence of fear.

NOC Outcomes
Fear Self-Control; Social Support; Coping

NIC Interventions
Anxiety Reduction; Emotional Support; Preparatory Sensory Information; Teaching: Disease Process/Treatment; Support System Enhancement

Ongoing Assessment

Actions/Interventions	Rationales
■ Assess for source of fear.	Related factors represent common sources of fear in this population. Accurate assessment of fear guides intervention.
■ Evaluate past coping mechanisms and their effectiveness.	Knowledge of past coping strategies can serve as a basis for adopting or adapting prior strategies.

Therapeutic Interventions

Actions/Interventions	Rationales
Inpatient:	
■ Encourage patient to talk about fears.	Talking about feelings helps the patient focus on fear as a real and actual part of life. Patients may have heard exaggerated accounts of being shocked.
■ Explain electrophysiology and implantation procedures ahead of time.	Answering all concerned questions will reduce the patient's anxiety level. The patient will be able to use problem-solving abilities effectively if anxiety level is low.
▲ Administer medication as prescribed.	Medications may be indicated for relief of anxiety.
■ Maintain a calm and tolerant manner while interacting with the patient, especially during frightening procedures.	The presence of a trusted person makes the patient feel secure.
■ Rehearse with the patient what it feels like when an ICD device fires.	Talking through the event may help patients cope with their fears. There will be several practice trials with the ICD in the procedure laboratory.
Outpatient:	
■ Assist the patient in developing his or her problem-solving abilities.	Guidance with a less stressful problem-solving situation will provide the base for more complex situations.
■ Assist the patient in providing emotional support to the family.	An ICD shock can be a frightening experience for all family members, especially if the member is touching the patient when the ICD fires. They require assurance that they will not be harmed and that proper firing is a positive experience.
■ Assist the patient with an ICD in understanding that not firing does not mean the ICD is defective.	Many patients receive the ICD prophylactically; therefore months or even years may go by without its firing. Periodic laboratory checks will verify accurate function.
■ Encourage use of support groups for patient and family.	Knowing what changes in lifestyle might occur helps to prepare for such situations and facilitates problem solving.

Related Care Plan

Disturbed body image, p. 24

■ = Independent   ▲ = Collaborative

Percutaneous Balloon Valvuloplasty

Percutaneous balloon valvuloplasty is a procedure that uses a balloon-tipped catheter to dilate the opening of a narrowed valve and split the valve leaflets apart. Valves become stenotic from either congenital defects or acquired diseases. Balloon valvuloplasty is most commonly used to repair mitral and aortic valves in adults. It is indicated for symptomatic patients who no longer respond to medical therapy and for those who are not candidates for valve replacement surgery. It is often used for older patients when surgery poses too great a risk. Successful balloon valvuloplasty may improve the patient's hemodynamic state sufficiently to reduce the risks associated with valve replacement surgery. This procedure can be performed in a catheterization laboratory under fluoroscopy and without the use of general anesthesia. A percutaneous retrograde approach through the femoral artery is most commonly used for aortic valves. The femoral vein is used in the antegrade approach across the atrial septum to the left atrium for the mitral valve.

NANDA-I NDx **Deficient Knowledge**

Common Related Factors

Unfamiliarity with procedure
Information misinterpretation
Cognitive limitation
Lack of exposure/recall

Defining Characteristics

Request for more information
Multiple questions
Verbalized misconceptions

Common Expected Outcome

Patient verbalizes understanding of balloon valvuloplasty and the care associated with it.

NOC Outcomes

Knowledge: Disease Process; Knowledge: Treatment Procedure

NIC Interventions

Teaching: Disease Process; Teaching: Procedure

Ongoing Assessment

Actions/Interventions	Rationales
■ Assess patient's knowledge of heart anatomy, valve disease, balloon valvuloplasty procedure, and possible risks or complications.	Patients must have correct information to give informed consent. This information provides an important starting point for education.

Therapeutic Interventions

Actions/Interventions	Rationales
■ Provide information about the following:	This information provides the patient with knowledge for understanding the need for the procedure.
• Patient's heart problem (most commonly mitral or aortic stenosis)	Mitral stenosis is associated with fibrous valve leaflets that reduce the valve orifice. Aortic stenosis is associated with thickened, fibrous cusps and valve calcification.

Actions/Interventions

- Specifics about procedure:
  - Conscious sedation
  - Insertion of catheter under fluoroscopy
  - Balloon inflation at several atmospheres of pressure for 12 to 30 seconds; repeated inflations are usually required
  - Monitoring of pressure gradients across valve to verify results
- Immediate postvalvuloplasty care:
  - Activity restrictions: lying flat with affected site straight until femoral introducer or sheath is removed and usually for several hours after removal
  - Routine vital sign monitoring
  - Increased oral fluid intake
  - Monitoring for complications: bleeding at site, valve tear or rupture, left-to-right shunt, embolism, restenosis
- Recovery:
  - May resume normal activities in 1 week per physician's order
  - Notifying physician of weight gain, dyspnea, edema (signs of valve dysfunction)
  - Medications
- Follow-up care

- ■ Be in room when physicians discuss risk and complications of procedure so that the patient's subsequent questions can be answered accurately.

Rationales

Anxiety can be reduced when the patient knows what to expect.

Patients need to be aware of postprocedure activities and instructions so they can participate in care.

Information enables the patient to reduce risk for or seek help for postprocedure complications.

Restenosis can occur post procedure. Early assessment facilitates prompt treatment.
It is important that the nurse know what the patient has been told by other health care providers in order to provide accurate answers to the patient's questions. Patients are often hesitant to ask questions and seek clarification of information from the physician.

Risk for Decreased Cardiac Output

Common Risk Factors

Fluid volume deficit related to radiographic dye and restricted oral intake before procedure
Valve tear or rupture leading to valvular insufficiency
Dysrhythmia
Pulmonary artery pressures and pulmonary vascular resistance secondary to left-to-right shunt with transseptal approach

Common Expected Outcome

Patient maintains adequate cardiac output as evidenced by strong peripheral pulses, systolic BP within 20 mm Hg of baseline, HR 60 to 100 beats/min with regular rhythm, urinary output ≥30 mL/hr, warm and dry skin, normal level of consciousness, and normal pulmonary artery diastolic pressure (PADP) and pulmonary capillary wedge pressure (PCWP).

NOC Outcomes

Cardiac Pump Effectiveness; Circulation Status; Fluid Balance

NIC Interventions

Invasive Hemodynamic Monitoring; Hemodynamic Regulation; Fluid Resuscitation

---

■ = Independent   ▲ = Collaborative

Ongoing Assessment

Actions/Interventions	Rationales
■ Assess patient's hemodynamic status.	The first few hours post procedure are crucial to recovery. Declining systolic blood pressure and increasing pulse may indicate decreased cardiac output and decompensation.
▲ Assess the following parameters as available: PADP, PCWP, central venous pressure, cardiac output.	Hemodynamic parameters provide information for differentiating decreased cardiac output resulting from fluid overload vs. deficit. PADP and PCWP are elevated with new mitral insufficiency, which is a common complication of the procedure.
■ Monitor ECG for rate, rhythm, and dysrhythmia.	Electrocardiography is necessary to assess myocardial changes and to monitor potential dysrhythmias.
■ Assess heart sounds for change in murmur.	A blowing high-pitched murmur denotes valvular insufficiency, a complication of the procedure.
■ Assess breath sounds.	Crackles may occur with increased fluid in pulmonary circulation as a result of decreased cardiac output.
■ Monitor fluid intake and urine output closely. Report if urine output is less than 30 mL/hr.	Alterations in the patient's fluid balance may develop after the procedure. Hypovolemia commonly occurs because the patient may be on NPO status from 6 to 12 hours before the procedure. The radiographic contrast media used during the procedure are hypertonic solutions that increase renal excretion of water. Fluid retention may develop as a compensatory mechanism for decreased cardiac output.
■ Assess for increased restlessness, fatigue, confusion, and disorientation.	Neurological changes can indicate hypoxia caused by decreased cardiac output. Stroke may occur as a complication of procedure.
▲ Monitor arterial blood gases or pulse oximetry as necessary.	These measures provide information on oxygen status. Changes in oxygen saturation of mixed venous blood is one of the earliest indicators of decreased cardiac output. Venous oxygen saturation will be more than 70% with left-to-right shunt. This shunt may occur secondary to the transseptal approach for mitral balloon valvuloplasty.

Therapeutic Interventions

Actions/Interventions	Rationales
■ If signs of hemodynamic compromise are observed, institute treatment for decreased cardiac output, p. 33.	Maintaining an adequate cardiac output is a priority.
• If cardiac output is decreased secondary to fluid volume deficit, anticipate fluid resuscitation.	Administration of IV fluid increases circulatory extracellular fluid volume to raise cardiac output.
• If cardiac output is decreased secondary to valve rupture or tear: • Administer afterload reducers (e.g., sodium nitroprusside).	Medications that reduce afterload contribute to improved cardiac output by decreasing ventricular workload and myocardial oxygen demand.
• Anticipate emergency open heart surgery for valve replacement.	Emergency replacement of a torn or ruptured valve may be the only option to restore cardiac output.
• If cardiac output is decreased secondary to pulmonary hypertension, anticipate use of vasodilators (nitrates, hydralazine).	These medications reduce pulmonary vascular resistance.
■ Administer oxygen therapy as prescribed.	Supplemental oxygen is necessary to increase arterial oxygen saturation above 90%.

Risk for Ineffective Peripheral Tissue Perfusion

Common Risk Factors

Mechanical obstruction from arterial and venous sheaths
Arterial vasospasm
Thrombus formation
Embolization of calcium debris
Bleeding or hematoma
Arterial dissection

Common Expected Outcome

Patient maintains optimal peripheral tissue perfusion in affected extremity as evidenced by strong, palpable pulse, reduction in/absence of pain, warm and dry extremities, and adequate capillary refill.

NOC Outcomes
Circulation Status; Tissue Perfusion: Peripheral

NIC Interventions
Circulatory Care: Arterial Insufficiency; Bleeding Precautions

Ongoing Assessment

Actions/Interventions	Rationales
Preprocedure:	
■ Assess and document presence or absence and quality of all distal pulses.	Risk for arterial occlusion is high. Distal pulses provide baseline for serial assessments.
■ Obtain Doppler ultrasonic reading for faint, nonpalpable pulses. Indicate if pulse check is with Doppler. Mark location of faint pulses with an X.	Marking the pulse site ensures consistency in assessing peripheral pulses during postprocedure monitoring.
■ Assess and document skin color and temperature, presence or absence of pain, numbness, tingling, movement, and sensation of all extremities.	Knowledge of baseline circulatory status of extremities will assist in monitoring for postprocedure changes.
Postprocedure:	
■ Assess presence and quality of pulses distal to arterial cannulation site.	Embolization from the femoral insertion site may cause distal acute arterial occlusion.
■ Check cannulation site for bleeding, swelling, and hematoma.	Lack of hemostasis at the arterial cannulation site contributes to the development of compartment syndrome by constricting vessels and compressing nerves.

Therapeutic Interventions

Actions/Interventions	Rationales
Postprocedure:	
■ Ensure safety measures to prevent displacement of arterial and venous sheaths.	Significant changes in position cause sheath to bend or move, which fosters potential bleeding and dislodgment.
• Maintain bed rest.	
• Keep cannulated extremity in neutral position at all times. Apply knee or leg immobilizer or soft restraint.	
• Do not elevate head of bed more than 30 degrees.	
• Assist with meals, use of bedpan, and position changes appropriate to activity limitations.	
▲ Continue prescribed dose of heparin infusion. Check partial thromboplastin time (PTT) and activated clotting time (ACT) 4 hours after start of infusion and after change in dose.	PTT is usually kept at 1½ to 2 times control. ACT can assist in determining when the sheath can be removed (ACT less than 150 to 180 sec).

■ = Independent   ▲ = Collaborative

Cardiac and Vascular Care Plans

Actions/Interventions

- Do passive range-of-motion exercises to unaffected extremities every 2 to 4 hours as tolerated.
- Instruct patient to immediately report presence of pain, numbness, tingling, and decrease or loss of sensation and movement.
- Immediately report to physician decrease or loss of pulse, change in skin color and temperature, presence of pain, numbness, tingling, delayed capillary refill, and decrease or loss of sensation and motion.
- If ineffective tissue perfusion is noted, anticipate removal of the catheter sheath.
- ▲ Prepare for possible embolectomy.

Rationales

ROM exercises prevent venous stasis and joint stiffness.

The patient needs to understand the meaning these symptoms represent for quick assessment, diagnosis, and treatment of complications.

Signs of compartment syndrome require immediate intervention to prevent tissue ischemia.

Presence of catheter sheath may obstruct blood flow and cause further complications.

Embolectomy is indicated to remove a blood clot obstructing or compromising circulation.

NANDA-I NDx **Risk for Bleeding**

Common Risk Factors

Treatment related to side effects
   Presence of large catheter sheaths usually left in place until clotting times are back to normal)
   Medications (heparinization/antiplatelets)
Arterial trauma
Abnormal blood profiles

Common Expected Outcomes

Patient does not experience bleeding.
Patient maintains therapeutic blood level of anticoagulant, as evidenced by PTT/PT/INR within desired ranges.

NOC Outcome
Blood Coagulation
NIC Interventions
Bleeding Precautions; Bleeding Reduction: Wound

Ongoing Assessment

Actions/Interventions

- Assess cannulation site for evidence of bleeding. Note amount of drainage if fresh blood is noted on the dressing. Circle or outline the size of any hematoma.

- Assess for signs of retroperitoneal bleeding.

- Postprocedure, monitor vital signs until stable.

- ▲ Monitor INR, prothrombin time, PTT, ACT, and platelets as appropriate.

Rationales

Fresh blood on dressing, oozing from cannulation site, pain, tenderness, swelling, and hematoma are all signs of bleeding. Identifying the size of the hematoma allows for serial comparisons.

Signs of retroperitoneal bleeding may include abdomen, flank, or thigh pain, loss of lower extremity pulse, or drop in hemoglobin level and hematocrit.

Increased heart rate and decreased blood pressure are initial compensatory mechanisms commonly noted with bleeding.

Laboratory tests provide information on coagulation status. Usually PTT is kept at 1½ to 2 times control for patients receiving heparin. Sheaths are usually removed when ACT is less than 150 to 180 seconds, depending on policy.

Actions/Interventions

- If significant bleeding occurs:
  - Monitor vital signs at least every 15 minutes until bleeding is controlled, and hold pressure above the site until hemostasis is restored.
  - Observe for neurovascular compromise in the affected extremity.

Rationales

Vigilant monitoring reduces risk for further complications.

Therapeutic Interventions

Actions/Interventions

Before removal of catheter sheaths:

- Maintain bed rest with patient in supine position with affected extremity straight.
- Do not elevate head of bed more than 30 degrees. Observe appropriate positioning for meals, bowel and bladder elimination, and position changes.
- Avoid sudden movement of affected extremity.

- Instruct patient to apply light pressure on dressing when coughing, sneezing, or raising head off pillow.
- Instruct patient to notify nurse immediately of signs of bleeding from cannulation site (e.g., feeling of wetness, warmth, "pop" at catheter sheath site, feeling of faintness).
- ▲ Administer heparin drip through infusion pump.

- ▲ If significant bleeding occurs:
  - Turn off heparin drip, and notify the physician immediately.
  - Remove dressing, and apply manual pressure or mechanical clamp directly above bleeding site or over artery.
  - Anticipate fluid challenge.

  - Administer protamine sulfate as ordered.
  - Anticipate removal of catheter sheaths.

After removal of catheter sheaths:

- ▲ Maintain occlusive pressure dressing on cannulation site for 20 to 30 minutes.
- Maintain bed rest in supine position with affected extremity straight for prescribed time.
- Instruct patient to avoid sudden movement of affected extremity.
- ▲ Resume mobilization and ambulation as prescribed.

Rationales

Length of time for sheath insertion varies according to type of procedure, institutional policy, and any procedural complications.

This position facilitates clot formation to preserve hemostasis and minimizes the risk for bleeding from cannulation site.

Significant changes in position cause catheter to bend or move, which interferes with clot formation and can facilitate bleeding.

Gradual and controlled position changes prevent this prevents displacement of catheter sheaths (may cause bleeding).

These measures facilitate clot formation.

Educating patients of such interventions can prevent complications from clot being dislodged.

Heparin anticoagulation is initiated during the procedure and for at least 4 to 6 hours afterward to prevent thrombus formation. Institutional policies may vary.

Rapid, efficient intervention is required.

Pressure devices provide temporary hemostasis and halt bleeding.

Fluid resuscitation expands blood volume and raises blood pressure.

Protamine sulfate reverses effect of heparin.

Sheath removal facilitates more optimal sealing of insertion site.

Care is guided by institutional protocols. Ice packs, sandbags, and mechanical clamps may be used to stop initial bleeding.

This position promotes clot formation.

This restriction facilitates clot formation and wound closure at the insertion site.

Protocols may vary according to institutional policy and type of procedure.

Related Care Plans

Anxiety, p. 18
Deficient fluid volume, p. 72
Fear, p. 69
Impaired physical mobility, p. 133

■ = Independent ▲ = Collaborative

Percutaneous Coronary Intervention: Percutaneous Transluminal Coronary Angioplasty (PTCA), Atherectomy, Stents

Intracoronary Stenting; Drug-Eluting Stents; Directional Atherectomy (DCA); Intracoronary Radiation; Brachytherapy

These interventions provide a means to nonsurgically improve coronary blood flow and revascularize the myocardium. A variety of procedures have been developed, although percutaneous transluminal coronary angioplasty (PTCA) remains the mainstay. Unfortunately, restenosis remains a critical problem with all techniques. Interventional procedures may be performed in combination with the diagnostic coronary angiogram, electively after diagnostic evaluation, or urgently if there is suspicion of coronary artery blockage in the setting of unstable angina or acute myocardial infarction (MI).

PTCA: This procedure uses a balloon-tipped catheter that is positioned at the site of the lesion. Multiple balloon inflations are performed until the artery is satisfactorily dilated to restore blood flow. The number of PTCA procedures performed annually continues to rise, especially among the older population, particularly older women, because of the risks associated with coronary artery bypass graft surgery for these patients.

Coronary atherectomy: This term refers to removal of plaque material by excision. It may be performed in conjunction with PTCA or stenting and continues to be applied to a wider patient domain that includes patients with multivessel disease and complex coronary anatomy. Atherectomy may be more effective than PTCA for more calcified lesions. Two types of devices have been developed:

1. *Directional:* has a rotating cutter blade that shaves the plaque. The tissue obtained is collected in a cone for removal. It is indicated for lesions with calcification or thrombus and for those at the ostium of a vessel.
2. *Rotational:* uses a burr at the tip of the catheter, which rotates at high speeds to grind up hard plaque. The removed pulverized microparticles are released into the distal circulation rather than collected as in directional atherectomy.

Intracoronary stents: These metallic coils are inserted after balloon dilation or atherectomy, or they are used alone, to provide structural support ("internal scaffolding") to the vessel. The stent remains in place as the catheter is removed. Because of the thrombogenic nature of the stent, anticoagulation and antiplatelet therapy are indicated for an indefinite period of time. These stents have reduced restenosis rates significantly. The newest models are "drug-eluding" stents that have an imbedded amount of medication, sometimes in a thin polymer for time release, and that inhibit new cell and tissue growth and prevent neointimal hyperplasia and restenosis. They have reduced typical restenosis rates to single digits. Additional antiplatelet therapy is needed for a year or more.

Brachytherapy: This technique uses intracoronary radiation to treat in-stent stenosis. It uses either gamma or beta radiation isotopes. The use of drug-eluting stents has reduced the need for this therapy.

Coronary laser angioplasty: This technique uses laser energy to treat in-stent stenosis.

NANDA-I NDx Deficient Knowledge

Common Related Factors	Defining Characteristics
Unfamiliarity with procedure	Requests for more information
Information misinterpretation	Statement of misconception
Cognitive limitation	Verbalization of problem
Lack of exposure/recall	Increase in anxiety level

Common Expected Outcome

Patient verbalizes understanding of heart anatomy and physiology, coronary artery disease (CAD), anticipated procedure, and follow-up therapies.

NOC Outcomes
Knowledge: Disease Process; Knowledge: Treatment Procedure

NIC Interventions
Teaching: Disease Process; Teaching: Procedure or Treatment

Ongoing Assessment

Actions/Interventions	Rationales
■ Assess patient's knowledge of cardiac anatomy and physiology, CAD, and anticipated procedure.	Patients must have correct information to give informed consent. This may be a first-time procedure for some or a repeat procedure for others because of high restenosis rates and the progressive nature of atherosclerosis.

Therapeutic Interventions

Actions/Interventions	Rationales
■ Encourage patient to verbalize questions and concerns.	Patients are anxious about the procedure and the possible outcomes and may have difficulty asking questions and interpreting information. Even patients who have undergone prior procedures may be fearful of the possible outcome with this procedure. A lower anxiety level will enable patient to cooperate better during the procedure.
■ Provide information about the following:	
• Heart anatomy and physiology; CAD	This knowledge helps the patient understand the rationale for procedure.
• Indications for interventional procedure	Patients with significant obstruction (70% to 100%) in areas reachable by catheterization are the best candidates.
• Type of procedure: PTCA versus atherectomy and use of stents	Some patients want to be involved in decision making regarding the type of procedure to be performed. However, they may lack knowledge regarding technical aspects and complications that guide such decision making.
• Vessels requiring intervention	These may be single lesions or vessels or multiple lesions and vessels; the vessels may be calcified or not calcified.
• Success rate	The success rate is greater than 90% in most cardiac centers.
• Procedure room environment: catheterization laboratory	Anxiety can be reduced when patient knows what to expect.
• Expected length of procedure	Patients need to understand that the length of the procedure depends on the number of vessels attempted, vessel anatomy, complications, and number of catheters required.
• Sensations that may be experienced during the procedure: • Warm, flushing, nauseous feeling and metallic taste when dye is injected • Pressure or skipped heartbeats as the catheter is advanced • Chest pain while balloon is inflated • Slow heart rate (HR) or low blood pressure (BP) because of vasovagal response or injection of contrast medium • Tachycardia and rapid pulse also possible	Patients may have less anxiety during the procedure when they know expectations and understand that these sensations are normal.

■ = Independent   ▲ = Collaborative

Actions/Interventions

- Patient will be awake during the procedure.
- Postprocedure expectations:

  - Expected discomfort

  - Frequent monitoring of vital signs and peripheral pulses
  - Possible complications: abrupt closure of artery, acute MI, bleeding, pseudoaneurysm, retroperitoneal bleeding, arteriovenous (AV) fistula, stroke, dissection requiring emergency coronary artery bypass graft surgery
- Immediate postprocedure care as follows:
  - Activity restrictions: lying flat with affected site straight until femoral introducer sheath is removed, vessel has sealed, and hemostasis is achieved
  - Importance of drinking fluids

  - Monitoring for complications

- Recovery:
  - Avoidance of lifting heavy objects for 1 week

  - No tub baths for 3 days
  - Possible return to work within 1 week per physician's discretion
  - When to notify physician (e.g., chest pain, bleeding, infection)
  - Medications, especially aspirin and Plavix

- Include cardiac clinical nurse specialist, catheter laboratory nurse, coronary care nurses, and dietitian as resource persons.

Rationales

Maintaining consciousness facilitates any reporting of chest pain and assists in the patient being able to vigorously cough and breathe deeply at designated times to circulate dye, position the catheter, and increase HR and BP.

Local anesthetic is used to reduce discomfort at insertion site. The patient may be uncomfortable when the PTCA balloon is inflated secondary to reduced coronary blood flow. Patients often report discomfort from lying on the hard radiograph table with restricted movement for a prolonged period (1 to 4 hours).

Data assist in detecting possible hemodynamic complications.

Patients need to be aware of potential complications so they can evaluate risk/benefit when giving informed consent.

This sheath is usually left in the artery until the activated clotting time (ACT) is within acceptable range (less than 180 seconds) or per institution policy.

Patients are allowed nothing by mouth before the procedure and may experience hypovolemia secondary to dye-induced diuresis and the effects of vasodilator medications. Fluids flush dye from the system, reduce risk for renal complications, and promote hydration. Older patients may be more susceptible to the hypovolemic effects of the procedure.

Common complications include bleeding at site, especially with the use of several simultaneous antiplatelet medications before, during, and after the procedure, and restenosis of vessel.

Most patients are discharged the same day. Patients need to be aware of potential complications to facilitate prompt intervention in case of an emergency.

Baths can increase risk for infection at the insertion site.

A variety of medication regimens are used depending on type of percutaneous coronary intervention performed and whether the procedure was related to an acute coronary syndrome. The primary medication focus post procedure centers on antiplatelets to prevent restenosis. Compliance with prescribed antiplatelets is key to preventing restenosis, especially when drug-eluting stents are used. Other medications can include calcium channel blockers, nitrates, angiotensin-converting enzyme inhibitors, and β-blockers.

Specialty expertise may be needed to achieve successful outcomes.

Acute Chest Pain

Common Related Factors

Myocardial ischemia caused by abrupt closure of affected coronary artery, coronary artery spasm, and possible MI
Residual pain from manipulation or dilation of coronary artery
Pain resulting from medical treatment

Defining Characteristics

Patient reports pain
Guarding behavior
Self-focused
Restlessness and apprehension
Facial mask of pain
Increased BP and increased HR
ST-segment and/or T-wave changes

Common Expected Outcomes

Patient reports satisfactory pain control at a level less than 3 to 4 on a 0 to 10 rating scale.
Patient exhibits increased comfort such as baseline levels for BP, pulse, respirations, and relaxed muscle tone or body posture.

NOC Outcomes
Pain Control; Comfort Status; Medication Response

NIC Interventions
Cardiac Care: Acute: Analgesic Administration; Pain Management

Ongoing Assessment

Actions/Interventions

■ Assess for chest pain characteristics associated with myocardial ischemia.
■ Monitor electrocardiogram for signs of ST-T wave changes reflective of myocardial ischemia or spasm.
■ Assess HR and BP during episode of pain.

▲ Obtain serial creatine kinase–MB (CK-MB) measurements (6 to 8 hours and 16 to 24 hours postprocedure).

■ Monitor patient response to effectiveness of treatment.

Rationales

Abrupt closure usually has a presenting symptom pattern similar to pain before the interventional procedure.
ST-segment elevation is commonly seen with abrupt closure of the coronary artery.
Attention to hemodynamic signs may help the nurse in evaluating pain; occurrence of pain after the procedure can be very frightening for the patient.
Elevated CK-MB levels of 5 to 8 times the upper normal limit is considered to be an MI and should be treated as such. A downward trend is expected.
The effects of both oral and intravenous (IV) medications must be monitored. IV medications can be further titrated to relieve pain.

Therapeutic Interventions

Actions/Interventions

■ Instruct the patient to report pain immediately.

■ Notify the physician of chest pain immediately.

▲ Administer medications as ordered:
• Nitroglycerin

• Calcium channel blockers

Rationales

Abrupt closure results from elastic recoil of the vessel and/or thrombosis. It is important that relief measures be initiated before additional myocardium is jeopardized.
It is important to differentiate expected residual pain from coronary dilation and manipulation from pain related to vessel closure. The physician needs to make the distinction.

Nitroglycerin is useful for arterial spasm that is a common postprocedure complication.
Calcium channel blockers are useful for arterial spasm.

■ = Independent ▲ = Collaborative

Actions/Interventions

- Morphine sulfate

- Antiplatelets and glycoprotein IIB/IIIA or adenosine diphosphate (ADP) inhibitors
■ Anticipate the need for possible emergency cardiac catheterization and repeat procedure.
■ Stay with the patient during pain.

Rationales

Morphine is useful for analgesic effect and for reducing myocardial ischemia by decreasing preload.

These medications are used to reduce clotting and prevent microembolization.

Abrupt closure occurs most often in the catheterization laboratory or during the first 24 hours.

Nursing presence provides emotional support and reassurance.

Risk for Bleeding

Common Risk Factors

Treatment related to side effects
- Presence of large catheter sheaths usually left in place until clotting times are back to normal
- Medications (heparinization/antiplatelets)
Arterial trauma
Abnormal blood profiles

Common Expected Outcomes

Patient does not experience bleeding.
Patient maintains therapeutic blood level of anticoagulant, as evidenced by PTT within desired range.

NOC Outcome
Blood Coagulation
NIC Interventions
Bleeding Precautions; Bleeding Reduction: Wound

Ongoing Assessment

Actions/Interventions

■ Assess cannulation site for evidence of bleeding. Note amount of drainage if fresh blood is noted on the dressing.

■ Assess for signs of retroperitoneal bleeding.

■ After procedure, monitor vital signs until patient's condition is stable.
▲ Monitor partial thromboplastin time (PTT), ACT, and platelets as appropriate.

■ Assess circle or outline of hematoma. Circle or outline the size of any hematoma.
■ If significant bleeding occurs:
- Monitor vital signs at least every 15 minutes until bleeding is controlled.
- Observe for neurovascular compromise in the affected extremity.
- Hold pressure above the site over the artery until hemostasis is achieved.

Rationales

Fresh blood on dressing, oozing, pain, tenderness, swelling, and hematoma are all signs of bleeding. Identifying the size of the hematoma allows for serial comparisons.

Signs of retroperitoneal bleeding may include abdominal, flank, or thigh pain; loss of lower extremity pulses; or drop in hemoglobin.

Increased HR and decreased BP are initial compensatory mechanisms commonly noted with bleeding.

These laboratory results provide information on coagulation status. Usually PTT is kept at 1½ to 2 times control. Sheaths can usually be removed when the ACT is less than 150 to 180 seconds depending on policy.

Presence of hematoma indicates bleeding under the skin that can compress nerves and decrease tissue perfusion.

Vigilant monitoring reduces risk for further complications.

Therapeutic Interventions

Actions/Interventions	Rationales
Before removal of catheter sheaths:	Length of time for sheath insertion varies according to type of procedure (i.e., stents require longer anticoagulation and longer insertion times), institutional policy, and any procedural complication.
■ Maintain bed rest with patient in supine position with affected extremity straight.	This position facilitates clot formation to preserve hemostasis and minimizes risk for bleeding from cannulation site.
■ Do not elevate head of bed more than 30 degrees. Observe appropriate positioning for meals, bowel and bladder elimination, and position changes.	Significant changes in position cause catheter to bend or move, which interferes with clot formation and can facilitate bleeding. Comfort issues need to be addressed by nursing staff.
■ Avoid sudden movement of affected extremity.	Gradual and controlled position changes prevent displacement of catheter sheaths (may cause bleeding).
■ Instruct patient to apply light pressure on dressing when coughing, sneezing, or raising head off pillow.	These measures facilitate clot formation and prevent dislodgment.
■ Instruct patient to notify nurse immediately of signs of bleeding from cannulation site (e.g., feeling of wetness, warmth, "pop" at catheter sheath site, feeling of faintness).	Educating patients on such intervention can prevent complications from clot being dislodged.
▲ Administer antiplatelet agents.	Antiplatelet therapies are especially required after stent placement. This area is receiving much research because a balance must be achieved between aggressive therapy to reduce restenosis and the risk for bleeding. Current agents include glycoprotein IIB/IIIA receptor inhibitors (e.g., abciximab [ReoPro], tirofiban [Aggrastat], and eptifibatide [Integrilin]). Research has shown these agents to decrease ischemic complications.
▲ If significant bleeding occurs: • Notify physician immediately. • Remove dressing, and apply manual pressure or mechanical clamp directly above bleeding site or over artery. • Anticipate fluid challenge. • Anticipate removal of catheter sheaths.	Rapid, efficient intervention is required. This procedure provides temporary hemostasis and halts bleeding. Fluid resuscitation expands blood volume and raises BP. Sheath removal may facilitate more optimal sealing of insertion site.
After removal of catheter sheaths:	
■ Maintain occlusive pressure dressing on cannulation site for 20 to 30 minutes.	Ice packs, sandbags, and mechanical clamps may be used to stop initial bleeding. Selection of adjunct device depends on physician preference and policy.
■ Maintain bed rest in supine position with affected extremity straight for prescribed time.	This positioning promotes clot formation.
■ Instruct patient to avoid sudden movement of affected extremity.	This facilitates clot formation and wound closure at the insertion site.
▲ Resume mobilization and ambulation as prescribed.	Protocols may vary according to institutional policy and type of procedure performed.
▲ Prepare for diagnostic imaging (computed tomography [CT] scan of abdomen, ultrasound).	Testing confirms assessment of complications such as fistula, retroperitoneal bleed, and pseudoaneurysm.

Cardiac and Vascular Care Plans

■ = Independent   ▲ = Collaborative

NANDA-I NDx ## Ineffective Peripheral Tissue Perfusion

Common Related Factors

Mechanical obstruction from arterial and venous sheaths
Arterial vasospasm
Thrombus formation
Embolization
Immobility
Swelling of tissues
Bleeding or hematoma
Arterial dissection

Defining Characteristics

Decrease or loss of peripheral pulses
Decrease in skin temperature of extremity
Presence of mottling, pallor, cyanosis, and rubor in skin of distal affected extremity
Delayed capillary refill in affected extremity
Decrease or loss of sensation and motion

Common Expected Outcome

Patient maintains optimal peripheral tissue perfusion in affected extremity, as evidenced by strong palpable pulse, reduction in/absence of pain, warm and dry extremities, and adequate capillary refill.

NOC Outcomes

Circulatory Status; Tissue Perfusion: Peripheral

NIC Interventions

Circulation Care: Arterial Insufficiency; Bleeding Precautions

---

Ongoing Assessment

Actions/Interventions

Preprocedure:
- Assess and document presence or absence and quality of all distal pulses.
- Obtain Doppler ultrasonic reading for faint, nonpalpable pulses. Indicate whether pulse check is with Doppler ultrasound. Mark location of faint pulses with an X.
- Assess and document skin color and temperature, presence or absence of pain, numbness, tingling, movement, and sensation of all extremities.

Postprocedure:
- Assess presence and quality of pulses distal to arterial cannulation site (radial for brachial artery, dorsalis pedis, and/or posterior tibial pulses for femoral artery) until stable.
- Check cannulation site for bleeding, swelling, and hematoma.

- Assess for pseudoaneurysm (pulsatile mass, systolic bruit, groin pain).

- Assess for arteriovenous (AV) fistula (pulsatile mass, groin pain, continuous bruit).
- Assess for retroperitoneal bleed.

Rationales

Risk for arterial occlusion is high. Distal pulses provide baseline for serial assessments.
Marking site of pulse ensures consistency in assessing peripheral pulses.

Knowledge of baseline circulatory status of extremities will assist in monitoring for postprocedure changes.

Arterial thrombosis at puncture site may lead to occlusion of artery or distal thrombosis into extremity.

Lack of hemostasis at the arterial cannulation site contributes to the development of compartment syndrome by constricting vessels or compressing nerves. Large hematomas can dissect into the retroperitoneum and be life threatening.
Pseudoaneurysm is an extraluminal cavity in communication with the adjacent femoral artery. Its presence is best confirmed by Doppler ultrasound.
AV fistula is a communication between an artery and vein. Its presence is best assessed by Doppler ultrasound.
Bleeding behind retroperitoneal cavity is best confirmed by stat CT scan of abdomen. Clinical picture includes abdominal/flank pain with increased pulse and decreased hemoglobin.

Therapeutic Interventions

Actions/Interventions	Rationales
Postprocedure:	
■ Ensure safety measures to prevent displacement of arterial and venous sheaths: • Maintain bed rest. • Keep cannulated extremity in neutral or slightly flexed position. • Apply knee or leg immobilizer or soft restraint. • Do not elevate head of bed more than 30 degrees. • Assist with meals, use of bedpan, and position changes appropriate to activity limitations.	Significant changes in position cause the sheath to bend or move, which fosters potential bleeding and dislodgment. Researchers continue investigating benefits of early sheath removal and early ambulation.
▲ Continue prescribed dose of antiplatelets. Check clotting times periodically after start of infusion and after change in dose.	Antiplatelets reduce ischemic complications and systemic clot formation. Patients with stent implantation require more aggressive anticoagulation until endothelialization occurs around the stent.
■ Do passive range-of-motion exercises to unaffected extremities every 2 to 4 hours as tolerated.	ROM exercises prevent venous stasis and joint stiffness.
■ Instruct patient to report presence of pain, numbness, tingling, and decrease or loss of sensation and movement immediately.	The patient needs to understand the meaning these symptoms represent for quick assessment, diagnosis, and treatment of complications.
▲ Immediately report to physician decrease or loss of pulse, change in skin color and temperature, presence of pain, numbness, tingling, delayed capillary refill, and decrease or loss of sensation and motion.	Signs of compartment syndrome require immediate intervention.
■ If ineffective tissue perfusion is noted, anticipate removal of catheter sheath.	Presence of catheter sheaths may obstruct blood flow and cause further complications.
▲ Prepare for possible embolectomy.	Embolectomy is indicated to remove blood clot obstructing or compromising circulation.

Related Care Plans

Anxiety, p. 18
Deficient fluid volume, p. 72
Impaired physical mobility, p. 133

Peripheral Arterial Revascularization

Femoral Popliteal Bypass; Percutaneous Transluminal Angioplasty (PTA)

Chronic peripheral arterial occlusive disease (PAD) is most commonly caused by atherosclerosis resulting in reduced arterial blood flow to peripheral tissues. Complications associated with arterial insufficiency include pain in the leg(s), ulcers or wounds that do not heal, and progressive amputation of the affected extremity. Revascularization is indicated when medical management is ineffective. Revascularization procedures are available to treat PAD of the femoral arteries with the goals of improving tissue perfusion, preventing tissue necrosis, reducing pain, and limb salvage. This care plan focuses on preoperative teaching and postprocedure care.

Femoral Popliteal Bypass Surgery: This procedure involves a surgical opening of the upper leg to directly visualize the femoral artery. It is performed to bypass the occluded arterial segment in the femoral artery using another blood vessel such as the saphenous vein or a synthetic material such as Dacron or Gore-Tex that is attached to the popliteal artery either above or below the knee. This allows rerouting the blood flow around the obstruction to optimize peripheral circulation. The distal vessel must be at least 50% patent for the grafts to remain patent. Additional locations along the arterial system can be bypassed. An aortoiliac endarterectomy can also be performed whereby the atheromatous plaque is removed and the vessel is sutured to restore circulation.

Percutaneous transluminal angioplasty (PTA): This minimally invasive endovascular procedure uses balloon-tipped catheters that are positioned at the site of the lesion or blockage. Multiple balloon inflations are performed until the atherosclerotic plaque is compressed and the artery is satisfactorily dilated. A stent (tiny, expandable metal coil) may be inserted into the newly opened area to provide structural support to the vessel. The stent remains in place as the deflated balloon catheter is removed. These stents can reduce restenosis rates.

 Deficient Knowledge

Common Related Factor

New procedure

Defining Characteristics

Multiple questions
Lack of questions
Misconceptions of health status
Request for information
Display of anxiety and/or fear
Noncompliance
Inability to verbalize health maintenance regimen
Development of complications

Common Expected Outcome

Patient verbalizes understanding of anticipated procedure and related care.

NOC Outcomes
Knowledge: Disease Process; Knowledge: Treatment Procedure

NIC Interventions
Teaching: Disease Process; Teaching: Procedure or Treatment

Ongoing Assessment

Actions/Interventions	Rationales
■ Assess knowledge regarding revascularization procedure being planned and the postprocedure management.	Thorough understanding of indications for care related to the revascularization procedure is necessary for informed consent to be given.

Therapeutic Interventions

Actions/Interventions	Rationales
■ Provide information about the etiology and physiology of peripheral arterial disease and indications for the procedure at this time.	Atherosclerosis is a progressive disease. Once medical management has not improved symptoms and patient exhibits ischemic pain at rest or significant disability or may be in danger of losing the limb from reduced peripheral circulation, then invasive revascularization measures are indicated.

Actions/Interventions	**Rationales**
■ Provide information on the revascularization procedure selected for patient: Femoral-popliteal bypass versus percutaneous transluminal angioplasty/stenting.	Some patients want to be involved in decision making regarding type of procedure to be performed. However, they may lack knowledge regarding the technical aspects and complications that guide such decision making. Not all disease can be treated with PTA, and not all patients may be candidates for a surgical procedure. The best procedure is based on individual circumstances.
■ Provide information regarding the specifics of the planned procedure:	Anxiety can be reduced when patients know what to expect.

■ Provide information regarding the specifics of the planned procedure:
  • PTAs/stents are mostly done as outpatient procedures.
  • The patient is allowed nothing by mouth (NPO) before and immediately after the procedure
  • Bypass surgery may be performed with general anesthesia (with tracheal intubation) or conscious sedation/local anesthesia; PTA is performed with conscious sedation and local anesthesia.
  • For surgical procedures the incision will be sutured together. For PTA the insertion site will be held with manual pressure or a closure device may be used.

■ Provide information on postprocedure expectations:	
• Frequent circulatory assessments below the surgical/PTA site	This information relieves patient anxiety about staff's need for frequent pulse checks.
• Activity restrictions: lying flat with affected and arteriotomy sites straight until hemostasis is achieved	Crossing legs may facilitate thrombus formation and graft closure or bleeding from the surgical site.
• Expected discomfort (encourage patient to notify staff when anesthetic effect wears off)	The site will be tender and sore for several days after the procedure, so early reports of discomfort will facilitate pain management.
• Need to notify nurse of any change in sensation in lower extremities or any bleeding or swelling	This information prevents delay in detecting changes in circulation or any postprocedure complications and allows prompt treatment of any occlusion.
■ Instruct in any medications ordered for postprocedure care (e.g., anticoagulants, antiplatelet medication, vasodilators, antibiotics).	A variety of medication regimens are used depending on the type of revascularization procedure performed. Post-PTA patients require long-term aspirin therapy. Short-term antiplatelet therapy with medications such as clopidogrel to prevent restenosis.
■ Instruct in the following signs or symptoms to report after discharge:	Information enables the patient to assume control during recovery.

  • Increased pain, redness, swelling, or bleeding or other discharge from leg incision
  • Coolness in leg or foot
  • Pain, discomfort, tingling, or numbness
  • Fever/chills

■ Instruct in the need for follow-up appointments and vascular testing to ensure vessel patency.	Duplex ultrasound provides verification of improved blood flow.
■ Clarify that atherosclerosis is a progressive disease and although symptoms have been relieved, the disease has not been cured.	Living with a chronic disease is challenging. Atherosclerosis is a systemic disease and may likewise affect other vital organs like the heart and cerebral circulation.
■ Explain the importance of lifestyle management (e.g., smoking cessation, hypertension management, exercise, low-fat diet) as appropriate.	Information provides rationale for therapy and aids patient in assuming responsibility for required lifestyle changes.

Cardiac and Vascular Care Plans

■ = Independent   ▲ = Collaborative

Risk for Ineffective Peripheral Tissue Perfusion

Common Risk Factors

Graft occlusion
Edema
Hypotension
Hematoma or bleeding
Compartment syndrome
Thrombus formation
Embolization
Arterial vasospasm
Restenosis
Arterial dissection

Common Expected Outcome

Patient maintains optimal peripheral tissue perfusion in affected extremity, as evidenced by adequate arterial pulsation distal to graft/PTA; no increase in limb pain; resolution of edema/warm skin in affected extremity, and evidence of normal wound healing.

NOC Outcomes
Circulation Status; Tissue Perfusion: Peripheral
NIC Interventions
Circulatory Care; Arterial Insufficiency; Lower Extremity Monitoring; Circulatory Status: Venous

Ongoing Assessment

Actions/Interventions	Rationales
■ Mark distal pulses (pedal and posterior tibial) with skin marker, and check every hour. Note pulse presence and strength. Compare with the side that was not operated on. Use Doppler ultrasound if needed for nonpalpable pulses.	Risk for arterial occlusion is high in the immediate postoperative period. Distal pulses indicate arterial patency.
■ Assess the patient's level of pain in affected limb. Signs of occlusion include the following: pain, pulselessness, poikilothermia (coolness), pallor, paralysis, or paresthesia.	Compartment syndrome can occur from local swelling around the fascial compartment of the leg. Signs include severe pain, decreased sensation, and hard, swollen leg. Saphenous nerve damage may occur as a result of dissection or trauma. Patients with acute arterial occlusion may report pain unrelieved by analgesics. Rapid intervention is critical to preserve circulation to limb.
■ Monitor blood pressure (BP).	Hypotension can reduce blood flow to the periphery. An increased BP can cause bleeding or hematoma.
■ During dressing changes, assess for presence of bleeding, swelling, and/or hematoma. Notify physician immediately if present.	These complications may hinder peripheral circulation by constricting vessels or compressing nerves. Large hematomas can dissect into the retroperitoneum and can be life threatening.

Therapeutic Interventions

Actions/Interventions	Rationales
■ Gently reposition patient every 1 to 2 hours. Instruct in importance of keeping affected extremity in neutral or slightly flexed position.	Ninety-degree flexion of hip can cause kinking in graft, which may precipitate clot formation or impair blood flow.

Actions/Interventions

■ Initiate prescribed activity according to institutional policy and patient's condition.

▲ Maintain adequate fluid intake.

■ Ensure that the incisional site is easily visualized; instruct patient or family to notify staff if bleeding is noted.
■ Administer anticoagulation therapy as ordered.
■ If bleeding is noted, administer intravenous fluids, colloids, and blood products as prescribed.

Rationales

The leg is not usually elevated in bed unless limb edema is evident. When the patient is sitting in a chair, elevate the leg to prevent edema. Progressive ambulation is typically initiated 1 day after the procedure.
Fluids promote effective circulating volume throughout the arterial system.
Vigilant monitoring helps reduce complications.

Risk for graft occlusion by thrombosis and restenosis is high.
Specific deficiencies guide treatment therapy.

NANDA-I NDx **Acute Pain**

Common Related Factors
Incision
Occlusion
Restenosis
Compartment syndrome

Defining Characteristics
Patient reports pain
Guarding behavior, protective self-focusing, and narrowed focus
Facial mask of pain
Alteration in muscle tone (rigid, tense)

Common Expected Outcome
Patient reports satisfactory pain control at a level less than 3 to 4 on a 0 to 10 rating scale.
Patient exhibits increased comfort such as baseline levels for BP, pulse, respirations and relaxed muscle tone or body posture.

NOC Outcome
Pain Level
NIC Intervention
Pain Management

Ongoing Assessment

Actions/Interventions

■ Assess pain characteristics.

■ Monitor effectiveness of analgesic and/or therapies used to reduce pain.

Rationales

The description of pain can help differentiate between incisional pain and pain from graft occlusion, restenosis, or compartment syndrome.
Pain caused by more than incisional discomfort may not respond to analgesics and may require emergency intervention.

Therapeutic Interventions

Actions/Interventions

▲ Anticipate the need for analgesics, and respond immediately to report of pain.

■ If pain is a result of bypass graft occlusion, anticipate immediate evaluation by the physician or surgeon. Prepare patient for surgical intervention.
■ If pain is caused by acute restenosis after PTA, anticipate need for repeat procedure.

Rationales

Patients have a right to effective pain relief. Patient-controlled analgesia devices may facilitate the patient's sense of control and promote increased comfort.
Rapid intervention is critical to preserve the limb.

Abrupt closure occurs most often during the first 24 hours after procedure. Repeat balloon inflations have longer-lasting benefit.

■ = Independent   ▲ = Collaborative

Actions/Interventions

■ If pain is caused by compartment syndrome, anticipate need for fasciotomy.

Rationales

Rapid intervention is needed to preserve the limb.

Related Care Plans

Peripheral arterial occlusive disease, Chronic, p. 308
Risk for impaired skin integrity, p. 185
Risk for infection, p. 114

Peripheral Arterial Occlusive Disease, Chronic

Intermittent Claudication; Arterial Insufficiency; Arteriosclerosis Obliterans; Percutaneous Transluminal Angioplasty (PTA)

Chronic peripheral arterial occlusive disease is most commonly caused by atherosclerosis resulting in reduced arterial blood flow to peripheral tissues, causing decreased nutrition and oxygenation at the cellular level. It can be characterized by four stages: asymptomatic, claudication, rest pain, and necrosis. Management is directed at removing vasoconstricting factors, improving peripheral blood flow, and reducing metabolic demands on the body. Because atherosclerosis is a progressive disease, older patients experience an increased incidence of this disease. Diabetes mellitus and tobacco use are significant risk factors in the development of chronic arterial insufficiency. Complications associated with arterial insufficiency include necrotic skin ulcers and progressive amputation of the affected extremity. Peripheral arterial disease (PAD) is a major cause of disability, significantly affecting quality of life. It is also a significant predictor of future cardiac and cerebrovascular events and is considered a cardiovascular disease risk equivalent.

NANDA-I NDx Ineffective Peripheral Tissue Perfusion

Common Related Factors

Atherosclerosis
Vasoconstriction secondary to medications and tobacco
Arterial spasm

Defining Characteristics

Pain, cramping, and ache in extremity
Intermittent claudication (cramping pain or weakness in one or both legs, relieved by rest)
Numbness of toes on walking, relieved by rest
Foot pain at rest
Tenderness, especially at toes
Cool extremities
Pallor of toes or foot when leg is elevated for 30 seconds
Dependent rubor (20 seconds to 2 minutes after leg is lowered)
Prolonged capillary refill
Difference in blood pressure (BP) in opposite extremity
Diminished or absent arterial pulses
Shiny skin
Loss of hair
Thickened, discolored nails
Ulcerated areas and gangrene
Bruits

Common Expected Outcome

Patient maintains optimal peripheral tissue perfusion in affected extremity, as evidenced by strong palpable pulse, reduction in/absence in absence of pain, warm and dry extremities, adequate capillary refill, and prevention of ulceration.

NOC Outcomes
Circulation Status; Tissue Perfusion: Peripheral
NIC Interventions
Circulatory Precautions; Circulatory Care;
   Arterial Insufficiency

Ongoing Assessment

Actions/Interventions	Rationales
■ Assess extremities for pain, pallor, paresthesia, poikilothermia (coolness), pulselessness, and paralysis.	This disease occurs primarily in the legs. The extremities manifest pain, numbness and tingling, coolness and pallor, with shiny hairless skin.
■ Assess quality of peripheral pulses, noting presence and strength; assess for bruits in lower extremities. Note capillary refill. If no pulses are noted, assess arterial blood flow using Doppler ultrasonic instrumentation.	Arterial occlusions signify reduced peripheral blood flow and diminished or obliterated peripheral pulses. Routine examination should include palpation of femoral, popliteal, posterior tibial, and dorsalis pedis pulses. The posterior tibial pulse is the most sensitive indicator, in that the dorsalis pedis pulse is absent in approximately 10% of healthy people without disease.
■ Assess skin color changes on elevation and dependent positioning.	In advanced disease, the lower extremities become pale when the leg is elevated as a result of reduced capillary blood flow, and they become red (rubor) when placed in a dependent position.
■ Assess pain, numbness, and tingling for causative factors, time of onset, quality, severity, and relieving factors.	Intermittent claudication is the most common symptom of peripheral vascular disease. It is muscle pain that is precipitated by exercise or activity and is relieved with rest. It commonly occurs in the calf muscles or buttocks. Claudication may not be experienced if patients, especially older patients, have limited their physical activity secondary to cardiac or pulmonary disorders or other contributing problems. Pain that occurs at rest signifies more extensive disease requiring immediate attention. Tingling or numbness represents impaired perfusion to nerve tissue cells.
■ Assess segmental limb pressure measurements such as ankle-brachial index (ABI).	Normally the BP readings in the lower extremities are higher than in the upper extremities. Normal ratio of ankle systolic pressure divided by brachial systolic pressure is 0.9 or greater. An ABI ratio of less than 0.9 in either leg is diagnostic of PAD. A ratio of 0.4 or greater signifies severe disease.
■ Assess for ulcerated areas on the skin.	Ulcers develop from ischemia and are commonly seen over bony prominences and on the toes and feet. Because of impaired tissue perfusion the ulcers become infected easily. If not treated, they can lead to gangrene.
▲ Monitor results of diagnostic tests: pulse volume recordings, vascular stress testing, magnetic resonance angiography, conventional arteriography, and digital subtraction angiography.	These tests are used to identify location and severity of disease; arteriography is useful for patients requiring surgical intervention. Exercise stress testing helps in reproducing claudication and provides data for evaluating the effectiveness of any treatment.

■ = Independent   ▲ = Collaborative

Cardiac and Vascular Care Plans

Therapeutic Interventions

Actions/Interventions	Rationales
■ Maintain affected extremity in a dependent position.	Gravity can increase peripheral blood flow. However, if edema is present in the lower legs, the feet should be elevated.
■ Keep extremity warm (socks or blankets).	Warmth promotes vasodilation and comfort.
■ Encourage need for progressive activity program, noting claudication.	During exercise, tissues do not receive adequate oxygenation from obstructed arteries and convert to anaerobic metabolism, of which lactic acid is a byproduct. Accumulation of lactic acid causes muscle spasm and discomfort. However, gradual progressive exercise helps promote collateral circulation. Patient should be encouraged to walk to the point of claudication, stop and rest, and continue walking.
■ Provide meticulous foot care.	Cleanliness is important to preventing infection. Toenails should be trimmed straight across. Minor trauma can result in skin breakdown.
▲ Administer analgesics as ordered.	The pain caused by chronic PAD is difficult to treat. Analgesics may provide some relief, but antiplatelet and hemorrheologic agents, exercise, and percutaneous or surgical procedures may be more effective.
▲ Provide drug therapy as ordered: • Antiplatelets (aspirin, dipyridamole, clopidogrel)	These medications reduce platelet aggregation and may increase pain-free walking distance and resting limb blood flow.
• Cilostazol (Pletal)	This medication is stronger than routine antiplatelets and causes direct arterial dilation, inhibits platelet aggregation, and improves pain-free walking distance. It should not be used in patients with heart failure. Pentoxifylline is less effective and not used as frequently.
• Lipid-lowering agents	For patients with PAD, the low-density lipoprotein (LDL) lipid goal is <100 mg/dL, and lower for patients with additional risk factors for heart attack and stroke.
■ Explain more-invasive therapies as indicated: percutaneous transluminal angioplasty/stenting, laser-assisted angioplasty, atherectomy, surgical revascularization.	These therapies are appropriate for symptomatic patients for pain relief, to promote ulcer healing, and for limb salvage.

NANDA-I NDx Deficient Knowledge

Common Related Factors
New condition
Lack of resources
Complexity of lifestyle changes expected

Defining Characteristics
Questioning members of health care team
Inaccurate follow-through of instruction
Verbalizing inaccurate information

Common Expected Outcome
Patient verbalizes understanding of self-care measures required to treat disease and prevent complications.

NOC Outcomes
Knowledge: Disease Process; Knowledge: Treatment Regimen
NIC Interventions
Teaching: Disease Process; Teaching: Prescribed Medication; Teaching: Prescribed Activity or Exercise

Ongoing Assessment

Actions/Interventions	Rationales
■ Assess knowledge of physiology of disease and treatment or preventive techniques prescribed.	PAD is a lifelong condition. Patients need to understand the self-care strategies for which they are responsible. Attention should be directed toward treating peripheral disease and reducing risk for cardiovascular and cerebrovascular atherosclerosis.

Therapeutic Interventions

Actions/Interventions	Rationales
■ Instruct in the physiology of blood supply to tissues.	Knowledge of causative factors helps patient understand rationale for therapies.
■ Instruct in prescribed diagnostic tests.	Explaining expected events ahead of time reduces anxiety and facilitates appropriate follow-through.
■ Instruct in how to prevent progression of disease:	The risk factors for atherosclerosis are smoking, hyperlipidemia, hypertension, diabetes mellitus, obesity, sedentary lifestyle, and family history of atherosclerosis. Atherosclerosis is not confined just to the lower extremities; it may occur in the coronary, cerebral, and renal vessels. Risk factor modification early in the disease may slow progression.
• Smoking: • Advise patient to avoid all tobacco. Consider referral to smoking-cessation clinics. • Dietary modification:	Nicotine is a vasoconstrictor and increases blood viscosity, further decreasing already compromised circulation. Smoking is the single risk factor most commonly implicated in the disease and is said to triple the risk for developing claudication.
• Provide diet counseling on need for reduction in saturated fats.	The National Heart, Lung and Blood Institute's Therapeutic Lifestyle Changes diet is an example of a heart-healthy diet plan to reduce lipids and obesity. Because patients with PAD are considered high risk for systemic atherosclerotic disease, their low-density lipoprotein cholesterol goal is less than 100 mg/dL with a goal of less than 70 mg/dL for patients with additional risk factors. Lipid-lowering medications may be required.
• If patient is overweight, provide diet counseling regarding attainment of ideal body weight. • Instruct patients with diabetes in appropriate diet. • Hypertension management	Obesity is a risk factor for PAD and cardiovascular disease. The correlation between diabetes control and the severity of PAD is high. Control of hypertension can improve systemic tissue perfusion.
■ Provide information on a daily exercise program: • Walk on flat surface to reduce calf pain. • Walk about half a block after intermittent claudication is experienced, unless otherwise ordered by the physician. • Stop and rest until all discomfort subsides. • Repeat same procedure for total of 30 minutes two to three times daily.	Exercise is an essential treatment for PAD. When the patient walks to the point of claudication, this ischemic stimulus (buildup of lactic acid) serves to promote enhanced collateral circulation. Once the lactic acid clears from the local blood system with rest, the pain should subside. Repetition serves to increase progress in improving walking ability.

■ Instruct in prevention of complications:
• Effects of temperature:
  • Keep extremities warm. Wear stockings to bed.
  • Keep house or apartment as warm as possible.
  • Wear warm clothes during winter.
  • Never apply hot water bottles or electric heating pads to feet or legs.
  • Avoid local cold applications and cold temperatures.
	Warmth promotes vasodilation. External heating devices must be used with caution, because burns may occur secondary to impaired nerve function. Cold causes vasoconstriction and reduced blood flow.

■ = Independent   ▲ = Collaborative

Cardiac and Vascular Care Plans

Actions/Interventions	Rationales

• Foot care:
  • Inspect daily.
  • Wash feet daily with warm soap and water. Dry thoroughly by gentle patting. Never rub dry.
  • File or trim toenails carefully and only after soaking in warm water. File or trim straight across. See podiatrist as needed.
  • Lubricate skin.
  • Wear clean stockings.
  • Do not walk barefoot.
  • Wear correctly fitting shoes.
  • Inspect feet often for signs of ingrown toenails, sores, blisters, and other concerns.
• Discuss available drug treatment.
	Poor peripheral circulation can result in tissue damage. Early assessment of potential problems reduces complications. Currently, several types of antiplatelet drugs are available. They need to be taken on a long-term basis; thus patient compliance is key to success. Patients with diabetes are at increased risk. In addition, patients with diabetic neuropathy may have no perception of pain or injury. Ulceration or gangrene of the toe or foot may follow mild trauma.

■ Explain that medicines do not replace other preventive or treatment measures.	Exercise, appropriate positioning, and hygienic foot care measures, along with invasive and noninvasive interventions, are required for optimal treatment.
■ Provide information on more-invasive therapies as indicated: • PTA/stents	PTA is a nonsurgical procedure using a balloon catheter to dilate an obstructed artery. Stents are used in conjunction with PTA and atherectomy to maintain patency of blood vessel.
• Atherectomy	Atherectomy uses a special catheter to "shave" away plaque.
• Surgical revascularization	This surgical procedure bypasses atherosclerotic lesion using autogenous saphenous vein or graft made from synthetic material.
• Amputation	Amputation is required if gangrene is present.

NANDA-I NDx Impaired Skin Integrity

Common Related Factors
Pressure over bony prominences
Decreased peripheral tissue perfusion
Trauma to skin

Defining Characteristics
Ulceration over bony prominences, primarily toes and feet
Presence of gangrene
Atrophic skin

Common Expected Outcome
Patient's skin will be intact without signs of ulcers, redness, or infection.
Patient experiences healing of ulcers.

NOC Outcomes
Tissue Integrity: Skin and Mucous Membranes;
  Wound Healing: Secondary Intention
NIC Interventions
Skin Care: Topical Treatments; Wound Care

Ongoing Assessment

Actions/Interventions	Rationales
■ Assess lower extremity circulation: • Skin temperature and color • Pulses and capillary refill • Sensation • Hair and nail growth patterns	Patients with significant arterial insufficiency are at greater risk for the development of skin ulcers. Decreased sensation associated with arterial insufficiency reduces patients' ability to recognize pressure and traumatic injuries. These injuries may go unnoticed until the wound becomes infected.
■ Assess skin for signs of redness, open wounds, and vascular ulcers: • Location • Pain • Ulcer characteristics • Condition of surrounding tissue	Arterial ulcers usually develop over bony prominences of toes and feet or any point of trauma. Patient may report pain that is burning or sharp. Ulcers have a well-defined border with a pale tissue bed. Eschar may be present. Ulcers may have drainage if infection is present. Surrounding tissue is usually pale on elevation or may have dependent rubor.

Therapeutic Interventions

Actions/Interventions	Rationales
■ Protect skin from trauma and prolonged pressure.	The poor peripheral circulation of PAD combined with decreased sensation places the patient at high risk for injury.
■ Cover noninfected wounds with appropriate dressings.	A variety of dressing materials are available to protect arterial ulcers during the healing process. Hydrocolloid dressings that can be left in place for several days have the benefit of reducing skin trauma and infection associated with frequent dressing changes. The wound healing process is often prolonged.
■ Use sterile technique when caring for broken skin or vascular ulcers.	Patient is at risk for wound infections because of decreased arterial blood flow to the tissue.
▲ Prepare for debridement of necrotic tissue from ulcer:	Removal of necrotic tissue from the ulcer is necessary to prevent infection and allow for healing of the wound.
• Surgical debridement	Surgical debridement involves use of instruments to manually cut away necrotic tissue. This procedure may be done at the bedside. The patient usually does not experience pain because tissue is dead. Bleeding will occur when healthy tissue is reached.
• Mechanical debridement	Mechanical debridement is usually accomplished with the application of sterile, wet-to-dry dressings. The wet gauze dressing adheres to the wound surface. Necrotic tissue is pulled away from the wound when the dressing is removed several hours after application.
• Pharmacological debridement	Pharmacological debridement involves the use of enzyme ointments to necrotic tissue in the wound. A sterile dressing is applied.
▲ Administer antibiotics as prescribed.	Antibiotics may be used for infected wounds or to prevent bacteremia. Route of administration may be oral, intravenous, or topical to the wound itself.
■ Measure wound with each dressing change.	Wound should decrease in size as it heals. Regular measurement will aid in evaluating the effectiveness of treatment measures.

Related Care Plans

Peripheral arterial revascularization, p. 303
Pressure ulcers, p. 946

■ = Independent   ▲ = Collaborative

Pulmonary Edema, Acute

Pulmonary Congestion; Cardiogenic Pulmonary Edema; Acute Heart Failure

Pulmonary edema is a pathological state in which there is an abnormal/excessive, diffuse accumulation of fluid in the alveoli and interstitial spaces of the lung. This fluid causes impaired gas exchange by interfering with diffusion between the pulmonary capillaries and the alveoli. It is commonly caused by left ventricular failure, altered capillary permeability of the lungs, adult respiratory distress syndrome, neoplasms, overhydration, and hypoalbuminemia. Acute pulmonary edema is considered a medical emergency.

 NANDA-I NDx **Impaired Gas Exchange**

Common Related Factors

Alveolar-capillary membrane changes
Ventilation-perfusion mismatch

Defining Characteristics

Abnormal arterial blood gases
Hypercapnia
Hypoxemia/hypoxia
Abnormal breathing pattern (rate, rhythm, depth)
Dyspnea
Tachypnea
Cough
Pink, frothy sputum
Crackles
Pulmonary capillary wedge pressure (PCWP) greater than 25 to 30 mm Hg (in intensive care unit setting)
Cyanosis or pallor
Irritability
Restlessness and apprehension
Tachycardia
Diaphoresis

Common Expected Outcome

Patient maintains optimal gas exchange, as evidenced by arterial blood gases (ABGs) within the patient's usual range, oxygen saturation of 90% or greater, alert response mentation or no further reduction in level of consciousness, relaxed breathing, and baseline heart rate (HR) for patient.

NOC Outcomes
Respiratory Status: Gas Exchange; Respiratory Status: Ventilation
NIC Interventions
Respiratory Monitoring; Ventilation Assistance; Medication Administration

Ongoing Assessment

Actions/Interventions

■ Assess respiratory rate and depth, presence of shortness of breath, and use of accessory muscles.

Rationales

Patients will adapt their breathing pattern over time to facilitate gas exchange. In the early stages, there is mild increase in respiratory rate. As it progresses, severe dyspnea, gurgling respirations, use of accessory muscles, and extreme breathlessness, as if "drowning" in one's own secretions, are noted.

Actions/Interventions

- Assess character of any secretions.

- Assess breath sounds in all fields, noting aerations and presence of wheezes and crackles in lung bases. Document precise location.
- Assess for diaphoresis, headache, and change in level of consciousness.

- Monitor vital signs.

- ▲ Use pulse oximeter to monitor oxygen saturation.

- ▲ Monitor serial arterial blood gases, and note changes.

- Assess skin, nail beds, and mucous membranes for pallor or cyanosis.

- ▲ Monitor chest x-ray reports.

Rationales

Frothy, blood-tinged sputum is characteristic of pulmonary edema.

Bubbling wheezes and crackles are easily heard over the entire chest, reflecting fluid-filled airways. The level of fluid ascends as the pulmonary edema worsens.

These are early nonpulmonary signs of hypoxia. Lethargy and somnolence are late signs. Cognitive changes may occur with chronic hypoxia.

With initial hypoxia and hypercapnia, blood pressure (BP), HR, and respiratory rate all rise. As the hypoxia and/or hypercapnia becomes severe, BP and HR will drop and dysrhythmias may occur. Respiratory failure may ensue when the patient is unable to maintain the rapid respiratory rate.

Pulse oximetry is useful to detect changes in oxygenation. Oxygen saturation should be maintained at 90% or greater.

In early stages, there is a decrease in both Po_2 and Pco_2 secondary to hypoxemia and respiratory alkalosis from tachypnea. In later stages, the Po_2 continues to drop while the Pco_2 may increase, reflecting respiratory acidosis.

Cool, pale skin may be secondary to a compensatory vasoconstrictive response to hypoxemia. As oxygenation and perfusion become impaired, peripheral tissues become cyanotic.

As interstitial edema accumulates, the x-ray films show cloudy, white lung fields.

Therapeutic Interventions

Actions/Interventions

- Position patient for optimal breathing patterns (high-Fowler's position with feet dangling at bedside).
- Encourage slow, deep breaths as appropriate.

- Assist with coughing or suctioning as needed.

- ▲ Provide oxygen as needed to maintain Po_2 at an acceptable level.
- ▲ Anticipate endotracheal intubation and use of mechanical ventilation.

- ▲ If arterial blood gases are expected to be drawn more often than at four 1-hour intervals, suggest appropriateness of an arterial line.
- ▲ Administer prescribed medication carefully, as follows:
  - Morphine sulfate

  - Sodium nitroprusside (Nipride)

  - Nitrates
  - Diuretics

Rationales

Upright position allows for increased thoracic capacity and full descent of diaphragm.

Slow, deep breathing reduces tachypnea and alveolar collapse.

Excessive secretions can interfere with gas exchange in the bronchopulmonary tree. Suctioning removes secretions to maintain patent airway, thereby enhancing oxygenation.

Supplemental oxygen may be required for the patient with pulmonary edema to maintain Po_2 at an acceptable level.

Early intubation and mechanical ventilation are recommended to prevent full decompensation of patient. Bilateral positive airway pressure (BiPAP) may also be indicated.

Arterial cannulation is indicated for the patient's comfort and for ease in obtaining necessary arterial blood gases.

Morphine reduces preload by vasodilation, decreases respiratory rate, and reduces anxiety.

Sodium nitroprusside reduces afterload and is required if systemic vascular resistance is high.

Nitrates reduce preload by dilating venous vessels.

Diuretics reduce intravascular fluid volume and decrease preload.

■ = Independent   ▲ = Collaborative

Actions/Interventions	**Rationales**
• Inotropic agents	Inotropic medications may be required to support BP and optimize cardiac output.
• Aminophylline	Aminophylline dilates bronchioles and dilates venous vessels. However, it is also a cardiac stimulant. Patients must be observed for cardiac dysrhythmias.

NANDA-I NDx Decreased Cardiac Output

Common Related Factors
Increased preload
Increased afterload
Impaired contractility
Altered heart rate or rhythm
Decreased oxygenation

Defining Characteristics
Variations in hemodynamic parameters
Dysrhythmias or electrocardiogram (ECG) changes
Weight gain, edema, and ascites
Abnormal heart sounds (S_3, S_4)
Abnormal breath sounds (crackles)
Anxiety and restlessness
Dizziness, weakness, and fatigue
Decreased peripheral pulses
Pallor, clammy skin
Oliguria
Dyspnea
Prolonged capillary refill

Common Expected Outcome
Patient maintains adequate cardiac output, as evidenced by strong peripheral pulses, systolic BP within 20 mm Hg of baseline, HR 60 to 100 beats/min with regular rhythm, urinary output ≥30 mL/hr, warm and dry skin, and normal level of consciousness.

NOC Outcomes
Cardiac Pump Effectiveness; Circulation Status
NIC Interventions
Invasive Hemodynamic Monitoring; Hemodynamic Regulation; Cardiac Care

Ongoing Assessment

Actions/Interventions	**Rationales**
■ Assess skin color, temperature, and moisture.	Cool, pale, clammy skin is secondary to compensatory increase in sympathetic nervous system stimulation and low cardiac output and desaturation.
▲ Assess HR, BP, and pulse pressure. Use direct intraarterial monitoring as ordered.	Sinus tachycardia and increased arterial BP are seen in early stages to maintain an adequate cardiac output.; BP drops as condition deteriorates. Auscultatory BP may be unreliable secondary to vasoconstriction. Pulse pressure (systolic minus diastolic) decreases in shock. Older patients have a reduced response to catecholamines; thus their response to decreased cardiac output may be blunted, with less increase in HR.
■ Assess peripheral pulses, including capillary refill.	Pulses are weak with reduced stroke volume and cardiac output. Capillary refill is slow, sometimes absent.
■ Assess for mental status changes.	Hypoxia and reduced cerebral perfusion are reflected in restlessness, anxiety, and irritability. Older patients are especially susceptible to reduced perfusion to vital organs.
■ Assess respiratory rate, rhythm, and breath sounds.	Crackles, rhonchi, and wheezes develop as fluid overload worsens. Rapid, shallow respirations are characteristic of reduced cardiac output.

Actions/Interventions

■ Assess fluid balance and weight gain.

■ Assess urine output.

■ Assess heart sounds for gallops (S_3, S_4).

■ Assess cardiac rhythm and ECG.

▲ Use pulse oximetry to monitor oxygen saturation; assess arterial blood gases.

▲ If hemodynamic monitoring is in place, assess central venous pressure (CVP), pulmonary artery pressure, PCWP, and cardiac output/cardiac index (CO/CI).

Rationales

Compromised regulatory mechanisms may result in fluid and sodium retention. Body weight is a more sensitive indicator of fluid retention than intake and output.

The renal system compensates for low BP by retaining water. Oliguria is a classic sign of inadequate renal perfusion from reduced cardiac output.

S_3 denotes reduced left ventricular ejection and is a classic sign of left ventricular failure. S_4 occurs with reduced compliance of the left ventricle, which impairs diastolic filling.

Cardiac dysrhythmias may occur from low perfusion, acidosis, or hypoxia, as well as from side effects of cardiac medications used to treat this condition. The 12-lead ECG may provide evidence of myocardial ischemia (ST-segment and T-wave changes).

Pulse oximetry is a useful tool to detect changes in oxygenation. Oxygen saturation should be kept at 90% or greater. As condition worsens, aerobic metabolism ceases and lactic acidosis ensues, raising the level of carbon dioxide and decreasing pH.

CVP provides information on filling pressures of the right side of the heart; pulmonary artery diastolic pressure and PCWP reflect left-sided fluid volumes. Cardiac output provides an objective number to guide therapy.

Therapeutic Interventions

Actions/Interventions

▲ Anticipate need for hemodynamic monitoring.

■ Position the patient for optimal reduction of preload (high-Fowler's position, dangling feet at bedside).
■ Anticipate prescribed medications:
 • Positive inotropic agents (e.g., dopamine, dobutamine, milrinone)
 • Vasodilators (e.g., nitrates, nitroprusside; angiotensin-converting enzyme inhibitor)
 • Diuretics

 • Morphine

 • Anticoagulants

Rationales

Swan-Ganz catheter provides pulmonary artery and PCWP measurements that guide therapy.
This position reduces preload by pooling blood in the lower extremities and decreasing venous return.

Inotropic medications augment myocardial contractility, increase BP, and increase CO/CI.
Vasodilators reduce preload, reduce afterload, and improve oxygenation.
Diuretics reduce intravascular fluid volume, reduce PCWP, and enhance sodium excretion.
Morphine reduces pulmonary congestion and relieves dyspnea.
Anticoagulant medications prevent venous thromboembolism.

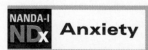 **Anxiety**

Common Related Factors
Change in environment (excessive monitoring equipment)
Change in health status
Threat of death

Defining Characteristics
Sympathetic stimulation
Restlessness
Focus on self
Uncooperative behavior
Vigilant watch on equipment
Tachypnea

■ = Independent   ▲ = Collaborative

Common Expected Outcomes

Patient demonstrates reduced anxiety, as evidenced by calm manner and cooperative behavior.

Patient describes a reduction in the level of anxiety experienced.

NOC Outcomes
Anxiety Self-Control; Coping

NIC Interventions
Anxiety Reduction; Calming Technique; Emotional Support

Ongoing Assessment

Actions/Interventions

■ Assess anxiety level (mild, severe). Note signs and symptoms, especially nonverbal communication.

■ Assess prior coping patterns/methods.

Rationales

Acute pulmonary edema can progress to an acute life-threatening situation that will produce high levels of anxiety in the patient as well as in significant others.

Anxiety and ways of decreasing perceived anxiety are highly individualized. Interventions are most effective when they are consistent with the individual's established coping pattern or previously successful coping mechanisms.

Therapeutic Interventions

Actions/Interventions

■ Acknowledge awareness of the patient's anxiety.

■ Maintain confident, assured manner. Assure the patient and significant others of close, continuous monitoring that will ensure prompt intervention.

■ Encourage verbalization of thoughts and feelings.
■ Reduce unnecessary external stimuli.

■ Explain all procedures as appropriate, keeping explanations basic.
▲ Administer antianxiety medication as appropriate.

▲ Refer to other support persons (e.g., clergy, social worker) as appropriate.

Rationales

Acknowledgment validates the feelings and communicates acceptance of those feelings.

The presence of a trusted person helps the person feel less threatened. The staff's anxiety may be easily perceived by the patient. The patient's feeling of stability increases in a calm, nonthreatening atmosphere.

Expressing emotions provides clarification of patient's perceptions and enhances coping.

Anxiety may escalate with excessive conversation, noise, and equipment around the patient.

Information helps allay anxiety. Patients who are anxious may not be able to comprehend anything more than simple, clear, brief instructions.

Short-tem use of antianxiety medication can enhance patient coping and reduce physiological manifestations of anxiety. Additional specialty expertise may be required.

Related Care Plans

Insomnia, p. 117
Dysrhythmias, p. 249
Excess fluid volume, p. 75
Ineffective breathing pattern, p. 30
Mechanical ventilation, p. 418

Pulmonary Arterial Hypertension

Right Ventricular Dilation, Right Atrial Dilation; Right-Sided Failure

The World Health Organization classified pulmonary hypertension into five categories as discussed below. Distinguishing the group is important, because treatment is different for each.

Group 1 pulmonary arterial hypertension (PAH) is the inability of the right ventricle to pump adequate blood into the lungs for oxygenation. PAH is characterized by progressive elevation of the pulmonary artery pressure and vascular resistance. Injury to the vascular bed impairs the function in the endothelium, vascular smooth muscle, and potassium channel, causing vasoconstriction. As the disease progresses, plexiform lesions, in situ thrombosis, and cell proliferation result in irreversible disease. Patients are limited by shortness of breath, dyspnea on exertion, presyncope/syncope, chest pain, edema, and ascites. PAH often leads to right ventricular failure and death. Etiology is broken down into two categories: idiopathic (primary) pulmonary hypertension, either sporadic or familial; and secondary PAH related to collagen vascular disease, congenital systemic-to-pulmonary shunts, portal hypertension, human immunodeficiency virus (HIV) infection, anorexigens, and persistent pulmonary hypertension of the newborn.

Diagnosis is made by an echocardiogram, electrocardiogram (ECG), physical examination, and heart catheterization. The right heart pressures during heart catheterization will show a mean pulmonary artery pressure of greater than 25 mm Hg at rest and greater than 35 mm Hg with exercise, with a normal wedge pressure. The echocardiogram will show a dilated right ventricle and right atrium with a normal left ventricle function and size; the left ventricle will, however, be underfilled. Right axis deviation and right ventricular hypertrophy will be documented on ECG. On physical examination jugular venous distention, reduced carotid volume, right ventricular heave, right-sided fourth heart sound, loud pulmonic valve closure (P_2), and tricuspid regurgitation murmur will be present. Peripheral edema and/or ascites may be present.

Treatment goals are to increase cardiac output, dilate the pulmonary artery, decrease complications, manage symptoms, recognize early signs of right ventricular failure, reduce hospitalizations through teaching, increase life expectancy, and improve quality of life.

The basis of current treatment is to affect one or more of the three molecular vascular pathways (prostacyclin-cAMP pathway, the nitric oxide-cGMP pathway, or the endothelin pathway) by medications that reduce vessel tone and inhibit proliferation of cells. Additional medications are prescribed in conjunction with the PAH medications to decrease symptoms, reduce side effects, and improve quality of life. In a very select few patients with advanced PAH, atrial septostomy (AS) may result in significant improvement in symptoms. The shunt created in this procedure may decompress the heart and alleviate right ventricular failure. Long-term survival post AS has not been determined. Some pulmonary hypertension centers may use it as a bridge to lung transplant.

Lung transplantation is considered based on the patient's stage of PAH, comorbidities, and underlying disease. To qualify there must be symptomatic progression of disease despite optimal treatment with a prostacyclin, cardiac index less than 2 liters/min/m², right atrial pressure greater than 15 mm Hg, and a mean pulmonary pressure greater than 55 mm Hg. The lung allocation score is calculated using the waiting-list urgency measure and posttransplant survival measure. Survival for PAH patients at 1, 3, and 5 years is reported as 75%, 60%, and 48%, respectively. Right ventricular function and size has been shown to return to normal by 3 months following lung transplantation.

Group 2 pulmonary venous hypertension is the result of left ventricular diastolic dysfunction. The left ventricle cannot relax, causing a rise in pressures on the right side. Treatment is focused on the underlying cause (e.g., obesity, hypertension, diabetes, diet [salt intake]). Treating with PAH medications may cause pulmonary edema and a worsening of patients' symptoms.

Group 3 pulmonary hypertension is associated with disorders of the respiratory system and/or hypoxemia. Patients may respond to phosphodiesterase (PDE)-5 inhibitors (e.g., sildenafil [Revatio]) or an endothelin antagonist (bosentan, ambrisentan); however, a ventilation-perfusion (VQ) mismatch may occur, causing a worsening of patients' hypoxemia.

Group 4 pulmonary hypertension caused by chronic thrombotic and/or embolic disease (chronic thromboembolic pulmonary hypertension [CTEPH]) may respond to PDE-5 inhibitors or low-dose prostacyclins. VQ scans and computed tomography (CT) scans of the chest are required to determine if the patient is a surgical candidate for pulmonary endarterectomy. A successful surgery can improve hemodynamics, functional class, quality of life, and survival.

Group 5 pulmonary hypertension caused by disorders directly affecting the pulmonary vasculature (e.g., pulmonary venoocclusive disease) rarely responds to any treatment. Lung transplant may be the only treatment choice.

Decreased Cardiac Output

Common Related Factors
Decreased or increased preload
Alteration in heart rhythm and rate
Impaired contractility
Decreased oxygenation
Low flow state to other organs

Common Expected Outcome
Patient maintains adequate cardiac output as evidenced by strong peripheral pulses, systolic BP within 20 mm Hg of baseline, HR 60 to 100 beats/min with regular rhythm, no presyncope/syncope events, oxygen saturation greater than 90%, urinary output ≥30 mL/hr, warm and dry skin, and normal level of consciousness.

Defining Characteristics
Low blood pressure (BP)
Presyncope/syncope
Oxygen saturation less than 90%
Decreased urine output
Dyspnea (at rest or with exertion)
Fatigue
Edema (ascites, peripheral)
Dysrhythmia
Reduced carotid volume

NOC Outcomes
Circulatory Status; Cardiac Pump Effectiveness

NIC Interventions
Hemodynamic Regulation; Dysrhythmia Management

Ongoing Assessment

Actions/Interventions	Rationales
■ Assess rate and quality of apical pulse.	Most patients have compensatory tachycardia in response to low cardiac output, fever, or worsening disease. Dysrhythmias may occur (e.g., atrial tachycardia or atrial fibrillation), and the pulse will be irregular and rapid.
■ Assess BP, including any related light-headedness with exertion.	Most patients will have a systolic pressure greater than 90 mm Hg. BP lower than 90 mm Hg or a mean arterial pressure less than 60 mm Hg needs to be reported. Patients are unable to raise their own cardiac output with activity; presyncope/syncope may occur.

Actions/Interventions

■ Assess respiratory rate, rhythm, and breath sounds.

■ Assess for complaints of fatigue, and determine physical activity classification.
  • Class I: Not limited by physical activity
  • Class II: Have a slight limitation in physical activity and are comfortable at rest
  • Class III: Limited by physical activity; are comfortable at rest but experience symptoms with minimal physical activity
  • Class IV: Have an inability to carry out any physical activity, experiencing symptoms even at rest and showing signs of right heart failure

■ Assess for signs of infection.

■ Assess for jugular venous distention.

■ Assess for liver congestion.

■ Assess urine output.

■ Determine changes in level of consciousness.

▲ Use pulse oximetry both at rest and with ambulation.

▲ Monitor serum electrolytes.

▲ Monitor lactate levels.

▲ Assess B-type natriuretic peptide (BNP) or N-terminal pro-BNP (pro-NT BNP).

■ Weigh patient daily, and evaluate trends in weight.

Rationales

Lungs will be clear in the absence of left-sided heart failure. Orthopnea and paroxysmal nocturnal dyspnea (PND) are signs of left-sided failure.

Fatigue and shortness of breath are classic signs of pulmonary hypertension caused by low cardiac output and right ventricular failure. Patients are further classified based on symptoms. According to the National Institutes of Health (NIH) registry, the life expectancy of a class III untreated patient is 2.6 years and a class IV untreated patient is 6 months.

PAH patients have no cardiac reserve; infections need to be treated early and aggressively.

A mean jugular venous pressure greater than 10 cm H_2O usually indicates volume overload, whereas a low jugular venous pressure usually indicates hypovolemia.

The liver may be pulsatile and enlarged. Liver enzymes may be elevated because of congestion. Ascites may be present.

Oliguria or inadequate urine output are signs of low renal perfusion. Oral diuretics may not be absorbed. Intravenous diuretics may be needed.

Hypoxia and reduced cerebral perfusion will present with restlessness, irritability, and sleepiness.

Pulse oximetry is a useful tool to detect changes in oxygenation that may be related to fluid status or severity of disease. Oxygen saturation should be at least 90% or greater.

Hypokalemia may cause dysrhythmias from chronic diuretic use. Hyponatremia may occur from chronic or high diuretic use. Sodium bicarbonate drop may signal the beginning of warm cardiogenic shock.

Signs of an increased lactate level need to be reported. This is a signal of cardiac shock. Patient may need treatment in an intensive care unit with intravenous (IV) phenylephrine or dopamine to increase cardiac output.

B-type natriuretic peptide is elevated with right or left ventricular distress.

A weight gain of 2 to 3 pounds indicates retention of approximately 1 liter of fluid. The patient may need increasing doses of diuretic, the addition of other diuretics, or the change to IV (e.g., metolazone [Zaroxolyn]). During diuresis weight should drop daily with adequate doses of diuretics.

Therapeutic Interventions

Actions/Interventions

■ Administer or evaluate patient's home compliance with prescribed medications.

Rationales

Pulmonary hypertension requires strict attention to doses and compliance with medications.

■ = Independent   ▲ = Collaborative

Cardiac and Vascular Care Plans

Actions/Interventions	Rationales
• Prostacyclins (epoprostenol, treprostinil, iloprost)	Prostacyclins affect the prostacyclin-cAMP pathway. They increase cardiac output, cause direct vasodilation of the vascular bed, decrease platelet aggregation, and inhibit cell growth. They are effective in increasing life expectancy and improving symptoms and quality of life. They are titrated up at a slow rate as an outpatient according to side effects and patient tolerance. Side effects include flushing, jaw pain (biting a lemon), diarrhea, and leg or foot pain. They are given continuously intravenously via an external pump or subcutaneously via an insulin pump, or they are inhaled. These medications cannot be stopped for any reason.
• Endothelin receptor antagonists (ERAs) (bosentan, ambrisentan)	These medications affect the endothelin pathway, affecting the endothelin type A (ETA) and endothelin type B (ETB) receptors known to be the most potent vasoconstrictor agents. They may cause increased liver enzymes, anemia, or birth defects, so monthly liver testing, pregnancy test, and complete blood count (CBC) every 3 months are mandated by the Food and Drug Administration (FDA). They may also cause peripheral edema, requiring an increase in the patient's furosemide (Lasix) dose.
• Phosphodiesterase or PDE-5 inhibitors (Viagra, Revatio, tadalafil)	These medications affect the nitric oxide-cGMP pathway, causing potent dilation of the pulmonary artery. Side effects include nasal congestion or headache. Do not hold for low blood pressure.
• Diuretics	Diuretics reduce volume and enhance sodium and water excretion.
• Positive inotropes (e.g., midodrine, phenylephrine, dopamine)	Positive inotropes improve myocardial contractility. They may be needed to raise blood pressure and cardiac output for diuretics to be effective.
• Antidysrhythmics (e.g., potassium, amiodarone)	Antidysrhythmics correct dysrhythmias such as atrial fibrillation or atrial tachycardia. Control of dysrhythmias is vital to patient survival. Ablation may be needed. Spironolactone may be added for its potassium-sparing effects.

NANDA-I NDx Excess Fluid Volume

Common Related Factor

Decreased cardiac output, causing the following:
  Decreased renal perfusion, which stimulates the renin-angiotension-aldosterone system and causes release of antidiuretic hormone
  Altered renal hemodynamics (diminished medullary blood flow), which results in decreased capacity of nephron to excrete water

Defining Characteristics

Weight gain
Edema (peripheral and or ascites)
Jugular vein distention
Shortness of breath/dyspnea
Decreased urine output
Elevated pulmonary capillary wedge pressure
Hepatomegaly and or pulsatile liver

Common Expected Outcome

Patient maintains optimal fluid balance, as evidenced by maintenance of stable weight, absence or reduction in edema, decreased shortness of breath, and oxygen saturations above 90%.

NOC Outcome
Fluid Balance
NIC Interventions
Fluid Monitoring; Fluid Management

Ongoing Assessment

Actions/Interventions	Rationales
■ Monitor daily weight. Verify patient's technique of weighing in the mornings around the same time, just after voiding, using the same scale every day.	Body weight is a more sensitive indicator of fluid or sodium retention than intake and output measurement. Consistent practice ensures accuracy of information for treatment. A weight change of 3 to 4 pounds over 1 to 2 days is significant for fluid weight gain.
■ Evaluate nutritional status.	As with heart failure, decreased appetite with weight loss accompanied by fluid retention will mask the true amount of fluid gained. Using other signs for edema are necessary (e.g., shortness of breath, swelling, tight clothing).
■ Assess for presence of edema by palpating ankles, feet, legs, and abdomen. Grade edema on a four-point scale.	Edema occurs when fluid accumulates in the extravascular spaces. Some pulmonary hypertension patients will retain fluids only in the abdomen. The lungs will be clear in PAH patients.
■ Assess for jugular vein distention, ascites, pulsatile liver, pain over liver, nausea.	Right heart failure affects venous pressure, causing hepatic congestion and changes in the abdominal system.
■ Assess sodium restriction with diet.	Excess sodium intake will result in fluid retention. Patients are instructed to keep sodium intake less than 2000 mg/day.
■ Monitor response to diuretics.	Oral diuretics do not work during low flow states. Intravenous diuretics or continuous IV doses may be required. The addition of inotropes (phenylephrine and dopamine) will improve response to diuretics.
▲ Monitor laboratory tests for side effects to diuretics such as hypokalemia, hyponatremia, and increased creatinine.	The electrolyte imbalances related to diuretic therapy can cause significant problems.
■ Monitor oxygen saturation levels.	Increased fluid retention will result in shortness of breath and lowered oxygen saturations. Supplemental oxygen may be required to keep oxygen saturation greater than 90%.

Therapeutic Interventions

Actions/Interventions	Rationales
■ Teach patients how to avoid foods high in sodium, including how to read food labels for sodium content: • Eliminate use of table salt and salt while cooking. • Restrict sodium intake to less than 2000 mg/day. • Teach about hidden salt in soups, restaurant meals, and spices. • Recommend use of salt substitutes.	Information is key for patients who will be comanaging fluids and sodium levels.
■ Instruct patients in prescribed diuretics.	Diuretics aid in the excretion of excess body fluids. Many different diuretics may be used. In some cases metolazone may be added. Taking it 30 minutes before the diuretic will enhance its effect. Maintaining a low-sodium diet and proper diuretics will reduce the need to urinate all day long, and compliance will be increased.
■ Instruct patient in signs of fluid retention and when to seek assistance from a medical provider.	Patient should weigh daily and watch for 3 to 4 pounds of weight gain over 1 to 2 days, which is a sign to call the physician's office.
■ Instruct patients in electrolyte imbalances. Teach patients to take potassium supplements and foods high in potassium during increased use of diuretics. Teach the signs of low potassium, such as muscle cramping and fatigue.	Electrolyte imbalances can contribute to dysrhythmias. Frequent laboratory testing may be required to maintain electrolyte balance.

■ = Independent   ▲ = Collaborative

NANDA-I NDx **Activity Intolerance**

Common Related Factors
Decreased cardiac output
Deconditioned state
Sedentary lifestyle
Lack of motivation/depression

Common Expected Outcomes
Patient reports increased activity from baseline, less short-ness of breath, and no syncope/presyncope.

Defining Characteristics
Verbal report of fatigue/weakness
Exertional discomfort/increasing shortness of breath
Syncope/presyncope
Inability to perform daily activities

NOC Outcomes
Activity Tolerance; Energy Conservation
NIC Interventions
Energy Management; Exercise Therapy

Ongoing Assessment

Actions/Interventions	**Rationales**
■ Assess patient's current activity level. Determine reasons for limiting activity.	Changes in functional capacity are related to disease progression. As the disease progresses, patients may eliminate some activities to avoid symptoms. Assessing daily activity, walking ability, showering, and stairs will give an assessment of activity tolerance.
▲ Document the functional capacity with a 6-minute walk test or a treadmill test.	Drops in oxygen during these tests and a drop in test results can indicate worsening of disease. A baseline assessment will be useful to assess medication response and worsening process.
■ Evaluate the need for oxygen during activity and sleep.	Supplemental oxygen may be required during increased activity or sleep when the demand for oxygen increases. A sleep study will rule out sleep apnea and drops in oxygen saturations during sleep.
■ Evaluate PAH symptoms, and teach signs of overexertion.	Common PAH symptoms include fatigue, shortness of breath, and syncope/presyncope. Changes in symptoms can be a symptom of worsening disease, lack of medication response, infection, and fluid retention. To avoid syncope, instruct patient to stop activity and rest at signs of light-headedness and not to lift more than 10 pounds.
▲ Consult cardiac rehabilitation or pulmonary rehabilitation programs.	Patients may benefit from one of these programs. They may do low weights with rapid repetitions but need to keep under the 10-pound weight limit.
■ Provide emotional support and encouragement while increasing activity levels.	Patients may be fearful of overexertion, especially if they have encountered episodes of presyncope or syncope. Appropriate supervision and support during efforts can enhance confidence. Participating in local support group meetings may be beneficial.

Deficient Knowledge

Common Related Factors
Unfamiliarity with pathology, treatment, and prognosis of PAH

Misinformation from unreliable sources

New medications

Emotional state affecting learning, such as depression

Defining Characteristics
Verbalizes lack of knowledge or inaccurate information

Questioning members of the health care team

Inaccurate follow-through of instructions

Common Expected Outcome
Upon discharge patient and significant other understand and verbalize pathology, treatment, medication regimen, and prognosis of PAH.

NOC Outcomes
Knowledge: Disease Process; Knowledge: Treatment Regimen

NIC Interventions
Teaching: Disease Process; Teaching: Prescribed Medications; Teaching: Prescribed Diet; Teaching: Prescribed Activity

Cardiac and Vascular Care Plans

Ongoing Assessment

Actions/Interventions

■ Assess knowledge of causes, treatment, and care of PAH. Identify educational needs and follow-up.

■ Identify existing misconceptions regarding care.

Rationales

Asking questions about the disease and continued treatment will assist in identifying educational needs.

This medical condition is less publicized in the media, leaving the patient less informed.

Therapeutic Interventions

Actions/Interventions

■ Educate the patient and significant others before discharge. Use a variety of educational materials, Internet sites, and support persons.
  • Normal heart circulation
  • PAH disease process and progression
  • Diagnostic testing and follow-up testing
  • Compliance to therapy
  • Symptoms of disease
  • Side effects of PAH medications
  • Diet
  • Psychosocial aspects of a fatal disease
  • Resources

■ Teach medication care and side effects before discharge.
  • Prostacyclin (epoprostenol [Flolan], trepostinil [Remodulin], iloprost)
    • Instruct to call physician's office for increase in the dose of prostacyclins. Some centers increase the dose weekly according to symptoms and side effects. Coordinate with specialty pharmacy nurses to coordinate continued home teaching for prostacyclins.

Rationales

Patients are better able to ask questions and seek assistance when they have basic information about their disease and its treatment. Encouraging questions will increase comfort level and may decrease complications. Using current patients to reach out and teach new patients may reduce the feeling of aloneness.

Compliance is enhanced when patients understand "why" and "how" to take medications.

■ = Independent   ▲ = Collaborative

Cardiac and Vascular Care Plans

Actions/Interventions	Rationales

Actions/Interventions

- Inform of side effects:
  - Flushing—cheeks, chest, hands, and feet
  - Jaw pain—(feels like biting a lemon) occurs with first bite of food, may use warm liquids or gum to reduce frequency
  - Diarrhea—use of over-the-counter medications such as Imodium to control
  - Leg or foot pain—elevate legs, use warm compresses, may need pain medications or medications for neuropathy
- Teach care of Hickman catheter for IV prostacyclins:
  - Dressing changes
  - Signs of infection (e.g., low-grade fever, redness, drainage, flulike symptoms)
- Instruct regarding subcutaneous sites for trepostinil, changing sites every 3 weeks, and measures to control pain. Pain may subside after 2 months on drug.
  - Ice or warm compresses
  - Neuropathic medications
  - Pain medications
  - Pluronic lecithin organogel (PLO) gels (from specialty pharmacy)
  - Lidocaine (Lidoderm) patches
- Instruct to never stop these medications (sudden withdrawal can result in worsening of PAH or death).
- ERAs (bosentan, ambrisentan)
- Instruct and give prescription for mandatory monthly liver and pregnancy testing and quarterly CBC.
- PDE-5 inhibitors (Viagra, Revatio, tadalafil)
- Teach side effects (e.g., stuffy nose, headache, and flushing).
- Inhaled prostacyclins (iloprost)
- Teach frequency of treatments and technique depending on the delivery system.
- Instruct to take the last treatment at bedtime and the first as soon as the patient wakes up.

■ Instruct in need for frequent exercise testing and repeat right heart catheterizations.

■ Provide information on potential lung transplantation.

■ Provide information on ways to enhance self-management efforts: recognizing changes in one's condition and their importance; decisions regarding appropriate treatment and evaluation of effectiveness; coping with depression.

Rationales

These tests are used to assess disease progression and need for added therapy.

Lung transplantation is considered based on the patient's stage of PAH, comorbidities, and underlying disease.

The burden of living with chronic PAH rests with the patient and caregiver. Living with a fatal disease and expensive medications can be depressing and cause a great deal of fear. Support systems and antidepressants can improve quality of life.

Related Care Plans

Powerlessness, p. 162
Shock, Cardiogenic, p. 331
Disturbed body image, p. 24
Risk for infection, p. 114
Death and dying: End-of-life issues, p. 969
Caregiver role strain, p. 36

Shock, Anaphylactic

Allergic Reaction; Distributive Shock; Vasogenic Shock

Anaphylactic shock is a potentially life-threatening situation characterized by massive vaso-dilation and increased capillary permeability triggered by a release of histamine. It is the most severe systemic form of hypersensitivity (antigen-antibody interaction); it occurs with-in seconds to minutes after contact with an antigenic substance and progresses rapidly to respiratory distress, vascular collapse, systemic shock, and possibly death if emergency treat-ment is not initiated. Causative agents include severe reactions to a sensitive substance such as a drug, vaccine, food (e.g., eggs, peanuts, shellfish), insect venom, dyes or contrast media, or transfused blood or blood products.

Ineffective Breathing Pattern

Common Related Factors

Facial angioedema
Bronchospasm
Laryngeal edema

Defining Characteristics

Dyspnea
Wheezing
Coughing
Hoarseness
Tachypnea
Stridor
Use of accessory muscles
Tightness of chest
Cyanosis
Respiratory distress

Common Expected Outcome

The patient will maintain an effective breathing pattern, as evidenced by relaxed breathing at normal rate and depth and improved breath sounds.

NOC Outcome
Respiratory Status: Ventilation
NIC Interventions
Respiratory Monitoring; Ventilation Assistance; Airway Management

Ongoing Assessment

Actions/Interventions	**Rationales**
■ Assess respiratory rate, rhythm, and depth, and observe for changes (e.g., increased shortness of breath, tachypnea, dyspnea, wheezing, stridor, hoarseness, coughing, use of accessory muscles).	Histamine is the primary chemical mediator of anaphylaxis. Through stimulation of histamine receptors (H_1), it causes smooth muscle contraction in the bronchi. As the anaphy-lactic reaction progresses, the patient develops wheezing, dyspnea, and increased pulmonary secretions. Vascular to interstitial fluid shifts contribute to respiratory distress through swelling in the upper airways.
■ Assess patient for the sensation of a narrowed airway.	Antigen-antibody reactions result in severe bronchial airway narrowing, edema, and obstruction. As airways narrow, patients demonstrate an increase in respiratory effort.

■ = Independent   ▲ = Collaborative

Actions/Interventions

■ Auscultate breath sounds, and report changes.

■ Assess presence of angioedema.

▲ Use pulse oximetry to monitor oxygen saturation; assess arterial blood gases.

■ Observe color of tongue, mucosa, and skin for changes.
■ Assess level of anxiety.

Rationales

Wheezing may be heard over the entire chest. However, as the bronchial constriction worsens, audible wheezing will decrease. Therefore it is important to note decreasing air movement, not just adventitious breath sounds.

Angioedema is noticeable in the eyelids, lips, tongue, hands, and feet, resulting from capillary fluid shifts.

Pulse oximetry is a useful tool to detect changes in oxygenation. Oxygen saturation should be kept at 90% or greater. As shock increases, aerobic metabolism ceases and lactic acidosis ensues, raising the level of carbon dioxide and decreasing pH.

Central cyanosis represents a medical emergency.

Respiratory distress and shock are life-threatening situations that produce high levels of anxiety in the patient and significant others.

Therapeutic Interventions

Actions/Interventions

■ Position the patient upright.

■ Instruct the patient to breathe deeply and slow down respiratory rate.
▲ Administer oxygen as prescribed.

■ Provide reassurance and allay anxiety by staying with the patient during acute distress.
■ Maintain patent airway. Anticipate emergency intubation or tracheostomy if stridor occurs.

▲ Administer medications as ordered:
  • Epinephrine

  • Corticosteroids

  • H_1-receptor blockers/antihistamines

  • Bronchodilators (intravenous [IV] isoproterenol [Isuprel]/inhaled β-adrenergic agonists [e.g., albuterol])
▲ Provide intravenous fluids.

■ Maintain a calm, assured manner. Assure the patient and significant others of close, continuous monitoring that will ensure prompt intervention.

Home care:
■ Assist patient/family in identifying factors that precipitate/exacerbate crises.
■ Provide information about emergency medications and plan should crisis reoccur.

Rationales

This position provides for optimal diaphragmatic and lung excursion and chest expansion.

Focusing on breathing may help calm the patient, and the increased tidal volume facilitates improved gas exchange.

Oxygen increases arterial saturation. Oxygen saturation that is less than 90% leads to tissue hypoxia, acidosis, dysrhythmias, and changes in level of consciousness.

Air hunger can produce an extremely anxious state that leads to rapid and shallow respirations.

Respiratory distress may progress rapidly. If laryngeal edema is present, endotracheal intubation will be required to maintain a patent airway.

Epinephrine is the cornerstone of treatment for anaphylaxis. It is fast acting and relaxes pulmonary vessels to improve air exchange and stabilizes cellular permeability.

Steroids stabilize the cell membrane and reduce cellular permeability, vasomotor response, and inflammation.

These medications block the action of histamine and reduce cellular edema.

These medications reduce bronchospasm and open airways by relaxing smooth muscles of the bronchioles.

Hypotension caused by vasodilation and distributive shock responds to fluid resuscitation.

The staff's anxiety may be easily perceived by the patient. The patient's feeling of stability increases in a calm, nonthreatening environment. The presence of a trusted person can help a patient feel less threatened.

Knowledge can reduce episodes or facilitate early action to treat.

Adequate preparation reduces risks.

NANDA-I NDx

Decreased Cardiac Output

Common Related Factors

Generalized vasodilation (decreased preload and afterload)
Increased capillary permeability (fluid shifts)

Defining Characteristics

Hypotension
Tachycardia or irregular heartbeats
Decreased peripheral pulses
Dizziness
Decreased central venous pressure (CVP)
Decreased pulmonary pressures
Oliguria
Anxiety/restlessness

Common Expected Outcome

Patient has adequate cardiac output, as evidenced by strong peripheral pulses; systolic blood pressure (BP) within 20 mm Hg of baseline; heart rate (HR) 60 to 100 beats/min with regular rhythm; urine output greater than 30 mL/hr; warm, dry skin; and alert, responsive mentation.

NOC Outcomes
Cardiac Pump Effectiveness; Circulation Status; Immune Status

NIC Interventions
Hemodynamic Regulation; Invasive Hemodynamic Monitoring; Allergy Management; Shock Management: Vasogenic; Intravenous Therapy

Ongoing Assessment

Actions/Interventions	Rationales
▲ Monitor vital signs with frequent monitoring of BP; specifically direct intraarterial monitoring as ordered.	The intense vasodilation results in severe hypovolemia and hypotension. Auscultatory BP may be unreliable.
■ Assess skin temperature and signs of any cyanosis, and assess peripheral pulses.	The massive vasodilation and increased capillary permeability eventually lead to reduced peripheral blood flow and tissue perfusion. Pulses are weak with reduced stroke volume and cardiac output.
■ Assess for changes in level of consciousness.	Early signs of cerebral hypoxia are restlessness and anxiety, with confusion and loss of consciousness occurring in later stages. Older patients are especially susceptible to reduced perfusion to vital organs.
■ Monitor urine output.	The renal system compensates for low BP by retaining water. Oliguria is a classic sign of inadequate renal perfusion.
■ Monitor cardiac rhythm for dysrhythmias.	Cardiac dysrhythmias may occur from the low perfusion state, acidosis, or hypoxia.
■ Assess breath sounds	Crackles and decreased breath sounds occur with fluid shifts and bronchospasm.
▲ Use pulse oximetry to determine oxygen saturation.	Pulse oximetry is a useful tool to detect changes in oxygenation. Oxygen saturation should be kept at 90% or greater.
▲ Monitor arterial blood gas results.	In the early compensatory stage of shock, the patient may develop respiratory alkalosis, as indicated by a decreased Pco_2 and an elevated pH. As the shock state progresses, the patient will develop respiratory acidosis as a result of hypoventilation and metabolic acidosis as a result of poor tissue perfusion and lactic acidosis.

■ = Independent ▲ = Collaborative

Actions/Interventions

▲ If hemodynamic monitoring is in place, monitor CVP, pulmonary artery pressure, pulmonary capillary wedge pressure, and cardiac output/cardiac index.

Rationales

Hemodynamic parameters provide information aiding in differentiation of decreased cardiac output secondary to fluid deficit (fluid shifts) or fluid overload (aggressive IV therapy). CVP provides information on filling pressures of the right side of the heart; pulmonary artery pressure and pulmonary capillary wedge pressure reflect left-sided fluid volumes.

Therapeutic Interventions

Actions/Interventions

▲ Place patient in the physiological position for shock: head of bed flat, with the trunk horizontal and lower extremities elevated 20 to 30 degrees with knees straight.

▲ Administer parenteral fluids using a large-bore needle. Avoid fluid overload in older patients.

▲ Anticipate administration of volume expanders.

▲ Administer medications as prescribed, noting responses:
  • Epinephrine

  • H_1-Receptor blockers/antihistamine (diphenhydramine)

  • Corticosteroids

  • Glucagon

▲ If transfused blood or blood products are the cause of the reaction, immediately stop the infusion and keep the vein open with normal saline solution; immediately notify the physician.

Rationales

This position promotes venous return. Do not use Trendelenburg's (head down) position because it causes pressure against the diaphragm.

Volume therapy may be required to maintain adequate filling pressures and optimize cardiac output.

Volume expanders may be indicated to correct hypovolemia.

Epinephrine is an endogenous catecholamine with both α- and β-receptor stimulating actions that provide rapid relief of hypersensitivity reactions. It is unknown whether epinephrine prevents mediator release or whether it reverses the action of mediators on target tissues, but its early administration is critical. For prolonged reactions, it may be necessary to repeat the dose.

Antihistamines reduce circulating histamines and reverse their adverse effects.

Steroids may be used to suppress immune and inflammatory responses and reduce capillary permeability.

Glucagon reverses hypotension in patients taking β-blocker medications who do not respond to fluid administration and epinephrine.

Safety measures reduce further injury. Eliminating causative factor can reduce worsening of symptoms.

NANDA-I NDx Deficient Knowledge: Allergens

Common Related Factors

Lack of exposure
Misinterpretation of information
Lack of recall

Defining Characteristics

Recurrent allergic reactions
Inability to identify allergens
Inaccurate follow-through of instructions

Common Expected Outcomes

Patient or significant others verbalize understanding of allergic reaction, prevention, and treatment.
Patient and significant others verbalize understanding of need to inform health care providers of allergies, need to wear medical alert bracelet/necklace, need to carry emergency components for intervention, and the importance of seeking emergency care.

NOC Outcomes

Knowledge: Disease Process; Knowledge: Treatment Regimen

NIC Interventions

Allergy Management; Teaching: Disease Process; Health Education

Ongoing Assessment

Actions/Interventions	Rationales
■ Assess knowledge of condition and exposure to allergens.	Not all allergies occur in youth. Adult-onset experiences may find the patient unaware.

Therapeutic Interventions

Actions/Interventions	Rationales
■ Instruct the patient or significant others about factors that can precipitate a recurrence of shock and ways to prevent or avoid these precipitating factors.	The patient is at high risk for developing anaphylactic shock in the future if exposed to the same antigenic substance and needs self-help information to prevent anaphylactic shock.
■ Explain factors that may increase risk for anaphylaxis (e.g., certain drugs, blood products, insect venom, food) and environmental control measures to be instituted.	Information enables the patient to take control and make needed lifestyle modifications. For example, if trigger is food, patient needs to be able to correctly read food label ingredients.
■ Instruct the patient in use of insect sting kits (containing a chewable antihistamine), epinephrine in prefilled syringe, and instructions for use as appropriate, and indicate how they are to be obtained.	In situations in which the patient cannot completely avoid exposure to allergens, he or she needs to have access to emergency treatment resources for immediate administration. These can be self-administered or given by someone else. The EpiPen is injected into the thigh muscle.
■ Instruct the patient with known allergies to wear medical alert identification.	In case of emergency, those providing care will be aware of this significant history.
■ Provide instruction in self-care measures to be performed at home during initial attack:	During initial attacks, patient should be prepared to stay calm and follow preset instructions. Although not all reactions are life threatening, true anaphylaxis is a medical emergency.
• Reduce exposure to trigger if possible.	
• Take an oral antihistamine (diphenhydramine [Benadryl]) if swallowing is intact.	
• For wheezing, use prescribed inhaled bronchodilator.	
• For drop in BP (dizziness), lie down with feet elevated.	
• For severe reaction, inject self (or instruct someone else) with epinephrine from kit (EpiPen, Ana-Kit).	
• Call 9-1-1 for help, or have someone drive to hospital before attack escalates.	
■ Ensure that the patient or significant others are made aware that when giving medical history they should include all allergies (e.g., latex, medications, contrast dyes, blood products).	Safety measures reduce potential injury. Health care providers need to be aware of both history of the reaction, causative factors, symptoms, and severity and the level of treatment required.
■ For allergens that are difficult to avoid, discuss referral to an allergist.	In some situations skin testing can be used to identify the specific allergen. Patients may also benefit from desensitization therapy.

Shock, Cardiogenic

Pump Failure; Acute Pulmonary Edema

Cardiogenic shock is an acute state of sustained decreased tissue perfusion caused by the impaired pumping of the heart. It is usually associated with myocardial infarction, cardiomyopathies, dysrhythmias, valvular stenosis, massive pulmonary embolism, cardiac surgery, or cardiac tamponade. It is a self-perpetuating condition because coronary blood flow to the myocardium is compromised, causing further ischemia and ventricular dysfunction. Patients with massive myocardial infarctions involving 40% or more of the left ventricular muscle mass are at highest risk for developing cardiogenic shock. The mortality rate for cardiogenic shock often exceeds 80%. This care plan focuses on the care of an unstable patient in a shock state.

■ = Independent ▲ = Collaborative

NANDA-I NDx Decreased Cardiac Output

Common Related Factors

Mechanical:
- Impaired left ventricular contractility
- Cardiac muscle disease
- Increased or decreased preload/afterload
- Dysrhythmias

Structural:
- Valvular dysfunction
- Septal defects

Defining Characteristics

Changes in level of consciousness
Variations in hemodynamic parameters (BP, HR, central venous pressure [CVP], pulmonary artery pressure [PAP])
Sustained hypotension with narrowing of pulse pressure
Pale, cool, clammy skin
Cyanosis and mottling of extremities
Oliguria/anuria
Pulmonary congestion/dyspnea/crackles
Respiratory alkalosis or metabolic acidosis

Common Expected Outcome

Patient maintains adequate cardiac output as evidenced by strong peripheral pulses, systolic BP within 20 mm Hg of baseline, HR 60 to 100 beats/min with regular rhythm, urinary output ≥30 mL/hr, warm and dry skin, and normal level of consciousness.

NOC Outcomes

Cardiac Pump Effectiveness; Circulation Status; Tissue Perfusion: Cardiac, Renal, Cerebral

NIC Interventions

Cardiac Care: Acute; Invasive Hemodynamic Monitoring; Hemodynamic Regulation; Dysrhythmia Management; Circulatory Care: Mechanical Assist Device; Shock Management: Cardiac

Ongoing Assessment

Actions/Interventions	Rationales
■ Assess skin color, temperature, and moisture.	Cool, pale, clammy skin is secondary to compensatory increase in sympathetic nervous system stimulation and low cardiac output and desaturation.
▲ Assess HR, BP, and pulse pressure. Use direct intraarterial monitoring as ordered.	Sinus tachycardia and increased arterial BP are seen in early stages to maintain an adequate cardiac output. BP drops as condition deteriorates. Auscultatory BP may be unreliable secondary to vasoconstriction. Pulse pressure (systolic minus diastolic) decreases in shock. Older patients have a reduced response to catecholamines; thus their response to decreased cardiac output may be blunted, with less increase in HR.
■ Assess peripheral and central pulses, including capillary refill.	Pulses are weak with reduced stroke volume and cardiac output. Capillary refill is slow, sometimes absent.
■ Assess for changes in level of consciousness.	Early signs of cerebral hypoxia are restlessness and anxiety, with confusion and loss of consciousness occurring in later stages. Older patients are especially susceptible to reduced perfusion to vital organs.
■ Assess respiratory rate, rhythm, and breath sounds.	Rapid, shallow respirations and presence of crackles and wheezes are characteristic of shock.
■ Assess urine output.	The renal system compensates for low BP by retaining water. Oliguria is a classic sign of inadequate renal perfusion from reduced cardiac output.

Actions/Interventions

■ Assess fluid balance and weight gain.

■ Assess heart sounds for gallops (S_3, S_4).

■ Assess cardiac rate, rhythm, and electrocardiogram (ECG).

▲ Use pulse oximetry to monitor oxygen saturation; assess arterial blood gases.

▲ If hemodynamic monitoring is in place, assess CVP, pulmonary artery pressure, pulmonary capillary wedge pressure (PCWP), and cardiac output/cardiac index (CO/CI).

■ Assess serum electrolytes, especially potassium and magnesium.

Rationales

Compromised regulatory mechanisms may result in fluid and sodium retention. Body weight is a more sensitive indicator of fluid or sodium retention than intake and output.

S_3 denotes reduced left ventricular ejection and is a classic sign of left ventricular failure. S_4 occurs with reduced compliance of the left ventricle, which impairs diastolic filling.

Cardiac dysrhythmias may occur from low perfusion, acidosis, or hypoxia, as well as from side effects of cardiac medications used to treat this condition. The 12-lead ECG may provide evidence of myocardial ischemia (ST-segment and T-wave changes) or pericardial tamponade (decreased voltage of QRS complexes).

Pulse oximetry is a useful tool to detect changes in oxygenation. Oxygen saturation should be kept at 90% or greater. As shock increases, aerobic metabolism ceases and lactic acidosis ensues, raising the level of carbon dioxide and decreasing pH.

CVP provides information on filling pressures of the right side of the heart; pulmonary artery diastolic pressure and PCWP reflect left-sided fluid volumes. CO/CI provides an objective number to guide therapy.

Hypokalemia and hypomagnesemia are causative factors for dysrhythmias, which can further reduce cardiac output.

Therapeutic Interventions

Actions/Interventions

■ Place patient in optimal position, usually supine with head of bed slightly elevated.

▲ Administer oxygen as prescribed.

▲ Maintain optimal fluid balance. For patients with decreased preload, administer intravenous fluids.

▲ If increased preload is a problem, restrict fluids and sodium as ordered.

▲ Initiate and titrate drug therapy as ordered:
• Inotropic agents:
  • Dopamine

  • Dobutamine

  • Milrinone
• Vasodilators:
  • Sodium nitroprusside (Nipride)

  • Intravenous nitroglycerin

• Diuretics

• Antidysrhythmics

Rationales

This position promotes venous return and increases cardiac output.

Oxygen may be required to maintain oxygen saturation above 90% or as indicated by order or protocol.

Optimal fluid status ensures effective ventricular filling pressure. Too little fluid reduces circulating blood volume and ventricular filling pressures; too much fluid can cause pulmonary edema in a failing heart. PCWP guides therapy.

Fluid restriction decreases extracellular fluid volume and reduces cardiac workload.

Therapy is more effective when initiated early. The goal is to maintain systolic BP greater than 90 to 100 mm Hg.

Dopamine is an inotrope and vasopressor that has varying effects at different doses. Low doses increase renal blood flow. Higher doses increase systemic vascular resistance and contractility.

Dobutamine is an inotrope that increases contractility with slight vasodilation.

Milrinone is a cyclic AMP-specific PDE inhibitor that has inotropic and vasodilator effects

Nitroprusside increases cardiac output by decreasing afterload and produces peripheral and systemic vasodilation by direct action to the smooth muscles of blood vessels.

Nitroglycerin may be used to reduce excess preload contributing to pump failure, and to reduce afterload.

Diuretics are used when volume overload is contributing to pump failure.

Antidysrhythmics are used when cardiac dysrhythmias are further compromising a low-output state.

■ = Independent   ▲ = Collaborative

Cardiac and Vascular Care Plans

Actions/Interventions

- Vasopressors (e.g., epinephrine, norepinephrine, phenylephrine)

- Morphine

▲ Provide electrolyte replacement as ordered.

▲ If mechanical assistance by counterpulsation is indicated, institute intraaortic balloon pump (IABP) or ventricular assist device (VAD).

▲ Prepare for surgical intervention as needed.

Rationales

Vasopressors increase the force of myocardial contraction and constrict arteries and veins. They augment the vasoconstriction that occurs with shock to increase perfusion pressure. They are not routinely used unless aforementioned medications have failed to improve coronary perfusion.

Morphine reduces pulmonary congestion and relieves dyspnea.

Electrolyte imbalance may cause dysrhythmias or other pathological states. Laboratory results guide therapy.

Mechanical assist devices such as VAD or IABP provide temporary circulatory support to improve cardiac output. These devices are used in cardiogenic shock when the patient does not respond to pharmacological interventions. IABP increases myocardial oxygen supply and reduces myocardial workload through increased coronary artery perfusion. The patient's stroke volume increases and thus improves perfusion of vital organs. The nurse needs to follow unit protocols for the management of the patient with a mechanical VAD.

Acute valvular problems or septal defects may require surgical treatment.

NANDA-I NDx   Impaired Gas Exchange

Common Related Factors

Alveolar capillary membrane changes
Altered oxygen supply
Ventilation-perfusion mismatch

Defining Characteristics

Abnormal breathing (rate, rhythm, depth)
May have Cheyne-Stokes respirations
Crackles
Hypoxia/hypoxemia
Hypercapnia
Tachycardia
Changes in level of consciousness
Headache
Pale/dusky color
Confusion/somnolence
Abnormal arterial blood gases

Common Expected Outcome

Patient maintains optimal gas exchange, as evidenced by arterial blood gases (ABGs) within the patient's usual range, oxygen saturation of 90% or greater, alert responsive mentation or no further reduction in level of consciousness, relaxed breathing, and baseline HR for patient.

NOC Outcomes

Respiratory Status: Gas Exchange; Tissue Perfusion

NIC Interventions

Respiratory Monitoring; Airway Insertion and Stabilization; Airway Management; Oxygen Therapy

Ongoing Assessment

Actions/Interventions	Rationales
■ Assess HR, BP, and rate, rhythm, and depth of respiration.	In the early stages of shock, with initial hypoxia and hypercapnia, the patient's respiratory rate will be rapid. As shock progresses, the respirations become shallow, and the patient will begin to hypoventilate. BP and HR will decrease and dysrhythmias may occur. Respiratory failure develops as the patient experiences respiratory muscle fatigue and decreased lung compliance.
■ Assess lungs, noting areas of decreased ventilation and the presence of adventitious sounds.	Moist crackles are caused by increased pulmonary capillary permeability and increased intraalveolar edema.
■ Assess skin, nail beds, and mucous membranes for pallor or cyanosis.	Cool, pale skin may be secondary to a compensatory vasoconstrictive response to hypoxemia. As oxygenation and perfusion become impaired, peripheral tissues become cyanotic.
■ Assess for restlessness, diaphoresis, headache, and changes in level of consciousness.	These are early nonpulmonary signs of hypoxia.
▲ Use pulse oximeter to monitor oxygen saturation.	Pulse oximetry tool is useful to detect changes in oxygenation. Oxygen saturation should be maintained at 90% or greater.
▲ Monitor arterial blood gases, and note changes.	Increasing $Paco_2$ and decreasing Pao_2 are signs of hypoxemia and respiratory acidosis. As the patient's condition begins to fail, the respiratory rate will decrease and $Paco_2$ will continue to increase.

Therapeutic Interventions

Actions/Interventions	Rationales
■ Place the patient in optimal position for ventilation.	Slightly elevated head of bed facilitates diaphragmatic movement.
▲ Initiate oxygen therapy as prescribed, attempting to maintain oxygen saturation at 90% or greater.	Supplemental oxygen may be required to maintain Po_2 at an acceptable level.
■ Assist with coughing, and suction as needed.	Suction removes secretions if the patient is unable to effectively clear the airway.
▲ Prepare patient for mechanical ventilation if noninvasive oxygen therapy is ineffective: • Explain need for mechanical ventilation. • Assist in intubation procedure. • Institute mechanical ventilation.	Early intubation and mechanical ventilation are recommended to prevent full decompensation of patient. Mechanical ventilation provides supportive care to maintain adequate oxygenation and ventilation to the patient.

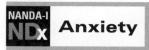

Anxiety

Common Related Factors	Defining Characteristics
Guarded prognosis; mortality rate 80% Fear of death Change in health status Unfamiliar environment	Sympathetic stimulation Verbalized anxiety Restlessness/agitation Increased awareness Increased questioning Uncooperative behavior Avoids looking at equipment or keeps vigilant watch over equipment

■ = Independent　▲ = Collaborative

Common Expected Outcomes

Patient uses effective coping mechanisms.
Patient describes reduction in level of anxiety experienced.

NOC Outcomes

Anxiety Self-Control; Coping

NIC Interventions

Anxiety Reduction; Support System Enhancement; Calming Technique

---

Ongoing Assessment

Actions/Interventions	Rationales
■ Assess anxiety level (mild, severe). Note signs and symptoms, especially nonverbal communication.	Shock can result in an acute life-threatening situation that will produce high levels of anxiety in the patient as well as in significant others.
■ Assess coping techniques commonly used.	Anxiety and ways of decreasing perceived anxiety are highly individualized. Interventions are most effective when they are consistent with the individual's established coping pattern. However, in the acute care setting these techniques may no longer be feasible.

Therapeutic Interventions

Actions/Interventions	Rationales
■ Acknowledge awareness of the patient's anxiety.	Acknowledgment of the patient's feelings validates the feelings and communicates acceptance of those feelings.
■ Encourage verbalization of feelings.	Talking about anxiety-producing situations and anxious feelings can help the person perceive the situation in a less-threatening manner.
■ Maintain confident, assured manner while interacting with patient. Assure patient and significant others of close, continuous monitoring that will ensure prompt intervention.	The staff's anxiety may be easily perceived by the patient. The patient's feeling of stability increases in a calm and non-threatening atmosphere. The presence of a trusted person may help the patient feel less threatened.
■ Reduce unnecessary external stimuli by maintaining a quiet environment. Keep "threatening" equipment out of sight as much as feasible.	Anxiety may escalate with excessive conversation, noise, and equipment around the patient.
■ Explain all procedures as appropriate, keeping explanations basic.	Information helps allay anxiety. Patients who are anxious may not be able to comprehend anything more than simple, clear, brief instructions.
▲ Refer to other support persons (e.g., clergy, social worker) as appropriate.	Additional specialty expertise may be required.

Related Care Plans

Imbalanced nutrition: Less than body requirements, p. 142
Ineffective coping, p. 49
Spiritual distress, p. 189
Mechanical ventilation, p. 418

Cardiac and Vascular Care Plans

Shock, Hypovolemic

Hypovolemic shock is an emergency situation that occurs from decreased intravascular fluid volume, resulting from either internal fluid shifts or external fluid loss. This fluid can be whole blood, plasma, or water and electrolytes. Losing about one-fifth of total blood volume can produce this condition, resulting from circulatory dysfunction and inadequate tissue perfusion. Common causes include hemorrhage (external or internal), severe burns, vomiting, and diarrhea. Hemorrhagic shock often occurs after trauma, gastrointestinal bleeding, or rupture of organs or aneurysms. Internal fluid losses occur in clinical conditions associated with increased capillary permeability and resulting shifts in fluid from the vascular compartment to interstitial spaces or other closed fluid compartments (e.g., peritoneal cavity). This third-spacing of fluids in the body is seen in patients with extensive burns or with ascites and leads to hypovolemic shock.

Hypovolemic shock can be classified according to the percentage of fluid loss. Mild shock (stage 1) is up to 15% blood volume loss, moderate shock (stage 2) is 15% to 30% blood volume loss, stage 3 is 30% to 40% blood volume loss, and severe shock is a greater than 40% loss. Older patients may exhibit signs of shock with smaller losses of fluid volume because of their compromised ability to compensate for fluid changes. Treatment focuses on prompt fluid/blood replacement, identification of causative factors/bleeding sites, control of bleeding, and prevention of complications. If aggressive treatment is not prompt, further collapse can cause irreversible brain and kidney damage and eventual cardiac arrest and death.

Deficient Fluid Volume

Common Related Factors

Inadequate fluid intake/severe dehydration
Active fluid volume loss (diuresis, abnormal bleeding or drainage, diarrhea)
Internal fluid shifts
Trauma
Failure of regulatory mechanisms

Defining Characteristics

Mild to moderate anxiety
Tachycardia/weak rapid heart rate
Hypotension/orthostasis
Capillary refill slow or greater than 3 seconds
Narrowing pulse pressure
Tachypnea
Urine output may be normal (greater than 30 mL/hr) or as low as 20 mL/hr
Cool, clammy skin
Decreased skin turgor
Thirst
Dry mucous membranes
Light-headedness or dizziness
Changes in level of consciousness

Common Expected Outcome

Patient is normovolemic as evidenced by systolic blood pressure (BP) greater than or equal to 90 mm Hg (or patient's baseline), absence of orthostasis, heart rate (HR) 60 to 100 beats/min, urinary output greater than 30 mL/hr, and normal skin turgor.

NOC Outcomes
Fluid Balance; Hydration; Vital Signs
NIC Interventions
Fluid Monitoring; Invasive Hemodynamic Monitoring; Fluid Resuscitation; Bleeding Precautions; Bleeding Reduction: Gastrointestinal; Shock Management: Volume; Emergency Care; Hypovolemia Management

■ = Independent   ▲ = Collaborative

Ongoing Assessment

Actions/Interventions	Rationales
■ Assess for early warning signs of hypovolemia, including changes in level of consciousness.	Mild to moderate anxiety, tachycardia, restlessness, headache, change in level of consciousness may be the first signs of impending hypovolemic shock; these may be easily overlooked or attributed to pain, psychological trauma, and fear.
▲ Assess HR, BP, and pulse pressure. Use direct intraarterial monitoring as ordered.	Sinus tachycardia and increased arterial BP are seen in early stages to maintain an adequate cardiac output; BP drops as condition deteriorates. In young adults, compensatory mechanism responses maintain a normal BP until major blood loss occurs.
■ Monitor for orthostasis.	Postural hypotension is a common manifestation in fluid loss. Note the significance of the following levels of orthostatic hypotension: • Greater than 10 mm Hg drop—circulating blood volume is decreased by 20% • Greater than 20 to 30 mm Hg drop—circulating blood volume is decreased by 40%
■ Monitor for possible sources of fluid loss: diarrhea, vomiting, profuse diaphoresis, polyuria, burns, ruptured organs, trauma, and wound drainage.	Specific manifestations/etiologies guide therapy.
■ Record and evaluate intake and output.	Accurate measurement is essential in detecting negative fluid balance and guiding therapy. Concentrated urine denotes fluid deficit.
■ Assess fluid balance, noting skin turgor and mucous membranes.	Loss of interstitial fluid causes loss of skin turgor.
■ If trauma has occurred, evaluate and document extent of patient's injuries; use primary survey (or another consistent survey method) or ABCs: airway with cervical spine control, breathing, circulation.	Primary survey helps identify imminent or potentially life-threatening injuries. This is a quick initial assessment.
■ Perform secondary survey after all life-threatening injuries are ruled out or treated.	Secondary survey uses methodical head-to-toe inspection. Anticipate potential causes of shock state from ongoing assessment.
■ If the only visible injury is obvious head injury, look for other causes of hypovolemia (e.g., long-bone fractures, internal bleeding, external bleeding).	Hypovolemic shock following trauma usually results from hemorrhage.
▲ If hemodynamic monitoring is in place, assess central venous pressure (CVP), pulmonary artery diastolic pressure (PADP), pulmonary capillary wedge pressure (PCWP), and cardiac output/cardiac index (CO/CI).	CVP provides information on filling pressures of the right side of the heart; PADP and PCWP reflect left-sided fluid volumes. CO/CI provides an objective number to guide therapy.
■ If patient is postsurgical, monitor blood loss (weigh dressings to determine fluid loss, monitor chest tube drainage, mark skin area).	It is important to note expanding hematoma or swelling or increased drainage to detect bleeding/coagulopathy.
▲ Obtain spun hematocrit, and reevaluate every 30 minutes to 4 hours, depending on stability.	Hematocrit decreases as fluids are administered because of dilution. As a rule of thumb, hematocrit decreases 1% per liter of lactated Ringer's or normal saline solution used. Any other hematocrit decrease must be evaluated as an indication of continued blood loss.
▲ Monitor coagulation studies, including INR, prothrombin time, partial thromboplastin time, fibrinogen, fibrin split products, and platelet counts, as appropriate.	Specific deficiencies guide treatment therapy.

Therapeutic Interventions

Actions/Interventions	Rationales
■ Prevent blood volume loss by controlling source of bleeding. If external, apply direct pressure to the bleeding site.	External bleeding is controlled with firm, direct pressure on the bleeding site, using a thick dry dressing material. Prompt, effective treatment is needed to preserve vital organ function and life.
■ Provide oral hygiene, and encourage oral fluid intake if able.	Oral hygiene promotes sensation of thirst/desire for oral intake. Oral route assists in maintaining fluid balance.
▲ Initiate intravenous (IV) therapy. Start two shorter, large-bore peripheral IV lines.	Maintaining an adequate circulating blood volume is a priority. The amount of fluid infused is usually more important than the type of fluid (crystalloid, colloid, blood). The amount of volume that can be infused is inversely affected by the length of the IV catheter; it is best to use shorter, large-bore catheters.
▲ Prepare to administer a bolus of 1 to 2 liters of IV fluids as ordered. Use crystalloid solutions for adequate fluid and electrolyte balance.	The patient's response to treatment depends on the extent of blood loss. If blood loss is mild (15%), expected response is a rapid return to normal BP. If IV fluids are slowed, the patient remains normotensive. If the patient has lost 20% to 40% of circulating blood volume or has continued uncontrolled bleeding, fluid bolus may produce normotension, but if fluids are slowed after bolus, BP will deteriorate. Extreme caution is indicated in fluid replacement in older patients. Aggressive therapy may precipitate left ventricular dysfunction and pulmonary edema.
▲ If hypovolemia is a result of severe burns, calculate fluid replacement according to the extent of the burn and patient's body weight.	Formulas such as the Parkland formula, which follows, guide fluid replacement therapy: % BSA (body surface area) burned × Weight in kg × 4 mL lactated Ringer's = Total fluid to be infused over 24 hours: half given intravenously over 8 hours and half given over next 16 hours
▲ Administer blood products (e.g., packed red blood cells, fresh frozen plasma, platelets) as prescribed. Transfuse patient with whole blood–packed red blood cells.	Preparing fully crossmatched blood may take up to 1 hour in some laboratories. Consider using uncrossmatched or type-specific blood until crossmatched blood is available. If type-specific blood is unavailable, type O blood may be used for exsanguinating patients. If available, Rh-negative blood is preferred, especially for women of childbearing age. Autotransfusion may be used when there is massive bleeding in the thoracic cavity.
▲ If hypovolemia is a result of severe diarrhea or vomiting, administer antidiarrheal or antiemetic medications as prescribed, in addition to IV fluids. NOTE: Disease pathology must be ruled out first (e.g., *Clostridium difficile*, norovirus).	Treatment is guided by cause of problem.
■ If bleeding is secondary to surgery, anticipate or prepare for return to surgery.	Surgery may be the only way to correct the problem.
▲ For trauma victims with internal bleeding (e.g., pelvic fracture), military antishock trousers (MAST) or pneumatic antishock garment (PASG) may be used.	These devices are useful to tamponade bleeding. Hypovolemia from long-bone fractures (e.g., femur or pelvic fractures) may be controlled by splinting with air splints. Hare traction splints or MAST/PASG trousers may be used to reduce tissue and vessel damage from manipulation of unstable fractures.

Cardiac and Vascular Care Plans

■ = Independent   ▲ = Collaborative

Cardiac and Vascular Care Plans

Decreased Cardiac Output

Common Related Factors

Fluid volume loss of 30% or more
Late uncompensated hypovolemic shock
Decreased ventricular filling (preload)
Alterations in heart rate and rhythm

Defining Characteristics

Tachycardia
Hypotension
Capillary refill greater than 3 seconds
Decreased pulse pressure
Decreased peripheral pulses
Cold, clammy skin
Change in level of consciousness
Decreased urinary output (less than 30 mL/hr)
Abnormal arterial blood gases: acidosis and hypoxemia
Fatigue
Cardiac dysrhythmias

Common Expected Outcome

Patient maintains adequate cardiac output, as evidenced by strong peripheral pulses, systolic BP within 20 mm Hg of baseline, HR 60 to 100 beats/min with regular rhythm, urinary output ≥30 mL/hr, warm and dry skin, and normal level of consciousness.

NOC Outcomes

Cardiac Pump Effectiveness; Circulation Status; Tissue Perfusion

NIC Interventions

Invasive Hemodynamic Monitoring; Hemodynamic Regulation; Emergency Care; Shock Management: Hypovolemia

Ongoing Assessment

Actions/Interventions	Rationales
■ Assess skin color, temperature, moisture, presence of cyanosis.	Cool, pale, clammy skin is secondary to compensatory increase in sympathetic nervous system stimulation and low cardiac output and desaturation.
▲ Assess HR, BP, and pulse pressure. Use direct intraarterial monitoring as ordered.	Sinus tachycardia and increased arterial BP are seen in early stages to maintain an adequate cardiac output. BP drops as condition deteriorates. Auscultatory BP may be unreliable secondary to vasoconstriction. Pulse pressure (systolic minus diastolic) decreases in shock. Older patients have a reduced response to catecholamines; thus their response to decreased cardiac output may be blunted, with less increase in HR.
■ Assess peripheral and central pulses, including capillary refill.	Pulses are weak with reduced stroke volume and cardiac output. Capillary refill is slow, sometimes absent.
■ Assess for changes in level of consciousness.	Early signs of cerebral hypoxia are restlessness and anxiety, with confusion and loss of consciousness occurring in later stages. Older patients are especially susceptible to reduced perfusion to vital organs.
■ Assess urine output.	The renal system compensates for low BP by retaining water. Oliguria is a classic sign of inadequate renal perfusion from reduced cardiac output.
■ Assess respiratory rate, rhythm, and breath sounds.	Rapid, shallow respirations and presence of crackles and wheezes are characteristic of shock.
■ Assess cardiac rhythm for dysrhythmias.	Cardiac dysrhythmias may occur from low perfusion, acidosis, or hypoxia, as well as from side effects of cardiac medications used to treat this condition.

Actions/Interventions

▲ Use pulse oximetry to monitor oxygen saturation; assess arterial blood gases.

▲ If hemodynamic monitoring is in place, assess CVP, pulmonary artery pressure, PCWP, and CO/CI.

Rationales

Pulse oximetry is a useful tool to detect changes in oxygenation. Oxygen saturation should be kept at 90% or greater. As shock increases, aerobic metabolism ceases and lactic acidosis ensues, raising the level of carbon dioxide and decreasing pH. The ability of the patient to attain high oxygen delivery parameters correlates with improved chance of survival.

CVP provides information on filling pressures of the right side of the heart; PADP and PCWP reflect left-sided fluid volumes. Cardiac output provides an objective number to guide therapy.

Therapeutic Interventions

Actions/Interventions

▲ Administer fluid and blood replacement therapy as described in prior nursing diagnosis, Deficient Fluid Volume.

▲ If possible, use a fluid warmer or rapid fluid infuser.

▲ Provide electrolyte replacement as ordered.

▲ If the patient's condition progressively deteriorates, initiate cardiopulmonary resuscitation or other lifesaving measures according to Advanced Cardiac Life Support guidelines, as indicated.

Rationales

Maintaining an adequate circulating blood volume is a priority.

Fluid warmers keep core temperatures warm. Infusion of cold blood is associated with myocardial dysrhythmias and paradoxical hypotension. Macropore filtering IV devices should also be used to remove small clots and debris.

Electrolyte imbalance may cause dysrhythmias and other pathological states.

Shock unresponsive to fluid replacement can deteriorate to cardiogenic shock. Depending on etiological factors, inotropic agents, antidysrhythmics, vasopressors, or other medications can be used.

NANDA-I NDx Anxiety

Common Related Factors

Health status change
Unfamiliar environment
Threat of death

Defining Characteristics

Verbalized anxiety
Restlessness and agitation
Apprehensive
Increased pulse and BP
Increased respirations
Focus on self
Difficulty concentrating

Common Expected Outcomes

Patient uses effective coping mechanisms.
Patient describes a reduction in level of anxiety experienced.

NOC Outcomes

Anxiety Self-Control; Coping

NIC Interventions

Anxiety Reduction; Presence; Calming Technique

Cardiac and Vascular Care Plans

■ = Independent   ▲ = Collaborative

Ongoing Assessment

Actions/Interventions	Rationales
■ Assess anxiety level (mild, severe). Note signs and symptoms, especially nonverbal communication.	Shock can result in an acute life-threatening situation that will produce high levels of anxiety in the patient as well as in significant others.
■ Assess coping techniques commonly used.	Anxiety and ways of decreasing perceived anxiety are highly individualized. Interventions are most effective when they are consistent with the individual's established coping pattern.

Therapeutic Interventions

Actions/Interventions	Rationales
■ Acknowledge awareness of the patient's anxiety.	Acknowledgment of the patient's feelings validates the feelings and communicates acceptance of those feelings.
■ Encourage verbalization of feelings.	Talking about anxiety-producing situations and anxious feelings can help the person perceive the situation in a less-threatening manner.
■ Maintain confident, assured manner. Assure patient and significant others of close, continuous monitoring that will ensure prompt intervention.	The staff's anxiety may be easily perceived by the patient. The patient's feeling of stability increases in a calm and non-threatening atmosphere. The presence of a trusted person may help the patient feel less threatened.
■ Reduce unnecessary external stimuli by maintaining a quiet environment.	Anxiety may escalate with excessive conversation, noise, and equipment around the patient.
■ Explain all procedures as appropriate, keeping explanations basic.	Information helps allay anxiety. Patients who are anxious may not be able to comprehend anything more than simple, clear, brief instructions.
■ Provide a quiet, private place for significant others to wait.	A quiet environment can reduce anxiety.
■ Offer Therapeutic Touch and related techniques (imagery, music)	These techniques provide comfort and support and decrease tension/anxiety.
▲ Refer to other support persons (e.g., clergy, social worker) as appropriate.	Additional specialty expertise may be required.

Related Care Plans

Acute respiratory distress syndrome, p. 358
Burns, p. 933
Gastrointestinal bleeding, p. 589
Imbalanced nutrition: Less than body requirements, p. 142
Impaired gas exchange, p. 78
Shock, Cardiogenic, p. 331

Shock, Septic

Distributive Shock; Sepsis; Bacteremia; Endotoxic Shock; Disseminated Intravascular Coagulation (DIC); Multiple Organ Failure

Septic shock is associated with severe infection and occurs after bacteremia of gram-negative bacilli (most common) or gram-positive cocci. Septic shock is mediated by a complex interaction of hormonal and chemical substances through an immune system response to bacterial endotoxins. In the early stages of sepsis, the body responds to infection by the normal inflammatory response. As the infection progresses, sepsis becomes more severe and leads to decreased tissue perfusion and oxygen delivery and multiple-organ dysfunction. Septic shock occurs as an exaggerated inflammatory response that leads to hypotension even with adequate fluid resuscitation. The primary effects of septic shock are massive vasodilation, maldistribution of blood volume, and myocardial depression. The maldistribution of circulatory volume results in some tissues receiving more than adequate blood flow and other tissues receiving less than adequate blood flow. As shock progresses, disseminated intravascular coagulation (DIC) may occur, resulting in a serious imbalance between clotting and bleeding.

Older patients are at increased risk for septic shock because of factors such as impaired immune response, impaired organ function, chronic debilitating illnesses, impaired mobility that can lead to pneumonia, decubitus ulcers, and loss of bladder control requiring indwelling catheters. The mortality rate from septic shock is high (30% to approximately 50%), especially in older patients. Immunocompromised patients and those with chronic diseases are also at increased risk. Patients are usually treated in an intensive care unit. Treatment is focused on providing fluid volume resuscitation and antibiotic therapy based on causative bacteria/cocci and supporting major organ dysfunction.

NDx Infection

Common Related Factors

An infectious process of either gram-negative or gram-positive bacteria

The most common causative organisms and their related factors are as follows:

- *Escherichia coli:* commonly occurs in genitourinary tract, biliary tract, intravenous (IV) catheter, or colon or intraabdominal abscesses
- *Klebsiella:* occurs in the lungs, gastrointestinal tract, IV catheter, urinary tract, or surgical wounds
- *Proteus:* occurs in the genitourinary tract, respiratory tract, abscesses, or biliary tract
- *Bacteroides fragilis:* occurs in the female genital tract, colon, liver abscesses, or decubitus ulcers
- *Pseudomonas aeruginosa:* occurs in the lungs, urinary tract, skin, or IV catheter
- *Candida albicans:* occurs in line-related infections, especially hyperalimentation infusion and pulmonary and urinary abscesses

Defining Characteristics

Changes in level of consciousness: lethargy or confusion
Fever or chills
Ruddy appearance with warm, dry skin
Leukocytosis
Positive blood cultures

Common Expected Outcome

The patient is free of infection, as evidenced by normal body temperature, normal white blood cell count, negative cultures, absence of chills, and normal level of consciousness.

NOC Outcomes
Vital Signs; Thermoregulation; Infection Severity
NIC Interventions
Vital Sign Monitoring; Medication Administration; Temperature Regulation

■ = Independent ▲ = Collaborative

Ongoing Assessment

Actions/Interventions	Rationales
■ Monitor heart rate (HR) and blood pressure (BP).	Septic shock can present in two phases. During the early, more treatable phase (high-output shock), there is an increase in cardiac output reflected by tachycardia and normal or elevated BP. However, as shock continues and the septic phase ensues, blood vessels dilate, causing hypovolemia and hypotension. Refractory hypotension despite optimal fluid therapy is a criterion for diagnosing septic shock.
■ Assess for presence of chills and febrile state.	Chills often precede temperature spikes. Temperature provides information about the patient's response to invading organisms. Temperature may be higher than 38° C or lower than 36° C.
■ Assess skin turgor, color, temperature, and peripheral pulses.	In early septic shock, warm, dry, flushed skin and bounding pulses are evident as a result of initial vasodilation (warm shock). As shock state continues, skin becomes cool, clammy, and cyanotic with reduced peripheral pulses.
■ Assess level of consciousness. Use neurological checklist, such as Glasgow Coma Scale.	Altered cerebral tissue perfusion may be the first sign of compensatory response to septic state. The patient may experience fatigue, malaise, anxiety, or confusion. Mild disorientation is common in older adults.
▲ Use pulse oximetry to assess oxygen saturation.	Pulse oximetry is a useful tool to detect changes in oxygenation. Oxygen saturation should be kept at 90% or greater.
▲ Assess arterial blood gases (ABGs). Note presence of respiratory alkalosis from tachypnea and hyperventilation.	Initially, respiratory alkalosis from hyperventilation may be evident. As shock increases, aerobic metabolism ceases and lactic acidosis ensues, raising the level of carbon dioxide and decreasing pH.
■ Assess related factors of infection thoroughly: • *Lungs:* Assess lung sounds and presence of sputum, including color, odor, and amount. Note presence of crackles and decreased breath sounds. • *Genitourinary:* Monitor urinalysis reports, assess color and opacity of urine, and assess for presence of drainage or pus around Foley catheter. • *Gastrointestinal:* Check for abdominal distention, and assess for bowel sounds and abdominal tenderness. • *IV catheters:* Assess all insertion sites for redness, swelling, and drainage. • *Surgical wounds:* Assess all wounds for signs of infection, including redness, swelling, and drainage. • *Pain:* Obtain patient's subjective statement of location and description of pain or discomfort. This may help localize a site.	Cause of shock guides treatment plan. Initial antibiotics are selected depending on the most likely site of infection. As culture reports are obtained, the most effective antibiotics will be selected.
▲ Obtain culture and sensitivity (C&S) samples as ordered.	Evidence of infection through a positive blood culture is a criterion for diagnosis. C&S reports show which antibiotic will be effective against the invading organism.
▲ Draw peak and trough antibiotic titers as needed.	Serum drug levels help ensure an appropriate level of antibiotic for the patient.
▲ Monitor white blood cell count.	White blood cell count provides data on progression of sepsis and response to treatment.
▲ Monitor for toxicity from antibiotic therapy, especially in patients with hepatic and/or renal insufficiency or failure and in older patients.	Aminoglycosides should be followed with urinalysis and serum creatinine levels at least three times per week. Chloramphenicol should be restricted in patients with liver disease.

Therapeutic Interventions

Actions/Interventions	Rationales
▲ Initiate early administration of antibiotics as prescribed.	Antibiotic therapy is begun with broad-spectrum antibiotics after the C&S is obtained but before the actual C&S report is received. After the C&S report is received, the physician should be notified if the organism is not sensitive to the present antibiotic coverage. The antibiotic may then be changed or supplemented. Common treatment for gram-positive organisms includes vancomycin; for gram-negative organisms, expanded penicillin and aminoglycosides are commonly used.
■ Remove any possible source of infection (e.g., urinary catheter, IV catheter).	Infection prevention begins with removing possible sites for bacterial entry into the body. Invasive catheters disrupt skin and mucous membranes and interfere with the body's first line of defense against infection.
▲ Maintain temperature in optimal range: • Administer antipyretics as prescribed. • Apply cooling mattress. • Administer tepid sponge baths. • Limit number of blankets/linens used to cover patients.	Normothermia prevents stress on the cardiovascular system and promotes comfort.
▲ Initiate appropriate isolation measures.	Isolation prevents the spread of infection.
▲ Assist with the incision and drainage of wounds, irrigation, and sterile application of saline-soaked 4 × 4s as indicated.	Early treatment promotes recovery.
▲ Manage the cause of infection, and anticipate surgical consult as necessary.	Surgical treatment may be indicated to drain pus or abscess, resolve obstruction, or repair a perforated organ.
▲ If signs of DIC occur, refer to the nursing care plan for Disseminated Intravascular Coagulation.	

Deficient Fluid Volume

Common Related Factors
Early septic shock
Decrease in systemic vascular resistance
Increased capillary permeability
Increased metabolic rate (fever, infection)
Failure of regulatory mechanisms

Defining Characteristics
Hypotension
Tachycardia/weak pulse
Decreased urine output (less than 30 mL/hr)
Concentrated urine
Decreased skin turgor
Dry mucous membranes
Weakness

Common Expected Outcome
Patient experiences adequate fluid volume as evidenced by urine output greater than 30 mL/hr, HR less than 100 beats/min, systolic BP greater than or equal to 90 mm Hg (or patient's baseline), and normal skin turgor.

NOC Outcomes
Fluid Balance; Electrolyte and Acid/Base Balance; Vital Signs; Hydration
NIC Interventions
Fluid Monitoring; Fluid Resuscitation; Invasive Hemodynamic Monitoring; Hemodynamic Regulation; Shock Management: Vasogenic

■ = Independent   ▲ = Collaborative

Ongoing Assessment

Actions/Interventions	Rationales
■ Assess for hypotension and tachycardia.	During the early phase of shock, tachycardia and normal BP are evident, but as shock progresses with subsequent vasodilation, hypotension ensues.
■ Assess urine output.	The renal system compensates for low BP by retaining water. Oliguria is a classic sign of inadequate renal perfusion from reduced cardiac output. As shock continues and the kidneys fail, urine output may stop, resulting in buildup of metabolic waste products.
■ Assess fluid balance, noting skin turgor and mucous membranes.	Compromised regulatory mechanisms may result in fluid and sodium retention. Loss of interstitial fluid causes loss of skin turgor. As sepsis continues, toxins cause leakage of fluid into tissues and cause swelling.
▲ If hemodynamic monitoring is in place, assess central venous pressure (CVP), pulmonary artery pressure, pulmonary capillary wedge pressure (PCWP), and cardiac output/cardiac index (CO/CI).	CVP provides information on filling pressures of the right side of the heart; pulmonary artery diastolic pressure and PCWP reflect left-sided fluid volumes. CO/CI provides an objective number to guide therapy.
▲ When initiating fluid challenges, closely monitor patient.	Close monitoring prevents iatrogenic volume overload. However, septic patients usually have refractory hypotension despite aggressive fluid therapy.

Therapeutic Interventions

Actions/Interventions	Rationales
▲ Perform fluid resuscitation aggressively as ordered. Use caution in fluid replacement in older patients.	Fluid administration is necessary to support tissue perfusion. Infusion rates will vary depending on clinical status. The fluid needs in septic patients may exceed 8 to 20 liters in the first 24 hours. Older patients may be more prone to congestive heart failure. In these patients, monitor closely for signs of iatrogenic fluid volume overload.
▲ Adjust fluid as ordered.	The optimal PCWP is usually 12 mm Hg in the absence of myocardial infarction and 14 to 18 mm Hg if myocardial infarction has occurred.
▲ If there is poor or no response to fluid resuscitation, administer vasoactive substances, such as phenylephrine hydrochloride (Neo-Synephrine), norepinephrine bitartrate (Levophed), or dopamine as prescribed.	In early septic shock the cardiac output is high or normal. At this point, the vasoactive agents are administered for their α-adrenergic effect to raise BP.

Decreased Cardiac Output

Common Related Factors	Defining Characteristics
Late septic shock: a decrease in tissue perfusion leads to increased lactic acid production and systemic acidosis, which causes a decrease in myocardial contractility	Decreased peripheral pulses
	Cold, clammy skin
	Hypotension
Gram-negative infections may cause a direct myocardial toxic effect	Agitation or confusion
	Decreased urinary output less than 30 mL/hr
Hypovolemia	Abnormal ABGs: acidosis and hypoxemia

Common Expected Outcome

Patient maintains adequate cardiac output, as evidenced by strong peripheral pulses; systolic BP within 20 mm Hg of baseline, HR 60 to 100 beats/min with regular rhythm; urine output greater than 30 mL/hr; warm and dry skin, and normal level of consciousness.

NOC Outcomes
Cardiac Pump Effectiveness; Circulation Status
NIC Interventions
Invasive Hemodynamic Monitoring; Hemodynamic Regulation; Acid/Base Management: Metabolic Acidosis; Shock Management: Vasogenic

Ongoing Assessment

Actions/Interventions	Rationales
■ Assess skin warmth and peripheral pulses.	Compensatory peripheral vasoconstriction in late stages of septic shock causes cool, pale, diaphoretic skin. Pulses are weak with reduced stroke volume and cardiac output.
■ Assess for any changes in level of consciousness.	Early signs of cerebral hypoxia are restlessness and anxiety, leading to agitation and confusion. The patient may become lethargic and comatose.
▲ Assess HR, BP, and pulse pressure. Use direct intraarterial monitoring as ordered.	Sinus tachycardia and increased arterial BP are seen in early stages to maintain an adequate cardiac output. However, as sepsis progresses, toxins are produced by the bacterial cells in the body, resulting in release of cytokines that cause extensive vasodilation and dangerously low blood pressures. The lowered BP compromises perfusion to vital organs. Auscultatory BP may be unreliable secondary to vasoconstriction. Pulse pressure (systolic minus diastolic) decreases in late septic shock.
■ Assess urine output.	The renal system compensates for low blood pressure by retaining water. Oliguria is a classic sign of inadequate renal perfusion from reduced cardiac output. As shock continues and the kidneys fail, urine output may stop, resulting in buildup of metabolic waste products.
■ Assess cardiac rhythm for dysrhythmias.	Cardiac dysrhythmias may occur from the low perfusion state, acidosis, or hypoxia, as well as from side effects of cardiac medications used to treat this condition.
▲ If hemodynamic monitoring is in place, assess CVP, pulmonary artery pressure, PCWP, and CO.	CVP provides information on filling pressures of the right side of the heart; pulmonary artery diastolic pressure and PCWP reflect left-sided fluid volumes.

Therapeutic Interventions

Actions/Interventions	Rationales
▲ Place patient in the physiological position for shock: head of bed flat with trunk horizontal and lower extremities elevated 20 to 30 degrees with knees straight.	This position promotes venous return.
▲ Administer inotropic agents: dobutamine hydrochloride, dopamine, digoxin, or milrinone. Continuously monitor their effectiveness. Administer sodium bicarbonate to treat acidosis.	Inotropic medications improve myocardial contractility and cardiac output. Sodium bicarbonate buffers the excess lactic acid released by anoxic tissues.

■ = Independent   ▲ = Collaborative

NDx Risk for Ineffective Breathing Pattern

Common Risk Factors

Progressive shock state
Lactic acidosis

Common Expected Outcome

Patient will maintain an effective breathing pattern, as evidenced by relaxed breathing at normal rate.

NOC Outcome
Respiratory Status: Ventilation

NIC Interventions
Respiratory Monitoring; Ventilation Assistance

Ongoing Assessment

Actions/Interventions	Rationales
■ Assess respiratory rate, rhythm, and depth.	Rapid, shallow respirations may occur from hypoxia or from acidosis with sepsis. As shock continues, lung function deteriorates, causing fluid to accumulate in the lungs. Development of hypoventilation indicates that immediate ventilator support is needed.
■ Assess for any increase in work of breathing: shortness of breath, and use of accessory muscles.	As septic shock progresses, patients may experience acute respiratory distress syndrome.
■ Assess lungs, noting areas of decreased ventilation and the presence of adventitious sounds.	Moist crackles are caused by increased pulmonary capillary permeability and increased intraalveolar edema. Older patients, who most commonly experience septic shock, may have difficulty clearing their airways, resulting in atelectasis and pneumonia.
▲ Use pulse oximetry to monitor oxygen saturation; assess ABGs.	Oxygen saturation should be kept at 90% or greater. As shock increases, aerobic metabolism ceases and lactic acidosis ensues, raising the level of carbon dioxide and decreasing pH.

Therapeutic Interventions

Actions/Interventions	Rationales
■ Position the patient with proper body alignment for optimal breathing pattern.	If not contraindicated, a sitting position allows for adequate diaphragmatic and lung excursion.
■ Suction as needed.	Productive coughing is the most effective way to remove moist secretions. If patient is unable to perform, suctioning may be needed to promote airway patency.
■ Provide reassurance and allay anxiety by staying with patient during episodes of respiratory distress.	Anxiety can result in rapid, shallow respirations and increase noneffective breathing efforts.
▲ Administer oxygen as prescribed.	Oxygen may be required to maintain oxygen saturation at 90% or greater. Desaturation leads to tissue hypoxia, acidosis, dysrhythmias, and decreased level of consciousness.
■ Anticipate need for intubation and mechanical ventilation if patient is unable to maintain adequate gas exchange.	Rapid, efficient intervention is critical to preserve vital organ function and life.

NANDA-I NDx Deficient Knowledge

Common Related Factors

New condition
Emotional state affecting learning (anxiety)

Defining Characteristics

Increased frequency of questions posed by patient and significant others
Inability to respond correctly to questions asked

Common Expected Outcome

Patient or significant others verbalize understanding of disease process and treatments used.

NOC Outcomes
Knowledge: Disease Process; Knowledge: Infection Control

NIC Interventions
Teaching: Disease Process; Infection Protection

Ongoing Assessment

Actions/Interventions	Rationales
■ Evaluate understanding of septic shock and patient's overall condition.	Information guides starting point for educational intervention.

Therapeutic Interventions

Actions/Interventions	Rationales
■ Keep the patient or significant others informed of disease process and present status of the patient.	Septic shock results in a critically ill patient with a tenuous baseline for recovery. The death rate depends on the cause of the infection, how early it is identified and treated, and how many organs have failed.
■ Explain common factors that placed the patient at risk for septic shock: • Advanced age with declining immune system • Malnourishment/poor hydration • Debilitating chronic illnesses • Insertion of indwelling catheter • Surgical and diagnostic procedure • Decubitus ulcer or wounds • Cross-contamination or exposure to resistant organisms	Knowledge is critical, especially in older patients and those who are immunosuppressed and already at greater risk for infection and sepsis.
■ Instruct regarding general hygiene measures to reduce risk for infection.	Practices such as good personal hygiene, hand washing, adequate rest, balanced diet, exercise, and oral care all promote reduced infection risks.

Related Care Plans

Acute renal failure, p. 790
Acute respiratory distress syndrome, p. 358
Disseminated intravascular coagulation, p. 698
Fear, p. 69
Shock, hypovolemic, p. 337
Imbalanced nutrition: Less than body requirements, p. 142
Ineffective tissue perfusion, p. 199

Deep Vein Thrombosis

Venous Thromboembolic Disease; Phlebitis; Phlebothrombosis

Thrombophlebitis is the inflammation of the wall of a vein, usually resulting in the formation of a blood clot (thrombosis) that may partially or completely block the flow of blood through the vessel. Venous thrombophlebitis usually occurs in the lower extremities. It may occur in superficial veins, which although painful, is not life threatening and does not require hospitalization, or it may occur in a deep vein, which can be life threatening because clots may break free (embolize) and cause a pulmonary embolism. Three factors contribute to the development of deep vein thrombosis (DVT): venous stasis, hypercoagulability, and endothelial damage to the vein. Prolonged immobility is the primary cause of venous stasis. Hypercoagulability is seen in patients with deficient fluid volume, oral contraceptive use, smoking, and certain malignancies. Venous wall damage may occur secondary to intravenous (IV) infusions, certain medications, fractures, and contrast x-ray studies. DVT most commonly occurs in lower extremities, where it is often asymptomatic and resolves in a few days. More proximal DVTs are associated with greater symptomatology and carry a higher risk for dislodgment and migration. Treatment is supportive, usually with anticoagulant therapy. Goals are to reduce risk for complications and prevent reoccurrence.

NANDA-I NDx Ineffective Peripheral Tissue Perfusion

Common Related Factors

Venous stasis
Injury to vessel wall
Hypercoagulability of blood

Common Expected Outcomes

Patient maintains optimal peripheral tissue perfusion in effected extremity, as evidenced by strong palpable pulses, reduction of/absence in pain, warm and dry extremities, and adequate capillary refill.
Patient does not experience pulmonary embolism, as evidenced by normal breathing, normal heart rate, and absence of dyspnea and chest pain.

Defining Characteristics

Usually involves changes in femoral, popliteal, or small calf veins
 • Pain
 • Edema (unilateral)
 • Tenderness
 • Increased warmth in leg
 • Pain during palpation of calf muscle
May be asymptomatic

NOC Outcomes

Tissue Perfusion: Peripheral; Blood Coagulation

NIC Interventions

Embolus Care: Peripheral; Teaching: Disease Process

Ongoing Assessment

Actions/Interventions

■ Assess for signs and symptoms of deep vein thrombosis.

■ Assess for contributing factors: immobility, leg trauma, intraoperative positioning (especially in older patients), dehydration, smoking, varicose veins, pregnancy, obesity, surgery, malignancy, and use of oral contraceptives.

■ Measure circumference of affected leg with a tape measure.

Rationales

DVT can be challenging to diagnose, especially if involving a distal vein.

Many patients are asymptomatic. Knowledge of high-risk situations aids in early detection. Venous stasis is a leading factor in the development of DVT.

Measurement is to document progression or resolution of swelling. The affected leg will be larger. In some patients, unequal leg circumference may be the only sign of DVT.

Actions/Interventions

▲ Monitor results of diagnostic tests:

- Duplex ultrasound

- D-dimer assay

- Impedance plethysmography

- Contrast venography

▲ Monitor coagulation profile (prothrombin time [PT]/ international normalized ratio [INR]/partial thromboplastin time [PTT]).

Rationales

These tests are used to document location of clot and status of affected vein.

Ultrasound uses a Doppler probe to document reduced flow, especially in popliteal and iliofemoral veins.

D-dimer is a marker for clot lysis. It does not provide any information about the site of the problem.

This test uses blood pressure cuffs to record changes in venous flow.

This test uses radiopaque contrast media injected through a foot vein to localize thrombi in the deep venous system.

The results of coagulation studies are used to measure the effectiveness of anticoagulant therapy. The PTT is used for patients receiving intravenous heparin. The PT/INR is used for patients receiving warfarin. Baseline values are obtained before the first dose of anticoagulant is administered. Repeated tests are done at prescribed intervals to adjust drug dosages to achieve desired changes in coagulation.

Cardiac and Vascular Care Plans

Therapeutic Interventions

Actions/Interventions

■ Encourage and maintain bed rest with affected leg elevated (depending on size and location of clot) as indicated.

▲ Administer/instruct in use of anticoagulant therapy as ordered (heparin/warfarin [Coumadin]).

▲ Administer analgesics as indicated.
■ Maintain adequate hydration.

■ Provide warm, moist heat to affected site.
▲ Apply below-knee compression stockings as prescribed. Ensure that stockings are of correct size and are applied correctly.
▲ With massive DVT severely compromising tissue perfusion, anticipate thrombolytic therapy.

▲ If the patient shows no response to conventional therapy or if the patient is not a candidate for anticoagulation, anticipate surgical treatment:
- Thrombectomy

- Placement of a vena cava filter

Rationales

Bed rest, the cornerstone of past treatments, may not be required for clots in the lower leg, because these are less likely to embolize. It may be required for upper extremity clots. Elevation of the leg will reduce venous pooling and edema.

Therapy will prevent further clot formation by decreasing normal activity of the clotting mechanism. Heparin IV or subcutaneous low-molecular-weight heparin is started initially. Oral anticoagulant therapy (warfarin) will be initiated while patient is still receiving heparin because the onset of action for warfarin can be up to 72 hours. Heparin will be discontinued once the warfarin reaches therapeutic levels.

Analgesics relieve pain and promote comfort.

Hydration prevents increased viscosity of blood, which contributes to venous stasis and clotting.

Heat relieves pain and inflammation.

These stockings promote venous blood flow and decrease venous stagnation. Inaccurately applied stockings can serve as a tourniquet and can facilitate clot formation.

Thrombolytic therapy is reserved for severe cases. Clot lysis carries a higher risk for bleeding than anticoagulation because it dissolves both undesired and therapeutic clots. Therefore use is restricted to patients with severe embolism that significantly compromises blood flow to tissues. Therapy must be initiated soon after the onset of symptoms (within 5 days).

Thrombectomy is a procedure to excise the clot if a major vein is occluded.

This filter traps any migrating clots and prevents pulmonary embolism It is recommended for patients who cannot take anticoagulants or those with recurrent DVT despite anticoagulant therapy.

■ = Independent   ▲ = Collaborative

Risk for Bleeding

Common Risk Factors

Anticoagulation therapy for DVT
Abnormal blood profiles

Common Expected Outcomes

Patient maintains therapeutic blood level of anticoagulant, as evidenced by PTT/PT/INR within desired range.
Patient does not experience bleeding.

NOC Outcome
Blood Coagulation
NIC Interventions
Bleeding Precautions; Bleeding Reduction

Ongoing Assessment

Actions/Interventions	**Rationales**
▲ Monitor platelet counts, coagulation test results (INR, PT, partial thromboplastin time [PTT]).	Effects of anticoagulation therapy must be closely monitored to reduce risk for bleeding. Type of test depends on anticoagulation medication administered.
■ Assess for signs and symptoms of bleeding.	Early assessment facilitates prompt treatment.
▲ Monitor platelets and heparin-induced platelet aggregation (HIPA) status.	Severe platelet reduction can occur with heparin use, especially unfractionated heparin therapy, and is known as heparin-induced thrombocytopenia (HIT). HIT is less commonly seen with the use of low-molecular-weight heparin.

Therapeutic Interventions

Actions/Interventions	**Rationales**
▲ Administer anticoagulant therapy as prescribed (continuous IV heparin/subcutaneous low-molecular-weight heparin; oral warfarin).	Anticoagulants are given to prevent further clot formation. The type of medication varies per protocol and severity of clot
▲ If bleeding occurs while on IV heparin: • Stop the infusion. • Recheck PTT level stat. • Administer protamine sulfate as ordered. • Reevaluate dose of heparin on basis of PTT result	Laboratory data guide further treatment. The guide for PTT level is 1.5 to 2 times normal. Protamine sulfate is a heparin antagonist.
▲ Convert from IV anticoagulation to oral anticoagulation after appropriate length of therapy. Monitor INR, PT, and PTT levels.	PT or INR levels should be in an adequate range for anticoagulation before discontinuing heparin.
▲ If HIPA is positive, stop all heparin products and anticipate a hematology consult.	Continuation of heparin products further complicates the situation.

Deficient Knowledge

Common Related Factor

Unfamiliarity with pathology, treatment, and prevention

Defining Characteristics

Multiple questions to health care team
Inaccurate follow-through
Inaccurate information

Common Expected Outcome

Patient and/or significant others verbalize understanding of disease, management, and prevention.

NOC Outcomes
Knowledge: Disease Process; Knowledge: Treatment Regimen

NIC Interventions
Teaching: Disease Process; Teaching: Prescribed Medications

Ongoing Assessment

Actions/Interventions	Rationales
■ Assess understanding of causes, treatment, and prevention plan for DVT.	This information provides an important starting point in education. DVT requires preventive action to reduce risk for reoccurrence.

Therapeutic Interventions

Actions/Interventions	Rationales
■ Explain the following conditions that place people at risk for blood clots: • Varicose veins • Pregnancy • Obesity • Surgery (especially pelvic or abdominal) • Immobility • Advanced age • Oral contraceptives	Knowledge of causative factors provides direction for subsequent treatment. Preventing thrombus formation is an ongoing concern.
■ Explain the rationale for treatment of deep vein thrombosis.	DVT may range from mild to life threatening and may require additional treatment with anticoagulation.
■ Explain the need for activity restriction and elevation of leg.	Activity restriction and elevation of leg prevent embolization with more significant DVT.
■ Instruct the patient in correct application of compression stockings.	Stockings applied incorrectly can act as a tourniquet and facilitate clot formation.
■ Instruct the patient to avoid rubbing or massaging calf.	Avoidance will prevent breaking off clot, which may circulate as embolus.
■ Instruct the patient to take medications as prescribed, explaining their actions, dosages, and side effects.	Accurate knowledge reduces future complications. Analgesics and antiinflammatory medications may be needed for short-term symptom relief. Patients may require anticoagulation for weeks or long term, depending on risks.
■ Discuss and give the patient a list of signs and symptoms of excessive anticoagulation: easy bruising, severe nosebleed, black stools, blood in urine or stools, joint swelling and pain, coughing up of blood, severe headache.	Patients need to self-manage their condition. Early assessment facilitates prompt treatment.
■ Inform the patient of the need for routine laboratory testing while on oral anticoagulation.	Continued regular assessment of anticoagulation is necessary to prevent both reoccurrence of clots and active bleeding.
■ Discuss the following measures to prevent recurrence: • Avoiding staying in one position for long periods; when traveling, moving feet/legs often	Avoidance will prevent venous stasis (at home, on train or plane, at desk).
• Not sitting with legs crossed	The patient should avoid any position that compresses the veins and limits venous return.
• Maintaining healthy body weight	Obesity contributes to venous insufficiency and venous hypertension through compression of the main veins in the pelvic region.

■ = Independent   ▲ = Collaborative

Actions/Interventions	Rationales
• Maintaining adequate fluid status	Adequate hydration prevents hypercoagulability.
• Wearing properly sized, correctly applied compression stockings as prescribed	Patients with DVT are at high risk for redevelopment and may need to wear stockings over the long term.
• Avoiding constricting garters or socks with tight bands	Wearing constricting clothing reduces optimal blood flow and promotes clotting.
• Quitting smoking	Nicotine is a vasoconstrictor that promotes clotting.
• Participating in an exercise program	Walking, swimming, and cycling help promote venous return through contraction of the calf and thigh muscles. These muscles act as a pump to compress veins and support the column of blood returning to the heart.
■ For patients with DVT, instruct in the following signs of pulmonary embolus: • Sudden chest pain • Tachypnea • Tachycardia • Shortness of breath • Restlessness	These symptoms can be caused by a clot that breaks off from the original clot in the leg and travels to the lungs.
■ Discuss safety or precautionary measures to use while on anticoagulant therapy: need to inform dentist or other caregivers before treatment, use of electric razor, use of soft toothbrush.	These measures help prevent bleeding.

Related Care Plan

Pulmonary embolism, p. 439

Venous Insufficiency, Chronic

Postphlebitic Syndrome; Peripheral Venous Hypertension; Venous Stasis Ulcer

Chronic venous insufficiency occurs from a disruption in the venous system that results in the pressure from the venous blood column no longer being supported toward the heart. This pressure is directed as backflow to the ankle area. The most common causes are congenital venous valve insufficiency, acquired valve incompetence from venous valve prolapse (often from history of deep vein thrombosis or varicose veins), venous obstruction from tumor or fibrosis, or calf muscle pump malfunction from sedentary lifestyle or muscle wasting disease. The increased backflow and pressure cause dilation of the venules of the skin, primarily in the ankle area, with resulting movement of fluid from the vascular bed to the tissue bed. Because the endothelium of the venules is subjected to higher than normal pressures, red blood cells move across the vessel wall into the interstitial spaces. When these red blood cells break down, they deposit hemosiderin in the tissues. The presence of hemosiderin in the tissues produces the characteristic skin color changes in venous insufficiency. The clinical manifestations of chronic venous insufficiency include dull aching, tenderness, pain in leg; leg pain getting worse when standing or when legs are raised; edema; skin color changes; dermatitis; and venous stasis ulcers. Once skin ulceration occurs, it is difficult to heal. Ulcers may recur with minimal skin trauma.

Risk for Ineffective Peripheral Tissue Perfusion

Common Risk Factors

Increased venous pressure
Dependent edema

Common Expected Outcomes

Patient maintains optimal peripheral tissue perfusion in effected extremity, as evidenced by strong palpable pulse, reduction in/absence of pain, warm and dry extremities, and adequate capillary refill.

Patient demonstrates measures to increase venous return and decrease leg edema.

NOC Outcomes
Tissue Perfusion: Peripheral; Circulation Status

NIC Interventions
Circulatory Care: Venous Insufficiency; Lower Leg Monitoring

Ongoing Assessment

Actions/Interventions	Rationales
■ Assess lower extremities for the following:	
• Edema by measuring leg circumference	Edema of chronic venous insufficiency may not be relieved with elevation of the extremity.
• Skin color	Skin may have a dark brown discoloration caused by deposition of hemosiderin in the tissues. This condition is sometimes referred to as brawny edema.
• Pain	Patient may report a dull aching or heaviness in the legs.
• Skin changes	Patient may have areas of induration as a result of liposclerosis. Areas of skin may be thinned or scarred from previous stasis ulcers.
▲ Monitor results of Doppler flow studies.	This diagnostic test assesses venous flow and any obstruction.

Therapeutic Interventions

Actions/Interventions	Rationales
■ Encourage patient to keep legs elevated when not ambulating. Patient may benefit from placement of the foot of the bed on 6-inch blocks to enhance venous return while sleeping.	Goal of treatment is to reduce venous hypertension and reduce tissue edema. Elevation uses effects of gravity to promote venous return.
▲ Apply appropriate venous compression devices such as support hose or pneumatic compression.	Prescription support hose are worn below the knee to support venous return. Hosiery should apply about 40 mm Hg of compression. Above-the-knee hosiery is not needed because the thigh muscle pump is usually adequate. Also, patients are less compliant with thigh-high compression because of difficulty with application and discomfort. Full-leg pneumatic compression devices may be used for short-term management of severe edema.
■ Encourage the patient to avoid standing for prolonged periods.	Standing in one position for a long time without walking will increase venous pressure and edema.
■ Teach the patient to change positions at frequent intervals.	Remaining in one position for more than a couple of hours contributes to venous stasis by compressing veins.
■ Teach the patient to avoid crossing legs at the knee when sitting.	The patient should avoid any position that compresses the veins and limits venous return.
■ Encourage weight reduction for overweight patients.	Obesity contributes to venous insufficiency and venous hypertension through compression of the main veins in the pelvic region.

■ = Independent ▲ = Collaborative

Actions/Interventions

- Encourage the patient to begin an exercise program.

▲ Administer prescribed diuretics.

Rationales

Walking, swimming, and cycling help promote venous return through contraction of the calf and thigh muscles. These muscles act as a pump to compress veins and support the column of blood returning to the heart.

Diuretic therapy may be used as an adjunct treatment to help mobilize fluid and reduce tissue edema.

NANDA-I NDx Impaired Skin Integrity

Common Related Factors

Venous stasis ulcers
Stasis dermatitis

Defining Characteristics

Loss of epidermis and dermis in areas of chronic edema around medial malleolus or tibial area
Irregular-bordered ulcer with granulation tissue at base or soft yellow necrosis

Common Expected Outcome

Patient will have intact skin without signs of infection.

NOC Outcomes

Circulation Status; Wound Healing: Secondary Intention; Knowledge: Treatment Regimen

NIC Interventions

Circulatory Care: Venous Insufficiency; Wound Care; Skin Care: Topical Treatments; Teaching: Procedure/Treatment; Teaching: Prescribed Activity/Exercise

---

Ongoing Assessment

Actions/Interventions

- Assess ulcer characteristics:
  - Location

  - Size

  - Tissue bed

  - Surrounding tissue

- Measure surface of ulcer area at regular intervals; use pictures as appropriate.
- Monitor for signs of infection.

▲ Obtain specimens for culture of any wound drainage.

Rationales

Venous stasis ulcers are usually located around the medial malleolus or in the pretibial and laterotibial areas of the ankle.

Initially a venous stasis ulcer will be small, but it increases in size over time. The borders of venous ulcers tend to be irregular.

New ulcers will have a beefy red color consistent with the presence of granulating tissue. Older ulcers may have soft tissue necrosis at the base of the ulcer. This tissue may be yellowish green and have a stringy consistency.

Tissue surrounding the ulcer will be edematous. Skin may have a dark brown color and may be dry and flaky (chronic stasis dermatitis). Patient may report severe itching.

Assessment provides data on response to therapy.

Many ulcers are already colonized. Aggressive wound care is indicated at first sign of infection or breakdown.

If the ulcer is infected, cultures need to be obtained before appropriate antimicrobial therapy can be started.

Therapeutic Interventions	
Actions/Interventions	**Rationales**
■ Maintain bed rest with leg elevation.	Reducing venous hypertension and edema is important for healing.
■ Cleanse wound using saline or noncytotoxic cleanser before any dressing change.	Preparation of the wound bed is necessary to promote healing; necrotic tissue may require removal before treatment is started.
▲ Apply appropriate dressings to protect ulcer during healing:	These ulcers heal through secondary intention. Use of long-term dressings with compression allows patient to be ambulatory.
• Unna boot	The Unna boot is the mainstay of treatment of venous ulcers. This traditional dressing covers the ulcer and provides compression. It is made of gauze dressing impregnated with zinc oxide, calamine lotion, and glycerin. Once applied, it forms a soft cast from the toes to just below the knee. The boot is covered with an elastic wrap. It can remain in place for 7 days or longer. Disadvantages include discomfort, limitations on bathing, and odor if drainage leaks through the dressing.
• Hydrocolloid (DuoDerm) or vapor-permeable dressing (Op-Site, Tegaderm)	These dressings promote wound debridement and healing. Do not use with heavy exudate–producing wounds.
• Hydrogels (Aqua Skin, Carrasyn V)	These dressings are used for shallow ulcers without exudates. They promote wound debridement and healing.
• Alginates (Kalginate, Kaltostat, Sorbsan)	These dressings are for ulcers with exudates or moderate drainage; avoid in dry or heavily bleeding ulcers.
• Gauze with sodium chloride solution	These dressings maintain a moist environment but requires multiple dressing changes.
▲ If the ulcer is not healing, anticipate surgical intervention.	Nonhealing ulcers may require debridement and skin grafting. For patients with repeated stasis ulcers, removal of veins with incompetent valves may be indicated. In some cases, valve transplantation may be used.
▲ Administer prescribed antibiotics.	Antibiotics are indicated if cellulitis is present in the affected area.
■ Once the ulcer is healed, teach the patient about measures to prevent new ulcer development:	Once the skin integrity has been compromised in venous insufficiency, it is less resistant to trauma. With the slightest trauma, the skin will break. An ulcer forms as a way to relieve pressure in the chronically edematous tissue.
• Continue wearing external compression hosiery as prescribed.	Maintaining compression to reduce venous hypertension is important in preventing new ulcers. Stockings should be applied when first getting up in the morning and removed at bedtime.
• Replace compression hosiery every 3 to 6 months.	Even without signs of wear, the compression effectiveness is lost with long-term use.
• Inspect skin around ankles daily.	Venous stasis ulcers usually develop around the perforator veins in the pretibial and medial malleolar areas of the ankles. The first sign may be a small reddened area that is tender to the touch.
• Keep skin clean and well lubricated.	The patient should avoid moisturizers that contain alcohol because of the drying effect on the skin.
• Exercise care when ambulating.	Even minor trauma to the skin can result in ulcer formation.

■ = Independent   ▲ = Collaborative

Pulmonary Care Plans

Acute Respiratory Distress Syndrome (ARDS)

Shock Lung; Noncardiogenic Pulmonary Edema; Adult Respiratory Distress Syndrome, Stiff Lung; Wet Lung

Acute respiratory distress syndrome (ARDS) is a form of respiratory failure characterized by noncardiogenic pulmonary edema and a refractory hypoxemia. The pathology results from damage to the alveolar-capillary membrane. This damage is caused by cytokines released by primed neutrophils during a massive immune response (systemic inflammatory response syndrome). These cytokines increase vascular permeability to such an extent that a massive noncardiac pulmonary edema develops. This edema not only interferes with gas exchange but also damages the pulmonary cells that secrete surfactant. Loss of surfactant allows alveoli to collapse and results in very stiff, noncompliant lungs. Fibrin and cell debris build up, forming a membrane (hyaline) and further decreasing gas exchange. The combined edema, loss of surfactant, alveoli collapse, and hyaline membrane formation lead to a progressive refractory hypoxemia and eventually death.

Anyone with a recent history of severe cell damage or sepsis is at risk for developing ARDS. Examples include individuals who have aspirated or who have suffered trauma, burns, multiple fractures, severe head injury, pulmonary contusions, near drowning (salt water aspiration seems to be slightly higher risk than fresh water aspiration), smoke inhalation, carbon monoxide exposure, drug overdose (narcotics, salicylates, tricyclic antidepressants and other sedative drugs, tocolytic agents, hydrochlorothiazide, protamine, interleukin-2), oxygen toxicity, shock, and so on.

Even with outstanding care, the mortality rate for ARDS is 40% to 60%, and even those who survive may have permanent lung damage. With such a high mortality rate, it is clear that early detection and prevention are critical as is treatment of any causal factors. Thus careful assessment of all at-risk individuals for early warning signs of developing respiratory distress is a nursing responsibility. Unfortunately, the only early warning sign may be labored breathing and tachypnea. Once ARDS develops, nursing care focuses on maintenance of pulmonary functions. Despite evidence that ARDS is the result of an inflammatory response, antiinflammatory therapy is not effective, and with time, respiratory failure with severe respiratory distress usually results. Research is focused on identifying new pharmacological treatments to halt the progressive downward cycle of ARDS, including human recombinant interleukin-1 receptor antagonist surfactant replacement therapy, corticoid steroids, and the like.

This care plan focuses on acute care in the critical care setting where the patient is typically managed with intubation and mechanical ventilation.

Ineffective Breathing Pattern

Common Related Factors

Decreased lung compliance:
- Low amounts of surfactant
- Fluid transudation

Fatigue and decreased energy:
- Increased work of breathing
- Primary medical problem
- Buildup of fibrin and cellular debris (hyaline membrane development)

Common Expected Outcomes

Patient maintains an effective breathing pattern, as evidenced by relaxed breathing at normal rate and depth, absence of dyspnea, and blood gas results within patient's normal parameters.

Patient verbalizes ability to breathe comfortably without sensation of dyspnea, anxiety, or fear related to a sensation of shortness of breath.

Defining Characteristics

Dyspnea/shortness of breath
Restlessness/change in level of consciousness
Tachypnea
Cough
Use of accessory muscles
Respiratory depth changes
Cyanosis
Arterial pH less than 7.35
Decreased Po_2 level (less than 50 to 60 mm Hg)
Increased PCo_2 level (50 to 60 mm Hg or higher)

NOC Outcomes

Respiratory Status; Airway Patency; Respiratory Status: Ventilation; Respiratory Status: Gas Exchange

NIC Interventions

Respiratory Monitoring; Airway Management; Mechanical Ventilation; Oxygen Therapy

Ongoing Assessment

Actions/Interventions	Rationales
■ Assess respiratory rate, rhythm, and depth.	Respiratory rate and rhythm changes are early warning signs of impending respiratory difficulties. Breathing pattern is essentially an unconscious response to a perceived threat or to impaired gas exchange. With a stiff, noncompliant, wet (pulmonary edema) lung, gas exchange is decreased, leading to hypoxemia, which leads to an increase in the depth and rate of ventilations.
■ Assess for use of accessory muscles.	Work of breathing increases greatly as lung compliance decreases. Moving air in and out of the lungs becomes more and more difficult, and passive ventilation is no longer adequate to meet oxygenation needs. The breathing pattern alters to include use of the accessory muscles to increase chest excursion to facilitate effective breathing.
■ Assess lungs for normal or adventitious breath sounds.	As pulmonary edema increases and fluid moves into the alveoli, adventitious breath sounds (crackles) are heard throughout the lung fields.
■ Assess sensation of dyspnea.	The sensation of dyspnea is associated with hypoxia and may cause anxiety, which leads to increased oxygen demand and may further affect breathing patterns.
■ Assess for cyanosis of tongue, oral mucosa, and skin.	Cyanosis of the tongue, oral mucosa, and skin indicates increased concentration of deoxygenated blood and that the breathing pattern is no longer effective to maintain adequate oxygenation of tissues.

■ = Independent ▲ = Collaborative

Actions/Interventions	Rationales
▲ Use pulse oximetry to monitor oxygen saturation; assess arterial blood gases (ABGs).	Pulse oximetry and ABGs provide an objective indication of oxygenation status (and therefore effectiveness of breathing pattern). With ARDS, oxygen saturation decreases. It should be kept at 90% or greater. The ABGs will indicate developing respiratory acidosis and hypoxemia.
■ Assess for cough.	Increased pulmonary edema and fibrin buildup stimulate cough reflex.
■ Assess energy level.	As compliance decreases and breathing patterns alter to include use of accessory muscles, the work of breathing increases dramatically, leading to patient fatigue. Energy expenditure increases oxygen demand. Eventually the patient may be incapable of adequately maintaining oxygenation needs.
■ Assess for changes in level of consciousness.	Increased restlessness, confusion, and/or irritability are early indicators of insufficient oxygenation of the brain and requires further intervention.

Therapeutic Interventions

Actions/Interventions	Rationales
■ Provide reassurance and allay anxiety by staying with patient during acute episode of respiratory distress.	The presence of a trusted person may help the person feel less threatened and can reduce anxiety, thereby reducing oxygen requirements.
▲ Position the patient to optimize ventilation: • Although for most patients with ineffective breathing patterns the upright position is most effective because it facilitates lung expansion, for the ARDS patient the prone position may be recommended. Follow physician orders and ensure patient comfort, and observe for changes in oxygen saturation levels with position changes. If saturation drops or fails to return promptly to baseline, reposition the patient for optimal oxygenation.	Prone positioning is a technique used to improve oxygenation in patients with ARDS who are receiving mechanical ventilation. The exact mechanism leading to improvement of oxygenation in this position is unknown. Proposed mechanisms include recruitment of collapsed alveoli, redistribution of ventilation from the ventral (collapsed in the prone position) to dorsal regions (recruited in the prone position), and mobilization of secretions.
■ Plan activity and rest to maximize the patient's energy.	Fatigue is common with the increased work of breathing. Activity increases metabolic rate and oxygen requirements. Rest helps mobilize energy for more effective breathing and coughing efforts.
▲ Maintain oxygen saturation at or above 90%.	Oxygen saturation below 90% leads to tissue hypoxia, anaerobic cellular metabolism, acidosis, electrolyte shifts, dysrhythmias, decreased level of consciousness, increasing hypoxia, and ultimately death. Use caution with FIO_2 greater than 40% because of the increased risk for oxygen toxicity.
▲ Administer medications as indicated (e.g., steroids, antibiotics, bronchodilators, antianxiety medications).	Steroids may help reduce the inflammation; antibiotics may be necessary to treat the underlying cause of the inflammatory response; the bronchodilators may be useful to decrease the work of breathing and provide airway clearance. Antianxiety drugs relieve anxiety and may increase cooperation with ventilatory efforts and procedures.
■ Provide suctioning as needed.	Suctioning cleans secretions from pulmonary congestion and reduces the work of breathing. Its use should be guided by objective data, not preset time intervals.
■ Keep all team members informed of respiratory status.	To be successfully treated, ARDS requires aggressive intervention by multiple team members. The nurse is often the first team member to recognize changes in effective breathing patterns that may require other team members to intervene.

Actions/Interventions

▲ Anticipate the need for intubation and mechanical ventilation.

Rationales

Early intubation and mechanical ventilation are recommended to prevent full decompensation of the patient. Mechanical ventilation provides supportive care to maintain adequate oxygenation and ventilation.

NANDA-I
NDx **Impaired Gas Exchange**

Common Related Factors

Diffusion defect:
- Abnormal A-a gradient (greater difficulty for oxygen and carbon dioxide to cross alveolar-capillary membrane) from:
  - Hyaline membrane formation from cellular debris and fibrin
  - Damaged alveolar-capillary membrane
- Increased shunting leading to an abnormal $\dot{V}/\dot{Q}$ ratio from:
  - Collapsed alveoli
  - Fluid-filled alveoli
- Increased dead space (areas with decreased pulmonary circulation) from:
  - Microembolization in the pulmonary vasculature
  - Increased shunting (shutdown of capillaries to alveoli that are not ventilated)

Defining Characteristics

Hypoxia resulting in:
- Restlessness, irritability, anxiety, and decreasing level of consciousness
- Fear of suffocation or death (feeling of "not being able to breathe")

Hypercapnia
Inability to move secretions
Pale, dusky skin color
Tachycardia
Cyanosis

Common Expected Outcome

Patient maintains optimal gas exchange as evidenced by ABGs within patient's usual range; alert, responsive mentation or no further reduction in level of consciousness; relaxed breathing; and baseline heart rate for patient.

NOC Outcomes

Respiratory Status: Gas Exchange; Respiratory Status: Ventilation

NIC Interventions

Respiratory Monitoring; Oxygen Therapy; Mechanical Ventilation

---

Ongoing Assessment

Actions/Interventions

■ Assess respiratory rate, rhythm, and depth.

■ Assess for changes in level of consciousness.

■ Assess lungs for areas of decreased ventilation and the presence of adventitious sounds.

▲ Use pulse oximetry to monitor oxygen saturation.

Rationales

Respiratory rate and rhythm changes are early warning signs of impending respiratory difficulties. Rapid, shallow breathing patterns affect gas exchange. Hypoxia is associated with increased breathing effort.

Restlessness and irritability are early indicators of development of further hypoxia and decreased perfusion to the brain.

As pulmonary edema increases and fluid moves into the alveoli, adventitious breath sounds (crackles) are heard throughout the lung fields, indicating increased hypoxia; decreased breath sounds are indicative of collapsed alveoli.

Pulse oximetry is a useful tool in the clinical setting to detect changes in oxygenation. Oxygen saturation should be maintained at 90% or greater.

■ = Independent ▲ = Collaborative

Actions/Interventions

▲ Closely monitor ABGs, and note changes.

▲ Assess cardiac rhythm for dysrhythmias.

▲ Monitor chest x-ray reports, noting improvement or worsening.

▲ Assess pulmonary artery pressure (PAP) and pulmonary capillary wedge pressure (PCWP), if present.

▲ Assess pulmonary function tests.

▲ Assess lactic acid levels.

▲ Assess fluid balance.

Rationales

A progressive hypoxemia is apparent on serial ABGs despite increased concentrations of inspired oxygen. Initially, hypocapnia (a decrease in $Paco_2$) may be present as a result of hyperventilation. However, respiratory acidosis with increase in $Paco_2$ occurs in later stages as a result of increase in dead space and decrease in lung compliance and alveolar ventilation.

Electrolyte shifts, hypoxia, and mechanical ventilation, especially with positive end-expiratory pressure (PEEP), place patient at risk for cardiac dysrhythmias and decreased cardiac output.

Chest x-ray studies will show bilateral diffuse infiltrates with normal cardiac silhouette to complete whiteout of both lung fields; x-ray studies of lung edema lag behind clinical presentation.

Initially PAP will be normal, but with PEEP and continuing deterioration, PAP may increase, leading to further pulmonary edema.

Decreased vital capacity, minute volume, functional residual capacity; decreased pulmonary compliance of greater than 50 mL/cm H_2O; increased shunt fraction greater than 15% to 20% (normal 3% to 4%) are indicative of worsening lung status.

Increasing lactic acid levels are indicative of anaerobic cellular metabolism.

Overhydration or dehydration places the patient at further risk. Tight fluid control is essential to maintaining hydration without increasing edema.

Therapeutic Interventions

Actions/Interventions

▲ Use a team approach in planning care with the physician, respiratory therapist, patient, family, and other team members.

■ Plan activity and rest to maximize the patient's energy. Temporarily discontinue activity if saturation drops, and make any necessary Fio_2, PEEP, or sedation changes to improve saturation.

■ Elevate head of bed; change the patient's position every 1 to 2 hours.

■ Institute prone positioning as indicated.

■ Provide suctioning as needed.

Rationales

Timely and accurate communication of assessments is required to keep pace with needed change in Fio_2, PEEP, and activity levels.

Activity increases metabolic rate and oxygen requirements. Rest helps mobilize energy for more effective breathing and coughing efforts.

Increasing the head of bed to more than 30 degrees prevents aspiration and ventilator-associated pneumonia. Repositioning facilitates movement and drainage of secretions, increases patient comfort, and maintains skin integrity.

Prone positioning is a technique used to improve oxygenation in patients with ARDS who are receiving mechanical ventilation. The exact mechanism leading to improvement of oxygenation in this position is unknown. Proposed mechanisms include recruitment of collapsed alveoli, redistribution of ventilation from the ventral (collapsed in the prone position) to dorsal regions (recruited in the prone position), and mobilization of secretions.

Suctioning clears secretions and increases airway patency to improve gas exchange. Its use should be guided by objective data, not preset time intervals.

Actions/Interventions

▲ Administer medication as indicated (e.g., steroids, sedation, antibiotics, bronchodilators).

▲ Anticipate the need for intubation and mechanical ventilation.

■ If patient is intubated, anticipate (assess for) need for PEEP or continuous positive airway pressure (CPAP).

Rationales

Steroids may help reduce the inflammation; sedation may be ordered to decrease the patient's energy expenditure during mechanical ventilation and to allow for adequate synchrony of the ventilator so that the patient can be adequately ventilated. Antibiotics may be necessary to treat the underlying cause of the inflammatory response. Bronchodilators may be useful to decrease the work of breathing and provide airway clearance.

Early intubation and mechanical ventilation are recommended to prevent full decompensation of the patient. Mechanical ventilation provides supportive care to maintain adequate oxygenation and ventilation to the patient.

Hypoxemia leads to tissue damage, causing an increased release of inflammatory mediators, which leads to further lung damage. Artificial positive pressure (PEEP or CPAP) assists in keeping alveoli open. Treatment with low tidal volumes and increased respiratory rates has been shown to be effective in counteracting decreased lung compliance seen in ARDS.

 NANDA-I NDx **Risk for Decreased Cardiac Output**

Common Risk Factors

Mechanical ventilation
Positive-pressure ventilation

Common Expected Outcome

Patient maintains adequate cardiac output (CO), as evidenced by strong peripheral pulses, systolic BP within 20 mm Hg of baseline, HR 60 to 100 beats/min with regular rhythm, urine output greater than 30 mL/hr, warm dry skin, and normal level of consciousness.

NOC Outcomes
Cardiac Pump Effectiveness; Tissue Perfusion: Peripheral; Tissue Perfusion: Abdominal Organs; Circulation Status

NIC Interventions
Hemodynamic Regulation; Mechanical Ventilation

Ongoing Assessment

Actions/Interventions

▲ Obtain CO measurement after positive-pressure ventilation changes.

▲ Assess vital signs and level of consciousness every hour, and with changes in positive-pressure ventilation and inotrope administration.

Rationales

Artificial positive pressure (PEEP or CPAP) assists in keeping alveoli open; however, the positive pressure compresses the great vessels returning to the heart, which, in turn, decreases the CO.

Mechanical ventilation can cause decreased venous return to the heart, resulting in decreased BP, compensatory increases in HR and decreased CO. This may occur abruptly with ventilation changes: rate, tidal volume, or positive-pressure ventilation. The level of consciousness will decrease if CO is severely compromised. Therefore close monitoring during ventilation changes is imperative.

■ = Independent   ▲ = Collaborative

Actions/Interventions

■ Assess peripheral pulses, capillary refill, and skin temperature.

■ Monitor fluid intake and urine output.

Rationales

Cold, clammy skin is secondary to compensatory increase in sympathetic nervous system stimulation and low CO and oxygen desaturation. Peripheral pulses are weak with reduced stroke volume and CO. Capillary refill is slow with reduced CO.

Optimal hydration status is needed to maintain effective circulating blood volume and counteract the ventilator's effect on cardiac output. With positive-pressure ventilation, pressure from the diaphragm decreases blood flow to the kidneys and could result in a drop in urine output. The brain is very sensitive to a decrease in blood flow and may respond by releasing antidiuretic hormone (to increase water and sodium retention), further reducing urinary output.

Therapeutic Interventions

Action/Interventions

▲ Administer medications as prescribed, noting response and observing for side effects.

▲ Administer intravenous (IV) fluids, as prescribed.

■ Anticipate need to decrease level of PEEP to a range that facilitates improved CO, if fluid administration and inotropes are not successful.

Rationales

Inotropic medications may be used to increase CO. Sedatives and analgesics are used to relieve pain and agitation. Neuromuscular blocking agents are given to promote synchronous breathing with mechanical ventilation.

Volume therapy may be required to maintain optimal fluid balance and increase CO without causing edema.

An "optimal PEEP" level is one that achieves maximal oxygenation benefits without causing a decrease in CO.

Risk for Ineffective Protection

Common Risk Factors

Decreased pulmonary compliance
Dependency on ventilator
Improper ventilator settings
Improper alarm settings
Positive-pressure ventilation
Increased secretions

Common Expected Outcomes

Patient remains free of injury, as evidenced by appropriate ventilator settings and ABGs within normal limits for patient.

Potential for injury from ventilator-associated pneumonia and barotrauma is reduced by ongoing assessment and early intervention.

NOC Outcomes
Respiratory Status: Ventilation; Risk Detection
NIC Intervention
Mechanical Ventilation

Ongoing Assessment

Actions/Interventions	Rationales
▲ Check ventilator settings every hour. Ensure that ventilator alarms are on. Notify respiratory therapist of discrepancy in ventilator settings immediately.	Patient safety is a priority. Assessment ensures that the patient is receiving correct mode, rate, tidal volume, FIO_2, PEEP, and pressure support. Immediate attention to details can prevent problems.
▲ Use pulse oximetry to monitor oxygen saturation; assess ABGs, as appropriate.	Pulse oximetry is a useful tool to detect changes in oxygenation; oxygen saturation should be at 90% or greater. ABGs provide additional information about developing respiratory acidosis and hypoxemia.
■ Assess rate and rhythm of respiratory pattern, including work of breathing.	It is important to maintain the patient in synchrony with the ventilator and not permit "fighting" it.
▲ Assess for signs of pulmonary infection.	Ventilator-associated pneumonia occurs in up to 25% of patients on ventilators. Mortality rates of up to 40% to 50% have been reported for these patients. Most ventilator-associated infections are caused by bacterial pathogens, with gram-negative bacilli being common.
■ Assess for signs of barotrauma every hour: crepitus, subcutaneous emphysema, altered chest excursion, asymmetrical chest, change in ABGs, shift in trachea, restlessness, evidence of pneumothorax on chest x-ray film. Notify physician of signs immediately.	Barotrauma is damage to the lungs from positive pressure, as seen in ARDS when high pressures are needed to ventilate the stiff lungs or when PEEP is used. Frequent assessments are needed because barotrauma can occur at any time and the patient will not show signs of dyspnea, shortness of breath, or tachypnea if heavily sedated to maintain ventilation. Being prepared for an emergency helps prevent further complications.
▲ Monitor chest x-ray film reports daily, and obtain a stat portable chest x-ray film if barotrauma is suspected.	Vigilant monitoring helps reduce complications.
▲ Monitor plateau pressures with the respiratory therapist.	Monitoring for barotrauma can involve measuring plateau pressure, which is the pressure after delivery of the tidal volume but before the patient is allowed to exhale. The ventilator is programmed so that after delivery of the tidal volume the patient is not allowed to exhale for half a second. Therefore pressure must be maintained to prevent exhalation. Elevation of plateau pressures increases both the risk and incidence of barotrauma when a patient is on mechanical ventilation.

Therapeutic Interventions

Actions/Interventions	Rationales
▲ Institute measures to reduce ventilator-associated pneumonia (VAP).	Nosocomial infections such as VAP are a leading cause of hospital mortality. Prevention of VAP is a national initiative to promote quality and safety
• Wash hands before and after suctioning, touching ventilator equipment, and/or coming into contact with respiratory secretions.	An artificial airway bypasses the normal protective mechanisms of the upper airways. Hand washing reduces transmission of microorganisms.
• Use a continuous subglottic suction ET tube for intubation expected to be longer than 24 hours.	This intervention prevents accumulation of secretions that can be aspirated.
• Keep head of bed elevated to 30 to 45 degrees or perform subglottic suctioning unless medically contraindicated.	Elevation promotes better lung expansion. It also reduces gastric reflux and aspiration.
• Brush teeth two or three times per day with a soft toothbrush. Chlorhexidine-based rinses may also be incorporated into oral care protocols.	Oral care reduces colonization of oropharynx with respiratory pathogens that can be aspirated into the lungs.
• Use sterile suctioning procedures.	This technique decreases the introduction of microorganisms into the airway.

■ = Independent   ▲ = Collaborative

Actions/Interventions

- Listen for alarms. Know the range in which the ventilator will set off alarm.
- ▲ Anticipate need for chest tube placement, and prepare as needed.

Rationales

The ventilator is a lifesaving treatment that requires prompt response to alarms.

If barotrauma is suspected, intervention must follow immediately to prevent tension pneumothorax while the patient is on the ventilator.

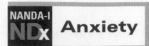

Anxiety

Common Related Factors

Inability to breathe adequately without support
Inability to maintain adequate gas exchange
Unknown outcome
Inability to communicate verbally

Defining Characteristics

Restlessness
Fear of sleeping at night
Uncooperative behavior
Withdrawal
Tachypnea
Vigilant watch on equipment
Facial tension
Focus on self

Common Expected Outcomes

Patient uses effective coping mechanisms.
Patient describes a reduction in level of anxiety experienced.

NOC Outcomes
Anxiety Self-Control; Coping
NIC Intervention
Anxiety Reduction; Presence; Emotional Support

Ongoing Assessment

Actions/Interventions

- Assess for signs of anxiety.

- Assess patient's understanding of ARDS and treatment.

Rationales

Anxiety can affect respiratory rate and pattern, resulting in rapid, shallow breathing and leading to ABG abnormalities and the patient "fighting" the ventilator.

ARDS is an acute, life-threatening problem for which most patients have not had prior experience.

Therapeutic Interventions

Actions/Interventions

- Display a confident, calm manner and an understanding attitude. Keep the patient or significant others informed of current patient status.

- Orient the patient and significant others to intensive care unit (ICU) surroundings, routines, equipment alarms, and noises. Explain all procedures to the patient before performing them.

Rationales

The presence of a trusted person may be helpful during periods of anxiety. ARDS is a serious syndrome with a high mortality rate. Significant others must be informed of changes. These patients are typically managed with intubation and mechanical ventilation and require critical care nursing in an acute care setting. Many causal factors are related to ARDS, and the patient or significant others should be informed of the need to treat the underlying cause.

The ICU is a busy environment that can be very upsetting and scary to the patient or significant others. Information helps decrease the patient's anxiety. Fear of the unknown can make the patient anxious or uncooperative.

Actions/Interventions	Rationales
■ Reduce distracting stimuli. Explain that alarms may periodically sound, which may be normal, and that the staff will be in close proximity.	Reducing stimuli provides a quiet environment that enhances rest. Anxiety may escalate with excessive noise, conversations, and equipment around the patient.
■ Explain the need for frequent assessments (i.e., vital signs, auscultation of lung sounds, ventilator checks).	This explanation helps reduce anxiety by providing a basis for actions.
■ Explain the need for suctioning as needed.	Information can help reduce the anxiety associated with the procedure.
■ Encourage visiting by family and friends.	The presence of significant others reinforces feelings of security for the patient.
■ Encourage sedentary diversional activities (e.g., television, reading, being read to, writing, occupational therapy).	These activities enhance the patient's quality of life and help pass time.
■ Provide relaxation techniques (e.g., tapes, imagery, progressive muscle relaxation).	Using anxiety-reduction techniques enhances the patient's sense of personal mastery and confidence.
■ If impaired communication is the problem, provide the patient with word-and-phrase cards, writing pad and pencil, or picture board.	These tools broaden the opportunity for communicating, which may reduce frustration.
■ Refer to psychiatric liaison clinical nurse specialist, psychiatrist, or hospital chaplain, as appropriate.	Specialty expertise may provide a wider range of treatment options and may be needed to achieve successful outcomes.

Related Care Plans

Respiratory failure, Acute, p. 445
Decreased cardiac output, p. 33
Insomnia, p. 117
Imbalanced nutrition: Less than body requirements,
    p. 142
Impaired physical mobility, p. 133
Impaired verbal communication, p. 39
Mechanical ventilation, p. 418
Powerlessness, p. 162
Risk for impaired skin integrity, p. 185
Tracheostomy, p. 461

Asthma

Bronchial Asthma; Status Asthmaticus

Asthma is a chronic inflammatory disorder that is characterized by airflow obstruction. This inflammatory response causes bronchoconstriction, increased mucus production, and hyperresponsiveness of the airways to a variety of stimuli. Although the stimuli for this exaggerated bronchoconstrictive response are individually defined, respiratory infection, cold weather, physical exertion, some medications, and allergens are common triggers. When a hypersensitive individual is exposed to a trigger, a rapid inflammatory response with subsequent bronchospasm occurs. Proinflammatory cells, primarily mast cells, signaled by immunoglobulin E, release inflammatory mediators that produce swelling and spasm of the bronchial tubes. This causes adventitious sounds (wheezing), coughing, increased mucus production, and feelings of "not being able to breathe" (dyspnea). Eosinophils and neutrophils rush to the area, and additional cytokines are released, some of which are long acting and result in epithelial damage, late-phase airway edema, continued mucus hypersecretion, and additional hyperresponsiveness of the bronchial smooth muscle. Reversal of the airflow obstruction usually occurs spontaneously or with treatment. Status asthmaticus occurs when the asthma attack is refractory to the usual treatment, with clinical manifestations that are

■ = Independent ▲ = Collaborative

more severe, prolonged, and life threatening. With repeated attacks, remodeling of the airway occurs through hypertrophy and hyperplasia of normal tissues.

Although this care plan focuses on acute care in the hospital setting, current thinking is to prevent the hypersensitivity reaction and thus keep airway remodeling at a minimum. For this reason, an asthma plan individualized for each patient and for optimal outpatient management is emphasized.

 NANDA-I NDx Ineffective Breathing Pattern

Common Related Factor

Swelling and spasm of the bronchial tubes in response to allergies, drugs, stress, infection, inhaled irritants

Defining Characteristics

Dyspnea/orthopnea
Respiratory depth changes
Tachypnea
Prolonged expiratory phase
Cyanosis
Cough
Nasal flaring
Wheezing
Use of accessory muscles

Common Expected Outcome

Patient maintains optimal breathing pattern, as evidenced by relaxed breathing, normal respiratory rate or pattern, and absence of dyspnea.

NOC Outcomes
Respiratory Status: Ventilation; Vital Signs Status
NIC Interventions
Respiratory Monitoring; Vital Signs Monitoring; Medical Administration

Ongoing Assessment

Actions/Interventions	Rationales
■ Assess respiratory rate, rhythm, and depth.	Respiratory rate and rhythm changes can be early warning signs of impending respiratory difficulties.
■ Assess relationship of inspiration to expiration.	Reactive airways allow air to move into the lungs more easily than out of the lungs. If the patient is gasping and frantically trying to "get air," an intervention to assist the patient in developing a more effective breathing pattern may be necessary.
■ Assess for conversational dyspnea.	Shortness of breath during normal conversation indicates respiratory distress.
■ Assess for dyspnea, retractions, flaring of nostrils, and use of accessory muscles	These signs signify an increase in respiratory effort. As moving air into and out of the lungs becomes more difficult, the breathing pattern alters to include use of accessory muscles.
■ Assess breath sounds, and note wheezes or other adventitious sounds.	Adventitious breath sounds may indicate a worsening condition or an additional developing pathology such as pneumonia. Wheezing occurs as a result of bronchospasm. Diminishing wheezing and inaudible breath sounds are ominous findings and indicate impending respiratory failure.

Actions/Interventions	Rationales
▲ Use by pulse oximetry to monitor oxygen saturation.	Pulse oximetry is a useful, noninvasive tool to detect early changes in oxygenation. Oxygen saturation should be at 90% or higher, with oxygen applied as ordered by the physician.
▲ Monitor arterial blood gases (ABGs).	During a mild to moderate asthma attack, patients may develop a respiratory alkalosis. Hypoxemia leads to increased respiratory rate and depth, and carbon dioxide is blown off. An ominous finding is respiratory acidosis, which usually indicates that respiratory failure is pending and that mechanical ventilation may be necessary.
▲ Monitor peak expiratory flow rates and forced expiratory volumes as obtained by the respiratory therapist.	The severity of the exacerbation can be measured objectively by monitoring these values. The peak expiratory flow rate (PEFR) is the maximum flow rate that can be generated during a forced expiratory maneuver with fully inflated lungs. It is measured in liters per second and requires maximal effort. When done with good effort, it correlates well with forced expiratory volume in 1 second (FEV_1) measured by spirometry and provides a simple reproducible measure of airway obstruction.
■ Assess level of anxiety.	Hypoxia and the sensation of being "not able to breathe" is frightening and may cause anxiety.
■ Assess for fatigue and the patient's perception of how tired he or she feels.	Fatigue may indicate increasing distress, leading to respiratory failure.
■ Assess the patient's vital signs as needed while in distress.	With initial hypoxia and hypercapnia, blood pressure (BP), heart rate (HR), and respiratory rate increase. As the hypoxia and/or hypercapnia become severe, BP and HR drop and respiratory failure may ensue.
■ Assess for the presence of pulsus paradoxus of 12 mm Hg or greater.	Pulsus paradoxus is an accentuation of the normal drop in systolic arterial BP with inspiration. Normally the difference in systolic BP at expiration and inspiration is less than 10 mm Hg. A pulsus paradoxus of 12 mm Hg or greater with asthma is a predictor of severe airflow obstruction.

Therapeutic Interventions

Actions/Interventions	Rationales
■ Keep head of bed elevated.	This position allows for adequate diaphragm excursion and lung expansion.
■ Encourage slow deep breathing. Instruct the patient to use pursed-lip breathing for exhalation. Instruct the patient to time breathing so that exhalation takes two to three times as long as inspiration.	Pursed-lip breathing during exhalation produces a positive distending pressure within the bronchioles, which facilitates expiratory airflow by helping to keep the bronchioles open. Prolonged expiration prevents air trapping.
■ Plan activity and rest to maximize the patient's energy.	Fatigue is common with the increased work of breathing from the ineffective breathing pattern. Activity increases metabolic rate and oxygen requirements.
▲ Use β_2-agonist drugs by metered-dose inhaler (MDI) or nebulizer (per respiratory therapist) as prescribed.	Short-acting β_2-adrenergic agonist drugs (SABAs) relax airway smooth muscle and are the treatment of choice for acute exacerbations of asthma. These inhaled short-acting inhaled bronchodilators work quickly to open the air passages, making it easier to breathe and decrease bronchoconstriction.

■ = Independent   ▲ = Collaborative

Actions/Interventions

▲ Administer other medications as ordered or instruct patient in methods.

▲ Anticipate the need for alternative therapies if life-threatening bronchospasm continues:

- Magnesium infusion

- Heliox (a helium-oxygen mixture)

- General anesthesia

Rationales

Corticosteroids are the most effective antiinflammatory drugs for the treatment of reversible airflow obstruction. They may be given parenterally, orally, or inhaled, depending upon the severity of the attack. Inhaled steroids should be administered after β-adrenergic agonists. During severe attacks, anticholinergics (e.g., ipratropium bromide [Atrovent]) may be effective when used in combination with β-adrenergic agonists. They produce bronchodilation by reducing intrinsic vagal tone to the airway and have been found to be synergistic in their effect with β-adrenergic agonists. Clinical practice guidelines from the National Asthma Education and Prevention Program (National Institutes of Health [NIH]) recommend inhaled β-adrenergic agonists and oral corticosteroids to manage severe attacks.

Magnesium possesses bronchodilating properties, but the role in acute asthma still remains controversial.

Helium is less dense than nitrogen and lessens functional resistance when gas flow is turbulent because of bronchospasm. This decreases the work of breathing. Heliox is not available in all institutions.

General anesthesia is used when there is both severe dynamic hyperinflation and profound hypercapnia that cannot be corrected by increasing minute ventilation.

 Ineffective Airway Clearance

Common Related Factors

Bronchospasm
Excessive mucus production
Ineffective cough and fatigue

Defining Characteristics

Abnormal lung sounds (rhonchi, wheezes)
Changes in respiratory rate or depth
Dyspnea
Verbalized chest tightness
Cough
Cyanosis
Abnormal ABGs

Common Expected Outcome

Patient will maintain clear open airways, as evidenced by normal or improved breath sounds, normal rate and depth of respirations, ability to effectively cough up secretions, and normal ABGs or oxygen saturation of 90% or greater on pulse oximeter.

NOC Outcomes

Respiratory Status: Airway Patency; Symptom Control

NIC Interventions

Airway Management; Cough Enhancement; Ventilation Assistance; Calming Technique; Airway Suctioning

Ongoing Assessment

Actions/Interventions	Rationales
■ Auscultate lungs for adventitious breath sounds (rhonchi and wheezes).	Assessment allows for early detection and correction of abnormalities. Rhonchi suggest secretions in the lower airways. Wheezing may indicate partial obstruction or resistance.
■ Assess secretions, noting color, viscosity, odor, and amount.	Thick, tenacious secretions increase airway resistance and the work of breathing and may be indicative of dehydration. Colored or odorous secretions may indicate bleeding (brown, red) or infections (green, yellow, salmon-colored).
■ Assess respiratory rate, rhythm, and depth.	Respiratory rate and rhythm changes are warning signs of impending respiratory difficulties. An increase in respiratory rate may be compensation for airway obstruction.
■ Assess cough for effectiveness and productivity.	Coughing is the most helpful way to remove most secretions. Possible causes of an ineffective cough are respiratory muscle fatigue; severe bronchospasm; and thick, tenacious secretions.
■ Assess for color changes in lips, buccal mucosa, nail beds.	Cyanosis indicates increased concentration of deoxygenated blood, and that breathing is no longer effective to maintain adequate oxygenation of tissues.
■ Use pulse oximetry to monitor oxygen saturation.	Pulse oximetry is a useful tool to detect changes in oxygenation. Oxygen saturation should be maintained at 90% or greater.
▲ Monitor laboratory work as ordered:	
• Theophylline level (if on theophylline)	Theophylline increases anxiety and causes tachycardia. It has a narrow window of therapeutic effectiveness, placing the patient at risk for subtherapeutic levels or toxicity.
• ABGs	Carbon dioxide retention occurs as the patient becomes fatigued from the increased work of breathing caused by the bronchoconstriction. Once the patient is intubated and mechanically ventilated, permissive hypercapnia may be used to maintain plateau pressure less than 30 to 35 cm H_2O.
• Complete blood count with special attention to white blood cell (WBC) count	An increased WBC count is associated with infection.
• Serum potassium level	β-adrenergic agonists cause potassium to shift intracellularly and can result in decline in serum potassium levels.
▲ Monitor chest x-ray reports.	The chest x-ray report provides information about lung hyperinflation, presence of infiltrates, or presence of barotrauma.

Therapeutic Interventions

Actions/Interventions	Rationales
■ Keep the patient as calm as possible.	Anxiety during an asthma attack can further potentiate the exacerbation.
■ Pace activities.	Fatigue can increase the work of breathing and decrease cough effectiveness.
▲ Ensure that respiratory treatments are given as prescribed; notify respiratory therapist as the need arises. Obtain PEFR or FEV_1 before and after treatments.	PEFR is the fastest airflow rate reached at any time during exhalation. It should improve with effective therapy. FEV_1 is the volume of air expired in 1 second.
■ Encourage the patient to cough, especially after treatments. Teach effective coughing techniques.	Controlled coughing techniques help mobilize secretions from smaller airways to larger airways because the coughing is done more effectively.

■ = Independent   ▲ = Collaborative

Actions/Interventions

▲ Maintain oxygen as prescribed.

▲ Administer medications and intravenous (IV) fluids as prescribed.

■ Anticipate the need for intubation and mechanical ventilation if ABGs begin to deteriorate (Pco_2 greater than or equal to 55 mm Hg), work of breathing continues to increase, PEFR is less than 40% of baseline with failure of PEFR to improve after treatment, and patient has subjective feelings of doom and/or decreasing alertness.

■ Encourage increased fluid intake (up to 3000 mL/day) if there are no contraindications such as cardiac or renal disease.

Rationales

Oxygen therapy decreases the risk for hypoxia. Oxygen saturation should be maintained at 90% or greater.

In severe exacerbations, IV access is needed for the administration of IV corticosteroids and for emergency medication administration. Although aggressive hydration is no longer recommended, fluid administrations may be necessary for those who present with dehydration.

Being prepared for an emergency helps prevent further complications. Intubation may be needed to facilitate removal of tenacious secretions and provide sources for augmenting oxygenation.

Fluids are lost from mouth breathing and oxygen therapy. Mucous membranes dry out. Maintaining hydration increases ciliary action to remove secretions and decreases viscosity of secretions.

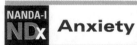

NANDA-I NDx Anxiety

Common Related Factors	**Defining Characteristics**
Respiratory distress	Complaints of inability to breathe
Hypoxia	Alterations in respiratory rate and depth
Change in health status	Increased heart rate
Change in environment	Uncooperative behavior
	Restlessness
	Apprehensiveness
	Frequent requests for someone to be in room
	Insomnia
	Diaphoresis

Common Expected Outcomes	**NOC Outcome**
Patient uses effective coping mechanisms.	Anxiety Self-Control
Patient describes a reduction in level of anxiety experienced.	**NIC Interventions**
	Anxiety Reduction; Calming Technique

Ongoing Assessment

Actions/Interventions

■ Assess for signs of anxiety (e.g., tachycardia, alterations in breathing pattern/rate, restlessness, apprehension).

▲ Use pulse oximetry to monitor oxygen saturation.

▲ Assess theophylline level if the patient is on theophylline.

Rationales

Anxiety increases as breathing becomes more difficult. Also, anxiety can affect respiratory rate and rhythm, causing rapid, shallow breathing.

Anxiety increases with increasing hypoxia and may be an early warning sign that the patient's oxygen levels are decreasing.

Theophylline increases anxiety and causes tachycardia. Therapeutic serum levels range from 10 to 20 mcg/mL. This narrow window of therapeutic effectiveness places the patient at risk for subtherapeutic or toxic levels. Short-acting β-agonists may also cause anxiety.

Pulmonary Care Plans

Therapeutic Interventions

Actions/Interventions	Rationales
■ Stay with the patient, and encourage slow, deep breathing. Assure the patient and significant others of close, continuous monitoring that will ensure prompt intervention.	The presence of a trusted person may help the patient feel less threatened.
■ Explain all procedures to the patient before starting; be simple and concise.	An informed patient who understands the treatment plan will be more cooperative and less anxious.
■ Explain importance of remaining as calm as possible.	Maintaining calmness will decrease oxygen consumption and work of breathing.
■ Keep significant others informed of the patient's progress. Avoid excessive reassurance.	Anxiety may be readily transferred to the patient from family members. Information can help relieve apprehension. Excessive reassurance may actually increase anxiety for many people.
■ Encourage expression of feelings.	Talking about anxiety-producing situations and anxious feelings can help the person perceive the situation in a less-threatening manner. Expressing emotions can enhance the patient's coping strategies.
■ Teach relaxation techniques such as progressive muscle relaxation if the patient's condition permits.	Although anxiety as the result of hypoxia requires correcting the hypoxic condition, some patients will experience anxiety as a learned response to the asthma attack. If this is the case, relaxation techniques may be effective in decreasing the anxiety.

NANDA-I

NDx Deficient Knowledge

Common Related Factors
Chronicity of disease
Long-term medical management

Defining Characteristics
Absence of questions
Inability to answer questions properly
Ineffective self-care

Common Expected Outcome
Patient or significant others verbalize knowledge of disease and its management and community resources available to assist the patient in coping with chronic disease.

NOC Outcomes
Knowledge: Health Behaviors; Knowledge: Medication; Asthma Control

NIC Interventions
Teaching Disease Process; Prescribed Medication

Ongoing Assessment

Actions/Interventions	Rationales
■ Assess knowledge of asthma triggers and of asthma medications: • Ability to distinguish between rescue medications and controllers • Correct use of metered-dose inhaler (MDI) and spacers • Use of spacers with MDI • Sequence to use medications • Treatment for status asthmaticus	Patient will need to learn to manage exposure to asthma triggers. Correct use of medications is important to control and reduce the frequency of acute attacks. Improper use of MDI will result in the medications not getting deep enough to influence the tracheobronchial tree.
■ Assess past and present therapies, as well as the patient's response to them.	Knowledge of what has been successful/unsuccessful in the past guides selection of interventions.

■ = Independent   ▲ = Collaborative

Actions/Interventions	Rationales
■ Evaluate self-care activities: preventive care and home management of acute attack.	The patient is living with a chronic disease and will be required to self-manage the disease.
■ Assess knowledge of care for status asthmaticus, as appropriate.	Adequate preparation on how to handle this potential emergency can be life-saving.
■ Assess tobacco use.	Although assessment of tobacco use is critical for all patients, it is especially important for patients suffering from lung disease. If the patient is a tobacco user, smoking cessation interventions need to be offered.

Therapeutic Interventions

Actions/Interventions	Rationales
■ Explain disease to the patient and significant others.	Asthma self-management education reduces use of health care resources (hospitalizations, urgent care visits) and morbidity. A common misconception held by patients and families is that asthma attacks can be averted without medication through self-control and discipline.
■ Instruct patient how to avoid asthma triggers (e.g., cigarette smoke, aspirin, air pollution, allergens, seasonal variations).	Information enables patient to take control. Environmental trigger control can reduce frequency of attacks and improve patient's quality of life.
■ Instruct in use of peak flow meters and develop an individualized plan on how to adjust medications and when to seek medical advice. Establish the patient's "personal best" PEFR.	Peak flow meters are the standard against which future measurements are evaluated. Use the zone system, individualized to the patient. Personal best is established by having the patient obtain and document peak flow each morning before medication use and in late afternoon for 2 weeks. Personal best is the highest peak flow reading regularly blown, which is then used to calculate the patient's zone. Monitoring peak flow is particularly important for those who cannot accurately perceive worsening airflow obstruction ("poor perceivers") and more severe levels of asthma. • GREEN ZONE: 80% to 100% of personal best. • YELLOW ZONE: 50% to 80% of personal best; this signals caution, and an acute exacerbation may be present. A temporary increase in medication may be indicated. • RED ZONE: Below 50% of personal best; this signals a medical alert. A β_2-adrenergic agonist should be taken, and if there is no improvement in PEFR to yellow or green zones, the physician should be notified.
■ Reinforce need for taking controller medications as prescribed.	Asthma is a chronic condition that is present even when attacks are not occurring. Medications, including antiinflammatory agents and bronchodilators, reduce incidence of attacks.
■ Review all medications with the patient including review of zones and dosage of each medication in each zone.	Short-acting β-agonists are the rescue medication of choice. Long-acting β_2-adrenergic agonists take too long to act in an emergency. Antiinflammatory medications, such as mast cell stabilizers or leukotriene-blocking agents, are designed to prevent the release of inflammatory mediators. Once an attack is present, the inflammatory mediators are already at work, and blocking release is not immediately effective. β_2-adrenergic agonists should be used before inhaled steroids because they open the airways and allow the antiinflammatory medication to reach deeper into the lung fields. Rinsing the mouth after using an inhaled steroid prevents a yeast infection. Increase each medication's effectiveness by correct use of spacers; slow, deep inhalation; and breath holding after inhalation.

Actions/Interventions	Rationales
■ Teach how to administer nebulizer treatments, MDIs, spacers, dry powder capsules, or Diskus with correct technique. Instruct patients to rinse their mouth with water after using inhalants containing a steroid component to avoid oral yeast infection.	Return demonstrations on techniques are necessary to ensure appropriate delivery of the medication.
■ Teach warning signs and symptoms of an asthma attack and importance of early treatment of impending attack. Provide written copy of daily and exacerbation management.	Patients need to have their own written treatment plan to reinforce information that is taught. Early treatment within 6 hours of onset may reduce hospitalizations.
■ Reinforce what to do in an asthma attack: • Home management • When to go to emergency department • Prevention	Information enables the patient to take control and reduce life-threatening situations. Medical help should be sought for severe exacerbations, ineffective response to treatment, and deteriorations in condition.
■ Instruct the patient to keep emergency phone numbers readily available.	Advance planning avoids delay in securing assistance.
■ Address long-term management issues.	Environmental controls, control of allergens, avoidance of precipitators, controlling air pollutants (avoidance of smoke, perfumes, aerosol sprays, powder, or talc), and good health habits help avoid attacks.
■ Discuss the need for the patient to obtain vaccines for pneumococcal pneumonia and yearly vaccine for influenza.	Regular immunizations decrease occurrence or severity of these diseases.
■ Discuss use of medical alert bracelet or other identification.	These forms of identification alert others to asthma history to facilitate the delivery of safe, effective medical care.
▲ Refer to support groups, as appropriate.	Community resources can provide support for patients as they learn disease management and appropriate health behavior changes such as smoking cessation.

Chest Trauma

Pneumothorax; Tension Pneumothorax; Flail Chest; Fractured Ribs; Pulmonary Contusion; Hemothorax; Myocardial Contusion; Cardiac Tamponade

Chest trauma is a blunt or penetrating injury of the thoracic cavity that can result in a potentially life-threatening situation secondary to hemothorax, pneumothorax, tension pneumothorax, flail chest, pulmonary contusion, myocardial contusion, and/or cardiac tamponade. This care plan focuses on acute care in the hospital setting.

 NANDA-I NDx Ineffective Breathing Pattern

Common Related Factors	Defining Characteristics
Pain	Shortness of breath/dyspnea
Simple pneumothorax	Tachypnea/shallow respirations
Tension pneumothorax	Decreased breath sounds on affected side
Flail chest	Asymmetrical chest expansion
Simple hemothorax (less than 400 mL blood)	Tracheal deviation
Massive hemothorax (1500 mL blood)	Paradoxical chest movements (flail chest)
Pulmonary contusion	Tachycardia

■ = Independent ▲ = Collaborative

Chest pain
Abnormal arterial blood gases (ABGs)
Oxygen saturation less than 90%
Cyanosis
Anxiety, restlessness

Common Expected Outcome

Patient maintains effective breathing pattern, as evidenced by relaxed breathing at normal respiratory rate and pattern, absence of dyspnea, and normal blood gas values within patient parameters.

NOC Outcome
Respiratory Status: Ventilation
NIC Interventions
Respiratory Monitoring; Airway Management; Ventilation Assistance

Ongoing Assessment

Actions/Interventions	Rationales
■ Assess respiratory rate, rhythm, and depth.	Respiratory rate and rhythm changes are early warning signs of impending respiratory difficulties.
■ Assess lungs for adventitious and decreased breath sounds; percuss lungs to note changes.	Decreased breath sounds may be evident on affected side. Hyperresonance to percussion on affected side is present with pneumothorax. Dullness is present with hemothorax.
■ Assess for use of accessory muscles.	As moving air in and out of lungs becomes more difficult, the patient uses accessory muscles to increase chest excursion and facilitate effective breathing.
■ Assess for changes in level of consciousness.	Restlessness, confusion, and/or irritability are early indicators of hypoxia to brain tissue.
■ Assess skin color and temperature.	Cool, pale skin may be secondary to a compensatory vasoconstrictive response to hypoxia.
▲ Use pulse oximetry to monitor oxygen saturation; assess ABGs.	Pulse oximetry is a useful tool to monitor oxygen saturation and detect early changes in oxygenation. Increasing $Paco_2$ and decreasing Pao_2 are signs of respiratory failure.
■ Assess chest excursion.	Paradoxical movement is a sign of flail chest. Decreased chest expansion on affected side is a sign of pneumothorax/hemothorax.
■ Assess for pain quality, location, and severity and whether it increases with inspiration.	Pain that increases with inspiration can be a sign of rib fracture.
■ Assess position of trachea.	Tracheal deviation from midline to unaffected side is a sign of tension pneumothorax.
■ Assess and inspect chest wall for obvious injuries that allow air to enter pleural cavity. Assess for presence of contusions, abrasions, and bruising on chest.	Air entering the pleural cavity would cause pneumothorax. Wound size and location may be the cause of the ineffective breathing pattern. Further injuries may have occurred beneath these integumentary manifestations of trauma (e.g., fractured ribs, pulmonary contusion, myocardial contusion).
▲ Monitor chest x-ray films.	The chest x-ray film will confirm correct placement of chest tubes, indicate signs of improvement of pneumothorax or hemothorax, and indicate the presence of rib fractures.
■ Palpate chest for subcutaneous emphysema or crepitus.	Emphysema is a sign of air escaping into the subcutaneous tissues.
■ Assess for tension pneumothorax: respiratory distress, tachycardia, cyanosis, tachypnea, hypotension, mediastinal shift (toward unaffected side), changes in breath sounds, distant heart sounds, subcutaneous emphysema.	Tension pneumothorax is a medical emergency. As pressure within the thorax increases, the great vessels and the lung become compressed, resulting in severe cardiovascular and pulmonary compromise that can quickly become fatal. Immediate identification of the problem is essential.

Actions/Interventions	Rationales
▲ Assess history of traumatic event: what happened, when, pain, and so forth.	History of traumatic event will assist in alerting the health care team to injury not immediately visible that may be causing the ineffective breathing pattern.

Therapeutic Interventions

Actions/Interventions	Rationales
■ Place in sitting position, if not contraindicated.	A sitting position allows for adequate diaphragmatic and lung excursion and chest expansion.
▲ Provide pain relief.	Pain interferes with deep breathing and effective ventilation. Pain relief enhances the ability to deep breathe and cough.
▲ Provide oxygen therapy.	Supplemental oxygen may be needed to maintain oxygen saturation of 90% or greater for adequate oxygenation.
■ Encourage patient to clear own secretions with effective coughing, helping to splint chest as needed. If not effective, suction as needed.	Productive coughing is the most effective way to remove secretions. If patient is unable to perform independently/effectively, suctioning may be needed.
■ If flail chest is present, tape flail segment or place manual pressure over the flail segment.	Patients with increasing respiratory distress may require external pressure to stabilize the chest until more definitive treatment (intubation, surgical stabilization) is initiated. This will prevent the outward motion of flail chest. The flail segment will still move inward with respirations, but stopping the outward motion will help decrease the pendelluft motion to the mediastinum and great vessels.
■ If open pneumothorax is present, cover chest wall defect with 4 × 4 dressing. Tape on three sides with waterproof tape.	An untaped side allows air to escape from the pleural cavity (flutter-valve effect) so that tension does not continue to increase.
▲ If the patient is not in severe respiratory distress, prepare for chest x-ray examination.	The chest x-ray film is used to determine pneumothorax or hemothorax size and/or to confirm suspected diagnosis. Patients with small pneumothoraces, hemothoraces, and minimal symptoms may not require a chest tube. However, if the patient's condition deteriorates with the need to be intubated or mechanically ventilated, a chest tube will be required, even with small pneumothoraces, because of the high risk for developing a tension pneumothorax in that circumstance.
▲ If tension pneumothorax is suspected, prepare for needle thoracostomy.	A needle thoracostomy reduces a tension pneumothorax to a pneumothorax.
▲ If severe respiratory distress or respiratory status is steadily deteriorating, prepare for chest tube placement. Connect the chest tube to water seal drainage.	Chest tubes are inserted to assist in reinflating the lung. Larger chest tubes are inserted for hemothorax than for pneumothorax to help alleviate chest tube clotting.
▲ Prepare for intubation if the patient's condition warrants.	Patients with flail chest may be stable initially because of compensatory mechanisms (e.g., splinting of flail segment and shallow respirations). As these compensatory mechanisms fail, increasing respiratory distress develops. Intubation and positive-pressure ventilation are a means of stabilizing the flail segment by preventing the patient from breathing independently, resulting in inward movement of the flail segment.

■ = Independent   ▲ = Collaborative

Pulmonary Care Plans

Deficient Fluid Volume

NANDA-I NDx

Common Related Factors

Trauma
Active fluid loss (hemothorax)
Chest tube drainage

Defining Characteristics

Decreased urine output
Decreased skin turgor
Thirst
Dry mucous membranes
Tachycardia
Hypotension
Cool, clammy skin
Pallor
Changes in level of consciousness
Weakness
Hemoconcentration

Common Expected Outcome

Patient is normovolemic, as evidenced by urine output greater than 30 mL/hr, systolic blood pressure (BP) greater than or equal to 90 mm Hg (or patient's baseline), heart rate less than 100 beats/min, normal skin turgor, and moist mucous membranes.

NOC Outcomes
Fluid Balance; Blood Loss Severity; Vital Signs; Tissue Integrity: Skin and Mucous Membranes
NIC Interventions
Fluid Monitoring; Fluid Management; Fluid Resuscitation; Bleeding Reduction; Blood Products Administration; Shock Management: Volume

Ongoing Assessment

Actions/Interventions	Rationales
■ Assess vital signs.	Tachycardia is an early indication of fluid volume deficit and a compensatory mechanism to maintain cardiac output. Blood pressure is not a good indicator of early shock.
▲ Assess central venous pressure (CVP).	Changes in CVP will distinguish hypotension caused by hypovolemia (low CVP reading of less than 6 cm H_2O) versus hypotension caused by pericardial tamponade/tension pneumothorax (high CVP reading of greater than 10 cm H_2O).
■ Assess for jugular venous distention (JVD).	JVD may occur with cardiac tamponade as a result of the increased heart pressures, or with tension pneumothorax from the shifting of the mediastinum toward the unaffected side.
■ Assess for restlessness and anxiety level.	Mild to moderate anxiety may be the first early warning sign before vital sign changes. Anxiety may also indicate pain and/or psychological traumas.
■ Monitor and document fluid intake and urine output.	Urine output of less than 30 mL/hr may indicate early acute tubular necrosis and acute renal failure secondary to hypovolemia.
▲ Monitor laboratory test results for complete blood count (CBC), electrolytes, blood urea nitrogen (BUN), creatinine levels, blood type and crossmatch, and urine specific gravity.	Serum sodium, BUN/creatinine ratio, and hematocrit are elevated with decreased fluid volume because they are measures of concentration. Increasing urine specific gravity reflects increased urine concentration.

Actions/Interventions

- If chest tube is in place:
  - Assess, measure, and document amount of blood in chest tube collection chamber.
  - Monitor chest tube drainage every 10 to 15 minutes until blood loss slows to less than 25 mL/hr.
  - Maintain and check tube patency; avoid dependent loops.
  - Maintain prescribed fluid level within collection system.
- Assess for orthostatic hypotension and weakness.

Rationales

Excessive chest tube drainage may indicate hemorrhage. Obstruction of drainage from chest tubes interferes with lung expansion. Accumulated drainage in dependent loops obstructs tube drainage and increases pressure within the lungs. Maintaining prescribed water seal and suction levels helps prevent complications.

Orthostatic hypotension is an early sign of hypovolemia.

Therapeutic Interventions

Actions/Interventions

▲ Provide oral fluids as ordered and tolerated.

■ Assist the patient in sitting or standing if orthostatic hypotension is present.

■ Attempt to control bleeding source by using direct pressure with sterile 4 × 4 dressing.

▲ Insert one to two large-bore peripheral intravenous (IV) lines. Administer crystalloid or colloid fluids as prescribed.

▲ Prepare the patient for transfusions, if prescribed, with typed and crossmatched blood if it is available and time permits.

▲ Prepare the patient for autotransfusion.

■ Prepare the patient for possible surgery as condition warrants.

Rationales

Oral fluid replacement is indicated for mild fluid deficit or as a supplement to IV fluids.

Hypotension may produce lightheadedness and dizziness that puts the patient at risk for fall. Orthostasis is especially evident in older patients.

Significant pressure may be required to halt bleeding.

Parenteral fluid replacement is indicated to prevent or treat hypovolemic complications. Rule for fluid replacement: infuse 3 mL IV fluid/1 mL blood volume lost.

Blood transfusion may be required to correct fluid loss. Type-specific blood may be used if unable to obtain type and crossmatch. Type O-negative blood may be used as last resort.

Autotransfusion is used in cases of blunt or penetrating injuries isolated to the chest area.

An open thoracotomy may be required to correct source of bleeding.

NANDA-I NDx Decreased Cardiac Output

Common Related Factors

Acute pericardial tamponade
Tension pneumothorax
Severe volume loss
Decreased ventricular filling (preload)

Defining Characteristics

Hypotension
Narrow pulse pressure
Diminished peripheral pulses
Pulsus paradoxus (systolic pressure falls more than 15 mm Hg during inspiration)
Tachycardia
Electrical alternans (decreased QRS voltage during inspiration)
Equalization of pressures (CVP, pulmonary artery pressure [PAP], and pulmonary capillary wedge pressure [PCWP])
Jugular venous distention
Distant or muffled heart tones
Change in level of consciousness
Cool, clammy skin

■ = Independent ▲ = Collaborative

Decreased urine output
Fall in hemoglobin and hematocrit
Decreased arterial or venous oxygen saturation
Acidosis
Nonspecific electrocardiogram (ECG) changes

Common Expected Outcome

Patient maintains adequate cardiac output (CO) as evidenced by BP within normal limits for patient, heart rate (HR) 60 to 100 beats/min with regular rhythm, urine output greater than or equal to 30 mL/hr, strong peripheral pulses, absence of JVD, absence of pulsus paradoxus, warm and dry skin, and normal level of consciousness.

NOC Outcomes
Vital Signs; Cardiac Pump Effectiveness; Circulation Status
NIC Interventions
Vital Sign Monitoring; Invasive Hemodynamic Monitoring; Hemodynamic Regulation

Ongoing Assessment

Actions/Interventions	Rationales
■ Assess for classic signs associated with acute pericardial tamponade:	Pericardial tamponade can decrease CO as the pericardial sac fills with blood to the point that it compresses the myocardium, causing decreased ability of the heart to pump blood out and take blood in.
• Low arterial BP with narrowing pulse pressure	An initial elevation in BP may occur with compensatory vasoconstriction. However, as venous return is compromised from the cardiac compensation, a significant drop in CO occurs.
• Pulsus paradoxus	Pulsus paradoxus is an accentuation of normal drop in systolic arterial blood pressure with inspiration. Normally the difference in systolic blood pressure at expiration and inspiration is less than 10 mm Hg.
• Distant or muffled heart sounds	Muffled heart sounds are caused by distention in pericardial sac, creating a cushion between stethoscope and heart sounds.
• Sinus tachycardia	Sinus tachycardia is related to compensatory catecholamine release.
• Distended neck veins	The jugular neck veins become distended as a result of impaired venous return to the heart.
■ Assess for changes in level of consciousness.	Restlessness, irritability, and anxiety are early indicators of hypoxia and reduced cerebral perfusion.
■ Assess peripheral pulses, capillary refill, and skin temperature.	Cool, pale, clammy skin is secondary to compensatory increase in sympathetic nervous system and low cardiac output. Peripheral pulses are weak with reduced stroke volume and cardiac output. Capillary refill is slow.
▲ Assess ECG changes.	A slowly developing tamponade may present like heart failure with nonspecific ECG changes. Low voltage of ECG complexes is also a common finding.
■ Monitor chest tube drainage for increase or decrease in drainage.	Sudden cessation of chest tube drainage suggests a clot.
▲ Assist with performance of echocardiogram if time permits.	An echocardiogram provides the most helpful diagnostic information. Effusions seen with acute tamponade are usually smaller than with chronic tamponade. However, to prevent circulatory collapse, treatment may be indicated before the echocardiogram can be performed.

Actions/Interventions

▲ If the patient is in the intensive care unit, assess the hemo-dynamic profile using pulmonary artery catheter; assess for equalization of pressure.

▲ Monitor serial chest x-ray films.

■ Assess for midline shift of trachea.

Rationales

The right atrial pressure, right ventricular diastolic pressure, pulmonary artery diastolic pressure, and PCWP are all elevated in tamponade and are within 2 to 3 mm Hg of each other. These pressures confirm the diagnosis.

The chest x-ray film is used to evaluate for widened mediastinum or increased heart size.

Tension pneumothorax will cause a midline shift of the trachea and mediastinum to the opposite side with compression of the great vessels, causing a decrease in CO.

Therapeutic Interventions

Actions/Interventions

▲ Keep the patient and significant others informed.

■ Place the patient in optimal position to increase venous return.

▲ Initiate oxygen therapy.

▲ Establish large-bore IV access. Maintain aggressive fluid resuscitation as ordered.

▲ Anticipate blood product replacement.

■ Have emergency resuscitative equipment and medications readily available.

▲ Assemble pericardiocentesis tray or open chest tray for bedside intervention of pericardial tamponade, or prepare the patient for transport to surgery.

▲ If repeated pericardiocentesis fails to prevent recurrence of acute tamponade, anticipate surgical correction.

▲ Assemble thoracentesis tray or chest tube drainage system for treatment of tension pneumothorax.

▲ Administer vasopressor agents (dopamine, norepineph-rine bitartrate [Levophed]), as ordered.

Rationales

With a tamponade, a patient may be feeling well and suddenly develop restlessness and feelings of doom. This can be confusing and frightening for the patients and their loved ones.

Positioning is guided by the extent of the chest trauma injuries.

Supplemental oxygen will maximize oxygen saturation at 90% or greater.

Fluids may be required to raise venous pressure above pericardial pressure and optimize CO. IV access provides for rapid fluid resuscitation and blood administration.

Blood replacement therapy corrects existing hematological or coagulation factor alterations.

Pericardiocentesis is the emergency treatment of choice. Vasopressor medications maximize systemic perfusion pressure to vital organs.

Acute tamponade is a life-threatening complication, but immediate prognosis is good with fast, effective treatment. Tamponade must be relieved to improve CO. It is indicated when systolic BP is reduced more than 30 mm Hg from baseline. Bedside pericardiocentesis can be a high-risk lifesaving procedure. Complications include pneumothorax and myocardial or coronary artery lacerations. If the patient's condition can be stabilized, drainage of fluid should be delayed until surgical or open resection and drainage can be performed. Pericardiocentesis should be performed under sterile conditions.

Surgical pericardiotomy (pericardial window) or resection of a portion of the pericardium may be indicated.

If tension pneumothorax is suspected, intervention must be rapid to lessen the compression of the mediastinum and great vessels, which results in decreased CO and shock.

These medications maximize systemic perfusion pressure to vital organs.

■ = Independent   ▲ = Collaborative

Acute Pain

Common Related Factors

Rib fractures
Chest tube incision
Contusions or abrasions
Penetrating wounds
Pleural irritation

Defining Characteristics

Verbalization of pain
Wincing, grimacing
Shallow respirations to minimize pain
Guarding behavior
Tachycardia
BP changes
Diaphoresis
Agitation/restlessness

Common Expected Outcomes

Patient reports satisfactory pain control at a level less than 3 to 4 on a 0 to 10 rating scale.
Patient exhibits increased comfort such as baseline levels for pulse, BP, respirations, and relaxed muscle tone or body position.

NOC Outcomes
Comfort Status; Pain Control; Medication Response

NIC Interventions
Pain Management; Analgesic Administration; Distraction

Ongoing Assessment

Actions/Interventions

- Assess pain level and characteristics.

- Evaluate effectiveness of all pain management, including medication and nonpharmacological interventions.

- Assess how the patient has successfully dealt with pain in the past.
- Assess the patient's cultural beliefs about reporting pain.

Rationales

Assessment is important to determine the type of pain the patient is experiencing to aid in the diagnosis and appropriate treatment.

All chest trauma patients will need some type of pain medication. Unlike other body fractures, rib fractures cannot be casted to reduce pain. The rib cage is in continuous motion; therefore the pain is more difficult to manage. Pain management is easiest if the pain is not allowed to peak but is consistently controlled. If one medication or complementary technique is not effective, other interventions will need to be implemented.

Patient responses to pain are highly varied and must be explored with each patient.

Many factors influence a patient's willingness to report pain. Some are afraid of addiction to pain medications and will need reassurance that addiction is not a problem in treatment of acute pain. Others believe "toughing it out" is the way to handle pain. This knowledge deficit would need to be addressed. Finding out how the patient has dealt with pain in the past gives insight as to how best to effectively relieve current pain.

Therapeutic Interventions

Actions/Interventions	Rationales
▲ Anticipate the need for analgesics, and respond immediately to complaint of pain.	In the midst of painful experiences, a patient's perception of time may become distorted. Prompt responses to complaints may result in decreased anxiety in the patient.
■ Assist the patient in splinting the chest with a pillow.	Splinting minimizes discomfort and assists with effective coughing and deep breathing.
▲ Give the patient as much control over pain management as the condition allows.	The ability to actively participate and control pain management may decrease the patient's fear of pain.
▲ Assist with insertion or maintenance of epidural catheter or intercostal nerve block, as appropriate.	A variety of measures may be used to effectively manage pain.
■ Plan care activities for times when the patient is most pain-free, if possible.	This facilitates more active participation by the patient.
■ Use distraction techniques.	Distraction techniques heighten one's concentration upon nonpainful stimuli to decrease one's awareness and experience of pain.
■ Teach additional nonpharmacological interventions such as massage therapy, music therapy, heat or cold therapy, imagery, controlled breathing, and so on when pain is relatively controlled.	Chest trauma results in significant pain. Offering a variety of alternative therapies, such as cutaneous stimulation or cognitive-behavioral strategies, may be useful.
■ Eliminate additional stressors or sources of discomfort whenever possible.	Patients may experience an exaggeration in pain or a decreased ability to tolerate painful stimuli when environmental, intrapersonal, or intrapsychic stressors are present.

 Anxiety

Common Related Factors

Acute injury
Unfamiliar environment
Hypoxia
Threat of death

Defining Characteristics

Apprehensive
Restlessness
Agitation
Difficulty concentrating
Irritability
Increased blood pressure
Tachycardia

Common Expected Outcomes

Patient uses effective coping mechanisms.
Patient describes a reduction in level of anxiety experienced.

NOC Outcomes

Anxiety Self-Control; Coping

NIC Interventions

Anxiety Reduction; Emotional Support;
Presence

Ongoing Assessment

Actions/Interventions	Rationales
■ Assess anxiety level (mild, severe). Note signs and symptoms, especially nonverbal communication.	Chest trauma can result in an acute life-threatening injury that will produce high levels of anxiety in the patient as well as in significant others.

■ = Independent   ▲ = Collaborative

Actions/Interventions

■ Assess coping factors.

Rationales

Anxiety and way of decreasing perceived anxiety are highly individualized. Interventions are most effective when they are consistent with the individual's established coping patterns.

Therapeutic Interventions

Actions/Interventions

■ Acknowledge awareness of the patient's anxiety; encourage the patient to express fears.

■ Maintain a confident, assured manner. Assure the patient and significant others of close, continuous monitoring that will ensure prompt interventions.

■ Reduce unnecessary external stimuli (e.g., clear unnecessary personnel from room; decrease volume of cardiac monitor).

■ Reduce the patient's or significant others' anxiety by explaining all procedures and treatment. Keep explanations basic.

■ Support the patient's use of coping strategies that have been effective in past.

▲ Refer to other support systems (e.g., clergy, social workers, other family and friends) as appropriate.

Rationales

Acknowledgment validates the feelings and communicates acceptance of those feelings.

The presence of a trusted person may help the patient feel less threatened. The staff's anxiety may be easily perceived by the patient. The patient's feeling of stability increases in a calm, nonthreatening atmosphere.

Anxiety may escalate with excessive conversation, noise, and equipment around the patient.

Information helps allay anxiety. Patients who are anxious may not be able to comprehend anything more than simple, clear, brief instructions.

Using anxiety-reduction strategies enhances the patient's sense of personal mastery and confidence.

Specialty expertise may be needed to achieve successful outcomes.

Related Care Plans

Respiratory failure, Acute, p. 445
Impaired gas exchange, p. 78
Risk for infection, p. 114
Thoracotomy, p. 455

Chronic Obstructive Pulmonary Disease (COPD)

Chronic Bronchitis; Emphysema; Chronic Airway Limitation

Chronic obstructive pulmonary disease (COPD) refers to a group of diseases, including chronic bronchitis and emphysema, that cause a reduction in expiratory outflow. It is usually a slow, progressive, debilitating disease, affecting those with a history of heavy tobacco abuse and prolonged exposure to respiratory system irritants such as air pollution, noxious gases, and repeated upper respiratory tract infections. It is also regarded as the most common cause of alveolar hypoventilation with associated hypoxemia, chronic hypercapnia, and compensated acidosis. This care plan focuses on exacerbation of COPD in the acute care setting, as well as chronic care in the ambulatory setting or chronic care facility.

NANDA-I NDx **Ineffective Airway Clearance**

Common Related Factors

Hyperplasia and hypertrophy of mucus-secreting glands
Increased mucus production in bronchial tubes
Thick secretions
Decreased ciliary function
Alveolar wall destruction
Decreased energy and fatigue
Impaired exhalation
Bronchospasm
Smoking

Defining Characteristics

Coarse lung sounds/wheezing
Changes in respiratory rate or depth
Persistent cough for months
"Smoker's cough"
Ineffective cough
Excessive secretions
Loud, prolonged expiratory phase
Dyspnea
Altered arterial blood gases (ABGs) (compensated hypercapnia)

Common Expected Outcomes

Patient will maintain clear open airway, as evidenced by normal breath sounds, normal rate and depth of respirations, and ability to cough up secretions.
Patient demonstrates effective coughing techniques.

NOC Outcome
Respiratory Status: Airway Patency
NIC Interventions
Cough Enhancement; Airway Management

Ongoing Assessment

Actions/Interventions	Rationales
■ Auscultate lungs after coughing as needed to note and document significant change in breath sounds:	Patients with COPD have hypertrophy and hyperplasia of goblet cells with increased mucus production. Impaired ciliary movement contributes to retained secretions and less effective coughing. These patients have decreased breath sounds in varying degrees depending on their stage of illness.
• Decreased or absent breath sounds	Decreased or absent breath sounds may indicate presence of mucus plug or other major airway obstruction.
• Coarse sounds	Coarse sounds indicate presence of fluid along larger airways.
• Presence of fine rales (crackles)	Fine crackles may indicate cardiac involvement or secretion trapping.
■ Assess for changes in respiratory rate, depth, and use of accessory muscles or tripod positioning.	Respiratory rate and rhythm changes are early signs of respiratory compromise. As compromise becomes greater, use of accessory muscles becomes evident and the patient assumes a tripod posture to facilitate breathing.
■ Assess characteristics of or changes in secretions: consistency, quantity, color, odor.	A sign of infection is discolored sputum; an odor may be present. Thick, tenacious secretions increase hypoxemia and may be indicative of dehydration.
■ Note any color changes in lips, buccal mucosa, or nail beds.	Cyanosis is more common in patients with chronic bronchitis. The patient with emphysema develops cyanosis in the later stages of this disease.
■ Assess hydration status: skin turgor, mucous membranes, tongue.	Airway clearance is impaired with inadequate hydration and subsequent secretion thickening.
▲ Use pulse oximetry to monitor oxygen saturation; assess ABGs.	Hypoxia can result from increased pulmonary secretions and respiratory fatigue. Oxygen saturation should be maintained at 90% or greater.
■ Assess the patient's physical capabilities with activities of daily living (ADLs), including ability to expectorate sputum. Note if patient has conversational dyspnea.	Fatigue can limit cough effectiveness. Hypoxemia can limit activity tolerance.

■ = Independent ▲ = Collaborative

Actions/Interventions

▲ Assess lung function spirometry results as available.

Rationales

Lung function parameters define disease severity prognosis and response to therapy.

Therapeutic Interventions

Actions/Interventions

▲ Administer β_2-adrenergic agonists (e.g., albuterol, levalbuterol) by metered-dose inhaler (MDI) or nebulizer, as prescribed.

▲ Administer anticholinergics such as ipratropium bromide (Atrovent) by MDI or nebulizer or tiotropium (Spiriva) dry powder inhalation only in conjunction with β_2-adrenergic agonist.

▲ Anticipate administration of intravenous (IV) corticosteroids (followed by oral steroids) during the acute exacerbation.

■ Encourage the patient to cough out secretions.

■ Assist with effective coughing techniques:
  • Splint chest.
  • Have patient use abdominal muscles.
  • Use cough techniques as appropriate (e.g., quad, huff).

▲ Assist in mobilizing secretions to facilitate airway clearance:
  • Increase room humidification.

  • Administer mucolytic agents as prescribed.
  • Perform chest physiotherapy: postural drainage, percussion, and vibration.
  • Encourage 2 to 3 liters of fluid intake unless contraindicated.
  • Encourage activity and position changes every 2 hours.

■ Perform nasotracheal suctioning as indicated if the patient is unable to effectively clear secretions. Use a well-lubricated soft catheter.

▲ Anticipate intubation and mechanical ventilation, if needed, with transfer to acute care setting.

Rationales

These short-acting inhaled bronchodilators work quickly to open the air passages, making it easier to breathe and decreasing bronchoconstriction.

These medications have been shown to work synergistically with β_2-adrenergic agonists to relieve bronchoconstriction.

Corticosteroids reduce swelling and inflammation in the airways.

Coughing is the most helpful way to remove most secretions.

Controlled cough techniques help mobilize secretions from smaller airways to larger airways because coughing is done more effectively. Forced expiratory coughing through an open airway (while saying "huh") may be effective to move the trapped mucus into the larger airways for the patient to cough up.

Increasing humidity of inspired air will decrease viscosity of secretions and facilitate their removal.

These agents help liquefy secretions.

Chest physiotherapy helps to loosen and mobilize secretions in smaller airways that cannot be removed by coughing.

Fluids prevent dehydration from increased insensible loss and keep secretions thin.

Activity helps mobilize secretions and prevents pooling in the lungs.

Suctioning is indicated when patients are unable to remove secretions from the airways by coughing because of weakness, thick mucus plugs, or excessive secretions. It can also stimulate a cough. Suctioning with a lubricated catheter minimizes irritations.

Early intubation and mechanical ventilation may be needed to prevent full decompensation and a potentially life-threatening situation.

NANDA-I NDx **Impaired Gas Exchange**

Common Related Factors

Increase in dead space caused by the following:
  • Loss of lung tissue elasticity
  • Atelectasis
  • Increased residual volume

Defining Characteristics

Altered inspiratory/expiratory (I/E) ratio (prolonged expiratory phase)

Active expiratory phase: use of accessory muscles of breathing

Increased upper and lower airway resistance caused by the following:
- Overproduction of secretions along bronchial tubes
- Bronchoconstriction

Increase in rate and depth of respiration
Hypoxemia/hypercapnia
$Paco_2$ greater than 55 mm Hg
Pao_2 less than 55 mm Hg
Tachycardia
Anxiety
Restlessness/irritability
Confusion/somnolence
Pale, dusky skin color (pale)/cyanosis
Increase in blood pressure (BP)

Common Expected Outcome

Patient maintains optimal gas exchange, as evidenced by arterial blood gases (ABGs) within the patient's usual range, oxygen saturation of 90% or greater, alert response mentation or no further reduction in level of consciousness, relaxed breathing, and baseline HR for patient.

NOC Outcomes
Respiratory Status: Gas Exchange; Vital Signs; Knowledge: Treatment Regimen
NIC Interventions
Respiratory Monitoring; Oxygen Therapy; Teaching: Psychomotor Skill

Ongoing Assessment

Actions/Interventions

- Assess for altered breathing patterns:
  - Increased work of breathing
  - Abnormal rate, rhythm, and depth of respiration
  - Use of accessory muscles
  - Abnormal chest excursions

- Assess generalized appearance.

- Assess for restlessness and changes in level of consciousness.

- Monitor vital signs.

- Assess level of anxiety.

- ▲ Use pulse oximetry to monitor oxygen saturation; assess ABGs.

- If the patient is on theophylline, monitor for therapeutic levels and side effects.

Rationales

The patient with COPD has hyperinflation of the alveoli. This change leads to an increased anterior-posterior chest diameter (barrel chest) and flattening of the diaphragm. As a result the patient may have decreased chest excursion and increased accessory muscle use. Patients will adapt their breathing patterns over time to facilitate gas exchange. Both rapid, shallow breathing patterns and hypoventilation affect gas exchange. Hypoxia is associated with increased breathing efforts.

Posture, upright positioning and mental alertness cue the nurse to the severity of the COPD exacerbation. The patient with COPD may adopt a tripod sitting position, with the forearms resting on the thighs. This position decreases the work of breathing.

Restlessness is an early signs of hypoxia. Lethargy and somnolence are late signs.

Hypoxia or hypercarbia may cause initial hypertension, tachycardia, and increased respiratory rate.

Dyspnea often increases anxiety, and anxiety increases oxygen use by tissues. Anxiety may be an indication of worsening hypoxemia.

Increasing $Paco_2$ and decreasing Pao_2 are signs of respiratory failure. As the patient's condition begins to fail, the respiratory rate will decrease and $Paco_2$ will begin to rise. The COPD patient has a significant decrease in pulmonary reserves, and any physiological stress may result in acute respiratory failure. Noninvasive measurement of oxygen saturation by pulse oximetry provides early recognition of impaired oxygenation status.

Theophylline increases anxiety and causes tachycardia. Therapeutic serum levels range from 10 to 20 mcg/mL. This narrow window of therapeutic effectiveness places the patient at risk for subtherapeutic or toxic levels.

■ = Independent   ▲ = Collaborative

Therapeutic Interventions

Actions/Interventions	Rationales
▲ Promote more effective breathing pattern for better gas exchange:	
• Instruct in positioning for optimal breathing.	Upright and high-Fowler's positions favor better lung expansion; the diaphragm is pushed downward. If the patient is bedridden, turning from side to side at least every 2 hours promotes better aeration of all lung lobes, thus minimizing atelectasis.
• Teach the patient pursed-lip breathing.	Pursed-lip breathing promotes positive airway pressure during exhalation. This breathing technique decreases CO_2 retention, allows for increased tidal volume, decreases breath rates, allows for longer period of time for O_2/CO_2 diffusion and increases alveolar ventilation. It is especially useful during activity or exertion.
• Teach the patient to use abdominal and other accessory muscles.	Use of abdominal muscles facilitates movement of the diaphragm, and use of the accessory muscles increases chest excursion.
• Teach the patient to take bronchodilators and anticholinergics as prescribed.	These drugs decrease work of breathing by decreasing airway resistance.
▲ Administer low-flow oxygen therapy as indicated (e.g., 2 liters/min by nasal cannula). If insufficient, switch to high-flow oxygen apparatus (e.g., Venturi mask) for more accurate oxygen delivery.	COPD patients who chronically retain carbon dioxide depend on "hypoxic drive" as their stimulus to breathe. When applying oxygen, close monitoring is imperative to prevent unsafe increases in the patient's Pao_2, which could result in apnea.
▲ If the Pao_2 level is significantly lower or if the $Paco_2$ level is higher than the patient's usual baseline (varies from patient to patient), anticipate the following:	Signs of respiratory failure include increasing $Paco_2$ and decreasing Pao_2, paradoxical breathing, fatigue, somnolence, and increased respiratory rate. Treatment centers on airway management, oxygen therapy, and more aggressive therapy using mechanical ventilation as needed to correct acidosis and hypoxemia.
• Vigorous pulmonary toilet and suctioning	
• Increase in Fio_2 with use of controlled high-flow system	
• Possible need for intubation and mechanical ventilation with placement in acute care setting	
▲ Use caution in administration of respiratory depressants such as narcotics and tranquilizers.	These medications reduce respiratory drive, thereby promoting hypoxemia.
▲ Plan activity with interspersed rest periods and after bronchodilator treatments. Work with respiratory therapist for best time sequence of pulmonary treatment.	Activities will increase oxygen consumption and should be planned so that the patient does not become hypoxic. Pacing activities will help the patient conserve energy.
▲ Administer bronchodilators, expectorants, antiinflammatories (steroids), and antibiotics, as ordered.	These medications reduce airway resistance, treat infection, and facilitate secretion removal.
▲ Work with the rehabilitation team and patient to establish discharge planning.	COPD is a chronic debilitating disease that requires a multidisciplinary approach to assist the patient in maximizing quality of life.

NANDA-I NDx Imbalanced Nutrition: Less Than Body Requirements

Common Related Factors	Defining Characteristics
Increased metabolic need caused by increased work of breathing	10% to 20% below ideal body weight
Poor appetite resulting from fever, dyspnea, and fatigue	Caloric intake inadequate for metabolic demands of disease state
Indifference to food	Muscle wasting
	Abnormal laboratory values (e.g., low serum albumin level)

Common Expected Outcome

Patient's optimal nutritional status is maintained as evidenced by stable body weight and adequate caloric intake; hemoglobin and albumin levels return to normal.

NOC Outcomes

Nutritional Status: Food and Fluid Intake;
  Knowledge: Diet

NIC Intervention

Nutrition Management

Ongoing Assessment

Actions/Interventions

▲ Compile nutritional history, including preferred foods and dietary habits. Consult with dietitian.

▲ Verify ideal body mass index, and compare the patient's weight to ideal.

■ Assess the patient's physical ability to eat (i.e., energy level).

■ Assess oral cavity.

▲ Monitor laboratory values that indicate nutritional status: serum albumin, total protein, ferritin, transferrin.

■ Assess weight weekly.

Rationales

The dyspnea of COPD may make it hard for patients to eat sufficient calories. Eating meals may increase dyspnea. Excessive mucus and coughing may decrease the appetite and alter the taste of foods. The dietitian can estimate the patient's daily caloric requirements.

Patients may be unaware of their actual weight. Objective data guide treatment plan.

Work of breathing may allow little energy for other activity, including eating.

Dry mucous membranes and poor dentition may contribute to decreased appetite and nutritional status.

Serum prealbumin and albumin levels reflect protein status, ferritin and transferrin reflect iron status. Decreased values may be indicative of poor nutritional status or other pathology.

During aggressive nutritional support, the patient can gain up to ½ pound/day.

Therapeutic Interventions

Actions/Interventions

■ Encourage small feedings of nutritionally dense, soft food or liquids. Add nutritional supplements as appropriate.

■ Instruct the patient to avoid very spicy foods, gas-producing foods, and carbonated beverages.

■ Instruct the patient to eat high-calorie foods first and have favorite foods available.

■ Avoid fluid intake with meals, and instead encourage fluids between meals.

■ Instruct the patient to plan activities.

■ Instruct the patient to eat slowly, use pursed-lip breathing between bites, and use bronchodilators before meals.

■ Reinforce the need to substitute nasal prongs for oxygen mask during mealtime.

■ Stress importance of frequent oral care.

■ Provide companionship at mealtime.

■ Assist with meals as needed, and cut up food if patients take longer than 1 hour to complete a meal.

■ Encourage the patient to sit up during meals.

Rationales

Small feedings are easier to digest and require less chewing.

Avoidance prevents possible abdominal distention. Cold foods may give less sense of fullness than hot foods.

When anorexia is a problem, these strategies can be useful to maintain nutrition. In addition, adding butter, mayonnaise, margarine, sauces, or gravies to food can add calories.

Fluid intake gives a sense of fullness with meals, thereby reducing desire for solid foods.

Planning activities allows rest before eating.

These techniques decrease dyspnea.

This change in oxygen delivery equipment will maintain the patient's oxygenation.

Oral care promotes mouth comfort and can enhance one's appetite.

Attention to the social aspects of eating is important in both the hospital and home settings.

These measures facilitate optimal intake.

This position reduces hypoxia and the danger of aspiration.

■ = Independent   ▲ = Collaborative

Pulmonary Care Plans

 Risk for Infection

Common Risk Factors

Retained secretions (good medium for bacterial growth)
Poor nutrition
Impaired pulmonary defense system secondary to COPD
Use of respiratory equipment
Chronic disease

Common Expected Outcome

The patient remains free of infection as evidenced by normal temperature, negative sputum cultures, normal WBC count, and breath sounds clear to auscultation.

NOC Outcomes
Risk Control; Knowledge: Infection Control
NIC Intervention
Infection Protection

Ongoing Assessment

Actions/Interventions	Rationales
■ Auscultate lungs to monitor for significant changes in breath sounds.	Bronchial breath sounds and rales (crackles) may indicate pneumonia.
■ Assess for any of the following significant changes in sputum: • Sudden increase in production • Change in color (rusty, yellow, greenish) • Change in consistency (thick)	These signs may indicate presence of infection.
■ Assess for other signs and symptoms of infection: fever, chills, increase in cough, elevated white blood cell (WBC) count, shortness of breath, nausea, vomiting, diarrhea, anorexia.	Prompt assessment of infection facilitates early intervention.
■ Assess the patient's understanding of techniques to prevent infection, such as careful hand washing, adequate rest and nutrition, and avoidance of crowds.	This knowledge helps the patient understand the rationale for interventions to reduce infection risk.
■ Assess vaccination status (flu and pneumococcal vaccines).	These vaccines prevent some types of infection and are recommended by such organizations as the American Lung Association and the American Thoracic Society.

Therapeutic Interventions

Actions/Interventions	Rationales
■ Encourage an increase in fluid intake, unless contraindicated.	Fluid intake maintains good hydration. Insensible loss is markedly increased during infection because of fever and increase in respiratory rate.
■ Ensure that oxygen humidifier is properly maintained. Reinforce not to add new water to old water.	Stagnant old water is a medium for bacterial growth.
■ Minimize retained secretions by encouraging the patient to cough and expectorate secretions frequently. If the patient is unable to cough and expectorate, instruct the patient or caregiver in nasotracheal oropharyngeal suctioning.	Retained secretions provide bacterial growth medium.
■ Follow standard precautions, including proper hand washing techniques, to minimize microorganism transmission.	Friction and running water effectively remove microorganisms from hands.

Deficient Knowledge

Common Related Factors
Recent diagnosis
Ineffective past teaching or learning
Unfamiliarity with resources

Common Expected Outcome
Patient verbalizes understanding of disease process and treatment.

Defining Characteristics
Noncompliance
Inability to verbalize health maintenance regimen
Repeated acute exacerbations
Development of complications
Misconceptions about health status
Multiple questions or no questions

NOC Outcomes
Knowledge: Disease Process; Knowledge: Health Behaviors; Knowledge: Medication; Knowledge: Treatment Regimen

NIC Interventions
Teaching: Disease Process; Teaching: Prescribed Medications; Teaching: Prescribed Activity/Exercise; Teaching: Psychomotor Skill

---

Ongoing Assessment

Actions/Interventions	Rationales
■ Assess knowledge base of COPD.	Patients need to understand the COPD is a progressive disease that requires self-management to reduce episodes of dyspnea, hypoxia, and acidosis.
■ Assess environmental, social, cultural, and educational factors that may influence the teaching plan.	To be effective, interventions need to be specific to the patient and address individual influences.
■ Assess cognitive function and emotional readiness to learn.	Cognitive impairments need to be assessed so an appropriate teaching plan can be designed. Patients with chronic hypoxia may have learning challenges.

Therapeutic Interventions

Actions/Interventions	Rationales
■ Allow the patient to identify what is most important to him or her.	This information clarifies learner expectations and helps the nurse match the information to be presented to the individual's needs. Adult learning is problem oriented.
■ Instruct the patient in basic anatomy and physiology of respiratory system, with attention to structure and airflow.	Information helps patients understand the complexities of their airway problems.
■ Discuss the relation of the disease process to signs and symptoms that the patient experiences.	Recognition of key signs prevents delays in seeking help and facilitates appropriate self-management.
■ Discuss purpose and method of administration for each medication.	Return demonstrations on MDI spacers, dry powder capsules, or Diskus techniques are necessary to ensure appropriate delivery of the medications. If a steroid component is used, teach the patient to rinse the mouth after use to avoid fungal mouth infections.
■ Instruct patient to avoid central nervous system depressants.	Depressants can depress respiratory drive.

■ = Independent ▲ = Collaborative

Actions/Interventions	Rationales
■ Discuss appropriate nutritional habits, including supplements, as appropriate.	COPD patients have increased nutritional needs because of work of breathing.
■ Discuss the concept of energy conservation. Encourage resting as needed during activities, avoiding overexertion and fatigue, sitting as much as possible, alternating heavy and light tasks, carrying articles close to the body, organizing all equipment at the beginning of activity, and working slowly.	Patients need to learn self-management skills to reduce dyspnea from fatigue.
■ Discuss signs and symptoms of infection and when to contact the health care provider.	Respiratory infections can increase the work of breathing and precipitate respiratory failure.
■ Discuss common factors that lead to exacerbations of lung problems: smoking, environmental temperature, and humidity.	Chemical irritants and allergens can increase mucus production and bronchospasm.
■ Refer the patient or significant others to smoking cessation support groups as appropriate.	Smoking or chronic exposure to tobacco smoke is the leading cause of COPD. Supportive groups provide emotional support and information.
■ Instruct in indoor or outdoor air quality:	Patients need to learn how to control air quality to promote effective breathing. Smoke and other factors resulting in poor air quality can cause bronchospasm. Similarly, cold air can induce bronchospasm.
• Avoid smoke-filled rooms, sudden changes in temperature, aerosol sprays.	
• Use air conditioning in hot weather.	
• Stay indoors when pollen counts are high or when outdoor air quality is poor or during ozone alerts.	
• Use scarves or masks over face in cold weather.	
■ Discuss the importance of specific therapeutic measures:	
• Breathing exercises	
• Exercise 1—TECHNIQUE:	This exercise strengthens muscles of respiration.
1 Lie supine with one hand on chest and one hand on abdomen.	
2 Inhale slowly through mouth, raising abdomen against hand.	
3 Exhale slowly through pursed lips while contracting abdominal muscles and moving abdomen inward.	
• Exercise 2—TECHNIQUE:	This exercise develops slowed, controlled breathing.
1 Walk; stop to take deep breath.	
2 Exhale slowly while walking.	
• Exercise 3—TECHNIQUE:	This exercise decreases air trapping and airway collapse.
1 For pursed-lip breathing, inhale slowly through nose.	
2 Exhale twice as slowly as usual through pursed lips.	
• Cough: Lean forward; take several deep breaths with pursed-lip method. Take last deep breath, cough with open mouth during expiration, and simultaneously contract abdominal muscles.	Controlled cough techniques help mobilize secretions.
• Teach forced expiratory technique: Instruct to take a deep breath, exhale forcefully without coughing through an open mouth while saying "huh." Repeat as many times as needed.	This technique moves the trapped mucus into the larger airways for the patient to cough up.
• Chest physiotherapy or pulmonary postural drainage: Demonstrate correct methods for postural drainage: positioning, percussion, vibration.	Chest physiotherapy facilitates expectoration of secretions and prevents waste of energy.
• Hydration: Discuss importance of maintaining good fluid intake. Recommend 1.5 to 2 liters/day.	Hydration decreases viscosity of secretions.
• Humidity: Discuss various forms of humidification.	Humidity prevents drying of secretions.

Actions/Interventions

- Discuss home oxygen therapy:
  - Type and use of equipment (compressed O_2 in tanks; liquid O_2; O_2 concentrator):
    - Demonstrate how to start oxygen flow and regulate flowmeter.

  - Discuss flow rate of oxygen at rest, at night, and with activity, as individualized to the patient.

  - Discuss use of portable oxygen system for ambulating in and outside of the home.
  - Discuss use of oxygen-conserving devices, as appropriate.

- Safety precautions:
  - Do not use around a stove or gas space heater.
  - Do not smoke or light matches around cylinder when oxygen is in use.
  - Post "No Smoking" sign, and call to visitors' attention.
- Discuss the need for periodic reevaluation to determine or substantiate oxygen needs.
- ▲ Discuss available resources:
  - Arrange for oxygen delivery or maintenance, as appropriate.
  - Arrange for home care nurse to check patient, as appropriate.
  - Refer to local lung association if available for support groups.
- ▲ Discuss or arrange for the patient to participate in a pulmonary rehabilitation program.

- Discuss the need for the patient to obtain vaccines for pneumococcal pneumonia and yearly vaccine for influenza.
- Discuss use of medical alert bracelet or other identification.
- Provide written instructions and reliable Internet resources.

Rationales

Medicare guidelines for reimbursement for home oxygen require a Pa_{O_2} less than 58 mm Hg and/or oxygen saturation of 88% or less on room air.

Patient or others who are primarily responsible for oxygen therapy at home should be able to demonstrate the process.

Oxygen delivery should be titrated to maintain an oxygen saturation of 90% or more. This will help improve the patient's exercise tolerance and reduce pulmonary hypertension.

This therapy can reduce activity-related hypoxia.

A variety of measures are appropriate to conserve energy, such as pacing activities, avoiding working with arms raised, or reorganizing home items so that most frequently used ones are within easy reach.

Oxygen is not combustible itself but can feed a fire if one occurs.

Objective data guide ongoing management.

Home care agencies and patient support groups provide patients with resources to maintain compliance with a treatment program.

Pulmonary rehabilitation improves on baseline physical conditioning, increases optimal capabilities, and teaches the patient techniques to control breathing and energy conservation.

Vaccines decrease occurrence or severity of these diseases.

These forms of identification alert others to COPD history.

These help the patient follow plan and maintain access to current therapies.

Related Care Plans

Activity intolerance, p. 8
Insomnia, p. 117
Ineffective therapeutic regimen management, p. 194
Self-care deficit, p. 170

■ = Independent   ▲ = Collaborative

Cystic Fibrosis

Cystic fibrosis (CF) is an autosomal recessive, profoundly life-shortening genetic disease. It occurs most commonly in whites of northern European descent but has been identified in most ethnicities. Genetic abnormalities in the seventh chromosome result in impaired function of CF transmembrane conductance regulator (CFTR) protein present in the mucus-secreting cells of the body, primarily affecting the respiratory and gastrointestinal tracts. The hallmark characteristics of CF are chronic, progressive lung disease resulting from secretion of dehydrated mucus with airway obstruction, and malnutrition from pancreatic insufficiency. However, there is a wide range of disease severity; respiratory symptoms can range from nearly asymptomatic disease with undetectable changes in lung function to severe obstructive disease early in childhood, whereas gastrointestinal (GI) symptoms may range from mild constipation, normal liver function, and intermittent pancreatitis to severe loss of pancreatic function, malabsorption with subsequent malnutrition, CF-related diabetes and end-stage liver disease. Nonetheless, with improved understanding and treatment, the majority of affected individuals now live well into adulthood. The sweat glands and the reproductive glands are also affected; almost all males with CF are sterile because of absence or impairment of the vas deferens, whereas females have reduced fertility. The impact on the sweat gland gives rise to abnormally high chloride secretion; a simple analysis of sweat chloride content continues to be the gold standard for CF diagnosis.

Lung disease accounts for most disease morbidity and remains the primary cause of death in CF. The cycle of lung disease in CF is caused by inflammation, infection, and impaired airway clearance. Daily lifelong airway clearance, attention to infection prevention, and early, aggressive treatment of pulmonary exacerbations are the mainstays of therapy aimed at slowing decline and preserving lung function. In addition, supporting normal growth and nutrition over the life span is associated with improved respiratory health, longevity, and quality of life in the adult patient. Lung transplant may be a treatment option for some patients. This care plan focuses on acute care treatment of pulmonary exacerbation.

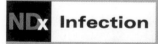

NDx Infection

Common Related Factors
New acquisition of common CF airway pathogens
Growth plume of known colonized CF airway pathogens
Invading viral organism

Defining Characteristics
Increased or new cough
Increased sputum
Dyspnea/wheezing
Decline in pulmonary function testing (spirometry)
Fever
Malaise
Elevated WBC count
Pathogenic microbes on airway culture

Common Expected Outcome
Patient experiences improvement in infection and suppression of bacterial growth, as evidenced by decrease in cough, mucous production to baseline, normothermia, and normal white blood cell (WBC) count.

NOC Outcome
Infection Status

NIC Interventions
Infection Control; Infection Protection

Ongoing Assessment

Actions/Interventions	Rationales
■ Assess for general signs/symptoms of infection: fever, malaise, cough/wheezing, increased sputum, weight loss, tachypnea, and tachycardia.	Pulmonary infections are associated with general symptoms of infection, along with increase in respiratory rate and heart rate.
■ Use pulse oximetry to monitor oxygen saturation.	Oxygen requirements can increase during acute respiratory infections or in response to fever.
▲ Obtain sputum specimen for culture and sensitivity as ordered.	Acquisition of new pathogens is often associated with CF pulmonary exacerbation. Common CF pathogens include *Pseudomonas aeruginosa, Staphylococcus aureus*/methicillin-resistant *S. aureus* (MRSA), *Haemophilus influenzae, Stenotrophomonas maltophilia, Burkholderia cepacia,* and *Achromobacter xylosoxidans.* Airway culture and sensitivities guide infection control measures, as well as antimicrobial selection.
▲ Monitor pending culture and sensitivity results for drug resistance.	Drug resistance may necessitate a change in antibiotics. A new organism may alter infection control precautions.
▲ Monitor white blood count (WBC) as ordered.	WBC count can be elevated in response to pulmonary exacerbation or infection with new organism.
▲ Monitor immunoglobulin E (IgE) as ordered.	CF pulmonary exacerbations can result from allergic bronchopulmonary aspergillosis (ABPA), an allergic response to *Aspergillus* in the airways. IgE will be significantly elevated.
▲ Monitor viral studies as ordered.	Pulmonary exacerbations can occur in response to or concurrently with viral illness.
▲ Monitor antibiotic levels as ordered.	Inadequate dosing can result in resistance and/or poor therapeutic response. Toxicity can result in poor outcomes or adverse events.

Therapeutic Interventions

Actions/Interventions	Rationales
▲ Institute appropriate infection control precautions.	Many CF pathogens require patients to be in contact isolation based on Centers for Disease Control and Prevention (CDC) and Cystic Fibrosis Foundation (CFF) Consensus Guidelines.
■ Ensure that patients with CF are not cohorted.	Cohorting of patients with CF is not recommended based on published CF Infection Control Consensus Guidelines.
▲ Administer intravenous (IV) antibiotics as ordered in timely manner.	Benchmark institutions set the standard for first dose of IV antibiotics within 4 hours of admission.
▲ Administer antipyretic as ordered for fever, avoiding nonsteroidal antiinflammatory drugs (NSAIDs) in patients receiving IV aminoglycosides.	Antipyretics maintain normothermia and reduce metabolic needs. Aminoglycosides and NSAIDS in combination can cause renal toxicity.
▲ Consider audiology evaluation in patients who have history of frequent IV aminoglycoside use.	Ototoxicity is a common adverse effect of aminoglycoside use.

Ineffective Airway Clearance

Common Related Factor	Defining Characteristics
Increased sputum production and mucous plugging in response to new or increased bacterial growth in airways	New or increased purulent sputum production Ineffective cough Dyspnea/tachypnea Increased work of breathing

■ = Independent ▲ = Collaborative

Abnormal breath sounds (rales, rhonchi, reduced breath sounds)
Fatigue
Chest pain
Abnormal chest x-ray film
Decline in pulmonary function testing (spirometry)

Common Expected Outcomes

Patient maintains clear, open airways as evidenced by normal breath sounds, normal rate and depth of respirations, and an airway free of secretions, with effective cough.

Patient will be proficient in using effective airway clearance therapies to clear secretions on a daily basis, as evidenced by decreased work of breathing and improved pulmonary function.

NOC Outcome
Respiratory Status: Airway Patency
NIC Interventions
Airway Management; Cough Enhancement

Ongoing Assessment

Actions/Interventions	Rationales
■ Assess respiratory rate, work of breathing, use of accessory muscles, and presence of retractions.	Infection, inflammation and mucous plugging will cause an increase in respiratory effort to compensate for airway obstruction.
■ Assess cough for effectiveness.	Habitual cough suppression is common in patients with CF; an effective mucus-clearing cough is essential for adequate airway clearance.
■ Assess lungs for adventitious sounds, degree of aeration.	Rales, rhonchi, and decreased aeration signify ongoing infection and inflammation.
■ Assess chest wall for equal chest expansion.	Unequal chest expansion can indicate pneumothorax—a complication of CF.
▲ Use pulse oximetry to monitor oxygen saturation.	Hypoxemia may result from impaired gas exchange and from buildup of secretions and bronchial constriction.
■ Assess comfort level with and adherence to recommended airway clearance therapy (ACT).	Patient satisfaction and proficiency with selected ACT regimen is essential for adherence.
■ Assess for barriers to ongoing airway clearance.	Identification of barriers to ACT can guide interventions to improve adherence.
▲ Monitor pulmonary function testing.	Improvement in spirometry signifies improved airflow and aeration, effective airway clearance, and treatment of infection.
▲ Observe sputum for amount, consistency, and color.	Decreasing amount and frequency of sputum production, lighter color, and thinner consistency of sputum indicate improvement in exacerbation. Scant amounts or streaking of blood in sputum can occur from airway inflammation; however, major hemoptysis can occur and is a life-threatening emergency.

Therapeutic Interventions

Actions/Interventions	Rationales
▲ Collaborate with patient and staff to determine preferred ACT. Options include: • Traditional chest physiotherapy • Mechanical chest wall percussion (vest) • Handheld oscillating devices • Autogenic or postural drainage	The CFTR defect causes mucus to become dehydrated. Secretions in CF are generally thick, sticky, and more difficult to clear. Frequent airway clearance is a mainstay in the treatment of acute exacerbations, as well as an integral part of health maintenance in CF. Individualized care and patient choice in therapy will impact adherence and effectiveness of treatment. A variety of supportive devices are available. Respiratory therapists can be helpful in these selections.

Actions/Interventions

▲ Collaborate with patient and staff to ensure that schedule for therapy is amenable to all and does not interfere with meals, rest times, or medications.

▲ Administer bronchodilators as ordered before ACT.

▲ Administer prescribed mucolytics as ordered in concert with ACT.

■ Encourage frequent and effective cough—particularly around ACT.

■ Provide opportunity for exercise and/or physical therapy.

▲ Administer pain medication as needed.

Rationales

ACT is time consuming and must be part of a balanced treatment plan. ACT should not be done immediately after meals, nor should it interfere with rest or other required therapies (i.e., medications, physical therapy); it therefore requires careful scheduling.

Relief of any bronchoconstriction present before ACT will optimize airway clearance.

Mucolytics assist in the breakdown of mucus and promote effective clearance of cellular debris in the airways.

Habitual cough suppression results in retention of mucus; patients should be encouraged to actively and intentionally use effective coughing to clear airway mucus.

Exercise supports the goal of airway clearance by loosening mucus and facilitating effective coughing. It also improves overall physical conditioning and recovery.

Attention to pain relief facilitates patient being able to cooperate comfortably with ACT and exercise/physical therapy.

Impaired Gas Exchange

Common Related Factors

Inflammation of airways and alveoli
Infection with lung consolidation, alveolar collapse.
Bronchiectasis with decreased surface area for gas exchange and loss of lung function

Defining Characteristics

Hypoxemia
Hypercapnia
Dyspnea
Cough
Tachypnea
Tachycardia
Restlessness/ irritability
Activity intolerance
Pale, dusky/cyanotic skin color

Common Expected Outcome

Patient maintains optimal gas exchange as evidenced by arterial blood gases (ABGs) within the patient's usual range, oxygen saturation of 90% or greater, alert response mentation and no further reduction in level of consciousness, relaxed breathing, and baseline HR for patient.

NOC Outcome

Respiratory Status: Gas Exchange

NIC Interventions

Respiratory Monitoring; Oxygen Therapy

Ongoing Assessment

Actions/Interventions

■ Assess for change in respiratory status, as evidenced by increased work of breathing, tachypnea, changing level of consciousness, increasing anxiety or restlessness, pallor or cyanosis.

■ Monitor changes in HR, respiratory rate.

Rationales

Patients will adapt their breathing pattern over time to facilitate gas exchange. Abnormalities may indicate respiratory compromise, hypoxia, or hypercarbia.

Respiratory rate and heart rate increase to compensate for early hypoxia.

■ = Independent ▲ = Collaborative

Actions/Interventions

▲ Use pulse oximetry to monitor oxygen saturation; assess ABGs if ordered.

▲ Monitor transcutaneous CO_2 as ordered.

Rationales

Increasing $Paco_2$ and decreasing Pao_2 are signs of respiratory failure. Severe hypoxemia and hypercarbia can lead to hypotension, arrhythmias, and falling respiratory effort.

Chronic hypercarbia can be present in patients with moderate to severe CF lung disease; increasing levels can indicate progression of acute infection and pending respiratory failure.

Therapeutic Interventions

Actions/Interventions

▲ Administer oxygen as prescribed, avoiding high concentrations of oxygen in patients with chronic CO_2 retention.

■ Provide for adequate rest between activities during the day, with minimal nighttime interruptions in sleep.

▲ Collaborate with respiratory care personnel in administration and monitoring of noninvasive ventilation as ordered.

Rationales

Supplemental oxygen maintains adequate oxygenation, decreases work of breathing and calorie expenditure, and relieves dyspnea, increasing level of comfort. Goal is oxygen saturation greater than 90%.

Activity increases oxygenation needs and should be paced appropriately to prevent fatigue.

Noninvasive ventilation (bilevel positive airway pressure [Bi-PAP]) is a therapy option for patients with severe lung disease and a superimposed acute illness, or for assistance with nighttime ventilatory needs.

 NANDA-I NDx # Imbalanced Nutrition: Less Than Body Requirements

Common Related Factors

Poor nutritional status resulting from anorexia
Chronic malabsorption
Increased caloric needs

Defining Characteristics

Weight loss, weight plateau
Abnormal eating behaviors
Low fat-soluble vitamin levels
Anemia
Hypoalbuminemia
Chronic abdominal discomfort
Abnormal stool patterns (diarrhea or constipation)
Gastroesophageal reflux

Common Expected Outcomes

Patient will maintain adequate nutritional status or demonstrate weight gain on trajectory to adequate nutritional status.
Patient will be free of signs/symptoms of malabsorption.

NOC Outcome
Nutritional Status: Food and Fluid Intake
NIC Interventions
Nutritional Monitoring; Nutritional Therapy; Nutritional Management

---

Ongoing Assessment

Actions/Interventions

▲ Collaborate with registered dietitian in obtaining full nutritional evaluation.

Rationales

Multidisciplinary input and collaboration will optimize therapeutic interventions. Patients with CF usually have a long history of impaired nutrition, and interventions need to be guided by baseline data.

Actions/Interventions

- Assess skin turgor, color, integrity.

- Assess abdomen for bloating, fullness, bowel sounds, palpable stool mass. Monitor stool patterns for frequency, consistency, odor, presence of oil/grease.

- ▲ Monitor serum chemistry as ordered.

- Monitor for excessive thirst, urination, hunger. Obtain bedside blood glucose as ordered.

- Monitor for increase in weight and appetite.

Rationales

Malnutrition can be associated with alteration in skin integrity. CF-related liver disease can result in jaundice.

Undertreated malabsorption is common in CF; symptoms may be normalized by patients and families; adjustments in pancreatic enzyme supplementation are warranted with signs/symptoms of malabsorption.

Hypoalbuminemia, elevation in liver enzymes, hyperglycemia, and alterations in electrolyte balances can all represent complications in CF.

CF-related diabetes occurs in up to 30% of adolescents and adults with CF; glucose intolerance can be present intermittently with pulmonary exacerbations.

Increasing trends in weight and appetite accompany resolution of pulmonary exacerbations.

Therapeutic Interventions

Action/Interventions

- Provide high-calorie, high-protein diet.

- Encourage liberal use of salt or salty food intake.

- ▲ Administer pancreatic enzymes before all meals and snacks containing fat/protein as ordered.
- Administer all fat-soluble vitamins with meals and enzymes.

- Encourage liberal hydration and high fiber intake.

Rationales

Patients with CF have increased caloric needs as much as 1.2 to 1.5 of the daily recommended amounts.

Hyponatremic dehydration and salt loss occur easily in the CF patient as sequelae to CF defect in the sweat glands.

Patients with CF require pancreatic enzyme supplementation to adequately digest food containing fat or protein.

Fat-soluble vitamin deficits are common in CF because of fat malabsorption. Vitamin supplements must be taken with pancreatic enzymes to be absorbed.

Chronic constipation can result from mucus secretion and dehydration in the intestinal lumen (especially when malabsorption is adequately treated and stool consistency is normalized).

NANDA-I NDx ## Deficient Knowledge

Common Related Factors

First exacerbation/hospitalization experience
Ineffective or incomplete education in past
Rapidly expanding clinical knowledge base with new interventions available

Defining Characteristics

Inability to verbalize treatment regimen or rationale
Verbalized misconceptions regarding outcomes in CF
Uncertainty and/or questions regarding treatment recommendations and goals
Nonadherence to therapy
Frequent exacerbations
Anxiety related to hospitalization

Common Expected Outcome

Patient and family can verbalize understanding of disease process, treatment recommendations, and goals of therapy.

NOC Outcome
Knowledge: Disease Process
NIC Interventions
Knowledge: Treatment Regimen; Teaching: Disease Process

■ = Independent   ▲ = Collaborative

Ongoing Assessment

Actions/Interventions	Rationales
■ Assess knowledge of genetics of CF.	CF is caused by a defect in the CFTR gene, a gene that makes a protein that controls the movement of salt and water into and out of body cells. Children who inherit a defective CFTR gene from each parent will have CF.
■ Assess baseline knowledge of disease pathophysiology.	CF is a disease of the secretory glands, including mucus and sweat glands, and affects many organs, especially the lungs and pancreas.
■ Assess knowledge of medications and airway clearance therapies, equipment.	Complex treatment regimens in CF can be difficult to maintain, and regular assessment of knowledge can identify gaps in therapy and sources of nonadherence.
■ Assess knowledge of nutritional needs.	Understanding of nutritional needs and options for meeting those needs promotes self-management.
■ Assess knowledge of diagnostic testing, including laboratory evaluations, pulmonary function testing, airway cultures, and pathogens	Patient understanding of individual baseline lung function and usual airway pathogens helps with understanding of treatment recommendations and goals of therapy.
■ Assess knowledge of infection control recommendations for individuals with CF.	Individuals with CF should have good understanding of infection prevention recommendations for their own protection and that of the greater CF community.

Therapeutic Interventions

Actions/Interventions	Rationales
■ Provide basic information on CF pathophysiology and treatment goals using reliable resources (e.g., www.CFF.org).	Currently there is no cure for CF. Goals of treatment are to prevent lung infections, remove thick mucus from the lungs, prevent intestinal blockage, enhance nutrition, and reduce risks for dehydration. With meticulous self-management and medical care, patients are living longer—many into their 40s and 50s.
■ Review ACT and breathing techniques to dislodge mucus.	Chest physical therapy is one of the mainstays of treatment. Patients often find it difficult to perform; strategies or adjunct aids to assist in effective performance need to be discussed.
■ Review pulmonary medications and nutritional/digestive medications and their rationale.	Complex medication regimens in CF change over time, and frequent review helps to clarify purpose and supports adherence. Pulmonary medications may include antibiotics, antiinflammatory medications, bronchodilators, and/or mucus thinners. Nutritional medications may include pancreatic enzymes, vitamin supplements, and salt.
■ Review pulmonary function testing and individual trends.	Data provide guide for progression or improvement in disease.
■ Review infection control recommendations.	Care providers have responsibility to ensure patients and families are informed about infection control strategies for optimal prevention of new pathogen acquisition.
■ Provide information about support groups.	Living with a chronic disease can be emotionally challenging. Groups that share common experiences can be helpful.

Additional Care Plans

Ineffective coping, p. 49

Head and Neck Cancer: Surgical Approaches

Radical Neck Surgery; Laryngectomy

Head and neck cancer accounts for approximately 3% of new cancers in the United States annually but is much more prevalent in developing nations. Ninety percent of head and neck cancers are squamous cell carcinomas, with the remaining 10% divided among lymphomas and minor salivary gland tumors. The primary risk factors for head and neck cancer are tobacco and alcohol. Although alcohol does not appear to be risk factor in and of itself, it has proven to have a synergistic effect with tobacco. New research is strongly linking human papillomavirus (HPV) infection to the development of head and neck cancer, specifically in the oral cavity and tonsil. This will be an area of continuing study over the next few years to evaluate the potential use of HPV vaccines. Head and neck cancer is often diagnosed at later stages when a patient presents with a mass in the neck, hoarseness, or respiratory distress. A computed tomography (CT) scan of the head and neck, along with a fine-needle biopsy, are the most common diagnostic tools. Treatment consists of combined modalities, such as surgery, radiation, and/or chemotherapy, in hopes of achieving the best outcome possible. The focus of this care plan is the surgical management of patients with head and neck cancer.

NANDA-I NDx **Ineffective Airway Clearance**

Common Related Factors

Presence of artificial airway: tracheostomy tube/laryngectomy tube
Thick, copious secretions
Pain
Edema
Decreased energy and fatigue
Inability/refusal to cough

Defining Characteristics

Adventitious breath sounds (rhonchi, wheezes, crackles)
Ineffective cough
Dyspnea
Changes in respiratory rate or depth
Orthopnea
Excessive secretions

Common Expected Outcome

Patient maintains clear, open airways, as evidenced by normal breath sounds, normal rate and depth of respirations, and ability to effectively cough up secretions after treatment and deep breaths.

NOC Outcome
Respiratory Status: Airway Patency
NIC Interventions
Airway Management; Cough Enhancement; Airway Suctioning

Ongoing Assessment

Actions/Interventions	Rationales
■ Assess respiratory rate, rhythm, and effort.	Respiratory rate and rhythm changes may be a compensatory response for airway obstruction and are early warning signs of impending respiratory difficulties.
■ Assess effectiveness of cough.	Pain may interfere with coughing. Thick, tenacious secretions may be difficult to expectorate.

■ = Independent   ▲ = Collaborative

Actions/Interventions

- Assess color, consistency, and quantity of secretions.

- Auscultate lungs after coughing for normal and abnormal sounds, as in the following: decreased or absent breath sounds, wheezing, coarse crackles.
- ▲ Use pulse oximetry to maintain oxygen saturation; assess arterial blood gases (ABGs).

- Assess color of skin, nail beds, and mucous membranes.

- Assess changes in level of consciousness.

- Assess for pain.

Rationales

Abnormalities may be the result of infection, smoking history, or other abnormalities. A sign of infection is discolored sputum.

Diminished breath sounds or the presence of adventitious sounds may indicate an obstructed airway.

Increasing $Paco_2$ and decreasing Pao_2 and pulse oximetry readings can result from increased pulmonary secretions and respiratory fatigue.

Color changes such as cyanosis indicate increased concentration of deoxygenated blood and that inadequate oxygenation of tissues is occurring.

Increasing confusion, restlessness and/or irritability are early signs of cerebral hypoxia.

Postoperative pain can result in shallow breathing and an ineffective cough.

Therapeutic Interventions

Actions/Interventions

- Maintain humidified oxygen through the tracheostomy collar.

- Encourage the patient to deep breathe every 2 hours while awake and to cough. Encourage effective coughing after taking deep breaths.
- Suction tracheostomy or stoma with sterile technique if the patient is unable to clear own secretions.

- Position the patient with the head of bed elevated.

- Encourage and assist the patient in changing position every 2 hours, and increase activity as tolerated.
- If a disposable inner cannula is used, change the tracheostomy inner cannula every 8 hours; if a nondisposable inner cannula is used, cleanse the inner cannula at least every 8 hours and as needed (prn).
- Maintain secure tracheostomy ties.

- Keep the same size sterile tracheostomy tube at the bedside.
- ▲ Consult respiratory therapy staff as needs arise.

Rationales

Humidification thins secretions for easier expectoration with coughing. With radical neck surgery, a total laryngectomy may be done, in which the entire larynx and preepiglottic region are removed and a permanent stoma is created. In other surgical procedures a tracheostomy may be performed to avoid potential airway complications in the immediate postoperative period.

Deep breathing prevents atelectasis and enhances gas exchange. Coughing is the most helpful way to remove most secretions, especially when combined with deep breathing.

A patent airway is a priority. Suctioning is indicated when patients are unable to remove secretions by coughing. Sterile technique is important because patients with impaired immune systems as a result of cancer and surgery are at risk for infection.

This position decreases surgical edema and increases lung expansion.

Frequent position changes facilitate mobilization of secretions.

Retained secretions can obstruct the airway.

Tracheostomy tube dislodgment may be prevented when the tube is securely tied.

This standby tube is for insertion if dislodgment should occur.

Specialty expertise may be required to guide therapy.

NANDA-I NDx **Impaired Verbal Communication**

Common Related Factors

Laryngectomy (results in permanent loss of voice)
Tracheostomy (may temporarily cause inability to create sound)

Defining Characteristics

Inability to speak
Difficulty vocalizing words
Difficulty maintaining usual communication pattern.

Common Expected Outcome

Patient uses a form of communication to get needs met and to relate effectively with persons and his or her environment.

NOC Outcome
Communication: Expressive

NIC Intervention
Communication Enhancement: Speech Deficit

Ongoing Assessment

Actions/Interventions	Rationales
■ Assess patient's communication ability.	With total laryngectomy, the vocal cords are removed, so sound is not produced. Assessment of the best nonverbal method for communication guides subsequent efforts. With a tracheostomy the majority of air bypasses the vocal cords. In some patients, no sound is made. In others, sound is "breathy" or weak. Patient should be evaluated by speech pathology staff to see if use of a speaking valve is appropriate.
■ Assess for additional obstacles to communication (e.g., the patient is hard of hearing, has low literacy, or has arthritis of the hands).	Accurate assessment of the full scope of limitations guides selection of appropriate communication aids.
■ Frequently assess the patient's need to communicate.	Early recognition of and prompt response to the patient's need to communicate decreases anxiety and helps establish trust.
■ Assess effectiveness of nonverbal communication methods.	Patient may use hand signals, facial expressions, and changes in body posture to communicate with others. However, others may have difficulty in interpreting these nonverbal techniques. Each new method needs to be assessed for effectiveness and altered as necessary.

Therapeutic Interventions

Actions/Interventions	Rationales
■ Ensure that unit personnel are aware of patient's inability to speak.	Knowledge may reduce patient's sense of frustration when attempting to communicate with unit staff.
■ Keep the call light within reach at all times. Answer the call light promptly.	Patient response decreases anxiety and feelings of helplessness.
■ Allow the patient time to communicate needs.	The nurse should set aside enough time to attend to all of the details of patient care. Care measures may take longer time to complete in the presence of a communication deficit.
■ Provide emotional support to the patient and significant others.	Difficulties communicating are a source of frustration to all involved.
■ Instruct the patient and significant others in alternative methods of communication: hand gestures, writing tablet with pen, picture board, word board, electronic communication system, electronic voice box.	Providing a variety of communication aids allows the patient more channels through which information can be communicated and broadens the group of people with whom the patient can communicate.

■ = Independent   ▲ = Collaborative

Pulmonary Care Plans

Actions/Interventions	Rationales
▲ Consult the speech therapy staff regarding alternate forms of speech. The following may be used for the patient:	
• For tracheostomy only: speaking valve	The speaking valve is "one-way," allowing air to enter through the tracheostomy, then forcing exhalation via the upper airway. As air flows over the vocal cords, the vibrations create sound. Patient's oxygen saturation must be monitored at 30 minutes following initial placement. Always remove for sleeping.
• Voice prosthesis (tracheoesophageal prosthesis [TEP])	The voice prosthesis is inserted into a fistula made between the esophagus and trachea. The prosthesis prevents aspiration but allows air from the lungs to enter the esophagus and out of the mouth with speech being produced by movement of the tongue and lips.
• Electrolarynx	The electrolarynx is a battery-operated, handheld device that uses sound waves to create speech while being held against the neck. The pitch is low, and the sound is electronic in nature.
• Esophageal speech	Esophageal speech is a method of swallowing air and "belching" it to create sound.
■ Encourage the patient to obtain an audiotape for home use that can be played when emergency service is called.	Patient will feel more secure in the home environment with a means for rapid communication in an emergency.
■ Encourage patient to wear medical alert bracelet to inform emergency personnel; "neck breather" is generally used.	This form of communication may be helpful in times of stress and emergency.

Risk for Ineffective Tissue Perfusion

Common Risk Factors
Tissue edema
Malfunction of wound drainage tubes
Preoperative radiation to surgical area
Extensive surgical dissection of blood vessels
Infection of surgical area

Common Expected Outcome
Patient maintains adequate tissue perfusion, as evidenced by normal incisional healing, gradual decrease in edema, gradual decrease in wound drainage, and no signs and symptoms of infection.

NOC Outcomes
Tissue Perfusion: Peripheral; Wound Healing: Primary Intention
NIC Interventions
Wound Care: Closed Drainage; Wound Care

Ongoing Assessment

Actions/Interventions	Rationales
■ Assess surgical wound drainage system for amount and color of drainage.	An abrupt cessation of drainage can indicate a clogged tube. Excessive drainage can indicate a leaking vessel in the area. Purulent drainage can indicate infection. White or "milky" drainage may indicate a chyle leak. Any of these *may* constitute a medical emergency.

Actions/Interventions	**Rationales**
■ Assess edema at the surgical wound.	Excessive edema can impede blood flow to or from the area and result in necrosis or infection.
■ Assess color of wound and surrounding skin for signs of decreased circulation: pale, blue, or dark in color.	Changes in perfusion can compromise skin flap integrity.
■ Assess wound edges for approximation.	Wound edges should be proximate (next to each other). Wound dehiscence can occur with excessive edema, necrosis, and infection.
■ Assess for hematoma formation: oozing from skin edges, swelling, increase in bruising, airway compromise.	Bleeding into the subcutaneous tissue may indicate a vessel leak and can result in a surgical emergency.
■ Monitor body temperature.	Fever is a sign of infection.

Therapeutic Interventions

Actions/Interventions	**Rationales**
▲ Gently compress drainage tubes as needed. Maintain suction as prescribed (e.g., Jackson-Pratt drain).	These procedures maintain patency and prevent buildup of fluid at the surgical site, which would cause excessive edema and possible infection or necrosis.
■ Keep head of bed elevated.	This position decreases local edema.
■ Perform tracheostomy tube and site cleaning as needed.	This keeps respiratory secretions away from the surgical wound.
■ Promptly change tracheostomy or wound dressings when wet.	Attention to tube and dressing changes prevents maceration of skin.

NANDA-I NDx

Imbalanced Nutrition: Less Than Body Requirements

Common Related Factors
Nothing by mouth (NPO) status
Decreased appetite
Dysphagia
Radiation therapy
Chemotherapy
Edema

Defining Characteristics
Weight loss
Documented inadequate caloric intake

Common Expected Outcome
Patient has adequate caloric intake, as evidenced by body weight greater than or equal to admission weight.

NOC Outcomes
Nutritional Status: Food and Fluid Intake; Nutritional Intake

NIC Intervention
Nutrition Management

Ongoing Assessment

Actions/Interventions	**Rationales**
■ Monitor weight at regular intervals.	These data provide encouragement when eating habits are impaired as well as identifying ineffective interventions.
▲ Monitor laboratory test results: serum albumin, protein, electrolytes, glucose.	These test results provide data on extent of nutritional deficiency.
■ Assess types of foods that the patient enjoys.	Selection of favorite foods may enhance interest in eating and improve caloric intake.

■ = Independent   ▲ = Collaborative

Actions/Interventions

■ Observe the patient during initial oral feeding.

Rationales

In tracheostomy patients, signs of aspiration of food or fluid from tracheostomy, such as choking, may occur when oral feeding is started. Postlaryngectomy, patients may have difficulty swallowing because of edema or surgical reconstruction. There is no longer any common pathway for food and air following a laryngectomy, so aspiration is a risk only for patients undergoing partial laryngectomies or other surgeries in which a tracheostomy is performed.

Therapeutic Interventions

Actions/Interventions

■ Instruct the patient in importance of adequate caloric intake.

▲ Consult with a dietitian.

■ Instruct in need for enteral feedings if prescribed. Instruct in procedure for administration of home enteral feedings if prescribed.

■ Assist the patient in performing oral hygiene.

▲ Consult speech therapy staff for swallowing evaluation as needed.

■ Encourage oral intake of soft foods when allowed.

■ Maintain suction setup at bedside for safety. Stay with the patient during initial oral feedings.

Rationales

Patient may not understand importance of caloric intake to promote incisional healing as well as to enhance overall nutritional status.

The dietitian will determine caloric requirements specific to the patient, assess caloric intake, and suggest enteral feedings, as appropriate.

Enteral feedings are initially used postoperatively until suture lines have healed. The feeding tube is put in place during surgery.

Oral hygiene keeps the mouth fresh and promotes interest in eating.

If a total laryngectomy is performed, swallowing should not be a problem because there is no connection between the esophagus and trachea. If a supraglottic laryngectomy is done, swallowing is more difficult because the epiglottis has been removed.

Soft foods and thicker liquids are easier to swallow than thin liquids. If aspiration is suspected, instruct patient in aspiration precautions and consult speech pathology staff or occupational therapy staff for a swallowing evaluation.

Suction may be needed during or after feedings to keep the airway patent.

NANDA-I NDx Disturbed Body Image

Common Related Factors

Visible incision
Facial and neck edema
Tracheostomy or laryngectomy stoma
Alteration in verbal communication
Dysphagia
Diagnosis of cancer

Defining Characteristics

Verbalization of negative feelings about body
Preoccupation with change
Refusal to look at face and neck
Withdrawal
Change in social behavior
Decreased motivation for self-care

Common Expected Outcome

Patient begins to adjust to body changes, as evidenced by ability to look at and talk about body changes, planning for discharge, showing interest in learning, and using alternative communication methods.

NOC Outcome
Body Image
NIC Interventions
Body Image Enhancement; Support System Enhancement

Ongoing Assessment

Actions/Interventions	Rationales
■ Assess the patient's mood and behavior for signs of difficulty in coping with changes in body appearance or function.	There is a broad range of behaviors associated with body image disturbance, ranging from totally ignoring the altered structure to preoccupation with it.
■ Assess the patient's perception of life changes precipitated by cancer treatments (i.e., occupational, interpersonal).	This assessment may give some perspective on any perceived misconceptions that could affect recovery.

Therapeutic Interventions

Actions/Interventions	Rationales
■ Encourage the patient to view the tracheostomy or stoma site.	Looking at the site is often the first indication that the patient is ready to deal with the change in appearance.
■ Suggest the use of a loose scarf or shirt over the stoma to camouflage it.	Decreasing the visibility of the tracheostomy or stoma site may promote enhanced self-esteem.
■ Encourage the patient and significant others to communicate fears or concerns regarding diagnosis of cancer treatment.	Misconceptions may need to be clarified.
■ Encourage visits, both in the hospital and at home, from significant others.	Visitors help the patient feel accepted and promote communication and support.
■ Refer to support services (e.g., Lost Cords, American Cancer Society, and International Association of Laryngectomees).	Rehabilitation after radical neck surgery is a long process, and support services can have a positive impact on the patient's recovery.
■ Arrange for a visit from a person who has had a laryngectomy.	Laypersons in similar situations offer a different type of support that is perceived as helpful.

Deficient Knowledge: Preoperative and Postoperative

Common Related Factors
New cancer diagnosis
New testing and treatment procedures
Expectations for follow-up care
Unfamiliarity with information resources
Emotional state affecting learning

Defining Characteristics
Questioning heath care team
Verbalizing inaccurate information
Expressing heed for more information

Common Expected Outcome
Patient demonstrates an understanding of diagnostic process; treatment plan options; surgical procedures; tracheostomy and stoma care/suctioning techniques; and individualized course of postoperative treatment (e.g., radiation therapy).

NOC Outcomes
Knowledge: Disease Process; Knowledge: Treatment Regimen

NIC Interventions
Teaching: Disease Process; Teaching: Psychomotor Skill

Ongoing Assessment

Actions/Interventions	Rationales
Preoperative:	
■ Assess knowledge of the diagnosis and treatment options.	This information provides the starting point for educational session. This type of cancer is less publicized in the media and is one with which many patients have no experience.

■ = Independent   ▲ = Collaborative

Actions/Interventions

Postoperative:

■ Assess knowledge of postoperative care and follow-up cancer treatment.

■ Assess support systems.

Rationales

Lack of knowledge of postoperative care can compromise patient's ability to care for self at home, especially with a tracheostomy or laryngectomy stoma. The following treatment plan depends on several factors, including the exact location of the tumor, the cancer stage, and other comorbid conditions.

Living with a serious disease is challenging and carries an emotional burden. Assessment helps determine home care needs.

Therapeutic Interventions

Actions/Interventions

■ Encourage questions, and provide information on the nature of the cancer and the usual methods for diagnosis.

■ Provide information about the selected treatment plan and its implications.

■ Provide information on postoperative procedures and treatments (e.g., regarding drainage tubes, dressings, feeding tube).

■ Teach the patient and caregiver as appropriate:
  • Signs and symptoms of infection and when to notify the health care provider
  • Indications for suctioning

  • Procedure for tracheal suction. Use a mirror for teaching; include return demonstration.
  • Procedure for cleaning inner cannula

  • Procedure for changing and securing tracheal ties

▲ Once healing has occurred, consult with speech therapy staff for appropriate intraluminal device for individual patients. The area around the stoma should be washed at least daily.

■ Instruct the patient to cover the stoma when coughing to expectorate. The stoma should also be covered to prevent inhalation of foreign materials (e.g., when shaving or applying makeup). Swimming is contraindicated to prevent aspiration of water through the stoma.

▲ Arrange for home health nurse care or visit as needed.

■ Discuss plans for radiation therapy, including what to expect, probable time schedule for the series, and possible side effects.

■ Teach importance of adequate calorie intake.

Rationales

Questioning facilitates open communication between patient and health care provider and allows verification of understanding of given information. Besides usual physical examination and routine laboratory tests, examination of tissue by biopsy is needed to confirm the diagnosis.

Treatment is individualized but usually consists of a combination of surgery, radiation, and/or chemotherapy. Head and neck surgery usually affects the patient's ability to chew, swallow, or talk. Radiation causes side effects such as redness to the face, dry mouth and thick saliva, changes in taste, and difficulty swallowing. The side effects of chemotherapy depend on the agents being used.

An understanding of the importance of caring for these devices may increase patient cooperation.

Early assessment facilitates prompt treatment.

A patent airway is a priority. Retained secretions can lead to a mucous plug.

Patients may need visual reinforcement to be successful with this procedure.

Information decreases the incidence of a clogged tracheostomy tube.

Information decreases the incidence of tracheostomy dislodgment.

Washing keeps stoma clean and reduces the risk for infection. Speech therapists can work with patients to develop best plan for lifestyle.

Covering the stoma helps reduce transmission of pathogens. Covering the stoma at other times helps prevent inhalation of foreign materials and reduces aspiration risk.

Continuity of care is facilitated through support services.

Postoperative radiation therapy may be used to control the patient's metastasis.

Caloric intake facilitates optimal nutritional balance.

Actions/Interventions

- Teach exercises after radical neck surgery for strengthening shoulder and neck muscles.
- Discuss medications.

- Discuss the use of a medical alert bracelet or other identification to alert others to the disease process or stoma.

Rationales

Restricted movement affects ability to perform many activities of daily living.

The patient may require follow-up treatment for cancer-related problems.

Patient safety is a priority.

Related Care Plans

Grieving, p. 82
Anxiety, p. 18
Impaired verbal communication, p. 39
Ineffective coping, p. 49
Risk for aspiration, p. 21
Risk for impaired skin integrity, p. 185

Lung Cancer

Squamous Cell; Small Cell; Non–Small Cell; Adenocarcinoma; Large Cell Tumors

Lung cancer is the second most commonly occurring cancer among men and women, and despite all available therapies, lung cancer remains the leading cancer-related cause of death for men and women. Lung cancer causes more deaths than breast, prostate, and colorectal cancers combined. It is also one of the most preventable cancers. Lung cancer occurs most often in persons older than 50 years who have long histories of cigarette smoking. The American Cancer Society estimates that more than 90% of all lung cancers are related to cigarette smoking.

Lung cancer is divided into two major cell types: non–small cell lung cancer (NSCLC) and small cell lung cancer. NSCLC accounts for more than 80% of cases with adenocarcinomas being most common (approximately 40%), then squamous cell carcinoma, large cell carcinoma, and mixed cell tumors. Small cell lung cancer is biologically and clinically distinct from the other histological types and accounts for approximately 15% of cases. The diagnosis and stage of lung cancer subtype are critical to the determination of appropriate treatment. Non–small cell cancer can be surgically resected in the early stages and treated with chemotherapy and/or radiation therapy based upon stage. Small cell cancer cannot be surgically resected and is always treated with chemotherapy and radiation therapy.

Prevention is essential. Providing smoke-free environments, testing for radon, and educational programs remain the most powerful interventions. Smoking cessation interventions are a part of all care plans for patients who smoke. Nurses can improve clinical outcomes (efficacy of treatments and quality of life) through smoking-cessation interventions.

Although there are currently no effective screening tests for lung cancer, it is hoped that genetic markers will soon be available to help identify people at high risk for developing cancer. Other promising research focuses on making the immune system and chemical messenger more effective in responding to early cellular changes of lung cancer. Currently work is being completed in the development of chemical messengers that control and stop abnormal cell growth (antioncogene therapy), the use of monoclonal antibodies that recognize and destroy only abnormal lung cells, and stimulation of the immune system by learning to control cytokines such as interleukin-2 (IL-2) and the interferons. In the future, systemic treatment (chemotherapy and targeted therapy) may be selected based on patients' cellular mutation status.

This care plan focuses on the educational aspects of lung cancer.

■ = Independent ▲ = Collaborative

Deficient Knowledge

Common Related Factors

New condition
Unfamiliarity with causes, diagnostic evaluation, and treatment
Emotional state affecting learning

Defining Characteristics

Questions to health care team
Verbalized misconceptions
Denial of diagnosis

Common Expected Outcomes

Patient describes probable cause of his or her cancer.
Patient describes the diagnostic evaluation for lung cancer.
Patient explains the treatment regimen for own type of lung cancer.
Patient verbalizes resources available for additional information and support.

NOC Outcomes

Knowledge: Disease Process; Knowledge: Treatment Procedures

NIC Interventions

Teaching: Disease Process; Teaching: Procedure/Treatment; Smoking Cessation Assistance

---

Ongoing Assessment

Actions/Interventions	Rationales
■ Assess patient's understanding of causes, diagnostic evaluation, and treatment interventions for lung cancer.	Educational programs are individualized to meet the patient's level of previous knowledge. Many patients are exposed to someone with lung cancer, yet many misconceptions continue to exist.
■ Assess readiness to learn.	Some patients are ready to learn soon after they are diagnosed; others cope better by denying or delaying the need for instruction. Learning also requires energy, which patients may not be ready to use. Physical and emotional pain, grieving, denial, anxiety, and anger are barriers to learning, and information presented may not be learned.
■ Assess the family's and significant other's willingness to participate in the teaching and learning process.	Often during the acute stages, the family or significant others may require the most teaching. This can assist them in providing support to the patient. Individuals do have a right to refuse educational services.

Therapeutic Interventions

Actions/Interventions	Rationales
■ Involve the patient in developing the teaching plan.	Allowing the patient to actively participate in the teaching plan increases motivation and helps ensure that the information most significant to the patient is presented first and in a comfortable format.
■ Involve significant others in development and implementation of the teaching plan.	Chronic illness and potentially fatal illnesses involve not only the patient but also the patient's loved ones.

Actions/Interventions	Rationales
■ Identify and communicate to the patient community resources, websites, and additional sources of information and support.	The American Lung Association (www.lungusa.org), the American Cancer Society (www.cancer.org), the National Cancer Institute (1-800-4-CANCER, http://cancernet.nci.nih.gov), the National Comprehensive Cancer Network (NCCN) (www.nccn.org), and many other sources have numerous teaching aids available to support and reinforce learning. Support groups can assist in the learning process by reinforcing learning and increasing motivation to learn. Warn the patient about resources that do not provide correct information (e.g., "Dr. Rob's Lung Cancer Cure Website").
■ Explain possible causes of lung cancer: tobacco use; passive exposure to smoke, radon, asbestos; air pollution containing benzpyrenes and hydrocarbons; and exposure to occupational agents such as petroleum, chromates, and arsenic.	The patient may benefit from understanding the broad range of causes of lung cancer.
■ If the patient is a smoker:	
• Discuss tobacco-dependence treatment for smoking cessation, such as use of pharmacological cessation aids, nicotine-replacement therapies, behavior modification, and smoking-cessation support groups.	Smoking cessation following the diagnosis of lung cancer will improve clinical outcomes. However, the perceived pressure to stop smoking is an added stressor to the patient with newly diagnosed lung cancer.
• Communicate information on the risk to children and nonsmokers caused by environmental second-hand tobacco smoke.	Second-hand passive smoke is a known carcinogen in individuals with long-term exposure. Children exposed to smoke also have an increased incidence of respiratory complications or disease.
■ Discuss evaluation of home for detection of radon and inexpensive removal, if necessary.	By its own action and by its interaction with cigarette smoking, radon is considered the second leading cause of lung cancer in the United States.
■ Discuss the diagnostic evaluation:	
• Chest x-ray film	Chest x-ray films are repeated at frequent intervals and may be the initial test performed when new symptoms are reported.
• Collection of sputum for cytological evaluation	Sputum cytological examination may help identify tumors that involve the bronchial wall.
• Bronchoscopy	Brush biopsies and multiple bronchial washings are performed to obtain a tissue diagnosis. Bronchoscopy is mandatory for small cell cancer.
• Percutaneous transthoracic needle aspiration or biopsy under fluoroscopy, and/or computed tomography (CT)	This procedure is indicated for non–small cell cancer. It is done if bronchoscopy has not yielded an adequate tissue diagnosis or if the lesion is not central and accessible by bronchoscopy.
• Mediastinoscopy	Mediastinoscopy is performed if the previous two procedures have not yielded a tissue diagnosis. It is used to sample lymph nodes and is mandatory for staging non–small cell cancer if surgery is being contemplated.
• Pulmonary function tests	These tests predict whether lung function is sufficient to tolerate a surgical resection. Most patients with lung cancer are long-term smokers with poor lung function.
• Imaging tests	Imaging tests use x-rays, magnetic fields, sound waves, or radioactive substances to find cancer. Monoclonal antibodies tagged with technetium concentrate in areas of tumor cells and are detected by single-photon emission computed tomography (SPECT).
• Positron emission tomography (PET) scan	PET scan is done to identify mediastinal and distant metastases. It is recommended for staging all NSCLC.

■ = Independent   ▲ = Collaborative

Actions/Interventions	Rationales
• Blood tests	Serum blood tests are done to determine whether there is liver or bone metastasis.
■ Describe the following tests for patients with small cell cancer:	
• Brain or head CT and magnetic resonance imaging (MRI) scans	These scans determine the presence of brain metastases.
• Liver and abdominal CT scans	These scans evaluate the liver and adrenals for signs of metastasis.
• Bone scan	These scans are done if the patient has bone pain (optional if PET scan obtained).
■ Discuss staging classifications for the following: *For small cell cancer:*	
• Limited stage	*Limited* usually means one lung and lymph nodes on the same side of the chest that can be encompassed in a single radiation therapy port. Port refers to the anatomical location designated to receive radiation therapy.
• Extensive stage	The *extensive* stage includes all other disease and means that cancer has spread to the other lung, to lymph nodes on the other side, or to distant organs.
For non–small cell cancer:	
• Tumor, node, metastasis (TNM) staging classification	The clinical diagnostic stage is based on pretreatment scans, radiographs, biopsies, and mediastinoscopy and is used to determine extent of disease and resectability. The postsurgical pathological stage is based on analysis of tissue obtained at thoracotomy and is used to determine prognosis as well as the need for additional treatment. Tumor size, spread to lymph nodes, and metastasis to distant organs are staged from 0 to IV. The lower the number, the less the cancer has spread. Tumor staging classification is helpful to determine the optimal treatment plan.
■ Explain "Performance Status Assessment."	This assessment probably is the most important prognostic factor for nonresectable cases.
• Fully ambulatory patients tolerate therapy better and live longer.	
• Patients with restricted activities and out of bed more than 50% of the day survive longer than more restricted patients.	
• Totally bedridden patients tolerate all forms of therapy poorly and have short survival.	
■ Explain treatments for non–small cell cancer:	The 5-year survival rate for all newly diagnosed lung cancer patients remains 15%, primarily because the disease has spread beyond the scope of surgical therapy before a diagnosis is made.
• Chemotherapy: systemic treatment with platinum-based combination therapy	Chemotherapy offers palliation of symptoms.
• Radiation therapy for regional inoperable tumor	Radiation relieves symptoms in a significant percentage of patients, especially those with superior vena cava syndrome, dyspnea, cough, hemoptysis, and pneumonia secondary to obstruction.
• Molecular targeted therapy	These agents (gefitinib, erlotinib) stop tumor growth by blocking molecules essential to the growth and progression of tumors.
• Describe radiation therapy protocol:	
• Radiation therapists carefully mark radiation ports before initiating therapy.	The treatment area must be identified before therapy.
• Do not remove skin markings.	Markings serve as "landmarks" for therapy doses.

Actions/Interventions	Rationales
• Use gentle soap and water cleansing on skin within treatment ports.	Keeping the skin clean and dry and using a water-soluble moisturizer as needed will promote skin integrity and reduce the risk for wet desquamation.
• Keep skin dry, and wear loose-fitting clothing to avoid friction. Do not apply tape to the treatment sites, and do not expose treatment sites to direct sunlight or temperature extremes.	Pressure from tight or irritating clothing will increase skin irritation and the risk for skin breakdown. The skin in the treatment area is more vulnerable to the effects of heat, cold, and ultraviolet light from sunlight or artificial sources.
• Follow a treatment schedule; for example, 5 days per week for 6 weeks.	Each treatment plan is individualized.
• Report the following treatment effects: shortness of breath, fatigue, sore throat, or altered sensation associated with spinal cord damage.	Early assessment promotes early intervention. Fatigue is common in patients undergoing radiation therapy.
• Address any misconceptions or fears the patient may have about radiation therapy.	Patients may worry about becoming radioactive, being a danger to loved ones, or learning that the treatment is not working.
• Surgery for resectable disease (stages I to IIIA)	Surgical resection offers the best chance for long-term survival. Selection of the type of operation is determined by tumor location and size.
• Pneumonectomy	Removal of the affected lung is reserved for extensive disease that is technically resectable.
• Lobectomy	Lobectomy is performed when the tumor is contained within a lobe and adequate margins can be obtained or when lymph node extension is limited to lobar nodes totally encompassed in the en bloc dissection.
• Wedge resection	Wedge resection is performed for small (less than 2 cm) peripheral nodules without lymph node or other extensive involvement.
■ Explain treatments for small cell cancer: • Chemotherapy	Because small cell cancer more often spreads from the primary site and because of its increased sensitivity to chemotherapy, combination chemotherapy is the major treatment and has improved survival fivefold.
• Prophylactic cranial irradiation (PCI)	PCI can improve both disease-free and overall survival in patients in complete remission. PCI should be considered after chemotherapy in stage I patients who have had a complete resection.
■ Explain any treatment options or potential clinical trials the physician may feel would be beneficial to the patient and how the patient can get additional information about these other therapies.	Gene therapy, the use of cytokines, and enhanced immune system therapy are topics in the national news. Patients may have questions about the appropriateness of these therapies for their cancer.

 Cancer-Related Fatigue

Common Related Factors	Defining Characteristics
Tumor and metastatic disease Chemotherapy/targeted therapy Radiation Pain Distress (spiritual or emotional) Anxiety/fear Malnutrition Anemia	A sense of physical or emotional tiredness that is not proportional to recent activity or treatment and interferes with the individual's daily functioning. Inability to restore energy, even after sleep Verbalization of an overwhelming lack of energy

■ = Independent   ▲ = Collaborative

Common Expected Outcomes

Patient reports reduction in fatigue, as evidenced by reports of increased energy and ability to perform desired activities.
Patient reports use of energy-conservation principles.

NOC Outcomes
Activity Tolerance; Endurance; Energy Conservation; Self-Care: Activities
NIC Interventions
Energy Management; Nutrition Management; Sleep Enhancement; Exercise Promotion

Ongoing Assessment

Actions/Interventions	Rationales
■ Assess for fatigue regularly using 0 to 10 scale and defining characteristics.	Fatigue has become the most common and distressing complaint for cancer patients, especially during treatment. Regular assessment allows the nurse to evaluate the fatigue and response to interventions and to develop and alter the plan accordingly.
■ Refer to Fatigue (p. 66).	

Therapeutic Interventions

Actions/Interventions

Rationales

In addition to the Fatigue care plan in Chapter 2, consider the following:

■ Educate patient regarding these treatments:

• Energy-conservation strategies	Conserving energy will allow the patient to achieve most desired goals and feel a sense of accomplishment. Energy conservation may include setting priorities, delegating tasks, frequent rest periods, work simplification, and use of assistive devices.
• Limiting naps to 20 to 30 minutes	Limiting the amount of sleep during naps will help the individual to sleep at night.
• Use of psychostimulants after ruling out other causes	These medications have been used cautiously and demonstrate improved symptoms of fatigue in some patients.
• Treatment for anemia as indicated	Cancer patients' anemia results from the disease itself and treatment. Correcting the anemia may improve the patient's energy level.
• Cognitive behavioral therapy (CBT)	Fear and anxiety associated with the patient's response to cancer and its treatment requires expenditure of energy. CBT facilitates psychological adjustment by helping certain patients recognize and change their maladaptive thoughts.
• Nutrition consultation	Protein caloric malnutrition may contribute to weakness and fatigue. Dietitian can counsel patient and family on how to maximize the patient's intake during treatment for optimal nutritional needs.

NANDA-I NDx Ineffective Protection

Common Related Factors

Cancer
Chemotherapy/targeted therapies
Radiation
Myelosuppression

Common Expected Outcome

Risk for ineffective protection is reduced by early assessment of complications and appropriate treatment.

Defining Characteristics

Paraneoplastic syndromes
Oncological emergencies
Decrease in number of circulating neutrophils, red blood cells, and/or platelets

NOC Outcomes

Immune Status; Blood Loss Severity; Neurologic Status: Consciousness

NIC Interventions

Surveillance; Bleeding Precautions; Neurologic Monitoring; Electrolyte Monitoring; Respiratory Monitoring

Ongoing Assessment

Actions/Interventions	Rationales

■ Assess for common paraneoplastic syndromes:
Endocrine: Caused by secretion of a hormone-like substance by the tumor
Hematological: Decreased neutrophils and decreased hematocrit and hemoglobin
Hypercalcemia: Seen most often with squamous cell cancer
  • Lethargy, polyuria, nausea, vomiting, abdominal pain, and constipation
  • Syndrome of inappropriate antidiuretic hormone (SIADH) with associated hyponatremia
  • Ectopic adrenocorticotropic hormone and Cushing's syndrome
Neurological: Most common extrathoracic manifestations of lung cancer characterized by the following:
  • Weakness of muscles, especially of pelvis and thighs
  • Eaton-Lambert syndrome, myasthenic syndrome
  • Peripheral neuropathy
  • Cerebellar degeneration
  • Polymyositis
  • Hematological
    • Migratory thrombophlebitis
    • Nonbacterial thrombotic endocarditis
    • Disseminated intravascular coagulation (DIC)
	These syndromes are extrapulmonary clinical manifestations of lung cancer that affect multiple body systems.

■ Assess for common oncological emergencies:
Neurological:
  • Headache, vomiting, papilledema
  • Stroke and seizures
Cardiovascular:
  • Cardiac tamponade:
    • Signs: chest pain, apprehension, dyspnea
	These emergencies can be life threatening and lead to permanent damage.
	These are caused by increased intracranial pressure.
	Strokes and seizures are caused by central nervous system metastases, infection, or metabolic consequences.
	Cardiac tamponade is caused by accumulation of fluid-containing tumor cells in the pericardial sac and by encasement of the heart by the tumor.

■ = Independent ▲ = Collaborative

Actions/Interventions

- Superior vena cava syndrome (SVCS):
  - SIGNS: facial and upper extremity edema, tracheal edema, cough, shortness of breath, dizziness, visual changes, hoarseness

Rationales

This syndrome is caused by partial or complete obstruction of blood flow through the SVC to the right atrium.

Therapeutic Interventions

Actions/Interventions

▲ Anticipate appropriate treatment for each type of paraneoplastic syndrome:
- For hypercalcemia: hydration and bisphosphonates
- For neuromyopathies: first, treatment of the primary tumor; then, steroids and physical therapy
- For DIC: heparin, cryoprecipitates, platelets, and packed red blood cells

▲ Anticipate treatment for neurological, oncological emergencies:
- Glucocorticoids
- Brain irradiation
- For seizures: maintenance of airway, anticonvulsant drug therapy

▲ Anticipate the following treatment for cardiovascular oncological emergencies:
- For cardiac tamponade: decompression of the heart either surgically or by pericardiocentesis
- To prevent reaccumulation of effusions:
  - Catheter drainage with instillation of sclerosing agent
  - Radiation therapy
  - Surgical intervention with creation of pericardial window
- For SVCS: radiation therapy, chemotherapy, surgery, anticoagulation, corticosteroids, diuretics

Rationales

A variety of systemic effects called paraneoplastic syndromes occur with this type of cancer. Specific manifestations guide treatment.

Being prepared for an emergency helps prevent further complications.

These are life-threatening problems that require immediate treatment.

NANDA-I NDx ## Acute Pain

Common Related Factors

Original tumor and metastatic disease
Chemotherapy and/or targeted therapy
Radiation

Defining Characteristics

Reports of pain
Moaning or crying
Grimacing
Restlessness
Irritability
Self-focused

Common Expected Outcomes

Patient reports satisfactory pain control at a level less than 3 to 4 on a 0 to 10 rating scale.
Patient exhibits increased comfort such as baseline levels for BP, pulse, respirations, and relaxed muscle tone or body posture.

NOC Outcomes

Pain Control; Medication Response; Comfort Status

NIC Interventions

Pain Management; Analgesic Administration

Ongoing Assessment

Actions/Interventions	**Rationales**
■ Assess for pain severity using 0 to 10 scale and defining characteristics.	Each individual may exhibit slightly different pain presentation.
■ Determine the patient's pain management goal.	Some patients may be content to have pain decreased; others may expect complete elimination of pain. This affects their perception of the effectiveness of the treatment modality and their willingness to participate in additional treatment.
■ Monitor effectiveness of pain-relief therapies.	Patients have a right to effective pain relief. Use of visual analog scales may provide objective data. Evidence of relaxed appearance and baseline HR, BP, and respiration support achievement of comfort goals.
■ Assess concerns and fears related to pain medication.	There remain many myths about pain. Some patients fear addiction to medication or incomplete pain relief. These concerns may enhance the perception of pain or decrease the patient's use of safe, effective, pain-relieving medications.
■ Assess side effects of pain therapies, including constipation.	Analgesics produce side effects. These side effects should be monitored and appropriate interventions taken. Constipation is preventable and should be anticipated and appropriate interventions planned.

Therapeutic Interventions

Actions/Interventions	**Rationales**
▲ Administer prescribed medications as follows (based on World Health Organization [WHO] analgesic ladder and NCCN guidelines for cancer pain):	Various medications may be given by a variety of routes, including patient-controlled analgesia (PCA), in which the patient can control the amount of medication delivered.
• Nonsteroidal antiinflammatory drugs (NSAIDs)	NSAIDs are used to treat muscle spasm associated with progressive tumor spread.
• Short- and long-acting opioid analgesics	These opioid medications are used for acute and chronic cancer pain, including bone metastases. It is essential to work for pain relief and patient comfort and not fear escalating doses as opioid tolerance develops or patients manifest symptoms of disease progression.
• Transdermal opioids	Transdermal administration may be indicated for patients unable to take oral medications.
■ Teach nonpharmacological interventions for pain relief.	Massage, distraction, music therapy, and support groups may enhance pharmacological interventions.
■ Consult pain specialist as needed.	Specialty expertise may be required to manage severe chronic or intractable pain.

Related Care Plans

■ = Independent   ▲ = Collaborative

Mechanical Ventilation

Ventilator; Respirator; Endotracheal Tube; Intubation

Mechanical ventilation can be a temporary or chronic lifesaving therapy. Its purpose is to maintain adequate ventilation by delivering preset concentrations of oxygen at an adequate tidal volume while reducing the work of breathing. The patient who requires mechanical ventilation must have an artificial airway (endotracheal [ET] tube) or tracheostomy. It is used most often in patients with hypoxemia and alveolar hypoventilation. Although the mechanical ventilator will facilitate movement of gases into and out of the pulmonary system (ventilation), it cannot ensure gas exchange at the pulmonary and tissues levels (respiration). It provides either partial or total ventilatory support for patients with respiratory failure. Mechanical ventilation may be used short-term in the acute care setting (e.g., after surgery; during general anesthesia) or long-term in the subacute, rehabilitation, or home care setting. Ventilator-associated pneumonia (VAP) is a significant nosocomial infection that is associated with endotracheal intubation and mechanical ventilation. Prevention of VAP is a primary focus of the 100,000 Lives Campaign to promote quality care and patient safety. This care plan focuses on patient care in a hospital setting.

NANDA-I NDx Impaired Spontaneous Ventilation

Common Related Factors

Metabolic factors
Respiratory muscle fatigue
Acute respiratory failure

Defining Characteristics

Arterial pH less than 7.35
Decreased Po_2 level (less than 50 to 60 mm Hg)
Increased Pco_2 level (50 to 60 mm Hg or greater)
Decreased oxygen saturation (Sao_2 less than 90%)
Apprehension
Increased restlessness
Increased or decreased respiratory rate
Dyspnea
Apnea
Decreased tidal volume
Forced vital capacity less than 10 mL/kg
Inability to maintain airway (i.e., depressed gag, depressed cough, emesis)
Adventitious breath sounds
Diminished lung sounds

Common Expected Outcomes

Patient maintains spontaneous gas exchange resulting in normal arterial blood gases (ABGs) within patient parameters, return to normal pulse oximetry, and decreased dyspnea.
Patient demonstrates no complications from the ventilation.

NOC Outcomes

Respiratory Status: Ventilation; Respiratory Status: Gas Exchange

NIC Interventions

Respiratory Monitoring; Ventilation Assistance; Airway Insertion and Stabilization; Artificial Airway Management; Mechanical Ventilation; Oxygen Therapy

Ongoing Assessment

Actions/Interventions	Rationales
Before intubation:	
■ Assess BP and HR.	Hypotension and tachycardia may result from hypoxia and/or hypercarbia.
■ Assess lungs for normal or adventitious breath sounds.	Changes in lung sounds are important in making an accurate diagnosis. Assessment allows for early detection of deterioration or improvement.
• Listen closely for rhonchi, rales (crackles), wheezing, and diminished lung sounds in each lobe, assessing side to side.	
• Reassess lung sounds after coughing or suctioning.	
■ Assess respiratory rate, pattern, and depth; note position assumed for breathing.	Respiratory rate and rhythm changes are early signs of impending respiratory difficulties. As moving air in and out of the lungs becomes more difficult, the breathing pattern alters to include use of accessory muscles to increase chest excursion.
▲ Use pulse oximetry, as available, to monitor oxygen saturation.	Pulse oximetry is useful in detecting early changes in oxygenation. Oxygen should be at 90% or greater.
■ Assess ABGs as appropriate.	Increasing $Paco_2$ and decreasing Pao_2 are signs of respiratory failure. If the patient's condition begins to fail, the respiratory rate/depth decreases and $Paco_2$ begins to rise.
■ Assess for changes in level of consciousness.	Restlessness, confusion, and irritability can be early signs of hypoxia. Lethargy and somnolence are later signs.
■ Assess skin color, checking nail beds and lips for cyanosis.	Cyanosis indicates increased concentration of deoxygenated blood and that the breathing pattern is no longer effective to maintain adequate oxygenation of tissues.
After intubation:	
■ Assess for ET tube position:	
• Inflate cuff until no audible leaks are heard.	Cuff pressure should not exceed 30 mm Hg. Cuff overinflation increases incidence of tracheal erosions.
• Auscultate for bilateral lung sounds while the patient is being manually ventilated by Ambu bag.	Assessment ensures good ET tube position. If diminished sounds are present over the left lung field, the ET tube is most likely below the carina in the right main stem bronchus and must be pulled back.
• Observe for abdominal distention.	Distention may indicate gastric intubation and can also occur after cardiopulmonary resuscitation when air is inadvertently blown or bagged into the esophagus, as well as the trachea.
• Ensure that chest x-ray evaluation is obtained.	Correct ET tube placement is necessary for effective mechanical ventilation.
• Ensure that ET tube is secure and centimeter markings show placement.	Securing the ET tube prevents it from accidentally being removed.
■ Assess ventilator settings and alarm system every hour.	Assessment ensures that settings are accurate and alarms are functional.
■ Assess patient comfort and ability to cooperate with therapy.	Patient discomfort may be related to incorrect ventilator settings that result in insufficient oxygenation. Once intubated and breathing on the mechanical ventilator, the patient should be breathing easily and not "fighting" the ventilator.

Therapeutic Interventions

Actions/Interventions	Rationales
Before intubation:	
■ Maintain the patient's airway:	
• Encourage the patient to breathe deeply and cough.	Deep breathing facilitates oxygenation. Coughing is the most helpful way to remove most secretions.

■ = Independent   ▲ = Collaborative

Actions/Interventions	Rationales
• If coughing and deep breathing are not effective, use nasotracheal suction as needed.	Suctioning is indicated when patients are unable to remove secretions from airway by coughing. It can also stimulate a cough.
• Use oral or nasal airway as needed.	An artificial airway is used to prevent the tongue from occluding the oropharynx. A patent airway is a priority.
• Provide oxygen therapy as prescribed and indicated.	Increasing oxygen tension in the alveoli may result in more oxygen diffusion into the capillaries.
■ Place the patient in high-Fowler's position, if tolerated. Check position often.	This position promotes lung expansion and improved air exchange. Do not let the patient slide down; this causes the abdomen to compress the diaphragm, which would cause respiratory change.

Prepare for endotracheal intubation:

Actions/Interventions	Rationales
▲ Notify respiratory therapist to bring mechanical ventilator.	A variety of ventilator types are available, depending on extent and type of the patient's problem. Positive-pressure ventilators are used most frequently.
■ If possible, before intubation, explain to the patient the need for intubation, the steps involved, and the temporary inability to speak because of the ET tube passing through the vocal cords.	Preparatory information can reduce anxiety and promote cooperation with intubation.
■ Prepare equipment:	
• ET tubes of various sizes, noting size used	Adult sizes range from 7 to 9 mm. Selection is based on size of patient.
• Benzoin and waterproof tape or other methods	These materials secure the ET tube.
• Syringe	A syringe is used to inflate the balloon (cuff) after the ET tube is in position.
• Local anesthetic agent (e.g., benzocaine [Cetacaine] spray, cocaine, lidocaine [Xylocaine] spray or jelly, and cotton-tipped applicators)	These agents suppress the gag reflex and promote general comfort.
• Sedation as prescribed	Sedation decreases combative resistance to intubation.
• Stylet	A stylet makes the ET tube firmer and gives additional support to direction during intubation.
• Laryngoscope and blades	These facilitate opening of the upper airway and visualization of the vocal cords for placement of oral ET tubes.
• Ambu bag and mask connected to oxygen	These provide assisted ventilation with 100% oxygen before intubation.
• Suction equipment	Suction maintains a clear airway. Yankauer suction device should be available.
• CO_2 detector	This device is attached to the ET tube immediately after intubation to verify tracheal intubation. Other capnography devices that provide numerical measurements of end-tidal CO_2 (normal value is 35 to 45 mm Hg) and capnograms may also be used.
• Oral airway/bite block if patient is being orally intubated	Oral airway/bite block prevents occlusion or biting of ET tube.
• Bilateral soft wrist restraints	These restraints may prevent self-extubation of ET tube.
■ Administer sedation as prescribed.	Sedation facilitates comfort and ease of intubation.

Assist with intubation:

Actions/Interventions	Rationales
■ Place the patient in supine position, hyperextending neck (if not contraindicated) and aligning the patient's oropharynx, posterior nasopharynx, and trachea.	This position is necessary to promote visualization of landmarks for accurate tube insertion.
▲ Oxygenate and ventilate the patient as needed before and after each intubation attempt. If intubation is difficult, the physician will stop periodically so that oxygenation is maintained with artificial ventilation by Ambu bag and mask.	Patent airway and oxygenation are priorities.

Actions/Interventions	Rationales
▲ Apply cricoid pressure as directed by physician.	Pressure is used to occlude esophagus and allow easier intubation of trachea. It may also prevent vomiting and aspiration.
After intubation:	
▲ Assist with verification of correct ET tube placement through: • Auscultation of bilateral breath sounds • Observation of symmetrical rise of both sides of chest • Observation of the purple to yellow color range on the CO_2 detector • Chest x-ray confirmation (after ET tube is taped)	Correct placement is needed for effective mechanical ventilation and to prevent complication associated with malpositioning, such as gastric distention, vomiting, lung trauma, and hypoxia.
■ Continue with manual Ambu bag ventilation until the ET tube is stabilized. Assist in securing the ET tube once tube placement is confirmed.	Stabilization is necessary before initiating mechanical ventilation.
■ Document ET tube position, noting the centimeter reference marking on ET tube.	Documentation provides a reference for determining possible tube displacement, usually 23 cm at the lips for men and 21 cm for women.
▲ Institute mechanical ventilation with settings as prescribed.	Modes for ventilating (assist/control, synchronized intermittent mandatory ventilation), tidal volume, rate per minute, fraction of inspired oxygen (FIO_2), pressure support, positive end-expiratory pressure, and the like must be preset and carefully evaluated for response.
■ Insert oral airway/bite block for orally intubated patient.	Oral airway/bite block prevents the patient from biting down on the ET tube.
■ Institute aseptic suctioning of airway.	Suctioning procedures should be based on need rather than preset time intervals to reduce risk for infection and airway trauma.
■ Apply bilateral soft wrist restraints as needed, explaining reason for use.	Although all patients do not require restraints to prevent extubation, many do.
▲ Administer muscle-paralyzing agents, sedatives, and narcotic analgesics as indicated.	These medications decrease the patient's work of breathing, decrease myocardial work, and may facilitate effective gas exchange.
■ Anticipate need for nasogastric/oral gastric suction.	Suction prevents abdominal distention. Oral gastric suctioning may also reduce the risk for sinusitis.
■ Respond to alarms, noting that high-pressure alarms may be from patient resistance or the patient's need for suctioning. A low-pressure alarm may be a ventilator disconnection. If the source of the alarm cannot be located, ventilate the patient with an Ambu bag until assistance arrives.	The key is that the patient receives oxygenation support at all times until mechanical ventilation is no longer required.

Risk for Ineffective Protection

Common Risk Factors

Dependency on ventilator
Improper ventilator settings
Improper alarm settings
Disconnection of ventilator
Positive-pressure ventilation
Decreased pulmonary compliance
Increased secretions

■ = Independent ▲ = Collaborative

Common Expected Outcomes

Patient remains free of injury as evidenced by appropriate ventilator settings and ABGs within normal limits for patient.

Potential for injury from ventilator-associated pneumonia and barotrauma is reduced by ongoing assessment and early intervention.

NOC Outcome
Respiratory Status: Ventilation; Risk Detection

NIC Intervention
Mechanical Ventilation

Ongoing Assessment

Actions/Interventions	Rationales
▲ Check ventilator settings every hour. Notify respiratory therapist of discrepancy in ventilator settings immediately.	Assessment ensures that the patient is receiving correct mode, rate, tidal volume, FIO_2, positive end-expiratory pressure (PEEP), and pressure support. Immediate attention to details can prevent problems.
• Mode:	
• Synchronized intermittent mandatory ventilation (SIMV)	SIMV ensures preset rate in synchronization with patient's own spontaneous breathing.
• Controlled mandatory ventilation (CMV)	CMV ensures preset rate with no sensitivity to patient's respiratory effort. The patient cannot initiate breaths or alter pattern.
• Assist control (AC)	AC ensures that the preset rate is sensitive to the patient's inspiratory effort. It delivers a preset tidal volume for each patient-initiated breath.
• Rate of mechanical breaths	Although patient dependent, the usual rate is between 10 and 14 breaths/min.
• Tidal volume (TV)	Typical ranges for TV are 6 to 8 mL/kg of ideal body weight. Research supports lower standard TVs to reduce barotrauma.
• FIO_2	The amount of oxygen prescribed depends on patient condition and ABG results.
• Positive end-expiratory pressure (PEEP)	PEEP serves to improve gas exchange and prevent atelectasis.
• Pressure support (PS)	Pressure support provides positive airway pressure during the inspiratory cycle of a spontaneous inspiratory effort.
■ Ensure that ventilator alarms are on.	Alarms alert caregiver to ventilation problems. Prompt response to alarms ensures correction of problems and maintenance of adequate ventilation.
▲ Use pulse oximetry to monitor oxygen saturation; assess ABGs, as appropriate.	Objective data guide ventilator settings and appropriate intervention.
■ Assess rate or rhythm of respiratory pattern, including work of breathing.	It is important to maintain the patient in synchrony with the ventilator and not permit "fighting" it.
▲ Assess for signs of pulmonary infection.	Ventilator-associated pneumonias occur in up to 25% of patients on ventilators. Mortality rates of 40% to 50% have been reported for these patients. Most ventilator-associated infections are caused by bacterial pathogens, with gram-negative bacilli being common.
▲ Assess for signs of barotrauma: patient with crepitus, subcutaneous emphysema, altered chest excursion, asymmetrical chest, abnormal ABGs, shift in trachea, restlessness, evidence of pneumothorax on chest x-ray studies.	Barotrauma is damage to the lungs from positive pressure as seen in acute respiratory patients when high pressures are needed to ventilate stiff lungs or when PEEP is used. Frequent assessments are needed because barotrauma can occur at any time and the patient will not show signs of dyspnea, shortness of breath, or tachypnea if heavily sedated to maintain ventilation.

Actions/Interventions

▲ Monitor chest x-ray reports daily and obtain a stat portable chest x-ray film if barotrauma is suspected.

▲ Monitor plateau pressures with the respiratory therapist.

Rationales

Vigilant monitoring helps reduce complications.

Monitoring for barotrauma can involve measuring plateau pressure, which is the pressure after delivery of the tidal volume but before the patient is allowed to exhale. The ventilator is programmed so that after delivery of the tidal volume the patient is not allowed to exhale for a half second. Therefore pressure must be maintained to prevent exhalation. Elevation of plateau pressures increases both the risk and incidence of barotrauma when a patient is on mechanical ventilation. There has been less occurrence of barotrauma since guidelines have recommended lower standard tidal volumes.

Therapeutic Interventions

Actions/Interventions

■ Institute measures to reduce VAP.

- Wash hands before and after suctioning, touching ventilator equipment, and/or coming into contact with respiratory secretions.
- Use a continuous subglottic suction ET tube for intubation expected to be longer than 24 hours.
- Keep head of bed elevated to 30 to 45 degrees or perform subglottic suctioning unless medically contraindicated.
- Brush teeth two to thee times a day with a soft toothbrush. Chlorhexidine-based rinses may also be incorporated into oral care protocols.
- Use sterile suctioning procedures.

▲ Listen for alarms. Know the range in which the ventilator will set off the alarm.
- *High peak pressure alarm*
  - If patient is agitated, give sedation as prescribed.
  - Empty water from water traps as appropriate.
  - Auscultate breath sounds; institute suctioning as needed. Notify respiratory therapist and physician if high-pressure alarm persists.
- *Low-pressure alarm*
  - If disconnected, reconnect patient to mechanical ventilator.
  - If malfunctioning, remove patient from mechanical ventilator and use Ambu bag.
  - Notify the respiratory therapist to correct malfunction.
- *Low exhale volume*
  - Reconnect patient to ventilator if disconnected, or reconnect tubing to the ventilator. If the problem is not resolved, notify the physician and respiratory therapist.

Rationales

Nosocomial infections are a leading cause of hospital mortality.

An artifical airway bypasses the normal protective mechanisms of the upper airways. Hand washing reduces germ transmission.

Intervention prevents accumulation of secretions that can be aspirated.

Elevation promotes better lung expansion. It also reduces gastric reflux and aspiration.

Oral care reduces colonization of oropharynx with respiratory pathogens that can be aspirated into the lungs.

This technique decreases the introduction of microorganisms into the airway.

The ventilator is a life-sustaining treatment that requires prompt response to alarms.

The high peak pressure alarm indicates bronchospasm, retained secretions, obstruction of ET tube, atelectasis, acute respiratory distress syndrome (ARDS), or pneumothorax, among others.

Low-pressure alarm indicates possible disconnection or mechanical ventilator malfunction.

Low exhale alarm indicates that the patient is not returning delivered TV (through leak or disconnection).

■ = Independent   ▲ = Collaborative

Pulmonary Care Plans

Actions/Interventions

- Check cuff volume by assessing whether the patient can talk or make sounds around the tube or whether exhaled volumes are significantly less than volumes delivered. To correct, slowly reinflate the cuff with air until no leak is detected. Notify the respiratory therapist to check cuff pressure.
- *Apnea alarm*
  - If disconnected, reconnect patient to ventilator.
  - If apnea persists, use Ambu bag to ventilate; notify physician.
- ▲ Notify physician of signs of barotrauma immediately; anticipate the need for chest tube placement, and prepare the patient as needed.

Rationales

Cuff pressure should be maintained at 20 to 30 mm Hg. Maintenance of low-pressure cuffs prevents many tracheal complications formerly associated with ET tubes. Notify the physician if leak persists. The ET tube cuff may be defective, requiring the physician to change the tube.

Apnea alarm is indicative of disconnection or absence of spontaneous respirations.

If barotrauma is suspected, intervention must follow immediately to prevent tension pneumothorax.

 NANDA-I NDx **Ineffective Airway Clearance**

Common Related Factors
Endotracheal intubation
Copious secretions
Decreased energy and fatigue

Defining Characteristics
Excessive secretions
Ineffective cough
Abnormal breath sounds
Dyspnea
Anxiety
Restlessness
Increased peak airway pressure

Common Expected Outcome
Patient will maintain clear, open airways, as evidenced by normal breath sounds after suctioning.

NOC Outcome
Respiratory Status: Airway Patency
NIC Interventions
Airway Management; Airway Suctioning

Ongoing Assessment

Actions/Interventions

- Assess lung for presence of normal or adventitious breath sounds.
- Observe quantity, color, consistency, and odor of sputum.
- ▲ Assess ABGs.

- ▲ Monitor for peak airway pressures and airway resistance.

- Assess the patient's tolerance of suctioning procedure.
- Assess oxygen saturation before and after the suctioning procedure.

Rationales

Diminished lung sounds or the presence of adventitious sounds may indicate an obstructed airway.
Changes in sputum characteristics may indicate infection.
Signs of respiratory compromise include decreasing Pao_2 and increasing $Paco_2$.
Increases in these parameters signal accumulation of secretions or fluid and potential for ineffective ventilation.
Many patients find suctioning to be stressful.
This assessment provides evaluation of effectiveness of therapy.

Therapeutic Interventions

Actions/Interventions

- Explain suctioning procedure to the patient; give reassurance throughout the procedure.

Rationales

Suctioning can be frightening to the patient. Reinforce the need to maintain a patent airway. Provide sedation and pain relief as needed.

Actions/Interventions

- Institute suctioning of airway "as needed" based on the presence of adventitious breath sounds and/or increased ventilatory pressure.

- Avoid saline instillation before suctioning.

- Use closed in-line suction.

▲ Hyperoxygenate as ordered.

▲ Administer pain medications, as appropriate, before suctioning.
- Silence ventilator alarms during suctioning. Reset alarms after suctioning.

▲ Administer adequate fluid intake (intravenous [IV] and nasogastric, as appropriate).
■ Turn the patient every 2 hours.

▲ Consult a respiratory therapist for chest physiotherapy as indicated.

Rationales

Frequency of suctioning should be based on the patient's clinical status, not on a preset routine such as every 2 hours. Oversuctioning can cause hypoxia and injury to bronchial and lung tissue.

Saline instillation before suctioning has an adverse effect on oxygen saturation.

This technique decreases infection rate, may reduce hypoxia, and is often less expensive. Sterile technique is a priority.

Hyperoxygenation before, during, and after endotracheal suctioning decreases hypoxia and cardiac dysrhythmias related to the suctioning procedure.

These medications decrease peak periods of pain and assist with effective cough.

Silencing alarms decreases the frequency of false alarms during suctioning and reduces stressful noise to the patient. Alarms need to be turned on again after suctioning to ensure safety.

Fluids promote patient's hydration and keep secretions liquid.

Turning mobilizes secretions and helps prevent ventilator-associated pneumonia.

Chest physiotherapy includes the techniques of postural drainage and chest percussion to loosen and mobilize secretions.

NANDA-I NDx   Risk for Decreased Cardiac Output

Common Risk Factors
Mechanical ventilation
Positive-pressure ventilation

Common Expected Outcome
Patient maintains adequate CO, as evidenced by strong peripheral pulses; systolic blood pressure within 20 mm Hg of baseline; heart rate 60 to 100 beats/min with regular rhythm; urine output >30 mL/hr, warm, dry skin; and normal level of consciousness.

NOC Outcomes
Cardiac Pump Effectiveness; Circulation Status; Respiratory Status: Ventilation
NIC Interventions
Hemodynamic Regulation; Mechanical Ventilation

Ongoing Assessment

Actions/Interventions

▲ Assess vital signs, level of consciousness, and hemodynamic parameters, if in place (central venous pressure, pulmonary artery diastolic pressures/pulmonary capillary wedge pressure, CO).

Rationales

Mechanical ventilation can cause decreased venous return to the heart, resulting in decreased BP, compensatory increased HR, and decreased CO. This may occur abruptly with ventilator changes: rate, tidal volume, or positive-pressure ventilation. The level of consciousness will decrease if CO is severely compromised. Therefore close monitoring during ventilator changes is imperative.

■ = Independent   ▲ = Collaborative

Pulmonary Care Plans

Actions/Interventions

- Assess peripheral pulses, capillary refill, and skin temperature.

- Monitor fluid balance and urine output.

- Monitor for dysrhythmias.

▲ Notify the physician immediately of signs of decrease in CO, and anticipate possible ventilator setting changes.

Rationales

Pulses are weak with reduced stroke volume and CO. Capillary refill is slow with reduced CO. Cold, pale, clammy skin is secondary to compensatory sympathetic nervous system stimulation and associated with low CO and oxygen desaturation.

Optimal hydration status is needed to maintain effective circulating blood volume and counteract the ventilatory effects on CO. With positive pressure ventilation, pressure from the diaphragm decreases blood flow to the kidneys and could result in a drop in urine output. The brain is very sensitive to a decrease in blood flow and may respond by releasing ADH (to increase water and sodium retention), further reducing urinary output. After the initial decrease in venous return to the heart, volume receptors in the right atrium signal a decrease in volume, which triggers an increase in the release of antidiuretic hormone from the posterior pituitary and retention of water by the kidneys.

Cardiac dysrhythmias may result from the low perfusion state, acidosis, or hypoxia.

Vigilant monitoring reduces risk for complications. Hypotension and decreased CO may be related to positive-pressure ventilator itself or use of PEEP mode.

Therapeutic Interventions

Actions/Interventions

▲ Maintain optimal fluid balance.

▲ Administer medications (diuretics, inotropic agents) as ordered.

Rationales

Volume therapy may be required to maintain adequate filling pressures and optimize CO. However, if pulmonary artery diastolic/pulmonary capillary wedge pressure rises and CO remains low, fluid restriction may be necessary.

Diuretics may be useful to help maintain fluid balance if fluid retention is a problem. Inotropic agents may be useful to increase CO.

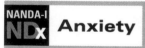 **Anxiety**

Common Related Factors

Inability to breathe adequately without support
Inability to maintain adequate gas exchange
Inability to communicate verbally
Unknown outcome

Defining Characteristics

Restlessness
Fear of sleeping at night
Uncooperative behavior
Withdrawal
Tachypnea
Vigilant watch on equipment
Facial tension
Focus on self

Common Expected Outcomes

Patient uses effective coping mechanisms.
Patient describes a reduction in level of anxiety experienced.

NOC Outcomes
Anxiety Self-Control; Coping
NIC Interventions
Anxiety Reduction; Presence; Emotional Support

Ongoing Assessment

Actions/Interventions	Rationales
■ Assess for signs of anxiety.	Anxiety can affect respiratory rate and pattern, resulting in rapid, shallow breathing and leading to ABG abnormalities and patient "fighting" the ventilator.
■ Assess understanding of need for mechanical ventilation.	Accurate appraisal can facilitate development of appropriate treatment strategies.

Therapeutic Interventions

Actions/Interventions	Rationales
■ Display a confident, calm manner and understanding attitude.	The presence of a trusted person may be helpful during periods of anxiety.
■ Reduce distracting stimuli. Inform the patient of alarms on ventilatory system, and reassure the patient about close proximity of health care personnel to respond to alarms.	Reducing stimuli provides a quiet environment that enhances rest. Anxiety may escalate with excessive noise, conversation, and equipment around the patient. An informed patient who understands the treatment plan will be more cooperative.
■ Be available to the patient or significant others and offer support, as well as explanations of the patient's care and progress.	An ongoing relationship establishes a basis for comfort in communicating anxious feelings.
■ Encourage visiting by family and friends.	The presence of significant others reinforces feelings of security for the patient.
■ Encourage sedentary diversional activities (e.g., television, reading, being read to, writing, occupational therapy).	These activities enhance the patient's quality of life and help pass time.
■ Provide relaxation techniques (e.g., tapes, imagery, progressive muscle relaxation).	Using anxiety-reduction techniques enhances the patient's sense of personal mastery and confidence.
■ If impaired communication is the problem, provide the patient with word-and-phrase cards, writing pad and pencil, or picture board.	These tools broaden the opportunity for communicating, which may reduce frustration.
▲ Refer to psychiatric liaison clinical nurse specialist, psychiatrist, or hospital chaplain, as appropriate.	Specialty expertise may provide a wider range of treatment options and may be needed to achieve successful outcomes.

NANDA-I NDx **Deficient Knowledge**

Common Related Factors

New treatment
New environment
Cognitive limitation
Decreased motivation to learn

Defining Characteristics

Questioning members of health care team
Expressing inaccurate information
Anxiety

Common Expected Outcome

Patient or significant others demonstrate knowledge of mechanical ventilation and care involved.

NOC Outcome
Knowledge: Treatment Procedure
NIC Intervention
Teaching: Individual

■ = Independent   ▲ = Collaborative

Ongoing Assessment

Actions/Interventions	Rationales
■ Assess the patient's perception and understanding of mechanical ventilation.	This information provides an important starting point in education.
■ Assess the patient's readiness and ability to learn.	Educational interventions must be designed to meet the learning limitations, motivation, and needs of the patient. Acute care patients may not be able to take in much information because of fatigue, pain, sensory overload, hypoxemia, and the like.

Therapeutic Interventions

Actions/Interventions	Rationales
■ Encourage the patient or significant others to express feelings and ask questions.	Questions facilitate open communication between patient and health care professionals and allow verification of understanding and the opportunity to correct misconceptions.
■ Explain that the patient will not be able to eat or drink while intubated but assure him or her that alternative measures (i.e., IV fluids, gastric feedings, or hyperalimentation) will be taken to provide nourishment.	Risk for aspiration is high if the patient eats or drinks while intubated. In long-term care settings, patients may be allowed to eat and drink after a swallow evaluation.
■ Explain to the patient the reason for the inability to talk while intubated. Explain alternative efforts for communicating.	The ET tube passes through the vocal cords, and attempts to talk can cause more trauma to the cords. However, patients must understand how to use supplementary methods for communication (paper, pen, pictures).
■ Explain that alarms may periodically sound off, which may be normal, and that the staff will be in close proximity.	Explaining expected events can help reduce anxiety.
■ Explain the need for frequent assessments (i.e., vital signs, auscultation of breath sounds, ventilator checks).	This information also helps reduce anxiety by providing a basis for actions.
■ Explain the need for suctioning as needed.	Information can help reduce the anxiety associated with the procedure.
■ Explain the weaning process, and explain that extubation demonstrated adequate respiratory function and a decrease in pulmonary secretions.	Information aids the patient in maintaining some control.
■ If long-term ventilation is anticipated, discuss or plan for long-term ventilator care management and use appropriate referrals: long-term ventilator care facilities versus home care management.	Continuity of care is facilitated through the use of specialty resources.

Related Care Plans

Insomnia, p. 117
Dysfunctional ventilatory weaning response, p. 205
Imbalanced nutrition: Less than body requirements, p. 142
Impaired gas exchange, p. 78
Impaired physical mobility, p. 133
Impaired verbal communication, p. 39
Powerlessness, p. 162
Tracheostomy, p. 461

Pneumonia

Pneumonitis; Community-Acquired Pneumonia (CAP); Hospital-Acquired Pneumonia (HAP); Aspiration Pneumonia

Pneumonia is caused by a bacterial or viral infection that results in an inflammatory process in the lungs. It is an infectious process that is spread by droplets or by contact and is one of the most common causes of death in older adults. Risk factors include upper respiratory infection, excessive alcohol ingestion, central nervous system depression, cardiac failure, any debilitating illness, chronic obstructive pulmonary disease (COPD), endotracheal (ET) intubation, and postoperative effects of general anesthesia. Pneumonia is a particular concern in persons older than 65 years or anyone who is bedridden, immunosuppressed, malnourished, or hospitalzedand patients exposed to MRSA, as well as the very young and very old. Pneumonia may be nosocomial or community-acquired (CAP).

Types of pneumonia include the following:
- Gram-positive pneumonias: pneumococcal pneumonia, staphylococcal pneumonia, streptococcal pneumonia (these account for most community-acquired pneumonias)
- Gram-negative pneumonias: *Klebsiella* pneumonia, *Pseudomonas* pneumonia, influenzal pneumonia, legionnaires disease (these account for most hospital-acquired pneumonias)
- Anaerobic bacterial pneumonias (usually caused by aspiration)
- *Mycoplasma* pneumonia
- Viral pneumonias (most common in infants and children; influenza A is the primary causative viral agent in adults)
- Parasitic pneumonia (opportunistic infection)

The Joint Commission has identified National Quality Improvement Goals as standardized performance measures that hospitals can use to measure the overall quality of care provided to pneumonia patients. In healthy people with responsive immune systems, treatment can be administered in the outpatient setting. This care plan focuses on acute care treatment of pneumonia.

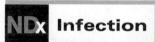 **Infection**

Common Related Factor	**Defining Characteristics**
Invading bacterial or viral organisms	Fever
	Chills
	Elevated WBC count
	Positive sputum culture report
	Tachypnea
	Dyspnea
	Cough with purulent sputum
	Tachycardia

Common Expected Outcomes

Patient experiences improvement in infection as evidenced by normal body temperature, normal white blood cell (WBC) count, and negative sputum culture report.
Patient demonstrates hygiene measures such as hand washing and control of infectious sputum.

NOC Outcomes
Medication Response; Thermoregulation
NIC Interventions
Infection Protection; Medication Administration

Ongoing Assessment

Actions/Interventions

■ Assess the patient's description of current illness.

Rationales

Classic signs of pneumonia include chills, fever, pleuritic chest pain, cough, dyspnea, sputum changes.

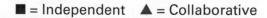
■ = Independent ▲ = Collaborative

Actions/Interventions	Rationales
■ Assess for predisposing risk factors: recent exposure to illness; alcohol, tobacco, or drug abuse; chronic illness; immunosuppressive therapy; malnutrition; prolonged immobility; tube feedings.	Patients are at risk from a variety of sources. Both etiology and causative organisms relate to the setting. For example, an intubated immobilized patient will have different pathogenic risk and treatment than a patient with CAP.
■ Assess immunization status.	Immunizations with pneumococcal vaccine and seasonal influenza vaccine are recommended by the CDC for high-risk groups, especially older adults, to reduce risk for developing pneumonia.
■ Assess temperature, closely monitoring for fluctuations.	Continued fever may be caused by drug allergy, drug-resistant bacteria, superinfection, or inadequate lung drainage.
■ Monitor breath sounds.	Bronchial breath sounds are evident in areas of lung consolidation. Egophony (often called E to A changes) is a simple technique to identify areas of consolidation in the lungs. Wheezing is evident if inflammation or narrowing of airways occurs. Crackles are evident if fluid is present in interstitial or alveolar lung areas.
▲ Obtain fresh sputum for Gram stain and for culture and sensitivity, as prescribed. Assess for drug resistance. • Instruct patient to expectorate into a sterile container. Be sure the specimen is coughed up and is not saliva. • If the patient is unable to cough up a specimen effectively, use sterile nasotracheal suctioning with a sputum trap.	This testing determines correct antibiotic coverage for the patient. Blood culture obtained before the initial antibiotic is given is an indicator or benchmark used to measure quality of care in hospitals. In the outpatient setting, patients will often be treated empirically.
▲ Monitor WBC count and blood culture.	Rising WBC count indicates the body's efforts to fight pathogens. Patients admitted to the emergency department or intensive care unit should have a blood test for presence of bacteria in their blood within 24 hours of hospital arrival (National Patient Safety Goal).
■ Assess hydration status.	Water loss is increased with fever.
▲ Use pulse oximetry to monitor oxygen saturation; assess arterial blood gases (ABGs) as indicated.	Pulse oximetry and ABGs provide an objective indication of oxygenation status. It should be 90% or greater. The ABGs will indicate developing respiratory acidosis and hypoxemia. Oxygenation assessment is a National Patient Safety Goal.
▲ Monitor serial chest x-ray reports.	Pneumonia causes increased areas of density on chest x-ray film, occurring in an isolated segment or lobe, either unilaterally or bilaterally. Serial changes guide subsequent treatment.

Therapeutic Interventions

Actions/Interventions	Rationales
▲ Administer prescribed antimicrobial agents within 4 hours of hospital arrival (e.g., cephalosporins, penicillins, vancomycin).	This timeline is an indicator or benchmark used to measure quality of care in hospitals—the focus is on giving an antibiotic early. As culture results become available, patients with community-acquired pneumonia should be receiving appropriate antibiotic within 24 hours of hospital arrival. Parenteral intravenous (IV) antibiotics are usually given for the first few days of acute cases and then changed to oral antibiotics, which may be adequate for milder cases from the first day. To prevent a relapse of pneumonia, the patient needs to complete the course of antibiotics as prescribed. Antiviral drugs (e.g., amantadine, rimantadine) are available for parenteral administration for viral respiratory infections. Antibiotics are not effective against viral pneumonia but may be used when concurrent viral and bacterial pneumonias are present. In CAP, patients are frequently started on oral antibiotics.

Actions/Interventions

▲ Use appropriate therapy for elevated temperatures: antipyretics, cold therapy.

■ Provide tissues and waste bags for disposal of sputum.

■ Wash hands frequently.

■ Keep the patient away from other patients who are at high risk for developing pneumonia by careful room assignment when patients are in semiprivate rooms.

■ Isolate patients as necessary after review of culture and sensitivity results.

Rationales

This treatment maintains normothermia and reduces metabolic needs.

Careful disposal of contaminated tissues reduces transmission of microorganisms.

Hand washing is the most effective method for preventing spread of infection.

Immunocompromised patients are at high risk for developing nosocomial pneumonia.

Isolation prevents potential spread of the disease. If the patient is positive for methicillin-resistant *Staphylococcus aureus* (MRSA), a private room with isolation is required.

Ineffective Airway Clearance

Common Related Factors

Increased sputum production in response to respiratory infection
Decreased energy and increased fatigue
Aspiration

Defining Characteristics

Abnormal breath sounds (e.g., rhonchi, bronchial lung sounds, egophony)
Decreased breath sounds over affected lung areas
Ineffective cough
Purulent sputum
Dyspnea, tachypnea
Change in respiratory status
Infiltrates seen on chest x-ray film
Hypoxemia

Common Expected Outcome

Patient will maintain clear, open airways, as evidenced by eupnea and normal breath sounds after coughing or suctioning, and normal rate and depth of respirations.

NOC Outcomes
Respiratory Status: Airway Patency
NIC Interventions
Airway Management; Cough Enhancement

Ongoing Assessment

Actions/Interventions

■ Assess respirations, noting rate, rhythm, depth, and use of accessory muscles.

■ Assess cough for effectiveness and productivity. Observe characteristics of sputum: color, amount, and odor; report significant changes.

■ Assess hydration status.

■ Auscultate lungs, noting areas of decreased ventilation and presence of adventitious sounds.

▲ Use pulse oximetry to monitor oxygen saturation; assess ABGs.

Rationales

An increase in respiratory rate and depth may be a compensatory response for airway obstruction. The breathing pattern may alter to include use of accessory muscles to increase chest excursion to facilitate effective breathing.

Patients may have ineffective cough because of fatigue or thick tenacious secretions. A sign of infection is discolored sputum. An odor may be present.

Airway clearance is impaired with inadequate hydration and thickening of secretions. Thick, tenacious secretions increase hypoxemia.

Bronchial lung sounds are commonly heard over areas of lung density or consolidation. Crackles are heard when fluid is present.

Oxygenation assessment is a National Patient Safety Goal.

■ = Independent   ▲ = Collaborative

Therapeutic Interventions

Actions/Interventions	Rationales
■ Assist patient with coughing, deep breathing, and splinting, as necessary.	Coughing is the most helpful way to remove most secretions. Deep breathing improves productivity of cough. Frequent nonproductive coughing can result in hypoxemia. Splinting the abdomen promotes more effective coughing by increasing abdominal pressure and upward diaphragmatic movement. If coughing is painful, medicate for pain.
■ Assist with suctioning if necessary.	If coughing is ineffective, nasotracheal suctioning may be required to remove secretions. However, suctioning can cause increased hypoxemia, especially without hyperoxygenation before, during, and after suctioning.
■ Encourage ambulation.	Ambulation mobilizes secretions and reduces atelectasis.
■ Maintain adequate hydration.	Fluids are lost by diaphoresis, fever, and tachypnea and are needed to aid in the mobilization of secretions.
■ Use humidity (humidified oxygen or humidifier at bedside).	Increasing the humidity of inspired air will loosen secretions. Clean the humidifier according to instructions to inhibit a reservoir for bacterial growth.
■ Assist the patient with use of incentive spirometer.	Incentive spirometry serves to improve deep breathing and prevent atelectasis.
■ For patients with reduced energy, pace activities.	Effective coughing is hard work and may exhaust an already compromised patient. Fatigue is a contributing factor to ineffective coughing.
■ Provide oral care.	Secretions from pneumonia are often foul tasting and smelling. Providing oral care may decrease nausea and vomiting associated with the taste of secretions.
▲ Consult the respiratory therapist for chest physiotherapy and nebulizer treatments, as appropriate and as ordered.	Chest physiotherapy includes the techniques of postural drainage and chest percussion to loosen and mobilize secretions in smaller airways that cannot be removed by coughing or suctioning. A nebulizer may be used to humidify the airway to thin secretions to facilitate their removal.
▲ Administer medication such as antibiotics and expectorants for productive coughs and cough suppressants for hacking nonproductive coughs as prescribed, noting effectiveness; administer inhaled bronchodilators and inhaled steroids, as prescribed, to open airway and decrease inflammation.	A variety of medications are available to treat specific problems. Most promote clearance of airway secretions and may reduce airway resistance. If treating the patient in the outpatient setting, review medication administration, timing, and adverse effects with the patient.
▲ Assist with bronchoscopy and thoracentesis, as appropriate.	Bronchoscopy is done to obtain lavage samples for culture and sensitivity and to remove mucous plugs; thoracentesis is done to drain associated pleural effusions.
▲ Anticipate possible need for supplemental oxygen or intubation if patient's condition deteriorates.	Oxygen may be needed to correct associated hypoxemia. Intubation may be needed to facilitate deep suctioning efforts and to provide source for augmenting oxygenation.

NANDA-I NDx Impaired Gas Exchange

Common Related Factors	Defining Characteristics
Collection of mucus in airways	Dyspnea
Inflammation of airways and alveoli	Hypoxemia/hypercapnia
Fluid-filled alveoli	Pale, dusky, cyanotic skin color

Ventilation-perfusion mismatch (especially with bacterial pneumonia)

Lung consolidation with decreased surface area available for gas exchange

Tachypnea

Tachycardia

Hypotension

Restlessness/irritability

Disorientation or confusion

In older patients, functional decline with or without fever

Common Expected Outcome

Patient maintains optimal gas exchange as evidenced by arterial blood gases (ABGs) within the patient's usual range, oxygen saturation of 90% or greater, alert response mentation or no further reduction in level of consciousness, relaxed breathing, and baseline HR for patient.

NOC Outcome
Respiratory Status: Gas Exchange

NIC Interventions
Respiratory Monitoring; Oxygen Therapy

Ongoing Assessment

Actions/Interventions	Rationales
■ Assess respirations: note quality, rate, rhythm, depth, dyspnea on exertion, use of accessory muscles, position assumed for easy breathing.	Patients will adapt their breathing patterns over time to facilitate gas exchange. Both rapid, shallow breathing patterns and hypoventilation affect gas exchange. Hypoxia is associated with signs of increased breathing effort. Conversational dyspnea and tripod posturing are evidence of significant dyspnea. Respiratory failure may ensue with the patient unable to maintain the rapid respiratory rate.
■ Monitor for changes in HR and BP.	With initial hypoxia and hypercapnia, BP and HR rise. As the hypoxia and/or hypercapnia becomes more severe, BP may drop, HR tends to continue to be rapid with arrhythmias.
■ Assess skin, nail beds, and mucous membranes for pallor or cyanosis.	Cool, pale skin may be secondary to a compensatory vasoconstrictive response to hypoxemia. As oxygenation and perfusion become impaired, peripheral tissues become cyanotic.
■ Assess for restlessness and changes in level of consciousness.	Increased restlessness, confusion and/or irritability are early indicators of insufficient oxygenation of the brain and requires further intervention. Always check the pulse oximetry results with any mental status changes in older adults.
▲ Use pulse oximetry to monitor oxygen saturation; assess ABGs.	Pulse oximetry is a useful tool to detect changes in oxygenation. Oxygen saturation should be at 90% or greater. The ABGs provide information about developing hypoxemia and respiratory acidosis. Increasing $Paco_2$ and decreasing Pao_2 are signs of respiratory failure. Oxygen assessment is a National Patient Safety Goal.

Therapeutic Interventions

Actions/Interventions	Rationales
▲ Maintain oxygen administration device as ordered. Avoid high concentrations of oxygen in patients with COPD.	Supplemental oxygen therapy maintains oxygen saturation of 90% or greater to provide for adequate oxygenation. Careful administration of low liter flow oxygen is indicated because hypoxia stimulates the drive to breathe in the patient who chronically retains carbon dioxide.
■ Plan activity and rest to minimize the patient's energy.	Activities increase metabolic rate and oxygen consumption and should be planned so the patient does not become hypoxic. Rest helps mobilize energy for more effective breathing and coughing efforts.

■ = Independent　▲ = Collaborative

Pulmonary Care Plans

Actions/Interventions

■ Anticipate need for intubation and possibly mechanical ventilation if condition worsens.

Rationales

Early intubation and mechanical ventilation are recommended to prevent full decompensation of the patient and a potentially life-threatening situation.

NANDA-I NDx **Acute Pain**

Common Related Factors

Pain resulting from disease
Coughing

Defining Characteristics

Reports of discomfort
Guarding behavior
Self-focused
Moaning/restlessness
Facial mask of pain
Irritability
Tachycardia
Increased BP
Tachypnea

Common Expected Outcomes

Patient reports satisfactory pain control at a level less than 3 to 4 on a 0 to 10 scale.
Patient verbalizes understanding of nonpharmacological interventions for pain relief.
Patient exhibits increased comfort such as baseline levels for pulse, BP, and respirations, and relaxed muscle tone or body posture.

NOC Outcomes
Pain Control; Medication Response
NIC Interventions
Pain Management; Analgesic Administration

Ongoing Assessment

Actions/Interventions

■ Assess complaints of pain with breathing or coughing.

■ Determine how the patient has effectively dealt with pain in the past.

Rationales

Assessment of pain/discomforting experience is the first step in planning pain management strategies. Pain can result in shallow breathing and poor cough effort.

This evaluation provides opportunity to consider the patient's reactions to and expectations for pain relief.

Therapeutic Interventions

Actions/Interventions

▲ Administer appropriate medications to treat the cough:

• Do not suppress a productive cough; use moderate amounts of analgesics to relieve pleuritic pain.

• Use cough suppressants and humidity for dry, hacking cough.

▲ Administer analgesics as prescribed and as needed. Encourage the patient to take analgesics before discomfort becomes severe. Evaluate medication effectiveness.

■ Use additional measures, including positioning and relaxation techniques.

Rationales

Careful balancing of dosage is needed to prevent reduction in respirations seen with some analgesics.

Coughing is necessary to mobilize secretions. Cough suppression will cause retained secretions and delay the resolution of infection.

An unproductive hacking cough irritates airways and should be suppressed.

Medications allow for pain relief and the ability to deep breathe and cough. Analgesics prevent peak periods of pain.

These measures facilitate effective respiratory excursion.

NANDA-I NDx

Deficient Knowledge

Common Related Factors

New condition and procedures
Unfamiliarity with disease process and transmission of disease

Common Expected Outcome

Patient and caregiver demonstrate understanding of disease process and compliance with treatment regimen and isolation procedures.

Defining Characteristics

Questions to health care team
Confusion about treatment
Inability to comply with treatment regimen, including appropriate isolation procedures

NOC Outcomes

Knowledge: Disease Process; Knowledge: Treatment Regimen

NIC Interventions

Teaching: Disease Process; Teaching: Prescribed Medication; Immunization/ Vaccination Administration

---

Ongoing Assessment

Actions/Interventions

■ Determine understanding of pneumonia complications and treatment.
■ Assess potential home care needs.

Rationales

This information provides an important starting point in education.
Therapy will continue after hospital discharge. Home care needs will depend on availability of supportive persons, the patient's energy level and cognitive level.

Therapeutic Interventions

Actions/Interventions

■ Teach the patient deep breathing exercises and techniques to cough effectively.
■ Discuss with the patient or caregiver the need to complete the full course of antibiotics, as prescribed, and for adequate rest for recuperation.
■ Provide information about need to do the following:
  • Maintain natural resistance to infection through adequate nutrition, rest, and exercise.
  • Avoid contact with people with upper respiratory infections.
  • Obtain chest x-ray examination 2 weeks after completion of therapy.
  • Obtain immunizations against influenza if older and chronically ill.
■ Provide smoking-cessation advice as indicated.

Rationales

These techniques facilitate clearance of secretions and prevent atelectasis.
Full antibiotic course is needed to prevent a relapse or development of a resistant organism. A prolonged period of convalescence may be needed for older patients.
These are preventive measures to reduce recurrence of disease and promote a healthy immune system. Chest x-ray examination after therapy completion ensures the resolution of the pneumonia and verifies the absence of other lung pathology obliterated by the pneumonia. One of the National Patient Safety Goals measures how often pneumonia patients in the hospital during the flu season were given flu vaccine if needed.

One of the National Patient Safety Goals is to provide advice about stopping smoking to patients while hospitalized.

Related Care Plans

Activity intolerance, p. 8
Anxiety, p. 18
Impaired gas exchange, p. 78
Imbalanced nutrition: Less than body requirements, p. 142
Mechanical ventilation, p. 418

■ = Independent   ▲ = Collaborative

Pulmonary Care Plans

Pneumothorax With Chest Tube

Collapsed Lung; Tension Pneumothorax

Presence of air in the intrapleural space can cause partial or complete collapse of the lung. The air causes disruption of the normal negative pressure that exists in the pleural space. Pneumothorax can be iatrogenic, spontaneous, or the result of injury. Several methods are available for treating pneumothorax, ranging from observation for collapses of less than 20% or needle or chest tube insertion for larger collapses. This case plan describes a chest tube drainage system used to reestablish negative pressure in the intrapleural space to facilitate lung reexpansion.

 NANDA-I NDx **Ineffective Breathing Pattern**

Common Related Factors

Partially or completely collapsed lung
Pain
Inadequate chest expansion

Defining Characteristics

Shallow respirations
Tachypnea
Decreased breath sounds on affected side
Dyspnea, shortness of breath
Asymmetrical chest expansion
Use of accessory muscles
Anxiety/restlessness
Tachycardia
Oxygen saturation less than 90%
Abnormal arterial blood gases (ABGs)

Common Expected Outcome

Patient maintains effective breathing pattern, as evidenced by relaxed breathing at normal rate and depth, clear and equal lung sounds bilaterally, and absence of dyspnea.

NOC Outcomes
Respiratory Status: Ventilation; Pain Level
NIC Interventions
Airway Management; Tube Care: Chest; Pain Management

Ongoing Assessment

Actions/Interventions	Rationales
■ Assess respiratory rate, rhythm, depth, effort, and use of accessory muscles.	Respiratory rate and rhythm changes such as an increase in respiratory rate with a decreased tidal volume (rapid, shallow respirations) are early warning signs of impending respiratory difficulties. Asymmetrical chest expansion may be evident. The breathing pattern may alter to include use of accessory muscles to increase chest excursion to facilitate effective breathing.
■ Auscultate lungs for area of diminished or absent breath sounds.	Breath sounds may be diminished in areas of partial collapse. Complete collapse of the lungs will result in all absent breath sounds on affected side.

Actions/Interventions

■ Assess heart rate.

▲ Use pulse oximetry to monitor oxygenation status; assess ABGs.

■ Assess pain quality, location, and severity.

■ Assess chest tube drainage system for the following:

• Secure connections

• Intact water seal
• Fluctuation (or tidaling) of fluid caused by pressure changes in the intrapleural space during inspiration and expiration
• Presence of air leak or bubbling in the water seal

• Amount of fluid in drainage collection chamber
• Tube patency, free of dependent loops

• Fluid levels

▲ Monitor serial chest x-ray films.

Rationales

Tachycardia is associated with increased work of breathing and hypoxia.

Pulse oximetry is a useful tool to monitor oxygen saturation and detect early changes in oxygenation. Rapid, shallow respirations result in respiratory alkalosis, as noted on ABGs. Increased $Paco_2$ and decreased Pao_2 are signs of respiratory failure.

Sudden, sharp chest pain occurs on the same side as the affected lung. It can result in shallow breathing.

Chest tubes are required to allow for reexpansion of the collapsed lung and must be carefully set up and monitored to reduce complications.

A loose connection can allow air entry and positive pressure into the intrapleural space, resulting in further lung collapse.

Water seal prevents air entry into the intrapleural space.

Cessation of fluctuating (or tidaling) of fluid can indicate lung reexpansion or, if abrupt, can indicate clogged or kinked tube.

Bubbling indicates air removal from the intrapleural space, especially during expiration or coughing. Cessation of bubbling can indicate lung reexpansion. Continuous bubbling can indicate air leak within the patient's chest or within the system.

Excessive drainage may indicate hemorrhage.

Obstruction of drainage from the chest tube interferes with lung expansion and increases pressure within the lung.

Maintaining prescribed water seal and suction levels helps prevent complications.

The chest x-ray film is used to document lung reexpansion.

Therapeutic Interventions

Actions/Interventions

■ Explain the procedure for chest tube insertion.

■ Maintain the chest tube drainage system:
• Secure connections.
• Maintain proper water levels in water seal and suction control chamber.

• Secure chest drainage system to an intravenous (IV) pole with wheels. Keep below level of chest.
■ Encourage deep breathing, and coughing after deep breathing, as needed.
■ Instruct the patient in splinting the chest tube site with a pillow during coughing and with movement.
■ Assist the patient in repositioning every 2 to 3 hours.
■ Administer pain medication as prescribed before activity: deep breathing, coughing, and physical mobility. Instruct the patient to notify the nurse of pain before it gets severe.

Rationales

Chest tubes are required to allow for reexpansion of the collapsed lung by maintaining negative pressure in the intrapleural space. Explanation prepares the patient and decreases fear.

Secure connections prevent dislodgment of tubing.
The amount of suction is determined by the depth of the tubing in the suction control chamber. As water evaporates, additional water is added to each chamber.
This maneuver allows mobility while preventing accidental knock over of the system.
These actions decrease atelectasis and enhance gas exchange.

Providing support to the insertion site will decrease discomfort associated with deep breathing and coughing.
Repositioning promotes improved lung expansion.
Effective pain management will enhance the patient's willingness to participate in care.

■ = Independent   ▲ = Collaborative

NANDA-I NDx **Deficient Knowledge**

Common Related Factors

Change in health status
Complexity of treatment
Emotional state affecting learning (e.g., anxiety)
Unfamiliarity with information resources

Defining Characteristics

Verbalizing inaccurate information
Questioning members of health care team

Common Expected Outcome

Patient verbalizes understanding of physical condition, reason for chest tube, importance of deep breathing, follow-up care, and signs and symptoms to report.

NOC Outcomes
Knowledge: Disease Process; Knowledge:
Treatment Regimen

NIC Interventions
Teaching: Disease Process; Teaching:
Procedure/Treatment

Ongoing Assessment

Action/Intervention	Rationale
■ Assess knowledge of pneumothorax and its treatment.	The suddenness of the medical problem may have overwhelmed the patient and served as a barrier to learning.

Therapeutic Interventions

Actions/Interventions	Rationales
■ Instruct the patient and significant others regarding the following:	
• Pneumothorax (etiology)	Pneumothorax may be iatrogenic, spontaneous, or the result of injury.
• Purpose of chest tube in lung reexpansion	Chest tube serves to reestablish negative pressure in the intrapleural space to facilitate lung reexpansion.
• Importance of keeping chest drainage unit below level of chest	Correct positioning prevents backup of drainage or air into intrapleural space.
• Chest tube insertion site care	Meticulous wound care decreases incidence of infection.
• Importance of deep breathing, coughing, and gradually increasing physical activity	These maneuvers enhance lung expansion.
• Pain medication actions and side effects	Medications promote comfort, which can enhance effective breathing patterns and early mobilization.
• Signs and symptoms to report	The patient needs to report fever, purulent drainage from insertion site, reddened wound edges, and signs of lung collapse: chest pain, dyspnea, shortness of breath.
▲ Collaborate with physician to determine likelihood of recurrence of pneumothorax. Instruct patient as appropriate.	In healthy patients who have experienced a spontaneous pneumothorax, recurrence is 10% to 50% for a second incident and 60% for a third incident. The patient needs to be aware of signs and symptoms of recurrence, as well as appropriate emergency medical treatment measures (planned in advance).
■ Instruct the patient in use of the Heimlich valve if used for home care.	The Heimlich valve is a one-way flutter valve that allows air from the pleural space to flow out through the tube with exhalation but prevents air from flowing into the chest during inhalation.
■ Instruct the patient in the importance of follow-up with a health care provider and the need for a repeat chest x-ray study.	Chest x-ray film confirms lung reexpansion.

Related Care Plan

Impaired gas exchange, p. 78

Pulmonary Embolism

Thromboembolism

Pulmonary embolism (PE) occurs when a thrombus (blood clot) originating in the venous system or the right side of the heart obstructs blood flow in the pulmonary artery or one of its branches. The clinical picture varies according to the size and location of the embolus, making diagnosis challenging. Careful analysis of risk factors aids in diagnosis; these include prolonged immobility, deep vein thrombosis, recent surgery, postpartum state, trauma to vessel walls, hypercoagulable states, and certain disease states such as heart failure and trauma. Treatment approaches vary depending on the degree of cardiopulmonary compromise associated with the PE. They can range from thrombolytic therapy in acute situations to anticoagulant therapy and general care measures to optimize respiratory and vascular status (e.g., oxygen, compression stockings). PE is a frequent hospital-acquired condition, and one of the most common causes of death in hospitalized patients, resulting from a variety of factors that predispose one to intravascular clotting. Prevention of thrombus formation is a critical nursing role. This care plan focuses on acute care treatment for PE.

 NANDA-I NDx

Ineffective Breathing Pattern

Common Related Factors
Hypoxia
Chest pain
Anxiety

Defining Characteristics
Dyspnea
Tachypnea
Use of accessory muscles
Tachycardia
Hypoxemia
Cyanosis

Common Expected Outcome
Patient will maintain an effective relaxed breathing pattern at normal rate and depth, and absence of dyspnea.

NOC Outcome
Respiratory Status: Ventilation
NIC Interventions
Airway Management; Respiratory Monitoring

Ongoing Assessment

Actions/Interventions

■ Assess respiratory rate, rhythm, and depth. Assess for any increase in work of breathing: shortness of breath, use of accessory muscles.

■ Assess lungs for adventitious sounds.

Rationales

Respiratory rate and rhythm changes are early warning signs of impending respiratory difficulties. Tachypnea is a typical finding of PE. The rapid, shallow respirations result from hypoxia. Development of hypoventilation (a slowing of respiratory rate) without improvement in the patient's condition indicates respiratory failure.

Breath sounds may be normal, though crackles are common in at least half of patients.

■ = Independent ▲ = Collaborative

Actions/Interventions

▲ Monitor arterial blood gases (ABGs), and note changes.

▲ Use pulse oximetry to monitor oxygen saturation.

■ Assess characteristics of pain, especially in association with the respiratory cycle.

Rationales

ABGs of the PE patient typically exhibit hypoxemia and respiratory alkalosis from a blowing off of carbon dioxide. Development of respiratory acidosis in this patient indicates respiratory failure, and immediate ventilator support is indicated.

Pulse oximetry is a useful tool to detect early changes in oxygenation. Goal is oxygen saturation levels greater than 90% on room air.

Pain is usually sharp or stabbing and gets worse with deep breathing and coughing. It can result in shallow respirations, further impairing effective gas exchange.

Therapeutic Interventions

Action/Interventions

■ Position patient with proper body alignment. Change position every 2 hours.

▲ Ensure that the oxygen delivery system is properly applied to the patient.

■ Provide reassurance and allay anxiety by staying with the patient during acute episodes of respiratory distress.

■ Prepare patient for diagnostic tests (e.g., chest x-ray examination, ABGs, D-dimer assay, computed tomography [CT] scan, ventilation-perfusion [V̇/Q̇] scan, and pulmonary arteriogram).

■ Assist patient with coughing and deep breathing. Suction as needed.

■ Anticipate the need for intubation and mechanical ventilation.

Rationales

If not contraindicated, a sitting position allows good lung excursion and chest expansion. Repositioning facilitates movement and drainage of secretions.

The appropriate amount of oxygen needs to be continuously delivered so the patient does not become desaturated.

Anxiety can result in rapid, shallow respirations and increase dyspnea.

Common tests like chest x-ray examination and D-dimer assay (marker for clot lysis) are readily available in acute care settings, especially to rule out PE. If there is high suspicion for PE, then CT scan and V̇/Q̇ scan are added to make diagnosis. Pulmonary arteriogram is the definitive test.

These maneuvers help keep airways open by clearing secretions.

Intubation and positive-pressure ventilation are a means to stabilize breathing and ventilation and prevent decompensation of the patient.

NANDA-I NDx Impaired Gas Exchange

Common Related Factors

Decreased perfusion to lung tissues caused by obstruction in pulmonary vascular bed by embolus

Increased alveolar dead space

Increased physiological shunting caused by collapse of alveoli resulting from loss of surfactant

Defining Characteristics

Confusion/somnolence

Restlessness/irritability

Hypoxemia

Hypercapnia

Tachycardia

Dyspnea

Pale, dusky skin color

Common Expected Outcome

Patient maintains optimal gas exchange, as evidenced by arterial blood gases (ABGs) within the patient's usual range, oxygen saturation of 90% or greater, alert response mentation or no further reduction of level of consciousness, relaxed breathing, and baseline HR for patient.

NOC Outcomes

Respiratory Status: Gas Exchange; Tissue Perfusion: Pulmonary

NIC Interventions

Respiratory Monitoring; Oxygen Therapy; Acid-Base Management

Ongoing Assessment

Actions/Interventions	Rationales
■ Monitor vital signs, noting any changes.	In initial hypoxia and hypercapnia, blood pressure (BP), heart rate (HR), and respiratory rate all rise. As the hypoxia and/or hypercapnia becomes more severe, BP may drop, HR tends to continue to be rapid and includes dysrhythmias, and respiratory failure may ensue, with the patient unable to maintain the rapid respiratory rate.
■ Auscultate lung sounds noting areas of decreased ventilation and presence of adventitious sounds.	Common clinical findings with PE include crackles.
■ Assess skin color, nail beds, and mucous membranes for color changes.	Cool, pale skin may be secondary to a compensatory response to hypoxemia. As oxygen and perfusion become impaired, peripheral tissues become cyanotic.
■ Assess for signs and symptoms of hypoxia.	Hypoxia results from increased dead space (ventilation without perfusion) that reduces effective gas exchange. Signs include tachycardia, restlessness, diaphoresis, headache, lethargy or confusion, and skin color changes.
■ Assess for presence of signs and symptoms of pulmonary infarction.	A large pulmonary embolus or multiple small clots in a specific area of the lung can cause an ischemic necrosis/infarction of the lung area. Signs include cough, hemoptysis, pleuritic pain, consolidation, pleural effusion, bronchial breathing, pleural friction rub, fever.
▲ Monitor ABGs, and note changes.	ABG analysis can be normal or show hypoxemia and hypocapnia because of tachypnea. Later signs of respiratory failure include low Pao_2 and elevated $Paco_2$. Metabolic acidosis results from lactic acid buildup from tissue hypoxia.
▲ Use pulse oximetry, as available, to continuously monitor oxygen saturation.	Pulse oximetry is a useful tool in the clinical setting to detect changes in oxygenation. Oxygen saturation should be at 90% or greater.
■ Assess for calf tenderness, swelling, redness, and/or hardened area.	PE often arises from a deep vein thrombosis and may have been previously overlooked.

Therapeutic Interventions

Actions/Interventions	Rationales
▲ Administer oxygen as needed.	Supplemental oxygen may be required to maintain Po_2 at an acceptable level.
■ Position the patient properly to facilitate ventilation-perfusion matching.	Upright and sitting positions optimize diaphragmatic excursions and lung perfusion. When the patient is positioned on one side, the affected area should not be dependent.
▲ Anticipate the need to start anticoagulant therapy and, if there is massive thromboembolism, the use of thrombolytic therapy.	Heparin or enoxaparin (Lovenox) is used to prevent recurrence of emboli. These medications do not dissolve clots that already exist. If a massive thrombus is present or the patient is hemodynamically unstable, then thrombolytic therapy (e.g., alteplase or reteplase [Retavase]) is used to directly lyse or dissolve the clot.

Risk for Bleeding

Common Risk Factors	Defining Characteristics
Anticoagulant or thrombolytic therapy	Altered clotting
Abnormal blood profiles	Bleeding

■ = Independent   ▲ = Collaborative

Common Expected Outcomes

Patient does not experience bleeding.
Patient maintains PTT/PT/INR within desired range.

NOC Outcomes

Blood Coagulation; Risk Control

NIC Interventions

Bleeding Precautions; Bleeding Reduction

Ongoing Assessment

Actions/Interventions	Rationales
■ Assess for history of a high-risk bleeding condition: liver disease, kidney disease, severe hypertension, cavitary tuberculosis, bacterial endocarditis, and heparin-induced thrombocytopenia.	Because anticoagulation therapy is the hallmark treatment for PE, prior patient experiences with bleeding or anticoagulants must be assessed before treatment. Risk versus benefit of treatment must be assessed.
▲ Monitor intravenous (IV) dosage and delivery system (tubing or pump).	IV anticoagulation is administered using an electronic infusion pump. This device reduces risk for overcoagulation or undercoagulation.
▲ Monitor platelet counts, coagulation test results (international normalized ratio [INR], prothrombin time, activated partial thromboplastin time [aPTT]), and hemoglobin and hematocrit. Notify physician immediately if higher or lower than designated range occurs.	Effects of anticoagulation therapy must be closely monitored to reduce risk for bleeding. Type of test depends on anticoagulation medication administered.
▲ Monitor platelets and heparin-induced platelet aggregation (HIPA) status.	Severe platelet reductions can occur with heparin use, especially unfractionated heparin therapy, and are known as heparin-induced thrombocytopenia (HIT). HIT is less commonly seen with the use of low-molecular-weight heparin.
■ Assess for signs and symptoms of bleeding: petechiae, purpura, hematoma; bleeding from catheter insertion sites; gastrointestinal or genitourinary bleeding; bleeding from respiratory tract; bleeding from mucous membranes; decreased hemoglobin and hematocrit.	Early assessment facilitates prompt administration of the appropriate antidote.

Therapeutic Interventions

Actions/Interventions	Rationales
▲ Administer anticoagulant therapy as prescribed (bolus, continuous IV heparin/subcutaneous low-molecular-weight heparin), oral warfarin [Coumadin]).	Anticoagulants are given to prevent further thrombus formation. The type of medication varies per protocol. New nonheparin agents are also available for patients who cannot tolerate heparin.
▲ If the patient is HIPA positive, stop all heparin products and consult a hematologist.	Continuation of heparin products is contraindicated in the patient who is HIPA positive.
▲ If bleeding occurs while on heparin, anticipate the following: • Stop the infusion. • Recheck aPTT level stat. • Administer protamine sulfate as ordered. • Take vital signs often. • Reevaluate dose of heparin on basis of aPTT result. • Notify blood bank to ensure blood availability if needed.	Laboratory data guide further treatments; aPTT guide is 1.5 to 2 times normal. Protamine is a heparin antagonist.
▲ Convert from IV anticoagulation to oral anticoagulation after appropriate length of therapy. Monitor INR, prothrombin time (PT), and aPTT levels.	The onset of anticoagulation with warfarin is 2 to 3 days. There needs to be an overlap of these medications to ensure adequate PT levels or INR levels for anticoagulation before discontinuing heparin.

Actions/Interventions	Rationales
▲ Administer thrombolytic therapy as prescribed.	Lytic agents are indicated for patients with massive PE that results in hemodynamic compromise. Be aware of the following contraindications for thrombolytic therapy to minimize complications: recent surgery, recent organ biopsy, pregnancy, recent stroke, or recent or active internal bleeding.
▲ Institute precautionary measures for thrombolytic therapy: • Use only compressible vessels for IV sites. • Compress IV sites for at least 10 minutes and arterial sites for 30 minutes. • Limit physical manipulation of patients. • Provide gentle oral care. • Avoid intramuscular injections. • Draw all laboratory specimens through an existing line: arterial line or venous heparin-lock line. • Send specimen for type and crossmatch as prescribed.	These measures reduce the risk for bleeding.

 NANDA-I NDx Deficient Knowledge

Common Related Factors
New medical condition
New treatment

Defining Characteristics
Inaccurate information
Questioning members of health team
Inaccurate follow-through of instruction

Common Expected Outcome
Patient verbalizes understanding of desired content: importance of medications, signs of excessive anticoagulation, and means to reduce risk for bleeding and recurrence of emboli.

NOC Outcomes
Knowledge: Disease Process; Knowledge: Medication

NIC Interventions
Teaching: Disease Process; Teaching: Prescribed Medication

Ongoing Assessment

Actions/Interventions	Rationales
■ Assess knowledge of pulmonary embolus: severity, prognosis, risk factors, therapy.	Assessment provides an important starting point in education. Knowledge serves to correct faulty ideas.

Therapeutic Interventions

Actions/Interventions	Rationales
■ Provide information on the cause of the problem, common risk factors, and effects of PE on body functioning.	Preventing thrombus formation is an ongoing concern. An informed patient is more likely to avoid common risk factors.

■ = Independent   ▲ = Collaborative

Actions/Interventions

- Discuss with and give the patient a list of measures to minimize recurrence of emboli:
  - Take anticoagulants as prescribed.
  - Keep medical checkup and blood test appointments.
  - Perform leg exercises as advised, especially during long automobile and airplane trips.
  - Do not cross legs at knees.
  - Use elastic stockings as prescribed.
  - Maintain adequate hydration.
- Instruct the patient about medications, their actions, dosages, and side effects.

- Discuss with and provide the patient with a list of what to avoid when taking anticoagulants:
  - Do not use a blade razor (electric razors preferred).
  - Do not take new medications without consulting the physician, pharmacist, or nurses.
  - Do not change diet of foods high in vitamin K (e.g., dark-green vegetables, cauliflower, cabbage, bananas, tomatoes).
  - Discuss drug, herb, alcohol, and food interactions with medication. Emphasize that significant diet changes and all over-the-counter medications and complementary therapies need to be discussed with the physician or nurse practitioner before initiation.
- Inform the patient of the need for routine laboratory testing while on oral anticoagulation.

- Discuss and give the patient a list of signs and symptoms of excessive anticoagulation: easy bruising, severe nosebleed, black stools, blood in urine or stools, joint swelling and pain, coughing up of blood, severe headache.
- Discuss safety or precautionary measures to use while on anticoagulant therapy: need to inform dentist or other caregivers before treatment, use of electric razor, use of soft toothbrush.
- If the patient is heparin-induced platelet aggregation (HIPA) positive, instruct about the importance of avoiding heparin.
- Explain the need for a vena cava filter device if clotting is a chronic problem.

Rationales

These measures reduce potential for thrombus formation.

Patients may require anticoagulation for weeks, months, or more, depending on their risks. Accurate knowledge reduces future complications.

These safety measures reduce risk for bleeding. Many medications and foods interact with warfarin, altering the anticoagulation effect.

Continued regular assessment of anticoagulation is necessary to prevent both reoccurrence of clots and active bleeding

Patients need to self-manage their condition. Early assessment facilitates prompt treatment.

These measures help prevent bleeding.

Heparin use can result in formation of antiheparin antibodies, which puts the patient at risk.

In high-risk patients this filter/interruption device can trap a thrombus migrating from a deep vein thrombosis in the leg.

Related Care Plans

Decreased cardiac output, p. 33
Anxiety, p. 18

Respiratory Failure, Acute

Ventilatory Failure; Oxygenation Failure

Acute respiratory failure is a life-threatening inability to maintain adequate pulmonary gas exchange. Persons with acute respiratory failure cannot carry out the two major functions of gas exchange: delivery of adequate amounts of oxygen into the arterial blood (oxygenation failure) or removal of a corresponding amount of CO_2 from the mixed venous blood (ventilatory failure). Respiratory failure can result from obstructive disease (e.g., emphysema, chronic bronchitis, asthma), restrictive disease (e.g., atelectasis, acute respiratory distress syndrome [ARDS], pneumonia, multiple rib fractures, postoperative abdominal or thoracic surgery, central nervous system [CNS] depression), or ventilation-perfusion abnormalities (e.g., pulmonary embolism). This care plan focuses on acute care management of respiratory failure.

NANDA-I NDx Impaired Spontaneous Ventilation

Common Related Factors

Respiratory muscle fatigue
Metabolic factors
CNS depression
Drug overdose

Defining Characteristics

Shortness of breath/dyspnea
Tachypnea
Increased $Paco_2$ level (50 to 60 mm Hg or greater)
Decreased Pao_2 level (less than 50 to 60 mm Hg)
Arterial pH less than 7.35
Decreased oxygen saturation (Sao_2 less than 90%)
Decreased tidal volume
Decrease in level of consciousness
Restlessness
Tachycardia
Cyanosis

Common Expected Outcome

Patient maintains spontaneous gas exchange resulting in normal arterial blood gases (ABGs) within parameters for patient, return to normal pulse oximetry, and decreased dyspnea.

NOC Outcomes

Respiratory Status: Gas Exchange; Respiratory Status: Ventilation; Vital Signs

NIC Interventions

Respiratory Monitoring; Ventilation Assistance; Mechanical Ventilation; Oxygen Therapy

Ongoing Assessment

Actions/Interventions	Rationales
■ Assess respiratory rate, pattern, and depth; note position assumed for breathing.	Respiratory rate and rhythm changes are early warning signs of impending respiratory difficulties. A three-point position or orthopnea is associated with breathing difficulty.
■ Assess for use of accessory muscles.	Work of breathing increases greatly as lung compliance decreases. As moving air into and out of lungs becomes more difficult, the breathing pattern alters to include use of accessory muscles to increase chest excursion to facilitate breathing.

■ = Independent   ▲ = Collaborative

Actions/Interventions

- Assess HR and BP.

- Assess for changes in level of consciousness.

- Assess for presence of cough and, if effective, amount expectorated, frequency, and color.
- Auscultate lungs for normal and adventitious sounds: wheezing, rales (crackles), or rhonchi.
- Monitor for dysrhythmias.

- Use pulse oximetry to monitor oxygen saturation.

- ▲ Monitor ABGs carefully, and notify physician of abnormalities.

Rationales

Hypotension plus tachycardia may result from hypoxia and/or hypercarbia.

Increased restlessness, confusion, and/or irritability are early indicators of insufficient oxygenation of the brain and requires further intervention.

These may be indicative of an etiology for the alteration in breathing pattern.

Changes in lung sounds may reveal specific problems that guide treatment.

Cardiac dysrhythmias may result from hypoxia, catecholamine release in response to low oxygen levels, and acidosis.

Pulse oximetry provides an objective indication of oxygen saturation. It should be kept at 90% or greater.

Increasing $Paco_2$ and/or decreasing Pao_2 is a sign of respiratory failure. However, ABG values may be acceptable initially, and the patient's work of breathing may be too extreme. As the patient's condition begins to fail, respiratory rate will decrease.

Therapeutic Interventions

Actions/Interventions

- Position patient to optimize ventilation.

- Plan activity and rest to maximize the patient's energy.

- ▲ Administer oxygen as needed. For patients with severe chronic obstructive pulmonary disease (COPD), give oxygen cautiously, preferably with a Venturi device.

- Assist with ventilatory support measures as appropriate:
  - Bilevel positive airway pressure (BiPAP)
  - When necessary, prepare for intubation and mechanical ventilation:

  - Position the patient appropriately, and have necessary equipment readily available.
  - Instruct the patient who is awake and alert.

  - Institute suctioning through an endotracheal (ET) tube as necessary.
  - After intubation, auscultate lungs for bilateral sounds.

  - Obtain chest x-ray study after intubation.

Rationales

If not contraindicated, a sitting position allows for adequate diaphragmatic and lung excursion and chest expansion.

Fatigue is common with increased work of breathing. Activity increases metabolic rate and oxygen requirements. Rest helps mobilize energy for more effective breathing and coughing efforts.

The Venturi device is a high-flow oxygen delivery system with a stable F_{IO_2} that is unaffected by the patient's respiratory rate or tidal volume. COPD patients who chronically retain carbon dioxide depend on "hypoxic drive" as their stimulus to breathe. When applying oxygen, close monitoring is imperative to prevent unsafe increases in the patient's Pao_2, which could result in apnea.

BiPAP is a noninvasive form of positive-pressure ventilation.

Early intubation and mechanical ventilation may be needed to maintain adequate oxygenation and ventilation and to prevent full decompensation of the patient and a potentially life-threatening situation.

Proper positioning facilitates alignment for successful intubation.

Explanation is essential to prepare the patient and reduce anxiety.

Airway patency is a priority.

This assessment ensures that the ET tube is not in the right main stem bronchus or the esophagus.

X-ray film confirms ET tube placement.

NANDA-I NDx **Risk for Ineffective Airway Clearance**

Common Risk Factors

Copious and tenacious tracheobronchial secretions
Inability to cough
Tracheobronchial infection
Presence of artificial airway (ET tube)
Fatigue/decreased energy
Impaired respiratory function

Common Expected Outcome

Patient will maintain clear, open airways, as evidenced by normal breath sounds, normal rate and depth of respiration, and ability to cough up secretions.

NOC Outcome
Respiratory Status: Airway Patency
NIC Interventions
Airway Suctioning; Airway Management

Ongoing Assessment

Actions/Interventions	Rationales
■ Assess lungs for adventitious breath sounds (e.g., rhonchi, wheezes).	Airway obstruction from fluid accumulation produces crackles and rhonchi. Wheezes are caused by bronchospasm.
■ Assess respiratory rate, rhythm, and depth.	An increase in respiratory rate and rhythm may be a compensatory response for airway obstruction. Hypoxia is associated with increased breathing effort.
■ Assess characteristics of sputum: color, consistency, amount, odor.	Abnormalities may be a result of infection, bronchitis, chronic smoking, or other conditions. A sign of infection is discolored sputum (no longer clear or white); an odor may be present. Thick, tenacious secretions increase hypoxemia and may be indicative of dehydration.
■ Assess cough for effectiveness and productivity.	Patients may have an ineffective cough because of respiratory muscle fatigue, severe bronchospasm, or thick, tenacious secretions.

Therapeutic Interventions

Actions/Interventions	Rationales
■ Use upright position (if tolerated, head of bed at 45 degrees). Instruct patient or assist in changing position every 2 hours.	This position provides better lung expansion and improved air exchange. Position changes mobilize secretions.
▲ Maintain humidified oxygen as prescribed.	Increasing humidity of inspired air will reduce viscosity of secretions and facilitate removal.
■ Instruct the patient to deep breathe adequately, to cough effectively, and to use incentive spirometry, as ordered.	These measures improve lung capacity and gas exchange. Coughing is the most effective way to remove most secretions.
▲ If cough is ineffective, use nasotracheal suction as ordered.	Suctioning is indicated when patients are unable to remove secretions from the airway by coughing because of weakness, thick mucous plugs, or excessive or tenacious mucous production. It can also stimulate a cough.
After intubation:	
▲ Institute suctioning of airway as needed (not routinely).	Frequency of suctioning should be based on presence of adventitious sounds and/or increased ventilatory pressure, not time intervals. Oversuctioning can cause hypoxia and injury to bronchial and lung tissues.

■ = Independent ▲ = Collaborative

Risk for Infection

Common Risk Factors

Increased secretions
Suctioning of airway
Endotracheal intubation

Common Expected Outcome

Patient remains free of infection, as evidenced by normal body temperature, normal white blood cell (WBC) count, negative cultures, normal vital signs, and absence of purulent drainage from tubes.

NOC Outcomes
Immune Status; Risk Detection; Risk Control
NIC Intervention
Infection Protection

Ongoing Assessment

Actions/Interventions	Rationales
■ Assess for fever.	Fever may be a manifestation of an infection or an inflammatory process. If the patient is receiving steroid therapy, detecting infections may be more difficult.
▲ Monitor WBC count.	Rising WBC count indicates body's efforts to combat pathogens.
■ Observe the patient's secretions for color, consistency, quantity, and odor.	Increased amounts of sputum and changes in color may indicate infection.
■ Monitor sputum cultures and sensitivities.	Identification of the infecting microorganism is important to determine antibiotic coverage.

Therapeutic Interventions

Actions/Interventions	Rationales
■ Practice conscientious bronchial hygiene, good hand-washing techniques, and sterile suctioning.	Many infections are transmitted by hospital personnel.
■ Administer mouth care (e.g., mouthwash, mouth swabs, mouth spray) every 2 hours and as needed; brush the patient's teeth at least every 12 hours.	Mouth care helps limit oral bacterial growth and promotes patient comfort.
■ Institute airway suctioning as needed.	Accumulation of secretions provides a medium for bacterial growth.
■ If patient was placed on mechanical ventilator, keep head of bed elevated greater than 30 degrees.	Upright positioning helps prevent ventilator-associated pneumonia (VAP). VAP occurs in up to 25% of patients on ventilators and carries a high mortality rate. Most infections are caused by bacterial pathogens, with gram-negative bacilli being common.
■ Institute measures to reduce VAP.	Nosocomial infections such as VAP are a leading cause of hospital mortality. Prevention of VAP is a national initiative to promote quality and safety.
• Wash hands before and after suctioning, touching, ventilator equipment, and/or coming into contact with respiratory secretions.	An artificial airway bypasses the normal protective mechanisms of the upper airways. Hand washing reduces transmission of microorganisms.
• Use a continuous subglottic suction ET tube for intubation expected to be longer than 24 hours.	This intervention prevents accumulation of secretions that can be aspirated.
• Keep head of bed elevated to 30 to 45 degrees or perform subglottic suctioning unless medically contraindicated.	Elevation promotes better lung expansion. It also reduces gastric reflux and aspiration.

Actions/Interventions

- Brush teeth two to three times per day with a soft toothbrush. Chlorhexidine-based rinses may also be incorporated into oral care products.
- Use sterile suctioning procedures.

Rationales

Oral care reduces colonization of oropharynx with respiratory pathogens that can be aspirated into the lungs.

This technique decreases the introduction of microorganisms into the airway.

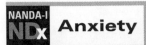

NANDA-I NDx Anxiety

Common Related Factors
Unknown outcome
Change in health status
Change in environment
Inability to speak if intubated
Inability to maintain adequate gas exchange

Defining Characteristics
Restlessness
Uncooperative behavior
Withdrawal
Vigilant watch on equipment
Tachypnea
Facial tension

Common Expected Outcome
Patient demonstrates reduced anxiety, as evidenced by calm manner and cooperative behavior.
Patient uses effective coping mechanisms.
Patient describes a reduction in level of anxiety experienced.

NOC Outcomes
Anxiety Self-Control; Coping
NIC Interventions
Anxiety Reduction; Presence; Emotional Support

Ongoing Assessment

Actions/Interventions

■ Assess for signs of anxiety.

Rationales

Respiratory failure is an acute life-threatening condition that will produce high levels of anxiety in the patient as well as significant others. Anxiety can affect respiratory rate and pattern, resulting in rapid, shallow breathing and leading to ABG abnormalities.

Therapeutic Interventions

Actions/Interventions

■ Display a confident, calm manner and understanding attitude. Assure the patient and significant others of close, continuous monitoring that will ensure prompt interventions. Reassure patient of the staff's presence.

■ Encourage visiting by family or significant others.

■ Anticipate questions. Provide explanations of mechanical ventilation and alarm systems on monitors and ventilators.

■ If impaired communication is the problem, provide patient with word-and-phrase cards, writing pad and pencil, or picture board.

▲ Use other supportive measures (e.g., medications, psychiatric liaison, clergy, social services) as indicated.

Rationales

The presence of a trusted person may be helpful during periods of anxiety. The staff's anxiety may be easily perceived by the patient. The patient's feeling of stability is increased in a calm, nonthreatening atmosphere.

The presence of significant others may reinforce feelings of security for the patient.

The ICU is a busy environment that can be scary and upsetting to patient and significant others. Information helps reduce anxiety. An informed patient who understands the treatment plan will be more cooperative and relaxed.

These tools provide a channel through which information can be communicated.

Medication and supportive resources may be used if the patient's anxiety continues to escalate. Specialty expertise may provide a wider range of treatment options.

■ = Independent ▲ = Collaborative

Pulmonary Care Plans

NANDA-I NDx Deficient Knowledge

Common Related Factors
Unfamiliarity with disease process and treatment
Cognitive limitation
Decreased motivation to learn

Defining Characteristics
Questioning members of health team
Anxiety
Expressing inaccurate information

Common Expected Outcome
Patient verbalizes understanding of disease process, procedures, and treatment.

NOC Outcomes
Knowledge: Disease Process; Knowledge: Treatment Regimen

NIC Interventions
Teaching: Disease Process; Teaching: Individual

Ongoing Assessment

Actions/Interventions

- Assess the patient's perception and understanding of the disease process that led to respiratory failure, and of oxygen therapy and deep breathing and coughing techniques.

Rationales

This provides an important starting point in education. Teaching interventions must be designed individually to meet specific patient needs. Acute care patients may not be able to take in much information because they may need to focus efforts on effective breathing rather than on the educational session.

Therapeutic Interventions

Actions/Interventions

- Explain the disease process to the patient or significant others, and correct misconceptions. Include family and significant others in the plan of care.

- Explain all tests and procedures before they occur.
- Explain the necessity of oxygen therapy, including its limitations.
- Instruct the patient to deep breathe and cough effectively.
- Instruct the patient in preventive measures as appropriate (e.g., avoidance of exposure to smoke and fumes, cold air, and allergens such as pollens, dust, and dander).
- Provide guidelines for activities and advancement of activities, the need for home oxygen, and timing for follow-up visits with health care providers.
- Discuss with the patient and significant others reversibility of condition, advance directives, and medical power of attorney.

Rationales

During the acute phase, family or significant others may require the most teaching. This will reduce their feelings of helplessness and assist them in supporting the patient. Acute respiratory failure is a serious condition.
An informed patient is more cooperative.
Oxygen is used to support arterial saturation.

These techniques facilitate clearance of secretions.
These efforts serve to prevent further respiratory difficulties.

Information aids in the transition from hospital to home.

Patients must make very clear what they want regarding life-sustaining treatments.

Related Care Plans

Sleep-Disordered Breathing

(Obstructed Sleep Apnea)

Sleep-disordered breathing (SDB) affects at least 20 million people in the United States and is defined as a cessation of breathing during sleep that is caused by repetitive partial or complete obstruction of the airway and pharyngeal structures. There are two types: the most common form, obstructive sleep apnea (OSA), and central sleep apnea. The prevalence in the general population is 2% to 4%. The manifestations of OSA include episodes of loud snoring, decreased oxygen saturation, brief periods of apnea, and arousal from sleep. These episodes may occur several times during sleep. OSA is strongly linked to cardiovascular diseases—especially hypertension and coronary artery disease, which eventually leads to heart failure—so the prevalence in heart failure patients rises to approximately 50%. Consequences of OSA include altered alertness, daytime somnolence, cognitive impairment, and increased morbidity and mortality. Common screening methods include pulse oximetry, blood gas analysis, and/or ambulatory airflow measurements, but the diagnosis of OSA is confirmed by overnight sleep laboratory studies.

Treatment for mild OSA includes conservative measures such as weight loss, abstaining from the use of alcohol and sedatives, avoiding the supine position during sleep, and sometimes oropharyngeal appliances or surgery. However, continuous positive airway pressure (CPAP) is the most consistently effective treatment for clinically significant OSA and appears to substantially improve the condition. Unfortunately, some patients complain that the CPAP mask or nasal device (BiPAP) is uncomfortable, so compliance with the treatment is often low. As technology advances, the treatment of OSA will become more comfortable and less cumbersome. Patients must be encouraged to try different equipment to adapt to their own facial structure, because patients who use CPAP report less fatigue, better blood pressure control, and improved quality of life.

 NANDA-I NDx **Ineffective Breathing Pattern**

Common Related Factors

Obesity
Enlarged tonsils and adenoids
Narrowing of respiratory passages
Decreased airway muscle tone during sleep

Defining Characteristics

Bradypnea/periods of apnea
Snoring

Common Expected Outcomes

Patient maintains effective breathing pattern, as evidenced by relaxed breathing at normal rate and depth and decreased snoring and apneic episodes.
Patient adheres to CPAP/BiPAP device regimen as prescribed.

NOC Outcomes

Respiratory Status: Airway Patency; Respiratory Status: Ventilation

NIC Interventions

Airway Management; Respiratory Monitoring

Ongoing Assessment

Actions/Interventions

- Assess current sleep pattern and sleep history.

Rationales

Periodic changes in sleep pattern need to be differentiated from true obstructive sleep disorder/apnea.

■ = Independent ▲ = Collaborative

Actions/Interventions

- Ask the patient's partner or significant other whether the patient snores or has apneic episode during the night.

- Assess for characteristics of SDB: loud snoring, apneic episodes (5 to 10 per hour), jerky or restless leg movement during sleep, daytime somnolence and fatigue.
- Assess for contributing factors to OSA: obesity (body mass index greater than 30), short thick neck circumference, age, large uvula, enlarged tonsils or adenoids, small recessive jaw, oropharyngeal edema, alcohol abuse.

- Assess physiological effects resulting from comorbidities affected by OSA.

Rationales

Most patients are unaware of their own snoring and apnea. The partner may have complained about loud snoring followed by stopping breathing and a loud gasp or snort when the patient is aroused by the apnea.

Although a variety of manifestations may occur, patients may only be aware of the daytime fatigue and sleepiness.

Research has shown that body type affects diagnosis. Excess body weight can result in accumulation of fat on the sides of the upper airway, causing it to become narrow. Increasing neck size has been correlated with severity of apnea. Aging causes loss of muscle mass replaced by fat, again leaving the airway narrow and soft. Anatomical abnormalities affect upper airway musculature. Alcohol use results in excessive relaxation of muscles in the upper airway during sleep.

During sleep apneic periods, there is a fall in PaO_2 levels with a buildup of $PaCO_2$. The immediate "arousal" to breathe causes surges in sympathetic activity that affects many organ systems, especially the cardiovascular system. The sympathetic stimulation can lead to cardiac arrhythmias, systemic vascular resistance, and reduced cardiac output in compromised heart failure patients. Research has demonstrated a high prevalence of OSA in patients with heart failure, hypertension, coronary artery disease, and stroke, although the exact relationship is unclear. OSA can aggravate conditions such as heart failure because of the increased physiological demands put on the heart during sleep.

Therapeutic Interventions

Actions/Interventions

- Suggest referral for nighttime sleep study if not already performed.

- In diagnosed patients, explain the mechanisms by which sleep apnea occurs:
  - Relaxation of muscles of the soft palate during sleep results in reduced airway size and partial or complete closure.
  - This closure causes cessation of breathing (apnea).
  - During the apneic period, the body struggles to breathe and is aroused to awaken, which reopens the airway.
  - The obstructive periods are associated with reduced oxygen saturation.
  - This sleep apnea–arousal–awaken cycle repeats on an ongoing basis, preventing the patient from reaching the deep stages of rapid eye movement (REM) sleep.

Rationales

The most definitive test is the overnight sleep study—polysomnography. Using electrodes, it records the type and depth of sleep, eye movement observations, respiratory effort and movement, oxygen saturation, and muscle movement. Patients can use simpler "screening" techniques such as home sleep monitoring (although it is difficult to maintain equipment during sleep) or overnight pulse oximetry to document drops in oxygen saturation during the apneic periods.

The more the patient understands the condition, the better he or she is able to participate in the treatment plan.

Actions/Interventions

■ Teach the patient about nonsurgical therapies to treat OSA:
- Weight loss—indicated for mild sleep apnea

- Nonsupine positioning—indicated for mild sleep apnea

- Oral appliances resembling mouth guards (tongue-retaining or mandibular advance devices)—indicated for mild sleep apnea
- CPAP—indicated for mild to severe apnea. CPAP uses a nasal or facial mask held in place with secure straps. Appropriate mask fitting is key to success.

- Nasal trumpets—indicated to bypass any nasal, soft palate, or sometimes tongue obstructions and commonly used in postanesthesia settings
- BiPAP—a variation of CPAP that delivers a lower amount of positive pressure during exhalation
- Supplementary oxygen
■ Emphasize compliance issues, especially related to CPAP.

■ Instruct patients to bring their CPAP/BiPAP devices to the hospital for personal use while hospitalized. Notify the hospital team, especially the anesthesiologist, of OSA problems so that ventilation needs can be correctly assessed.
■ Instruct the patient to reduce or avoid drinking alcohol.

■ Instruct the patient regarding possible surgical technique (uvulopalatopharyngoplasty), as indicated.

■ Refer to sleep specialist as needed.

Rationales

Weight loss has been shown to improve this condition, although the amount of weight loss required varies among patients.
Supine sleeping causes the most significant relaxation of upper airway muscles, causing the tongue to more easily fall back and occlude the airway or airway muscles and tissues like the tonsils to relax and block the airway. Turning on one's side can reduce episodes of apnea. Suggested techniques include sewing or attaching a sock filled with tennis balls lengthwise down the back of a pajama top. This reminds the patient to stay positioned on the side.
Repositioning the muscles may prevent the apneic episode. These devices should be fitted by a specialty dentist. The devices are more appropriate for milder forms of OSA.
The positive pressure serves to "stabilize" the airway and maintain patency. The mask is connected to a small air compressor that delivers preset positive pressure to the upper airway. The mask is usually worn for at least 4 hours during the night's sleep. It should be used daily, although patients with milder levels may need the device only a few days a week. Side effects include dry mucous membranes, dermatitis, skin breakdown, nasal congestion, and feelings of claustrophobia. Humidification can be added to reduce problems associated with dryness.
These devices may reduce mucosal trauma but they are not readily tolerated by patients on a long-term basis.

Patients often find the BiPAP device more tolerable than CPAP.
Supplementary oxygen raises oxygen saturation.
Patients frequently have difficulty getting masks or nasal devices to fit properly, or they may feel claustrophobic while wearing the devices. The CPAP device is only effective while in use, making compliance a key issue. Many patients find the nasal device easier to tolerate than the mask. Patients can use more portable units. Patients need to take the device with them when they anticipate sleeping away from home, for example, on vacations, for work travel, or on long plane flights, especially if they already have heart failure.
It is more effective for patients to use their own face mask and devices that have been properly fitted. Use of the positive pressure aids ventilation, maintains tissue oxygen saturation, and reduces the workload of the heart.

Alcohol causes relaxation of the muscles of the upper airway and can aggravate the condition.
This procedure involves removal of part of the soft palate, uvula, and redundant peripharyngeal tissues to eliminate snoring. It does not always prevent the apneic periods. The procedure can be done surgically or with laser assistance. It is indicated for individuals who cannot tolerate CPAP.
Specialists may provide additional treatment strategies.

■ = Independent   ▲ = Collaborative

Sleep Deprivation

Common Related Factors

Sleep apnea
Sleep stage shifts
Cycle of sleep-apnea-arousal-sleep that interferes with REM sleep

Defining Characteristics

Daytime drowsiness
Decreased ability to function
Fatigue
Irritability
Slowed reaction
Inability to concentrate

Common Expected Outcome

Patient achieves optimal amounts of sleep, as evidenced by rested appearance, verbalization of feeling rested, and improvement in sleep pattern.

NOC Outcomes
Sleep; Rest

NIC Intervention
Sleep Enhancement

Ongoing Assessment

Actions/Interventions	Rationales
■ Assess for complaints of waking up feeling tired or fatigued and experiencing daytime somnolence.	The cycle of interrupted sleep results in reduced REM sleep, which the body requires for rest and to replenish itself. Interrupted sleep is associated with feelings of tiredness and often of complaints of feeling worse upon awakening than when retiring for sleep. Patients are often embarrassed by episodes of falling asleep such as in movie theaters, during work meetings, or while watching television.
■ Assess for safety issues at work and at home.	Memory and cognitive changes can significantly affect ability to perform activities of daily living and occupational activities. Decreased alertness and impaired concentration during the day places the patient at risk for accidents.
■ Assess history of automobile accidents.	The "drowsy driver syndrome," which has been linked to frequent automobile accidents, may be caused by OSA and lack of alertness and slowed reflexes while driving.
■ Assess for other factors that contribute to fatigue such as alcohol and medications.	It is critical that patients with OSA do not aggravate their condition through use of sedatives, analgesics, narcotics, tranquilizers, other prescribed medications, or alcohol that also contribute to reduced alertness and fatigue.
■ Assess whether interpersonal relationships and quality of life have been affected by chronic fatigue, irritability, or mood changes.	Lack of sleep can contribute to irritability and depression, making it difficult to maintain healthy personal relationships. Impotence is also related to OSA and may affect feelings of intimacy. The patient's sleep partner may experience disrupted sleep because of the patient's loud snoring. Many patients report remaining awake waiting for the partner to breathe again after a period of apnea.

Therapeutic Interventions

Actions/Interventions	Rationales
■ Explain the relationship of REM sleep and of feeling refreshed when awakening.	REM sleep is characterized by rapid eye movements and is essential to waking up feeling refreshed. It is the deepest level of relaxation. This level is not reached when patients are continually being aroused from sleep and restarting their sleep cycles.
■ Reinforce the importance of adhering to prescribed treatment.	Most treatments need to be initiated on a daily basis (weight management, positioning, use of CPAP). Knowledge of the physiological basis for restful sleep may provide the rationale for compliance with treatments.
■ Instruct the patient to consider alternative transportation (carpool, public transportation) until achieving a more restful sleep.	Daytime somnolence, reduced alertness, impaired concentration, and delayed reaction time place the patient at great risk for injuring self and others. Using alternative modes of travel reduces this risk.
■ Refer to social worker as needed for assistance with personal relationships.	Specialized expertise may be needed to help the patient gain insight into problems.

Related Care Plans

Ineffective therapeutic regimen management, p. 194
Obesity, p. 601
Fatigue, p. 66

Thoracotomy

Chest Surgery; Thoracic Surgery; Lobectomy; Pneumonectomy; Segmental Resection; Wedge Resection

Thoracotomy is a surgical opening into the thorax for biopsy, excision, drainage, and/or correction of defects. The surgical procedures done by thoracotomy correction may include the following:

- *Lobectomy:* Removal of one lobe of the lung; lobectomy is indicated for lung cancer, bronchiectasis, tuberculosis (TB), emphysematous bullae, benign lung tumors, or fungal infections.
- *Segmental resection:* Removal of one or more lung segments; segmental resection is indicated for bronchiectasis or TB.
- *Wedge resection:* Removal of a small localized lesion that occupies only part of a segment; wedge resection is indicated for excision of nodules or lung biopsy.
- *Endoscopic thoracotomy (thoracostomy):* Small incisions, useful for open lung biopsy to determine diagnosis, or for lymph node biopsy.
- *Pneumonectomy:* Removal of entire lung; indicated for lung cancer, extensive TB, bronchiectasis, or lung abscess.

This care plan focuses on postoperative care of the patient having a thoracotomy.

■ = Independent   ▲ = Collaborative

NANDA-I NDx Ineffective Breathing Pattern

Common Related Factors

Positive pressure in pleural space secondary to surgical incision
Collapse of lung on affected side (partial or complete)
Void in thoracic cavity if pneumonectomy performed
Pain
Decreased energy

Defining Characteristics

Dyspnea/shortness of breath
Tachypnea
Shallow respirations
Asymmetrical chest excursion
Use of accessory muscles
Restlessness
Tachycardia
Oxygen saturation less than 90%
Abnormal ABGs

Common Expected Outcome

Patient maintains effective breathing pattern, as evidenced by relaxed breathing at a normal rate and depth, clear lung sounds, and absence of dyspnea.

NOC Outcome
Respiratory Status: Ventilation
NIC Interventions
Tube Care: Chest; Airway Management

Ongoing Assessment

Actions/Interventions	Rationales
■ Assess respiratory rate, depth, effort and use of accessory muscles.	Respiratory rate and rhythm changes such as increase in respiratory rate with decreased tidal volume (rapid, shallow respirations) are early warning signs of impending respiratory difficulties. The breathing pattern may alter to include use of accessory muscles to increase chest excursion.
■ Assess pain quality, location, and severity.	Sources of pain after a thoracotomy include the chest wall incision and the chest tube in the pleural space. Pain can contribute to shallow breathing.
▲ Use pulse oximeter to monitor oxygen saturation; assess ABGs, if necessary.	Pulse oximetry is a useful tool to monitor oxygen saturation and detect early change in oxygenation. Oxygen saturation should be at 90% or greater. Increased $Paco_2$ and decreased Pao_2 are signs of respiratory compromise.
▲ Assess closed chest drainage system for the following:	The closed drainage system must be functioning correctly to promote lung reexpansion and effective breathing.
• Secure connections	A loose connection can allow air entry and positive pressure into the intrapleural space, resulting in lung collapse.
• Intact water seal	Sufficient fluid must be maintained in the water seal chamber to prevent air reflux into the pleural space.
• Fluctuation (or tidaling) of fluid	Cessation of fluctuation (or tidaling) can indicate clogged or kinked tube if abrupt or lung reexpansion.
• Presence of air leaks or bubbling in the water seal	Bubbling in water seal chamber indicates air leak, which may be present because the lung has not yet expanded or because of a persistent air leak. There may be a leak in the system before the water seal drainage (e.g., loose tubing connection or air leak around entrance site of tube).
• Tube patency; free of dependent loops	Obstruction of drainage from chest tube interferes with lung expansion. Drainage accumulating in dependent loops obstructs drainage flow and increases pressure in the lung.

Actions/Interventions	Rationales
• Fluid levels	Amount of suction (negative pressure) being applied to the pleural space is regulated by the amount of fluid in the suction control chamber, not the amount dialed on Emerson/wall suction.
• Amount of fluid in drainage collection system. Report drainage of bright red blood of 100 mL/hr for 2 hours consecutively.	Excessive drainage may indicate hemorrhage.
▲ Monitor serial chest x-ray films.	The chest x-ray film confirms chest tube placement and helps determine whether the lung has reexpanded.
■ Palpate area around chest tube insertion site for subcutaneous emphysema or crepitus.	Presence of a new air leak of crepitus should be reported immediately.

Therapeutic Interventions

Actions/Interventions	Rationales
■ Position patient for optimal breathing pattern. Reposition every 2 to 3 hours.	If not contraindicated, a sitting position allows for improved lung expansion and chest excursion. Repositioning reduces pooling of secretions. After pneumonectomy, position the patient on his or her back or with operative side dependent.
▲ Ensure that oxygen delivery system is applied to the patient.	Supplemental oxygen may be needed to maintain oxygen saturation at 90% or greater.
■ Encourage sustained deep breaths by emphasizing slow inhalation, holding end inspiration for a few seconds, and passive exhalation.	Controlled breathing techniques promote effective aeration and may also help slow respirations in patients who are tachypneic.
• Encourage use incentive spirometer.	Incentive spirometry enhances deep breathing, decreasing the potential for atelectasis.
▲ Maintain chest tube drainage system:	
• Position chest drainage system below the patient's chest level, in an upright position.	Gravity will aid in drainage and prevent backflow into chest. Postpneumonectomy patients generally do not have chest tubes. The space gradually fills with serosanguineous fluid.
• Place drainage unit in stand, tape to floor, or hang on bed to prevent tipping of unit.	This maneuver maintains integrity of system and prevents tube dislodgment.
• Make sure tubing is free of kinks and clots. Compress tubing from insertion site downward.	This promotes tube drainage.
• Set suction correctly to maintain a constant gentle bubbling in the suction control chamber.	The use of suction with a closed drainage system promotes drainage of fluid from the pleural space and reexpansion of the lung.
▲ Do not clamp chest tubes unless:	Clamping chest tubes is dangerous because a tension pneumothorax may occur.
• The physician has prescribed clamping	
• Closed chest drainage system is being changed to new system	
• System becomes disconnected or water seal is disrupted	

Ineffective Airway Clearance

Common Related Factors	Defining Characteristics
Incisional pain	Adventitious breath sounds (e.g., rhonchi, wheezes)
Thoracic surgery	Changes in respiratory rate or depth
Thick secretions	Ineffective cough
Fatigue	Dyspnea
	Excessive secretions
	Tachycardia

■ = Independent   ▲ = Collaborative

Common Expected Outcome

Patient will maintain clear, open airways, as evidenced by normal breath sounds, normal rate and depth of respiration, and ability to cough up secretions effectively after deep breaths.

NOC Outcome
Respiratory Status: Airway Patency
NIC Interventions
Cough Enhancement; Airway Suctioning

Ongoing Assessment

Actions/Interventions	Rationales
■ Auscultate lungs, noting areas of decreased ventilation and presence of adventitious breath sounds.	Diminished breath sounds or presence of adventitious sounds may indicate an obstructed airway.
■ Assess cough effectiveness and productivity. Observe characteristics of or changes in sputum.	Several factors can interfere with effective coughing, such as fatigue, pain, malpositioning, and thick, tenacious secretions. An ineffective cough leads to retained secretions and an increased risk for airway obstruction and infection. A sign of infection is discolored sputum (no longer clear or white).
■ Assess the patient for pain.	Postoperative pain can prevent the patient from taking deep breaths and from coughing effectively to clear the airway.
■ Assess for changes in HR, BP, and temperature.	Tachycardia and tachypnea may be related to increased work of breathing or hypoxia. Fever may develop in response to retained secretions or atelectasis.

Therapeutic Interventions

Actions/Interventions	Rationales
▲ Administer humidified oxygen as prescribed.	Humidity prevents drying of secretions and facilitates movement.
▲ Encourage fluid intake (oral or IV).	Adequate hydration promotes thinner mucus, which is easier for the patient to remove with coughing.
▲ Assist the patient in performing coughing and breathing maneuvers.	Coughing is the most helpful way to remove most secretions, especially when combined with deep breathing. The patient may be unable to perform independently. These maneuvers keep airways open by clearing secretions.
■ Instruct the patient in the following: • Use of pillow or hand splints when coughing • Use of incentive spirometry	Providing support, especially to insertion site, will reduce discomfort with deep breathing and coughing. Incentive spirometry facilitates deep breathing.
■ Use suctioning as needed to clear airway. Avoid deep tracheal suctioning in the postpneumonectomy patient.	Suctioning is needed when patients are unable to remove secretions from airways by coughing. Avoiding deep tracheal suctioning decreases the risk for bronchial stump suture line rupture.
▲ Administer pain medication as needed, offering it before the patient asks for it.	Medication prevents peak periods of pain and helps the patient participate in pulmonary therapy measures.
■ Assist the patient with ambulation or position changes.	Ambulation helps the patient maintain adequate lung expansion, thus preventing buildup of secretions or atelectasis. The patient with pneumonectomy should never be positioned with remaining lung in dependent position; this would compromise respiratory excursion of the remaining lung.

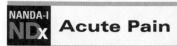

Acute Pain

Common Related Factors
Incisional pain
Chest tube insertion

Defining Characteristics
Verbalization of pain
Guarding behavior
Wincing, grimacing
Shallow respirations to minimize pain
Agitation, restlessness
Tachycardia
BP changes

Common Expected Outcomes
Patient reports satisfactory pain control at a level less than 3 to 4 on a 0 to 10 rating scale.
Patient exhibits increased comfort such as baseline levels for pulse, blood pressure (BP), respirations, and relaxed muscle tone or body posture.

NOC Outcomes
Pain Status; Comfort Level; Pain Control
NIC Interventions
Pain Management; Analgesia Administration; Distraction

Ongoing Assessment

Actions/Interventions	Rationales
■ Assess pain level and characteristics.	Assessment is important to determine type of pain patient is experiencing to aid in diagnosis and appropriate treatment.
■ Determine techniques that the patient considers useful in pain prevention or relief.	Patient responses to pain are highly varied and must be explored with each patient. The patient may have prior experiences with pain that can be useful in this situation.
■ Assess the degree to which pain interferes with the treatment plan.	Assessment guides level of treatment. Good pain control promotes increased feelings of well-being, increased ability to promote lung expansion, and increased mobility—all of which optimize recovery.

Therapeutic Interventions

Actions/Interventions	Rationales
■ Anticipate the need for pain medications and respond immediately to complaints of pain.	In the midst of pain, a patient's perception of time may become distorted. Prompt responses to complaints may reduce associated anxiety. Effective pain management facilitates ambulation and breathing exercises. Postoperative thoracotomy pain can be severe with the continued movement of respiratory muscles needed to maintain ventilation.
▲ Assist the patient as needed with patient-controlled analgesia (PCA) and assess its effectiveness.	The patient may be hesitant to use PCA effectively for fear of drug overdose. Likewise, the patient may not have full cognitive or manual ability to use PCA correctly.
■ Use nonpharmacological methods of pain management (e.g., positioning, distraction, touch).	These measures can promote comfort alone or in combination with medications.
■ Assist patient in splinting the chest with a pillow.	Splinting may promote comfort, reduce pain, and assist with effective coughing and deep breathing.
■ Provide scheduled rest periods.	Rest promotes comfort, sleep, and relaxation.

■ = Independent   ▲ = Collaborative

Deficient Knowledge

Common Related Factors

Unfamiliarity with postoperative thoracotomy care
Emotional state affecting learning

Defining Characteristics

Verbalizing inaccurate knowledge
Questioning members of health care team

Common Expected Outcome

Patient or significant others verbalize understanding of postoperative thoracotomy care.

NOC Outcomes
Knowledge: Disease Process; Knowledge: Treatment Regimen

NIC Interventions
Teaching: Disease Process; Teaching: Procedure/Treatment; Support System Enhancement

---

Ongoing Assessment

Actions/Interventions	Rationales
■ Assess knowledge of postoperative care and home recovery.	Postoperative patients may be overwhelmed by the amount of information for which they are responsible.
■ Determine knowledge of etiological factors of disease and need for behavior modification.	Changes in lifestyle (if needed) serve to protect remaining lung (e.g., avoidance of smoke, pollutants, inhalants).
■ Assess support system and knowledge of additional resources.	Specialized services may be required to meet specific needs.

Therapeutic Interventions

Actions/Interventions	Rationales
▲ Reinforce postoperative surgical routine and expected recovery course.	Information enables the patient to assume some control over events and enhances cooperation.
▲ Instruct to resume normal activities gradually (e.g., begin with short walks rather then stair climbing).	Information provides rationale for recovery plan and aids patient in assuming responsibility for care. An informed patient is more cooperative and successful.
■ Instruct the patient in administration, actions, and potential side effects of medications and/or home oxygen.	Medications promote comfort, which can enhance effective breathing patterns and early mobilization. Supplemental oxygen should be titrated to maintain an oxygen saturation of 90% or more. Oxygen is not combustible but can feed a fire if one occurs.
■ Instruct in use of Heimlich valve if used for home care.	The Heimlich valve is a one-way flutter valve that allows air from the pleural space to flow out through the tube with exhalation but prevents air from flowing into the chest during inhalation.
■ Instruct the patient or significant others to seek professional advice for dyspnea, fever, chills, unusual wound drainage, change in wound appearance, loss of appetite, or unintentional weight loss.	The patient needs to know when to seek health care advice for possible problems.
■ Refer the patient or significant others to smoking-cessation groups or support groups as appropriate.	Smoking cessation will improve clinical outcomes. Patient may be unaware of services available. Groups that come together for mutual support and information can be beneficial.

Actions/Interventions	Rationales
■ If surgery was treatment for lung cancer:	
• Instruct the patient or significant others about known causes of lung cancer and need for avoidance: cigarette smoking, air pollution, industrial pollutants.	Information helps in understanding environmental etiologies. Avoidance protects remaining lung and improves oxygenation. Respiratory irritants can cause bronchoconstriction with resultant irritating cough and rapid, shallow respiratory rate.
• Refer the patient to the American Cancer Society for informational support.	The ACS and many other sources have numerous teaching aids to support and reinforce learning. Patients may be unaware of services available for questions or problem resolution.

Related Care Plans

Anxiety, p. 18
Impaired physical mobility, p. 133
Lung cancer, p. 409
Pneumothorax with chest tube, p. 436
Risk for infection, p. 114

Tracheostomy

Artificial Airway; Tracheotomy

Tracheostomy is a surgical opening into the trachea that is used to prevent or relieve airway obstruction and/or to serve as an access for suctioning and for mechanical ventilation and other modes of oxygen delivery (i.e., tracheostomy collar, T-piece). A tracheostomy can facilitate weaning from mechanical ventilation by reducing dead space and lowering airway resistance. It also improves patient comfort by removing the endotracheal (ET) tube from the mouth or nose. The tracheostomy is preferred over an endotracheal tube when an artificial airway is needed for more than a few days. Methods can be instituted for the patient to eat and speak, as well. This care plan focuses on tracheostomy in the acute care setting, as well as the patient in a chronic care facility or with home care.

Ineffective Airway Clearance

Common Related Factors

Copious secretions
Thick secretions
Decreased energy and fatigue
Uncooperativeness
Confusion
Presence of artificial airway: tracheostomy

Defining Characteristics

Abnormal breath sounds (crackles, rhonchi)
Shortness of breath/dyspnea
Increased breathing effort: use of accessory muscles, intercostal retractions, nasal flaring
Ineffective cough
Tachypnea/changes in breathing pattern
Increasing restlessness and irritability
Change in level of consciousness
Pallor, cyanosis
Diaphoresis

■ = Independent   ▲ = Collaborative

Common Expected Outcome

Patient maintains a clear, open airway as evidenced by normal breath sounds, normal rate and depth of respiration, and ability to effectively cough up secretions.

NOC Outcome
Respiratory Status: Airway Patency
NIC Interventions
Airway Management; Cough Enhancement; Airway Suctioning; Artificial Airway Management

Ongoing Assessment

Actions/Interventions	Rationales
■ Assess for tachypnea, nasal flaring, and increased use of accessory muscles of respiration.	These abnormalities indicate respiratory compromise. An increase in respiratory rate and rhythm may be a compensatory response for airway obstruction. The breathing pattern may alter to include use of accessory muscles to increase chest excursion.
■ Assess changes in HR, BP, and temperature.	With initial hypoxia and hypercapnia, blood pressure (BP), heart rate (HR), and respiratory rate all rise. As the hypoxia and/or hypercapnia become severe, BP and HR drop. Fever may develop in response to retained secretions.
■ Auscultate lungs, noting areas of decreased ventilation and for presence of adventitious breath sounds.	Decreased or absent breath sounds may indicate the presence of a mucous plug or other airway obstruction; wheezing may indicate partial airway obstruction or narrowing; coarse crackles/rhonchi may indicate presence of secretions along larger airways.
■ Assess effectiveness of cough. Observe color, consistency, and quantity of secretions.	Abnormalities may be a result of infection, bronchitis, long-term smoking, or other conditions. A sign of infection is discolored sputum. Thick, tenacious secretions increase hypoxemia and may be indicative of dehydration.
■ Assess for changes in level of consciousness.	Increasing confusion, restlessness, and/or irritability can be early signs of cerebral hypoxia.

Therapeutic Interventions

Actions/Interventions	Rationales
▲ Provide warm, humidified air.	A tracheostomy bypasses the nose, which is the body area that humidifies and warms inspired air. A decrease in the humidity of the inspired air will cause secretions to thicken. Also, cool air may decrease ciliary function. Providing humidification of inspired air will prevent drying and crusting of secretions.
▲ Administer oxygen as needed.	Supplemental oxygen provides for adequate tissue oxygenation. Oxygen saturation should be kept at 90% or greater.
■ Encourage the patient to cough out secretions. If cough is ineffective, institute suctioning of airway as needed.	Coughing is the most helpful way to remove most secretions. The patient may be able to perform independently. Suctioning removes secretions if the patient is unable to effectively clear the airway. Frequent suctioning should be based on patient's clinical status, not on a present routine, such as every hour. Oversuctioning can cause hypoxia and injury to bronchial and lung tissue.
■ Transport the patient with portable oxygen, Ambu bag, suction equipment, and extra tracheostomy tube.	Being prepared for an emergency helps prevent future complications.

Risk for Impaired Gas Exchange

Common Risk Factors

Infection
Copious tracheal secretions
Inability to cough and deep breathe
Tracheostomy leak
Pneumothorax
Aspiration
Restricted lung expansion from immobility
Preexisting medical conditions

Common Expected Outcome

Patient maintains optimal gas exchange as evidenced by arterial blood gasses (ABGs) within the patient's normal range, oxygen saturation of 90% or greater, alert response mentation or no further reduction in level of consciousness, relaxed breathing, and baseline HR for patient.

NOC Outcome
Respiratory Status: Gas Exchange
NIC Interventions
Respiratory Monitoring; Oxygen Therapy

Ongoing Assessment

Actions/Interventions	Rationales
■ Assess HR and temperature, noting changes.	Tachycardia is associated with increased work of breathing or hypoxia. Fever may develop in response to retained secretions or atelectasis.
■ Assess respiratory rate, quality, rhythm, depth, and effort.	Patients will alter breathing patterns over time to facilitate gas exchange. Respiratory rate and rhythm changes are early warning signs of impending respiratory difficulties. Rapid, shallow breathing patterns affect gas exchange. Hypoxia is associated with increased breathing effort.
■ Assess for restlessness and changes in level of consciousness.	Increased restlessness, confusion, and/or irritability are early indicators of insufficient oxygenation of the brain and requires further intervention.
■ Auscultate lung sounds, noting areas of decreased ventilation or presence of adventitious sounds.	Changes in lung sounds may reveal the etiology of impaired gas exchange.
▲ Use pulse oximetry as appropriate to monitor oxygen saturation. Monitor ABGs, and note changes.	Pulse oximetry is a useful tool to detect changes in oxygenation. Oxygen saturation should be maintained at 90% or greater. Increasing $Paco_2$ and decreasing Pao_2 are signs of respiratory failure.
▲ Monitor effectiveness of tracheostomy cuff, and assess for signs of cuff leak (patient able to vocalize while cuff is supposed to be inflated, low pressure ventilator alarm sounding, loud upper airway noises audible, feeling air coming from around nose or mouth). Collaborate with the respiratory therapist, as needed, to determine cuff pressure.	Maximum recommended levels for cuff pressure range from 20 to 25 mm Hg (27 to 33 cm H_2O), or less, if the trachea can be sealed with less. Signs of cuff leak are caused by air escaping upward past the vocal cords instead of being directed to the lower airway.

■ = Independent   ▲ = Collaborative

Pulmonary Care Plans

Therapeutic Interventions

Actions/Interventions	Rationales
▲ If a leak is present: • Try to reinflate the cuff, checking the pilot tube and valve for leaks. • If unsuccessful, notify the physician. • If patient is being mechanically ventilated and is losing a large portion of the tidal volume because of a cuff leak, the tracheostomy tube will need to be replaced.	An intact cuff is required to ensure direction of air into bronchial airways.
■ Maintain adequate airway. If obstruction is suspected, troubleshoot as appropriate:	A patent airway is a priority.
• Move head and neck.	Moving head and neck corrects any kinking of the tube or malpositioning.
• Attempt to deflate cuff.	This maneuver is important if there is a possibility of a herniated cuff.
• Try to pass a suction catheter.	This is an attempt to aspirate a mucous plug and to assess for airway patency.
• Remove inner cannula, and replace with backup inner cannula.	A mucous plug can become lodged in the tube and obstruct the patient's airway.
• Remove and replace tracheostomy tube if all else is unsuccessful.	A new tube can restore airway patency.
■ Place the patient in semi-Fowler's to high-Fowler's position.	This position promotes full lung expansion and improved air exchange.
▲ Administer humidified oxygen as needed.	Humidification of oxygen. This maintains oxygenation and prevents drying of mucosal membranes.
■ If lung sounds are abnormal, use tracheal suction as needed.	Suctioning is indicated when patients are unable to remove secretions from airway by coughing because of weakness, thick mucus plugs, or excessive or tenacious mucus.
■ Ensure that smoke, aerosol spray, dust, whiskers, and so forth do not enter the trachea.	Chemical irritants and allergens can increase mucus production and bronchospasm.
▲ If pneumothorax is present, set up chest tube placement.	A chest tube evacuates air from the pleural cavity and reexpands the collapsed lung.

NANDA-I NDx **Risk for Infection**

Common Risk Factors

Surgical incision of tracheostomy
Increased secretions
Suctioning of airway

Common Expected Outcomes

Patient remains free of infection, as evidenced by normal temperature, normal sputum culture, normal WBC count, absence of purulent drainage around stoma, and breath sounds clear to auscultation.
Infection is recognized early to allow for prompt treatment.

NOC Outcomes

Immune Status; Risk Control; Tissue Integrity: Skin and Mucous Membranes

NIC Interventions

Infection Protection; Wound Care; Skin Surveillance

Pulmonary Care Plans

Ongoing Assessment

Actions/Interventions	Rationales
▲ Observe the stoma for erythema, exudates, odor, and crusting lesions. If present, culture stoma and notify the physician.	Culture and sensitivity reports guide antibiotic selection.
■ Assess skin integrity under tracheal ties.	This is a common site for infection and skin breakdown.
▲ Monitor white blood cell (WBC) count.	Rising WBC count indicates the body's efforts to combat pathogens.
■ Assess for fever.	Fever may be a manifestation of an infection or inflammatory process.

Therapeutic Interventions

Actions/Interventions	Rationales
■ Provide stoma care: • Clean area around stoma and under phalanges of tube with a swab of half-strength hydrogen peroxide. • If applicable, clean inner cannula with hydrogen peroxide; rinse with sterile water or saline solution. If disposable inner cannula is used, dispose of used inner cannula and replace with a new inner cannula of the correct size. • Keep stoma clean and dry by using a sterile gauze dressing around tracheostomy site. • Secure tracheostomy tube with twill tape, using a square knot on the side of the neck or specially designed foam tracheostomy ties.	Frequent stoma care is required for postoperative patients. Care for patients with long-term stoma placement is based on need.
■ Keep spare tracheostomy tube of same size and brand at bedside.	Being prepared for an emergency helps prevent future complications.
■ Keep tracheal obturator taped at head of bed for emergency use.	The tracheal obturator is used to reinsert the tracheostomy.
■ Maintain inflated tracheostomy cuff: • Immediately after operation • If patient is on mechanical ventilation • If patient is prone to regurgitate and aspirate; cuff should be deflated at other times to prevent tracheal erosion	Inflated cuff protects the airway and is required for mechanical ventilation. Patients are not able to vocalize while the cuff is properly inflated.
■ Do not allow secretions to pool around the stoma. Suction the area, or wipe with aseptic technique. Keep skin under tracheostomy ties and back of neck clean and dry.	These steps keep the stoma clean and dry. The back of the neck should be checked carefully in bedridden patients because secretions tend to flow to the back of the neck. Clean, dry skin helps prevent skin irritation.
■ Check tightness of tracheostomy ties.	Ties loose enough that one finger can be inserted between the patient and the ties help reduce skin breakdown.
▲ Use barrier creams or absorptive or hydrocolloid dressings around the tracheostomy and under its ties as needed.	These may be used to prevent or treat breakdown. Dressings that break apart when wet should not be placed near stoma to avoid particles entering the trachea.
▲ If signs of infection are present, apply topical antifungal or antibacterial agent, as ordered.	These agents are either toxic to the pathogen or retard its growth.

NDx Impaired Verbal Communication

Common Related Factor	Defining Characteristics
Tracheostomy	Difficulty in maintaining usual communication pattern Difficulty speaking Frustration

■ = Independent   ▲ = Collaborative

Common Expected Outcome

Patient uses a form of communication to get needs met and to relate effectively with persons and environment.

NOC Outcome
Communication: Expressive
NIC Intervention
Communication Enhancement: Speech Deficit

Ongoing Assessment

Actions/Interventions	Rationales
■ Assess the patient's communication ability.	Standard tracheostomy tubes allow the vocal cords to move, but no airflow passes over them if the cuff is inflated; therefore vocalization is not possible.
■ Assess for anxiety and fear of not being able to communicate needs.	The inability to communicate enhances a patient's sense of isolation and may promote a sense of helplessness.
■ Assess effectiveness of nonverbal communication methods.	Patient may use hand signals, facial expressions, and changes in body posture to communicate with others. However, others may have difficulty in interpreting these nonverbal techniques. Each new method needs to be assessed for effectiveness and altered as necessary.

Therapeutic Interventions

Actions/Interventions	Rationales
■ Provide a call light within easy reach at all times. Answer light promptly.	Prompt response decreases anxiety and feelings of helplessness.
■ Place patient in a room close to the nurse's station.	This ensures easy observation of the patient by nursing staff.
■ If patient is able to nod or speak "yes" or "no" answers, try to phrase questions so that patient can use these responses.	Patients can become easily frustrated when they cannot communicate in a simple manner.
■ Provide alternative methods for communicating, such as word-and-phrase cards, writing pad and pencil, hand gestures, or picture board for patients who are unable to write.	Providing a variety of communication aids allows the patient more channels through which information can be communicated.
■ Provide emotional support to patient and significant others.	Difficulties communicating are a source of frustration to all involved.
▲ Allow the patient time to communicate needs.	The nurse should set aside enough time to attend to all of the details of patient care. Care measures may take a longer time to complete in the presence of a communication deficit.
▲ Collaborate with the physician and speech therapist on possible use of "talking" tracheostomy tube (as appropriate).	The "talking" tracheostomy tube provides a port for compressed gas to flow in above the tracheostomy tube, allowing air for phonation.
▲ If the patient no longer requires mechanical ventilation, consider use of a Passy-Muir valve or fenestrated tracheostomy tube.	These adaptive devices can facilitate talking.

NDx Deficient Knowledge

Common Related Factor	Defining Characteristics
New procedure or intervention in hospital	Anxiety
	Lack of questioning
	Increased questioning
	Expressed need for more information

Common Expected Outcome

Patient or caregiver demonstrates knowledge and skills appropriate for tracheostomy care.

NOC Outcomes
Knowledge: Treatment Procedure; Knowledge: Treatment Regimen
NIC Interventions
Teaching: Disease Process; Teaching: Psychomotor Skill

Ongoing Assessment

Actions/Interventions	Rationales
■ Assess knowledge regarding purpose and care of a tracheostomy.	This information provides an important starting point in education.
■ Assess ability to manage care at home.	Both cognitive and technical skills are required for managing tracheostomy tubes.
■ Assess ability to respond to emergency situations.	This information is especially important, because lack of airway patency is a life-threatening problem.

Therapeutic Interventions

Actions/Interventions	Rationales
■ Discuss the patient's need of tracheostomy and its particular purpose.	Adults learn information that is important to them.
■ Provide instruction in sterile tracheostomy care and suctioning; include step-by-step care guidelines on the following: • How to suction • Use of twill tape and/or loop-and-pile fasteners • Cleaning of tracheostomy with or without disposable inner cannula • Cleaning around tracheostomy site	Information enables the patient to take control of his or her life. Long-term care may be the patient's responsibility. Clearly focused teaching allows the learner to concentrate more completely on material being discussed. The patient or caregiver can begin to acquire skills at a pace that is not overwhelming.
■ Provide information on reinsertion of tracheostomy tube.	The first tube change is done by the physician, usually at 7 days after the tracheostomy, because reinsertion may be difficult if the stoma is not mature or healed. Thereafter, the patient or caregiver should be taught step-by-step reinsertion instructions and should complete a return demonstration.
■ Instruct in the need to call health care provider if amount of secretions increases or change in color or characteristic occurs.	Changes could signify the presence of an infection.
■ Discuss the weaning process, as appropriate, with the use of fenestrated tracheostomy tubes, tracheostomy buttons, or progressively smaller tubes.	Preparation and explanation helps reduce anxiety.
■ Reinforce knowledge of the following emergency techniques: • Tracheostomy reinsertion (as appropriate) • Obtaining audiotape for home use that can be played when emergency service is called	Preparing ahead of time can reduce distress and complications. Patient will feel more secure in the home environment with a means for rapid communication in an emergency.
▲ Collaborate with case manager or social worker as appropriate to attain equipment and arrange for home care nurses.	Continuity of care is facilitated through the use of appropriate resources.

■ = Independent   ▲ = Collaborative

Actions/Interventions

■ Explain the process of decannulation, as appropriate.

■ Explain home care as follows:
- Stoma should be covered.

- Swimming is contraindicated.
- A loose scarf or shirt may be used over the tracheostomy site.

Rationales

When the patient's tracheostomy remains capped with the patient effectively maintaining own respirations and airway clearance, the tracheostomy tube can be removed. With removal, the stoma site is covered with a folded 4 × 4 bandage and tape. The opening will close in a few days. Until the site is healed, the patient should be instructed to cover the site with two fingers while attempting to cough or talk to prevent outward airflow through the stoma site.

Covering stoma prevents inhalation of foreign materials (e.g., shaving, makeup).
Aspiration is possible if water gets into the stoma.
This camouflages the area.

Related Care Plans

Disturbed body image, p. 24
Imbalanced nutrition: Less than body requirements, p. 142
Impaired verbal communication, p. 39
Pneumothorax with chest tube, p. 436
Risk for aspiration, p. 21

Tuberculosis

TB; Mycobacterium Tuberculosis

Patients infected with *Mycobacterium tuberculosis* (MTB) develop either latent TB infections or TB disease. Among adults, TB disease is usually confined to the respiratory tract. Everyone with TB disease needs antimicrobial therapy, as do people with latent TB infections who are at high risk for progressing to TB disease. Pulmonary TB disease is contagious, spread by airborne droplet nuclei that are produced when an infected person coughs or sneezes. Those at higher risk for development of clinical disease include the immunosuppressed (patients receiving cancer chemotherapy, patients infected with human immunodeficiency virus [HIV], patients with diabetes mellitus, adolescents, and patients younger than 2 years of age). Patients with latent TB infections may progress to TB disease. A reactivation can occur later in patients with decreased resistance, concomitant diseases, and immunosuppression. People are more likely to become infected with TB if they have consistent close contact with a person who has active disease. Crowded living arrangements contribute to disease transmission. Immigrants from countries where TB is common may have undiagnosed TB when they enter the United States. Other variables that increase the risk for infection with TB include older age, poverty, homelessness, and drug and alcohol abuse. There has been a recent resurgence of TB with the emergence of multidrug resistant TB (MDR-TB) and extremely drug-resistant (XDR-TB) strains of the bacillus. These drug-resistant strains of the disease are more common among people with HIV disease or inadequately treated TB or people who live in areas where these strains are endemic.

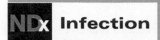 **Infection**

Common Related Factor

Pulmonary TB disease

Defining Characteristics

Purulent or bloody expectoration
Temperature spikes
Positive AFB culture report
Night sweats and chills
Cough, possibly nonproductive
Fatigue
Weight loss
Loss of appetite

Common Expected Outcomes

Patient's infection is effectively treated, as evidenced by negative acid-fast bacillus (AFB) culture report on reexamination and absence of fever.
Risk for spread of infection is reduced.

NOC Outcomes
Infection Status; Medication Response
NIC Interventions
Infection Control; Medication Administration

Ongoing Assessment

Actions/Interventions	Rationales
■ Assess color, consistency, and amount of sputum.	Yellow or yellow-green sputum is indicative of respiratory infection. Hemoptysis can be a sign of TB.
■ Monitor temperature.	Fever suggests infection. Patients with TB usually have low-grade fever with elevations in the late afternoon. Night sweats may accompany fever.
▲ Monitor AFB sputum cultures.	The MTB is an AFB. The AFB culture of sputum will be positive with active disease. Sputum cultures are repeated throughout treatment to determine whether antimicrobial drugs are effective based on drug-susceptibility testing.

Therapeutic Interventions

Actions/Interventions	Rationales
▲ Induce sputum with heated aerosol if needed to expedite diagnosis and start early treatment.	Precautions to prevent airborne transmission are important during and after procedures that stimulate coughing (e.g., sputum collection, bronchoscopy). These procedures need to be carried out in rooms designated for this with appropriate ventilation.
■ Maintain respiratory isolation.	Respiratory isolation is indicated until the patient responds to the medication (days to weeks). The Centers for Disease Control and Prevention (CDC) recommends airborne precautions to prevent transmission of TB. All health care workers who enter the patient's room should wear a National Institutes of Occupational Safety and Health (NIOSH) certified N95 or higher level respirator. The respirator needs to be properly fitted for each user to ensure a tight seal around the nose and mouth.

■ = Independent   ▲ = Collaborative

Actions/Interventions

- If available, use negative-airflow rooms for isolation.

- Keep tissues and sputum cups at bedside; dispose of secretions properly.
- Have patient cover mouth when coughing or sneezing.
- Use masks. Have anyone entering the patient's room wear a mask. If the patient is transported out of room for any reason, have the patient wear a mask.
- Keep the door to the patient's room closed at all times, and post an isolation sign where visible. Place respiratory isolation sticker on chart.
- Assist visitors with following appropriate isolation techniques.
- Teach patient hand-washing techniques to use after handling sputum.
- Provide a high-protein, high-calorie, increased-fluid diet.
- Refer patient contacts to be assessed for possible infection and for chemoprophylactic treatment.

▲ Administer medications as ordered.

▲ Monitor for side effects:

1. Isoniazid
   - Monitor baseline measurements of hepatic enzymes, and repeat measurements if baseline results are abnormal or if symptoms of adverse reactions occur. Ask about peripheral neuropathy.

Rationales

The MTB is a small droplet that remains infective over time and distance. Air currents leaving a standard patient room may be inhaled by persons who have not had direct contact with the infectious person. Negative-airflow rooms maintain the flow of air in the patient's room to prevent contaminated air from moving into hallways and surrounding areas. The room air is vented through special filters and eventually discharged to the outside, where it is rendered harmless by natural elements.

The disease spreads when droplets from the cough or sneeze are propelled in the air and deposited on nearby persons.

Covering mouth decreases airborne contaminants.

To be effective, the masks need to be designed to filter out droplet nuclei. Other masks are of limited value.

Private respiratory isolation rooms should be maintained with negative pressure to avoid spreading infected particles outward.

Following isolation techniques prevents spread of infection.

Friction and running water effectively remove microorganisms from hands.

This diet maintains optimal nutritional status.

Referral for TB testing helps prevent spread or development of infection. The area of induration of a Mantoux TB skin test that indicates a positive result depends on the patient's age, immune status, injection drug use, and HIV coinfection. Isoniazid (INH) prophylaxis is recommended for preventive TB therapy.

Anti-TB drug treatment should be promptly initiated for patients with TB disease. Choice of medications is based on drug-susceptibility testing. The primary drugs used are isoniazid (INH), rifampin (RIF), pyrazinamide (PZA), and ethambutol (EMB). Other drugs may be added for MDR-TB or XDR-TB strains. For patients taking anti-HIV drugs, rifabutin and rifapentine should replace rifampin.

Treatment of active disease usually consists of a combination therapy of these drugs in an attempt to increase the therapeutic effectiveness and decrease the development of resistant strains. Combination medications, such as Rifamate (isoniazid and rifampin) or Rifater (isoniazid, rifampin, and pyrazinamide) may improve adherence to therapy, but they make side effects and drug interactions more difficult to evaluate. Patients on anti-TB therapy should be monitored monthly for drug side effects, for infectiousness, and for clinical and bacteriological response to therapy.

Potential adverse reactions for this drug include hepatic enzyme elevation, hepatitis, peripheral neuropathy, mild effects on central nervous system, and drug interactions. Hepatitis risk increases with age and alcohol consumption. Pyridoxine can prevent peripheral neuropathy.

Actions/Interventions

2. Rifampin
   - Monitor baseline complete blood count, platelets, and hepatic enzymes. Repeat measurements if baseline is abnormal or if symptoms of adverse reaction occur. Ask about rash and GI symptoms.

3. Pyrazinamide
   - Monitor baseline uric acid and hepatic enzymes. Repeat measurements if baseline is abnormal or if symptoms of adverse reaction occur. Ask about joint pain.
4. Ethambutol
   - Monitor baseline and monthly tests for visual acuity and color vision.
▲ Monitor interactions with the patient's other medications.

■ Report all confirmed TB cases to the health department.

Rationales

Potential adverse reactions for this drug include gastrointestinal upset, drug interactions, hepatitis, bleeding problems, influenza-like symptoms, and rash. This drug colors body fluids orange and may permanently discolor soft contact lenses. There are interactions associated with oral contraceptives, which may be rendered ineffective by accelerating estrogen metabolism.

Adverse reactions include hepatitis, rash, gastrointestinal upset, joint aches, hyperuricemia, and gout.

Adverse reactions include optic neuritis.

Older patients are more susceptible to drug interactions because of decreased liver function and chronic conditions. People treated for HIV infection need careful monitoring to manage drug interactions.
Reporting enables coordination of follow-up care and contact investigation to facilitate prophylaxis for patient contacts.

NANDA-I NDx **Ineffective Breathing Pattern**

Common Related Factors
Frequent productive cough and hemoptysis
Decreased energy/fatigue
Decreased lung volumes
Inflammatory response
Increased metabolism as result of high fever

Defining Characteristics
Tachypnea
Dyspnea/orthopnea
Respiratory depth changes
Use of accessory muscles
Nasal flaring
Retractions
Tachycardia

Common Expected Outcome
Patient will maintain effective breathing pattern, as evidenced by relaxed breathing at normal rate and depth and absence of dyspnea.

NOC Outcome
Respiratory Status: Ventilation
NIC Intervention
Respiratory Monitoring

Ongoing Assessment

Actions/Interventions
■ Assess respiratory rate, rhythm, depth, and effort.

Rationales
Respiratory rate and rhythm changes are early warning signs of impending respiratory difficulties. Symptoms may be masked by chronic respiratory conditions common among older adults. Hypoxia is associated with increased breathing effort.

■ = Independent ▲ = Collaborative

Actions/Interventions

- Assess cough and effectiveness. Assess nature of secretions: color, amount, consistency.

- Auscultate lungs for presence of normal and adventitious breath sounds.
- Observe for retractions, flaring of nostrils, and use of accessory muscles with breathing.

- Monitor temperature, noting times of spikes.
- ▲ Use pulse oximetry to monitor oxygen saturation; assess arterial blood gases (ABGs) as indicated.

Rationales

The cough typically becomes frequent and productive; it may be accompanied by chest pain during coughing. Hemoptysis may be present in advanced cases.

Bronchial breath sounds and crackles may be present.

Work of breathing increases greatly as lung compliance decreases. As moving air in and out of lung becomes more difficult, the breathing pattern alters to include use of accessory muscles to increase chest excursion. Retractions or nasal flaring signify an increase in respiratory effort.

Low-grade fever occurs, especially in the afternoon.

Pulse oximetry is a useful tool to detect changes in oxygenation. Oxygen saturation should be at 90% or greater.

Therapeutic Interventions

Actions/Interventions

- ▲ Maintain oxygen saturation 90% or greater.

- Promote hydration and fluid balance.
- Maintain semi-Fowler's position.

- Assist the patient with coughing, changing position, and deep breathing.
- Plan activity and rest to maximize the patient's energy.

Rationales

Oxygen saturation less than 90% can lead to tissue hypoxia, acidosis, dysrhythmias, and change in level of consciousness.

Hydration liquefies secretions for easy expectoration.

A sitting position allows for adequate diaphragmatic and lung excursion and chest expansion.

These maneuvers improve productivity of the cough.

Activity increases metabolic rate and oxygen requirements. Rest helps mobilize energy for more effective breathing and coughing efforts.

NANDA-I NDx Ineffective Therapeutic Regimen Management

Common Related Factors

Complexity of therapeutic regimen
Knowledge deficit of prescribed regimen
Patient value system: health and spiritual beliefs, cultural beliefs, and cultural influences
Long-term therapy
Lack of motivation
Patient and provider relationship
Financial difficulty
Language barriers
Social support deficits

Defining Characteristics

Verbalized difficulty with prescribed regimen
Verbalization by patient that he or she did not follow prescribed regimen
Increased illness symptoms/resistance to treatment
- TB reactivation shown on chest x-ray and sputum examination
- Poor nutritional status: signs of malnutrition, not feeling well
- Drug-resistant organism seen on culture and sensitivity testing

Common Expected Outcomes

Patient verbalizes intention to follow prescribed regimen.
Patient demonstrates ongoing adherence to plan.
Patient identifies appropriate resources.

NOC Outcomes

Compliance Behavior; Knowledge: Treatment Regimen; Adherence Behavior

NIC Interventions

Health System Guidance; Surveillance; Teaching: Disease Process

Ongoing Assessment

Actions/Interventions	Rationales
■ Assess the patient for evidence of noncompliance: weight loss; increased coughing; thick, green-gray purulent sputum; drug-resistant organism on culture and sensitivity testing.	These are potential clues suggesting lack of improvement in condition that could be related to noncompliance.
■ Identify the cause of noncompliance, including understanding of treatment; importance of compliance; and financial, emotional, cognitive, and language barriers.	To be effective, interventions need to be patient specific and address individual concerns. Language barriers and cultural influences may be strong among foreign-born patients.
■ Conduct pill counts.	Pill counts provide some objective evidence of compliance.
■ Review laboratory results for expected changes associated with medication side effects.	Specific manifestations may alert health care providers to drug noncompliance.
■ Monitor for expected signs and symptoms, such as orange-stained urine associated with certain medication side effects.	This strategy provides some objective evidence of drug compliance for specific medications.

Therapeutic Interventions

Actions/Interventions	Rationales
■ Teach the patient the following:	A patient with knowledge of disease will be more likely to be compliant with the treatment regimen.
• Detection, transmission, signs, or symptoms of relapse	Individuals may experience relapse and so should be taught to recognize the possible recurrence of TB and to seek immediate medical attention.
• Treatment and length of therapy	Patients may require drugs for 6 months or longer.
• Prevention of spread of infection to others	Persons most susceptible are those in close contact during the infectious period. After 2 to 3 weeks of effective medication therapy, patients showing signs of clinical improvement may no longer be infectious.
• Importance of compliance with therapy	Compliance is key to halt progression of disease and promote suppression of infection.
• Health regimen to follow after discharge: clinic appointments, sources of free medication, resource telephone numbers	Long-term follow-up is required.
■ Discuss importance of following therapeutic regimen.	Most treatment failures result from patients prematurely stopping the medication, taking the medication irregularly, or failing to take the medication at all. If the patient cannot adhere to a medication regimen, a responsible person should be designated to administer the medication. The patient should be instructed in the likelihood of developing a multidrug-resistant strain of TB if medications are not taken as prescribed.
■ Suggest formulations that combine two to three medications to decrease pill burden.	The greater number of times during the day the patient needs to take medications, the greater the risk for not following through. Polypharmacy is a recognized barrier.
■ Refer noncompliant patients for directly observed therapy programs.	Such a program may be required as a means to enhance adherence and optimal management of TB.
■ Review potential side effects of treatment:	
• Drug side effects: nausea; loss of appetite; vomiting; persistent, dark urine; yellow skin; malaise; unexplained fever for more then 3 days; or abdominal tenderness.	All patients taking isoniazid, rifampin, or pyrazinamide need to report immediately any symptoms suggesting hepatitis.
• The need to abstain from alcohol while on isoniazid.	Alcohol increases the incidence of hepatitis.
• The need to obtain an eye examination monthly while on ethambutol.	The major side effect is reduced visual acuity.

■ = Independent ▲ = Collaborative

Actions/Interventions

- Rifampin may accelerate the clearance of drugs metabolized by the liver, including methadone, warfarin sodium (Coumadin), glucocorticoids, estrogens, oral hypoglycemic agents, digitalis, anticonvulsants, ketoconazole, fluconazole, a cyclosporine, and anti-HIV medications, especially protease inhibitors.
- Women taking rifampin should use an alternative birth control method other than oral contraceptives or contraceptive implants.
- Rifabutin and rifapentine cause harmless orange-stained tears, saliva, and urine.

■ Adapt respiratory isolation techniques to home environment:
- Have the patient cover mouth when coughing or sneezing.
- Teach appropriate use of tissues and to dispose of secretions properly.
- Teach the patient to wash hands after coughing or sneezing.

■ Explain the importance of good nutrition while taking TB medications.

■ Review possible individual risk factors that may reactivate TB (e.g., malnutrition, alcoholism, immunosuppression, diabetes mellitus, and cancer).

■ Encourage the patient to abstain from smoking. Provide smoking-cessation resources.

▲ Arrange for social service involvement for the patient and family.

Rationales

Persons co-infected with HIV may need alternative treatments or dosage adjustments of anti-TB and anti-HIV medications.

Rifampin may render oral contraceptives ineffective by accelerating estrogen metabolism.

Most family members at home have been exposed; however, respiratory safeguards are indicated until medication therapy suppresses the infectious phase.

Meeting the patient's metabolic needs will decrease fatigue and help the patient build resistance.

Any conditions that lower one's immune defenses can result in reactivation of the disease.

Continued smoking in the face of significant respiratory infection and disease may hasten the patient's death. There are numerous resources and supports to assist the patient in quitting smoking.

Continuity of care is facilitated through the use of these services.

Related Care Plans

Activity intolerance, p. 8
Imbalanced nutrition: Less than body requirements, p. 142

Neurological Care Plans

Alzheimer's Disease/Dementia

Multi-Infarct Dementia (MID); Dementia of the Alzheimer Type (DAT)

Dementia is characterized by a progressive impairment of cognitive function, personality, and behavior. The person with dementia experiences loss of memory, orientation, language skills, concentration, and judgment. In advanced stages, the person experiences behavior and personality changes such as aggressiveness, mood swings, wandering, and confusion. These changes interfere with the person's ability to carry out role responsibilities and activities of daily living. The causes of dementia are numerous and include degenerative disorders of the nervous system, vascular disorders, and autoimmune disorders. Multi-infarct dementia (MID) develops in people who have sustained brain injury from multiple strokes. This type of irreversible dementia occurs more often in men than women. People in the later stages of acquired immunodeficiency syndrome (AIDS) may develop dementia. Alcoholism and Parkinson's disease are known to contribute to dementia.

Alzheimer's disease (AD) is an irreversible disease of the central nervous system that manifests as a cognitive disorder. Onset is usually between 50 and 60 years and is characterized by progressive deterioration of memory and cognitive function. Disease progression begins with memory impairment, speech and motor difficulties, disorientation of time and place, impaired judgment, memory loss, forgetfulness, and inappropriate affect (lasts 2 to 4 years), followed by loss of independence, complete disorientation, wandering, hoarding, communication difficulties, complete memory loss (lasts up to 7 years), and the final stage with blank expression, irritability, seizures, emaciation, and absolute dependence (in the last year) until death. The estimated total duration of the disease is 14 years.

Although the cause is unknown, research has found specific genetic loci associated with the development of AD. Chronic inflammation, stroke, and cellular damage from free radicals have been identified as risk factors for AD. Drug therapy for Alzheimer's disease includes cholinesterase inhibitors and NMDA (N-methyl-D-aspartate) antagonists. These drugs have been shown to delay the progression of cognitive impairment in the patient. Some patients may experience improved memory function with these drugs.

This care plan addresses needs for patients with a wide variety of dementia, of which Alzheimer's is a type. Focus is on the home care setting.

Risk for Violence: Self-Directed or Other-Directed

Common Risk Factors

Impaired perception of reality
Impaired frustration tolerance
Decreased self-esteem
Perceived threat to self
Alteration in sleep or rest pattern
Impaired self-expression (verbal and nonverbal)
Anxiety
Impaired coping skills
Decreased sense of personal boundaries
Drug intoxication or idiosyncratic reaction
Physical discomfort
Overstimulation

Common Expected Outcomes

Patient avoids self-directed harm.
Patient does not harm others.

NOC Outcomes

Aggression Control; Cognitive Ability; Mood
Equilibrium; Risk Control

NIC Interventions

Mood Enhancement; Environmental Management: Violence Prevention

---

Ongoing Assessment

Actions/Interventions	Rationales
■ Assess cognitive factors that may contribute to development of violent behaviors, including the following: • Decreased ability to solve problems • Alteration in sensory and perceptual capacities • Impairment in judgment • Psychotic or delusional thought patterns • Impaired concentration or decreased response to redirection	Factors may indicate decline in cognitive condition. The patient may become overresponsive to environmental stimuli, leading to agitation and combativeness. The patient may have poor impulse behavior control. Decreased attention span and memory loss can contribute to the person's inability to respond to environmental stimuli.
■ Assess physical factors that may foster violence: physical discomfort, such as being wet or cold, and sensory overload (overstimulation), such as noise.	Correcting physical factors will decrease stimulation and may decrease confusion. Patients with Alzheimer's disease may experience increased confusion, restlessness, and agitation in the late afternoon and early evening. These changes are called sundowner's syndrome. The increased confusion may be related to anxiety that occurs in response to an accumulation of sensory stimuli during the day, fatigue, or an inability to see in the dark.
■ Assess emotional factors that can lead to violence: inability to cope with frustrating situations, expressions of low self-esteem, noncompliance with treatment plan, and history of aggressive behaviors as a means of coping with stress.	Thorough assessment of precipitating factors is needed so that preventive measures can be instituted.
■ Evaluate impact of medication regimen on behaviors in terms of contribution to agitation.	Neuroleptics (e.g., loxapine) and antipsychotics (e.g., haloperidol) may cause extrapyramidal side effects, manifested as restlessness.

Therapeutic Interventions

Actions/Interventions	Rationales
■ Involve the patient on a cognitive level as much as possible. Instruct the caregiver in the following techniques. Begin with least restrictive measures, and progress to most restrictive measures.	This approach allows the patient some measure of control over the environment and may increase the patient's co-operation with caregivers.

Level I:

Nonaggressive behaviors: may include wandering or pacing, restlessness or increased motor activity, climbing out of bed, changing clothes or disrobing, hand wringing or hand washing.

■ Give verbal feedback, and institute interpersonal approaches.	At this level of dementia, the patient may still have insight about the losses he or she is experiencing.
■ Initiate measures such as reorientation, reduced stimuli, and consistent schedules.	Sensory stimulation needs to be reduced. Frequent reorientation to one's environment increases one's ability to trust others. Consistency in schedules and the physical environment promotes orientation and reduces anxiety.
■ Speak in slow, clear, soothing tones. Make comments brief and to the point. Repeat as needed.	Attention to technique helps avoid communication conflicts. The patient may have declines in short-term memory that require frequent repetition of new information.
■ Use distraction.	Impaired short-term memory may allow introduction of new stimuli to calm agitated behavior.

Level II:

Verbally aggressive behaviors: may include cursing, yelling, screaming, unintelligible or repetitious speech, and threats or accusations.

■ Attempt verbal control; attempt feedback about behavior (for less cognitively impaired), distraction (for cognitively impaired), or limit setting (although this may increase agitation at times).	These techniques can decrease sensory stimuli.
■ If feasible, allow the patient more personal space.	If the patient's memory span is short, leaving the room briefly may decrease his or her agitation.
■ Acknowledge fear of loss of control; evaluate use of touch and hand holding.	Touch may be calming to some and aggravating to others.
■ If the patient wanders or paces, consider the need to provide visual supervision, especially if the patient expresses the need to leave.	Providing for safety is a priority. Doors to the outside may need to be locked to prevent the person from leaving.
■ Provide diversional activity (e.g., folding towels, handling worry beads, walking with the patient).	These activities may assist in increasing the patient's feelings of self-worth and meet his or her need for activity. Repetitive activities can reduce agitation and provide a release of energy.

Level III:

Physically aggressive behaviors: may include hitting, kicking, spitting or biting, throwing objects, pushing or pulling others, and fighting.

■ Permit verbalization of feelings associated with agitation.	Verbalization of feelings may diffuse aggressive behavior.
■ Offer acceptable alternatives to unacceptable behaviors, such as undressing in public, by allowing the patient to select his or her own clothing.	Providing the patient some control over the environment may diffuse perceptions of threats in the environment.
■ If the patient poses a potential threat of injury to self or others, consider use of soft physical restraints, such as cloth wrist, hand, leg, belt, or vest type restraints.	As initial measures become ineffective, more extreme measures may be indicated to ensure safety of the patient or caregiver.
■ Initiate safety measures such as drawer and cabinet locks in the bathroom and kitchen.	This action reduces the patient's access to hazardous items.
■ Use pharmaceutical restraints, such as antidepressants (amitriptyline) or antipsychotics (haloperidol), only if agitation has reached a point where soft restraints are inadequate to protect the patient from injury.	Medication may be indicated to decrease potential risk for injury.

■ = Independent ▲ = Collaborative

Neurological Care Plans

NANDA-I NDx Self-Care Deficit: Bathing, Grooming, Feeding

Common Related Factors

Impaired memory
Disorientation
Impaired judgment
Impaired sense of social self

Defining Characteristics

Requires assistance with at least one of the following: bathing, oral hygiene, dressing or grooming, feeding
Denies need for personal hygiene measures
Refuses to change clothes or wears more than one set of clothing
Unable to assist in personal care because of motor deficits or confusion

Common Expected Outcome

Patient participates in self-care activities, as evidenced by appropriately dressing, bathing, and feeding self.

NOC Outcome

Self-Care: Bathing, Grooming, Eating

NIC Intervention

Self-Care Assistance: Bathing, Grooming, Feeding

Ongoing Assessment

Actions/Interventions	**Rationales**
■ Assess cognitive deficits or behaviors that would create difficulty in bathing self, performing oral hygiene, selecting and putting on appropriate clothing, choosing food menu items, and feeding self. ■ Assess level of independence in completing self-care.	In the early stages of the disease, the patient may have problems with forgetfulness, information processing, and the retrieval of information necessary to make decisions about self-care activities. The patient with impaired thought processes is unable to self-monitor personal grooming, hygiene, and nutrition needs adequately. The nurse needs to reassess the patient's self-care ability at regular intervals to provide assistance for the patient and caregivers.

Therapeutic Interventions

Actions/Interventions	**Rationales**
Instruct the caregiver in strategies to facilitate self care activities as in the following:	
■ Stay with the patient during self-care activities if his or her judgment is impaired.	This approach promotes safety and provides necessary redirection.
■ Allow enough time in quiet environment; limit distractions.	Rushing promotes frustration and failure. Distractions interrupt the patient's concentration when performing an activity.
■ Follow established routines for self-care, if possible, or develop a routine that is consistently followed.	An established routine becomes rote and requires less decision making.
■ Provide a simple, easy-to-read, large-print list of self-care activities to complete each day (e.g., brush teeth, comb hair).	Reminders may enhance functional abilities.
■ Assist, as needed, with perineal care each morning and evening (or after each episode of incontinence).	Poor hygiene after elimination increases the risk for skin breakdown.
■ Assist, as needed, in selecting clothing. Allow the patient to choose if possible (e.g., put out two or three sets of clothing and allow a choice).	Giving the patient some control over the environment reduces anxiety.

Actions/Interventions

- Encourage the patient to dress as independently as possible. Provide easy-to-wear clothes (elastic waistbands, snaps, large buttons, loop-and-pile closures).
- Assist in selecting nutritious, high-bulk foods. Allow the patient to choose foods he or she prefers, if possible.
- Assist in setup of meal as needed (e.g., open containers, cut food).
- If judgment is impaired, cool down hot liquids to palatable temperatures before serving.
- Limit number of choices of food on plate or tray.

- Provide easy-to-eat finger foods if motor coordination is impaired. Provide nutritious between-meal snacks if nutritional intake is inadequate.
- If the patient has difficulty with complex tasks: break the task into smaller steps; use calm, unhurried voice to offer praise and encouragement.

Rationales

It is important for the patient to maintain functional ability for as long as possible.

These measures promote adequate intake.

Easy access promotes better nutritional intake.

This measure is necessary to avoid injury.

It is important to reduce the number of decisions that the patient is required to make.

This approach promotes meeting the patient's nutritional needs.

Disorientation and impaired memory can limit the person's ability to process information and respond appropriately to directions and environmental stimuli. These techniques make it easier for the person to participate in self-care activities.

NANDA-I NDx

Impaired Social Interaction

Common Related Factors

Impaired sense of social self
Memory deficits
Disturbed thought processes
Social isolation
Impaired judgment

Defining Characteristics

Dysfunctional interactions with others
Family reports of changes in interaction
Use of unsuccessful social interaction behaviors

Common Expected Outcome

Patient engages in social interaction, as evidenced by positive contacts with caregiver or significant others.

NOC Outcome
Social Involvement
NIC Intervention
Socialization Enhancement

Ongoing Assessment

Actions/Interventions

- Assess cognitive deficits or behaviors that interfere with forming relationships with others.
- Assess previous patterns of interaction.

- Assess potential to interact in a community day care situation.

Rationales

As disease progresses, ability to maintain attention and memory deteriorates. Behavior may be socially unacceptable.
Ability and/or willingness to interact may vary with the patient's mood, perceptions, and reality orientation.
Confusion, disorientation, and loss of social inhibitions may result in socially inappropriate and/or harmful behavior to self or others. Programs vary in capacity for handling patients in late stages of dementia of Alzheimer's type (DAT).

■ = Independent ▲ = Collaborative

Therapeutic Interventions

Actions/Interventions	Rationales
■ Within the context of the nurse-patient relationship, provide regular opportunity for frequent, brief contacts.	Being present demonstrates caring and provides the patient with an opportunity for social interaction.
■ Discuss subjects in which the patient is interested but which do not require short-term recall.	Interactions that require short-term recall become difficult and frustrating for the patient.
■ When discussing past experiences, assist the patient in connecting them with here-and-now.	Past coping strategies may assist with current situations. Reminiscence promotes long-term memory skills and can relieve depression.
■ Assist the caregiver in doing the following:	
• Support participation in social activities appropriate to the patient's level of cognitive functioning, such as small family parties.	Large gatherings become more problematic as symptoms intensify. The patient may not be able to tolerate excessive stimuli in large gatherings.
• Redirect the patient when behaviors become socially embarrassing or the patient expresses delusional ideas.	The patient's short-term memory loss allows the nurse to redirect the patient's behavior and thinking and promote reality orientation.
• Do not correct the patient's ideas or confront them as delusional.	Challenges to the patient's thinking can be perceived as threatening. The confused patient may become anxious and agitated.
• Consider impact of environment on social interaction. Avoid an overstimulating environment (noise, lights, activity).	Sensory overload aggravates impaired cognitive thinking.
• Involve the patient in developing a daily schedule that includes time for social activity, as well as quiet time.	The patient is more likely to participate in activities that match his or her talents, interests, and abilities. A schedule that includes activities interspersed with rest periods allows the patient to have energy for social interaction.
■ Provide information on community day care programs that will help the patient maintain social interaction.	Involvement with group activities is determined by various factors, including group size, activity level, and the patient's tolerance level. Fluctuations in mood and affect may influence ability to respond appropriately to others. Adult day care also provides needed respite for the caregiver.

NANDA-I NDx Impaired Home Maintenance

Common Related Factors

Impaired memory
Disorientation
Impaired judgment

Defining Characteristics

Disorientation in familiar surroundings
Need for supervision in potentially hazardous situations
Family caregiver concerns about caring for the patient at home

Common Expected Outcomes

Caregiver or family provides safe home environment.
Caregiver or family describes nursing or community resources available for home care.

NOC Outcomes

Family Functioning; Safety Behavior: Home Physical Environment; Self-Care: Instrumental Activities of Daily Living

NIC Interventions

Family Support; Self-Care Assistance; Home Maintenance Assistance

Ongoing Assessment

Actions/Interventions	**Rationales**
■ Assess cognitive deficits to determine safety needs.	Impaired judgment can limit the patient's ability to live without supervision.
■ Assess ability to recognize danger (smoke, fire).	Cognitive impairment limits the patient's ability to perceive potential threats in the environment.
■ Assess frequency of disorientation, wandering, becoming lost in familiar surroundings.	These behaviors are the most frequent reason given by family members for placing the patient in a closely supervised care setting.
■ Assess the family's or caregiver's understanding of the patient's needs or deficits, resources to provide adequate supervision and behavior management, the family's ability to cope, and internal or external support systems.	Thorough assessment is needed to determine potential problems and complications.
■ Determine adequacy of the home environment.	Social services agencies can provide help in determining whether patients can live in their home safely.

Therapeutic Interventions

Actions/Interventions	**Rationales**
■ Involve the patient, family, or caregiver in all home planning.	In initial stages, the patient will be able to contribute to care decisions and should not be excluded from home planning.
■ Discuss need to wear identification bracelet at all times.	This approach allows patients to be identified quickly if they become lost.
■ Suggest daily supervised exercise or a walking program.	Structured activity may decrease wandering behavior and meet the patient's need for exercise.
■ Identify and encourage correction of obstacles and hazards in the home.	Ensuring environmental safety is a priority.
■ Provide information about home security devices, such as keyed door locks and audible alarms.	Attention to security measures may decrease wandering behavior.
■ Recommend procedures for getting help (e.g., calling police, notifying neighbors) in case the patient becomes lost.	Caregivers need to have up-to-date photographs and physical description information readily available for people who will search for the lost patient.
■ Help the family identify and mobilize available support networks such as home health services, church groups, and senior citizens organizations.	A network of family members, friends, and community resources can facilitate home patient care. Using these services promotes independence and reduces caregiver burden.
■ Provide information about support groups available to family members.	Support groups often have the best practical tips and suggestions.
■ Provide literature and references related to caring for cognitively impaired persons in the home.	The Alzheimer Association has a broad range of resources to help families and caregivers.

NANDA-I NDx **Caregiver Role Strain**

Common Related Factors	**Defining Characteristics**
Knowledge deficit regarding management of care	Expresses difficulty in performing patient care
Personal and social life disrupted by demands of caregiving	Verbalizes anger with responsibility of patient care
Multiple competing roles	States that formal and informal support systems are inadequate
No respite from caregiver demands	Expresses problems in coping with patient's behavior
Unaware of available community resources	Expresses negative feeling about patient or relationship
Reluctant to use community resources	Neglects patient care
Community resources not available	
Community resources not affordable	

■ = Independent ▲ = Collaborative

Common Expected Outcomes

Caregiver demonstrates competence and confidence in performing the caregiver role by meeting care recipient's physical and psychosocial needs.

Caregiver verbalizes positive feelings about care recipient and their relationship.

Caregiver reports that formal and informal support systems are adequate and helpful.

NOC Outcomes
Caregiver Well-Being; Caregiver-Patient Relationship
NIC Intervention
Caregiver Support

Ongoing Assessment

Actions/Interventions	Rationales
■ Assess caregiver-care recipient relationship.	Mutually rewarding relationships foster therapeutic care-giving experience. Dysfunctional relationships can result in ineffective, fragmented care or even lead to neglect or abuse.
■ Assess family communication pattern.	Open communication among all family members creates a positive environment, whereas concealing feelings creates problems for the caregiver and care recipient.
■ Assess family resources and support systems.	Family and social support is related positively to coping effectiveness. Some cultures are more accepting of this responsibility. However, factors such as blended family units, aging parents, geographical distances between family members, and limited financial resources may hamper coping effectiveness.
■ Determine the caregiver's knowledge and ability to provide patient care, including bathing, skin care, safety, nutrition, medications, and ambulation.	Basic instruction may reduce caregiver anxiety and improve the relationship. Caregiver frustration can lead to anger directed toward the patient. These emotions may result in verbal or physical abuse or neglect of the patient.

Therapeutic Interventions

Actions/Interventions	Rationales
■ Provide information on disease process and management strategies.	Accurate information increases understanding of the care recipient's condition and behavior, including the knowledge that regardless of the quality of care, the disease will progress and care requirements will continually increase. Families need to understand the importance of consistency when caring for the person with dementia.
■ Encourage the caregiver to identify available family and friends who can assist with care giving.	Respite care helps family members cope with the burden of care. As the patient's cognitive function declines, he or she requires more hours of direct supervision. Nighttime wandering may keep family members from getting adequate sleep.
■ Suggest that the caregiver use available community resources such as respite care, home health care, adult day care, and Alzheimer's Association	Resources provide opportunity for multiple competent providers and services on a temporary basis or for a more extended period. Using these resources may allow family members to continue job responsibilities and other family activities.
▲ Consult a social worker for referral for community resources and/or financial aid, if needed.	The family may need guidance in planning for long-term care, estate planning, powers of attorney, and living wills for the patient.
■ Encourage the caregiver to set aside time for self.	The caregiver may need reminders to attend to own physical and emotional needs. Having own "respite" time helps conserve physical and emotional energy. Simple activities such as a relaxing bath, time to read a book, or going out with friends help to maintain physical and mental wellbeing.

Actions/Interventions

- Acknowledge to the caregiver his or her role and its value.

Rationales

Caregivers have identified how important it is to feel appreciated for their efforts. The patient may not be able to express this himself or herself.

Related Care Plans

Chronic confusion, p. 43
Insomnia, p. 117
Impaired memory, p. 130
Ineffective coping, p. 49

Carpal Tunnel Syndrome

Repetitive Stress Injury; Median Nerve Compression

Carpal tunnel syndrome develops when the median nerve is compressed as it passes through the wrist to the hand. The carpal tunnel is an anatomical canal that is located between the bones of the hand and a band of fibrous tissue. This tissue protects the tendons of the wrist during movement of the joint. Inflammation of the synovium of the joint causes swelling, pain, and paresthesia. The swelling contributes to narrowing of the tunnel and compression of the median nerve. The pain and paresthesia occurs most often in the thumb, index finger, middle finger, and radial aspect of the ring finger. Chronic median nerve compression may lead to progressive weakness and loss of fine motor control in the hand. Muscle atrophy may develop over time. This disorder has a high prevalence among people in occupations that involve repeated and prolonged flexion of the wrist. Carpal tunnel syndrome is becoming a common occupational repetitive stress injury. Other situations that are known to contribute to carpal tunnel syndrome include burn injuries of the hand, wrist fractures, rheumatoid arthritis, and diabetes mellitus. Women are more likely to develop carpal tunnel syndrome than men. This gender difference is thought to be related to the smaller size of the carpal tunnel in women. Medical management of carpal tunnel syndrome includes splinting of the joint, drug therapy to reduce inflammation and pain, and modification of activities to restrict harmful movement. Surgery is done when prolonged nerve compression is severe and associated with muscle atrophy and progressive loss of motor and sensory function.

 Acute Pain

Common Related Factors

Median nerve compression
Wrist inflammation
Repeated and prolonged joint flexion

Defining Characteristics

Pain relieved by shaking the hands
Pain at night
Numbness and tingling of the fingers
Burning sensation in the fingers

Common Expected Outcomes

Patient reports satisfactory pain control at a level of less than 3 to 4 on a 0 to 10 rating scale.
Patient uses pharmacological and nonpharmacological pain relief strategies.
Patient exhibits increased comfort such as baseline levels for pulse, blood pressure, respirations, and relaxed muscle tone or body posture.

NOC Outcomes

Comfort Status; Medication Response; Pain Control

NIC Interventions

Analgesic Administration; Pain Management

■ = Independent   ▲ = Collaborative

Ongoing Assessment

Actions/Interventions	Rationales

■ Assess pain characteristics:
  • Quality (e.g., sharp, burning, shooting)
  • Severity (scale of 0 [meaning no pain] to 10 [most severe pain]
  • Location and radiation
  • Onset (gradual or sudden)
  • Duration (how long; intermittent or continuous)
  • Associated or related symptoms
  • Precipitating or relieving factors
	The patient may report pain in the fingers, especially at night. The pain may be relieved initially by shaking the hands. As the nerve compression progresses, the patient may report numbness, tingling, and daytime pain. The patient may report pain radiating from the wrist to the shoulder. Weakness in the hand with decreased grip strength may occur with carpal tunnel syndrome. Activities that involve repeated flexion of the wrist may aggravate the pain and paresthesias. The patient may identify occupational activities such as using a computer keyboard that aggravate the pain. Household and recreational activities that involve prolonged wrist flexion may also aggravate the pain.

■ Assess for Tinel's sign by tapping the area over the patient's wrist.	The patient with carpal tunnel syndrome will report a tingling sensation in the hand and fingers.
■ Assess for Phalen's sign by having the patient hold his or her wrists together with the hands in a palmar-flexed position for 20 to 30 seconds.	The patient will complain of numbness and tingling with carpal tunnel syndrome.
■ Apply manual compression over the carpal tunnel canal for 30 seconds.	The patient will develop numbness in the fingers.
■ Ask the patient about measures used to relieve the pain.	A pain management plan will be based on the patient's previous use of pain relief measures and their perceived effectiveness.
▲ Refer the patient for ultrasound or electrodiagnostic procedures.	Ultrasound imaging and nerve conduction studies may be done to confirm a diagnosis of carpal tunnel syndrome and assess the degree of median nerve compression.

Therapeutic Interventions

Actions/Interventions	Rationales
■ Encourage the patient to rest the affected wrist.	Resting the affected area reduces repeated stress on the carpal tunnel and decreases pain. A splint may be used to keep the wrist in a neutral position. Splints may be worn at night only or during the day with activity.
■ Apply cold packs to wrist.	Cold therapy will reduce inflammation in the carpal tunnel and help relieve pain.
■ Suggest participation in yoga.	Current evidence indicates that yoga has contributed to reduced pain. Patients have experienced improved grip strength in the affected hand.
▲ Administer analgesics.	Nonsteroidal antiinflammatory drugs (NSAIDs), such as ibuprofen, are effective in managing the pain as part of conservative treatment for carpal tunnel syndrome.
▲ Administer pyridoxine (vitamin B_6).	Vitamin B_6 supplements have been found to be helpful in relieving pain and paresthesias from carpal tunnel syndrome.
▲ Prepare the patient for injection of corticosteroids into the joint.	Direct injection of corticosteroids into the carpal tunnel is used to reduce inflammation and relieve pain. The patient may require multiple injections at weekly or monthly intervals.
▲ Prepare the patient for surgical release of the carpal ligament.	Open or endoscopic procedures are done to cut the carpal ligament. This procedure enlarges the carpal tunnel and relieves pressure on the median nerve.
▲ Refer the patient to an occupational therapist.	The occupational therapist can design custom-fitted splints that keep the wrist in a neutral position or in slight extension. The patient may need adaptive equipment for work, household, or recreational activities. These devices limit the degree of wrist flexion with activity.

NANDA-I NDx Deficient Knowledge

Common Related Factors
New condition, procedure, treatment
Misinterpretation of information
Unfamiliarity with information resources
Lack of recall

Defining Characteristics
Verbalizing inaccurate information
Questioning members of health care team
Incorrect task performance
Expressing frustration or confusion when performing task

Common Expected Outcome
Patient verbalizes understanding of information about carpal tunnel syndrome, treatments, and methods to prevent repetitive injury.

NOC Outcomes
Knowledge (Carpal Tunnel Syndrome); Information Processing

NIC Interventions
Learning Facilitation; Teaching: Individual

Ongoing Assessment

Actions/Interventions	Rationales
■ Assess the patient's previous knowledge of carpal tunnel syndrome.	Adults learn best when teaching builds on previous knowledge or experience. This experience is the foundation for an individualized teaching plan.

Therapeutic Interventions

Actions/Interventions	Rationales
■ Teach the patient to implement preventive measures:	Prevention is important in relieving pressure in the carpal tunnel.
• Take frequent rest periods during repetitive activities that involve wrist flexion.	Short breaks (e.g., 30 seconds to 1 minute every 30 minutes) relieve pressure in the carpal tunnel. Rest breaks should include gentle stretching and bending exercises for the wrist and hand.
• Adjust work/activity areas to keep elbows at 90-degree angle with wrists straight during activities.	This position reduces pressure in the carpal tunnel and relieves nerve compression.
• Do not rest wrists on a hard surface for prolonged periods, especially with repetitive activity.	This position puts pressure on the median nerve as it passes through the carpal tunnel.
• Use large pens and pencils with soft grip adapters when writing.	These devices encourage the patient to relax his or her grip when holding the pen or pencil. This adaptation reduces stress on the carpal tunnel.
• Wear fingerless gloves if the work/activity area is cold.	Keeping the hands and wrists warm reduces pain and stiffness with activity. This adaptation is important if the patient is not able to control environmental temperature in the work setting.
■ Teach the patient that full recovery following medical or surgical treatment may take several months.	Accurate information corrects misperceptions or unrealistic expectations patients may have about carpal tunnel treatments. Patients may expect immediate and complete recovery of wrist function and pain relief.
■ Provide the patient with information about state and federal laws related to workplace requirements to prevent repetitive stress injury.	This information helps the patient talk with his or her employer about implementing workplace accommodations to prevent aggravation of carpal tunnel syndrome.

■ = Independent   ▲ = Collaborative

Neurological Care Plans

Actions/Interventions

▲ Refer the patient to an occupational therapist.

▲ Refer the patient to a physical therapist.

Rationales

The occupational therapist can help the patient learn new ways of doing familiar activities that reduce repetitive stress on the carpal tunnel. These adaptations can include adjusting the height of chairs or work surfaces to reduce wrist flexion with activity. The therapist may help the patient select ergonomically correct equipment such as desks, chairs, computer keyboards, or tool handles.

The physical therapist can teach the patient stretching, strengthening, and conditioning exercises to improve body mechanics and posture with repetitive activities of the hand and wrist.

Craniotomy

Craniectomy; Burr Hole; Cranioplasty; Cranial Surgery

Craniotomy is the surgical opening of the cranium to gain access to disease or injury affecting the brain, ventricles, or intracranial blood vessels. Craniectomy is removal of part of the cranium to treat compound fractures, infection, or decompression. Burr holes are drilled in the cranium and used for clot evacuation and decompression of fluid beneath the dura or in preparation for craniotomy. Cranioplasty is the application of artificial material to repair the skull to improve integrity and shape. Cranial surgery is either supratentorial—above the tentorium, involving the cerebrum; or infratentorial—below the tentorium, involving the brainstem or cerebellum.

NANDA-I NDx Decreased Intracranial Adaptive Capacity

Common Related Factors

Cerebral edema
Cerebral ischemia or infarction
Increased cerebral blood flow
Increased intracranial pressure (ICP)
Hypercapnia
Hydrocephalus
Systemic hypotension

Defining Characteristics

Decreased level of consciousness (LOC)
Changed pupillary size, reaction to light, deviation
Focal or generalized motor weakness
Presence of pathological reflexes (Babinski)
Seizures
Increased blood pressure (BP) and bradycardia
Changed respiratory pattern
Repeated increases in ICP greater than 10 mm Hg for more than 5 minutes
Disproportionate increase in ICP after a nursing activity
Elevated ICP waveforms
Baseline ICP greater than 10 mm Hg
Wide-amplitude ICP waveform

Common Expected Outcome

Patient maintains optimal cerebral tissue perfusion, as evidenced by NIHSS score less than 4, by Glasgow Coma Scale (GCS) score greater than 13, absence of new neurological deficit, and ICP of 10 mm Hg or less.

NOC Outcomes

Fluid Balance; Neurological Status: Consciousness; Medication Response

NIC Interventions

ICP Monitoring; Neurological Monitoring; Cerebral Edema Management

Ongoing Assessment

Actions/Interventions

- Assess baseline neurological status, using NIHSS and Glasgow Coma Scale (GSC); monitor vital signs.

- Evaluate contributing factors to change in responsiveness; reevaluate in 5 to 10 minutes to see whether change persists.

- Assess function of surgical drains.

- Evaluate function of catheter used to monitor ICP. Analyze monitored values.

- ▲ Monitor serum glucose, osmolarity, complete blood count (CBC), sodium, and arterial blood gases. Report the following:
  - Po_2 less than 80 mm Hg
  - $Paco_2$ greater than 45 mm Hg
  - Hematocrit less than 30%
  - Sodium less than 130 or greater than 150 mEq/liter
  - Glucose less than 80 or greater than 200 mg/dL
  - Osmolarities less than 185 or greater than 310 mOsm/liter

Rationales

Early detection of changes is necessary to prevent permanent neurological dysfunction. Cerebral edema occurs for 24 to 72 hours postoperatively. Early signs include change in LOC, pupillary asymmetry, blurred vision, diplopia, new focal deficits, respiratory changes, speech changes, increased complaint of headache, yawning, or hiccuping. Increased BP, one fixed and dilated pupil, and bradycardia are late signs usually associated with medullary ischemia or compression. Fever may be related to expected postoperative response; dehydration; infection; or surgery near the third and fourth ventricles, hypothalamus, or pons.

Factors such as anesthesia, medications, awakening from sound sleep, or not understanding a question can affect responsiveness. It is important to differentiate expected from unexpected changes that require treatment.

Intraventricular drains and self-contained bulb suction and drainage systems are most commonly used. All drains and catheters should be secured to the patient or bed to prevent negative-gravity suctioning, and increased risk for bleeding or dislodging the drain.

An ICP monitor is usually in place for 24 to 72 hours postoperatively. Elevated P_2 waves, ICP greater than 10 mm Hg, and wide-amplitude waveforms indicate increasing ICP.

A $Paco_2$ less than 20 mm Hg may decrease CBF because of profound vasoconstriction that produces hypoxia. $Paco_2$ greater than 45 mm Hg induces vasodilatation with increase in CBF, which may trigger increase in ICP. Decreasing serum osmolarity indicates increasing edema.

Therapeutic Interventions

Actions/Interventions

- ▲ Maintain core body temperature within normal range using antipyretics or hypothermia blanket as ordered. Turn blanket off at temperature of less than 38° C (100.4° F) rectally.

- Maintain head of bed (HOB) at 30 degrees unless contraindicated (e.g., if patient is hemodynamically unstable, following insertion of ventricle-peritoneal shunt, following drainage of chronic subdural hematoma, or following infratentorial surgery).

- Maintain head and neck in neutral alignment. Avoid neck flexion or rotation.
- Avoid Valsalva maneuver with position changes.

- Reorient the patient to the environment as needed.

- Limit direct care activities.

Rationales

Temperature greater than 39° C (102.2F) and shivering will increase metabolic demands, and increase ICP.

This position improves venous drainage and reduces ICP. Keeping the HOB flat will decrease risk for new or recurrent subdural hemorrhage, dizziness, and orthostatic hypotension. The HOB should be raised gradually over 24 hours. Patients who have supratentorial surgery will have the HOB elevated. The bed may be kept flat for a patient who had infratentorial surgery.

This position prevents venous outflow obstruction and increased ICP.

Valsalva maneuvers increase intrathoracic pressure and cerebral blood flow, thereby increasing ICP.

Reality orientation reduces anxiety. Increased anxiety can cause increased ICP.

Unnecessary nursing care activities (e.g., routine linen changes, bathing) stimulate brain metabolism, increase cerebral blood flow, and contribute to increased ICP.

■ = Independent   ▲ = Collaborative

Actions/Interventions

▲ Administer artificial tears (methylcellulose drops) every 2 hours. Cover the patient's eyes, or tape eyelids closed.

▲ Administer osmotic diuretic, as ordered.

Rationales

The exposed cornea needs to be protected to prevent dryness. The unconscious patient may have difficulty closing the eyes (cranial nerve VII palsy).

Osmotic diuretics reduce cerebral edema and decrease ICP.

Risk for Deficient Fluid Volume

Common Risk Factors

Neurogenic diabetes insipidus (DI)
Dehydration secondary to use of hyperosmotic agents, profuse diaphoresis, fluid restriction.

Common Expected Outcome

Patient is normovolemic, as evidenced by systolic BP greater than or equal to 90 mm Hg (or patient's preoperative baseline), absence of orthostasis, heart rate (HR) 60 to 100 beats/min, urine output greater than 30 mL/hr, normal serum sodium and serum osmolarity, and urine specific gravity between 1.005 and 1.025.

NOC Outcomes

Fluid Balance; Medication Response; Electrolyte and Acid-Base Balance

NIC Interventions

Fluid/Electrolyte Management; Medication Administration

Ongoing Assessment

Actions/Interventions

■ Monitor fluid intake and urine output. Report urine output greater than 200 mL/hr for 2 consecutive hours.

■ Assess urine specific gravity.

▲ Monitor serum and urine electrolytes and osmolality.

■ Assess for signs of dehydration (tachycardia, hypotension, poor skin turgor).

■ Weigh daily if possible.

Rationales

DI occurs when the renal tubules are unable to conserve water due to decreased antidiuretic hormone. Disruption of the neurohypophyseal system during surgery decreases production and release of antidiuretic hormone (ADH).

Specific gravity is decreased to less than 1.005 with DI. Supratentorial surgery (near the pituitary fossa) can cause temporary DI. A decrease in ADH secretion seems to be a common response to irritation at this site.

DI results in hypernatremia (greater than 135 mEq/liter, increased serum osmolality (greater than 295 mOsm/kg), decreased urine sodium, and decreased urine osmolality (less than 400 mOsm/kg).

The patient with DI will complain of unquenchable thirst and a preference for ice water or other cold beverages. Decreased circulatory volume causes hypotension and a compensatory tachycardia.

DI causes weight loss because of fluid loss.

Therapeutic Interventions

Actions/Interventions

▲ Replace fluid output as directed.

▲ Administer vasopressin as prescribed, noting adverse reactions.

Rationales

The patient who is alert can respond to thirst and increase oral fluid intake. Intravenous (IV) fluids may be indicated to replace fluids when oral intake is not sufficient.

Vasopressin is ADH replacement. The drug is administered intravenously or subcutaneously. The onset of action is within 1 to 2 hours with duration of 3 to 6 hours. Vasopressin can have vasopressor effects that increase risk for myocardial ischemia as an adverse reaction.

Risk for Excess Fluid Volume

Common Risk Factor

Syndrome of inappropriate antidiuretic hormone (SIADH)

Common Expected Outcome

Patient is normovolemic, as evidenced by urinary output greater than or equal to 30 mL/hr, stable weight, normal serum sodium, normal osmolarity, and urine specific gravity between 1.005 and 1.025.

NOC Outcomes
Fluid Balance; Electrolyte and Acid-Base Balance

NIC Intervention
Fluid/Electrolyte Management

Ongoing Assessment

Actions/Interventions	Rationales
▲ Monitor serum and urine electrolytes and osmolarity (at least every 6 hours if IV saline is being administered).	These tests provide information on fluid volume excess (usually determined by hyponatremia and lowering of serum osmolarity). SIADH occurs from persistently high levels of circulating ADH. The secretion of ADH is no longer regulated by changes in plasma osmolality.
■ Monitor fluid intake and urine output, daily weight.	Urine output will be significantly less than fluid intake. Urine volume may be less than 30 to 40 mL/hr. Weight gain occurs in SIADH without signs of peripheral edema.
■ Assess for signs of hyponatremia (confusion, headache, fatigue, vomiting, muscle twitching, or seizures).	These clinical manifestations are associated with hyponatremia. SIADH may cause cerebral edema and increased ICP.

Therapeutic Interventions

Actions/Interventions	Rationales
▲ Restrict oral or IV fluids as ordered. In a patient with a nasogastric tube and feedings, normal saline solution can be used for flush after feedings.	Fluid restriction of 1 to 1.2 liters/day usually corrects hyponatremia associated with SIADH. Intravenous D$_5$W is inappropriate because of excess free water and should not be used for piggyback medications.
▲ If fluid restriction fails to correct hyponatremia, anticipate orders for a 3% IV saline solution with the concurrent use of IV furosemide (Lasix) and potassium.	Administration of a hypertonic solution may cause cardiac problems from further fluid overload. Furosemide promotes diuresis. Potassium supplementation corrects diuretic-induced potassium excretion.

 Risk for Seizures

Common Risk Factors

Intracranial bleeding
Infarction
Tumor
Trauma

■ = Independent   ▲ = Collaborative

Common Expected Outcomes

Patient does not sustain injury during seizure activity.
Patient does not experience seizure activity.

NOC Outcomes
Risk Control; Risk Detection; Seizure Control; Medication Response

NIC Intervention
Seizure Precautions/Management

Ongoing Assessment

Actions/Interventions	Rationales

■ Observe for seizure activity. Record and report the following observations:
  • Time of onset.
  • Body parts involved: order of involvement and character of movement.
  • Tonic-clonic stages.
  • Incontinence.
  • Duration of seizure.
  • Postictal state (e.g., confusion, drowsiness, sleep).
	A record of activity will determine seizure type. Postoperative seizure activity may occur as a result of neuronal injury from decreased cerebral perfusion pressure. Hyponatremia from SIADH may precipitate seizure activity.

■ Monitor for signs of airway obstruction.	Loss of motor control during a seizure can compromise the airway if the tongue falls back into the upper airway.

Therapeutic Interventions

Actions/Interventions	Rationales
▲ Administer anticonvulsants preoperatively.	These drugs are given to patients considered at high risk for seizures, such as those with lesions near the motor cortex.
■ Keep bed in low position.	Patient safety is a high priority. Keeping the bed in the lowest position decreases the risk for falls during seizure activity.
■ Keep padded side rails up.	This measure reduces risk for injury during tonic-clonic seizure activity.
▲ If seizure occurs, remain with patient, do not attempt to introduce anything into the mouth during the seizure. Maintain airway. Turn patient on side, suction, and administer oxygen if needed. Administer anticonvulsants.	Inserting objects could result in increased risk for aspiration, broken teeth, or soft tissue injury. When phenytoin is given intravenously it should be administered in normal saline. It will precipitate in any dextrose solution. Infuse no faster than 50 mg/min to prevent hypotension. IV diazepam (Valium) is often used to control recurrent seizures and should not be administered any faster than 10 mg/min to prevent respiratory compromise.
■ Maintain minimal environmental stimuli: noise reduction, curtains closed, private room (when available or advisable), dim lights.	During the postictal phase of a seizure, the patient may be disoriented. The patient may sleep for several hours before returning to baseline LOC.

NANDA-I NDx Deficient Knowledge

Common Related Factor	Defining Characteristic
New procedure and treatments	Patient and significant others verbalize questions and concerns.

Common Expected Outcome

Patient and significant others verbalize understanding of diagnosis, surgical procedure, and expected results.

NOC Outcomes
Knowledge: Disease Process; Knowledge: Treatment Regimen

NIC Intervention
Teaching: Procedure/Treatment

Ongoing Assessment

Actions/Interventions

■ Assess the patient's or significant others' knowledge regarding surgery and postoperative expectations.

Rationales

The patient may have cognitive impairment that limits his or her ability to understand explanations. The family may need more detailed explanations. They may have misperceptions about the outcomes of surgery. A planned surgical intervention can usually allow for more structured patient preparation as compared with an emergent surgical event following a trauma.

Therapeutic Interventions

Actions/Interventions

■ Discuss post operative care issues with the patient and family. Include the following:
  • Need for monitoring equipment and frequent assessments
  • Change in body image related to head dressing, loss of hair at the surgical site, potential for and duration of facial edema

  • Wound care after the dressing is removed: antiseptic cleanser and antibiotic ointment
  • Long-term medications such as corticosteroids, anticonvulsants, antibiotics
■ Before discharge, discuss protecting the scalp and head from cold, sun, and injury.

▲ Obtain social work and/or case management assistance in transitioning the patient to a rehabilitation facility or home.

Rationales

Information helps the patient and family cooperate with the treatment plan.

Knowledge about equipment used postoperatively can reduce anxiety.

The edema usually peaks about 3 days after surgery and then gradually diminishes. Hair will regrow as part of the expected healing process. Patients and families need information about the short-term duration of most of these changes.

The patient and family need to learn how to prevent wound infection.

These medications reduce or prevent edema, seizure, and infection.

Protective garments should be worn until incision is completely healed and hair has regrown. If the patient has had only burr holes, these will heal relatively quickly with the bone regenerating and filling in the holes. A patient who has had a craniectomy (removal of a piece of the skull) will need greater protection from injury to the uncovered area of brain. Large pieces of the skull will not sufficiently regenerate. Plastic surgery can be done in many cases (depending on the primary diagnosis) to restructure the shape of the skull after craniectomy.

Depending on the patient's age, primary diagnosis, and level of function postoperatively, the patient may require rehabilitation or home care services.

Related Care Plans

Diabetes insipidus (see the **Evolve** website)
Syndrome of inappropriate antidiuretic hormone (see the **Evolve** website)

■ = Independent   ▲ = Collaborative

Head Trauma

Traumatic Brain Injury; Closed Trauma; Skull Fracture; Subdural Hematoma; Concussion

Head injury (craniocerebral trauma) is a leading cause of death in the United States for persons 1 to 42 years of age. An estimated 3 million people suffer head injuries every year. About one-half of all severe head injuries result from accidents involving automobiles, motorcycles, bicycles, and pedestrians. People who do not use appropriate safety equipment (e.g. seat belts, helmets) have a significant increase in head injury with accidents. Approximately 20 percent of head injuries are associated with violence, such as blunt force trauma and firearms. The severity of the head injury is defined by the traumatic coma data bank on the basis of the Glasgow Coma Scale (GCS): Severe head injury = GCS of 8 or less; moderate head injury = GCS of 9 to 12. Most head injuries are blunt (closed) trauma to the brain. Damage to the scalp, skull, meninges, and brain runs the gamut of skull fracture with loss of consciousness, concussion, and/or extracerebral or intracerebral pathological conditions. Patients with moderate to severe head trauma are usually observed in a critical care unit where immediate intervention can be achieved. Most deaths occur in the first few hours after head trauma as a result of internal bleeding or worsening cerebral edema. Patients with minor head trauma (scalp laceration or concussion) are most often treated and released to be observed at home with instructions to call or return if symptoms worsen. Older persons are most often affected with postconcussion syndrome, characterized by decreased neurological function 2 weeks to 2 months after the initial injury and often caused by a slow subdural bleed. This care plan focuses on moderate-to-severe head trauma in the acute care setting.

NANDA-I NDx Decreased Intracranial Adaptive Capacity

Common Related Factors

Cerebral edema
Increased intracranial pressure (ICP)
Decreased cerebral perfusion pressure (CPP)
Impaired autoregulation
Cortical laceration
Intracranial hemorrhage

Defining Characteristics

Decreased level of consciousness (confusion, agitation, inappropriate affect, disorientation, somnolence, lethargy, coma)
Headache
Vomiting
Pupillary asymmetry
Changes in pupillary reaction
ICP greater than 10 mm Hg
CPP less than 60 mm Hg

Common Expected Outcome

Patient maintains optimal cerebral tissue perfusion, as evidenced by GCS greater than 13, ICP less than 10 mm Hg, CPP 60 to 90 mm Hg, and absence of secondary neurological deficit.

NOC Outcomes
Neurological Status: Consciousness; Medication Response
NIC Interventions
Cerebral Edema Management; Neurological Monitoring; ICP Monitoring

Neurological Care Plans

Ongoing Assessment

Actions/Interventions	Rationales
■ Serially assess neurological status as follows:	Deteriorating neurological signs indicate increased cerebral ischemia and intracranial pressure.
• Level of consciousness (LOC), according to Glasgow Coma Scale (GSC)	A decreased LOC is the first sign of increased ICP. A GCS score of less than 13 indicates neurological dysfunction and possible damage.
• Orientation to person, place, and time	
• Motor signs: drift, decreased movement, abnormal or absent movement, increased reflexes	Focal signs of neurological dysfunction suggest structural versus metabolic abnormality.
• Pupil size, symmetry, and reaction to light	Pupillary changes indicate an increase in intracranial pressure.
• Extraocular movement, deviation	Changes in eye movement and gaze occur with cranial nerve injury.
• Speech, thought processes, and memory changes	Impaired cognitive function indicates injury to the cerebral cortex.
■ Report deteriorating neurological status immediately.	Surgical intervention may be necessary to preserve cerebral function.
■ Assess for rhinorrhea (cerebrospinal fluid [CSF] drainage from nose), otorrhea (CSF drainage from ear), battle sign (ecchymosis over the mastoid process), raccoon eyes (periorbital ecchymosis).	These signs may indicate frontal, orbital, or basal skull fractures.
■ Evaluate presence or absence of protective reflexes: corneal, gag, blink, cough, startle, grab, Babinski.	Changes in reflex responses are an indication of increased ICP. Absence of these reflexes indicates disruption of the brainstem. Loss of protective reflexes increases the patient's risk for injury.
■ Monitor vital signs with special attention to blood pressure, respiratory rate and rhythm, and body temperature.	Continually increasing ICP results in life-threatening hemodynamic changes; early recognition is essential to survival. Increased blood pressure associated with bradycardia is a late sign of increased ICP that suggests medullary ischemia or compression. Increase in core body temperature in the absence of infection usually indicates hypothalamic damage. Hyperthermia increases metabolic demands and contributes to increased ICP. Changes in breathing patterns occur as compensation for increased ICP or in response to specific patterns of brain injury.
▲ Monitor ICP through cranial catheter device. Report ICP greater than 10 mm Hg sustained for more than 5 minutes.	Normal ICP should be below 15 mm Hg with the patient at rest.
■ Calculate the CPP (CPP = Mean systemic arterial pressure – ICP).	CPP should be 80 to 100 mm Hg. There is little or no perfusion if CPP is less than 60 mm Hg.
▲ Use pulse oximetry to monitor oxygen saturation; assess ABGs as ordered.	Pulse oximetry is a useful tool to defect changes in oxygenation. Oxygen saturation should be at 90% or greater. $Paco_2$ greater than 45 mm Hg induces cerebral vasodilation and increased intracranial pressure. $Paco_2$ less than 60 mm Hg induces cerebral vasoconstriction and cerebral ischemia.
■ Monitor fluid intake and urine output. Assess urine specific gravity.	The use of hyperosmotics to manage cerebral edema and ICP will alter hydration and electrolytes. Decreased urine output may indicate decreased renal perfusion and a possible decrease in cerebral perfusion.
▲ Monitor serum electrolytes, blood urea nitrogen, creatinine, osmolarity, glucose, and hemoglobin and hematocrit.	Changes in these laboratory test results may be associated with treatment complications or neurologic injury to the hypothalamus or pituitary gland. Be aware that hemoconcentration will cause false "normal" hemoglobin levels and hematocrit.
■ Assess for pain, fever, and shivering.	These symptoms increase cerebral blood flow and ICP.

■ = Independent   ▲ = Collaborative

Neurological Care Plans

Therapeutic Interventions

Actions/Interventions	Rationales
■ If ICP is above 15 mm Hg, postpone nursing care activities that can be deferred (e.g., routine care, invasive procedures).	Limiting unnecessary care will prevent further ICP increases. Clustering of care in a short period of time is associated with increased ICP.
■ Elevate head of bed (HOB) 30 degrees with head in neutral position.	Raising the HOB minimizes cerebral edema by promoting venous blood flow from the brain.
■ If patient is intubated, ensure that neck tapes securing the endotracheal (ET) tube are not too tight.	Tight tape impedes jugular venous outflow.
▲ Assist with diagnostic testing (radiograph, computed tomography [CT], and magnetic resonance imaging [MRI]).	Patient safety is a priority during diagnostic testing to ensure safe head positioning, continued monitoring, and maintenance of stable ICP. Diagnostic evaluation is necessary to determine the exact location of brain injury.
■ Reorient the patient to the environment, and provide familiar objects and pictures.	These measures decrease anxiety and help maintain stable ICP levels.
▲ Administer osmotic diuretics, as ordered.	Osmotic diuretics reduce cerebral edema.
■ If neuromuscular blocking agents are used (pancuronium [Pavulon]), remember that cerebration is still intact and that pain is perceived.	These drugs may be used to control response to noxious stimuli (e.g., intubation and suctioning) to reduce effect on ICP.
■ Avoid neck and hip flexion.	Careful alignment when positioning the patient prevents venous obstruction and decreases cerebral edema.
■ Avoid Valsalva maneuvers.	Increased ICP can be caused by Valsalva maneuver when straining with defecation.
■ Hyperventilate and hyperoxygenate before suctioning ET tube or trachea.	This measure avoids hypoxemia, hypercapnia, and hypotension, which contribute to increased ICP.

NANDA-I NDx **Risk for Deficient Fluid Volume**

Common Risk Factors

Diabetes insipidus (DI)
Dehydration secondary to use of hyperosmotic agents, profuse diaphoresis

Common Expected Outcome

Patient remains normovolemic, as evidenced by systolic BP greater than or equal to 90 mm Hg (or patient's baseline), absence of orthostasis, heart rate (HR) 60 to 100 beats/min, urine output greater than 30 mL/hr, normal skin turgor, and urine specific gravity between 1.005 and 1.025.

NOC Outcomes
Fluid Balance; Electrolyte and Acid-Base Balance; Medication Response
NIC Intervention
Fluid/Electrolyte Management

Ongoing Assessment

Actions/Interventions	Rationales
■ Monitor fluid intake and urine output .Report urine output greater than 200 mL/hr for 2 consecutive hours.	DI occurs when the renal tubules are unable to conserve water due to decreased antidiuretic hormone. Disruption of the neurohypophyseal system may occur with head injury and decreases production and release of antidiuretic hormone (ADH).
■ Assess urine specific gravity.	A decrease in urine specific gravity less than 1.005 occurs with DI.

Actions/Interventions	Rationales
▲ Monitor serum and urine electrolytes and osmolarity.	DI causes hypernatremia, increased serum osmolality, and decreased urine osmolality and urine sodium concentration.
■ Monitor for signs of dehydration (decreased skin turgor, weight loss, increased heart rate, decreased blood pressure).	Polyuria causes decreased circulatory blood volume and weight loss.
■ Monitor daily weights.	Polyuria causes weight loss in the patient with DI.

Therapeutic Interventions

Actions/Interventions	Rationales
■ Replace fluid output as directed.	The patient with DI has intense thirst. Oral intake in response to thirst may correct the problem. IV fluid administration may be needed if the patient is unable to maintain oral fluid intake in response to thirst.
▲ Administer vasopressin as ordered.	Vasopressin is a synthetic antidiuretic hormone that will reduce urine concentration and decrease urine output. Careful monitoring of the urine output and serum sodium and osmolarity is mandatory when vasopressin is administered.

Risk for Excess Fluid Volume

Common Risk Factor

Syndrome of inappropriate antidiuretic hormone (SIADH)

Common Expected Outcome

Patient remains normovolemic, as evidenced by normal serum sodium, normal serum and urine osmolarity, stable weight, urine output greater than or equal to 30 mL/hr, HR less than 100 beats/min, lungs clear to auscultation, and urine specific gravity between 1.005 and 1.025.

NOC Outcomes
Fluid Balance; Electrolyte and Acid-Base Balance
NIC Intervention
Fluid/Electrolyte Management

Ongoing Assessment

Actions/Interventions	Rationales
■ Assess fluid intake and urine output, and monitor weight.	Urine output will be significantly less than fluid intake. Urine volume may be less than 30 to 40 mL/hr. Weight gain occurs in SIADH without signs of peripheral edema.
▲ Assess serum and urine electrolytes and osmolality.	These tests provide information on fluid volume excess (usually determined by hyponatremia and lowering of serum osmolarity). SIADH occurs from persistently high levels of circulating ADH. The secretion of ADH is no longer regulated by changes in plasma osmolality.
■ Assess for signs of hyponatremia (confusion, headache, fatigue, vomiting, muscle twitching, or seizures)	These clinical manifestations are associated with hyponatremia. SIADH may cause cerebral edema and increased ICP.

Therapeutic Interventions

Actions/Interventions	Rationales
▲ Restrict oral or IV fluids as ordered. In a patient with a nasogastric tube and feedings, normal saline solution can be used for flush after feedings.	Fluid restriction of 1 to 1.2 liters/day usually corrects hyponatremia associated with SIADH. Intravenous D_5W is inappropriate because of excess free water and should not be used for piggyback medications.

■ = Independent   ▲ = Collaborative

Actions/Interventions

▲ If fluid restriction fails to correct hyponatremia, anticipate order for 3% saline solution infusion given with furosemide (Lasix) and potassium.

Rationales

Administration of a hypertonic solution may cause cardiac problems from further fluid overload. Furosemide promotes diuresis. Potassium supplementation corrects diuretic-induced potassium excretion.

NDx Risk for Seizures

Common Risk Factors

Cortical laceration
Intracranial bleeding
Hyponatremia
Hypoxia
Multiple contusions
Penetrating injuries to brain

Common Expected Outcomes

Patient does not sustain injury with seizure activity.
Patient does not experience seizure activity.

NOC Outcomes

Seizure Control; Risk Detection; Risk Control; Medication Response

NIC Intervention

Seizure Precautions/Management

Ongoing Assessment

Actions/Interventions

■ Observe for seizure activity. Record and report the following observations:
  • Time of onset
  • Body part involved; order of involvement and character of movement
  • Tonic-clonic stages
  • Incontinence
  • Duration of seizure
  • Postictal state (e.g. confusion, drowsiness, sleep)
■ Monitor for signs of airway obstruction

Rationales

Any cerebral irritation puts the patient at risk for seizure activity. Seizures occur in about 5% of patients with nonpenetrating head trauma; the risk is greater with penetrating injuries. Seizures increase cerebral metabolism and oxygen demand. Ischemic injury from the primary trauma can be aggravated by seizure-induced hypoxia. Careful documentation of seizure activity helps in diagnosing the specific type of seizure. Generalized tonic-clonic seizures are more likely to occur with increased ICP.

Loss of motor control during a seizure can compromise the airway if the tongue falls back into the upper airway.

Therapeutic Interventions

Actions/Interventions

■ Implement seizure precautions: side rails up and padded, bed in low position, head protection if needed.
▲ Administer anticonvulsants as directed.

■ If seizure occurs, remain with the patient, do not attempt to put anything in the patient's mouth, maintain airway.
■ Turn the patient's head to the side, and suction, and administer oxygen if needed.

Rationales

Patient safety is a priority. These measures reduce risk of injury during seizure activity.

Phenytoin (Dilantin) can only be mixed in normal saline. Precipitation will be noted when mixed with D_5W. Infuse no faster than 50 mg/min to prevent hypotension.

Inserting objects will often cause more harm, such as broken teeth, soft tissue injury, and airway obstruction.

This position is used to maintain airway patency during the postictal state.

Risk for Imbalanced Nutrition: Less Than Body Requirements

Common Risk Factors

Facial trauma
Restriction of intake
Impaired LOC
Multisystem trauma

Common Expected Outcome

Patient weighs within 10% of ideal body weight.

NOC Outcome
Nutritional Status: Nutrient Intake
NIC Intervention
Nutrition Management

Ongoing Assessment

Actions/Interventions	Rationales
▲ Monitor albumin, protein, glucose, and electrolytes.	These laboratory tests are indicative of general nutritional states.
■ Assess skin color, turgor, and muscle mass.	Dry, flaky skin, tenting, and decreased muscle mass indicate decreased nutritional intake.
■ Assess rate and quality of wound healing.	Extra calories are needed to maintain basic metabolism plus wound healing.
■ Monitor daily weights.	Changes in weight will occur with nutritional changes. Daily fluctuations occur with shifts in fluid balance. Sustained changes over a week are reflections of nutritional status.
▲ Consult with speech therapist to evaluate for dysphagia.	Swallowing and gag reflexes may be impaired as a result of head trauma. Evaluation of swallowing needs to be done before initiating oral intake. This assessment is done to reduce risk for aspiration with oral intake.

Therapeutic Interventions

Actions/Interventions	Rationales
▲ Administer tube feedings.	Patients with head injury need about 2000 kcal/day. Patients with multiple trauma may need two to three times that (or more). The enteral route of nutritional support is preferred over the IV route. IV nutritional support requires placement of a central venous catheter. The central line increases the risk for infection. Hyperglycemia is a complication of total parenteral nutrition that requires frequent blood glucose monitoring and insulin administration.
■ Maintain HOB at 30 degrees.	This position prevents risk for aspiration with tube feedings.
■ Avoid insertion of feeding tube through the nose in a patient with head injury unless the possibility of a basal skull fracture has been excluded.	Basilar fractures often traverse the paranasal sinuses. A feeding tube could penetrate brain tissue through the fracture site.

■ = Independent ▲ = Collaborative

NDx Deficient Knowledge

Common Related Factor

Lack of prior experience with head injury

Defining Characteristics

Questioning members of health care team
Verbalization of incorrect information
Withdrawal from environment
Frustration with health care

Common Expected Outcome

Patient or family describes the type of head injury, treatment, and expected outcome.

NOC Outcomes
Knowledge: Disease Process; Knowledge: Treatment Regimen
NIC Interventions
Teaching: Disease Process; Teaching: Procedure/Treatment

Ongoing Assessment

Actions/Interventions	Rationales
■ Assess knowledge of injury, treatment, and expected outcome.	Knowledge will reduce the fear of the unknown. Because most head trauma occurs as an unexpected accident, the patient and family have no previous experience with this type of injury.
■ Assess the patient's cognitive function.	Head trauma can cause impaired short-term memory, decreased attention span, and decreased concentration. These changes can limit learning new information.

Therapeutic Interventions

Actions/Interventions	Rationales
■ Prepare the family for the intensive care unit (ICU) environment.	Head trauma can result in life-threatening injury that will produce high levels of anxiety. In addition, the ICU environment may be stressful at first visit. The presence of "high-tech" equipment is a source of anxiety to most patients and families. A brief explanation of the positive features of these monitoring devices and treatments may reduce their anxiety.
■ Explain treatments or procedures and equipment used, such as the following: • ICP monitor • IV lines and medications • Cardiopulmonary and oximetry monitors • Feeding tubes and pumps • Mechanical ventilator	The patient with cognitive impairment may have distorted perceptions of therapeutic equipment. The patient who is disoriented may perceive the equipment as threatening and attempt to remove it. Frequent explanations in simple terms may calm anxiety and promote reality orientation.
■ Reinforce information given to the patient or family about the following: • Type of head injury, where the injury is in the brain, and what brain functions will be affected by the injury • Results of CT scan, radiographs, MRI	Repetition may be beneficial in retaining new information. Daily updates and explanations can help the patient and family cope with the uncertainty they experience with the long-term rehabilitation.

Actions/Interventions	Rationales
• Care plan and changes in condition	The care plan varies depending on the type and extent of skull and brain injury. A patient with a mild contusion, nondisplaced skull fracture, and mild concussion can likely expect a full recovery. The plan will focus on reestablishing physical and mental function. A patient with a depressed skull fracture and severe brain injury may require long-term care as a result of permanent neurological deficits. The care plan will focus on prevention of complications resulting from chronic mobility, communication, and sensory and cognitive deficits.
■ If the patient has impaired LOC, instruct the family and significant others to avoid discussions at the bedside that they would not want the patient to hear.	Although the patient may be unresponsive, ability to hear may be intact.
■ Keep the family up-to-date with any new changes in condition.	Regular conferences with family caregivers help them become members of the rehabilitation team. They can provide insights about the patient's personality and behavior before the injury.
■ Discuss the role of physical, occupational, or speech therapist.	Specialized service may be required for recovery. Patient and family members need to understand the roles of members of the health care team.
■ Discuss the need for rehabilitation and home care support, if necessary.	Parents or spouses often become the primary caregivers when the patient is discharged from the rehabilitation setting. They need ongoing support to adapt to the changes in roles and responsibilities.
■ Prepare the patient and family for changes in personality and behavior.	It may take months for the patient to recover; some personality changes may be permanent.
■ Provide the family with names and numbers of local support groups, if available.	Groups that come together for mutual support can be beneficial.
■ Refer the family to social services or financial counselors, as appropriate.	The patient and family may need ongoing support for decisions about financial resources, guardianship, powers of attorney, and living wills. Resources for respite care may help families cope more effectively with responsibilities for patient care.

Related Care Plan

Decreased intracranial adaptive capacity, p. 119
Ineffective airway clearance, p. 11
Impaired physical mobility, p. 133
Self-care deficit, p. 170

Headache: Migraine, Cluster, Tension

Headache is defined as pain in the head or face, either "primary" or "secondary" in origin. Migraine, cluster, and tension headaches are classified as primary because the pain occurs without pathological cause. Secondary headaches are a result of a known pathology, such as cranial tumor or aneurysm. Migraine headache is a benign, recurring headache that can be unilateral or bilateral. Migraine headache is the most common type of vascular headache. Changes in the intracranial blood vessels are thought to be the cause of the pain, with vasospasm and ischemia being the primary mechanisms. Evidence suggests that neurological, vascular, and chemical factors are involved. Women are affected three times more often than men. Migraines may occur with an aura or without. The aura is a collection of neurological

■ = Independent ▲ = Collaborative

symptoms that precede the onset of pain by 10 to 30 minutes. These symptoms include changes in level of consciousness, vision, behavior, and motor or sensory function. A variety of precipitating events trigger migraine headaches, including stress, foods high in tyramine, hunger, sleep disturbances, and for women, alterations in reproductive hormone levels. Manifestations are associated with autonomic nervous system dysfunction. Migraines may begin in early childhood and adolescence, and 65% of patients with migraine headaches have a family history of migraine headache.

Tension headaches are the most common form of headache, occurring in women more often than men. The usual age of onset is 20-25 years old. The pain is usually mild to moderate and described as a tightening or sensation of pressure around the head. This type of headache is believed to be related to muscle tension in the jaw and neck with hypersensitivity of pain fibers in the trigeminal nerve. The exact mechanisms for the pain are unknown. Many patients may experience both migraine and tension headaches.

Cluster headaches are defined as pain episodes that occur for several days at a time followed by long periods of remission. The person may experience several short headaches in one day. Men are affected more often than women, with the age of occurrence between 20 and 50 years old. The pain is described as severe, with tearing, burning, and reddening of the eye on one side of the face. The mechanisms of cluster headaches are thought to be similar to those causing migraine headaches. The exact mechanisms remain unknown but may include vascular and neurogenic alterations of the hypothalamus associated with changes in serotonin transmission.

This care plan focuses on the classic migraine, which is believed to be a dysfunction of the hypothalamic and upper brainstem areas. Diagnosis, treatment, and follow-up care are usually accomplished in an outpatient setting.

Deficient Knowledge

Common Related Factor	**Defining Characteristics**
Unfamiliar with diagnosis and treatment plan	Verbalized lack of understanding Questions Noncompliance

Common Expected Outcomes

Patient will verbalize understanding of migraine headache etiological factors and treatment.
Patient will verbalize understanding of prevention protocol for recurrent headaches and successful prevention of recurrent headaches.

NOC Outcomes
Knowledge: Disease Process; Knowledge: Medication
NIC Interventions
Teaching: Disease Process; Teaching: Prescribed Medications

Ongoing Assessment

Actions/Interventions

- Assess the patient's current understanding of the cause of headache, prevention, and treatment.

Rationales

An individualized teaching plan is based on the patient's level of understanding, current knowledge, and need for new information. The patient needs to be open to learning ways to manage the headaches. The strategies may require lifestyle changes and new behaviors for managing headache triggers.

Therapeutic Interventions

Actions/Interventions	**Rationales**
■ Explain etiological factors of migraine headache:	Knowledge may reduce anxiety and clear up common misconceptions.
• The central pain mechanism in the brain is regulated by serotonin and norepinephrine level, usually in excess, that causes pain. Serotonin is believed to play a role in pain progression. Changes in neurotransmitter levels cause cerebral vasodilation and headache.	
• Serotonergic cells are hyperactive during migraine (can be seen on positron emission tomography [PET]), and serotonin levels are more easily manipulated than other neurotransmitters.	
▲ Explain and facilitate diagnostic testing (may include a computed tomography scan, PET scan, magnetic resonance imaging scan, and/or electroencephalogram).	These tests are done to rule out other possible diagnoses; results should be negative.
■ Discuss avoidance of foods known to precipitate migraine, such as caffeinated drinks, chocolate, most alcohol (especially red wine), citrus fruits or drinks, pickled or cured foods, some cheeses, and monosodium glutamate.	Migraine headaches may or may not have a precipitating event. For those that do, knowledge of one's individual "stressor" may guide treatment. Foods high in the amino acid tyramine are known to trigger migraine headaches. Tyramine stimulates release of epinephrine and norepinephrine.
■ Help the patient recognize and prevent situations that seem to cause headache, such as exhaustion, fatigue, stress, fever, or bright lights.	Changing lifestyle and behavior is usually the most difficult aspect of the treatment plan for migraine sufferers.
■ Ensure thorough understanding of prescribed medication therapy for prophylaxis of migraine headache. Prescriptive choices include the following:	Preventive medications are prescribed for patients who experience frequent or incapacitating headaches that are not controlled with acute pain management. Accurate knowledge helps the patient make decisions for achieving maximum benefit from drug therapy.
• Tricyclic antidepressants	The tricyclic antidepressants block uptake of serotonin and catecholamines; often used for migraines associated with muscle contraction.
• Calcium channel blockers	Calcium channel blockers are thought to prevent migraines by altering cerebral vessel constriction.
• Beta adrenergic blockers	Beta blockers are a commonly used drug for migraine prophylaxis. This group of drugs inhibits serotonin uptake and prevents vasodilation.
• Methysergide maleate (Sansert)	Methysergide maleate blocks the effects of serotonin on cerebral blood vessels.
• Divalproex sodium (Depakote)	This drug is an anti-epilepsy drug recently approved by the FDA for migraine prophylaxis. Women of childbearing age need complete information about risks and benefits of the drug because of its adverse effects on the fetus.
■ Provide support group information: • National Headache Foundation • American Council for Headache Education	These resources provide additional information about coping with headaches.

NANDA-I
NDx **Acute Pain**

Common Related Factor	**Defining Characteristics**
Cerebral artery vasoconstriction causing increased serotonin levels, followed by vasodilation	Aura (30% of sufferers) Premonition Unilateral (60%) or bilateral headache

■ = Independent ▲ = Collaborative

Neurological Care Plans

Nausea, vomiting
Scalp tenderness
Scalp and neck muscle contraction
Throbbing pain with activity
Exhaustion

Common Expected Outcomes

Patient reports satisfactory pain control at a level less than 3 to 4 on a 0 to 10 rating scale.

Patient uses pharmacological and nonpharmacological pain relief strategies.

Patient exhibits increased comfort such as baseline levels for pulse, blood pressure, respirations, and relaxed muscle tone or body posture.

NOC Outcomes
Pain Control; Medication Response
NIC Intervention
Analgesic Administration

Ongoing Assessment

Actions/Interventions	Rationales
■ Obtain thorough medical history and family history.	Migraines tend to occur in family members and can be related to stress or the physical environment. Headache may be attributed to a particular source such as head injury, sinus or dental infection, hypertension, eye problems, seizures, arthritis, or allergies.
■ Obtain detailed headache history, including the following:	Detailed information is necessary to differentiate from other serious neurological problems and to determine etiological factors and type of headache before a specific treatment protocol can be designed.
• Age of onset, frequency, and duration	Many patients experience their first migraine headache in early adolescence. Migraine headache pain may reach peak intensity an hour after onset. The pain may continue for several hours or even days.
• Typical location	The pain may begin on one side of the head and spread to include both sides.
• Type of pain	Patients may describe the pain as deep, steady, throbbing, or stabbing.
• Precipitating factors	Identifying headache triggers is important in developing a plan for prevention. Theses triggers may include foods, stress, weather changes, fatigue, or hormonal changes during the menstrual cycle.
• Aggravating factors	Bright lights and noise may intensify headache pain.
• Associated symptoms	Associated symptoms may occur before, during, or after the headache. The symptoms may include nausea, vomiting, numbness, visual disturbances, vertigo, and sensitivity to odors.
• Relief measures	Patients may have tried a variety of treatments to cope with headache pain. Those measures that have been successful should be included in the individualized care plan.
• Effect on activities of daily living	For some patients, migraine headaches are incapacitating. Headache episodes can disrupt the patient's ability to work and participate in family or social activities.

Actions/Interventions	Rationales
■ Assess for depression and suicide risk.	Many patients experience anxiety and depression with recurrent and disabling headaches. The treatment plan needs to include a holistic approach to support effective coping strategies.

Therapeutic Interventions

Actions/Interventions	Rationales
■ Encourage the patient to lie down in a quiet dark room.	Darkness diminishes photophobia, and quiet decreases neural stimulation. If implemented at the onset of pain, these measures may reduce the intensity and duration of the headache.
■ Provide gentle head massage if tolerated.	Massage may promote relaxation of scalp muscles and reduce pain intensity.
■ Apply cold packs.	Application of cold therapy to the forehead, temples, or back of the neck may decrease headache intensity.
■ Support head and neck with pillows.	Position changes reduce muscle tension, which aggravates pain.
▲ Administer attack-aborting medications, as prescribed.	These medications are taken at the earliest onset of a migraine headache to reduce the severity and duration of the headache. Selective serotonin receptor agonists (e.g. sumatriptan) and non-selective serotonin agonists (ergot alkaloids) act by constricting cerebral arteries. Opioid analgesics may be used in patients with hypertension when use of a vasoconstricting drug might be contraindicated. A variety of routes of administration are available to facilitate patient management of this approach to headache relief. The routes include oral, intranasal spray, and subcutaneous injection.
▲ Administer analgesics for mild to moderate pain.	Acetaminophen and nonsteroidal antiinflammatory drugs (e.g. aspirin, ibuprofen, naproxen) may be useful to relieve mild to moderate migraine pain. These drugs act on peripheral pain receptors and relieve inflammation. Many over-the-counter drugs marketed specifically for migraine headache contain these active ingredients. Opioid analgesics may be prescribed for relief of more severe headache pain.
■ Provide information on additional pain- or stress-relieving measures, including relaxation techniques, physical therapy, exercise, and biofeedback.	Patients can decrease the frequency of migraine headaches by avoiding precipitating events that trigger pain episodes. Regular sleep patterns, exercise, and stress management activities can reduce headache frequency.

Related Care Plan

Ineffective coping, p. 49

■ = Independent   ▲ = Collaborative

Neurological Care Plans

Intracranial Infection

Meningitis; Encephalitis; Brain Abscess, Empyema

Intracranial infection may be the result of meningitis, encephalitis, brain abscess, or empyema. Meningitis is an inflammation or infection of the membranes of the brain or spinal cord caused by bacteria, viruses, or other organisms. Bacterial meningitis is the most common form of the disorder. The infecting bacteria are often found in the nasopharynx and can be transmitted by sneezing or coughing. Pneumococcal meningitis is often secondary to pneumonia, sinusitis, alcoholism, and trauma (such as a basal skull fracture). The causative bacteria is *streptococcus pneumoniae*. Meningococcal meningitis is caused by *neisseria meningitides*. This form of meningitis is more common in children and young adults. Factors contributing to infection with meningitis include poor hygiene, high density living arrangements, and inadequate nutrition. Meningitis may occur as a complication of infection with *haemophilis influenzae*. Epidemics are seen in winter and spring months. Immunizations are available for both forms of meningitis. Antibiotic therapy is required. Viral illnesses are treated symptomatically. Viral meningitis is more likely to occur in summer months. Hydrocephalus often occurs secondary to viral meningitis.

Encephalitis is an inflammation/infection of the brain and meninges. The highest mortality rate is caused by herpes simplex virus (HSV), which is the most common form. An abscess is a localized purulent collection in the brain. Empyema is a type of brain abscess that forms in a preexisting space such as the subdural space of the brain, requiring surgical drainage and injection of antibiotics. Causes may be direct or indirect. Direct causes are a result of extension of infections from the ear, tooth, mastoid, or sinus. Indirect causes include bacterial endocarditis, skull fracture, or nonsterile procedures. Empyema may also form in the epidural space of the spine. Hospitalization is usually required for differential diagnosis, neurological monitoring, and treatment.

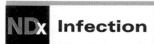 **Infection**

Common Related Factors	**Defining Characteristics**
Brain infection	Temperature greater than 39° C (102.2° F)
Encephalitis	Increased white blood cell (WBC) count
Brain abscess	Nuchal rigidity
	Altered level of consciousness (LOC)
	Irritability
	Motor-sensory abnormalities
	Chills
	Malaise
	Headache
	Localized redness and swelling (e.g., along a suture line or area of injury)

Common Expected Outcome

Source of infection is determined and treated.

NOC Outcomes
Thermoregulation; Medication Response

NIC Interventions
Fever Treatment; Medication Administration, Parenteral

Ongoing Assessment

Actions/Interventions	Rationales
■ Monitor temperature.	This provides information about the patient's response to invading organisms. Fever is a classic manifestation of meningitis. Fever is not common with a brain abscess.
▲ Monitor WBC count.	Elevated WBC counts occur in both bacterial and viral infections.
■ Evaluate LOC.	Alterations in LOC occur in most patients with intracranial infections. Changes may range from drowsiness to coma. Accumulation of infectious exudate with adhesion formation can lead to hydrocephalus, increased ICP, and further decreasing LOC.
■ Evaluate motor-sensory status. • Nuchal rigidity (neck stiffness) • Brudzinski's sign • Kernig's sign • Photophobia	Changes in nerve function are common manifestations of intracranial infections. Inflammation of affected nerve tissue or pooling of infectious exudate causes these changes. Meningeal or cerebral inflammation can produce nuchal rigidity, Brudzinski's sign (flexion of neck onto chest causes flexion of both legs and thighs), and Kernig's sign (resistance to extension of the leg at the knee with the hip flexed). The patient will report pain with both of the assessment maneuvers. The patient with meningitis will complain of sensitivity or even pain in brightly lit rooms or direct sunlight.
■ Evaluate for signs of cerebrospinal fluid (CSF) otorrhea/rhinorrhea.	After basal skull fracture, CSF leakage may lead to intracranial infection.
▲ Monitor peak or trough levels of antibiotics as prescribed.	These levels provide means to monitor effectiveness and prevent toxicity of medication.
■ Assess for headache.	Headache may be the only manifestation of a brain abscess. The pain may intensify with exertion.

Therapeutic Interventions

Actions/Interventions	Rationales
▲ Administer antibiotics as prescribed.	Consistent timing is required to maintain therapeutic blood levels, reduce virulence, eradicate pathogens, and prevent fluctuations in antibiotic blood levels.
▲ Administer antipyretics as prescribed; document patient response.	Fever increases cerebral metabolic demand.
■ Apply cooling blanket for temperature greater than 39.5° C (103.1° F).	High temperatures can add to neurological damage.
■ Implement respiratory precautions.	Respiratory isolation precautions are indicated for patients with meningococcal meningitis.

NDx Risk for Injury: Seizures

Common Risk Factors

Cerebral irritation
Cerebral edema

Common Expected Outcomes

Patient does not sustain injury during seizure activity.
Patient does not experience seizure activity.

NOC Outcomes
Risk Detection; Risk Control; Seizure Control; Medication Response
NIC Intervention
Seizure Precautions/Management

■ = Independent ▲ = Collaborative

Neurological Care Plans

Ongoing Assessment

Actions/Interventions	Rationales

■ Observe for seizure activity. Record and report the following observations:
  • Time of onset
  • Body parts involved: order of involvement and characteristic of movement
  • Tonic-clonic stages
  • Incontinence
  • Duration of seizure
  • Postictal state (e.g. confusion, drowsiness, sleep)
	A record if activity will determine seizure type. Seizure activity may occur as a result of inflammation of brain tissue.

■ Monitor for signs of airway obstruction.	Loss of motor control during a seizure can compromise the airway if the tongue falls back into the upper airway.

Therapeutic Interventions

Actions/Interventions	Rationales
▲ Administer anticonvulsants as ordered.	Anticonvulsants are administered intravenously to interrupt seizure activity. Long-term oral administration is given to prevent seizures.
■ Institute seizure precautions for high-risk patients, such as keeping bed in low position, side rails raised at all times, and padding rails.	Safety measures are implemented to prevent injury such as falls during seizure activity.
■ If seizure occurs, remain with patient, do not attempt to introduce anything into the mouth during the seizure. Maintain airway. Turn patient on side, suction, administer oxygen if needed.	Inserting objects could result in increased risk of aspiration, broken teeth, or soft tissue injury.
■ Maintain minimal environmental stimuli: noise reduction, curtains closed, private room (when available or advisable), dim lights.	During the postictal phase of seizure activity, the patient may be disoriented or sleep for several hours before returning to baseline LOC.

NANDA-I
NDx **Acute Pain**

Common Related Factors
Meningeal irritation
Increased ICP

Defining Characteristics
Headache
Photophobia
Nuchal rigidity
Irritability

Common Expected Outcomes
Patient reports satisfactory pain control at a level less than 3 to 4 on a 0 to 10 rating scale.
Patient uses pharmacological and nonpharmacological pain relief strategies.
Patient exhibits increased comfort such as baseline levels for pulse, blood pressure, respirations, and relaxed muscle tone or body posture.

NOC Outcomes
Pain Control; Medication Response
NIC Interventions
Analgesic Administration; Environmental Management: Comfort

Ongoing Assessment

Actions/Interventions	Rationales
■ Assess for headache, photophobia, restlessness, irritability.	Severe headache is the most common early symptom of intracranial infection. Headache is caused by irritation of dura and tension on vascular structures. The location of the headache helps determine the source of the infection. Headaches are usually intensified by movement or exertion. Photophobia (light sensitivity) may occur with meningeal irritation.

Therapeutic Interventions

Actions/Interventions	Rationales
■ Decrease external stimuli, such as restricting visitors as appropriate and reducing noise in the environment.	Stimulation can increase ICP, thereby aggravating pain.
■ Keep the patient's room darkened, or have the patient wear sunglasses.	Reducing visual stimuli can minimize effects of photophobia.
▲ Administer analgesics as prescribed.	NSAIDs are usually effective in managing pain.
■ Discourage the Valsalva maneuver (e.g., instruct the patient to exhale when moving up in bed; provide stool softeners).	Straining can cause increased cerebral blood flow and increased ICP. These changes can aggravate headache pain.
■ Explain that treatment of infection will also decrease pain.	Antibiotic and corticosteroid therapy reduce acute inflammation and thereby reduce pain.

NANDA-I NDx **Deficient Knowledge**

Common Related Factors
Unfamiliarity with disease process
New treatment (possible surgical drainage)

Common Expected Outcome
Patient or significant others verbalize understanding of current infection, possible causes, tests, treatment, and follow-up care.

Defining Characteristics
Verbalized questions or concerns
Incorrect or inaccurate information is conveyed

NOC Outcomes
Knowledge: Disease Process; Knowledge: Treatment Regimen
NIC Interventions
Teaching: Prescribed Medication; Teaching: Disease Process

Ongoing Assessment

Actions/Interventions	Rationales
■ Assess the patient's or significant others' knowledge base about current central nervous system infection, treatment, and follow-up care.	Intracranial infection is frequently an unfamiliar diagnosis. Assessing actual learning needs will provide guidance in designing a teaching plan.

Therapeutic Interventions

Actions/Interventions	Rationales
■ Provide explanations of disease process, cause if known, diagnostic testing (e.g., CT, MRI, lumbar puncture), and length of convalescence.	Information helps the patient and family become part of the health care team. Convalescence after an intracranial infection usually takes several weeks.

■ = Independent ▲ = Collaborative

Actions/Interventions	Rationales
■ Provide information about appropriate immunizations.	Vaccines for meningitis are recommended for high-risk patients such as children, college students living in dormitories, and older adults.
■ Instruct the patient or significant others in principles of antibiotic therapy, effects and possible side effects, maintenance of therapeutic levels, and duration of treatment. If the patient is to be discharged on medications (e.g., antibiotics, anticonvulsants), instruct in dose, frequency, route, and possible side effects. It is best to provide written instructions for reference at home.	Compliance with pharmacological therapy is necessary to promote effective outcomes and prevent reinfections.
■ Provide information about adjunct treatments that may be indicated: physical and occupational therapy, and speech therapy.	Physical and occupational therapy can assist in overcoming residual muscle rigidity from lengthy bed rest and can retrain in activities of daily living if infection caused memory loss or neurological dysfunction. Speech therapy may be necessary to assist with swallowing and articulation problems. Therapy required depends on diagnosis, promptness of treatment, and resultant recovery or disability.
■ Teach patient and family about measures to prevent transmission of meningitis.	Meningitis represents a community health concern. Prevention of transmission in improving hygiene such as frequent handwashing, and containing coughs and sneezes with tissues. Proper disposal of tissues is important.
■ Refer patient and family to social service agencies.	Social service agencies can assist families in managing high density or overcrowded living arrangements.

Related Care Plans

Acute pain, p. 151
Decreased intracranial adaptive capacity, p. 119
Deficient fluid volume, p. 72
Imbalanced nutrition: less than body requirements, p. 142

Low Back Pain/Herniated Intervertebral Disk

Slipped Disk; Ruptured Disk; Sciatica; Laminectomy

Herniated lumbar intervertebral disks are a common cause of severe back pain. Age of onset is typically between 30 and 50 years of age, with men affected more often than women. Etiological factors include trauma (50%), degenerative diseases (e.g., osteoarthritis and ankylosing spondylitis), and congenital defects (e.g., scoliosis). Weak back and abdominal muscles combined with strenuous activity and heavy lifting is a common scenario for disk herniation in the lumbar spine. In many cases the disk is spontaneously reduced or reabsorbed without treatment, but more often the problem becomes chronic with pain and disability depending on the location and severity of the herniation. The amount of disk pulposus herniated into the spinal canal affects the narrowing of the space and the degree of compression on the lumbar or sacral spinal roots. A variety of surgical procedures may be done to reduce nerve compression and relieve lower back pain. Conservative management (rest, heat or ice, and nonsteroidal antiinflammatory drugs [NSAIDs]) is usually accomplished in the ambulatory setting and is the focus of this care plan. Duration of treatment depends on location of herniation of symptoms. Hospitalization is necessary only if pain and sensorimotor deficits are incapacitating.

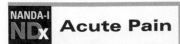

Acute Pain

Common Related Factors

Trauma
Muscle spasm
Nerve root compression

Defining Characteristics

Verbalized complaint of the following:
- Mild to excruciating lower back pain
- Radiating pain to buttock or leg
- Guarding behavior
- Change in sleep pattern
- Physical and social withdrawal

Common Expected Outcomes

Patient reports satisfactory pain control at a level less than 3 to 4 on a 0 to 10 rating scale.
Patient uses pharmacological and nonpharmacological pain relief strategies.
Patient exhibits increased comfort such as baseline levels for pulse, blood pressure, respirations, and relaxed muscle tone or body posture.

NOC Outcomes
Pain Control; Medication Response
NIC Interventions
Pain Management; Positioning; Medication Management

Ongoing Assessment

Actions/Interventions	Rationales
■ Identify the following changes in sensorimotor function: • Absent lumbar lordosis • Lumbar scoliosis • Limited movement or flexion • Slight motor weakness • Decreased knee and ankle reflexes • Paresthesia or numbness • Changes in bowel or bladder function	Decrease in motor function is often a guarding behavior, a protective action or inaction to control pain. The cervical spine is affected most often because it is the most flexible segment of the spine. A herniated disk can press against adjacent nerves, causing pain and paresthesias. The specific level of injury will determine the symptoms experienced by the patient. Alterations in gait and posture may represent nerve injury or adaptation to chronic pain.
▲ Facilitate diagnostic testing, if needed: spinal x-ray films, computed tomography, magnetic resonance imaging, lumbar puncture for cerebrospinal fluid (protein will be high with normal cell count), myelogram, and/or nerve conduction studies.	Serial testing may be done to determine progression of herniation.
■ Obtain detailed pain history, including the following: • Location and onset of pain • Presence of radiating pain • Recurrent (duration and frequency) or continuous pain • Precipitating factors • Relief factors (preference for standing or lying down) • Aggravating factors (sitting, jarring movements)	Remission and exacerbation of pain in the patient with a lumbar herniation often occur because of decreased edema and root compression, as well as spontaneous reduction of the disk into its normal position and reabsorption of disk exudate. Lumbar disk disease may cause pain that radiates along the path of the sciatic nerve into the leg and groin area. Muscle weakness may occur with the pain.
■ Evaluate effectiveness of previous treatments.	Patients may have tried multiple home remedies for pain relief before seeking professional care.

Therapeutic Interventions

Actions/Interventions	Rationales
■ Instruct the patient to do the following: • Begin bed rest on a firm mattress. • Use a pillow under the knees (lumbar).	Rest reduces pressure on nerve roots, relieves muscle spasms, and promotes comfort during the healing process. A firm mattress provides back support. A board can be placed underneath a soft mattress for support. Most patients

■ = Independent ▲ = Collaborative

Actions/Interventions

Rationales

find positioning in a semi-Fowler's position with knees flexed reduces pressure on nerve roots and promotes muscle relaxation. A supine position may aggravate pain. The use of appropriate sleep aids for body positioning will promote comfort and decrease stress on nerve roots.

▲ Initiate drug therapy, possibly including analgesics, muscle relaxants, antiinflammatory drugs, and/or sedatives as ordered.

These drugs reduce inflammation and muscle spasm. Medications and dosage depend on patient symptoms and amount of relief.

▲ Refer the patient for a physical therapy consult.

The physical therapist can provide a variety of treatments for muscle relaxation and pain relief, including ultrasound and thermal treatments. The physical therapist can help the patient learn exercises to strengthen back muscles and prevent further injury.

■ Instruct the patient in use of back braces, corsets, or traction therapy (pelvic belt).

These devices limit spinal movement and relieve pressure on nerve roots. Traction does not seem to have a direct effect on disk placement but does provide relief from spasms and decreases pressure on nerve roots, thereby providing pain relief.

■ Assist the patient in using additional pain control modalities, such as heat and cold applications, relaxation therapy, imagery, and anxiety reduction.

Nonpharmacological pain interventions will contribute to effective pain management. These strategies may reduce the development of problems associated with overuse of opioid analgesics. Cold packs or heat may be effective when used early in the acute pain episode by reducing inflammation and relieving muscle spasms.

NANDA-I NDx **Deficient Knowledge**

Common Related Factors
Unfamiliar diagnosis
New treatments

Defining Characteristics
Verbalized lack of understanding
Multiple questions
Noncompliance

Common Expected Outcome
Patient verbalizes understanding of treatment program and demonstrates skills necessary for protecting vertebrae.

NOC Outcomes
Knowledge: Disease Process; Knowledge: Treatment Regimen

NIC Interventions
Teaching: Disease Process; Teaching: Prescribed Activity/Exercise

---

Ongoing Assessment

Actions/Interventions

Rationales

■ Assess the patient's understanding of the diagnosis and treatment plan.

Patients often have misunderstandings about the cause of back pain and measures for effective management. The effectiveness of the treatment plans requires patient's cooperation and willingness to make necessary changes in lifestyle behaviors.

Therapeutic Interventions

Actions/Interventions	Rationales
■ Design a teaching plan specific to the patient's needs and treatment plan.	The patient needs information about treatment options to guide decision making. The long-term effectiveness of nonsurgical and surgical approaches to treatment is similar for patients with mild to moderate disease. Surgical therapy is associated with better outcomes for patients with moderate to severe disease.

Conservative treatment plan

• Remission and exacerbation	Patients experience periods of improvement and exacerbation of symptoms because of changes in the amount of inflammation at the level of herniation until the area is healed.
• Exercise program: muscle strengthening exercise is prescribed	Exercise helps support the spinal column. These exercises focus on strengthening abdominal and paravertebral muscles. The patient may need to continue specific back exercises for a lifetime.
• Proper body mechanics: instruction in proper lifting and avoidance of repetitive motion and body movements	Improper body mechanics can aggravate weakened disks. Extremes of spinal flexion and rotation are discouraged. The patient may need to learn ways to modify the home and work environment to protect the back during activities.
• Medications: analgesics, NSAIDs, muscle relaxants	Appropriate use of medications for pain relief will help the patient maintain desired activity levels.
• Application and use of support garments and traction equipment	The use of supportive back braces and corsets minimizes injury and relieves nerve root compression.
• Weight control	Obesity and increased abdominal adipose tissue adds to strain on the lumbar spine and paravertebral muscles. Weight reduction, as part of the treatment plan, decreases the risk of exacerbations.

Surgical intervention

• Type of surgery: • Diskectomy—partial removal of lamina • Laminectomy—excision of posterior arch of vertebra (lamina) • Spinal fusion—fusion of vertebrae with bone grafts, rods, plates, or screws	Surgery may be required for patients who suffer severe herniation resulting in cord compression, loss of function, and unrelenting pain. Laminectomy may also be done after poor response to conservative treatment.
• Pain: immediately postoperative (spasms, incisional)	Patients need to understand that incisional pain is part of the normal postoperative experience. This pain is managed with analgesics. Patients who have experienced long-term radiating pain and paresthesias may continue to have these symptoms for several postoperative weeks. This pain will diminish over time.
• Postoperative expectations: initial immobility, relearning how to move	Physical therapy will be required in the home and as an outpatient to strengthen muscles, to learn to move, and to protect the spine.
• Recurrent herniation: may occur near site of original herniation or at another location	Degenerative or other changes may predispose the patient to repeat herniation and repeat laminectomy, despite following prescribed treatment plan.

Related Care Plans

■ = Independent   ▲ = Collaborative

Multiple Sclerosis

Disseminated Sclerosis; Demyelinating Disease

Multiple sclerosis (MS) is a chronic progressive and degenerative nervous system disease characterized by scattered patches of demyelination and glial tissue overgrowth in the white matter of the brain and spinal cord. These structural changes in nerve tissue lead to decreased nerve conduction. As the inflammation or edema diminishes, some remyelination may occur, and nerve conduction returns. Among the clinical symptoms associated with MS are extremity weakness, visual disturbances, ataxia, tremor, incoordination, sphincter impairment, and impaired position sense. The clinical manifestations occur randomly with no predictable pattern of progression. Remissions and exacerbations are associated with the disease. Although the specific cause is unknown, etiological hypotheses include environmental, viral, and genetic factors. Infection with the Epstein-Barr virus in genetically susceptible individuals is thought to trigger an immune response that begins the inflammatory process causing demyelination. Loss of myelin disrupts nerve conduction. MS lesions are found in the cerebral white matter, optic nerves, brainstem, cerebellum, and cervical spinal cord. MS is considered the disease of young adults. Onset is typically between 15 and 50 years of age. Women are affected more often than men. This care plan focuses on maintenance care in the ambulatory care setting.

NDx Deficient Knowledge

Common Related Factor

Unfamiliarity with the disease process and management

Defining Characteristics

Verbalization of misconceptions
Questioning

Common Expected Outcome

Patient or significant others verbalize understanding of disease process, medications used, adverse effects, and follow-up care.

NOC Outcomes

Knowledge: Disease Process; Knowledge: Treatment Regimen

NIC Interventions

Teaching: Disease Process; Teaching: Procedures/Treatment; Teaching: Prescribed Medications

Ongoing Assessment

Actions/Interventions

■ Assess knowledge of disease, exacerbations, remissions, medical regimen, and resources.

Rationales

Lack of knowledge about MS and its progressive nature can compromise the patient's ability to care for self and cope effectively.

Therapeutic Interventions

Actions/Interventions

■ Discuss disease process in simple, straightforward manner, as follows:
  • MS is a chronic, slowly progressive nervous system disease that affects nerve conduction.

Rationales

Accurate information about MS reduces anxiety and allows the patient to comprehend the disease process. The patient and family members need to understand the disease process in order to make informed decisions concerning financial resources, long-term care, power of attorney, and living wills.

Actions/Interventions

- There is no definitive diagnostic test, but some tests are used in conjunction with a careful history and physical examination, such as magnetic resonance imaging; visual-evoked potentials (VEP); and cerebrospinal fluid analysis.

- There is no specific cure. Newest treatments include β-interferon administration to decrease the number of exacerbations and Copolymer 1 administration, a synthetic myelin basis protein, to replace the lost myelin. A variety of disease modifying drugs are available for patients to reduce relapses. These drugs are part of long-term therapy.
- MS can result in weakness, visual disturbance, walking unsteadiness, and sometimes urine or bowel problems.
- ■ Instruct the patient or significant others when to contact the health care team (e.g., urinary symptoms; motor, sensory, visual disturbances; exacerbations).
- ■ Instruct the patient or significant others about steroid therapy:
  - Side effects (e.g., sodium retention, fluid retention, pedal edema, hypertension, gastric irritation).
  - Measures to control side effects (e.g., low-sodium diet, daily weighing, leg elevation, support hose, blood pressure monitoring, antacids, adequate rest, and avoidance of contact with persons with infectious disease).
- ■ Teach about drugs used for muscle spasticity.

- ■ Instruct in the following:
  - Importance of maintaining the most normal activity level possible
  - Avoidance of hot baths
  - Sleeping in a prone position
  - Need to inspect areas of impaired sensation for serious injuries

  - Need to use energy conservation techniques

- ■ Instruct the patient to avoid potentially exacerbating activities: emotional stress, physical stress or fatigue, infection, pregnancy, physically "run down" condition.

- ■ Facilitate involvement with support groups and/or counseling, as desired.

Rationales

The diagnosis of MS is based on criteria from the Revised International Panel on MS Diagnosis (Revised McDonald Criteria). The patient needs to provide a detailed history to assist in accurate diagnosis of MS. Patients may experience symptoms for many months before a diagnosis is made. An MRI is used to detect the presence of MS plaques. VEP tests are useful in confirming a diagnosis of MS. The demyelination that occurs with MS results in a slowing of response time. Analysis of cerebrospinal fluid is done to detect increased immune cells indicative of MS.

Drug therapy is initiated to reduce disease activity and disease progression. The drugs work by modifying or suppressing immune system activity. Many of the drugs are administered as subcutaneous injections by the patient. The cost of treatment is expensive and may be covered by the patient's health insurance.

The patient and family need to plan strategies for management of exacerbations of MS.

Prompt treatment of exacerbations can be initiated when the patient and family know what to report.

Steroid therapy decreases edema and acute inflammatory response within evolving plaque. Prednisone and adrenocorticotropic hormone are used most often for acute exacerbations.

These measures reduce fluid retention and the risk for infection and gastric ulcers.

Muscle spasticity can be managed with muscle relaxants. The FDA has recently approved Botox for management of muscle spasticity. Drugs may be used for short-term or long-term therapy.

When the patient can have a normal activity pattern, it helps maintain functional ability and improve body image.

Heat increases metabolic demands and may increase weakness.

Good positioning during sleep decreases flexion spasms.

Careful attention to these areas decreases risk for injury. Patients may have decreased temperature sensation that increases risk for burns.

The fatigue in MS is from nerve demyelination not muscle fatigue. A balance of daily rest and exercise is indicated. Drugs such as amantadine or pemoline are helpful in treating fatigue.

Young female patients may choose to become pregnant. Symptoms of MS diminish during pregnancy, but exacerbation is common and sometimes severe during the postpartum period. Stress is the most common cause of exacerbations.

Support groups can assist with issues such as family process, work, parenting, and sexuality. Developmentally, this age-group is typically in its most productive years, therefore MS has the potential for causing major life cycle alterations. Depression and cognitive impairment are common problems for the patient with MS.

■ = Independent ▲ = Collaborative

Impaired Physical Mobility

Common Related Factors

Motor weakness
Tremors
Spasticity

Defining Characteristics

Unsteady gait
Limited range of motion (ROM)
Lack of coordination
Inability to move purposefully
Reluctance to attempt movement

Common Expected Outcomes

Patient performs physical activity independently or within limits of activity restrictions.
Patient demonstrates use of adaptive techniques that promote ambulation and transferring.
Patient is free of complications of immobility, as evidenced by intact skin, absence of thrombophlebitis, normal bowel pattern, and clear breath sounds.

NOC Outcomes
Ambulation; Mobility
NIC Interventions
Environmental Management; Teaching: Prescribed Activity/Exercise; Exercise Therapy: Stretching/Muscle Control

Ongoing Assessment

Actions/Interventions	Rationales
■ Assess the patient's gait, muscle strength, weakness, coordination, and balance.	Changes in these findings are a gauge to assess progression and remission of MS.
■ Assess endurance level and stamina (e.g., number of stairs the patient can climb, distance the patient can walk, ability to work, ability to perform activities of daily living [ADLs] independently).	Motor dysfunction contributes to weakness with MS. Cerebellar dysfunction causes tremors, poor coordination, and ataxia. These symptoms can interfere with ADLs and mobility. Restricted movement affects the ability to perform most ADLs. A variety of assessment tools are available, depending on the clinical setting. Such tools provide objective data for baselines. For example, the FIM measures 18 self-care items related to eating, bathing, grooming, dressing, toileting, bladder and bowel management, transfer, ambulation, and stair climbing. Fatigue and reduced functional ability may be more pronounced in the evening.
■ Determine the patient's ability to use assistive devices (cane, walker) and adaptive techniques (using larger muscle groups).	Proper use of assistive devices can promote activity and reduce risk for falls.

Therapeutic Interventions

Actions/Interventions	Rationales
■ Encourage self-care as tolerated and seeking assistance when necessary; arrange for home care when needed.	Exacerbations become more frequent and longer in duration as the disease progresses.
■ Suggest placing frequently needed items (cooking material, personal care items, cleaning supplies) within easy reach.	Home modifications can help the patient maintain a desired level of functional independence and reduce fatigue with activity.
■ Encourage stretching exercises and ROM daily. Suggest scheduled rest periods.	These activities promote venous return, prevent flexion contractures, and maintain muscle strength and endurance. Exercises and early ambulation require much energy. Rest periods help reduce the level of fatigue.

Actions/Interventions

▲ Instruct the patient in use of adaptive techniques and equipment. These may include wrist weights, adaptive equipment such as stabilized plates and nonspilling cups, stabilization of extremity, and training patient to use trunk and head. Consult a physical therapist and occupational therapist for use of assistive or ambulatory devices and ADL evaluation.

Rationales

Aids can compensate for impaired function and increase the level of activity. The goal for using adaptive devices is to promote safety, increase mobility, prevent falls, and conserve energy. Home environment evaluation may be necessary.

 NANDA-I NDx **Risk for Disturbed Sensory Perception: Visual**

Common Risk Factor

Optic nerve demyelination

Common Expected Outcome

Patient achieves optimal functioning within limits of visual impairment, as evidenced by ability to care for self, to navigate environment safely, and to engage in meaningful activities.

NOC Outcomes

Risk Control: Visual Impairment; Vision Compensation Behavior

NIC Intervention

Communication Enhancement: Visual Deficit

Ongoing Assessment

Actions/Interventions

■ Assess for visual impairment.

■ Ask patient about specifics such as ability to read or see television, history of falls, or ability to self-medicate.

■ Assess factors or aids that improve vision, such as glasses, contact lenses, or bright and/or natural light.

■ Evaluate the patient's ability to function within limits of visual impairment.

■ Evaluate psychological response to visual loss.

Rationales

Common symptoms include diplopia, blurred vision, nystagmus, visual loss, scotomas (blind spots), and impaired color perception.

Visual impairment can contribute to problems in daily activities. The risk for falls and medication errors increases if the person has diminished visual acuity.

Nursing interventions should include strategies that enhance the patient's adaptive abilities.

Personal appearance and condition of clothing and surroundings are good indicators of the patient's adaptation to visual loss.

Anger, depression, and withdrawal are common responses. Self-esteem is often negatively affected.

Therapeutic Interventions

Actions/Interventions

■ Encourage the patient to ask for orientation to new environments, such as location of bathrooms, stairs, and other features in unfamiliar homes, restaurants, and businesses.

■ Encourage the patient and family to place objects within reach. Do not change familiar home environments without informing the patient.

■ Provide an eye patch for diplopia; encourage alternating the patch from eye to eye.

Rationales

The patient may be embarrassed or hesitant to ask for assistance.

Consistent placement of belongings enhances independence.

Alternating the patch from one eye to another alleviates diplopia. Using adaptive techniques can help the patient cope with visual changes. Corrective lenses may be beneficial for changes in visual acuity.

■ = Independent   ▲ = Collaborative

Actions/Interventions

- Instruct the patient to rest eyes when fatigued.
- Advise the patient of the availability of large-type reading materials and talking books.
- If the patient is hospitalized, place the call light within reach with side rails up and bed in low position to prevent injury.
- Teach the patient to turn head from side to side when entering an unfamiliar environment.

Rationales

Fatigue can aggravate visual problems.

These resources allow the patient to retain desired activity for work and leisure.

Patient safety is a priority.

Visual scanning will help the patient who has decreased peripheral vision. This technique promotes safety in a new environment.

Risk for Urinary Retention/Incontinence

Common Risk Factor
Neurogenic bladder

Common Expected Outcomes
The patient maintains residual urine of less than 100 mL/hr.
The patient does not experience urinary tract infection (UTI).
The patient remains dry between voluntary voiding.

NOC Outcomes
Urinary Continence; Urinary Elimination
NIC Interventions
Urinary Retention; Urinary Incontinence Care

Ongoing Assessment

Actions/Interventions

- Inquire about symptoms of urinary retention, frequency, urgency, pain, and abdominal distention.

- Assess for signs of UTI.

- Assess pattern of fluid intake.

Rationales

Patients may experience either a spastic bladder, characterized by frequency and dribbling, or a flaccid bladder, in which an absence of sensation to void results in urine retention.

Retention predisposes to infection. Infection can trigger an exacerbation of MS.

Fluid intake is related to bladder filling and voiding. Patients may reduce fluid intake to control incontinence. Decreased intake increases the risk for UTI.

Therapeutic Interventions

Actions/Interventions

- Initiate individualized bladder training program. Instruct the patient about the Credé method and intermittent catheterization for residual urine if signs of retention are present.
- Encourage the patient to drink 2 to 3 liters of fluid daily.

- Instruct the patient about signs and symptoms of UTI.

- Explain prescribed medications.

- Recommend vitamin C and liberal intake of cranberry juice.

Rationales

Residual urine greater than 100 mL predisposes the patient to UTIs. Bladder Credé methods stimulate complete emptying of the bladder.

Increased fluid intake increases urine output and reduces the risk for infection.

Patients need to be able to recognize symptoms of UTI so that treatment can be started as soon as possible.

Cholinergic drugs are indicated for flaccid bladder, and anticholinergic drugs are indicated for spastic bladder

These nutrients acidify urine and reduce bacterial growth.

Risk for Impaired Skin Integrity

Common Risk Factors

Sensory changes
Immobility

Common Expected Outcome

Patient maintains intact skin, as evidenced by absence of breakdown, burns, or pressure ulcer formation.

NOC Outcome
Tissue Integrity: Skin and Mucous Membranes
NIC Intervention
Skin Surveillance

Ongoing Assessment

Actions/Interventions

■ Assess skin integrity and areas of body with decreased sensation.

Rationales

Sensory changes may result in hypoalgesia, paresthesia, and loss of position sense, which can lead to trauma, injury, and skin integrity changes.

Therapeutic Interventions

Actions/Interventions

■ Instruct the patient to avoid extremes in heat and cold (water and environmental) and prolonged physical pressure.
■ Instruct the patient to test bath water with unaffected extremity.
■ Instruct the patient to notice foot placement when ambulating.
■ Instruct the patient to change position every 2 hours, even when watching television or working at a desk.

Rationales

The patient needs knowledge to prevent thermal and pressure injury to the skin.
Decreased temperature sensation increases risk for burns.

This technique compensates for decreased position sense.

Normal protective mechanisms are absent, so a conscious decision must be made to change position.

Related Care Plans

Grieving, p. 82
Constipation, p. 46
Disturbed body image, p. 24
Ineffective sexuality patterns, p. 182
Powerlessness, p. 162
Self-care deficit, p. 170

Parkinson's Disease

Parkinsonism

Parkinson's disease (PD) is a movement disorder associated with dopamine deficiency in the brain. Other neurotransmitter alterations may also contribute to the disease process. This chronic neurological disorder affects the extrapyramidal system of the brain responsible for control and regulation of movement. There is no specific diagnostic test. A diagnosis of PD is based on thorough evaluation of presenting clinical manifestations. The four characteristic signs are tremor at rest, rigidity, postural instability, and slowness of movement. Other clinical manifestations include shuffling gait, masklike facial expressions, and muscle weakness affecting writing, speaking, eating, chewing, and swallowing. Onset is usually around 60 years of age; however, a significant number of young adults have PD. Secondary Parkinsonism is associated with traumatic brain injury and side effects of the phenothiazine drug group. Etiological hypotheses include exposure to environmental toxins and age-related degeneration of brain neurons. Some theories suggest gene mutation may play a role in the development of PD. Free radical formation has also been considered as a contributing factor. There is no cure for PD. Treatment is focused on slowing disease progression and symptom management. Drug therapy is the primary treatment for PD. As the disease progresses and tremors become more severe, surgical therapy may be used. Patient care is usually managed in the outpatient setting.

NANDA-I NDx   Impaired Physical Mobility

Common Related Factors
Neuromuscular impairment
Decreased strength and endurance

Defining Characteristics
Tremors
Muscle rigidity
Decreased ability to initiate movements (akinesis)
Impaired coordination of movement
Limited range of motion (ROM)
Impaired ability to carry out activities of daily living (ADLs)
Postural disturbances

Common Expected Outcomes
Patient performs physical activity independently or within limits of activity restrictions.
Patient demonstrates use of adaptive techniques that promote ambulation and transferring.
Patient is free of complications of immobility, as evidenced by intact skin, absence of thrombophlebitis, normal bowel pattern, and clear breath sounds.

NOC Outcomes
Ambulation; Mobility
NIC Interventions
Teaching: Prescribed Activity or Exercise; Environmental Management

Ongoing Assessment

Actions/Interventions	Rationales
■ Assess for rigidity:	Rigidity may be unilateral or bilateral
• Cogwheel	Cogwheel rigidity is an interrupted but rhythmic muscle movement.
• Plastic	Plastic rigidity represents more resistance to movement.
• Lead pipe	This type of rigidity is complete resistance to movement.
■ Assess extent of tremors.	Typically tremors are more prominent at rest and are aggravated by emotional stress. Hand tremors may present as a "pill-rolling" movement at rest. Tremors occur as a result of unopposed acetylcholine activity from the dopamine deficiency.
■ Assess posture, coordination, and ambulation.	Clinical manifestations may range from only a slight limp to the typical shuffling, propulsive gait with rigidity. These changes are more common in advanced PD.
■ Assess for bradykinesia.	The patient with PD will have difficulty initiating movement or changing direction of movement. This results from poor coordination of opposing muscle groups. The patient's movements will be slow and hesitant.

Therapeutic Interventions

Actions/Interventions	Rationales
■ Encourage patient to perform ROM to all joints daily.	Exercise reduces muscle rigidity, maintains joint mobility, and prevents muscle atrophy.
■ Provide tips for getting in and out of chair. Use sturdy, high-seated chair with arms.	This type of chair provides more support and reduces risk for falls with changes in position.
■ Reinforce need for regular activity and ambulation.	Activity is important to reduce hazards of immobility. Some patients have shown improvement with rhythmic exercise programs such as yoga or tai chi.
■ Encourage the family to supervise and assist with ambulation as needed.	Safety with ambulation is an important concern to prevent falls. The use of mobility aids such as canes and walkers promotes stability and reduces the risk for falls.
■ Encourage the patient to lift feet and take large steps while walking.	A broad-based gait helps improve balance and reduces shuffling.
■ Discuss the need for removing environmental barriers in the home.	Maintaining patient safety is a priority.
■ Instruct the family to allow sufficient time for ADLs.	The family often wants to perform the task rather than enabling the patient to do it.
▲ Consult physical and occupational therapists about aids to facilitate ADLs and safe ambulation and to promote muscle strengthening.	Aids can increase mobility and allow the patient some control over the environment.

NANDA-I NDx Imbalanced Nutrition: Less Than Body Requirements

Common Related Factors
Difficulty swallowing and dysphagia
Choking spells
Drooling
Regurgitation of food or fluids through nares

Defining Characteristics
Documented intake below required caloric level
Malnutrition
Weight loss
Constipation

Common Expected Outcome
Patient maintains optimal nutritional status, as evidenced by adequate oral intake, weight gain, weight within normal limits for height and age, and absence of constipation.

NOC Outcomes
Nutritional Status: Nutrient Intake; Respiratory Status: Airway Patency
NIC Interventions
Nutrition Management; Aspiration Precautions

Ongoing Assessment

Actions/Interventions	Rationales
■ Assess degree of swallowing difficulty with fluids, solids, and/or medications.	Swallowing difficulty accompanied by fatigue and fine motor impairment causes diminished appetite and poor nutritional intake. Swallowing problems are associated with the later stages of the disease.
■ Inquire about episodes of choking, drooling, and nasal regurgitations.	Poor muscle coordination and weakness in the mouth and throat increase the risk for aspiration. Drooling indicates inability to swallow saliva because of muscle weakness.
■ Assess overall nutritional status.	Bradykinesia, tremors, and rigidity may interfere with feeding self-care, chewing, and swallowing.
■ Monitor weight at each visit. Encourage the patient or family to keep a weight and/or diet log.	Weight loss is usually the result of decreased intake.

■ = Independent   ▲ = Collaborative

Therapeutic Interventions

Actions/Interventions	Rationales
■ Reinforce the need for high-Fowler's position for eating and drinking.	This position reduces the risk for aspiration.
■ Elicit family supervision during meals. Avoid distractions.	The patient needs to focus on swallowing in order to avoid aspiration.
■ Stress importance of allowing adequate time for meals; avoid rushing the patient.	It may be difficult for patients to swallow under pressure. Bradykinesia may require more time for feeding self-care.
■ Suggest high-calorie, low-volume supplements between meals.	Additional caloric intake may be required for optimal nutrition.
■ Suggest the patient take small bites of food. Encourage the patient to swallow two to three times after taking a bite of food.	Smaller bites may be easier to swallow.
■ Suggest appetizing foods that are easily chewed and fluids that are thickened rather than watery fluids.	Fluids are more difficult to control when swallowing.
■ Suggest four to five small meals per day and at least 2000 mL of fluids (if fluids are not restricted for another health reason).	Small meals may be tolerated with greater success than three meals daily. This meal plan is associated with improved nutritional intake.
■ Encourage oral hygiene after meals.	Toothbrushing and rinsing the mouth are useful in removing residual and pocketed food that can be aspirated later.
▲ Consult a dietitian for needed changes in food consistency, for caloric counts, and for diet suggestions to help avoid constipation.	The dietitian can recommend alterations in food selection to promote adequate calorie and nutrient intake.
▲ If swallowing difficulties worsen, consult a speech therapist.	A specialist may be needed to design plans to improve the patient's ability to swallow.
▲ Consult a physical therapist for wrist or hand brace.	Braces help control tremors and improve ability to feed self.

NANDA-I NDx **Impaired Verbal Communication**

Common Related Factor
Dysarthria/slurred speech

Defining Characteristics
Difficulty in articulating words
Monotonous voice tones
Slow, slurred speech
Stammered speech

Common Expected Outcomes
Patient communicates needs adequately.
Patient uses alternative methods of communication as indicated.

NOC Outcome
Communication Ability
NIC Intervention
Communication Enhancement: Speech Deficit

Ongoing Assessment

Actions/Interventions	Rationales
■ Evaluate the patient's ability to speak, as well as to understand spoken words, written words, and pictures.	As the disease progresses, cognitive abilities diminish. The patient with PD may have slurred speech as a result of dysarthria.
■ Assess voice quality.	As PD progresses, the patient's voice may become lower-pitched and softer.

Therapeutic Interventions

Actions/Interventions	Rationales
■ Maintain eye contact when speaking.	This approach promotes patient focus and attention.
■ Allow patient time to articulate.	The patient may be discouraged and give up if rushed. The patient needs time to organize thoughts before speaking.
■ Encourage face and tongue exercises.	Regular exercise can reduce rigidity and facilitate muscle relaxation.
■ Encourage the patient to practice reading aloud or singing.	Activities that involve the affected muscles help the patient practice muscle control.
■ Avoid speaking loudly unless the patient is hard of hearing.	Loud talking does not improve the patient's ability to understand.
▲ Consult a speech therapist if indicated.	The speech therapist can evaluate the patient's need for adaptive devices such as voice synthesizers or computers.
■ Provide alternative communication aids as needed, such as picture or word boards.	These aids reduce communication frustration.

Chronic Low Self-Esteem

Common Related Factors

Changes in body image, especially drooling, tremors, gait, slurred speech
Dependence on others

Defining Characteristics

Minimal eye contact
Self-deprecating statements
Anger
Expression of shame
Rejection of positive feedback

Common Expected Outcome

Patient recognizes self-maligning statements and begins to verbalize positive expression of self-worth.

NOC Outcomes
Body Image; Self-Esteem

NIC Interventions
Body Image Enhancement; Self-Esteem Enhancement

Ongoing Assessment

Actions/Interventions	Rationales
■ Assess the patient's perception of self. Note verbalizations regarding self.	Patients may attempt to hide tremors. Over time, they may withdraw from social interactions because they are embarrassed by their symptoms.
■ Assess the degree to which the patient feels loved and respected by others.	The manner in which one is treated by others influences self-esteem. Feeling loved and respected despite disabilities implies that one is valued by others and supports self-esteem.
■ Evaluate the patient's support system.	A positive social network can promote effective coping with the changes of PD.

Therapeutic Interventions

Actions/Interventions	Rationales
■ Encourage the patient to verbalize fears and concerns. Listen attentively.	Verbalization of actual or perceived threats can help reduce anxiety. Patients may express concern about increasing dependency on others for mobility and ADLs.

■ = Independent   ▲ = Collaborative

Neurological Care Plans

Actions/Interventions	Rationales
■ Discuss feelings about symptoms: tremors, drooling of saliva, slurred speech.	Patients may be ashamed about changes in their appearance and their inability to control symptoms.
■ Discuss the impact of alteration in health status on self-esteem.	Disturbances in self-esteem are natural responses to significant changes. Reconstruction of the individual's self-esteem occurs after grieving has taken place and acceptance has followed.
■ Instruct the family to avoid overprotection of the individual; promote social interaction as appropriate.	Patients should not be forced into uncomfortable situations. Overprotection by family members may reinforce the patient's feelings of unworthiness and dependence on others.
■ Instruct the family to provide privacy, if desired, especially when performing ADLs and eating.	The patient may be embarrassed about eating in public places because of swallowing difficulties; family meals should be encouraged.
■ Explore strengths and resources with the patient.	Attention to the patient's strengths will reinforce a more positive self-esteem.
■ Teach the patient necessary self-care measures related to the disease.	Each success will reinforce positive self-esteem.
■ Advise of the realistic need for additional support in coping with lifelong illness. Refer to support groups.	As this disease progresses, self-care and home care issues become more evident, especially for older persons who may live alone or with an equally elderly or frail spouse. Use of lay support groups or individuals may help the patient recognize positives even in the face of disease.
■ Refer to the American Parkinson's Disease Association.	Local chapters of the organization provide information and resources such as support groups.

NANDA-I
NDx **Deficient Knowledge**

Common Related Factor

Uncertainty about cause of disease and its treatment

Defining Characteristics

Multiple questions
Lack of questions
Apparent confusion over condition

Common Expected Outcome

Patient or caregiver verbalizes disability and special needs with regard to disease process, activity, exercises, ambulation, medication, diet, and elimination.

NOC Outcomes

Knowledge: Disease Process; Knowledge: Treatment Regimen

NIC Interventions

Teaching: Disease Process; Teaching: Prescribed Medication; Teaching: Activity/ Exercise

---

Ongoing Assessment

Actions/Interventions	Rationales
■ Evaluate the patient's and caregiver's understanding of the disease process, diagnostic tests, treatments, and outcomes.	An individualized teaching plan is based on the patient's previous knowledge and desire for additional information.

Therapeutic Interventions

Actions/Interventions	Rationales
■ Reinforce explanation of the disease and treatment: • Disease: has a gradual onset and progression; has no known cure. • Treatment: therapy aimed at relieving symptoms and preventing complications.	Knowledge of the disease process and treatment may assist with the patient's coping skills. Information helps the patient and family make decisions about long-term care, financial resources, living arrangements, power of attorney, and living wills.
■ Encourage independence and avoid overprotection by encouraging the patient to do things for self: feeding, dressing, ambulation.	In early stages and with medication therapy, most ADLs can be continued (driving, working), but as the disease progresses, assistance will be required.
■ Discuss with the patient, family, and caregiver the use and the potential side effects of the following:	Patients may find it challenging to find the right medications for PD that manage symptoms effectively with minimal side effects. Dosage of medication may need to be adjusted.
• Anticholinergics: benztropine mesylate (Cogentin), procyclidine (Kemadrin), cycrimine (Pagitane), trihexyphenidyl (Artane)	These drugs decrease tremors by blocking acetylcholine activity. Side effects include constipation, dry mouth, confusion, blurred vision.
• Dopaminergic drugs: • Dopamine precursors: levodopa, carbidopa/levodopa (Sinemet)	These drugs cross the blood-brain barrier, where they are converted to dopamine. The addition of carbidopa decreases peripheral conversion of levodopa and makes more of the drug available to the brain. Side effects include nausea, hypotension, confusion, and dyskinesia. The patient may develop a tolerance to these drugs, producing an "on-off" phenomenon. The management for this phenomenon is to reduce the dosage or give the patient a drug holiday.
• Dopamine agonists: bromocriptine (Parlodel), ropinirole (Requip), pergolide (Permax)	This class of drugs mimics the activity of dopamine on postsynaptic receptors. These drugs are used in combination with carbidopa/levodopa. Side effects are increased sleepiness, confusion, and hypotension.
• Monoamine oxidase B inhibitor: selegiline (L-deprenyl)	This drug potentiates the effect of carbidopa/levodopa. Patients may experience sleep problems as a side effect. Adverse interactions with meperidine have been reported.
• Indirect agonist: amantadine (Symmetrel)	This antiviral medication has both anticholinergic and dopaminergic effects in patients with PD. It also reduces the development of dyskinesia from other PD drugs. Side effects may include dry mouth, ankle swelling, and a reddish-blue mottling of the skin (livedo reticularis).
• Catechol-O-methyltransferase inhibitor (COMT): tolcapone (Tasmar), entacapone (Comtan)	These drugs block peripheral conversion of levodopa, making more of the drug available to cross the blood-brain barrier. They decrease the development of tolerance to levodopa. Liver toxicity is associated with the use of these drugs.
■ Discuss activity recommendations: • Encourage the family and significant others to participate in physical therapy exercises of stretching and massaging muscles.	As the disease progresses, muscles and joints become stiff. Exercise improves strength and decreases rigidity.
• Encourage daily ambulation outdoors but avoidance of extreme hot and cold weather.	Extremes in temperature exacerbate symptoms in the patient with PD and are not generally well tolerated by older persons whose physiological responses are impaired.
• Encourage the patient to practice lifting feet while walking, using heel-toe gait, and swinging arms deliberately while walking.	A wide base of support is best for balance.

■ = Independent   ▲ = Collaborative

Actions/Interventions	Rationales
• Encourage the patient to dress daily, avoiding clothing with buttons (use zippers or hook and loop fasteners instead) and shoes with laces or snaps.	These actions may increase the patient's self-esteem.
• Prevent falls by clearing walkways of furniture and throw rugs, and provide handrails on stairs.	Environmental modifications will facilitate patient safety.
■ Discuss potential surgical interventions for patients who develop severe tremors:	
• Stereotactic pallidotomy	Stereotactic pallidotomy involves the use of electrical stimulation of selected neuron centers to diminish rigidity or tremors by creating permanent lesions.
• Stereotactic thalamotomy to relieve tremors and rigidity	Stereotactic thalamotomy uses thermal coagulation of neuron centers to reduce tremors.
• Neurotransplantation of dopamine-producing cells and stem cell research	Transplantation of dopamine-producing cells from fetal tissue is considered an experimental procedure. Sources of fetal tissue are either human or porcine. The procedure is considered high risk, but many patients demonstrate symptomatic improvement.
• Deep brain stimulation	Deep brain stimulation using an implanted pulse generator, similar to a cardiac pacemaker, provides control of tremors in patients whose drug therapy has been unsuccessful.

Related Care Plans

Activity intolerance, p. 8
Caregiver role strain, p. 36
Constipation, p. 46
Diarrhea, p. 54
Risk for aspiration, p. 21
Self-care deficit, p. 170

Seizure Activity

Convulsion; Epilepsy; Seizure Disorder

A seizure is an occasional, excessive disorderly discharge of neuronal activity from the cerebral cortex causing behavioral and physical disturbances. Recurrent seizures (epilepsy) may be classified as partial, generalized, or partial complex. Onset is usually before 20 years of age, and there seems to be a genetic predisposition to idiopathic epilepsy. Patients with new onset of seizure activity after age 20 may have a history of brain injury or disease such as closed head trauma, brain tumor, or stroke. Fever, low blood glucose level, drug and alcohol abuse, acid-base imbalances, electrolyte imbalances, and medication side effects may also contribute to the onset of seizures. Seizure activity has three distinct phases. The preictal phase is that time before the actual seizure. The patient may experience symptoms that warn of an impending seizure. This is called an aura. During the ictal phase, the patient experiences a progression of neuromuscular changes as a result of the disorganized neuron activity. The postictal phase is the period immediately following seizure activity. This phase represents brain recovery and return to baseline status. A patient with new onset of seizures may require hospitalization for diagnosis and initiation of treatment. Follow-up care is in the outpatient setting. This care plan focuses on self-care in the ambulatory setting.

NANDA-I NDx Deficient Knowledge

Common Related Factors

Lack of exposure
Information misinterpretation
Unfamiliarity with information resources

Common Expected Outcome

Patient verbalizes understanding of the disease process, treatment, and safety measures.

Defining Characteristics

Verbalization of problem
Request for information
Statement of misconception

NOC Outcomes

Knowledge: Disease Process; Knowledge: Treatment Regimen; Seizure Control

NIC Interventions

Seizure Precautions/Management; Teaching: Disease Process; Teaching: Treatment/ Procedures

Ongoing Assessment

Actions/Interventions	Rationales
■ Assess knowledge concerning the disorder and treatment plan.	This information provides a baseline upon which to design an individualized teaching plan. Patient and family members may have misconceptions about the causes and treatment of seizures.
■ Assess frequency, duration, and type of seizure activity. Ask the patient and family about seizure history, and if precipitating factors are involved, such as odors, visual stimulation, fatigue, stress, febrile illness, menstruation, or alcohol consumption. Inquire about warnings before seizure (aura, prodromal signs).	Each individual may present with his or her own pattern of seizure activity. Understanding the pattern is necessary for planning appropriate treatments.
■ Determine physical effects of prior seizures, such as change in level of consciousness preceding seizure activity, body part in which seizure started, epileptic cry, automatism, length of seizure, head and eye turning, pupillary reaction, associated falls, oral secretions, urinary or fecal incontinence, cyanosis, postictal state, any postseizure focal abnormality (Todd's paralysis that can last for up to 24 hours).	Knowledge of changes that occur with each phase of seizure activity may help the patient and family plan appropriate care to prevent seizures and prevent injury during a seizure.

Therapeutic Interventions

Actions/Interventions	Rationales
■ Provide information about the patient's specific type of seizure.	Generalized seizures affect the entire brain and are bilateral and symmetrical. There is usually no aura, but there is loss of consciousness. Generalized seizures range from staring spells to the stiffening (tonic) and jerking (clonic) of extremities. Partial seizures, or focal onset seizures, affect a specific region of the cerebral cortex with physical effects depending on where the seizure originated. Partial (simple) seizures are typically just motor or sensory and do not cause loss of consciousness. Partial (complex) seizures are psychomotor like partial simple seizures but also involve changes in consciousness such as confusion and memory loss. This seizure can spread through the cerebrum and culminate in a generalized seizure.

■ = Independent   ▲ = Collaborative

Actions/Interventions	Rationales
■ Discuss the disease process, including aura and prodrome.	Knowledge of warnings facilitates use of safety measures that can be implemented, such as sitting or lying down or pulling over if driving.
■ Teach the patient and family about specific antiepilepsy drugs (AEDs).	Drug therapy is the primary approach to management of seizure activity. Patients may need to take a combination of medications to achieve effective seizure control.
• Hydantoins: phenytoin (Dilantin), fosphenytoin (Cerebyx)	This class of drugs is a mainstay of drug therapy for seizures. Patients need to implement routine dental care to decrease the development of gingival hyperplasia. This side effect occurs with long-term use of these drugs.
• Iminostilbenes: carbamazepine (Tegretol), oxcarbazepine (Trileptal)	These drugs are used for partial complex and generalized seizures. The side effects of these drugs include nausea, diplopia, hepatic toxicity, and leukopenia. The patient may need periodic blood work done to monitor for drug side effects.
• Phenobarbital	This drug is a long-acting barbiturate. It is used in combination with hydantoins in the management of partial complex and generalized seizures. The drug is a class IV controlled substance. Dependency can develop with long-term use.
• Valproates: valproic acid (Depakene), divalproex sodium (Depakote)	These drugs are used in the management of partial, partial complex, and generalized seizures. With long-term use the patient may develop weight gain, alopecia, hepatic toxicity, and thrombocytopenia. Periodic blood work needs to be done to monitor for side effects. The patient needs to implement safety precautions to prevent bleeding.
■ Review need for medication and optimal schedule. Discuss danger of seizure activity with abrupt withdrawal.	Patients sometimes believe they no longer need medication because they have not experienced a seizure in some time. Patients may be able to discontinue drug therapy if they are seizure-free for 2 to 5 years. Stopping medications should only be done under close supervision by a health care provider. Abrupt discontinuation of anticonvulsants may trigger seizure activity.
■ Discuss the need for periodic follow-up check on anticonvulsant blood levels and possible complete blood count check.	Anemia and other blood dyscrasias occur with anticonvulsant therapy.
■ Provide information for patients undergoing continuous video electroencephalogram (EEG) monitoring.	This assessment technique is used for patients who have new-onset seizures or seizures that do not respond to drug therapy. Documentation of the brain location of seizure activity and type of seizure will guide decisions about drug therapy and other treatment. The patient may be hospitalized for several days until a seizure is documented.
■ Reinforce information about surgical therapy for seizure management.	Patients who do not respond to drug therapy may be candidates for surgical intervention. Procedures range from destruction of a single seizure focus to a hemispherectomy. Surgery may be curative or palliative.
■ Explain to the patient, caregiver, or significant others what to do during a seizure:	
• If the patient is on the floor, remove furniture or other potentially harmful objects from the area.	Injury prevention is a priority during seizure activity.
• Do not restrain the patient during seizure. Loosen clothing.	Physical restraint applied during seizure activity can cause pathogenic trauma.
• Allow the seizure to run its course. Do not place a tongue blade or other objects in the patient's mouth.	Inserting objects often causes more harm, such as dislodging teeth, causing lacerations, and obstructing the airway.

Actions/Interventions	Rationales
• If the airway is occluded, open the airway, then insert an oral airway.	Airway patency is a priority.
• Roll the patient to the side after cessation of muscle twitching.	This position is important to promote gravity drainage of secretions and maintain airway patency.
■ If seizures persist longer than 30 to 60 seconds or are incessantly repetitive, instruct the caregiver or patient to call 9-1-1.	The patient may require intravenous phenytoin, phenobarbital, diazepam, or lorazepam to stop status epilepticus.
■ Educate about safety measures:	
• Driving	Laws vary from state to state; in most states, the patient must be seizure-free for 6 months to 2 years.
• Home safety—The patient should have someone else present when cooking and bathing to reduce the risk for injury	
• Work safety—Avoid construction work, ladder climbing, heavy equipment operation	Most states have laws prohibiting workplace discrimination against people with epilepsy.
• Personal safety—Dive or swim with a companion; wear medical alert identification; be aware of the effect of alcohol and drugs	There is an increased risk for seizures produced by interaction of alcohol with anticonvulsant drugs.
▲ Refer the patient to a dietitian if a ketogenic diet is prescribed.	This diet therapy is usually attempted only for severe, unrelenting seizure disorders. The diet is a high-fat, low-carbohydrate, low-protein diet, divided into several small meals per day. The diet is complex and requires education about careful selection of foods.
■ Refer to the Epilepsy Foundation of America.	This organization provides information and resources to support effective coping and seizure management.
■ Provide information, as appropriate, about specially trained animals for epileptics.	Some dogs are able to detect a seizure prodrome and warn the patient so safety measures can be implemented before the seizure begins.

NANDA-I NDx Risk for Chronic Low Self-Esteem

Common Risk Factors

Seizure activity
Dependence on medications
Social isolation
Discrimination
Misperceptions

Common Expected Outcome

Patient verbalizes positive statements about self in relation to living with a seizure disorder.

NOC Outcome
Self-Esteem
NIC Intervention
Self-Esteem Enhancement

Ongoing Assessment

Actions/Interventions	Rationales
■ Assess feelings about self, disorder, and long-term therapy.	Patients may express frustration, anxiety, and unrealistic expectations because of the unpredictability of their seizures. Many patients begin to identify themselves as chronically ill and express feelings of loss of independence.

■ = Independent ▲ = Collaborative

Actions/Interventions

- Assess perceived implications of the disorder and its effect on socialization.

Rationales

Patients may have a fear of or have experienced actual discrimination in jobs and schooling, as well as a fear of loss of control and embarrassment in public.

Therapeutic Interventions

Actions/Interventions

- Encourage ventilation of feelings.

- Incorporate the family and significant others in the care plan.
- Dispel common myths and fears about convulsive disorders.

- Refer to support group if possible.

- ▲ Consult a social worker to assist with financial and vocational issues.

- ▲ Consult a psychologist if anxiety, depression, and lifestyle changes become troublesome.

Rationales

Talking about feelings can support effective coping and improved insight.

A strong social support system may promote more effective coping and positive self-esteem for the patient.

Historically, epilepsy has been seen as a mental disorder with negative connotations, but with good health habits and maintenance of a medication schedule, most seizure disorders are controllable and have no relationship to mental capabilities or intellect.

These groups provide practical assistance in dealing with social and personal issues.

Human rights organizations and/or labor relations departments may need to be contacted if job security or discrimination is evident.

The patient may benefit from talk therapy to promote effective coping and support positive self-esteem.

Related Care Plans

Impaired home maintenance, p. 95
Risk for aspiration, p. 21

Spinal Cord Injury

Quadriplegia; Tetraplegia; Paraplegia; Neurogenic Shock; Spinal Shock

Spinal cord injury (SCI) is damage to the spinal cord at any level from C1 to L1 or L2, where the spinal cord ends. Injury may result in (1) concussion (transient loss of function), (2) complete cord lesion (no preservation of motor and sensory function below the level of injury; irreversible damage), (3) incomplete lesion (can be a partial transection); residual and mixed motor/sensory function below level of injury with some potential for improvement in function. Complete cord injury above C7 results in tetraplegia (formerly called quadriplegia); injury from C7 to L1 causes paraplegia.

Neurogenic (or spinal) shock often follows cervical and high thoracic SCI. Spinal shock can last for 7 to 10 days to weeks or months after injury. It temporarily results in (1) total loss of all motor and sensory function below the injury; (2) sympathetic disruption, resulting in loss of vasoconstriction and leaving parasympathetics unopposed, leading to bradycardia and hypotension; (3) loss of all reflexes below the injury; (4) inability to control body temperature, secondary to the inability to sweat, shiver, or vasoconstrict below the level of injury; (5) ileus; and (6) urinary retention. When neurogenic shock resolves, it is followed by a stage of spasticity.

Primary causes of SCI are motor vehicle accidents, followed by sporting accidents, falls, and penetrating injuries (gunshot or knife wounds). Motor vehicle accidents are the leading cause among people younger than age 65. Among people older than 65 years, falls is the leading cause of SCI. Approximately 50% of people who sustain SCI are men between 15 and 29 years of age. Approximately 11,000 new SCIs occur per year. This care plan focuses on the acute care of an SCI victim.

Risk for Ineffective Breathing Pattern

Common Risk Factor
High cervical SCI with neuromuscular impairment

Common Expected Outcome
Patient maintains an effective breathing pattern, as evidenced by relaxed breathing at normal rate and depth and absence of dyspnea.

NOC Outcomes
Respiratory Status: Airway Patency; Respiratory Status: Ventilation
NIC Interventions
Respiratory Monitoring; Airway Stabilization and Management

Ongoing Assessment

Actions/Interventions	Rationales
■ Monitor respiratory rate, depth, and effort.	Injury at C4 or above causes paralysis of the diaphragm, necessitating intubation. All patients with tetraplegia will have some degree of respiratory insufficiency as a result of intercostal muscle weakness or paralysis. If the patient has a C5 to T6 cord injury, abdominal and intercostal muscle innervation will be absent/diminished and the patient will be unable to take deep breaths and cough. This situation increases the patient's risk for atelectasis and respiratory infection.
■ Auscultate breath sounds.	Hypoventilation occurs with diaphragmatic respirations as a result of decreased vital capacity and tidal volume. Lung sounds will be diminished.
▲ Use pulse oximetry to monitor oxygen saturation; assess ABGs as ordered.	Pulse oximetry is a useful tool to detect changes in oxygenation. Oxygen saturation should be at 90% or greater. Spinal cord edema (even with an incomplete lesion at or below C4) and hemorrhage can affect phrenic nerve function and cause respiratory insufficiency. The patient may have a chronically low Pao_2 level and elevated $Paco_2$ level.
▲ Monitor vital capacity	Monitoring detects changes early so ventilatory support may be initiated before full decompensation occurs.

Therapeutic Interventions

Actions/Interventions	Rationales
▲ Administer oxygen as needed.	Initially, supplemental oxygen is necessary to maintain a high Pao_2 level.
▲ Assist with intubation and ventilatory support, if indicated.	Patients with high cervical cord injury (above C4 or C5) are at greatest risk for apnea and respiratory arrest. Blind nasotracheal intubation or fiberoptic endotracheal intubation without neck involvement will be performed. Duration of intubation depends on extent of spinal cord damage. Long-term airway management may require a tracheostomy. Mechanical ventilation may be needed for the tetraplegic patient who cannot maintain spontaneous respirations.
■ Suction the patient as needed. When stabilized, implement postural drainage and chest percussion.	These measures mobilize secretions to prevent pneumonia or atelectasis.

■ = Independent ▲ = Collaborative

Actions/Interventions

- Teach an assisted cough technique.

- Encourage use of an incentive spirometer.
- ▲ Apply an abdominal binder.

Rationales

The low tetraplegic and the paraplegic patient can use a coughing technique that employs manual abdominal pressure to support air movement with coughing.

This device promotes deep breathing.

A binder supports weak abdominal muscles used to promote diaphragmatic breathing.

 Risk for Decreased Cardiac Output

Common Risk Factor

Neurogenic shock (traumatic sympathectomy) as a result of spinal cord injury at T5 or above

Common Expected Outcome

Patient has adequate cardiac output as evidenced by systolic BP within 20 mm Hg of baseline; heart rate 60 to 100 beats/min with regular rhythm; urine output greater than or equal to 30 mg/hr; strong peripheral pulses; warm, dry skin; eupnea with absence of pulmonary crackles; and orientation to person, time, and place.

NOC Outcomes
Circulation Status; Vital Signs
NIC Interventions
Hemodynamic Regulation; Invasive Hemodynamic Monitoring

Ongoing Assessment

Actions/Interventions

- Assess heart rate and BP closely.

- Assess level of consciousness.

- Assess peripheral pulses and capillary refill.

Rationales

Loss of sympathetic innervation results in bradycardia and vasodilation of vessels below the injury resulting from an unopposed parasympathetic nervous system. The patient will be hypotensive.

Restlessness is an early sign of hypoxia and decreased cerebral perfusion from decreased cardiac output.

Peripheral vasodilation decreases venous return, further decreasing cardiac output and blood pressure.

Therapeutic Interventions

Actions/Interventions

- ▲ Administer intravenous (IV) fluids as ordered to maintain BP.

- Avoid elevating head of bed.

- ▲ Administer vasopressors if needed.

- ▲ Apply military antishock trouser (MAST) suit or sequential compression boots (SCBs).

Rationales

Patients with neurogenic shock secondary to SCI have a relative hypovolemia. Circulatory blood volume is unchanged but the space in the circulatory system is increased with decreased systemic vascular resistance. IV fluids need to be infused carefully to prevent fluid volume excess. Because of abnormal autonomic hemodynamics, overhydration may lead to pulmonary edema.

Because of sympathetic disruption and resultant loss of vasoconstrictor tone below the injury, head elevation will result in further drop of BP.

These drugs are titrated to maintain a mean arterial pressure of 80 mm Hg or higher. Atropine may be given to correct bradycardia,

These help compensate for lost muscle tone and decreases venous pooling.

Impaired Physical Mobility

Common Related Factors

SCI
Neurogenic (spinal) shock

Defining Characteristics

Inability to move purposely within environment
Limited range of motion (ROM)
Decreased muscle strength

Common Expected Outcomes

Patient performs physical activity independently or within limits of activity restrictions.
Patient demonstrates use of adaptive techniques that promote ambulation and transferring.
Patient is free of complications of immobility, as evidenced by intact skin, absence of thrombophlebitis, normal bowel pattern, and clear breath sounds.

NOC Outcomes

Mobility; Ambulation: Wheelchair; Immobility Consequences: Physiological

NIC Interventions

Positioning; Neurological Monitoring; Exercise Therapy: Joint Mobility

---

Ongoing Assessment

Actions/Interventions	Rationales
■ Perform neurological assessment to estimate level of injury.	This assessment provides baseline for future comparison.
• Evaluate movement of major muscle groups in upper and lower extremities: at toes, ankles, knees, hips, fingers, elbows, and shoulders.	The patient's functional ability will depend on the level of injury.
• Assess motor strength, checking for level of progression, symmetry and asymmetry, ascending and descending paralysis, paresthesia.	Injury to the corticospinal tracts results in loss of motor strength.
• Evaluate sensation to pinprick (spinothalamic tract). Start at toes and ascend gradually up to face. If sensation changes, mark skin.	The spinothalamic tracts transmit sensations of pain and temperature.
• Assess light touch (anterior spinothalamic track). Start at toes and ascend as described.	The anterior spinothalamic tract transmits sensations of light touch.
• Check for proprioception (joint position sense that reflects posterior columns). Ask the patient to close eyes. Move the toes and fingers up and down slowly to determine whether the patient can perceive motion.	Changes in proprioception are the result of injury to the dorsal column spinal tract.
• Evaluate deep tendon reflexes: biceps, triceps, knee, ankle.	Changes in reflexes will be related to the level of injury.
■ Serially monitor the patient for any deviation from initial baseline examination, noting signs of complete or incomplete injury.	If the patient has a worsening deficit or higher evolving sensory deficit, additional studies such as magnetic resonance imaging or myelography are indicated. A change from flaccid to spastic paralysis indicates resolution of spinal shock.

Therapeutic Interventions

Actions/Interventions	Rationales
■ Apply a low–air-loss mattress to bed before the patient is placed in bed. Immobilize the patient. Maintain the patient in a collar and on a backboard. Once all studies are completed and the patient is stabilized, remove the backboard.	Immobilization is necessary to prevent additional injury from active or passive movements of the spine. Early removal of the backboard reduces potential for pressure ulcer formation. Special mattresses promote even distribution of pressure to reduce risk for skin breakdown.

■ = Independent ▲ = Collaborative

Actions/Interventions	Rationales
▲ Insert nasogastric tube if appropriate.	This measure prevents vomiting and aspiration. Paralytic ileus is common after SCI. Vomiting will cause jerking movements that can further spinal injury. The immobilization of head and neck prevents the patient from protecting his airway if vomiting occurs.
■ If the spine is stable, logroll and reposition the patient at least every 2 hours.	Frequent turning relieves pressure and reduces risk for skin breakdown.
■ Perform ROM exercises.	These exercises reduce potential for contractures, which may occur once neurogenic shock advances to the next stage of spasticity.
■ Provide support to feet.	A high-top sneaker or special device may be helpful to prevent footdrop.
▲ Administer methylprednisolone as prescribed.	Methylprednisolone decreases spinal cord ischemia, improves impulse conduction, represses release of free fatty acids from the spinal cord, and restores extracellular calcium. Clinical practice guidelines recommend high-dose methylprednisolone be administered within 8 hours of injury to reduce the extent of permanent paralysis.
▲ Administer anticoagulants as prescribed.	Subcutaneous administration of low-dose or low-molecular-weight heparin may be indicated to reduce the risk for DVT.
▲ Consult and work with physical and occupational therapists.	An interdisciplinary approach needs to be initiated early in the patient's care to promote effective mobility in the rehabilitation phase of care. Splints and braces may be used to maintain joints and extremities in a position of anatomical function. Selection of a wheelchair is important to provide stability of the trunk, to maximize use of remaining function to propel the chair, and to prevent pressure ulcers. The physical therapist will help the patient learn safe transfer techniques.
■ Prepare the patient and family for possible surgical intervention.	Decompression, realignment, and/or stabilization can be accomplished with traction or surgery depending on the site and extent of damage. Early surgery to remove bone fragments, relieve cord compression, and repair open wounds improves chances for good recovery.

NANDA-I NDx Risk for Impaired Skin Integrity

Common Risk Factors

Impaired physical mobility
Complete bed rest
Sensory disturbance

Common Expected Outcome

Patient maintains intact skin, as evidenced by no redness over bony prominences and capillary refill less than 6 seconds over areas of redness.

NOC Outcome
Tissue Integrity: Skin and Mucous Membranes
NIC Intervention
Skin Surveillance

Ongoing Assessment

Actions/Interventions	Rationales
■ Assess skin integrity, noting color, moisture, texture, and temperature, especially at pressure points.	Pressure ulcers are a common complication of spinal cord injury. Early identification of stage I pressure ulcers allows for prompt initiation of pressure relief interventions.

Therapeutic Interventions

Actions/Interventions	Rationales
■ Keep skin clean and dry.	Moisture accumulation leads to skin maceration and skin breakdown over pressure points. Increased skin moisture, especially in skin folds, adds to the risk for development of fungal skin infection.
■ Apply thin dressing of DuoDerm or similar product to bony prominences.	A variety of dressings are available to protect and maintain intact skin.
■ Turn the patient every 2 hours. Use lift sheets when repositioning patient.	Because of sensory disturbance, the patient will be unable to detect painful pressure. Lift sheets reduce shear forces, which further contribute to skin breakdown.
■ Provide appropriate prophylactic use of pressure-relieving devices.	The use of pressure-relieving devices helps prevent skin breakdown. These devices should be used on the patient's bed and wheelchair.
■ Instruct the patient in a wheelchair to shift position every 20 to 30 minutes.	Frequent position changes prevent pressure areas from developing.
■ Provide adequate nutritional intake.	A high-protein, high-carbohydrate, and high-calorie diet is needed to counteract catabolic effects of injury and maintain healthy, intact skin. Enteral feedings may be necessary.
■ Teach the patient and caregivers to inspect skin daily. Provide a long-handled, angled mirror.	Skin breakdown is an ongoing, lifetime concern for the patient with a spinal cord injury. Use of a mirror allows the patient independence in doing skin inspection.

Disturbed Body Image

Common Related Factor

Paralysis secondary to SCI

Defining Characteristics

Verbalization of functional alteration of body part
Denial of injury outcome or refusal to look at body
Withdrawal, isolation
Focused behavior or verbal preoccupation with body part or function

Common Expected Outcome

Patient demonstrates enhanced body image and self-esteem, as evidenced by ability to look at, touch, talk about, and care for parts of body with reduced function.

NOC Outcomes
Body Image; Self-Esteem

NIC Interventions
Coping Enhancement; Body Image Enhancement

Ongoing Assessment

Actions/Interventions	Rationales
■ Assess perception of dysfunction.	The patient may perceive changes that are not present or real. The effects of neurogenic shock will seem permanent to the patient, even if the injury is an incomplete lesion.

■ = Independent ▲ = Collaborative

Actions/Interventions

- Assess perceived impact on activities of daily living (ADLs), personal relationships, and occupational activity.

- Inquire about coping skills used before injury.

- Assess the patient's social support system.

Rationales

The patient needs to understand that decisions about relationships and occupation need not be made immediately because prior knowledge and beliefs about disability may change during the rehabilitative stage of care.

Previous coping skills may not be sufficient or appropriate to help the patient adjust to the dramatic life changes from SCI.

The patient will have a new level of dependency. A strong social support network can help the patient achieve an appropriate level of functional independence that promotes self-esteem.

Therapeutic Interventions

Actions/Interventions

- Acknowledge normality of emotional response to change in body function. Allow the patient to grieve.

- Help the patient verbalize feelings regarding impairment.

- Help the patient identify helpful coping mechanisms (prayer, communication, perseverance, distraction).
- Encourage interaction with family and friends to enhance self-worth.
- ▲ Refer for counseling as needed.

Rationales

Stages of grief over loss of body function are normal (e.g., losing the function of one's legs is like a "death" of the body part as well as the "death" of future plans). The grieving process may take years.

Expression of feelings supports coping and the development of insights about the impact of the injury.

As a result of the overwhelming nature of SCI, prior coping skills may not be effective.

Family and friends will provide feedback as the patient integrates the impact of injury into a new perception of self.

Both the patient and caregivers may benefit from professional help in developing effective coping and adjustment.

NANDA-I NDx **Deficient Knowledge**

Common Related Factors

Lack of exposure
New injury
Misperceptions
Cognitive limitation

Defining Characteristics

Verbalized lack of knowledge
Request for information
Statement of misconception

Common Expected Outcome

Patient and caregivers verbalize understanding of the injury, prognosis, ongoing care measures, and rehabilitation expectations.

NOC Outcomes

Knowledge: Disease Process; Knowledge: Treatment Regimen

NIC Interventions

Teaching: Disease Process; Teaching: Treatment/Procedures; Discharge Planning

Ongoing Assessment

Actions/Interventions

- Assess the patient's knowledge of injury and prognosis.

- Assess understanding of treatment and rehabilitation process.

Rationales

An understanding of the prognosis is necessary to progress to rehabilitation.

An effective teaching plan will build on previous knowledge of treatment.

Therapeutic Interventions

Actions/Interventions	Rationales
■ Explain what is happening as care/tests (ventilatory support, x-ray films, laboratory tests) are performed.	Knowledge is power. This information will assist with eventual coping once the situation has stabilized. Many patients are young and may have no previous experience with illness or hospitalization.
■ Explain spinal cord function and effects of injury on body functions (respiration, mobility, bowel and bladder function). Expect to see a grieving process. Wait until the patient is ready for more information.	The patient and family need to develop realistic expectations about the patient's long-term needs for assistance with self-care activities and ADLs.
■ Encourage the patient and caregiver to participate in care while the patient is hospitalized. Explain about positioning, skin care, ulcer prevention, bowel and bladder management, nutrition, and medications.	Patients and caregivers need time to develop new skills for meeting ADLs and other dimensions of SCI care.
■ Initiate discussion concerning the caregiver's ability to provide long-term home care, especially if the patient requires mechanical ventilation, and if special equipment or transportation is required.	Family members need to learn to balance their desire to help the patient and the patient's need to achieve functional independence. The demands of supportive care may be perceived by family members as an overwhelming burden.
▲ Provide social service referral.	Although care at home is less costly, many third-party payers may not cover special equipment, supplies, home alterations, or utility costs. The patient and family may need help with financial resources to support long-term care.
■ Encourage participation in support groups.	Support groups assist the patient in coping with the disability.

Related Care Plans

Stroke

Brain Attack; Cerebrovascular Accident (CVA); Thrombotic Stroke; Embolic Stroke; Hemorrhagic Stroke; Ischemic Stroke

Stroke is a disease that affects the arteries leading to and within the brain. Strokes are classified as either ischemic (due to a cerebral thrombus or an embolus) or hemorrhagic (due to rupture of a cerebral blood vessel). Stroke is the leading cause of serious, long-term disability in the United States and Canada. It is the third leading cause of death in the United States; 72% of those affected are older than 65 years of age. African Americans have a higher incidence of stroke than whites or Hispanics. Risk factors for stroke include poorly controlled hypertension, diabetes mellitus, high cholesterol levels, smoking, cocaine use, alcohol abuse, obesity, high-dose estrogen drug therapy, and cerebral aneurysm. Acute ischemic stroke is a medical emergency requiring prompt treatment with thrombolytic therapy within 3 hours after symptom recognition ("time is brain"). Hemorrhagic stroke needs to be ruled out prior to treatment with thrombolytics. Stroke severity is determined using the NIH stroke scale (NIHSS). Much attention is directed to providing safe, efficient and quality care to stroke patients. National guidelines by the American Stroke Association and the Brain Attack Coalition

■ = Independent ▲ = Collaborative

provide direction for stroke care provided by hospitals. The Get With the Guidelines—Stroke continuous quality improvement program provides a mechanism for physicians and hospital staff to monitor their performance. The Joint Commission provides certification for Primary Stroke Centers.

The clinical manifestations of stroke and outcomes for the patient vary, depending on the area of the brain affected. The area of the brain supplied by the middle cerebral artery is the most common site for stroke. A stroke in the nondominant hemisphere often causes spatial-perceptual deficits, changes in judgment and behavior, and unilateral neglect. A stroke in the dominant right hemisphere typically causes dysphasia, dysarthria, left-sided sensory loss and homonymous hemianopsia, a decreased awareness of the left side of the body, left-sided paralysis and/or paresis, apraxia, impaired judgment, increased emotional lability, and deficits in handling new spatial information. A stroke in the dominant left hemisphere can cause repetitive or expressive dysphasia, dysarthria, right-sided sensory loss and homonymous hemianopsia, right-sided paralysis and/or paresis, increased emotional lability, and a deficit in handling new language information. In this type of stroke there is typically intact judgment, infrequent apraxia, and usually a normal awareness of both sides of the body. This care plan focuses on acute care management of ischemic stroke in the hospital.

Impaired Cerebral Tissue Perfusion

Common Related Factors

Intracranial hemorrhage
Ischemia (embolism or thrombosis)

Defining Characteristics

Altered mental status
Changes in motor response
Changes in papillary reactions
Behavioral changes
Speech abnormalities
Dysphagia
Headache

Common Expected Outcome

Patient maintains optimal cerebral tissue perfusion, as evidenced by National Institutes of Health Stroke Scale (NIHSS) score less than 4, Glasgow Coma Scale (GCS) score greater than 13, absence of new, neurological deficits, and stable blood pressure.

NOC Outcomes

Tissue Perfusion: Cerebral; Neurological Status; Blood Coagulation; Medication Response

NIC Interventions

Cerebral Perfusion Promotion; Neurological Monitoring; Medication Administration

Ongoing Assessment

Actions/Interventions

■ Assess neurological status (serially) using National Institutes of Health Stroke Scale (NIHSS) or Glasgow Coma Scale.

Rationales

This information is used to determine the effects of stroke and identify life-threatening complications such as increased intracranial pressure (ICP). The NIHSS is a standardized assessment of consciousness, vision, sensory and motor responses, speech and language function. Scores may range from 0 (no stroke) to 42 (severe stroke). Current practice guidelines recommend that patients with an initial score greater than 4 may benefit from thrombolytics. The Glasgow Coma Scale measures changes in level of consciousness based on verbal, motor, and pupillary responses. Scores range from 0 to 15. A score less than 13 is associated with a decreased level of consciousness.

Actions/Interventions

- Assess past history of cardiac dysrhythmias, hypertension, smoking.

- Monitor vital signs as needed.

▲ Monitor baseline electrocardiogram, and observe for changes.
- Monitor fluid intake and urine output.

▲ Use pulse oximetry to monitor oxygen saturation; assess ABGs as ordered.

Rationales

Cardiac workup is warranted if stroke is embolic; atrial fibrillation is a major cause of embolic stroke. Hypertension seems to be related to hemorrhagic stroke. Atherosclerosis and transient ischemic attacks are associated with thrombotic stroke.

Frequent assessment of blood pressure (BP) is essential. A normotensive state is desired to promote effective cerebral perfusion pressure.

Stroke can produce cardiac electrical changes and dysrhythmias.

A decrease in urine output may indicate decreased renal perfusion and an associated decrease in cerebral perfusion. Because of cerebral edema, fluid balance must be regulated. Fluids may be restricted if the patient has significant increase in ICP, or volume expanders may be used if the patient is hypotensive with decreased cerebral perfusion.

Oxygen saturation should be 90% or greater for adequate cerebral perfusion. $Paco_2$ greater than 45 mmHg induces cerebral vasodilatation and increases ICP.

Therapeutic Interventions

Actions/Interventions

▲ Administer the following medications:
- Thrombolytics

- Anticoagulants and antiplatelet drugs

- Antihypertensives

- Osmotic diuretics

- Raise head of bed no higher than 30 degrees.

- Keep the patient's head and neck in neutral position.

- Avoid unnecessary care activities.

▲ Control body temperature: administer antipyretics, initiate topical cooling methods, administer hypothalamic depressants, as prescribed.
▲ Maintain volume status by replacing or restricting fluids, as prescribed.

Rationales

Thrombolytics are given to dissolve clots in cerebral vessels. These drugs work best when administered within 3 hours of an ischemic stroke. Tissue plasminogen activator (tpa) is the first drug of choice. Early administration of tpa is associated with reduced neurologic damage and stroke severity.

Anticoagulants and antiplatelet drugs are given to reduce clot formation and prevent extension of existing clots.

Antihypertensives are given to control severe hypertension and maintain cerebral perfusion.

Osmotic diuretics are given to decrease ICP by reducing cerebral edema.

Current evidence suggests that elevating the head of bed reduces ICP by increasing cerebral venous outflow. This position may also reduce cerebral perfusion and contribute to increased risk for cerebral infarction.

This position promotes venous drainage from the brain and decreases ICP.

Frequent stimulation of the patient can serve as a noxious stimulus and increases brain activity and ICP. Clustering care activities in a short period of time also increases ICP.

Controlling fever reduces metabolic demands of the brain and reduces ICP.

Fluid balance will be adjusted to reduce cerebral edema and prevent a hypercoagulable state.

■ = Independent ▲ = Collaborative

NANDA-I NDx Risk for Ineffective Airway Clearance

Common Risk Factors
Neurological dysfunction
Obstruction
Secretions

Common Expected Outcome
Patient maintains clear, open airways, as evidenced by normal breath sounds, normal rate and depth of respirations, and ability to cough up secretions after treatments and deep breaths.

NOC Outcome
Respiratory Status: Airway Patency
NIC Intervention
Airway Management

Ongoing Assessment

Actions/Interventions	Rationales
■ Monitor respiratory rate and rhythm, breath sounds, and ability to handle secretions.	Maintaining the airway is always the first priority. Airway obstruction may occur with stroke as a result of impaired cranial nerve function leading to diminished airway protective reflexes and impaired chewing and swallowing. Weakness of the hypoglossal nerve may allow the tongue to fall back in the pharynx and obstruct the airway. Diminished cough and gag reflexes increase the risk for aspiration of oral secretions and food.
■ Check presence of gag reflex.	Brainstem strokes may diminish cranial nerve function and cause impaired function of airway protective reflexes. An impaired gag reflex increases the risk for atelectasis and airway obstruction.
■ Assess for dysphagia	Impaired swallowing may occur with stroke. The use of a formal dysphagia screening protocol significantly decreases the risk of aspiration pneumonia. The Joint Commission quality indicators for Stroke Center Certification include screening all stroke patients for dysohagia prior to oral intake. This is a safety issue to prevent aspiration pneumonia.

Therapeutic Interventions

Actions/Interventions	Rationales
■ Position the patient upright.	This position reduces the work of breathing and promotes more effective coughing.
■ If the patient is comatose, use an oropharyngeal airway.	An artificial airway keeps the tongue from obstructing the airway. Cranial nerve involvement (hypoglossal nerve) may cause unilateral weakness and tongue deviation.
■ Encourage deep breathing and coughing.	Coughing is the most helpful way to remove most secretions. The patient may be unable to perform independently. The sitting position and splinting the abdomen promote more effective coughing by increasing abdominal pressure and upward diaphragmatic movement.
■ Suction mouth and airways to remove secretions.	Impaired cranial nerve function may result in decreased cough effectiveness. Impaired swallowing may lead to aspiration of oral secretions and airway obstruction. Suctioning helps the patient manage airway secretions.

Actions/Interventions

▲ Provide respiratory support:
- Administer supplemental oxygen.
- Anticipate endotracheal or tracheal intubation.

Rationales

This measure reduces hypoxemia, which can cause cerebral vasodilation and increased ICP.

The patient with a persistent decreased LOC may require intubation to optimize airway clearance.

NANDA-I NDx Impaired Physical Mobility

Common Related Factors

Paresis or paralysis
Loss of balance and coordination
Increased muscle tone

Defining Characteristics

Inability to move purposefully within physical environment
Limited range of motion
Decreased muscle strength, control, and/or mass

Common Expected Outcomes

Patient performs physical activity independently or within limits of activity restrictions.
Patient demonstrates use of adaptive techniques that promote ambulation and transferring.
Patient is free of complications of immobility, as evidenced by intact skin, absence of thrombophlebitis, normal bowel pattern, and clear breath sounds.

NOC Outcomes

Mobility; Body Positioning: Self-Initiated; Transfer Performance; Ambulation

NIC Intervention

Exercise Therapy: Muscle Control

Ongoing Assessment

Actions/Interventions

- Assess degree of weakness in both upper and lower extremities.
- Assess ability to move and change position, to transfer and walk, for fine muscle movement, and for gross muscle movements.

- Assess ability to perform range of motion (ROM) to all joints.

- Observe for activities or situations that increase or decrease muscle tone.

- Monitor skin integrity for areas of blanching or redness.

Rationales

There may be differing degrees of involvement on the affected side.

Paralysis, paresis, and sensory loss are contralateral to the side of the brain affected by the stroke. In the early phase of stroke recovery the patient may be completely immobile. As brain recovery progresses, paresis or paralysis may be limited to one side of the body or just one extremity.

This assessment provides data on the extent of any physical problems with muscle paralysis or paresis from the stroke. The data will guide therapy to promote mobility. Testing by a physical therapist may be needed.

Initially muscles demonstrate hyporeflexia, which later progresses to hyperreflexia. Activities that cause spastic response can be postponed until later in recovery.

Impaired mobility increases the risk for skin breakdown.

Therapeutic Interventions

Actions/Interventions

- Change position of patient at least every 2 hours, keeping track of position changes with a turning schedule.

- Perform active and passive ROM exercises in all extremities several times daily. Increase functional activities as strength improves and the patient is medically stable.

- Perform activities in a quiet environment with few distractions.

Rationales

Position changes optimize circulation to all tissues and relieve pressure. Patients may not feel increases in pressure or have the ability to adjust position. Loss of motor control can contribute to abnormal posturing.

ROM activities preserve muscle strength and prevent contractures, especially in spastic extremities. Early mobilization and ROM exercises should begin as soon as the patient is stable and no longer requires intensive care.

Impaired cognitive function that occurs with stroke may decrease the patient's attention span and concentration. The patient may be easily distracted.

■ = Independent ▲ = Collaborative

Neurological Care Plans

Actions/Interventions

- Teach the patient and family exercises and transfer techniques.

- Use pressure-relieving devices on the bed and chair.
- Initiate rehabilitation techniques in the hospital setting as soon as medically possible.

For balance and coordination problems:
- Assist the patient in performing movements or tasks. Begin with tasks that require a small range of movements and encourage control (e.g., sitting upright and maintaining balance).

- Encourage focusing on proximal muscle control initially and then distal muscle control, such as beginning with limb positioning and progressing to self-feeding and writing.
- Ensure that the center of gravity is over the pelvis or equally distributed over stance for sitting and standing activities; provide a safe environment for these activities.
- Teach the patient and family exercises and techniques to improve balance and coordination.
- Reinforce safety precautions with the patient and family.

For increased muscle tone (spasticity):
- Instruct the family in concepts of spasticity and ways to reduce tone.

- Perform muscle stretching activities in gentle, rhythmical motions.
- ▲ Apply splinting devices to spastic extremities as prescribed, with ongoing assessment for increasing tone.

Rationales

Once medically stable, the patient may have long-term deficits such as altered perception and motor strength. Exercise will increase strength and endurance, promote use of the affected side, and promote transfer safety. Upon discharge, the patient and family will need to continue an exercise program to maintain the patient's mobility.

These devices decrease risk for pressure ulcer development.

Early rehabilitation in the medically stable patient prevents further systemic deterioration and facilitates transition to long-term rehabilitation.

Mobility interventions follow a pattern of progressive activity for the patient with a stroke. Activities to encourage balance are the first step and begin with the patient sitting on the side of the bed. As muscle tone improves and patient gains some voluntary muscle control, the focus shifts to activities that support transfer from the bed to a chair and finally ambulation.

Larger muscle groups are easier to focus on and control.

Patients may have impaired righting reflexes and wide base stance. Spatial deficits make it difficult for patients to determine their position in space.

Support from significant others will encourage compliance and success.

Spatial deficits, impaired judgment, and loss of motor function increase the patient's risk for falls, perceptual accidents (bumping into things), wandering, and impulsive behavior.

Spasticity is a sign of improvement. Muscles that remain flaccid are not likely to recover. Spasticity will gradually diminish as control of muscles is regained. As spasticity decreases, a phenomenon known as synergy often occurs. This is the involuntary movement of part of an extremity after an initial voluntary movement of the whole extremity.

This approach reduces stimuli that contribute to muscle spasticity.

Devices are used to prevent muscle shortening that occurs with chronic flexion. This approach helps prevent contractures.

 NANDA-I NDx **Risk for Impaired Verbal Communication**

Common Risk Factor
Left brain hemisphere stroke

Common Expected Outcomes
Patient effectively communicates basic needs.
Patient maximizes remaining communication ability.
Patient and family verbalize understanding of communication impairment.
Patient and family are involved in measures to promote communication.

NOC Outcome
Communication Ability
NIC Intervention
Communication Enhancement: Speech Deficit

Ongoing Assessment

Actions/Interventions	Rationales
■ Assess expressive ability.	The patient with expressive forms of dysphasia will have difficulty finding words. Speech will be non fluent with use of single words or short phrases to communicate ideas. Writing will be difficult. The patient with receptive forms of dysphasia will have fluent speech but produce meaningless language. Rhythm, cadence, and articulation are normal. The patient is unable to correct errors in speech, such as words that sound alike or have similar meaning.
■ Assess ability to comprehend language.	Verbal comprehension is usually intact with expressive dysphasia. Some patients with expressive dysphasia may experience changes in reading comprehension. The patient with receptive dysphasia has impaired verbal and reading comprehension.
■ Assess function of facial and hypoglossal cranial nerves.	Weakness of the tongue and facial muscles necessary for speech contribute to dysarthria. The patient will have difficulty forming clear sounds and have slurred speech.

Therapeutic Interventions

Actions/Interventions	Rationales
■ Acknowledge the patient's frustration with impaired communication	Inability to express needs or feelings is most distressing to patients. The staff needs to be sensitive to the dignity of the patient.
■ Minimize stimuli in the environment.	Communication can be facilitated and distractions minimized by turning off the television or radio, or by closing the door.
■ Provide clear, simple directions.	The patient with dysphasia requires directions to be repeated frequently. Tasks need to be explained in very simple steps and presented one at a time.
■ Incorporate multimodality input, such as music, song, and visual demonstration.	These different inputs enhance function in intact speech-language areas.
■ Use written materials (if appropriate).	These supplement auditory input (e.g., communication board with pictures, numbers, words, and/or alphabet). If the patient has homonymous hemianopsia, place material in the unaffected field of vision. Homonymous hemianopsia affects the field of vision in both eyes, opposite the side of the brain affected by stroke.
■ Use prompting cues, such as gestures or holding an object that is being discussed.	Visual cueing can enhance the patient's understanding of verbal messages.
■ Allow adequate time for patient response.	If the patient feels rushed, communication problems are worsened. The patient needs more time to cognitively process information and formulate a verbal response.
■ Provide opportunities for spontaneous conversation.	The patient needs frequent opportunities to talk without the expectation of a desired outcome. This method decreases the patient's anxiety about communication abilities.
■ Anticipate the patient's needs until alternative means of communication can be established.	The nurse should plan enough time to attend to all the details of patient care. Care measures may take longer to complete in the presence of a communication deficit.
■ Provide reality orientation and focus attention, but avoid constantly correcting errors.	Constant correction increases frustration, anxiety, and anger.
▲ Collaborate with a speech therapist.	A comprehensive multidisciplinary plan of care may be required to improve the patient's communication ability.

■ = Independent ▲ = Collaborative

Neurological Care Plans

Actions/Interventions

- Encourage the family to attempt communication with the patient; explain type of dysphasia and methods of communication that can be tried.
- Demonstrate to the patient any progress made.

Rationales

Consistency of approach by professional caregivers and family members promotes more effective communication for the patient.

Positive feedback increases confidence and facilitates the patient's ongoing efforts to communicate verbally.

NANDA-I NDx **Risk for Disturbed Sensory Perception (Tactile)**

Common Risk Factor

Stroke within the sensory transmission and/or integration pathways of the brain

Common Expected Outcome

Patient's skin remains free of injuries, including pressure ulcers.

NOC Outcomes
Risk Detection; Risk Control
NIC Intervention
Peripheral Sensation Management

Ongoing Assessment

Actions/Interventions

- Assess the patient's ability to sense light touch, pinprick, and temperature. Touch skin lightly with a pin, cotton ball, or hot/cold object, and ask him or her to describe the sensation and point to where the touch occurred.
- Using the patient's toes or fingers, assess position sense (ability to sense whether the joint is moved in an upward or downward position).

Rationales

Early assessment determines the level of alteration and identifies specific areas of risk. Tactile deficits increase risk for injury related to the patient's inability to sense pain or temperature.

Loss of position sense occurs in patients with strokes affecting the anterior cerebral artery, basilar artery, and posterior cerebral artery. Spatial-perceptual deficits increase the patient's risk for injury.

Therapeutic Interventions

Actions/Interventions

- Perform regular skin inspections, and instruct the patient in techniques to do the same. Explain consequences of prolonged pressure on the skin.
- Provide tactile stimulation to affected limbs using rough cloth or hand, and instruct the patient or family in methods used.
- Explain how a stimulus might feel (e.g., cool water, soft flannel).
- Teach the patient to check temperature of water with unaffected side before using water (thermal screening).
- Instruct the patient to regularly move affected limbs.

- Teach the patient and family strategies to modify home environment.

▲ Facilitate referral to a physical therapist or occupational therapist to learn adaptive skills.

Rationales

Pressure on the affected side should last no longer than 30 minutes. Inability to sense pressure increases risk for skin breakdown.

Frequent application of stimuli helps patients learn to recognize sensations.

Verbal descriptions improve patient understanding of the stimulus.

Diminished temperature sensation, especially for heat, increases the risk for accidental burn injury.

Movement promotes circulation. Impaired sensitivity to pain or numbness increases the likelihood of prolonged stationary positioning.

Optimal safety can be achieved by modification in the environment, by regulating the temperature setting on the hot water heater, by moving sharp-edged furniture, and by lighting hallways.

Patients and caregivers need to learn adaptive skills to reduce risk for injury.

Risk for Unilateral Neglect

Common Risk Factor

Stroke in the nondominant hemisphere or the dominant right side

Common Expected Outcomes

Patient incurs no injuries as a result of deficit.

Patient can cross midline with eyes and unaffected arm.

Patient observes and touches affected side during activities of daily living (ADLs).

Patient begins to wash, dress, and eat with attention to both sides.

Patient and family verbalize cognitive awareness of deficit.

NOC Outcomes
Body Positioning: Self-Initiated; Self-Care: Activities of Daily Living (ADL); Safety Behavior: Personal

NIC Intervention
Unilateral Neglect Management

Ongoing Assessment

Actions/Interventions	Rationales
■ Assess the patient's response to touch, pain, and temperature.	Assessment data determine the actual level of sensation for comparison with how the patient uses the affected side. Use may be different from actual ability.
■ Perform visual fields confrontation test.	The patient may not be able to see on the affected side (hemianopsia). The patient who complains of diplopia may benefit from patching one eye.
■ Observe the patient's performance of ADLs.	This information determines the patient's recognition of the affected side. The patient may not, for example, bathe the affected side, forgetting that it is there. Injury to the parietal lobe in the nondominant hemisphere makes it difficult for the patient to recognize the contralateral side of the body, even if visual fields are intact
■ Assess for distorted spatial relationships.	Impaired spatial awareness and proprioception interferes with the patient's awareness of the affected side of the body.

Therapeutic Interventions

Actions/Interventions	Rationales
■ Approach the patient from the unaffected side when the patient initially regains consciousness.	Approaching the patient from the unaffected side increases awareness of the presence of people in the environment and facilitates ability to interact with others.
■ As the patient becomes more alert, approach from the affected side while calling the patient's name.	This approach will enhance the patient's awareness of the affected side of the body.
■ Ensure a safe environment by placing a call light on the patient's unaffected side.	Hemianopsia limits the patient's ability to see objects in the affected visual field. If the patient cannot find the call light, he or she may attempt to get up without assistance. This behavior increases the risk for falls.
■ Provide tactile stimulation to the affected side.	Frequent stimulus application increases short-term memory of sensation.
■ Place all food in small quantities, arranged simply on a plate.	This approach diminishes spatial/visual deficits. Small quantities make it easier to delineate foods because of the space between food items.
■ Attach a watch or bright bracelet to the affected arm.	This technique draws the patient's attention to the affected side.

■ = Independent ▲ = Collaborative

Actions/Interventions

- Encourage the patient to wash the affected side of the body and to dress the affected side of the body first.

- Practice drawing and copying figures with the patient.

- Draw a bright mark on the sides of a newspaper or book when the patient is reading.

- Teach compensatory strategies such as visual scanning (turning head in order to visualize entire area).

- ▲ Initiate physical therapy or occupational therapy consults.

Rationales

This approach to ADLs increases the patient's awareness of the affected side of the body. Increased tactile and visual awareness of the affected side promotes neural perception and integration of external stimuli.

These activities help develop fine motor skills and relearn spatial relationships.

This technique cues the end of a line and the return for next line.

The patient needs to learn strategies to reduce the chance of injury and increase visual awareness of entire field of vision.

Physical and occupational therapists can help the patient learn adaptive skills to promote increased self-care and decrease risk for injury.

Deficient Knowledge

Common Related Factors
Unfamiliar with diagnosis
Unfamiliar with risk factors
Required rehabilitation

Defining Characteristics
Questions about diagnosis and outcomes
Concerns about follow-up

Common Expected Outcome
Patient and/or caregivers verbalize understanding of disease process and potential outcomes.

NOC Outcomes
Knowledge: Disease Process; Knowledge: Treatment Regimen; Knowledge: Medication; Knowledge: Personal Safety

NIC Interventions
Teaching: Disease Process; Teaching: Prescribed Activity/Exercise

---

Ongoing Assessment

Actions/Interventions

- Determine stroke-related deficits that may affect learning.

- Assess the patient's perception of the diagnosis and care needs.
- Determine readiness and ability to learn.

- Determine counseling and social service needs.

Rationales

Each stroke patient has different deficits and must be treated as an individual. These deficits may include emotional lability, loss of self-control, communication deficits, and cognitive changes.

Patients are more receptive to learning if their own identified needs and goals are being met.

The teaching plan will be individualized based on the patient's ability to comprehend and remember new information.

Some patients may not be ready to accept disability and will not want to learn. Further counseling may be necessary, as may be social services involvement to help facilitate care outside the hospital.

Therapeutic Interventions

Actions/Interventions	Rationales
■ Discuss type of stroke, progress, treatments, and preventive measures.	Explaining physical and mental changes that occur with stroke helps reduce anxiety and limit the onset of depression. Knowing what to expect during stroke recovery promotes effective coping and the motivation to participate in the rehabilitation process.
■ Prepare the patient and family for possible changes in patient behavior and judgment.	Patients may experience mood changes and depression within 6 months of the initial stroke injury. Emotional liability may continue for several months.
■ Include the caregiver in the rehabilitation process to learn and assist with care, as well as to provide emotional support for the patient's efforts.	Almost all stroke victims will have some degree of disability and will require assistance and emotional support. Family members need to understand how a stroke may influence their social and personal roles and activities.
■ Assist the spouse or family in obtaining the support they need.	Stroke victims are often older persons whose disabilities may be overwhelming to an equally elderly or frail spouse. The responsibility of caregiving can increase fear and stress for the family member.
■ Teach measures to manage or reduce risk factors for repeated stroke.	Knowing the risk factors is the first step in controlling them and decreasing the chance of further stroke. Risk factors include hypertension, heart disease, smoking, polycythemia, alcohol use, obesity, hypercholesterolemia, diabetes mellitus, and sedentary lifestyle.
■ Provide education concerning long-term medication use for stroke prevention.	Clinical practice guidelines from the American Heart Association/American Stroke Association recommend daily use of antiplatelet medications for recurrent stroke prevention. These medications may include low-dose aspirin combined with extended release dipyridamole, and clopidogrel. Oral anticoagulants, such as warfarin, may be indicated for patients with embolic strokes from atrial thrombi. Current evidence suggests that the addition of cholesterol-lowering statin drugs may benefit patients with thrombotic strokes from cerebral atherosclerosis.
■ Encourage the use of community resources and support groups.	The family needs information about how community resources can promote effective coping and decrease feelings of caregiving as a burden.

Related Care Plans

■ = Independent   ▲ = Collaborative

Transient Ischemic Attack

Transient Ischemic Attack (TIA); Carotid Endarterectomy; Carotid Artery Stent

A transient ischemic attack (TIA) is a cerebrovascular disorder that produces temporary neurological deficits. Atherosclerosis in the cerebral vessels is the primary cause of TIA. Emboli that originate in blood vessels outside the cerebral circulation also contribute to the occurrence of TIAs. A TIA is considered an early warning of the risk for an impending stroke. Clinical manifestations of a TIA depend on the location of the ischemia in the brain. Symptoms usually last no longer than 5 to 20 minutes and resolve within 24 hours of onset. The patient will not have any residual neurological deficits. Treatment of TIA includes measures to promote cerebral blood flow and manage risk factors for stroke. Long-term drug therapy to control coagulation is an important part of the treatment. Surgical interventions are used to improve carotid artery blood flow in patients at high risk for stroke. A carotid endarterectomy (CEA) is done to remove atherosclerotic plaques in the carotid arteries and improve blood flow to the brain. Carotid artery stenting (CAS) is a newer and less invasive procedure that is done to improve blood flow. A stent is threaded into the carotid artery. Once is place the stent is expanded to widen the area of blockage and capture any dislodged plaque. Recent clinical trials comparing CEA to CAS found that both procedures are safe and offer equal benefits for a diverse population of patients.

 NANDA-I NDx Deficient Knowledge

Common Related Factors
Unfamiliarity with disease process and treatment
Lack of exposure to information

Defining Characteristics
Lack of questions about problem
Multiple questions about problem
Misinformation about disease and its treatment

Common Expected Outcome
Patient verbalizes accurate knowledge about TIAs and their treatment.

NOC Outcomes
Knowledge: Disease Process; Knowledge: Medication; Knowledge: Treatment Procedure

NIC Interventions
Teaching: Disease Process; Teaching: Prescribed Medication; Teaching: Procedure/Treatment

Ongoing Assessment

Actions/Interventions

- Assess the patient's knowledge of TIAs, anticoagulant therapy, revascularization procedures, and risk factors for stroke.

Rationales

Patient education is based on the person's knowledge of the disorder. The patient needs to understand the cause of a TIA and the importance of risk factor management to prevent a stroke.

Therapeutic Interventions

Actions/Interventions	Rationales
■ Provide the patient and family with information about cerebrovascular disease and TIAs.	The patient and family need to understand the relationship between atherosclerosis, cerebrovascular disease, and TIAs to make appropriate decisions about seeking early treatment for TIAs and stroke prevention. Compliance with medical and surgical therapies will be enhanced if the patient and family have appropriate knowledge.
■ Teach the patient and family about managing risk factors for stroke.	Risk factors for TIA and stroke include poorly controlled hypertension, diabetes mellitus, obesity, smoking, and atrial fibrillation. Cardiac dysrhythmias such as atrial fibrillation are associated with the formation of atrial thrombi that can embolize to the carotid arteries and cerebral blood vessels.
■ Teach the patient about the use of medications to control coagulation.	Medications to reduce the formation of thrombi and embolizations of existing thrombi are given to decrease the risk for stroke.
• Low-dose aspirin	Administration of a single daily dose of aspirin (81 to 325 mg) is effective in reducing thrombus formation and embolization because of its antiplatelet activity.
• Platelet aggregation inhibitors	Dipyridamole (Persantine) decreases platelet aggregation. Ticlopidine (Ticlid) and clopidogrel (Plavix) are platelet aggregation inhibitors that have been shown to be as effective as aspirin in reducing thrombus formation. The use of low-dose aspirin combined with extended release dipyridamole has been shown to be highly effective in stroke prevention.
• Oral anticoagulants	Anticoagulants are used for patients with a history of atrial thrombosis related to atrial fibrillation.
■ Provide the patient and family with information about revascularization procedures.	Carotid endarterectomy has a high rate of success in restoring blood flow through narrowed carotid arteries. Complications include bleeding at the operative site, neurological deficits, and heart attacks. The results of clinical trials suggest that the patient having carotid artery stenting is less likely to experience heart attack as a complication compared to CEA but more likely to experience neurological deficits or stroke.

 Risk for Ineffective Cerebral Tissue Perfusion

Common Risk Factors

Edema from carotid endarterectomy
Hemorrhage
Hematoma formation
Hypotension

Common Expected Outcome

Patient maintains optimal cerebral tissue perfusion as evidenced by National Institutes of Health Stroke Scale (NIHSS) score less than 4, Glasgow Coma Scale (GCS) score greater than 13, absence of neurological deficits, and stable blood pressure.

■ = Independent ▲ = Collaborative

Ongoing Assessment

Actions/Interventions	Rationales
■ Assess neurological status using NIHSS or GCS.	Stroke is associated with both carotid endarterectomy and carotid artery stenting as a result of embolization of atherosclerotic plaque, and reduced cerebral perfusion. The NIHSS is a standardized assessment of consciousness, vision, sensory, and motor responses, and speech and language function. Scores range from 0 (no stroke) to 42 (severe stroke). The GCS measures changes in level of consciousness based on verbal, motor, and pupillary responses. Scores range from 0 to 15. A score less than 13 is associated with a decreased level of consciousness.
■ Monitor blood pressure (BP).	Stable systemic BP is necessary to maintain adequate cerebral perfusion.
■ Check for symmetry of neck. Check behind neck of supine patient.	Bleeding from the neck incision or hematoma formation in the neck may decrease blood flow through the carotid artery and reduce cerebral perfusion. External bleeding may pool behind the neck and not saturate a neck dressing. Frequent assessment of the area behind the neck is necessary even if the neck dressing appears dry and intact.

Therapeutic Interventions

Actions/Interventions	Rationales
■ Report sudden or progressive deterioration in neurological status.	Prompt intervention is necessary to minimize damage from inadequate cerebral blood flow. Current practice guidelines recommend that patients with an NIHSS score greater than 4 may benefit from thrombolytics.
▲ Administer medications as ordered to keep BP within desired range.	Extreme fluctuations in blood pressure reduce cerebral perfusion pressure and result in cerebral ischemia and stroke.

NANDA-I NDx **Ineffective Breathing Pattern**

Common Related Factors
Edema
Hematoma formation

Defining Characteristics
Tachypnea
Change in depth of breathing
Complaint of shortness of breath
Use of accessory muscles

Common Expected Outcome
Patient's optimal breathing pattern is maintained, as evidence by eupnea, regular respiratory rate/pattern, and verbalization of comfort with breathing.

NOC Outcomes
Respiratory Status: Ventilation
NIC Interventions
Respiratory Monitoring

Ongoing Assessment

Actions/Interventions	Rationales
■ Assess respiratory rate, rhythm, and depth.	Changes in breathing patterns can occur with hemispheric injury or brainstem injury.

Actions/Interventions

- Use pulse oximetry to monitor oxygen saturation; assess ABG's as ordered.

- Assess trachea for midline position, neck for symmetry.

Rationales

Pulse oximetry is a useful tool to detect changes in oxygenation. Oxygen saturation should be at 90% or greater. $Paco_2$ greater than 45 mm Hg induces cerebral vasodilatation and increased intracranial pressure. $Paco_2$ less than 60 mm Hg induces cerebral vasoconstriction and cerebral ischemia.

Swelling or hematoma can obstruct the airway.

Therapeutic Interventions

Actions/Interventions

- Elevate head of bed 30 to 40 degrees.

- Encourage deep breathing.

- Suction airway as needed.

- Provide reassurance and allay anxiety by staying with the patient during acute episodes of respiratory distress.
- ▲ Provide supplemental oxygen therapy.
- Notify the physician immediately of any change in neck symmetry or tracheal position.

Rationales

A sitting position can help reduce neck edema and promote effective lung expansion and chest excursion.

Deep inspiration increases oxygenation and prevents atelectasis.

Suctioning removes accumulated secretions and improves oxygenation.

Anxiety can result in rapid shallow respirations and increase dyspnea and respiratory rate.

Oxygen saturation is important to promote cerebral perfusion.

An expanding hematoma in the neck can be a life-threatening emergency.

Neurological Care Plans

■ = Independent   ▲ = Collaborative

Gastrointestinal and Digestive Care Plans

Abdominal Surgery

Gastrectomy; Splenectomy; Pancreatectomy; Cholecystectomy; Prostatectomy; Cystectomy; Appendectomy; Hysterectomy; Nephrectomy; Abdominal Aortic Aneurysm Resection; Bowel Resection; Exploratory Laparotomy

Open surgery of the abdomen may be done for the following: gastrectomy (removal of all or part of the stomach); splenectomy (removal of the spleen); pancreatectomy (partial or total removal of the pancreas); liver resection; cholecystectomy (removal of the gallbladder); removal of biliary stones or resection of biliary structures; prostatectomy (removal of the prostate gland); cystectomy (removal of the bladder); appendectomy (removal of the appendix); hysterectomy (removal of the uterus); nephrectomy (removal of a kidney); resection or repair of abdominal aortic aneurysms; small and large bowel resection; or repair of trauma to any abdominal structure resulting from blunt or penetrating injury. An exploratory laparotomy involves an open incision of the abdominal cavity. This procedure is done to inspect the abdominal organs for signs of injury, ischemia, or tumor. Tissue biopsy or repair may be done during a laparotomy. Nursing care interventions are similar for all patients having abdominal surgery, regardless of the type. This care plan addresses the major common diagnoses associated with open abdominal surgical procedures. Although most postoperative abdominal surgical patients remain in the hospital for 3 to 7 days, shorter stays (less than 24 hours) are becoming more common. As laparoscopic techniques and instrumentation continue to develop, less open abdominal surgery is being performed.

NANDA-I NDx Deficient Knowledge: Preoperative

Common Related Factors
Proposed surgical experience
Lack of previous similar surgical procedure
Anxiety/fear

Defining Characteristics
Questions
Lack of questions
Verbalized misconceptions

Common Expected Outcomes
Patient verbalizes understanding of proposed surgical procedure and realistic expectations for the postoperative course.
Patient demonstrates the ability to cough, deep breathe, use the incentive spirometer, and perform leg exercises.

NOC Outcome
Knowledge: Treatment Procedure(s)
NIC Intervention
Teaching: Preoperative

Ongoing Assessment

Actions/Interventions	Rationales
■ Assess the patient's knowledge of proposed surgical procedure.	The patient should be aware of the nature of the surgical procedure, as well as risks and benefits of the surgical procedure, the reason it is being done, location of the surgical incision, and expected length of recovery. The patient should have information provided for understanding of surgical procedure and postoperative care.
■ Assess the patient's previous experience with surgery.	Patients who have had surgery in the past may have negative feelings related to side effects of anesthesia and postoperative pain; they may recall longer hospitalizations than today's typical shorter stays.

Therapeutic Interventions

Actions/Interventions	Rationales
■ Explain and reinforce the surgeon's explanations regarding the proposed surgical procedure.	The patient may have questions and need clarification of information to have better understanding of the surgery.
■ Prepare patients having open abdominal surgery to expect the following:	
• An incision in the abdomen, either stapled or sutured closed, with a dressing in place	Size and location of the incision depend on the nature of the surgical procedure.
• Surgical drains near the surgical incision	Surgical drains promote drainage of fluid from the incisional site, decrease pressure on healing tissue, and reduce abscess formation.
• Intravenous (IV) lines	IV lines are inserted before surgery to provide fluid, electrolytes, and emergency IV access.
• Nasogastric (NG) tube	An NG tube may be placed during surgery to keep the stomach free of fluid and prevent distention, nausea, and vomiting. The NG tube is discontinued when normal peristaltic activity resumes, which is indicated by the patient having audible bowel sounds and passing flatus.
• Early ambulation, usually out of bed the first postoperative day	This activity helps prevent pulmonary atelectasis, deep vein thrombosis, and other complications of immobility.
• Postoperative leg exercises	Leg exercises help promote venous return and decrease the incidence of deep vein thrombosis.
• Antiembolic stockings or sequential compression devices for patients who remain on bed rest for more than 12 hours	These devices prevent deep vein thrombosis.
• Need for dynamic turning, coughing, deep-breathing exercises, and incentive spirometry; give opportunities for return demonstration	These techniques help prevent pulmonary atelectasis and stasis of secretions, which could lead to pneumonia.
• Need for pain management	Adequate pain management allows patients having abdominal surgery to participate actively in their care, to ambulate, and to breathe effectively. The patient has a right to be involved in selecting the type of pain management used.
• Measures used by the surgical team in the operating room, such as a time-out, to ensure the correct procedure is carried out.	Teaching the patient about expectations to promote safety during the procedure may reduce the person's level of anxiety. The Joint Commission patient safety goals include performance standards to promote communications among all members of the surgical team at all stages of preparation for the procedure. These standards include a time-out before the start of the procedure to conduct a final assessment that the correct patient, site, and positioning are identified and that all consents, relevant information, and equipment are available.

■ = Independent ▲ = Collaborative

NANDA-I NDx Ineffective Breathing Pattern

Common Related Factors
Abdominal incision pain
Abdominal distention compromising lung expansion
Sedation

Defining Characteristics
Dyspnea, tachypnea/bradypnea
Poor coughing effort
Shallow breathing
Splinting respirations
Altered chest excursion
Refusal/inability to use incentive spirometer

Common Expected Outcome
Patient maintains an effective breathing pattern as evidenced by relaxed breathing at a normal rate and depth and absence of dyspnea.

NOC Outcomes
Respiratory Status: Airway Patency; Respiratory Status: Ventilation

NIC Interventions
Respiratory Monitoring; Cough Enhancement

Ongoing Assessment

Actions/Interventions	Rationales
■ Assess rate, rhythm, and depth of respirations.	Respirations are typically shallow, because the least amount of excursion is less painful when an abdominal incision is present. Also, the higher the incision, the more the breathing is affected.
■ Auscultate breath sounds at least every 4 hours for the first 48 hours postoperatively.	The bases of the lungs are least likely to be ventilated; therefore breath sounds may be diminished over the bases.
■ Observe for splinting.	Splinting refers to the conscious minimization of an inspiration to reduce the amount of discomfort caused by full expansion of the lungs.
■ Assess ability to use incentive spirometer.	In incentive spirometry, the patient takes and holds a deep breath for a few seconds. Incentive spirometry encourages deep breathing, and holding the breath allows for full expansion of alveoli.
■ Assess for abdominal pain and distention.	Abdominal pain and distention can impair thoracic excursion and result in an ineffective breathing pattern.
■ Assess temperature according to postoperative policy.	Elevated temperature in the first 48 hours postoperatively may indicate atelectasis, which can lead to pneumonia.
■ Assess the amount and characteristics of sputum.	Increased amounts of sputum, as well as changes in color and a thicker consistency, may indicate pneumonia.

Therapeutic Interventions

Actions/Interventions	Rationales
▲ Manage pain using whatever plan for pain management has been prescribed.	Effective pain management allows for deeper breathing and coughing. Patients using patient-controlled analgesia (PCA) may need reinstruction or reminders to push the button during the early postoperative phase until they are fully recovered from anesthesia.
■ Position patient with head of bed (HOB) elevated 30 degrees.	This position puts the least strain on abdominal muscles and enhances diaphragmatic excursion.

Actions/Interventions

- Encourage or assist the patient to turn side to side every 2 hours; position with pillows or positioning devices as needed. Encourage ambulation as tolerated.
- Encourage the patient to do deep-breathing exercises a minimum of 10 times every hour. Encourage use of incentive spirometer every 1 to 2 hours.
- Encourage coughing every hour.
- Help the patient splint the abdominal incision by using hands or a pillow.
- ▲ Administer oxygen as prescribed.

Rationales

Breathing effectiveness and mobilization of secretions are enhanced by position change and an upright position.

Deep breathing keeps alveoli from collapsing. Incentive spirometry encourages deep breathing, and allows for the full expansion of alveoli.
Effective coughing clears the bronchial tree of secretions.
Splinting the incision eases the discomfort of coughing and taking deep breaths.
Promoting lung expansion and oxygenation of the tissues is a goal of the patient with atelectasis.

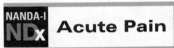

Acute Pain

Common Related Factors

Abdominal incision
Presence of drains, tubes

Defining Characteristics

Subjective complaint of pain
Guarded movement
Expressive behavior of pain

Common Expected Outcomes

Patient reports satisfactory pain control at a level less than 3 to 4 on a 0 to 10 rating scale.
Patient uses pharmacological and nonpharmacological pain relief strategies.
Patient exhibits increased comfort such as baseline levels for pulse, blood pressure, respirations, and relaxed muscle tone or body posture.

NOC Outcomes

Comfort Level; Pain Control; Pain Level

NIC Interventions

Analgesic Administration; Pain Management; Patient-Controlled Analgesia (PCA) Assistance; Positioning

---

Ongoing Assessment

Actions/Interventions

- Assess the location, quality, onset, frequency, radiation, and duration of pain. Have the patient rate pain intensity on a scale (0 to 10 or Faces).
- Assess for abdominal distention.

- Check abdomen for rigidity (hard, boardlike abdomen) and rebound tenderness (pain elicited when pressure is applied and then released on the abdomen).

Rationales

Some pain is expected after abdominal surgery; appropriate pain management will provide comfort and enable the patient to move and rest.
Distention of the abdomen by accumulation of gas and fluid occurs postoperatively because normal peristalsis does not return until the third or fourth day after surgery; distention stresses suture lines and causes pain.
Either of these may indicate peritonitis, a serious inflammation of the lining of the peritoneum that can result from intraabdominal leakage of organ secretions or visceral contents after abdominal surgery.

Therapeutic Interventions

Actions/Interventions

- Assist the patient to a comfortable position.

Rationales

A semi-Fowler's position is usually most comfortable, because stress on the suture line is relieved.

■ = Independent   ▲ = Collaborative

Actions/Interventions	**Rationales**
▲ Administer analgesics, or assist the patient in using PCA before pain becomes too severe.	It is more difficult to control pain once it becomes severe. Individualizing the pain-relieving regimen recognizes individual differences in pain perception and provides for more effective control. Nonsteroidal antiinflammatory drugs are used alone for mild pain and in combination with opioids for moderate or severe pain.
■ Use nonpharmacological treatment measures (e.g., distraction, music, relaxation).	These measures reduce perception and sensation of pain.
▲ Administer pain medication before painful procedures (e.g., dressing changes, ambulation).	Effective pain management maximizes the patient's ability to tolerate or participate in procedures.

Risk for Deficient Fluid Volume

Common Risk Factors

Nasogastric suctioning
Loss of fluid from intestinal or interstitial space drains
Wound drainage
Blood loss in surgery or postoperative bleeding
NPO (nothing by mouth) status
Vomiting

Common Expected Outcome

Patient is normovolemic, as evidenced by stable blood pressure (BP) at or above 90/60 mm Hg or patient's baseline, heart rate of 60 to 100 beats/min, urine output of at least 30 mL/hr, and good skin turgor.

NOC Outcomes
Fluid Balance; Hydration
NIC Interventions
Fluid/Electrolyte Management; Surveillance

Ongoing Assessment

Actions/Interventions	**Rationales**
■ Monitor and report any postoperative bleeding: • Intraabdominal	Bleeding may occur from any vessel in the dissected area; usually seen as increased bloody drainage on dressing.
• Intraluminal	This type of bleeding is usually from anastomosis; this is seen as increased bloody drainage from tubes.
• Incisional	Bleeding from an incision is usually from subcutaneous tissue; this is seen as increased bloody drainage on dressings.
■ Mark extension of drainage from incisions.	Outlining the stain on the surface of the dressing and indicating the time of the assessment allows staff to quantify the amount of drainage and severity of bleeding later.
■ Assess hydration status: • Monitor BP and heart rate.	Hypotension and/or tachycardia may indicate fluid volume deficit.
• Check mucous membranes, skin turgor, and thirst.	Increasing thirst and a coated tongue occur with fluid volume deficit. The patient may complain of a dry mouth. Tenting of the skin is associated with fluid volume deficit.
• Monitor urine output.	Output of 30 mL/hr or higher indicates adequate hydration.
• Monitor, record, and report output of emesis, NG tube output, output from surgical drains (check for drainage around drains also), and incisional drainage.	Wound drainage, tube drainage, and emesis can be sources of fluid loss from the body.

Actions/Interventions	Rationales
▲ Monitor hemoglobin (Hgb) and hematocrit (Hct) and coagulation profile.	Dropping Hgb and Hct may indicate internal bleeding. Excessive postoperative bleeding may result from coagulopathy.

Therapeutic Interventions

Actions/Interventions	Rationales
▲ Administer IV fluid as ordered; be prepared to increase fluids if signs of fluid volume deficit appear.	IV fluids are prescribed to correct fluid volume deficit and maintain fluid balance postoperatively.
▲ Provide oral fluids of patient's choice, as allowed.	Oral fluids are usually restricted until peristalsis returns (typically 72 to 96 hours) and NG tube is removed, because swallowed fluids will be sucked out by the NG tube along with electrolytes; this puts the patient at risk for electrolyte imbalance, especially hypokalemia. However, patients may be allowed ice chips or small sips of clear fluids.
▪ Provide oral hygiene every 4 hours.	NPO status and/or fluid volume deficit will cause a dry, sticky mouth. Oral care stimulates saliva secretion and relieves dry mouth.

NANDA-I NDx **Risk for Infection**

Common Risk Factors
Abdominal incision
Atelectasis
Indwelling urinary catheter
Venous access devices
Presence of tubes and drains
Inadvertent interruption of closed drainage systems
Obesity
Smoking history
Immunosuppression
Poor nutritional status
Diabetes

Common Expected Outcomes
Patient is free of infection, as evidenced by the following:
- Healing wound/incision that is clean, dry, well approximated, and free of redness, swelling, purulent discharge, and pain
- Normal body temperature within 72 hours postoperatively
- Venous access sites free of redness and purulent drainage
- Clear breath sounds without cough or sputum production

NOC Outcomes
Risk Detection; Wound Healing: Primary Intention
NIC Interventions
Infection Control; Tube Care; Tube Care: Urinary; Wound Care; Wound Care: Closed Drainage

Ongoing Assessment

Actions/Interventions	Rationales
▪ Monitor temperature.	For the first 48 to 72 hours postoperatively, temperatures of up to 38.5° C (101.3° F) are expected as a normal stress response after major surgery. Beyond 72 hours, temperature should return to patient's baseline. Temperature spikes, usually occurring in the later afternoon or night, are often indications of infection.

▪ = Independent ▲ = Collaborative

Actions/Interventions

▲ Monitor white blood cell (WBC) count.

■ Assess incision and wound for redness, drainage, swelling, and increased pain:
- Closed wounds or incisions

- Open wounds

■ Assess all peripheral and central IV sites for redness, swelling, warmth, purulent drainage, and pain.

■ Assess color, clarity, and odor of urine.

▲ Obtain specimens of wound drainage, sputum, blood, and urine in sterile containers.

■ Assess quality of breath sounds, cough, and sputum production.
■ Assess stability of tubes and drains.

Rationales

Elevated WBC count is typically an indication of infection; however, in older patients, infection may be present without an increase in WBC count because of normal age-related changes in the immune system.

Incisions that have been closed with sutures or staples should be free of redness, swelling, and drainage. Some incisional discomfort is expected. These incisions are usually kept covered by a dry dressing for 24 to 48 hours; beyond 48 hours there is no need for a dressing if the incision is not draining.

Wounds left open to heal by secondary intention should appear pink/red and moist and should have minimal serosanguineous drainage. These wounds are usually packed with sterile gauze moistened with sterile saline. Discomfort is expected upon packing.

IV lines disrupt skin integrity and provide a potential portal of entry for pathogens into the circulatory system. Continual monitoring for signs of inflammation or infection is essential.

Cloudy, foul-smelling urine is an indication of urinary tract infection, which can occur as the result of an indwelling catheter.

Specimens are sent for analysis to determine if pathogens are present. Identification of pathogens guides clinical decisions about selection of antimicrobial drugs.

Adventitious breath sounds can indicate a respiratory infection.

In-and-out motion of improperly secured tubes and drains allows access by pathogens through stab wounds where tubes and drains are placed.

Therapeutic Interventions

Actions/Interventions

■ Wash hands before contact with the postoperative patient.

■ Use aseptic technique during dressing change, wound care, or handling or manipulation of tubes and drains.
■ Ensure that closed drainage systems (urinary catheter, surgical tubes and drains) are not inadvertently interrupted (opened). Irrigate tubes and drains only by physician prescription; use aseptic technique and sterile irrigant.
■ Tape connectors and pin extension or drainage tubing securely to the patient's gown. Prevent kinking of drain tubing.

■ Provide aseptic site care to all peripheral and central venous access devices according to hospital policy.
■ Provide care for indwelling urinary catheters according to hospital policy.
■ Encourage adequate nutritional intake.

■ Educate the patient and family on the signs and symptoms of infection: elevated temperature, redness, swelling of the incisional area, and purulent or foul-smelling wound drainage.

▲ Administer antibiotics and antipyretics as prescribed.

Rationales

Hand washing remains the most effective method of infection control.

Aseptic technique for dressing changes and wound care limits the introduction of pathogens.

Opening of sterile systems allows access by pathogens and puts the patient at risk for infection.

Stabilizing and securing drain tubing minimizes tension on tubes and connection. Kinking of tubing prevents drainage of urine or wound exudate. Stasis contributes to the development of infection.

Aseptic technique prevents transmission of pathogens.

Frequent perineal hygiene reduces the number of pathogens around the urinary catheter entrance site.

Adequate intake of protein, vitamins, and minerals is essential to promote immune system function and wound healing.

Educating the patient and family assists in early recognition of adverse signs and symptoms.

These drugs are used to treat infections and the fever usually associated with infection.

NANDA-I NDx Risk for Impaired Tissue Integrity

Common Risk Factors

Delayed wound healing
Infection
Presence of seroma or hematoma
Increased intraabdominal pressure
Mechanical force (e.g., stress, tension against wound)

Common Expected Outcome

Patient has an intact wound without complications such as dehiscence, evisceration, or fistula.

NOC Outcomes
Wound Healing: Primary Intention; Tissue Integrity: Skin and Mucous Membranes
NIC Interventions
Skin Surveillance; Wound Care; Positioning

Ongoing Assessment

Actions/Interventions	Rationales
■ Assess wound for hematoma (collection of bloody drainage beneath the skin) or seroma (collection of serous fluid beneath the skin).	Presence of either type of fluid collection predisposes the wound to separation and infection.
■ Assess condition of stitches or staples and retention sutures, if present; report any closures that appear to have loosened or fallen out.	Wound edges should remain approximated, without tension, puckering, or open gaps between stitches or staples. An incision is most vulnerable to injury during the first 48 hours, before wound strength begins to develop. Retention sutures (large sutures placed in addition to routine closures) are used when obesity, extreme abdominal distention, intraabdominal infection, poor nutritional status, and/or a history of wound evisceration is present. Wound dehiscence (separation of the suture line or wound) occurs with excessive stress on a new incision. Obesity or improper techniques for mobility may add to stress on sutures and contribute to dehiscence. Wounds left open to heal by secondary intention are open only as deep as the subcutaneous tissue is deep; the fascia, muscle, and peritoneum have usually been closed. The deepest portion of the wound will come together, with the presence of tissue beneath being visible.
■ Assess open wounds for evidence of evisceration (protrusion of abdominal contents).	Evisceration of a surgical wound is a serious complication. The wound should be covered immediately with a sterile dressing moistened with normal saline. The patient is usually returned to the operating room for wound repair.
■ Assess wounds and dressings for suspicious drainage.	The presence of yellow, green, or brown fluid or material with an acrid or fecal odor indicates the presence of a fistula, a communication between some portion of the bowel and the incision or open wound.

■ = Independent   ▲ = Collaborative

Gastrointestinal and Digestive Care Plans

Therapeutic Interventions

Actions/Interventions	Rationales
■ Prevent strain on the abdominal incision or wound:	
• Keep HOB elevated 30 degrees.	Elevation relaxes abdominal muscles and reduces tension on the incision.
• Encourage patient to splint the incision with pillow or hands before coughing.	Excessive coughing and straining of abdominal muscles and skin can predispose the wound to dehiscence.
• Educate the patient to splint the incision when transferring from bed to chair or when getting up to ambulate.	These activities may strain abdominal muscles and increase tension on a suture line. Supporting the area with a pillow or hands when moving reduces the risk for wound separation.
• Ensure proper functioning of suction machine.	Malfunction of NG suctioning can cause nausea, which may lead to retching and increased strain on abdominal muscles.
▲ If dehiscence or evisceration occurs or is suspected (i.e., wound edges are separated and/or abdominal viscera are visible and protruding through the abdominal wound):	
• Place the patient in Fowler's position.	Positioning promotes relaxation of abdominal muscles and reduces strain on the incision.
• Cover area with saline solution–soaked sterile gauze.	Keeping viscera moist increases viability.
• Notify the physician of the need for wound evaluation.	This situation usually requires a return to surgery for repair.
▲ If a fistula is suspected, protect wound edges with petrolatum-based ointment or hydrocolloid.	Intestinal contents can be highly corrosive to skin, denuding it in a matter of hours; this causes pain and may interfere with later attempts to close or pouch the fistula.
▲ Consult with wound care specialist.	A nurse with advanced education in wound care may provide specialized interventions for management of incision complications.

NANDA-I NDx

Risk for Deep Vein Thrombosis (DVT)

Common Risk Factors

Prolonged time in operating room (OR)
Position in OR
Decreased postoperative activity
Dehydration

Common Expected Outcome

Patient remains free of thrombophlebitis and deep vein thrombosis, as evidenced by bilaterally equal calves and absence of calf pain.

NOC Outcome
Tissue Perfusion: Peripheral
NIC Intervention
Circulatory Care: Venous Insufficiency

Ongoing Assessment

Actions/Interventions	Rationales
■ Assess legs for swelling.	Except for minor differences, calves should have the same approximate circumference. Unilateral swelling could indicate thrombophlebitis or deep vein thrombosis (DVT).
■ Assess for changes in skin color, temperature, or vein distention in legs.	Redness, warmth, and edema over a vein is associated with superficial thrombophlebitis. These changes increase the risk for DVT.
■ Assess for pain on compression of calf or dorsiflexion of foot (Homans' sign).	Homans' sign may be an indication of deep vein thrombosis.

Therapeutic Interventions

Actions/Interventions	Rationales
■ Reinforce or encourage leg exercises taught preoperatively; strive for 10 repetitions each hour until fully ambulatory.	Contracting the leg muscles decreases venous stasis and encourages good venous return; both decrease the opportunity of thromboembolic developments.
▲ Use antiembolic stockings or sequential compression devices while the patient is in bed.	Both interventions promote venous blood flow and reduce venous stagnation.
■ Discourage gatching of the bed at the knee. Encourage the patient not to cross legs at the knee or ankle while in bed.	Compression on veins contributes to venous pooling in the legs and decreased venous return.
▲ Encourage ambulation by the patient as soon as possible according to physician's prescription.	Being fully upright is preferable to "dangling" or sitting in a chair because contracted muscles push against the leg vessels and improve venous return most effectively when the patient is upright and legs are straight.
▲ Administer prophylactic anticoagulant therapy as prescribed.	Low-dose or low-molecular-weight heparin are used to prevent thrombus formation.
▲ Administer IV fluids; encourage oral fluid intake as prescribed.	Adequate hydration reduces hemoconcentration, and reduces the risk for deep vein thrombosis.
■ Before discharge, instruct the patient and family about guidelines for resuming normal activity.	Providing guidelines promotes the return of activity at an appropriate level, which will help reduce the complications of immobility and promote a sense of well-being.

Deficient Knowledge

Common Related Factors

Lack of previous experience with abdominal surgery
Need for home management

Common Expected Outcome

Patient verbalizes understanding of and demonstrates ability to provide wound care, advance diet as tolerated, limit activities as appropriate, recognize signs and symptoms of wound infection or other surgical complications, and return for follow-up care with physician.

Defining Characteristics

Multiple questions
Lack of questions
Inability to provide self-care on discharge

NOC Outcomes

Knowledge: Diet; Knowledge: Treatment Regimen; Knowledge: Prescribed Activity

NIC Interventions

Teaching: Disease Process; Teaching: Prescribed Diet; Teaching: Prescribed Activity/Exercise; Teaching: Psychomotor Skill

Ongoing Assessment

Actions/Interventions	Rationales
■ Assess the patient's ability to perform wound care, verbalize appropriate activity, and verbalize appropriate diet.	A teaching plan will be based on an assessment of the patient's ability to care for wounds and knowledge of activity and diet. Physical limitations may compromise learning and must be considered when designing the educational approach. Teaching standardized content that the patient already knows wastes valuable time and hinders critical learning.

■ = Independent   ▲ = Collaborative

Actions/Interventions

- Assess the patient's understanding of the need for further therapy, if necessary.

- Assess the patient's understanding of the need for close follow-up observation.

Rationales

Patients who have had abdominal surgery for malignancies may require further therapy, such as chemotherapy, irradiation, or immunotherapy.

Patients who leave the hospital with sutures, staples, or drains in place need to return for their removal or arrange to have a home health caregiver remove them.

Therapeutic Interventions

Actions/Interventions

- Teach the patient to perform appropriate wound care:
Closed abdominal incision:
  - Staples or sutures and dressings are usually removed by the time of discharge, and Steri-Strips have been placed.
Open abdominal wounds:
  - Wounds require twice-daily wet-to-dry saline solution packings until the wound has granulated in enough to close.

- Teach the patient appropriate activity:
  - No lifting more than 10 pounds for 6 weeks

  - Mild exercise (e.g., walking)

  - Showering

  - No driving until anterior abdominal wound has healed

- Teach the patient that a well-balanced, high-calorie, high-protein diet is desirable for healing that continues over a period of weeks.

- Teach the patient the importance of any further cancer therapy planned (e.g., chemotherapy, radiation therapy, immunotherapy).
- Teach the patient that bowel function will return to preoperative baseline in 2 to 3 weeks.
- Instruct the patient to seek medical attention for any of the following: temperature of 38° C (100.4° F) or higher, foul-smelling wound drainage, redness or unusual pain in any incision, or absence of bowel movement.

Rationales

Steri-Strips maintain wound approximation and should be left in place until they fall off.

The primary purpose of a wet-to-dry dressing is to mechanically debride a wound. The moistened layer of the dressing increases the absorptive ability of the dressing to collect exudates and wound debris. As the dressing dries, it adheres to the wound and debrides the wound of the tissue when the dressing is removed.

This activity restriction minimizes risk for loss of wound integrity.

Exercise increases stamina and improves circulation and reduces risk for DVT.

When there is an open wound, which may take up to 8 weeks to heal completely, use of a handheld shower head is a good way to clean the wound.

Operating foot pedals while driving, especially the brake, increases abdominal pressure and muscle straining.

Patients who have undergone gastrectomy should be taught to eat small, frequent meals, because they no longer have the same preoperative gastric capacity. Small, frequent meals are less likely to cause "dumping syndrome," which results from too large an osmotic load.

These therapies are typically offered if the pathology report indicates that the tumor was not confined to the bowel or bowel wall.

Return to baseline function usually occurs after the patient has resumed a normal schedule and diet.

The patient needs to report and receive prompt treatment for postoperative complications such as infection or possible bowel obstruction.

Related Care Plans

Ineffective airway clearance, p. 11
Constipation, p. 46
Anxiety, p. 18
Imbalanced nutrition: Less than body requirements, p. 142

Bowel Diversion Surgery: Colostomy, Iliostomy

Fecal Diversion; Stoma

Bowel diversion surgery results in an opening into the small or large intestine for the purpose of diverting the fecal stream past an area of obstruction or disease, protecting a distal surgical anastomosis, or providing an outlet for stool in the absence of a functioning intact rectum. These procedures may be performed to promote wound healing of an intestinal injury such as a gunshot wound. Diverted fecal material is directed away from the wound to promote wound healing. Depending on the purpose of the surgery and the integrity and function of anatomical structures, stomas may be temporary or permanent. Peristomal irritation, body image, self-care, and knowledge deficit are important nursing concerns. This care plan focuses primarily on the person with a new stoma who is being cared for in the hospital environment.

NANDA-I NDx
Deficient Knowledge: Surgical Procedure

Common Related Factors
Lack of previous similar experience
Need for additional information
Previous contact with poorly rehabilitated ostomate

Defining Characteristics
Verbalized need for information
Verbalized misinformation/misconceptions
Multiple questions
Lack of questions

Common Expected Outcomes
Patient verbalizes understanding that loss or bypass of anal sphincter will result in the need to surgically create a stoma and wear a collection pouch.
Patient demonstrates correct techniques for care of stoma and collection pouch.

NOC Outcomes
Knowledge: Treatment Regimen; Knowledge: Treatment Procedures
NIC Interventions
Teaching: Procedures/Treatment; Teaching: Preoperative

Ongoing Assessment

Actions/Interventions

- Inquire regarding information from surgeon about ostomy formation (e.g., purpose, site). Ascertain (from chart, physician) whether stoma will be permanent or temporary.

- Explore previous contact that the patient has had with persons with a stoma.

- Identify any misinformation and misconceptions the patient has about the ostomy.

Rationales

The patient needs to understand the purpose of the surgical procedure in relation to the underlying GI problem. Learning readiness/adaptation is often delayed in patients with temporary stomas; individuals with temporary stomas may often feel that learning ostomy management is not necessary.

Previous experience, whether positive or negative, will have an impact on the patient's expectations and fears regarding this surgery and postoperative stoma care.

Providing factual information can ease the patient's anxiety and provide a basis for learning new knowledge and self-care skills.

■ = Independent   ▲ = Collaborative

Therapeutic Interventions

Actions/Interventions	Rationales
■ Reinforce and reexplain the proposed procedure.	Anxiety often makes it necessary to repeat instructions or explanations several times before patients are able to comprehend.
■ Use diagrams, pictures, and audiovisual equipment to explain anatomy and physiology of GI tract, pathophysiology necessitating ostomy, and proposed location of stoma. Show the patient the actual pouch or one similar to the one that the patient will wear after surgery.	Ileostomy stomas are located in the right lower quadrant; colostomy stomas may be in the upper right quadrant, midabdomen at waistline, or left upper or lower quadrant. Visualization of information serves to reinforce and enhance learning. Understanding the purpose and need for a pouch encourages the patient to participate in ostomy management.
■ Explain need for a pouch in terms of loss of sphincter.	Patients should be told that preoperative bowel habits may return after surgery but that control of defecation is lost, and therefore a pouch is necessary to collect or contain stool and gas. The location of the stoma in the GI tract determines stool frequency and consistency. Output from a sigmoid colostomy is soft to solid, frequency is similar to preoperative patterns, and output may be regulated by irrigation. With a transverse colostomy, the output is mushy, occurs after meals, and cannot be regulated. Output from an ileostomy is liquid.
■ Offer a visit from a rehabilitated ostomate.	Contact with another individual who has undergone the same procedure enhances factual information from health care personnel.

NANDA-I NDx

Risk for Self-Care Deficit: Toileting

Common Risk Factors

Presence of new stoma
Presence of poorly placed stoma
Presence of pouch
Poor hand-eye coordination

Common Expected Outcome

Patient performs self-care needs (emptying and changing pouch) independently or with minimal assistance.

NOC Outcome
Self-Care: Toileting
NIC Intervention
Ostomy Care

Ongoing Assessment

Actions/Interventions	Rationales
■ Assess for the following: presence of old abdominal scars, presence of bony prominences on the anterior abdomen, presence of creases or skinfolds on the abdomen, extreme obesity, scaphoid abdomen, pendulous breasts, and ability to see and handle equipment.	Stoma placement is easier for a patient who has a flat abdomen with no scars, bony prominences, or obesity. The stoma should be placed in a site that is visible and easily reached by the patient.

Actions/Interventions	Rationales
■ Assess for patient concerns about caring for stoma and collection pouch.	Patients may have many concerns that will influence their ability to successfully manage changes in toileting self-care associated with a stoma. These concerns may include the visibility of the stoma and collection pouch, handling the fecal-filled pouch, or a noticeable smell.

Therapeutic Interventions

Actions/Interventions	Rationales
▲ Consult an enterostomal therapy (ET) nurse or surgeon to indelibly mark the proposed stoma site that the patient can easily see and reach; scars, bony prominences, and skin-folds are avoided; hip flexion should not change contour.	Stoma location is a key factor in self-care. A poorly located stoma can delay or preclude self-care. ET nurses are commonly asked by surgeons to preoperatively mark stoma areas. The stoma location is determined ideally with the patient in a sitting position.
■ If possible, have the patient wear a pouch over the proposed site; evaluate effectiveness 12 to 24 hours after applying the pouch.	Stoma site selection is facilitated by observing the appliance faceplate on the person's body under normal wearing conditions (e.g., dressed in normal clothing, moving about).

NDx Risk for Ineffective Stoma Tissue Perfusion

Common Risk Factors

Surgical manipulation of bowel
Postoperative edema
Tightly fitted faceplate
Pressure from rod or other support device

Common Expected Outcome

Patient's stoma remains pink and moist.

NOC Outcome
Tissue Perfusion: Abdominal Organs
NIC Interventions
Ostomy Care; Surveillance

Ongoing Assessment

Actions/Interventions	Rationales
■ Assess the following at least every 4 hours for the first 24 hours after surgery, and notify the physician of changes:	
• Color of stoma	The stoma (a piece of intestine) should be pink and moist, indicating good perfusion and adequate venous drainage. Dusky or blue appearance may indicate venous congestion or poor blood supply, either of which could result in a necrotic stoma.
• Moist appearance of stoma	Healthy intestine continuously secretes mucus, which maintains the moisture of the stoma.
• Stomal edema	Edema is either caused by preoperative pathology or by manipulation of the bowel during surgery; the stoma can be quite swollen.
• Presence of rods or support devices	Transverse or loop stomas are often supported by a rod or other support device, which usually is removed several days after surgery; patients may be discharged with the support device in place.

■ = Independent ▲ = Collaborative

Actions/Interventions	Rationales
• Correctly fitted faceplate	The opening of the ostomy appliance should be 1/8-inch larger than the stoma itself. A faceplate that is too tight can constrict the venous return of the stomal circulation and result in edema or damage to the stoma.
• Abdominal distention	Abdominal distention may decrease blood flow to the distal bowel and stoma.

Therapeutic Interventions

Actions/Interventions	Rationales
■ Fit the patient with a correctly sized faceplate.	Proper fit protects the surrounding skin from contact with drainage.
■ Anticipate and prepare the patient for possible surgical stoma revision if signs or symptoms of compromised circulation are present.	Necrosis extending to the fascia may represent a surgical emergency because of threat of perforation and peritonitis.

Impaired Skin Integrity

Common Related Factors
Continuous contact of bowel secretions with skin
Fungal infection

Defining Characteristics
Patient complains of burning and itching
Skin is red and tender
Skin is excoriated

Common Expected Outcomes
Patient's skin is free of irritation caused by contact with fecal output from ostomy.
Patient's skin is free of infection.

NOC Outcomes
Tissue Integrity: Skin and Mucous Membranes;
Bowel Continence
NIC Interventions
Skin Care: Topical Treatments; Ostomy Care

Ongoing Assessment

Actions/Interventions	Rationales
■ Assess peristomal skin for redness, excoriation, tenderness, vesicles, papular rashes, or drainage.	Loss of peristomal skin integrity is associated with allergies, mechanical trauma, chemical reactions, and infection. Small bowel effluent contains proteolytic enzymes. Exposure of the skin to the effluent can cause skin irritation within hours. *Candida albicans* is a common cause of peristomal skin infection.

Therapeutic Interventions

Actions/Interventions	Rationales
■ Maintain intact peristomal skin using the pouch method. • Choose appropriate pouch by evaluating skin condition (pouch adhesives will not adhere to wet or moist skin), size and shape of abdomen, presence of current or recent sutures, stoma site, and characteristics of ostomy effluent.	The pouch opening should be no more than 1/8-inch larger in diameter than the stoma. Minimal gap between pouch opening and the stoma prevents leakage of effluent onto peristomal skin.

Actions/Interventions	Rationales
• Clean and prepare skin with mild soap and water.	Skin preparation is the most important step in pouching the stoma to prevent leakage.
• Prepare pattern as a guide to customize the fit of the pouch; apply hydrocolloid skin barrier. Apply collection pouch over skin barrier according to manufacturer's directions.	A correctly fitted pouch used with a skin barrier will promote skin integrity.
• Empty the pouch when it is 1/3 to 1/2 full. Keep the pouch emptied routinely. Change the skin barrier every 3 to 4 days.	More frequent changes of the skin barrier can cause mechanical trauma to the skin. Emptying the pouch when it is 1/3 to 1/2 full reduces the risk for leakage and odor. The weight of a full pouch can pull it away from the skin barrier.

 NANDA-I NDx

Risk for Disturbed Body Image

Common Risk Factors

Presence of stoma
Loss of fecal continence
Presence of pouch
Fear of offensive odor
Fear of appearing "different"
Primary disease (after cancer)

Common Expected Outcome

Patient demonstrates enhanced body image and self-esteem, as evidenced by ability to look at, touch, talk about, and care for stoma.

NOC Outcomes
Body Image; Psychosocial Adjustment; Life Change
NIC Interventions
Ostomy Management; Body Image Enhancement

Ongoing Assessment

Actions/Interventions	Rationales
■ Assess the patient's perception of change in body structure and function.	The patient may experience a period of grief about the loss of normal bowel elimination. The patient needs to recognize feelings before they can be dealt with effectively.
■ Assess the patient's perceived impact of change.	Changes in body image can have an impact on the person's ability to carry out daily roles and responsibilities. The patient's response to real or perceived changes in body structure and/or function is related to the importance that the patient places on the structure or function (e.g., a very fastidious person may experience the visual presence of a stool-filled pouch on the anterior abdomen as intolerable).
■ Note verbal and nonverbal references to the stoma.	Negative statements about the stoma may indicate limited ability to integrate the change into the patient's self-concept. Patients often "name" stomas as an attempt to separate the stoma from themselves. Others may look away or totally deny the presence of the stoma until they are able to cope.
■ Note the patient's ability and readiness to look at, touch, and care for the stoma and ostomy equipment.	Looking at the stoma is often the first indication that the patient is ready to participate in stoma care.

■ = Independent   ▲ = Collaborative

Therapeutic Interventions

Actions/Interventions	Rationales
■ Acknowledge normalcy of emotional response to perceived change in body structure and function.	Loss of control over bowel elimination may threaten the patient's developmental level. Because control of elimination is a skill/task of early childhood and is a socially private function, loss of control precipitates body image change and possible self-concept change. The patient needs to understand that grief is a normal response.
■ Assist the patient in looking at, touching, and caring for the stoma when ready.	The patient's readiness to learn may be judged by willingness to look at the stoma and ask questions. Some patients acknowledge the stoma with minimal emotional difficulty, whereas others have a more difficult time adjusting.
■ Assist the patient in identifying specific actions that could be helpful in managing the perceived loss or problems related to the stoma.	The most common concern is odor; helping patients gain control over odor will facilitate an acceptable body image.

NANDA-I NDx

Deficient Knowledge: Stoma Care

Common Related Factors

Presence of new stoma
Lack of similar experience

Defining Characteristics

Demonstrated inability to empty and change pouch
Verbalized need for information about diet, odor, activity, hygiene, clothing, interpersonal relationships, equipment purchase, or financial concerns

Common Expected Outcome

Patient or significant other is capable of ostomy care on discharge.

NOC Outcomes
Knowledge: Treatment Regimen; Knowledge: Prescribed Diet; Knowledge: Health Resources

NIC Interventions
Ostomy Management; Teaching: Psychomotor Skill; Teaching: Prescribed Diet

Ongoing Assessment

Actions/Interventions	Rationales
■ Assess the patient's ability to empty and change the pouch.	Most patients will be independent in emptying the pouch by time of discharge; some may still need assistance with pouch change and may require outpatient follow-up care by a home care nurse.
■ Assess the patient's ability to care for peristomal skin, and identify problems.	The patient needs to be able to maintain pouch integrity to prevent fecal material from coming into contact with the skin and causing breakdown.
■ Assess patient's concerns about diet, activity, hygiene, and clothing.	The teaching plan needs to provide information to allay the patient concerns about how the presence of the stoma may affect diet, activity, hygiene, and clothing selection.

Therapeutic Interventions

Actions/Interventions	Rationales
■ Provide psychomotor teaching during first and subsequent applications of the pouch. Include at least one caregiver as approved or desired by the patient.	Even before patients are able to participate actively, they can observe and discuss ostomy care. It is beneficial to teach others alongside the patient, as long as all realize that the goal is for the patient to become independent in ostomy self-care.
■ Gradually transfer responsibility for pouch emptying and changing to the patient.	Repeated practice by the patient with positive feedback from the nurse will help the patient gain confidence in self-care ability.
■ Allow at least one opportunity for supervised return demonstration of pouch change before discharge.	Ostomy care requires both cognitive and psychomotor skills. Postoperatively, learning ability may be decreased, requiring repetition and need for return demonstrations.
■ Teach the patient about resuming activity.	The patient should understand that activity should not be altered by the presence of the stoma or pouch.
■ Teach about bathing and showering.	Normal bathing or showering is acceptable; the patient should be prepared for the possibility that small amounts of stool may pass during bathing and showering. Some patients purchase small, disposable pouches for bathing and showering; others prefer removing the pouch for bathing and showering.
■ Teach about selecting clothing.	No special clothing or alterations in existing clothing should be required by the presence of the stoma or pouch.
■ Teach the patient the following regarding diet: • *For ileostomy:* Eat a balanced diet; use special care in chewing high-fiber foods (e.g., popcorn, peanuts, coconut, vegetables, string beans, olives); increase fluid intake during hot weather or vigorous exercise. • *For colostomy:* Eat a balanced diet; no foods are specifically contraindicated; certain foods (e.g., eggs, fish, green onions, cheese, asparagus, broccoli, leafy vegetables, carbonated beverages) may increase flatus and fecal odor.	Dietary intake will influence the consistency and frequency of fecal output from the stoma. Patients need to learn individual responses to foods. The patient must understand that not eating to minimize fecal output is detrimental and that the stoma will have output regardless.
■ Discuss odor control, and acknowledge that odor (or fear of odor) can impair social functioning.	Odor control is best achieved by eliminating odor-causing foods from the diet. Green leafy vegetables, eggs, fish, and onions are primary odor-causing foods. Oral deodorants and pouch deodorants may also help. Pouch filters help muffle sounds and deodorize flatus.
■ Teach the patient to report lack of stool output from the stoma.	Absence of ostomy output may be a sign of intestinal obstruction.
■ Discuss availability of ostomy support groups (e.g., United Ostomy Association, National Foundation for Ileitis and Colitis).	Contact with other people who have ostomies increases the perception of the colostomy being manageable and enhancing the patient's sense of control.
■ Instruct the patient to maintain contact with an ET nurse.	This provides an opportunity for follow-up and problem solving.

Related Care Plan

Risk for infection, p. 114
Ineffective sexuality patterns, p. 182

■ = Independent   ▲ = Collaborative

Cholecystectomy: Laparoscopic/Open, Postoperative Care

Cholecystitis is an inflammation of the gallbladder. Most patients who develop cholecystitis have cholelithiasis or gallstones. Right upper quadrant pain that occurs after eating a high-fat meal is the most common manifestation of acute cholecystitis. Although eating a fat-free diet will decrease the patient's symptoms temporarily, surgical removal of the gallbladder and gallstones (cholecystectomy) is usually recommended. The preferred method for cholecystectomy is laparoscopic surgery using small abdominal incisions in combination with telescopic visualization of the abdominal cavity. The abdominal cavity is inflated with carbon dioxide to facilitate visualization of the abdominal organs generally and the gallbladder specifically. Once the gallbladder is dissected away from surrounding tissue, it is removed through one of the puncture wounds. The carbon dioxide is evacuated, and the multiple puncture wounds are closed. If the surgeon is not able to successfully remove the gallbladder using a laparoscopic approach, a larger open incision is made in the right upper quadrant for direct visualization and removal of the gallbladder.

 NANDA-I NDx **Risk for Infection**

Common Risk Factors

Abdominal incisions
Presence of tubes and drains

Common Expected Outcome

Patient remains free of infection, as evidenced by healing wound or incision that is free of redness, swelling, purulent discharge, and pain, and by normal body temperature within 48 hours postoperatively.

NOC Outcomes

Knowledge: Infection Control; Tissue Integrity: Skin and Mucous Membranes; Wound Healing: Primary Intention

NIC Interventions

Infection Control; Teaching: Prescribed Medication; Wound Care

Ongoing Assessment

Actions/Interventions	Rationales
■ Monitor temperature.	For the first 48 to 72 hours postoperatively, temperatures of up to 38.5° C (101.3° F) are expected as a normal stress response to surgery. Beyond 72 hours, temperature should return to the patient's baseline. Temperature spikes, usually occurring in late afternoon or at night, are often indications of infection.
■ Assess incisions for redness, drainage, swelling, and increased pain.	Incisions that have been closed with sutures or staples should be free of redness, swelling, and drainage. Some incisional discomfort is expected. These incisions are usually kept covered by a large adhesive bandage for 24 to 48 hours; beyond 48 hours, there is no need for a dressing. Laparoscopic incisions may be covered with smaller adhesive bandages.

Actions/Interventions	Rationales
■ Assess stability of tubes and drains.	If an open cholecystectomy was performed, a wound drain may be placed and removed before discharge. In-and-out motion of improperly secured tubes and drains allows access by pathogens through stab wounds where tubes and drains are placed.

Therapeutic Interventions

Actions/Interventions	Rationales
■ Wash hands before contact with the postoperative patient.	Hand washing remains the most effective method of infection control.
■ Teach use of aseptic technique during dressing change, wound care, or handling or manipulating of tubes and drains.	Aseptic technique prevents transmission of pathogens to the area.
■ Ensure that surgical tubes and drains are not inadvertently interrupted (opened). Securely tape connectors, and pin extension or drainage tubing to the patient's clothing.	Opening sterile systems allows access by pathogens and puts the patient at risk for infection. Drains may be left in place until the first return visit to the surgeon (about 7 days), if not removed at the time of discharge.
■ Instruct the patient and caregiver in administration of antibiotics and antipyretics as prescribed.	Antibiotics are necessary for the treatment of abscess and infection. Antipyretics will reduce fever and promote comfort.

Risk for Ineffective Breathing Pattern

Common Risk Factors
Right upper quadrant abdominal incision
Presence of pain

Common Expected Outcome
Patient maintains effective breathing pattern as evidenced by relaxed breathing at normal rate and depth and absence of dyspnea.

NOC Outcomes
Respiratory Status: Ventilation; Comfort Level
NIC Interventions
Respiratory Monitoring; Pain Management; Cough Enhancement

Ongoing Assessment

Actions/Interventions	Rationales
■ Assess rate, rhythm, and depth of respirations.	The right upper quadrant incision and pain may limit the patient's ability to take a deep breath. Shallow breathing puts the patient at risk for atelectasis and pneumonia.
■ Auscultate breath sounds.	The base of the lungs are least likely to be ventilated; therefore breath sounds may be diminished over the bases.
■ Observe for splinting.	Splinting refers to the conscious minimization of an inspiration to reduce the amount of discomfort caused by full expansion of the lungs.

■ = Independent   ▲ = Collaborative

Gastrointestinal and Digestive Care Plans

Actions/Interventions

- Assess ability to use incentive spirometer.

- Assess for abdominal distention.

- Assess temperature according to postoperative policy.

- Assess the amount and characteristics of sputum.

- Monitor pain level and use of analgesics.

Rationales

In incentive spirometry, the patient takes and holds a deep breath for a few seconds. Incentive spirometry encourages deep breathing, and holding the breath allows for full expansion of alveoli.

Distention can impair thoracic excursion and result in an ineffective breathing pattern.

Elevated temperature in the first 48 hours postoperatively may indicate atelectasis, which can lead to pneumonia.

Increased amounts of sputum, as well as changes in color and a thicker consistency may indicate pneumonia.

Pain inhibits the ability to cough and deep breathe and use the incentive spirometer correctly.

Therapeutic Interventions

Actions/Interventions

- Encourage deep breathing, coughing, and use of incentive spirometer every hour while the patient is awake.
- Encourage the patient to splint the incision area when coughing and deep breathing.
- ▲ Administer analgesics at regular intervals.

Rationales

Increasing deep breathing will expand the alveoli and decrease the development of atelectasis.

Providing external support to the operative site will decrease discomfort associated with increased respiratory effort.

Controlling pain will help the patient feel more comfortable with deep breathing.

NANDA-I NDx Deficient Knowledge

Common Related Factors

Lack of previous experience with laparoscopic surgery
Need for home management

Common Expected Outcome

Patient verbalizes understanding of and demonstrates ability to perform postoperative care after discharge.

Defining Characteristics

Multiple questions
Lack of questions
Inability to provide self-care on discharge

NOC Outcomes

Knowledge: Treatment Regimen; Knowledge: Prescribed Activity

NIC Interventions

Wound Care; Teaching: Prescribed Activity; Teaching: Psychomotor Skills

Ongoing Assessment

Actions/Interventions

- Assess the patient's ability to perform wound care, verbalize appropriate activity, and describe appropriate diet.
- Assess the patient's understanding of the need for close follow-up observation.

Rationales

This information is the foundation for an individualized teaching plan.

Patients who leave the hospital with sutures, staples, or drains in place need to return for removal, usually about 1 week after surgery.

Therapeutic Interventions

Actions/Interventions	Rationales

■ Teach the patient to perform appropriate wound care:
  • Abdominal incisions
 	
  • Dressings
	Staples or sutures and dressings may be present at the time of discharge.
	Dressings are usually adhesive bandages. Most bandages can be removed within one to two days following laproscopic surgery.

■ Teach the patient appropriate activity: no lifting more than 10 pounds for 6 weeks, return to work in 3 or 4 days, showering and bathing are acceptable.	Activity restrictions reduce strain on abdominal muscles and promote healing. These restrictions reduce the risk for wound dehiscence.
■ Teach the patient about eating a well-balanced, high-calorie, high-protein diet.	Such a diet promotes healing. A high-fat meal may result in diarrhea because of the reduced availability of bile for fat digestion.
■ Teach the patient that bowel function will return to preoperative baseline in 2 to 3 days.	Bowel sounds will be hypoactive initially but should return to normal within the first 2 to 3 days postoperatively. The presence of flatus or stool signals the return of peristalsis.
■ Instruct the patient to seek medical attention for any of the following: temperature higher than 38° C (100.4° F), foul-smelling wound drainage, redness or unusual pain in any incision, or absence of bowel movement.	Signs and symptoms of infection should be reported to the physician.
■ Teach the patient that minor abdominal pain and shoulder pain are expected after laparoscopic surgery and should be managed with oral analgesic agents.	During abdominal laparoscopic surgery, the peritoneal cavity is filled with carbon dioxide; this facilitates visualization of structures by the surgeon. Until the gas is completely absorbed, some discomfort is typical in the shoulder area; this referred pain is caused by irritation of the nerves by the unabsorbed carbon dioxide gas.
■ Teach the patient to empty drainage collection devices.	Drains are left in place until drainage is less than 30 mL/24 hr; this usually occurs 3 to 7 days postoperatively. Patients may be discharged with drains in place. Patients should prepare a clean surface (e.g., clean paper towels) to work on and should wash hands under running water before emptying the collection device. These measures reduce risk for infection.

Cirrhosis

Laënnec's Cirrhosis; Hepatic Encephalopathy; Ascites; Liver Failure

Cirrhosis is an inflammatory disease of the liver. The inflammatory process results in irreversible fibrosis and scarring of hepatic tissue. Worldwide the most common cause of cirrhosis is viral infection such as hepatitis B and C. Alcohol abuse is the primary cause of Laënnec's cirrhosis. Other causes include biliary obstruction, prolonged right-sided heart failure, and metabolic defects such as alpha-1 antitrypsin deficiency. The incidence of cirrhosis is highest in men between 40 and 60 years old. The development of cirrhosis occurs over many years before the person presents with characteristic symptoms. Malnutrition contributes to the development of cirrhosis in people who abuse alcohol. The disruption of hepatic function in cirrhosis can lead to the development of end-stage liver disease with ascites, portal hypertension, hepatic encephalopathy, and liver failure.

■ = Independent   ▲ = Collaborative

NANDA-I NDx

Imbalanced Nutrition: Less Than Body Requirements

Common Related Factors

Poor eating habits
Excess alcohol intake
Lack of financial means
Altered hepatic metabolic function
Inadequate bile production
Nausea, vomiting, anorexia

Defining Characteristics

Documented inadequate dietary intake
Weight loss
Muscle wasting, especially in extremities
Skin changes consistent with vitamin deficiency (flaking, loss of elasticity)
Coagulopathies
Dark urine
Pale or clay-colored stool

Common Expected Outcome

Patient achieves adequate nutrient intake, as evidenced by consumption of 3000 kcal/day and by weight gain or stabilization.

NOC Outcomes

Nutritional Status: Nutrient Intake; Knowledge: Diet

NIC Interventions

Nutrition Therapy; Nutrition Monitoring; Teaching: Prescribed Diet

Ongoing Assessment

Actions/Interventions	Rationales
■ Assess for changes in body weight and muscle mass.	Actual weight may remain steady while muscle mass deteriorates and ascitic fluid accumulates. Muscle wasting and weight loss are common in advanced cirrhosis.
■ Document intake.	A diary kept by the patient or caregiver may facilitate nutritional assessment in the home.
▲ Monitor potassium levels and albumin/protein levels.	Hypokalemia (K^+ less than 3.5 mEq/liter) is common in cirrhosis as a result of increased aldosterone levels, which increase K^+ excretion. Serum albumin/protein levels are decreased secondary to decreased hepatic production of protein and loss of protein molecules to the peritoneal space.
▲ Monitor glucose levels.	Patients with cirrhosis may be hypoglycemic, because the liver fails to perform glycolysis (breakdown of stored glycogen) and gluconeogenesis (formation of glucose from amino acids).
▲ Monitor coagulation profile.	Several coagulation factors made by the liver require adequate amounts of vitamin K. Patients with cirrhosis commonly have hypovitaminosis that is severe enough to precipitate coagulopathy.

Therapeutic Interventions

Actions/Interventions	Rationales
■ Instruct the patient in the need for a diet high in calories from carbohydrate sources. Instruct the patient to have proteins in the diet up to 75 to 100 g/day. Protein restriction is needed in the later stages of cirrhosis.	Aberrant protein metabolism in the failing liver can cause hepatic encephalopathy because ammonia, which is normally metabolized into urea (which can be excreted), passes through the damaged liver unchanged and goes on to become a cerebral toxin.
■ Suggest small, frequent meals and assistance with meals as needed.	Fatigue is a common symptom in cirrhosis that can limit energy for eating. Meals should be planned for times when the person is least fatigued.

Actions/Interventions

▲ Provide dietary or pharmacological vitamin supplementation.

▲ Provide enteral or parenteral nutritional support as ordered, using carbohydrates as the calorie source.

▲ Administer prescribed medications:
  • Acid-suppressing agents
  • Antiemetics

Rationales

If bile production is impaired, absorption of fat-soluble vitamins A, D, E, and K will be inadequate. B vitamin supplements are needed for patients with alcoholic cirrhosis.

Nutritional support is typically provided during advanced stages of cirrhosis or if bleeding complications make the gut unsuitable for enteral nutrition.

Medications alleviate gastric distress and promote increased appetite and food intake.

Excess Fluid Volume, Extravascular (Ascites)

Common Related Factors

Increased portal venous pressure
Hypoalbuminemia
Low serum oncotic pressure
Aldosterone imbalance

Defining Characteristics

Increasing abdominal girth
Ballottement
Taut abdomen, dull to percussion
Dehydration

Common Expected Outcomes

Patient experiences a decrease in ascites formation and accumulation as evidenced by decreased abdominal girth.
Patient remains hydrated.

NOC Outcomes

Fluid Balance; Knowledge: Treatment Regimen; Nutrition Status: Food and Fluid Intake

NIC Interventions

Fluid Monitoring; Fluid/Electrolyte Management

Ongoing Assessment

Actions/Interventions

■ Assess for presence of ascites:

  • Measure abdominal girth, taking care to measure at the same point consistently.

  • Check the abdomen for dullness on percussion.

▲ Monitor serum albumin, serum protein, and globulin levels.

■ Assess for signs of portal hypertension: history of upper gastrointestinal (GI) bleeding from esophageal varices, hemorrhoids, and visible superficial veins.

Rationales

Ascites is a third-spacing collection of protein-rich fluid in the peritoneal cavity. Its volume may be so severe as to impair respiratory and digestive functions, as well as mobility.

Accumulation of fluid in the peritoneal cavity results in an increased abdominal girth. Measuring changes in abdominal girth can help assess the progression of ascites.

Fluid in the peritoneal cavity will produce a dull percussion sound.

Protein molecules act as fluid "magnets" that help maintain body fluid in correct compartments; low protein level allows shift of fluid to extravascular space from vascular and interstitial spaces.

Portal hypertension is high blood pressure within the portal vein and mesenteric vascular bed, which is usually a high-flow, low-resistance vascular system. As cirrhosis progresses, normally distensible hepatic tissue is replaced by nonelastic scar tissue; blood flowing through the hepatic vasculature is subjected to higher pressures, called portal hypertension. The higher pressure in this venous system leads to distention of superficial abdominal veins. The patient may develop prominent internal hemorrhoids. Esophageal varices may develop and rupture, leading to upper gastrointestinal bleeding.

■ = Independent   ▲ = Collaborative

Actions/Interventions

- Monitor intake, urinary output, and body weight.

- Assess breathing patterns.

Rationales

Although overall intake of fluid may be adequate, shifting of fluid out of the intravascular to the extravascular spaces may result in dehydration. The risk for this occurring increases when diuretics are given. Weight gain occurs with fluid retention.

Ascites may limit excursion of the diaphragm on inspiration. The patient may hypoventilate in a supine position.

Therapeutic Interventions

Actions/Interventions

- Instruct the patient and caregiver to:
  - Restrict fluid and sodium intake as ordered.

  - Take or administer spironolactone as prescribed.

  - Take or administer diuretics cautiously.

▲ For patients unresponsive to the aforementioned measures, assist with paracentesis as needed.

- For patients with a peritoneovenous shunt (LeVeen shunt, Denver shunt):

  - Apply abdominal binder.
  - Encourage use of incentive spirometer.

Rationales

Increased aldosterone levels contribute to aggressive sodium reabsorption, which enhances accumulation of ascitic fluid.

Spironolactone, a diuretic, antagonizes aldosterone. It causes excretion of sodium and water but spares potassium.

Excess fluid is extravascular; aggressive diuresis can lead to dehydration and acute tubular necrosis or hepatorenal syndrome.

A paracentesis is a bedside procedure to remove ascitic fluid from the peritoneal cavity. A trocar catheter is inserted into the abdomen using sterile technique. The procedure is done to obtain fluid for laboratory analysis or as a temporary measure to relieve abdominal pressure. Rapid removal of ascitic fluid may be necessary to improve breathing, appetite, mobility, and comfort; reaccumulation of the fluid is common.

Although paracentesis effectively removes ascitic fluid, it also wastes protein and is only a temporary measure. Peritoneovenous shunting returns ascitic fluid to the vascular space.

Inspiring against resistance and the use of an abdominal binder increase intraperitoneal pressures, causing the valve in the shunt to open and allowing ascitic fluid to shunt into the vascular space.

NANDA-I NDx

Risk for Deficient Fluid Volume

Common Risk Factors

Overly aggressive diuresis
GI bleeding
Coagulopathies

Defining Characteristics

Decreased urine output (less than 30 mL/hr)
Concentrated urine
Hypotension/orthostasis
Tachycardia
Dry mucous membranes

Common Expected Outcome

Patient maintains normal fluid volume as evidenced by systolic blood pressure (BP) greater than or equal to 90 mm Hg (or for patient's baseline), absence of orthostasis, heart rate 60 to 100 beats/min, urine specific gravity less than 1.030, urinary output greater than 30 mL/hr, and moist mucous membranes.

NOC Outcomes
Fluid Balance; Hydration

NIC Interventions
Fluid Monitoring; Hypovolemia Management

Ongoing Assessment

Actions/Interventions	Rationales
■ Monitor blood pressure and heart rate; check for orthostatic changes.	Changes from the patient's baseline vital signs can indicate shifts in fluid balance. Decreased blood pressure and elevated heart rate may occur with decreased circulatory blood volume. Orthostatic changes in blood pressure may be an early indicator of decreasing circulatory blood volume.
■ Measure urine specific gravity, amount, and color.	Decreased fluid volume is associated with decreased urine volume, increased specific gravity, and darker urine color.
■ Check moisture of mucous membranes.	Dry mucous membranes indicate dehydration.
■ Assess for hematemesis (vomited blood), hematochezia (bright red blood per rectum), and melena (dark, tarry stool). Test any emesis, gastric aspirate, or stool for blood.	As portal hypertension worsens and possible coagulopathies develop, patients with cirrhosis are at risk for bleeding. Esophageal varices, because of the close proximity of the hepatic vasculature and the venous drainage of the esophagus, are common among cirrhotic patients.

Therapeutic Interventions

Actions/Interventions	Rationales
▲ For signs of fluid volume deficit:	
• Hold diuretics	These drugs may deplete intravascular volume.
• Administer intravenous (IV) fluids as prescribed.	IV fluids may be administered at home, or patient may require hospital admission for severe dehydration.
▲ If GI bleeding occurs, administer IV fluids, volume expanders, or blood products.	If bleeding occurs, IV fluids and volume expanders expand intravascular fluid volume and prevent complications of hypovolemia (e.g., acute tubular necrosis, shock). Transfusion with blood products may be necessary.

Risk for Disturbed Sensory Perception

Common Risk Factors

Hepatic encephalopathy
Delirium tremens
Acute alcohol intoxication
Hepatic metabolic insufficiency

Common Expected Outcome

Patient remains arousable, oriented, able to follow directions, and free from injury caused by neurosensory changes.

NOC Outcomes
Cognitive Orientation; Neurological Status
NIC Interventions
Surveillance: Safety; Medication Administration; Delusion Management

Ongoing Assessment

Actions/Interventions	Rationales
■ Monitor or instruct caregiver to monitor for the following signs and symptoms: altered attention span; inability to give accurate history; inability to follow commands; disorientation to person, place, and/or time; delusions; inappropriate behavior; self-directed or other-directed violence; and inappropriate affect.	All signs and symptoms may be caused by alcohol intoxication, delirium tremens, or hepatic encephalopathy. Hepatic encephalopathy typically occurs in end-stage disease. Accumulation of ammonia and other neurological toxins can impair thinking and neuromuscular function.

■ = Independent   ▲ = Collaborative

Actions/Interventions

▲ For patients requiring hospitalization, monitor blood alcohol level on admission. Note time since last ingestion of alcohol.

▲ Monitor blood ammonia levels.

■ Assess for signs and symptoms of hepatic encephalopathy; note stage:
- *Stage I:* mild confusion, mood changes, inability to concentrate, sleep disturbances, and mild asterixis (rapid wrist flapping or liver flap)
- *Stage II:* confusion, apathy, aberrant behavior, asterixis, and apraxia (loss of ability to carry out familiar, purposeful movements)
- *Stage III:* severe confusion, incoherence, diminished responsiveness to verbal stimuli, and hyperactive deep tendon reflexes
- *Stage IV:* no reaction to stimuli, no corneal reflex, dilated pupils, and flexion or extension posturing

Rationales

It is important to determine whether changes in level of consciousness are related to acute alcohol intoxication or to hepatic encephalopathy. Delirium tremens can occur up to 7 days after last alcohol intake.

Normally, ammonia is produced in the colon by the interaction of amino acids and colonic bacteria, metabolized by the liver, and excreted. Cirrhotic patients may lack the hepatic ability to metabolize ammonia, which accumulates and acts as a cerebral toxin.

In the early stages, hepatic encephalopathy can be reversed with early intervention. Symptoms of encephalopathy may progress slowly. The patient may fluctuate among the four stages.

Therapeutic Interventions

Actions/Interventions

▲ Protect the patient from physical harm:
- Pad side rails.
- Keep bed in low position.
- Assist patient with ambulation.
- Restrain patient if necessary.
- Administer sedatives that require nonhepatic metabolism as prescribed, document effectiveness, and notify physician if dosage needs adjustment.
- Orient patient to time, place, and person; place calendar and clock in room, provide environmental stimulation (television, radio, newspaper, visitors).
- Provide emotional support by reassuring patient and family of physiological cause of confusion.

▲ Decrease intestinal bacteria content:
- Administer nonabsorbable antibiotics (neomycin, kanamycin) as prescribed.

- Administer lactulose as prescribed.

▲ Decrease sources of dietary ammonia: order low-protein diet (0 to 40 g/day). Limit ammonia-containing foods such as gelatin, onions, and string beans.

Rationales

Impaired sensory perception increases the patient's risk for injury and falls. Physical restraints and sedatives should be used only when all other interventions prove ineffective. Overmedication may precipitate coma.

Because ammonia is produced by the interaction of the colonic bacteria and amino acids, reduction of the bacteria colonies normally present in the colon will result in reduced production of ammonia.

This laxative alters colonic pH and stimulates evacuation. An acidic pH in the colon inhibits bacteria production; evacuation of colonic contents reduces the absorption of ammonia into the bloodstream and therefore improves encephalopathic states.

Protein makes amino acids available in the colon, which in turn enhances production of ammonia.

NANDA-I NDx ## Risk for Impaired Skin Integrity (Itching)

Common Risk Factors

Jaundice
Elevated bilirubin levels

Common Expected Outcomes

Patient has intact skin.
Patient verbalizes decreased itching or ability to tolerate itching without scratching.

NOC Outcomes

Tissue Integrity: Skin and Mucous Membranes; Self-Care: Hygiene

NIC Interventions

Skin Care: Topical Treatments; Medication Administration

Ongoing Assessment

Actions/Interventions	Rationales
■ Assess for jaundice, itchiness , and scratching.	In hepatic failure bilirubin cannot be excreted, and accumulates in the skin and other tissues (sclera of the eye). Unexcreted bilirubin moves by diffusion into subcutaneous and cutaneous structures and irritates the tissue, causing histamine release and itching. Excessive scratching can lead to skin breakdown.

Therapeutic Interventions

Actions/Interventions	Rationales
■ Emphasize importance of keeping skin clean and well moisturized. • Use tepid water. • Avoid alkaline soaps. • Apply emollient lotions.	Keeping the skin clean and moisturized reduces drying that can contribute to itching.
■ Discourage scratching; keep nails short. Suggest that the patient wear hand mitts if scratching cannot be discouraged by other means.	Nails can introduce pathogens and cause localized infection. Long fingernails may cause skin trauma from repeated scratching.
■ Keep room temperature cool. Encourage patient to wear loose-fitting, soft cotton clothing.	Cotton clothing allows for evaporation of perspiration and adds to the patient's comfort.
▲ Administer antihistamines as ordered.	These medications can reduce itching.

Related Care Plans

Disturbed body image, p. 24
Ineffective coping, p. 49
Ineffective health maintenance, p. 92

■ = Independent   ▲ = Collaborative

Colorectal Cancer

Large Bowel Cancer; Rectal Cancer; Bowel Resection; Hemicolectomy; Colectomy

Colorectal cancer is the second most common cancer death in the United States. Colon cancer occurs more often than rectal cancer. Risk factors for colorectal cancer include familial polyposis, family history of colorectal cancer, and a personal history of colorectal cancer, colorectal polyps, or chronic bowel inflammatory disease. Other risk factors include physical inactivity, obesity, and a diet that is high in fat and low in fiber, smoking, and alcohol consumption. Overall, men and women are affected about equally. Early colorectal cancer often has no symptoms, which is why screening is so important. Most colorectal cancers begin as a polyp, a small growth in the wall of the colon. However, over time some polyps grow and become malignant. Signs of colorectal cancer include bleeding from the rectum, blood in the stool or in the toilet after having a bowel movement, a change in the shape of the stool, cramping pain in the lower stomach, and a feeling of discomfort or an urge to have a bowel movement when there is no need to have one. The TNM staging system indicates tumor depth, node involvement, and presence of tumor metastasis, which have been shown to be the most significant variables in determining the prognosis of colon cancer. Colorectal cancer may metastasize through direct extension to adjacent tissues or by hematological-lymphatic spread. Surgical removal is the preferred treatment for colorectal cancer, although irradiation may be used preoperatively. Postoperative chemotherapy has proven beneficial in treatment of colon cancer. Irradiation and immunotherapy are used, but with limited success. This care plan addresses the preoperative stage, care of the patient who has undergone colon resection, and self-care teaching.

Deficient Knowledge: Preoperative

Common Related Factors
New disease
Preoperative preparation

Defining Characteristics
Questions
Lack of questions
Verbalized misconceptions
Inability to participate in making treatment decisions

Common Expected Outcomes
Patient verbalizes understanding of disease process.
Patient verbalizes understanding of proposed diagnostic and surgical procedures.

NOC Outcomes
Knowledge: Disease Process; Knowledge: Treatment Procedure(s)

NIC Interventions
Teaching: Disease Process; Teaching: Preoperative; Teaching: Procedure/Treatment

Ongoing Assessment

Actions/Interventions

- Assess knowledge of common signs/symptoms of colon cancer.

Rationales

Because many colon cancers are advanced by the time of diagnosis, patients may feel guilty about not having sought treatment sooner.

Actions/Interventions

■ Assess knowledge of necessary diagnostic procedures.

■ Assess knowledge of proposed method of treatment and possible outcomes.

Rationales

The patient may have had multiple diagnostic examinations at this point and may not understand the importance of repeating procedures or undergoing further diagnostic studies. Diagnostic tests may be repeated to determine the exact size and location of tumors before surgery. Scans of distant tissues may be done to identify possible metastasis at the time of surgery.

As with other cancers, patients may feel hopeless that "nothing can be done." Patients may have previous experience with people who had cancer. This knowledge may influence the patient's attitude and anxiety about learning.

Therapeutic Interventions

Actions/Interventions

■ Teach patient the following about colon cancer:
  • Risk factors

  • Signs and symptoms

  • Method of spread and relationship to treatment

■ Teach the patient about the following diagnostic procedures, as appropriate:
  • Colonoscopy with biopsy of lesions to confirm a diagnosis

  • Carcinoembryonic antigen (CEA)

  • Chest x-ray examination

  • Computed tomography (CT) scans

  • Complete blood count (CBC)

Rationales

Family history and a personal history of colorectal cancer, colorectal polyps, or chronic inflammatory bowel disease is the greatest risk for cancer. Other risk factors include the American diet (high calorie, high fat, low fiber) and history of other cancers, especially breast cancer in women.

Because the right side of the colon is distensible, tumors on the right side are usually asymptomatic until the disease is widespread. Symptoms at that time include weight loss, anemia, weakness, and fatigue. Tumors on the left side of the colon usually result in bleeding, constipation and/or diarrhea, increased abdominal cramping, decreased caliber of the stool (i.e., pencil or ribbon shaped), a feeling of incomplete evacuation, and sometimes complete obstruction.

Colon cancer spreads by direct extension into surrounding tissue, by lymphatic channels, and by seeding into the peritoneal cavity. Excision of the tumor and surrounding tissue is the only curative treatment, although radiation therapy, chemotherapy, and immunotherapy may help reduce the tumor and check the spread. Biopsies done by colonoscopy may indicate stage of a colon tumor, although only at operation will the full extent of the disease be known.

Colonoscopy is a procedure that uses a flexible scope instrument to visualize the entire colon directly. Although a tumor may have been identified by digital examination, the entire colon should be examined before surgery; the presence of more than one tumor is possible.

CEA is a blood test that gives an indication of ongoing cancer activity. Blood is drawn preoperatively so that progress can be monitored postoperatively.

A preoperative chest x-ray study is done to evaluate the lung for evidence of metastatic disease.

CT scans are done to determine distant metastatic spread. This information helps the surgeon decide how extensive a procedure is necessary.

CBC is determined to assess for anemia. Colon tumors, particularly advanced colon tumors, bleed; bleeding may result in significant anemia, which is corrected before surgery.

■ = Independent   ▲ = Collaborative

Actions/Interventions	Rationales
• Endoscopic ultrasound	An ultrasound identifies lesions within the layers of the bowel wall and distinguishes involved lymph nodes.
■ Teach the patient about types of surgical treatment	The type of surgery will be determined by the location of the tumor and whether or not there is metastasis. Right or left hemicolectomy (removal of the right or left half of the colon or large intestine) is done to remove tumors of the ascending, transverse, descending, and sigmoid colon. Tumors that are too close to the anus are treated with abdominoperineal resection (resection of a portion of the colon, along with the rectum); this procedure results in a permanent colostomy because the rectum is gone. Tumors that are in the lower rectosigmoid colon or in the rectum may be treated with a low anterior resection, in which the tumor and surrounding colon are removed and the colon is then anastomosed (no colostomy).
■ Teach the patient about steps taken to prepare the bowel for surgery:	
• Clear liquid diet	This diet reduces the residue in the bowel.
• Antibiotics	These drugs are not absorbed from the intestine and therefore reduce bacteria normally present in the colon to prevent postoperative peritonitis.
• Colyte, GoLYTELY, and/or other osmotic agents	These laxatives induce diarrhea and clean bowel before surgery; these may also be used before colonoscopy.
■ Prepare the patient for what to expect after surgery:	
• Incisions, drains	After colectomy, most patients have one midline incision. Patients who have had an abdominoperineal resection have an anterior midline incision, a perineal incision where the rectum was removed, and a colostomy. Anterior incisions are typically sutured or stapled closed; perineal incisions may be closed or may be packed and left to heal by secondary intention. All patients have small drains in the lower abdomen to drain lymphatic fluid from the operative area.
• Intravenous (IV) lines	Patients resume oral feedings when peristalsis resumes; therefore administration of IV fluids is necessary and continues until the patient can tolerate oral fluids.
• Activity	Patients should expect to get out of bed on the first postoperative day to prevent complications of immobility (e.g., deep vein thrombosis, atelectasis).
• Pain management	Patients should be involved in choice of postoperative pain management. Options include traditional intramuscular medications given as needed, medications given via intravenous patient-controlled analgesia, or bolus or continuous-infusion epidural analgesics.
• Thromboembolism precaution	Patients undergoing colon resection for cancer have a high incidence of venous thromboembolism, including deep vein thrombosis and pulmonary embolism. There is strong evidence that the use of low-molecular-weight heparin (e.g., Lovenox) reduces the risk. Intermittent pneumatic calf compression has been shown to be effective in reducing the risk for thromboembolism. Whether there is an additive effect by using more than one mode of prophylaxis for patients undergoing colonic resection is yet to be determined.

Altered Bowel Elimination: Postoperative Ileus

Common Related Factors

General anesthesia
Manipulation of bowel during surgery

Defining Characteristics

Abdomen silent on auscultation
No stooling or flatus
Report of bloated feeling
Nausea
Abdominal distention

Common Expected Outcome

Patient passes flatus and stool 48 to 72 hours postoperatively.

NOC Outcome
Bowel Elimination

NIC Interventions
Flatulence Reduction; Bowel Management

Ongoing Assessment

Actions/Interventions

■ Assess for bowel sounds, abdominal distention, presence of flatus or stool, and nausea.

Rationales

Bowel sounds will be hypoactive initially, but should return to normal 48 to 72 hours after surgery. The presence of flatus or stool indicates the return of peristalsis. The absence of bowel sounds, flatus, and stool with abdominal distention may indicate a postoperative paralytic ileus. Nausea may occur as a result of accumulation of intestinal content.

Therapeutic Interventions

Actions/Interventions

■ Maintain NPO (nothing by mouth) status until bowel sounds return and patient begins to pass flatus. Fluids will be administered intravenously.
■ Ensure patency of nasogastric tube, and provide good oral care.
■ Encourage and assist with ambulation beginning the first postoperative day.
■ Assist the patient with initial food and fluid selection.

Rationales

Until peristaltic activity returns, oral intake puts the patient at risk for nausea and vomiting.

Keeping the stomach empty reduces the risk for nausea, vomiting, and aspiration.
Increasing ambulation hastens resolution of ileus by stimulating peristalsis.
Low-fiber foods and easily digestible foods produce less gas and distention.

 Risk for Infection

NANDA-I

Common Risk Factors

Length of procedure
Intraoperative leakage of bowel contents
Insertion of circular staple gun through rectum to abdominal cavity
Postoperative wound contamination

■ = Independent ▲ = Collaborative

Common Expected Outcome

Patient remains free of infection as evidenced by temperature less than 38.5° C (101.3° F) and by a clean, dry, healing wound.

NOC Outcomes
Risk Control; Wound Healing: Primary Intention
NIC Interventions
Infection Control; Wound Care

Ongoing Assessment

Actions/Interventions	Rationales
■ Assess length of surgical procedure.	The longer the patient is in surgery, the greater the risk for postoperative infection.
■ Assess wound for redness, warmth, drainage, pain, swelling, or dehiscence.	These assessment findings are signs of wound infection.
▲ Obtain culture of suspicious drainage.	Normal drainage is clear, yellow, and odorless. Identification of infecting microorganisms is necessary to select appropriate antibiotic therapy.
■ Monitor temperature.	Temperature above 38.5° C (101.3° F) should arouse suspicion of infection.
▲ Monitor white blood cell (WBC) count.	An elevated WBC count is an indication of infection.

Therapeutic Interventions

Actions/Interventions	Rationales
■ Wash hands on entering room.	Hand washing remains the most effective means of infection control.
■ Use aseptic technique for dressing changes.	Aseptic technique prevents transmission of bacterial infections to the surgical wound.
▲ Administer antibiotics and antipyretics as prescribed.	These drugs treat infections and the fever associated with infections.
■ If stoma is present, maintain good skin seal.	While many patients will have a colon resection with end-to-end anastomosis, some patients may have extensive removal of large intestine that requires creation of a colostomy. A minimal gap between the stoma and collection pouch opening contains fecal drainage and prevents possible contamination of the incision.

NANDA-I NDx Deficient Knowledge: Postoperative

Common Related Factors
Lack of previous experience with colon surgery
Need for home management
Need for long-term follow-up care

Defining Characteristics
Multiple questions
Lack of questions
Inability to provide self-care on discharge

Common Expected Outcome
Patient or caregiver verbalizes knowledge and demonstrates ability to perform wound care, select appropriate diet, plan activity, report complications, and receive necessary follow-up care.

NOC Outcomes
Knowledge: Diet; Knowledge: Disease Process; Knowledge: Treatment Regimen
NIC Interventions
Teaching: Disease Process; Teaching: Psychomotor Skill; Teaching: Prescribed Activity/Exercise; Teaching: Prescribed Diet

Ongoing Assessment

Actions/Interventions	Rationales
■ Assess ability to perform wound care, verbalize appropriate activity, and describe appropriate diet.	Adults learn best when they are active participants. Active participation also facilitates changes needed to allow for discharge.
■ Assess understanding of expected bowel function.	Patient should understand that usual bowel pattern might not return until 2 to 3 weeks postoperatively.
■ Assess understanding of need for further cancer therapy close follow-up care.	Patients who have abdominal surgery for malignancies may require further therapy such as chemotherapy, irradiation, or immunotherapy. Ongoing surveillance is needed to detect recurrence of cancer.

Therapeutic Interventions

Actions/Interventions	Rationales
■ Teach patient or caregiver to perform appropriate wound care:	
• Anterior abdominal wound	Staples or sutures and dressings usually have been removed by the time of discharge, and Steri-Strips have been placed to maintain wound approximation. Steri-Strips should be left in place until they fall off.
• Perineal wound	The patient can take sitz baths twice daily for cleansing and comfort, after which the wound is repacked with saline solution–moistened gauze. Usually clean technique (hands washed; clean but not sterile gloves) is used.
■ If patient has a colostomy:	
• Teach patient or caregiver how to apply skin barrier around stoma.	This barrier promotes peristomal skin integrity and prevents irritation of skin from fecal output.
• Inform patient or caregiver that the barrier can remain on the skin for 3 to 4 days. It should be removed after the fourth day, and the skin around the stoma should be inspected.	Skin infections, irritation, and allergic reactions to barrier material can occur around the stoma.
• Clean the skin with warm water and mild soap. Dry the skin completely before applying a new barrier.	These measures promote skin integrity and reduce infection.
• Apply a clean collection bag (appliance) and empty the bag when it is about half full of stool.	Emptying the bag before it gets too full reduces the risk for leakage of fecal material and odor.
• Note amount, color, and consistency of stool.	Changes in the diet and infections can produce changes in the fecal output from the stoma.
• If there is no stool from the colostomy, check stoma with a gloved, lubricated finger. If there is still no stool or flatus, notify the physician.	An absence of colostomy output may be a sign of intestinal obstruction.
■ Teach the patient that bowel function may not return to preoperative baseline for several weeks.	The more colon that is resected, the longer the period of adaptation. During this time stool may be loose and stooling more frequent.
■ Teach patient appropriate activity guidelines:	
• No lifting more than 10 pounds for 6 weeks	This activity restriction reduces strain on abdominal muscles and the risk for stoma prolapse.
• Mild exercise (e.g., walking)	Exercise increases stamina and prevents deep vein thrombosis and pneumonia.
• Showering	The patient can usually shower once the incisions have healed.
• Bathing unless open perineal wound exists	It may take up to 8 weeks to heal completely. Using a hand-held shower head is a good way to clean the wound.
• No driving until anterior abdominal wound has healed	Operating foot pedals while driving, especially the brake pedal, increases strain on abdominal muscles.

■ = Independent   ▲ = Collaborative

Actions/Interventions	Rationales
■ Teach the patient the following about diet:	
• A well-balanced, high-calorie, high-protein diet.	This type of diet should continue over a period of weeks to promote effective healing.
• Fiber should be added to the diet.	Because the patient has already had colon cancer, the risk for future tumors is high. A high-fiber diet is associated with more frequent bowel movements and less time for suspected carcinogenic food by-products to be in contact with the colonic mucosa. Foods high in fiber include grains, fruits, and vegetables.
■ Teach the patient the rationale for any further cancer therapy planned (e.g., chemotherapy, radiation therapy, immunotherapy).	These therapies are typically offered if the pathology report indicates that the tumor was not confined to the bowel or bowel wall.
■ Teach the patient the importance of follow-up colonoscopies.	These procedures allow early detection of any recurrent tumors. They are usually scheduled every 6 months for persons with a history of colon cancer.
■ Discuss family risk with patients.	Parents, siblings, and adult children older than 40 years should be screened yearly for colon cancer.
■ Teach patients who have had removal of the rectum that phantom rectum sensations and a feeling of needing to have a normal bowel movement are normal and will subside over time.	These situations are related to remaining nerve fibers in the perineum.
■ Instruct the patient to seek medical attention for any of the following: temperature higher than 38° C (100.4° F), foul-smelling wound drainage, redness or unusual pain in any incision, or absence of bowel movement.	These signs and symptoms are indicative of an infection or possible bowel obstruction.

Related Care Plans

Acute pain, p. 151
Grieving, p. 82
Ineffective coping, p. 49
Bowel diversion surgery, p. 561

Enteral Tube Feeding

Enteral Hyperalimentation; G-Tube; Jejunostomy; Duodenostomy; PEG Tube; Dobhoff Tube

Enteral tube feedings provide nutrition using a nasogastric tube, a gastrostomy tube, or a tube placed in the duodenum or jejunum. Tubes may be inserted through the external nares or may be placed through a small incision into the stomach or small intestine. Enteral tube feedings are indicated for patients who have a functional gastrointestinal system but are unable to maintain adequate nutritional intake orally. Enteral tube feedings can be more cost effective than total parenteral nutrition (TPN). Critically ill patients receiving enteral tube feedings tend to have better outcomes and fewer complications. The problems associated with the administration of enteral tube feedings include pulmonary aspiration of feeding formula, diarrhea, and fluid and electrolyte imbalances. Feedings may be continuous or intermittent (bolus). Enteral feeding may occur in the hospital, in long-term care, or in home care. The focus of this care plan is the prevention and management of problems commonly associated with enteral feeding.

Imbalanced Nutrition: Less Than Body Requirements

Common Related Factor

Mechanical problems during feedings, such as clogged tube, inaccurate flow rate, stiffening of tube, delivery pump malfunction

Common Expected Outcome

Patient's nutritional status improves, as evidenced by gradual weight gain or stable weight and increased physical strength.

Defining Characteristics

Continued weight loss
Failure to gain weight
Weakness

NOC Outcomes

Nutritional Status: Nutrient Intake; Weight Control

NIC Interventions

Nutritional Monitoring; Enteral Tube Feeding; Gastrointestinal Intubation

Ongoing Assessment

Actions/Interventions	Rationales
■ Assess tubing for patency and free flow of enteral feeding.	A clogged feeding tube decreases the delivery of nutrients.
■ Assess equipment (pump) used for administration; ensure that proper flow rate is indicated and that pump is delivering enteral feeding at appropriate rate.	A feeding pump regulates formula delivery at a continuous rate. This method causes less diarrhea than with intermittent feedings.
■ Assess weight every other day or as ordered.	Weight gain is an indicator of improved nutritional status; however, sudden gain of more than 2 pounds in a 24-hour period usually indicates fluid retention. Most commercially available tube-feeding preparations contain 1 kcal/mL. An adult of average size and weight requires 1800 to 2400 kcal/24 hours.
■ Assess physical strength of patient; note improvement or deterioration.	Improved muscle strength and activity tolerance are indicators of sufficient calories.

Therapeutic Interventions

Actions/Interventions	Rationales
■ Instruct caregiver to:	
• Flush tubing with 20 mL of water after medication administration and any time the flow of solution is interrupted.	Flushing the tube is important to reduce the risk for clogging. Clogging of a feeding tube may require replacement of the tube. Any delay in the administration of the feeding formula decreases the patient's nutrient intake.
• Crush medications, and dilute with water.	Whenever possible, liquid forms of medication should be administered through a feeding tube to reduce the risk for clogging. Pills should be crushed to the finest consistency possible and mixed with water before being administered through the feeding tube.
• Keep pump alarms on.	Any interruption in the flow of solution is noted early when alarms sound.
■ In case flow is interrupted for more than 1 hour, instruct the caregiver how to recalculate amount to be given over 8 hours and reset the administration rate.	Rapid administration to "catch up" can precipitate a hyperglycemic crisis because the pancreas may not be able to produce adequate insulin for the increased carbohydrate load. The risk for diarrhea also increases when the rate is suddenly increased.

■ = Independent   ▲ = Collaborative

Actions/Interventions

▲ Consult dietitian.

Rationales

The dietitian ensures that ongoing nutritional needs are being met as the patient's condition or situation changes. The dietitian will calculate the patient's caloric and nutrient needs. Using this information, the dietitian provides guidance in selection of the appropriate feeding formulas and any additional nutrient supplements.

 Risk for Aspiration

Common Risk Factors

Depressed or lack of gag reflex
Poor positioning of tube at placement
Migration of the tube
Supine positioning of patient as feeding is administered
Increased gastric residual volume
Delayed gastric emptying

Common Expected Outcome

Patient maintains a patent airway, as evidenced by normal breath sounds, absence of coughing, no shortness of breath, and no aspiration.

NOC Outcomes
Aspiration Control; Respiratory Status: Ventilation
NIC Interventions
Aspiration Precautions; Enteral Tube Feeding; Respiratory Monitoring

Ongoing Assessment

Actions/Interventions

▲ Obtain an x-ray study immediately after tube insertion.

■ Assess correct position of tube before initiation of feeding by aspirating fluid from the tube and checking the color and pH of the fluid.

■ Assess level of consciousness (LOC) and gag reflex before administration of feeding.

■ Assess pulmonary status for clinical evidence of aspiration. Auscultate breath sounds for development of crackles and/or wheezes. Monitor chest x-ray results as ordered.

Rationales

Radiological confirmation of the feeding tube position should be obtained after placement of a nasoenteral tube.

pH readings of 0 to 5 usually indicate gastric placement of the tube. The color of the gastric fluid varies from off-white to grassy green or brown. Intestinal fluid is golden yellow to brownish green and has a pH of 6 or higher. A pH of 6 or higher in watery yellow fluid may indicate respiratory placement of the tube. This assessment is especially important for gastrostomy tubes because the potential for reflux is increased; duodenostomy and jejunostomy tubes carry somewhat less risk. Also, smaller-diameter, more flexible feeding tubes can easily enter the trachea during insertion.

A decreased level of consciousness is a prime risk factor for aspiration. High-risk patients are comatose, have decreased gag reflex, or cannot tolerate the head of bed (HOB) elevated. Nasoduodenal or gastroduodenal feeding tubes are preferred for high-risk patients.

Aspiration of small amounts of feeding can occur without coughing or sudden onset of respiratory distress, especially in patients with a decreased LOC. Pulmonary infiltrates on chest x-ray results indicate some level of aspiration has occurred. Coughing and shortness of breath may indicate aspiration.

Actions/Interventions

■ Assess for residual volume before feeding. If the patient is on continuous feedings, check residual every 4 hours.

■ Auscultate bowel sounds to evaluate bowel motility, and assess for abdominal distention and firmness.

Rationales

Feedings are held if residual volume is greater than 50% of the amount to be delivered in 1 hour. Gastric residuals should be checked frequently when feedings are initiated, and feedings should be held if residual volumes exceed 200 mL.

Decreased gastrointestinal motility increases the risk for aspiration because feeding formula accumulates in the stomach. When combined with a decreased LOC or diminished gag reflex, aspiration is a higher risk.

Therapeutic Interventions

Actions/Interventions

■ Elevate HOB to 30 degrees during and for 1 hour after each feeding.
■ If the patient has an endotracheal or tracheostomy tube, keep the cuff inflated during feedings and for 1 hour after feedings.
■ In case of aspiration:
  • Stop the feeding.
  • Keep the HOB elevated.
  • Suction airway as necessary.
  • Document time feeding was stopped, patient's appearance, and change in respiratory status.
  • Document adventitious breath sounds.

Rationales

This position facilitates gravity flow of feeding past the gastroduodenal sphincter and reduces the risk for aspiration.

This measure protects the airway from inadvertent entry of feedings into the trachea.

Respiratory aspiration requires immediate action by the caregiver to maintain the airway and promote effective breathing and gas exchange. Tracheal suctioning may be necessary to maintain airway patency.

NANDA-I
NDx **Risk for Diarrhea**

Common Risk Factor
Intolerance to tube feeding

Common Expected Outcome
Patient does not experience diarrhea during tube feedings.

NOC Outcomes
Bowel Elimination; Symptom Control
NIC Intervention
Diarrhea Management; Enteral Tube Feeding

Ongoing Assessment

Actions/Interventions

■ Assess bowel sounds, and for abdominal distention or cramping.
■ Assess number and character of stools.

■ Monitor intake and output. Measure volume of liquid or watery stools.

Rationales

Diarrhea is typically accompanied by hyperactive bowel sounds.

A patient diary can be useful for gathering data. Many factors contribute to the development of diarrhea in tube-fed patients. Sorbitol-based elixirs for liquid forms of medications may increase the incidence of diarrhea. *Clostridium difficile* has been found to occur more often in tube-fed hospitalized patients than in non–tube-fed patients.

Diarrhea can lead to profound dehydration.

■ = Independent   ▲ = Collaborative

Actions/Interventions	Rationales
■ Note osmolarity and fiber content of the feeding.	Hyperosmolar or high-fiber feedings draw fluid into the bowel and can cause diarrhea. Isotonic feedings are preferred.
■ Note history of lactose intolerance.	Milk-based feedings contain lactose, which is not tolerated by individuals with lactase deficiency.

Therapeutic Interventions

Actions/Interventions	Rationales
■ Begin feedings slowly; consider a dilute solution.	Large amounts of concentrated solutions may stimulate osmotic diarrhea. Gradual increase in rate will allow time for the gastrointestinal system to adapt to the increased volume and solutes.
■ Instruct the caregiver to increase both rate and strength to prescribed amounts, but not at the same time.	High-rate feeding combined with high osmolality may precipitate diarrhea.
■ Administer feedings at room temperature.	Cold stimulates peristalsis.
■ Do not allow formula to hang longer than 8 hours at room temperature.	The risk for bacterial contamination increases the longer a feeding formula remains at room temperature in the feeding delivery system.
■ Change feeding setup daily.	Use of a clean feeding delivery bag and tubing minimizes risk for bacterial contamination.

NANDA-I NDx Deficient Knowledge

Common Related Factor

New procedure and treatment

Common Expected Outcomes

Patient or caregiver verbalizes reasons for tube feedings and begins to participate in care.

Patient or caregiver demonstrates independence in enteral feeding administration.

Defining Characteristics

Verbalized inaccurate information

Inappropriate behavior

Questions

NOC Outcome

Knowledge: Treatment Procedure(s)

NIC Interventions

Teaching: Psychomotor Skill; Teaching: Procedure/Treatment

Ongoing Assessment

Actions/Interventions	Rationales
■ Assess patient's or caregiver's knowledge of: • Tube feeding purpose, expected length of therapy, and expected benefits. • Ability to administer own feedings. • Ability to use equipment related to feeding: measuring devices, feeding pump, and tubing. • Ability to minimize complications related to tube feedings: checking for residual volume, assuming sitting position, and maintaining a bacteria-free feeding.	Many patients require feedings well beyond hospitalization and can administer feedings to self. Teaching the patient and caregiver is based on their knowledge and ability to manage the equipment and minimize complications. Assessment of their understanding is the foundation for an individualized teaching plan.

Therapeutic Interventions

Actions/Interventions	Rationales
■ Demonstrate feedings and tube care. Allow return demonstration.	Supervised practice allows the patient and caregiver to use new information and skills immediately and enhances retention. Repeated practice helps the patient and caregiver gain confidence in their ability to manage the enteral feedings. Necessary alteration in teaching plan can be undertaken.
■ Arrange for home care nurse if the patient is unable to feed self.	Community resources provide support for the patient and caregiver as they learn new skills.

Related Care Plans

Risk for aspiration, p. 21
Diarrhea, p. 54
Deficient fluid volume, p. 72
Impaired oral mucous membrane, p. 148

Gastrointestinal Bleeding

Lower Gastrointestinal Bleed; Upper Gastrointestinal Bleed; Esophageal Varices; Ulcers

Loss of blood from the gastrointestinal (GI) tract is most often the result of erosion or ulceration of the mucosa, but it may also be the result of arteriovenous (AV) malformation or malignancies, increased pressure in the portal venous bed, or direct trauma to the GI tract. Alcohol abuse is a major etiological factor in GI bleeding. Varices, usually located in the distal third of the submucosal tissue of the esophagus or the fundus of the stomach, can also cause life-threatening GI hemorrhage. Upper GI bleeding may manifest as blood tinged, bright red, or coffee ground emesis. The patient with upper GI bleeding may also experience dark, tarry stools. Lower GI bleeding may occur as bright red blood from the rectum. This type of bleeding is often associated with the presence of hemorrhoids. Tumors of the colon may cause bleeding detected as occult blood in the feces rather than visible bleeding. Inflammatory bowel disease may cause lower GI bleeding characterized as bloody diarrhea. Factors that alter coagulation or cause generalized inflammation of the intestinal mucosa can contribute to bleeding anywhere in the GI tract. Treatment may be medical or surgical or may involve mechanical tamponade. Acute GI bleeding may be life threatening without prompt treatment. In patients with GI bleeding, stabilization of blood pressure and restoration of intravascular volume is the highest priority. The focus of this care plan is the acute hospital management phase of a patient with active GI bleeding.

NANDA-I NDx Deficient Fluid Volume

Common Related Factors	Defining Characteristics
Upper GI bleeding (mouth, esophagus, stomach, duodenum) caused by gastric ulcer, duodenal ulcer, gastritis, esophageal varices, Mallory-Weiss tear, blunt or penetration trauma, cancer Lower GI bleeding (small or large intestine, rectum, anus) caused by tumors, inflammatory bowel disease (diverticular disease, Crohn's disease, ulcerative colitis), AV malformations, blunt or penetrating trauma, hemorrhoids	Hematemesis (observed or reported) Melena Hematochezia (bright red blood per rectum) Coffee ground emesis (indicates slower upper GI bleed) Orthostatic changes Tachycardia Hypotension Change in level of consciousness (LOC)

■ = Independent   ▲ = Collaborative

Generalized GI bleeding: systemic coagulopathies; radiation therapy; chemotherapy; family history of GI bleeding; history of recent violent retching; history of alcohol use or abuse; altered coagulation profile; history of aspirin, anticoagulant therapy, steroid, nonsteroid, or ibuprofen use or abuse

Thirst
Dry mucous membranes
Weakness
Pallor

Common Expected Outcome

Patient is normovolemic as evidenced by no signs of active bleeding, systolic blood pressure (BP) greater than 90 mm Hg (or patient's baseline), absence of orthostasis, heart rate 60 to 100 beats/min, urine output greater than 30 mL/hr, and normal skin tugor and mucous membranes.

NOC Outcomes
Blood Coagulation; Fluid Balance
NIC Interventions
Bleeding Reduction: Gastrointestinal; Fluid Monitoring; Fluid Management; Fluid Resuscitation

Ongoing Assessment

Actions/Interventions	Rationales
■ Monitor color, amount, and consistency of hematemesis, melena, or rectal bleeding; encourage patient to describe unwitnessed blood loss accurately using common household measures (e.g., a cupful, a spoonful, a pint).	Careful assessment of GI bleeding can help determine the exact site of the bleeding.
■ Obtain history of use or abuse of substances known to predispose to GI bleeding: aspirin, aspirin-containing drugs, nonsteroidal antiinflammatory drugs, alcohol, steroids.	Drugs that cause ulceration of the GI mucosa contribute to the development of bleeding.
■ Monitor BP for orthostatic changes (from patient lying prone to high-Fowler's).	A drop in BP greater than 10 mm Hg indicates that circulating blood volume is decreased by 20%. A drop in BP greater than 20 to 30 mm Hg indicates that circulating blood volume is decreased by 40%.
■ Assess for tachycardia.	An increase in pulse rate indicates hypovolemia. This change in pulse is a compensatory mechanism to maintain cardiac output.
▲ Monitor coagulation profile, hemoglobin (Hgb), and hematocrit (Hct).	Many individuals with GI bleeding have longstanding nutritional deficits that result in an altered coagulation profile because of the liver's inability to produce adequate amounts of vitamin K, a precursor to many coagulation factors. Hgb and Hct are monitored as indicators of both blood loss and hydration status. Initially, Hgb and Hct will drop because of blood loss; as fluid resuscitation proceeds, hemodilution will result in further drop in Hgb and Hct.
■ Obtain diet history.	A history of inadequate or sporadically adequate nutrition is important in understanding hemopoietic capability.
■ Monitor urine output.	Urine output of at least 30 mL/hr is an indication of adequate renal perfusion.

Therapeutic Interventions

Actions/Interventions	Rationales
▲ For active bleeding, start one or more large-bore intravenous (IV) lines.	Rapid volume expansion is necessary to prevent or treat hypovolemia complications; IV medication and/or blood component administration is likely.
▲ Provide volume resuscitation with crystalloids or blood products as ordered.	Crystalloids are more commonly used, whereas blood products are selectively used to replace specific coagulation factors (e.g., platelets only, fresh-frozen plasma).

Actions/Interventions

- Monitor cardiopulmonary response to volume expansion.

▲ Insert nasogastric (NG) tube for stomach lavage. Lavage stomach until clots are no longer present and return is clear; use room-temperature saline solution.

▲ Assist with or coordinate diagnostic procedures performed to identify bleeding site:
  - Endoscopy

  - Sigmoidoscopy, proctoscopy, and colonoscopy

  - Barium studies:
    - Barium swallow

    - Barium enema
  - Small bowel follow-through

  - Angiography
    - After angiography: dress the site with pressure dressing; connect arterial line to pressure or flush system.

▲ Administer vasopressin drip as ordered. May be given IV continuous drip, piggyback bolus, or intraarterially if a line was placed during an angiographic procedure to a specific area (e.g., celiac artery for esophageal bleeding).
- Monitor for side effects of vasopressin.

▲ Administer vitamin K as ordered.
▲ Administer antacids and H2-receptor antagonists (e.g., cimetidine, Zantac).
- Guard against administration of drugs that may potentiate further bleeding, such as aspirin-containing compounds and anticoagulants.
▲ For the patient who is bleeding from esophageal or gastric varices and who is in a critical care area, prepare for insertion of a Sengstaken-Blakemore tube.

▲ Assist with preparation of the patient for surgical procedures such as sclerotherapy, endoscopic varicose ligation, or thermal coagulation.

Rationales

Amount of fluid administered will depend on rate of bleeding and patient's hemodynamic status. Patients with history of alcohol abuse may have alcohol-related cardiomyopathies. Elderly patients may experience cardiovascular difficulty with rapid fluid volume resuscitation because of diminished cardiac function, a normal phenomenon of aging.

The NG tube provides a way to monitor continuing blood loss closely and for medication administration. Iced saline solution may cause undesirable ischemic changes in gastric mucosa.

This procedure provides direct visualization of the esophagus, stomach, and duodenum. The procedure must precede x-ray films requiring barium ingestion to maximize visualization by the endoscopist.
These procedures provide direct visualization of the rectum and colon.

This x-ray procedure is an indirect visualization of the esophagus, stomach, and small intestine.
This x-ray procedure is an indirect visualization of colon.
This x-ray procedure is an indirect visualization of the small intestine.
This procedure may be diagnostic or performed for arterial line placement to infuse vasoconstrictive medications locally. Conclusive diagnosis is made only if bleeding is more than 0.5 mL/min.
Vasopressin is a commercial preparation of antidiuretic hormone that promotes vasoconstriction and reduces bleeding.

Side effects of vasopressin may include anginal pain, ST-segment changes on electrocardiogram, sinus bradycardia, tremors, sweating, vertigo, pounding in head, abdominal cramps, circumoral pallor, nausea and vomiting, flatus, urticaria, and fluid retention. Elevated BP can be the result of vasoconstriction from vasopressin.
This drug allows coagulation factor production.
These drugs suppress gastric and duodenal secretions.

Drugs that interfere with the coagulation mechanisms increase the risk for bleeding.

The Sengstaken-Blakemore tube has balloons that inflate in the esophagus and upper portion of the stomach to provide tamponade (pressure) against the vessels that are bleeding.
If esophageal varices are the source of the bleeding, surgical measures may be used to control the bleeding.

■ = Independent   ▲ = Collaborative

Deficient Knowledge

Common Related Factors

First GI bleed
Unfamiliar environment

Defining Characteristics

Multiple questions
Lack of questions
Verbalized misconceptions

Common Expected Outcome

Patient or significant other verbalizes understanding of causes and management of GI bleeding.

NOC Outcomes

Knowledge: Treatment Regimen; Knowledge: Treatment Procedures

NIC Interventions

Teaching: Procedures/Treatment; Teaching: Prescribed Medication; Substance Use Treatment

Ongoing Assessment

Actions/Interventions	Rationales
■ Assess understanding of the cause and treatment of GI bleeding.	A teaching plan is based on the patient's previous knowledge.
■ Assess understanding of the need for long-term follow-up, and possible lifestyle changes.	Prevention of recurrence of bleeding may require health behavior changes by the patient.

Therapeutic Interventions

Actions/Interventions	Rationales
■ Explain procedures necessary for diagnosis and/or treatment before they are performed.	Understanding the need for unpleasant procedures may help the patient comply or participate in and increase the effectiveness of treatment or procedure.
■ Explain the importance of avoidance of substances containing aspirin, alcohol, nonsteroidal antiinflammatory drugs, ibuprofen, and steroids.	Use of these products is known to damage the mucosal barrier and predispose to bleeding.
■ Teach the patient the dose, administration schedule, expected actions, and possible adverse effects of medications that may be prescribed for long periods.	Drugs given to decrease gastric acid production may be prescribed indefinitely; patients must understand that cessation of bleeding or other symptoms does not mean the need for medication has ended.
▲ Refer the patient to alcohol rehabilitation if indicated.	The patient may benefit from a formal treatment program to control alcohol use and prevent future bleeding episodes.

Related Care Plans

Diarrhea, p. 54
Fear, p. 69
Ineffective therapeutic regimen management, p. 194
Risk for impaired skin integrity, p. 185

Hepatitis

Serum Hepatitis; Infectious Hepatitis; Viral Hepatitis

Hepatitis is inflammation of the liver, usually caused by a virus. Hepatitis may also result from adverse drug reactions or other chemical ingestion. Hepatitis may develop in response to viral infections with rubella, varicella, Epstein-Barr, cytomegalovirus, and herpes simplex virus. Viral hepatitis types A and E are transmitted via the fecal-oral route or through poor sanitation; person-to-person contact; or consumption of contaminated food, water, or shellfish. Hepatitis E infections are associated with contaminated water and occur most commonly in developing countries. Cases of hepatitis E in the United States are seen in patients who have traveled to areas that are endemic for the virus. There is no specific treatment for this form of hepatitis, and immune globulin is not useful in prophylaxis after exposure. Types B and C (formerly called non-A, non-B) are transmitted by blood, semen, and vaginal secretions. They can be transmitted via contaminated needles and renal dialysis (parenterally) or through intimate contact with carriers. Hepatitis B and C may progress to a chronic active form of the disease. As a result, the patient is at risk for liver failure that may require liver transplantation. Hepatitis D occurs only in the presence of hepatitis B. Hepatitis D develops as a co-infection or superimposed infection with hepatitis B. A co-infection with hepatitis D tends to increase the severity of the hepatitis B infection. Vaccine for the prevention of hepatitis B is widely available. The Occupational Safety and Health Administration (OSHA) requires that employers offer the hepatitis B vaccine to health care workers who are at risk for all types of hepatitis. A vaccine is also available for hepatitis A, although its use is not as widespread as hepatitis B vaccine. Some cases of hepatitis remain subclinical, and most are managed in the home. Fulminant hepatitis can result in massive destruction of liver tissue and can be fatal. This care plan addresses nursing concerns that may be managed in the hospital or at home.

NDx   Deficient Knowledge

Common Related Factors

New condition
Unfamiliarity with disease course and treatment

Defining Characteristics

Lack of questions
Many questions
Noncompliance with infection control procedures

Common Expected Outcome

Patient or caregiver verbalizes and demonstrates knowledge of and compliance with treatment regimen and infection control procedures.

NOC Outcomes
Knowledge: Disease Process; Knowledge: Treatment Regimen
NIC Interventions
Teaching: Disease Process; Teaching: Procedures/Treatment

Ongoing Assessment

Actions/Interventions

- Determine the patient's understanding of the disease process, disease transmission, complications, treatment, and signs of relapse.

Rationales

An individualized teaching program is based on the patient's previous knowledge of hepatitis and its transmission and treatment. Noncompliance may be related to incomplete understanding of disease transmission and/or the treatment regimen.

■ = Independent   ▲ = Collaborative

Gastrointestinal and Digestive Care Plans

Therapeutic Interventions

Actions/Interventions	Rationales
■ Teach the patient or caregiver about disease transmission:	
• Hepatitis A	Fecal-oral transmission occurs as a result of crowded living conditions; poor personal hygiene; contaminated food, water, milk, or raw shellfish.
• Hepatitis B	Percutaneous and permucosal transmission occurs from needles, blood products, sex, and birth.
• Hepatitis C	Percutaneous transmission occurs from blood products and needles.
• Hepatitis E	Fecal-oral transmission occurs in developing countries with inadequate sanitation systems. The virus is known to be endemic in Central America, Africa, the Middle East, and Asia. People traveling in these countries should be careful to avoid consuming local tap water and uncooked foods.
■ Teach about treatment.	Adequate rest, nutrition, and prevention of complications are the mainstay of therapy for all types of hepatitis. Because the disease is typically viral, medications are not helpful.
■ Teach about infection control procedures.	Hand washing is the most effective method of preventing the transmission of type A. Patients usually do not need to be isolated unless they are incapable of or unwilling to participate in infection control measures. Personal care items (e.g., razors, toothbrushes) should not be shared because the risk for parenteral exposure exists. Safe sex should be discussed and encouraged.
■ Discuss future need to avoid blood donation.	Even after patients with hepatitis are well, they may carry the virus and should refrain from blood donation to prevent risk for disease transmission.
■ Teach about possible complications and long-term sequelae of hepatitis.	Hepatitis can lead to chronic hepatitis and/or fulminant hepatitis if liver cells do not regenerate. Chronic hepatitis can result in cirrhosis and liver failure.
■ Encourage family members to obtain hepatitis vaccines, as indicated.	Vaccines for hepatitis A and B can prevent transmission of the infection.

NANDA-I NDx **Activity Intolerance**

Common Related Factors

Decreased metabolism of nutrients
Increased basal metabolic rate caused by viral infection

Defining Characteristics

Verbal report of fatigue or weakness
Unable to endure or complete desired activities
Dyspnea associated with activity
Abnormal heart rate, BP, or respiratory response to activity

Common Expected Outcomes

Patient exhibits activity tolerance as evidenced by rating of perceived exertion of 3 or less (0 to 10 scale), heart rate less than or equal to 120 beats/min (or within 20 beats/min of resting heart rate), systolic blood pressure (BP) within 20 mm Hg increase over resting systolic BP, respiratory rate less than 20 breaths/min, absence of chest pain or dyspnea.
Patient reports ability to perform required activities of daily living.
Patient verbalizes and uses energy-conservation techniques.

NOC Outcomes

Activity Tolerance; Energy Conservation; Self-Care: Activities of Daily Living

NIC Intervention

Energy Management

Ongoing Assessment

Actions/Interventions	Rationales
■ Assess general energy levels and activity tolerance; note specific trends.	Fatigue may be the most profound manifestation of hepatitis. Some patients have peak energy levels early in the day or after naps.
■ Assess need for assistive devices.	The use of assistive devices can decrease exertion.
▲ Monitor liver enzyme levels.	Elevations in hepatic enzyme levels indicate damage or death of liver cells; new elevations or failure of enzyme levels to trend toward normal indicates continuing damage, which could result from premature activity or overexertion.
■ Assess emotional response to activity intolerance.	If the patient attempts activities but is too exhausted to participate meaningfully, then the patient may experience increased frustration about activity intolerance.

Therapeutic Interventions

Actions/Interventions	Rationales
■ Maintain or encourage bed rest until enzyme levels begin to normalize. Provide for long, uninterrupted periods of rest and relaxation.	Healing damaged liver cells and generating new ones requires metabolic expenditure; maintaining bed rest reduces the energy required for movement and increases the energy available for healing.
■ Encourage bathroom use, or provide a bedside commode.	Use of a bedpan requires more energy expenditure than getting up to use the bathroom or commode.
■ Provide or encourage a quiet environment and promote rest using strategies that the patient identifies as helpful (e.g., music, reading, dim lights).	The patient needs to be included in creating an environment that promotes effective rest.
■ Provide information on energy conservation techniques.	Setting priorities for activity and keeping frequently used objects within easy reach help conserve energy. Patients need to learn to delegate tasks to others during recovery.
■ Assist the patient in identifying realistic goals for engaging in activity.	The patient may need assistance in balancing the desire for activities with the reality of a need for rest and of the activity intolerance imposed by the disease process.
■ Assist the patient in planning the day.	Activities should be planned to coincide with the patient's peak energy level.

NANDA-I NDx

Risk for Imbalanced Nutrition: Less Than Body Requirements

Common Risk Factors

Inability to absorb or metabolize foods
Unwillingness to eat
Nausea and vomiting

Common Expected Outcomes

Patient or caregiver verbalizes and demonstrates selection of foods or meals that will maintain a stable weight.
Patient weighs within 10% of ideal body weight.

NOC Outcomes
Nutritional Status: Nutrient Intake; Knowledge: Prescribed Diet
NIC Interventions
Nutrition Management; Teaching: Prescribed Diet

■ = Independent   ▲ = Collaborative

Ongoing Assessment

Actions/Interventions	Rationales
■ Document the patient's actual weight, and encourage the patient to weigh self weekly.	A decrease in body weight over time is an indication of inadequate caloric intake.
■ Obtain nutritional history.	A complete nutritional history provides information about the patient's weight-loss history, food likes and dislikes, food intolerances, and food allergies. Anorexia is a major problem in hepatitis. Patients with hepatitis may experience aversion to specific foods such as meat.
■ Assess for nausea.	Nausea is a common manifestation in the preicteric phase of hepatitis. Food odors may contribute to the nausea.
▲ Monitor serum albumin level.	This test indicates degree of protein depletion (2.5 g/dL indicates severe depletion; 3.8 to 4.5 g/dL is normal)

Therapeutic Interventions

Actions/Interventions	Rationales
▲ Administer or teach use of antiemetics as prescribed before meals.	These drugs decrease nausea, increase food tolerance, and maximize intake.
▲ Consult dietitian as indicated.	Diet should be high in calories to provide a source for energy; high in carbohydrates because carbohydrates are easily metabolized and stored by the liver; and limited in fats, which may trigger nausea.
■ Provide or encourage small meals with frequent snacks.	This meal plan increases daily intake because less energy is required to eat smaller meals.
■ Provide or encourage largest meal at breakfast.	Anorexia tends to worsen later in the day.
■ Discourage the use of alcoholic beverages.	Alcohol damages liver cells and provides "empty calories" (calories without nutritional value).
▲ Administer or teach use of vitamin supplement as prescribed.	Liver damage may limit adsorption and metabolism of fat-soluble vitamins.

Related Care Plans

Nausea, p. 137
Fatigue, p. 66
Ineffective health maintenance, p. 92
Readiness for enhanced immunization status, p. 105

Inflammatory Bowel Disease

Crohn's Disease; Ulcerative Colitis; Diverticulitis

Inflammatory bowel disease (IBD) refers to a cluster of specific bowel abnormalities whose symptoms are often so similar as to make diagnosis difficult and treatment empirical. Crohn's disease is associated with involvement of all four layers of the bowel and may occur anywhere in the gastrointestinal (GI) tract, although it is most common in the small bowel at the terminal ileum. Ulcerative colitis occurs only in the colon and involves the mucosal and submucosal layers. Cause is unknown for both diseases, but a familial history of IBD is found in patients who develop Crohn's disease and ulcerative colitis. Specific genetic mutations have been identified in people with Crohn's disease. The incidence of Crohn's disease is higher in people of Ashkenazi Jewish heritage than other ethnic groups. Incidence is usually in the 15- to 30-year-old age-group. Both Crohn's disease and ulcerative colitis are associated with the development of diarrhea and nutritional deficiencies. Systemic manifestations can involve the liver, joints, skin, and eyes. Diverticulitis is inflammation of a diverticulum in the colon.

The diverticulum is a herniation of the mucosal layer of the colon through the muscle layer. Obstruction of the diverticulum with hardened fecal material or undigested food particles causes the inflammation. Diverticular disease often occurs in persons older than 40 years of age; it seems to be etiologically related to high-fat, low-fiber diets and occurs almost exclusively in the colon. IBD is treated medically. If medical management fails or if complications occur, surgical resection and, possibly, fecal diversion are undertaken. This care plan focuses on chronic, ambulatory care.

NANDA-I NDx

Acute Pain: Abdominal, Joint

Common Related Factors

Bowel inflammation and contractions of diseased bowel or colon
Systemic manifestations of IBD

Defining Characteristics

Reports of intermittent colicky abdominal pain associated with diarrhea
Abdominal rebound tenderness
Hyperactive bowel sounds
Abdominal distention
Pain and cramps associated with eating
Chronic joint pain

Common Expected Outcomes

Patient reports satisfactory pain control at a level less than 3 to 4 on a 0 to 10 rating scale.
Patient uses pharmacological and nonpharmacological pain relief strategies.
Patient exhibits increased comfort such as baseline levels for pulse, blood pressure, respirations, and relaxed muscle tone or body posture.

NOC Outcomes

Comfort Level; Medication Response; Symptom Control

NIC Interventions

Medication Administration: Oral; Medication Administration: Topical; Pain Management

Ongoing Assessment

Actions/Interventions	**Rationales**
■ Assess pain: intermittent, colicky abdominal pain; abdominal pain and cramping associated with eating; joint pain.	Although the exact mechanism is unclear, a strong autoimmune etiology is believed to exist in Crohn's disease and ulcerative colitis; systemic manifestations often include arthritis-like symptoms. The person with diverticulitis may complain of dull pain in the left lower quadrant of the abdomen. Changes in the severity and nature of the abdominal pain may indicate a life-threatening condition such as perforation of the GI tract.
■ Auscultate bowel sounds.	Inflammation of the intestines contributes to increased peristalsis and diarrhea. The intestinal hypermotility combined with the inflammation causes cramping abdominal pain. Hyperactive bowel sounds are typical with abdominal cramping pain.
■ Evaluate patient's perception of dietary impact on abdominal pain.	Many patients with IBD cannot tolerate dairy products and may not tolerate many other foods.
■ Assess presence of changes in bowel habits, such as diarrhea.	Cramping abdominal pain often increases with diarrhea. Patients with diverticular disease may have a history of constipation alternating with diarrhea.
■ Determine measures the patient has successfully used to control pain.	This information can be helpful in developing an effective pain management program.

■ = Independent   ▲ = Collaborative

Therapeutic Interventions

Actions/Interventions	Rationales
■ Instruct patient to take medications as prescribed.	The goal of medical treatment is to induce clinical remission while avoiding toxic medications.
• Sulfasalazine	Sulfasalazine (Azulfidine) is a salicylate that decreases inflammation and is typically used to bring the disease to remission.
• Corticosteroids	Corticosteroids are given to decrease inflammation. These drugs may be administered by a variety of routes including oral, IV, and rectal.
• Immunosuppressants/Immunomodulators	Drugs that suppress or modify immune system activity are initiated when patients do not respond to sulfasalazine and corticosteroids.
• Anticholinergics/Antidiarrheals	Anticholinergics and antidiarrheal drugs are given to manage diarrhea by decreasing smooth muscles spasms and intestinal motility and secretions.
■ Encourage patient to engage in usual diversional activities, hobbies, relaxation techniques, and psychosocial support systems as tolerated.	Distraction heightens the patient's concentration on non-painful stimuli to decrease awareness and experience of pain. Relaxation techniques bring about a state of physical and mental awareness and tranquility to reduce tension and pain. The patient's social support network can reduce the burden of suffering associated with pain.
■ Recommend necessary alterations in diet.	Small frequent meals tend to be better tolerated and cause less gastrointestinal distress. An increase in dietary fiber reduces constipation and abdominal discomfort for the patient with diverticular disease.

NANDA-I NDx Imbalanced Nutrition: Less Than Body Requirements

Common Related Factors
Malabsorption and diarrhea
Increased nitrogen loss with diarrhea
Decreased intake
Poor appetite and nausea

Defining Characteristics
Body weight more than 10% to 20% below ideal
Decreased serum calcium, potassium, vitamins K and B_{12}, folic acid, and zinc
Muscle wasting
Pedal edema
Skin lesions
Poor wound healing

Common Expected Outcome
Patient's nutritional status improves, as evidenced by weight gain or stabilization of weight; controlled diarrhea; and normal serum electrolyte, vitamin, and mineral profiles.

NOC Outcome
Nutritional Status: Nutrient Intake
NIC Interventions
Nutrition Monitoring; Nutrition Management

Ongoing Assessment

Actions/Interventions	Rationales
■ Document patient's actual weight (do not estimate).	Decreased body weight is a sign of poor nutrition.
■ Obtain nutritional history; monitor dietary intake.	This assessment information provides the basis for initiating diet therapy.

Actions/Interventions

- Assess for skin lesions, skin breaks, tears, decreased skin integrity, and edema of extremities.
- ▲ Assess serum electrolytes, calcium, vitamins K and B_{12}, folic acid, and zinc levels to determine actual or potential deficiencies.
- Assess patterns of elimination: color, amount, consistency, frequency, odor, and presence of steatorrhea (stools high in undigested fat).

Rationales

Protein malnutrition causes impaired skin integrity and tissue edema.

Patients may experience deficiencies related to altered food intake and/or inability of the bowel mucosa to absorb nutrients.

Diarrhea and steatorrhea are indications of nutrient malabsorption.

Therapeutic Interventions

Actions/Interventions

- ▲ Consult dietitian to review nutritional history, how to perform calorie count, and to assist in menu selection.

- Encourage patient or caregiver to evaluate factors that enhance appetite, and adjust environment accordingly.
- ▲ Encourage use of vitamin and mineral supplements as ordered.
- ▲ Anticipate need for total parenteral nutrition as prescribed.

- ▲ Administer or instruct the patient to take medications to control diarrhea.

Rationales

Dietitians can analyze the patient's nutritional intake and provide guidance in selecting foods to improve the patient's nutritional status. High-calorie, high-protein, low-residue diets are recommended to maximize calorie absorption and reduce diarrhea.

An environment free of distractions and unpleasant odors can promote increased intake.

These replacements compensate for deficiencies.

This therapy is for patients who cannot tolerate oral intake and/or require bowel rest during an acute exacerbation of the disease.

Antidiarrheals can reduce loose stools, urgency, and fecal soiling. Controlling diarrhea can contribute to increased nutrient absorption and improve patient's appetite.

Risk for Deficient Fluid Volume

Common Risk Factors

Presence of excessive diarrhea or nausea and vomiting
Blood loss from inflamed bowel mucosa
Poor oral intake

Common Expected Outcome

Patient remains adequately hydrated as evidenced by good skin turgor, urine output greater than 30 mL/hr, and moist mucous membranes.

NOC Outcomes
Fluid Balance; Coagulation Status
NIC Interventions
Bleeding Reduction: Gastrointestinal; Fluid Monitoring

Ongoing Assessment

Actions/Interventions

- Assess hydration status: skin turgor, mucous membranes, intake and output, weight, blood pressure, and heart rate.

Rationales

Tenting of the skin, dry mucous membranes, reduced urine output, weight loss, increased heart rate, and hypotension are signs of fluid deficit.

■ = Independent   ▲ = Collaborative

Actions/Interventions

▲ Document Hemoccult-positive stools or obvious presence of bloody diarrhea. Monitor hemoglobin and hematocrit if the patient is bleeding

■ Monitor urine output and specific gravity.

Rationales

Bleeding leads to decreased circulatory volume and fluid deficit. Blood loss is typically most severe in patients with ulcerative colitis, but patients with Crohn's disease also may have bloody diarrhea. Decreased hemoglobin and hematocrit occur with bleeding.

Decreased urine output and concentrated urine are an indication of fluid volume deficit.

Therapeutic Interventions

Actions/Interventions

■ Maintain fluid intake that equals output.

■ Instruct and encourage patient to take medications as ordered.

▲ Anticipate need for intravenous (IV) therapy.

Rationales

Oral fluid intake is the preferred method to maintain hydration and fluid balance.

A variety of drugs are used to reduce intestinal inflammation and control diarrhea. Decreasing diarrhea will limit fluid lost with stools.

IV fluids are used if patient's oral intake is inadequate to maintain normal fluid volume status.

NANDA-I NDx Deficient Knowledge

Common Related Factors

Need for continuous and long-term management of chronic disease
Change in health care needs related to remission or exacerbation of disease

Defining Characteristics

Multiple questions by patient or caregivers related to disease process and management
Noncompliance with therapy

Common Expected Outcome

Patient or caregiver verbalizes understanding of disease and management.

NOC Outcomes
Knowledge: Disease Process; Knowledge: Treatment Regimen

NIC Interventions
Teaching: Disease Process; Teaching: Prescribed Diet; Teaching: Prescribed Medication

Ongoing Assessment

Actions/Interventions

■ Assess patient's understanding of IBD and necessary management.

Rationales

Patients need to understand that IBD differs from individual to individual; some cases are managed successfully throughout the course of the disease on medications alone, whereas others progress to needing surgical intervention.

Therapeutic Interventions

Actions/Interventions

■ Discuss the disease process and its management. Explain that IBD is characterized by remissions and exacerbations.

Rationales

The chronic nature of IBD requires that the patient understand that remissions and exacerbations are the expected course of the disease; as such, medication and dietary management are typically ongoing, although adjustments may be required, depending on the stage of the disease. Careful medical management may eliminate or postpone the need for surgical intervention.

Actions/Interventions

- Discuss surgical interventions for IBD.

- Encourage contact with Crohn's and Colitis Foundation of America.

Rationales

Bowel resection with either anastomosis or bowel diversion with an ostomy may be done for patients with severe IBD. A total colectomy with an ileostomy can cure ulcerative colitis. Crohn's disease cannot be cured with surgery but bowel resections with anastomosis may be done to manage complications and severe symptoms of the disease. Colon resection may be indicated for management of severe diverticular disease.

Community resources provide the patient and caregiver with ongoing support and information.

Related Care Plans

Bowel diversion surgery, p. 561
Deficient fluid volume, p. 72
Diarrhea, p. 54
Ineffective therapeutic regimen management, p. 194
Risk for impaired skin integrity, p. 185
Total parenteral nutrition, p. 614

Obesity

Overweight; Bariatric Surgery

Overweight and obesity are common health problems in the United States, and their prevalence is growing globally. The prevalence of obesity in the United States continues to be high. Recent epidemiological studies conclude that this prevalence exceeds 30% in most sex and age groups. The increased prevalence of obesity in children and adolescents may add to a growing obesity problem as they reach adulthood. Overweight is defined as a body mass index (BMI) of 25 to 29.9 kg/m², and obesity is defined as a BMI of 30 kg/m² or more. Obesity is now classified as follows: class 1, BMI of 30 to 34.9 kg/m²; class 2, BMI of 35 to 39.9 kg/m², and class 3 (extreme obesity), BMI of 40 kg/m² or more. Excess weight accounts for significant health problems, including cardiovascular disease, type 2 diabetes mellitus, hypertension, stroke, dyslipidemia, osteoarthritis, respiratory problems, sleep disorders, and some cancers. Women are more likely to be obese than men. Obesity tends to coincide with age (older adults are more likely to be obese than younger adults), and obesity is more prevalent among African American and Hispanic individuals than among whites. Genetics are also thought to play a role in obesity. A sedentary lifestyle; physiological factors involved in appetite, satiety, and metabolism; and emotional factors associated with overeating all contribute to the complexity of obesity, which is best managed using a multifocused approach. Simple nutritional management, exercise, behavior modification, use of medications, and surgical procedures are all possible methods for managing obesity. Bariatric surgical procedures are usually used for those patients with a BMI greater than 40. These surgeries may restrict the volume of the stomach and therefore the amount of food consumed. Other procedures bypass portions of the intestine to reduce absorption of food intake. Most bariatric surgery programs include surgical therapy with a long-term program of lifestyle modifications such as eating habits and physical activity. The focus of this care plan is on the obese individual in the outpatient setting.

■ = Independent   ▲ = Collaborative

NDx Deficient Knowledge

Common Related Factors

Lack of familiarity with options to address obesity
Emotional state affecting learning (anxiety, denial, fear)

Defining Characteristics

Lack of knowledge regarding nutritional needs for height and frame
Lack of knowledge regarding food selection and preparation
Demonstrated inability to correctly read labels on food products
Lack of knowledge regarding role of exercise in weight management
Demonstrated inappropriate food selections
Demonstrated inability to plan an appropriate menu
Continued weight gain
Lack of knowledge regarding complications of unmanaged obesity
Lack of knowledge regarding surgical options

Common Expected Outcomes

Patient verbalizes measures necessary to achieve weight-reduction goals.
Patient demonstrates appropriate selection of meals or menu planning toward the goal of weight reduction.
Patient begins an appropriate program of exercise.
Patient verbalizes other measures (medications, surgery, behavior-modification programs) to consider if conservative management fails to achieve desired weight loss.
Patient verbalizes health consequences of continued obesity.

NOC Outcomes

Knowledge: Diet; Knowledge: Prescribed Activity; Knowledge: Surgical Options

NIC Interventions

Health Education; Teaching: Prescribed Activity/Exercise; Teaching: Prescribed Diet; Teaching: Surgical and Medication Alternatives

Ongoing Assessment

Actions/Interventions	Rationales
■ Assess knowledge regarding nutritional needs for height and level of activity or other factors (e.g., pregnancy).	A person's height, activity level, or other factors can influence his or her caloric needs. Obese individuals may underestimate their calorie intake and overestimate their activity level.
■ Assess ability to read food labels.	Food labels contain information necessary in making appropriate selections but can be misleading. Patients need to understand that "low-fat" or "fat-free" does not mean that a food item is calorie free. Serving sizes must also be understood to limit intake according to a planned diet.
■ Assess ability to plan a menu, making appropriate food selections.	Unplanned, impulsive eating can lead to overeating.
■ Assess ability to accurately identify appropriate food portions.	Obese people often underestimate portion sizes.
■ Assess usual activity level.	Patients may confuse routine activity with exercise necessary to enhance and maintain weight loss.
■ Assess or explore with the patient how social situations may contribute to overeating.	Overeating may be triggered by environmental cues unrelated to physiological hunger sensations.

Therapeutic Interventions

Actions/Interventions	Rationales
■ Include the family, caregiver, and food preparer in nutrition counseling.	The patient will be more likely to adhere to changes in food intake when family members are involved in those changes. Research has demonstrated that men whose wives diet with them are more likely to achieve goals than those for whom "special food" is prepared.
■ Review and reinforce basic nutrition information: • Four food groups or the food pyramid • Proper serving sizes (may need to teach use of gram scale) • Caloric content of food • Methods of preparation to avoid additional calories	The key principle of obesity therapy is to eat fewer calories than are expended in order to consume fat stores as fuel. Baking, boiling, broiling, poaching, and grilling are preferable to frying in oil.
■ Teach the patient to read food labels.	Portion size in relation to calories is important in food selection and meal planning. When using packaged foods portion size is often less than the entire package.
■ Teach the patient to plan a menu incorporating nutritional needs and food preferences.	Compliance with a diet is enhanced when the patient's preferences are incorporated into the planned diet.
■ Encourage the patient to see a physician before beginning an aggressive exercise program.	Patients need to understand that exercise without calorie reduction will not contribute to weight loss. Current recommendations are 30 minutes of moderate exercise most days of the week for weight loss maintenance. Overexertion should be avoided. Low-impact exercise, such as walking, is a good initial exercise plan.
▲ Refer the patient to commercial weight-loss program as appropriate.	Some individuals require the regimented approach or ongoing support during weight loss, whereas others are able to (and may prefer to) manage a weight-loss program independently.
▲ Refer the patient to specialized dietitians.	The dietitian can provide specialized information and ongoing support for weight loss. Some individuals require assistance only with meal preparation/choices and can handle other aspects of lifestyle changes.
■ Inform the patient about pharmacological agents for weight loss.	Because drugs do nothing to permanently alter eating behaviors, use of drugs for weight management often fails when the patient stops taking the medication. Drugs for weight loss include appetite suppressants (nonadrenergic and serotonin reuptake inhibitors), digestive inhibitors (interfere with digestion and absorption of fat), and fat substitutes as food additives.
■ Provide the patient with information about and referrals for bariatric surgical interventions for weight loss. Information may include:	Options depend on the patient's appropriateness for a procedure and usually according to extensive criteria, such as extent of obesity, existing complications of obesity, and likelihood of postprocedure compliance. Patients should be referred to their physicians to discuss the appropriateness of such procedures. The obese patient is at increased risk for cardiovascular and pulmonary complications with surgical procedures. Many procedures are done using minimally invasive techniques.
• Criteria for surgical therapy	Bariatric surgeries are considered for patients who are unable to achieve or maintain weight loss through diet and exercise. Specific criteria include severe obesity (BMI of 40 or higher) or obesity (BMI 35-39.9) with a weight-related health problem such as hypertension or type 2 diabetes mellitus.
• Types of procedures • Lipectomy/liposuction	These procedures involve removal of body fat and are considered cosmetic, body-shaping surgeries. The patient needs to understand that removing body fat does not result in long term weight loss.

■ = Independent ▲ = Collaborative

Actions/Interventions	Rationales
• Roux-en-Y gastric bypass	The Roux-en-Y procedure is a type of gastric bypass surgery. The volume capacity of the stomach is reduced. An anastomosis is created directly between the smaller stomach pouch and the jejunum. Weight loss occurs by decreased gastric capacity and some reduced intestinal absorption.
• Biliopancreatic diversion	The biliopancreatic diversion is another type of gastric bypass surgery recommended for patients with a BMI of 50 or higher. A variety of specific surgical techniques are used for this procedure. Approximately 70% of the stomach is removed. The remaining gastric tissue is formed into a sleeve or tube and anastomosed to a portion of the small intestine. Surgical channels are created to allow for passage of biliary and pancreatic secretions into the intestines. Weight loss occurs by decreased gastric capacity and significant reduction of intestinal absorption.
• Sleeve gastrectomy	Sleeve gastrectomy is the first part of the biliopancreatic diversion. Most of the stomach is removed and the remaining tissue is shaped into a sleeve or tube. This procedure may be performed to allow the patient to lose some weight before the biliopancreatic diversion is performed. Weight loss occurs through reduced gastric capacity.
• Gastric banding	Gastric banding use techniques to partition the stomach into a small upper portion and the larger lower portion. Techniques include inflated, adjustable gastric bands and vertical gastric stapling. Weight loss occurs through reduced gastric capacity. Weight loss tends to be less and occur at a slower rate than with gastric bypass procedures.
• Risks of weight loss surgery	The general risks with bariatric surgery are the same as with any major surgical procedure. Specific risks associated with bariatric surgery include vitamin and mineral deficiencies, fluid volume deficit, gastric ulcers, dumping syndrome, increased risk for cholelithiasis and renal calculi, food intolerances, and hypoglycemia.

NANDA-I NDx Imbalanced Nutrition: More Than Body Requirements

Common Related Factors
Lack of knowledge regarding weight-control measures
Poor dietary habits
Use of food as a coping mechanism
Metabolic disorders
Diabetes
Sedentary lifestyle
Inadequate exercise

Defining Characteristics
Weight 20% or more over ideal body weight for height and frame
Reported or observed dysfunctional eating patterns
Reported or observed noncompliance with recommended diet or exercise plan

Common Expected Outcome
Patient demonstrates understanding of and participates in planned dietary and exercise treatment program.

NOC Outcomes
Weight Control; Nutritional Status: Nutrient Intake

NIC Interventions
Nutritional Monitoring; Weight-Reduction Assistance; Self-Responsibility Facilitation

Ongoing Assessment

Actions/Interventions	Rationales
■ Obtain baseline weight, and weigh on routine schedule.	Daily weights are not recommended. Slight variations may unnecessarily encourage or discourage a patient; minor variations occur as the result of time of day. Adherence to diet and exercise programs will be reflected in gradual and consistent weight loss. Most experts suggest loss of 0.5 to 1 pound per week.
■ Determine BMI.	BMI describes relative weight for height and is significantly correlated with total body fat content. BMI should be used to assess the degree of overweight and obesity and to monitor changes in body weight. BMI is calculated as weight (in kilograms) divided by height squared (in square meters). Convenient conversion tables of heights and weights resulting in selected BMI units are commonly used in clinical practice.
■ Record weight history.	It is helpful to use milestones to help patients recall the history of their weight gain. Evaluate diet attempts to get a better perspective on medical/physical diet history. Questions such as, "How much did you weigh in high school?" "How much did you weigh when you got married?" "How much did you weigh after your first child was born?" may help establish when obesity became a problem.
■ Perform a nutritional assessment.	This should include types and amount of foods eaten, how food is prepared, the pattern of intake (time of day, frequency, and other activities the patient is engaged in while eating), amount of fast food consumed, and access to grocery store.
■ Assess the patient's activity patterns, including regular exercise program.	Increasing activity levels may need to begin at a slow pace if the person has a very sedentary lifestyle.
■ Explore the importance and meaning of food with the patient.	When food is used as a coping mechanism or as self-reward, the emotional needs being met by intake of food will need to be addressed as part of the overall plan for weight reduction.
■ Assess for behaviors that may affect success (smoking, drug/alcohol abuse).	This information may also be helpful in identifying psychosocial or emotional factors in the development of obesity.

Therapeutic Interventions

Actions/Interventions	Rationales
■ Encourage the patient to keep a diet diary (or daily food journal).	A food intake record provides a means for objectively discussing actual versus perceived intake.
▲ Arrange for consultation with a dietitian.	This will assist the patient in selecting appropriate types and amounts of foods, discussing food preparation, and planning nutritious meals.
■ Help the patient plan how to avoid or manage social situations that result in overeating.	The patient needs to learn new strategies to cope with settings that trigger overeating.
■ Encourage the patient to be more aware of nutritional habits that may contribute to or prevent overeating:	
• To realize the time needed for eating	Hurried eating may result in overeating because satiety is not realized until 15 to 20 minutes after ingestion of food.
• To focus on eating and avoid other diversional activities (e.g., reading, watching television, talking on the telephone)	Distractions at mealtime contribute to overeating.

■ = Independent   ▲ = Collaborative

Actions/Interventions

- To observe for cues that lead to eating (e.g., time of day, boredom, depression)
- To eat in a designated place (e.g., at the table rather than in front of the television or standing in front of the refrigerator)
- To recognize actual hunger versus desire to eat

■ Encourage the patient to set realistic goals for beginning an exercise program.

■ Encourage successes; assist the patient in coping with setbacks.

▲ Encourage patient to participate in local support groups.

Rationales

Awareness and recognition of cues can help the person substitute other activities for eating.

Limiting eating to a designated place can help reduce snacking and other impulse eating.

Eating when not hungry is a commonly recognized symptom among overeaters.

A balanced, reasonable diet and a modest exercise program will provide weight reduction for a great many patients. Remind patients that missing a day of planned exercise or occasional dietary indiscretion will inevitably happen and should not be construed as failure.

Positive feedback for weight loss encourages adherence to the treatment plan. The patient may experience temporary weight gains or weight plateaus. These changes can be discouraging to the patient's efforts to continue a weight loss program. Patients need to understand that these changes are expected and that slight modifications in diet or exercise can return the patient to a pattern of continued weight loss.

Social support is important in successful weight loss and long-term weight management.

 NANDA-I NDx **Disturbed Body Image**

Common Related Factors

Recent or longstanding change in appearance
Loss of social status

Common Expected Outcomes

Patient demonstrates enhanced body image and self-esteem as evidenced by ability to discuss the role weight plays in body image disturbance.
Patient verbalizes satisfaction with ability to begin managing obesity.

Defining Characteristics

Verbalized discontent with size and appearance
Withdrawal from social contact

NOC Outcomes

Body Image; Self-Esteem

NIC Interventions

Body Image Enhancement; Weight-Reduction Assistance

Ongoing Assessment

Actions/Interventions

■ Assess the patient's perception of the impact of being overweight.

■ Assess the degree to which body image disturbance is affecting the patient's overall self-esteem.

Rationales

These perceptions often include exclusion from social activities, being passed over for jobs or promotions, inability to find and purchase attractive clothing, and general disdain by a public that cherishes a "fit-and-trim" look. Research has shown that the morbidly obese (i.e., those 100% above ideal body weight) are subject to certain types of job discrimination.

Body image is a major component of self-esteem; as such, body image disturbance can and often does result in self-esteem disturbance, which can affect the person's overall ability to function.

Therapeutic Interventions

Actions/Interventions	**Rationales**
■ Acknowledge normalcy of feelings related to being overweight; encourage verbalization about the same.	Guilt about feelings can contribute to overeating. Discouragement and frustration can also contribute to overeating.
■ Demonstrate empathy and empower the patient to participate in a corrective plan.	Self-esteem is enhanced when the patient feels a sense of control.
■ Engage the patient in realistic goal setting.	Patients are easily discouraged when they cannot meet unrealistic goals. This sense of failure can lead to overeating. Patients need to be aware that surgical therapy does not produce immediate changes in body weight or shape.
■ Include significant others and caregivers in education, planning, and goal setting.	These people will be important sources of ongoing support for the patient facing a long-term weight-reduction plan.
■ Refer the patient to support groups, if desired.	Support groups can provide companionship, enhance motivation for weight loss, and decrease loneliness. Sharing may provide solutions to common problems.

Related Care Plans

Abdominal surgery, p. 550
Activity intolerance, p. 8
Sleep-disordered breathing, p. 451
Noncompliance, p. 139
Powerlessness, p. 162
Self-care deficit, p. 170

Pancreatitis, Acute

Pancreatitis is an inflammatory disorder of the pancreas that results in the self-destruction of the pancreas by its own enzymes, causing edema, necrosis, and hemorrhage. The mechanism responsible for causing abnormal enzyme activity in the pancreas is unknown. Activation of these proteases and lipases before they are excreted into the intestine causes inflammation and damage to the pancreatic tissue. The patient may develop jaundice from obstruction of the common bile duct by an edematous pancreas. Damage to insulin-secreting cells of the pancreas produces episodes of hyperglycemia. The two most common causes are alcohol abuse and biliary obstruction. In severe cases, pancreatitis can be complicated by acute respiratory distress syndrome (ARDS). Repeated episodes of acute pancreatitis can lead to the development of chronic pancreatitis and diabetes mellitus. The focus of this care plan is the care of the acutely ill person with pancreatitis.

NANDA-I NDx **Acute Pain**

Common Related Factors	**Defining Characteristics**
Inflammation of pancreas and surrounding tissue	Verbalized pain
Biliary tract disease	Guarding behavior
Biliary obstruction	Moaning
Excessive alcohol intake	Facial mask of pain
Abdominal trauma or surgery	
Infectious process	
Heavy metal poisoning	

■ = Independent ▲ = Collaborative

Common Expected Outcomes

Patient reports satisfactory pain control at a level less than 3 to 4 on a 0 to 10 rating scale.

Patient uses pharmacological and nonpharmacological pain relief strategies.

Patient exhibits increased comfort such as baseline levels for pulse, blood pressure, respirations, and relaxed muscle tone or body posture.

NOC Outcomes
Pain Control; Comfort Level; Symptom Control

NIC Interventions
Medication Administration; Pain Management; Positioning

Ongoing Assessment

Actions/Interventions	Rationales
■ Assess pain characteristics.	Epigastric pain or umbilical pain radiating to the back and/or shoulders, increasing pain in the supine position, abdominal distention with rebound tenderness, extreme restlessness, and pain aggravated by food intake are typical pain complaints related to pancreatitis.
■ Assess history of previous attacks.	Pancreatitis may be a chronic, relapsing disease.
■ Assess precipitating factors.	Often a bout of pancreatitis is precipitated by an alcoholic binge or consumption of a large meal that is high in fat content.
■ Auscultate bowel sounds; report decrease or absence of bowel sounds.	Extravasation of pancreatic enzymes causes paralytic ileus with decreased or absent bowel sounds.

Therapeutic Interventions

Actions/Interventions	Rationales
▲ Reduce pancreatic stimulus by maintaining patient NPO (nothing by mouth) or with nasogastric tube to low suction as ordered.	Oral intake causes vagally stimulated pancreatic secretion; the escape of pancreatic secretions into the pancreas causes pain and damage by autodigestion.
▲ Administer medication as prescribed.	Antispasmodics may be given to decrease intestinal motility and reduce secretion of pancreatic enzymes. Pain management is most effective when pain is treated before it becomes severe. Opioid analgesics are used for pain management.
■ Use repositioning, massage, and other nonpharmacological measures.	Many patients experience decreased pain by assuming positions that draw the knees to the abdomen. Side-lying positions or elevation of the head of the bed may contribute to pain relief. Other non-pharmacological measures may distract the patient's awareness of painful stimuli and promote relaxation.

NANDA-I NDx Risk for Deficient Fluid Volume

Common Risk Factors

Vomiting
Decreased intake
Shifting of fluids to extravascular space
Hemorrhage
Ileus

Common Expected Outcome

Patient maintains normal fluid volume, as evidenced by urine output greater than 30 mL/hr, good skin turgor, and stable blood pressure (BP) and heart rate.

NOC Outcomes
Fluid Balance; Electrolyte and Acid-Base Balance

NIC Interventions
Fluid Monitoring; Fluid and Electrolyte Management

Ongoing Assessment

Actions/Interventions	Rationales
■ Monitor BP and heart rate.	The release of enzymes and inflammatory kinins into the vascular system causes increased vascular permeability and vasodilation. These changes lead to hypovolemia. Fluid volume deficit occurs rapidly in pancreatitis; BP decreases and heart rate increases. Subtle vital sign changes may indicate profound fluid volume deficit.
■ Assess hydration status, including urine output, thirst, mucous membranes, skin turgor, and daily weight.	Decreased urine volume and concentrated color denotes fluid deficit. Loss of interstitial fluid causes loss of skin turgor. Increased thirst and dry mucous membranes occur with fluid volume deficit. Daily weight loss is a sign of fluid losses.
■ Observe for complications of dehydration.	The single most important element in preventing multiple organ failure is maintaining fluid balance. Oliguria and impaired renal function can occur rapidly as a result of the severity of fluid volume deficit.

Therapeutic Interventions

Actions/Interventions	Rationales
▲ Administer intravenous fluids as prescribed.	In acute pancreatitis, a patient may require several liters of fluid over the first 24 hours. Fluid resuscitation is essential to maintain hemodynamic stability. Since the patient is kept NPO to reduce pancreatic stimulation, intravenous fluid administration is required.

NANDA-I NDx Deficient Knowledge

Common Related Factor
Unfamiliarity with disease process

Defining Characteristics
Multiple questions
Misconceptions
Repeat admissions to hospital with recurrent bouts of pancreatitis

Common Expected Outcome
Patient verbalizes understanding of causative factors and disease process for pancreatitis.

NOC Outcomes
Knowledge: Disease Process; Knowledge: Substance Use Control

NIC Intervention
Teaching: Disease Process

■ = Independent   ▲ = Collaborative

Ongoing Assessment

Actions/Interventions

- Assess the patient's understanding of the disease process, particularly potentially controllable behaviors that may trigger episodes of pancreatitis.

Rationales

Continuation of precipitating behaviors can lead to a chronic form of pancreatitis.

Therapeutic Interventions

Actions/Interventions

- Teach about the relationship of alcohol consumption to pancreatitis and the recurrent nature of pancreatitis.
- Teach about relationship of biliary (gallbladder) disease to pancreatitis.
- Teach the patient that certain foods may precipitate a bout of pancreatitis.

Rationales

Eliminating alcohol use can reduce episodes of pancreatitis and their severity.

Patients with pancreatitis secondary to gallstones should undergo cholecystectomy during the same hospitalization.

Many patients with chronic pancreatitis tolerate fatty and spicy foods poorly, although other patients are intolerant to other foods best identified by the individual. Reduction of fat from the diet can reduce stimulation of the pancreas.

Peptic Ulcer Disease

Duodenal Ulcers; Gastric Ulcers; Stress-Induced Ulcers

Peptic ulcer disease (PUD) is characterized by mucosal erosions or ulcers that develop from a weakening in the lining of the mucosa that surrounds the upper gastrointestinal (GI) tract. These ulcerations may develop in the lower esophagus, stomach, or duodenum. PUD can be caused by hyperacidity, pepsin, bile salts, ischemia, aspirin, and nonsteroidal antiinflammatory drugs (NSAIDs). NSAIDs cause a weakening in the lining of the gastrointestinal tract by decreasing the protective layer. This decrease in the protective layer is attributed to the inhibition of mucosal prostaglandins caused by the NSAIDs. Prostaglandins stimulate the secretion of mucus and bicarbonate, which helps in making the mucosa more resistant to acid penetration. Prostaglandins also increase mucosal blood flow and play a role in healing. *Helicobacter pylori* is a common cause of duodenal ulcers, although the mechanism is not fully understood. Current evidence suggests that the bacteria produce enzymes that cause direct injury to the mucosal lining. Indirectly, the bacteria stimulate release of hydrogen ions that increase acidity and further contribute to mucosal erosion. Gastric ulcers develop when the protective mucousal layer becomes more permeable to hydrogen ions. This type of ulcer is associated with bile reflux and use of NSAIDs. Other factors that contribute to the development of peptic ulcer disease include altered gastric emptying (delayed or too rapid), bile reflux through an incompetent pyloric sphincter, or increased stress associated with critical illness, surgery, or acute trauma. Stress-induced ulers are thought to be caused by the effects of elevated cortical levels as part of the normal stress response. Ulcerative or erosive diseases in the upper GI tract can cause gastrointestinal bleeding, abdominal pain, anorexia, nausea and vomiting, or diarrhea.

Imbalanced Nutrition: Less Than Body Requirements

Common Related Factors	Defining Characteristics
Nausea, vomiting, anorexia	Weight loss
Alcohol intake	Inadequate dietary intake
Diarrhea	Malabsorption of iron, vitamins, and minerals
Gastrointestinal bleeding	
Abdominal pain	

Common Expected Outcomes

Patient or caregiver verbalizes and demonstrates selection of foods or meals that will achieve a cessation of weight loss.

Patient weighs within 10% of ideal body weight.

NOC Outcome
Knowledge : Diet Nutrition Intake

NIC Interventions
Nutrition Monitoring; Nutrition Therapy

Ongoing Assessment

Actions/Interventions	Rationales
■ Assess for changes in body weight.	Weight loss is an indication of inadequate nutritional intake. Gastric ulcers are more likely to be associated with loss of appetite, vomiting, and weight loss than duodenal ulcers.
■ Obtain a nutritional history.	Patients may often overestimate the amount of food eaten. The patient may not eat sufficient calories or essential nutrients as a way to reduce pain episodes with peptic ulcer disease. Because of this, patients are at high risk for malnutrition.
▲ Monitor laboratory values for serum albumin.	This test indicates the degree of protein depletion (2.5 g/dL indicates severe depletion; 3.8-4.5 g/dL is normal).

Therapeutic Interventions

Actions/Interventions	Rationales
■ Teach about the importance of eating a balanced diet with meals at regular intervals.	Specific dietary restrictions are no longer part of the treatment for PUD. During the symptomatic phase of an ulcer the patient may find benefit from eating small meals at more frequent intervals.
■ Assist patient with identifying foods that cause gastric irritation.	Patients need to learn what foods they can tolerate without gastric pain. Soft, bland, nonacidic foods cause less gastric irritation. The patient is more likely to increase food intake if the foods are not associated with pain. Foods that may contribute to mucosal irritation include spicy foods, pepper, and raw fruits and vegetables.
■ Encourage the patient to limit intake of coffee and other caffeinated beverages.	Caffeine stimulates the secretion of gastric acid. Coffee, even if decaffeinated, contains a peptide that stimulates the release of gastrin and increases acid production.
■ Instruct in the importance of abstaining from excessive alcohol.	Alcohol causes gastric irritation and increases gastric pain.

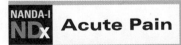

Acute Pain

Common Related Factors
Gnawing or cramping upper abdominal pain
Abdominal distention
Recent NSAID or acetylsalicylic acid (ASA) use

Defining Characteristics
Weight loss
Nausea and vomiting
Pain relieved by food or antacids
Early satiety

■ = Independent   ▲ = Collaborative

Gastrointestinal and Digestive Care Plans

Common Expected Outcomes

Patient reports satisfactory pain control at a level less than 3 to 4 on a 0 to 10 scale.

Patient uses pharmacological and nonpharmacological pain relief strategies.

Patient exhibits increased comfort such as baseline levels for pulse, blood pressure, and respirations and relaxed muscle tone or body posture.

NOC Outcomes
Pain Control; Comfort Status; Medication Response
NIC Interventions
Physical Comfort Promotion; Pain Management

Ongoing Assessment

Actions/Interventions

- Assess the patient's pain including location, characteristics, precipitating factors, onset, duration, frequency, quality, intensity, and severity.

Rationales

Patients with gastric ulcers typically demonstrate pain 1 to 2 hours after eating. The patient with duodenal ulcers demonstrates pain 2 to 4 hours after eating or in the middle of the night. With both gastric and duodenal ulcers the pain is located in the upper abdomen and is intermittent. Patients may report relief after eating or taking an antacid.

Therapeutic Interventions

Actions/Interventions

- Administer prescribed drug therapy:
  - Proton pump inhibitors
  - Antibiotics such as metronidazole, tetracycline, clarithromycin, or amoxicillin
  - H_2 histamine receptor antagonists
  - Prostaglandin analogues
  - Antacids
  - Sucralfate

- Teach use of nonpharmacological pain relief strategies such as guided imagery, relaxation, distraction, music therapy, or acupressure.

Rationales

The proton pump inhibitors block production and secretion of gastric acid and thereby reduce gastric pain. The antibiotics treat the *H. pylori* infection and promote healing of the ulcer. As the ulcer heals, the patient experiences less pain. H_2 histamine antagonists block secretion of gastric acid. The prostaglandin analogues reduce acid secretion and enhance the integrity of the gastric mucosa to resist injury. The antacids buffer gastric acid and prevent the formation of pepsin. This mechanism of action promotes healing of the ulcer. Sucralfate forms a barrier at the base of the ulcer crater to protect the healing ulcer from gastric acid.

Nonpharmacological relaxation techniques will decrease the production of gastric acid, which in turn will reduce pain.

NDx Risk for Deficient Fluid Volume

Common Risk Factors
Gastrointestinal bleeding
Nausea/vomiting

Common Expected Outcome
Patient is normovolemic as evidenced by systolic blood pressure greater than or equal to 90 mm Hg (or patient's baseline), absence of orthostasis, heart rate 60 to 100 beats/min, urine output greater than 30 mL/hr, and normal skin turgor.

NOC Outcomes
Fluid Balance; Hydration; Tissue Integrity; Skin and Mucous Membranes
NIC Interventions
Fluid Monitoring; Fluid Management; Fluid Resuscitation

Ongoing Assessment

Actions/Interventions	Rationales
■ Monitor vital signs, and check for changes in orthostatic blood pressure and pulse.	Gastrointestinal bleeding can cause anemia, which in turn if bleeding is brisk, can cause fairly rapid changes in vital signs and physical symptoms. A decrease in blood pressure with changes in position is an early indicator of decreased circulatory volume.
■ Monitor fluid intake and urine output.	The kidney will reabsorb water into circulation to support a decrease in blood volume. This compensatory mechanism results in decreased urine output. A decrease in circulatory blood volume leads to decreased renal perfusion and decreased urine output.
▲ Monitor hemoglobin and hematocrit laboratory values.	Erosion of the gastric mucosa by an ulcer results in GI bleeding. A decrease in hemoglobin and hemocrit occurs with bleeding.
■ Assess for sign of hematemesis or melena.	The patient with a bleeding ulcer may vomit bright red blood or coffee-ground emesis. Melena occurs when there is bleeding in the upper GI tract.

Therapeutic Interventions

Actions/Interventions	Rationales
■ Instruct the patient to report symptoms of nausea, vomiting, dizziness, shortness of breath, or dark tarry stool immediately.	These assessment findings are signs of GI bleeding and should be reported immediately.
▲ Administer IV fluids, volume expanders, and blood products as ordered	Isotonic fluids, blood products, and volume expanders such as albumin can restore or expand intravascular volume.

 NANDA-I NDx **Deficient Knowledge**

Common Related Factors

New condition, treatment
Lack of recall of previously learned information
Recurrent peptic ulcer disease
Recurrent episodes of GI bleeding

Defining Characteristics

Incorrect responses to questions about peptic ulcer disease
Inaccurate follow-through with treatment regimen and lifestyle modification
Multiple questions
Lack of questions

Common Expected Outcome

Patient verbalizes understanding of importance of compliance with medical regimen, knowledge of peptic ulcer disease, and commitment to self-care management.

NOC Outcomes

Knowledge: Disease Process; Knowledge: Diet; Knowledge: Medication; Information Processing

NIC Interventions

Learning Facilitation; Teaching: Individual

Ongoing Assessment

Actions/Interventions	Rationales
■ Assess for knowledge and misconceptions regarding peptic ulcer disease, lifestyle behaviors, and treatment regimen.	Patients may have inaccurate information about how lifestyle behaviors contribute to peptic ulcer disease. The patient needs accurate knowledge to make informed decisions about taking prescribed medications and modifying behaviors that contribute to peptic ulcer disease or gastrointestinal bleeding.

■ = Independent　▲ = Collaborative

Therapeutic Interventions

Actions/Interventions

- Explain pathophysiology of disease and how it relates to the functioning of the body.

- Discuss lifestyle changes required to prevent further complications or episodes of peptic ulcer disease.

- Instruct patient in what signs and symptoms to report to health care provider.
- Discuss therapy options and rationales for using these options.

Rationales

Understanding of the disease process helps to foster willingness to follow recommended treatment plan and modify behaviors to prevent recurrent episodes or related complications.

Modification of lifestyle behaviors such as alcohol use, coffee and other caffeinated beverages, and overuse of aspirin or other NSAIDs is necessary to prevent recurrent ulcer development and prevent complications during the healing phase.

Self-recognition of signs and symptoms can help ensure early initiation of treatment.

Correct use of antibiotics and acid suppression medications can promote rapid healing of an ulcer.

Related Care Plans

Abdominal surgery, p. 550
Gastrointestinal bleeding, 589
Acute pain, 151
Ineffective therapeutic regimen management, 194

Total Parenteral Nutrition

Intravenous (IV) Hyperalimentation

Total parenteral nutrition (TPN) is the administration of nutrients consisting of concentrated glucose and amino acid solutions via a central vein. A variety of central venous access devices may be used to deliver the TPN solution. TPN therapy is necessary when the gastrointestinal (GI) tract cannot be used or when oral intake is not able to meet the patient's nutritional needs. TPN solutions may contain 20% to 60% glucose and 3.5% to 10% protein (in the form of amino acids), in addition to various amounts of electrolytes, vitamins, minerals, and trace elements. These solutions can be modified, depending on the presence of organ system impairment and/or the specific nutritional needs of the patient. Fluid and electrolyte status require frequent monitoring while receiving TPN. To provide necessary amounts of essential fatty acids and the fat-soluble vitamins (A, D, E, and K), Intralipid is administered along with TPN. TPN is often used in hospital, long-term, and subacute care, but it is also commonly used in the home care setting. This care plan addresses nursing care needs that may occur in any of these settings.

NANDA-I NDx Imbalanced Nutrition: Less Than Body Requirements

Common Related Factors

Prolonged NPO (nothing by mouth) status
Alterations in GI tract function (e.g., GI surgery, fistulas, bowel obstruction, esophageal injury or disease, dysphagia, stomatitis, nausea, vomiting, or diarrhea)
Increased metabolic rate or other conditions necessitating increased intake (e.g., sepsis, burns, or chemotherapy)
Psychological reasons for refusal to eat

Defining Characteristics

Caloric intake less than body requirements
Weight loss (or weight 20% below ideal)
Poor skin turgor and wound healing
Decreased muscle mass
Decreased serum albumin, total protein, and transferrin levels
Electrolyte imbalances

Common Expected Outcome

Patient achieves an adequate nutritional status, as evidenced by stable weight or weight gain and by improved albumin levels.

NOC Outcome
Nutritional Status: Nutrient Intake
NIC Intervention
Nutritional Monitoring: TPN Administration

Ongoing Assessment

Actions/Interventions	Rationales
■ Obtain accurate intake and output, daily weights and calorie counts, including calories provided by TPN.	The composition of TPN is based on the individual's calculated needs. A comprehensive baseline assessment will be completed by an interdisciplinary team before TPN is initiated. Team members may include physicians, dietitians, and pharmacists. Changes in fluid balance, weight, and caloric intake are used to monitor the effectiveness of TPN. Daily weights are necessary to determine if nutritional goals are being met. Weight is also used to assess fluid volume status. Weight gain of more than ½ pound per day may indicate fluid retention.
■ Assess wound healing and skin integrity.	Delayed wound healing may indicate a need for TPN. Changes in skin integrity and wound healing will be used to monitor TPN effectiveness.

Therapeutic Interventions

Actions/Interventions	Rationales
▲ Assist with insertion and maintenance of central venous or peripherally inserted central venous lines.	The osmolality of TPN solutions requires infusion into a large central vein with high-volume blood flow.
▲ Administer prescribed rate of TPN solution via infusion pump.	Giving TPN at the prescribed rate is necessary to meet nutritional needs and prevent complications. Falling behind on TPN administration deprives the patient of needed nutrition; boluses (or too-rapid administration) can precipitate a hyperglycemic crisis because the hormonal response (i.e., insulin) may not be available to allow use of the increased glucose load.
■ Assist with or encourage oral intake if indicated.	Patients may be fed orally in addition to TPN to maximize nutritional support. Patients may benefit psychologically from having oral intake, especially at shared mealtimes with family members.
▲ Refer to or collaborate with appropriate resources: nutritional support team, dietitian, pharmacy, home health nurse.	The risk for most complications that occur in the hospital is decreased when the administration of parenteral nutrition is supervised by an experienced nutritional support team.

Risk for Deficient Fluid Volume

Common Risk Factors

Hyperglycemia
Inability to respond to thirst mechanisms because of NPO status
Low serum protein level

■ = Independent   ▲ = Collaborative

Common Expected Outcome

Patient is normovolemic as evidenced by systolic BP greater than or equal to 90 mm Hg (or patient's baseline), absence of orthostasis, heart rate 60 to 90 beats/min, urine output of at least 30 mL/hr and normal skin turgor.

NOC Outcome
Fluid Balance
NIC Interventions
Fluid Monitoring; TPN Administration

Ongoing Assessment

Actions/Interventions	Rationales
■ Assess for signs and symptoms of fluid volume deficit: decreased blood pressure, increased heart rate, skin dryness, loss of turgor, high urine specific gravity.	Early identification of changes in fluid balance facilitates prompt interventions.
■ Monitor intake and output.	An intake consistently lower than output indicates fluid volume deficit and need for additional fluid to prevent dehydration. An intake higher than output may indicate fluid overload and result in pulmonary complications.
▲ Monitor blood glucose levels.	Hyperglycemia, caused by infusion of glucose in the TPN solution, can lead to hyperosmolar, nonketotic coma with subsequent dehydration secondary to osmotic diuresis.
▲ Monitor serum protein levels according to protocol, usually every 3 to 7 days.	Low serum protein level may lead to loss of fluids from intravascular spaces, secondary to low colloidal pressures.
■ During the first week of TPN administration, weigh patient daily and record weight; weigh weekly thereafter.	Daily weights are necessary to determine if nutritional goals are being met. Weight is also used to assess fluid volume status. Weight gain of more the 1/2-pound per day may indicate fluid retention.

Therapeutic Interventions

Actions/Interventions	Rationales
▲ Administer TPN at prescribed, constant rate; if infusion is interrupted, infuse 10% dextrose in water until TPN infusion is restarted.	This substitute infusion provides needed fluid in addition to protecting the patient from sudden hypoglycemia; hypoglycemia can result when the high glucose concentration to which the patient has metabolically adjusted is suddenly withdrawn.
▲ Encourage oral intake of fluids unless contraindicated. Administer maintenance or bolus fluids as prescribed, in addition to TPN.	Patients who are NPO and only receiving TPN may not be receiving adequate amounts of fluids, especially because TPN is initiated in low administration rates; therefore additional fluid may be required.

NANDA-I NDx **Risk for Excess Fluid Volume**

Common Risk Factors
Overinfusion of TPN
Inability to tolerate increased vascular load

Common Expected Outcome
Patient maintains normal fluid volume, as evidenced by balanced intake and output, absence of edema, and absence of excessive weight gain.

NOC Outcome
Fluid Balance
NIC Interventions
Fluid Monitoring; TPN Administration

Ongoing Assessment

Actions/Interventions	Rationales
■ Assess for signs and symptoms of fluid volume excess: • Edema	Edema occurs when fluid accumulates in the extravascular spaces. Edema usually begins in the fingers, facial area, and presacral area. Generalized edema, called anasarca, occurs later and involves the entire body. Weight gain in excess of 1 pound per day is an indication of fluid volume excess.
• Shortness of breath and crackles	These respiratory changes are caused by accumulation of fluid in the lungs.
• Jugular venous distention	Elevated central venous pressure is noticed first as distention of the jugular veins.
▲ Monitor serum sodium level.	Hypernatremia may cause or aggravate edema by holding fluid in the extravascular spaces.

Therapeutic Interventions

Actions/Interventions	Rationales
▲ If signs and symptoms of fluid volume excess occur, administer diuretics as prescribed.	Diuretics aid in the excretion of excess body fluids.
■ Position the patient in a semi-Fowler's or high-Fowler's position.	Elevating the head of the bed allows for ease in breathing. This position promotes pooling of fluid in the bases and makes more lung tissue available for gas exchange.
■ Handle edematous extremities with caution.	Edematous skin is more susceptible to injury and breakdown.

 ## Risk for Altered Body Composition

Common Risk Factors
Electrolyte imbalances:
• Hypokalemia (K less than 3.5 mEq/liter)
• Hyponatremia (Na less than 115 mEq/liter)
• Hypocalcemia (Ca less than 6.8 mg/dL)
• Hypomagnesemia (Mg less than 1.5 mg/dL)
• Hypophosphatemia (PO_4 less than 2.5 mg/dL)
Essential fatty acid deficiency (EFAD)
Hyperglycemia (glucose greater than 200 mg/dL)
Hypoglycemia (glucose less than 60 mg/dL)

Common Expected Outcomes
Patient maintains normal serum electrolyte levels.
Patient has normal blood glucose level.

NOC Outcome
Electrolyte and Acid-Base Balance
NIC Intervention
Electrolyte Monitoring

■ = Independent   ▲ = Collaborative

Ongoing Assessment

Actions/Interventions	Rationales
▲ Assess for signs and symptoms of electrolyte imbalance: • Hypokalemia • Alteration in muscle function (e.g., weakness, cramping) • Electrocardiogram changes (e.g., ventricular dysrhythmias, ST-segment depression, or U-wave) • Changes in level of consciousness (e.g., confusion, lethargy) • Abdominal distention and loss of bowel sounds • Hyponatremia • Decreased skin turgor, weakness, tremors or seizures, lethargy, confusion, nausea, vomiting • Hypocalcemia • Paresthesias, tetany, seizures, positive Chvostek's sign, irregular heart rate • Hypomagnesemia • Muscle weakness, cramping, twitching, tetany, seizures, irregular heart rate • Hypophosphatemia • Muscle weakness, changes in level of consciousness	When patients are receiving TPN and no other nutrition, there is a risk, especially early in TPN therapy, that all electrolyte needs may not be met. As physiological condition changes, patients may have altered needs for electrolytes and will require adjustment of the TPN solution.
■ Assess for signs and symptoms of essential fatty acid deficiency.	TPN solutions contain no fat; fat is a nutritional requirement that allows essential fat-soluble vitamins A, D, E, and K to be absorbed. Patients commonly receive Intralipid (intravenous [IV] fat) solutions at the same time as TPN.
• Tendency to bruise and thrombocytopenia	These findings are caused by coagulopathy secondary to inadequate vitamin K levels.
• Dry, scaly skin	This change relates to vitamin D and E deficiencies.
• Poor wound healing	This change relates to vitamin A and E deficiencies.
▲ Monitor serum triglyceride level twice weekly if patient is receiving Intralipid.	Patients receiving an intravenous fat emulsion should have serum triglyceride monitored until levels are stable and when changes are made in the amount of fat administered.
■ For patients receiving Intralipid therapy, monitor for signs and symptoms of fat embolism dyspnea, cyanosis, headache, flushing.	Fat embolism is a rare but serious complication of Intralipid therapy.
▲ Assess for hyperglycemia or hypoglycemia; notify physician. • Hypoglycemia • Glucose level less than 60 mg/dL • Weakness, agitation, clammy skin, tremors • Hyperglycemia • Glucose level greater than 200 mg/dL • Glycosuria • Thirst, polyuria, confusion	Blood glucose should be monitored frequently upon initiation of TPN, after any changes in insulin dose, and until measurements are stable.

Therapeutic Interventions

Actions/Interventions	Rationales
▲ Administer electrolyte replacement therapy as prescribed.	Electrolytes are supplied based on the patient's calculated need.
▲ Administer 10% or 20% Intralipid as ordered.	It is recommended that patients who are NPO and/or receiving only TPN for more than 2 weeks receive IV fat emulsions or Intralipid. Intralipid can also be given in absence of EFAD to provide extra calories.
■ When discontinuing TPN therapy, taper rate over 2 to 4 hours.	This measure prevents hypoglycemic episode caused by abrupt TPN withdrawal.

Actions/Interventions

▲ Use corrective actions if TPN solution stops or must be stopped suddenly:
  - For clotted catheter or if subsequent TPN bags are not available, hang 10% dextrose and water at the rate of TPN infusion.
  - For hyperglycemia, administer insulin as prescribed.
  - For emergency or cardiac arrest situations, stop TPN infusion; administer bolus doses of 50% dextrose.

Rationales

This solution provides a higher concentration of glucose to prevent sudden hypoglycemia.

This measure facilitates metabolic use of glucose.
These measures prevent hypoglycemia during resuscitation.

Related Care Plan

Risk for infection, p. 114

■ = Independent   ▲ = Collaborative

CHAPTER

7

Musculoskeletal Care Plans

Amputation, Lower Extremity

Generally there are about 11 lower limb amputations for every upper limb amputation performed. The level of the amputation depends on the amount of affected tissue, the ability of the blood supply to promote healing, and the prognosis for fitting a functional prosthesis. The leading cause of amputation is vascular disease, with an equal prevalence rate in men and women, who are usually in the 61- to 70-year-old age range. Clinical conditions that predispose the patient to amputation include peripheral vascular disease, diabetes, arterial sclerosis, and Buerger's disease. Another cause of amputation is trauma, the second leading cause of amputation, in which the accident itself may sever the limb or in which the limb is so damaged that it must be removed after the accident. Primary bone tumors occur in 4.5% of all amputations, and about 33% of these occur in the 16- to 20-year-old age range. The surgical procedure for an uncomplicated amputation rarely requires hospitalization for more than 5 days, but often the clinical situations surrounding amputation make these patients medically unstable. The portion of the limb that remains intact after the surgery is referred to as the *residual limb* or *stump* and may be fitted with an artificial device called a *prosthesis* that is used to take the place of the severed limb. Under those circumstances, the hospital course may be longer. The vast majority of recovery takes place out of the hospital, either in a rehabilitation center or on an outpatient basis. This care plan primarily covers information about patient care before and immediately after lower extremity surgery. Because nurses will encounter patients in various stages of recovery and rehabilitation, references are made about posthospitalization rehabilitation.

NANDA-I NDx **Anxiety, Preoperative**

Common Related Factors

Change in health status
Stress associated with surgery
Situational crisis: surgery

Defining Characteristics

Expressed concern about amputation
Expressed fear of amputation of wrong extremity
Irritability, restlessness, insomnia
Increased blood pressure, pulse, respirations

Common Expected Outcomes

Patient uses effective coping mechanisms.
Patient describes a reduction in the level of anxiety experienced.
Patient maintains desired level of role function and problem solving.

NOC Outcomes

Anxiety Self-Control; Coping

NIC Interventions

Anxiety Reduction; Presence; Calming Technique; Emotional Support

Ongoing Assessment

Actions/Interventions	**Rationales**
■ Assess the patient's level of anxiety.	The level of preoperative anxiety will vary based on the patient's understanding of the surgery, perception of surgical outcomes, previous surgery experience, and personality. Reactions to anxiety may range from mild to severe. The patient may appear calm but express nervousness with mild anxiety. As the level of anxiety increases, the patient may experience increased vital signs and report feeling overwhelmed by the anticipated surgery.
■ Determine the patient's concerns about the anticipated amputation.	Patients facing extremity amputation may express fear about the wrong extremity being amputated. Other concerns may include postoperative pain, body image changes, and changes in role function.
■ Determine how the patient uses defense mechanisms to cope with anxiety.	Assessment of defense mechanisms helps determine the effectiveness of coping strategies used by the patient. Some defense mechanisms may be highly adaptive in managing anxiety. Other defense mechanisms may lead to less-adaptive behavior with long-term use.

Therapeutic Interventions

Actions/Interventions	**Rationales**
■ Acknowledge awareness of the patient's anxiety.	Acknowledgment of the patient's feelings validates the feelings and communicates acceptance of those feelings.
■ Assure the patient that he or she is safe. Stay with the patient as necessary during preoperative visits by members of the surgical team.	The presence of a trusted person may help the patient feel less threatened.
■ Assist the patient in verbalizing anxious feelings and assessing the situation realistically.	Talking about anxiety-producing situations and anxious feelings can help the patient perceive the situation in a less-threatening manner.
■ Support the patient's use of coping strategies that the patient has found effective in the past.	Using anxiety-reduction strategies enhances the patient's sense of personal mastery and confidence.
■ Use simple language and brief statements when teaching the patient about what to expect before surgery.	Patients experiencing moderate to severe anxiety may be unable to comprehend anything more than simple, clear, and brief explanations.
▲ Collaborate with the surgeon to accurately mark the extremity to be amputated before the patient is moved to the operating room.	Being present with the patient during marking of the extremity may lessen the patient's concern of the wrong extremity being amputated. The Joint Commission (TJC) developed patient safety goals for hospital staff to mark the surgical site without ambiguity. This marking should take place while the patient is awake and aware.
■ Review with the patient all surgical consent forms to ensure that the extremity to be amputated is accurately reported.	Including the patient in record review allows the person to have a sense of control for ensuring that the correct extremity is amputated.
■ Teach the patient about measures used by the surgical team in the operating room, such as a time-out, to ensure that the correct extremity is amputated.	Teaching the patient about expectations to promote safety during the procedure may reduce the person's level of anxiety. TJC patient safety goals include performance standards to promote communication among all members of the surgical team at all stages of preparation for the procedure. These standards include a time-out before the start of the procedure to conduct a final assessment that the correct patient, site, and positioning are identified and that all consents, relevant information, and equipment are available.

■ = Independent   ▲ = Collaborative

Impaired Skin Integrity

Common Related Factors

Surgical incision
Skin breakdown caused by immobility
Abnormal wound healing
Surgical drain

Defining Characteristics

Redness
Pain
Edema
Drainage/discharge
Incomplete closure of skin flap

Common Expected Outcome

Patient manifests signs of optimal wound healing, as evidenced by intact skin, absence of skin breakdown, and a properly fitting prosthesis.

NOC Outcomes
Tissue Integrity: Skin and Mucous Membranes;
Wound Healing: Primary Intention

NIC Interventions
Amputation Care; Incision Site Care; Skin
Surveillance

Ongoing Assessment

Actions/Interventions	Rationales
■ Assess wound for:	
• Normal healing	Wound should be clean and dry, with edges of incision approximated and intact. Patients with diabetes or with poor circulation, such as the elderly, may face considerable obstacles in healing, and the course of wound healing may be anything but normal.
• Bleeding and hemorrhage	As with other surgical dressings, there should be no frank bleeding from the incisional site. A small amount of oozing from the incision is normal. Documentation of drainage characteristics helps other caregivers assess status change. Initially most postamputation dressings are pressure or pressure cast dressings. A surgical drain may be placed to remove fluid or blood that might interfere with granulation.
• Proper fit of postsurgical cast or pressure dressing	A rigid dressing or a cast may be applied to the residual limb immediately after the surgery and will remain in place for 7 to 10 days, until the sutures are removed. After removal of the sutures, a new cast or rigid dressing may be applied. Occasionally these casts are fit with a primitive prosthetic device that allows for early ambulation.
■ Monitor the residual limb every hour for the first 24 hours; observe for symptoms indicative of infection.	Signs of inflammation may be present. Edema, redness, pain, and tenderness should decrease over the next 3 to 5 postoperative days.
■ Check residual limb for signs of impaired circulation. Check pulses above the amputation site.	The residual limb should be warm and dry with no discoloration reflective of impaired circulation. Many patients experienced circulatory compromise before the amputation; this problem may continue to represent a threat to the residual and unaffected limb. Preserving the health in the residual limb is of utmost importance. Adaptation to a properly fitting prosthesis is dependent on having an adequate residual limb remaining for a good prosthetic fit and stability of the joints above the residual limb.

Actions/Interventions	Rationales
■ Assess for prolonged pressure on tissues associated with immobility.	Nonblanching redness over areas of pressures is an early indicator of impaired skin integrity. Early ambulation is of great psychological benefit to the patient. It will also prevent development of pressure sores and contractures from prolonged inactivity.
■ Monitor and report complaints of unusual pain.	Pain may reflect the development of postoperative infection.
■ Monitor vital signs, including temperature, according to postoperative protocol.	Tachycardia, tachypnea, and fever are early signs of infection. It is normal for the temperature and heart rate to be elevated in the first few days after surgery. Temperature should not exceed 38.3° C (101° F), and the heart rate should not exceed 120 beats/min.

Therapeutic Interventions

Actions/Interventions	Rationales
■ Elevate the residual limb for the first 24 hours.	Elevation of the residual limb for the first 24 hours reduces edema and promotes venous return. Prolonged elevation of the residual limb increases the risk of hip flexion contractures that may delay or interfere with rehabilitation and mobility.
■ Reinforce or change the dressing as needed; use aseptic technique. Note drainage. If a rigid dressing is not used, remove bandage on residual limb, cleanse wound frequently, and reapply dressings using a smooth figure-eight wrap.	Daily cleansing helps prevent infection. The proper application of elastic bandages in the figure eight helps reduce edema and helps shape the residual limb.
■ Instruct the patient in how to wrap the residual limb with compression bandages.	Compression bandages aid in shaping the residual limb in preparation for prosthesis fitting. Wrapping the compression dressing around the waist seems to be essential in keeping the bandage firmly in place, and compressing the medial thigh encourages the residual limb to shrink in a fashion that will promote good interface with the prosthetic socket.
■ Assist the patient with wrapping the residual limb; use an elastic bandage and when indicated a residual limb shrinker if wrapping is too difficult.	Patients may need time to adjust to seeing their residual limb and may balk at assuming responsibility for its care until they are ready.
■ Instruct the patient to report slippage of the cast, rigid dressing, or compression dressing.	Slippage of the cast or rigid dressing may reflect underlying pathology such as infection or incomplete closure of skin flap, which would interrupt healing.
■ Discuss weight-bearing limitations and their importance.	These restrictions prevent skin breakdown and facilitate proper wound healing. The patient's limb may be non–weight bearing for 4 to 6 weeks after surgery; other patients will begin partial weight bearing on the residual limb soon after the surgery. Factors that influence how soon weight bearing takes place include the indications for the amputation, the level and the type of the amputation, and the repair/preparation of the residual limb.
■ Teach signs and symptoms of residual limb breakdown.	Early detection of residual limb breakdown allows for prompt treatment. Complications may jeopardize the patient's rehabilitation plan and make further amputation necessary.

■ = Independent   ▲ = Collaborative

Impaired Physical Mobility

Common Related Factors

Activity limitations caused by loss of body part
Change in center of gravity creating balance problems
Postoperative protocol
Difficulty in using assistive devices
Pain on mobility
Fatigue

Defining Characteristics

Inability to move purposefully within environment
Reluctance to attempt movement
Limited range of motion (ROM)

Common Expected Outcomes

Patient performs physical activity independently or within limits of amputation.
Patient is free of complications of immobility, as evidenced by intact skin, absence of thrombophlebitis, normal bowel pattern, and clear breath sounds.
Patient demonstrates use of adaptive techniques that promote ambulation and transfer.

NOC Outcomes

Mobility; Ambulation: Wheelchair; Coordinated Movement: Transfer Performance

NIC Interventions

Exercise Therapy: Ambulation; Energy Management; Exercise Therapy: Balance

Ongoing Assessment

Actions/Interventions	Rationales
■ Assess bed positioning and transfer skills.	Learning transfer techniques helps reestablish the patient's independence and promotes a feeling of security when moving in bed and ambulating.
■ Assess nutritional status.	Adequate calories and protein are needed for healing and energy for ambulation and transfer techniques. Performing transfer techniques and performing activities with a prosthetic device consume more calories and take a greater physical effort than normal ambulation.
■ Assess activity tolerance.	A patient who had normal activity tolerance before the amputation may find crutch walking and walking with a prosthesis more tiring and requiring strengthening of certain muscle groups to support movement.
■ Assess understanding of postoperative activity and exercise program.	Postoperatively, ROM exercises will be encouraged in all unaffected extremities. Some patients will begin to ambulate soon after surgery. Other patients will remain non–weight bearing until the temporary prosthesis is made 4 to 6 weeks after surgery. At that time physical therapists will implement a program of functional training with the patient and the prosthesis.
■ Assess the patient's knowledge of ambulating and moving with assistive devices.	Patients may already know how to crutch walk, but balance is significantly affected after an amputation. Attention must be paid to developing an awareness of new physical boundaries after the amputation.
▲ Monitor whether patient is a candidate for a prosthesis.	This decision involves consideration of type and level of amputation, age and strength of the patient, the type of function the patient is attempting to regain, and perhaps most of all the motivation of the patient. Older or debilitated patients may not be able to handle a prosthesis; a wheelchair may be more appropriate. On the other hand, no assumptions should be made about older patients being too old to adapt to a prosthesis.

Actions/Interventions	**Rationales**
■ Assess the impact of the loss of sensory information that was perceived via the amputated part.	The lack of sensory feedback may be the major limiting factor in the effective use of a prosthesis. Other factors that may exaggerate the effect of the sensory loss are the age of the patient and the existence of other sensory deficits (e.g., vision or hearing deficits, bilateral amputations).

Therapeutic Interventions

Actions/Interventions	**Rationales**
■ Reinforce and teach prevention of postoperative complications (flexion or abduction contracture, and external rotation of hip): avoid sitting for long periods; avoid use of pillows under residual limb; maintain proper alignment; avoid flexing residual limb while sitting or lying.	Patients often develop contractures of the affected extremity, which complicates rehabilitation and the recovery period.
■ Reinforce and teach proper positioning:	
• Have the patient lie on his or her back, keeping the pelvis level and the hip joint extended.	This positioning prevents contractions.
• Maintain neutral rotation. Use or teach the patient to use a trochanter roll to prevent external rotation.	The residual limb will have the tendency to externally rotate.
• Have the patient lie prone with lower extremity in extension for 30 minutes three or four times a day.	This activity prevents positioning deformities (flexion contraction).
■ Instruct the patient to perform ROM exercises:	Exercise therapy maintains and strengthens muscle groups. ROM exercises are directed toward maintaining normal joint mobility. Disuse can cause permanent shortening of the muscle, resulting in contractures. Quadriceps settings are performed for above- and below-the-knee amputations. Straight leg raises are performed with the knee fully extended for below-the-knee amputations. Hip adductions are done for above-the-knee amputations. Patients will need to continue the muscle-strengthening program throughout the rehabilitation program and beyond.
• Adduction exercises of lower extremity 10 times every 4 hours after the first 24 hours	
• Hamstring tightening exercises in prone position 10 times every 4 hours after the first 24 hours	
■ Instruct patient to be sitting up in chair two to three times a day after the first 24 hours.	This activity helps the patient develop skill with transfer techniques.
■ Encourage early ambulation with assistive devices. The patient should be able to stand within 48 hours. Ambulate with crutches at least three times daily.	Early ambulation promotes confidence about regaining independence. The patient may use a walker, crutches, or wheelchair as appropriate.
■ Teach crutch walking to patients with no previous experience with crutches. Instruct patients in the use of wheelchairs, walkers, support bars, and a trapeze.	Learning correct technique with assistive devices promotes safety and reduces the risk for falls.
■ Teach the patient not to bend knee over the bed or edge of the chair if the patient had a below-the-knee amputation.	Allowing the residual limb to hang in a dependent position decreases venous return and increases edema. Flexion contractures may occur if the residual limb remains bent.
■ Provide a trapeze bar in bed.	A trapeze bar increases mobility in bed and allows the patient to be more independent.
■ Assist the patient with transfers and ambulation until able to perform safely. Encourage the patient to ask for needed assistance.	Assistance may be required to prevent new injuries that would complicate recovery. Muscle weakness and impaired balance after a lower extremity amputation may result in an injury. The patient's center of gravity changes following a lower extremity amputation. Adjustment to the change in center of gravity initially requires conscious effort to maintain balance.

■ = Independent   ▲ = Collaborative

Actions/Interventions

■ Teach the patient to perform activities of daily living (ADLs) to foster independence. If the patient is not a candidate for a prosthesis, instruct in self-care activities from a wheelchair.

■ Instruct the patient awaiting a prosthesis regarding the need for a long-term functional training program.

Rationales

The nurse will coordinate activities of different disciplines to maximize the patient's return to optimal function. The disciplines involved will include (but not be limited to) occupational therapy and job training, rehabilitation and physical therapy, work of the prosthetic maker, ongoing medical care and psychological support services, and financial assistance programs.

It may take several months for a lower extremity to reach a point where a final device may be fitted. This period allows for the patient to adapt progressively to wearing a prosthesis and to work toward regaining function of the remaining limb.

NANDA-I NDx **Disturbed Body Image**

Common Related Factors

Loss of body part
Loss of independence
Inability to maintain prior lifestyle

Defining Characteristics

Verbal preoccupation with changed body part
Refusal to discuss change
Actual change in function
Change in social behavior

Common Expected Outcomes

Patient demonstrates enhanced body image and self-esteem, as evidenced by ability to look at residual limb and talk about amputation and the ability to provide self-care to the residual limb (as appropriate).
Patient reports increased independence in the performance of activities.
Patient reports resuming aspects of his or her life or role that may have necessitated relearning after the amputation.

NOC Outcomes

Acceptance: Health Status; Body Image; Grief Resolution

NIC Interventions

Amputation Care; Body Image Enhancement; Grief Work Facilitation

---

Ongoing Assessment

Actions/Interventions

■ Assess the patient's perception of change in structure or function from loss of body part.

■ Assess the patient's feelings about using a mechanical part to replace or substitute for a missing body part.

Rationales

The acute (versus chronic) nature of the factors requiring amputation, the patient's prior health and age, the feelings and responses of the significant others, and the patient's lifestyle and work impact the adjustment to amputation.

Artificial limbs are clearly mechanical devices that never feel or perform like a real body part. There is always some loss of function, and sensory changes are massive and may include some low-level noise that may draw further attention to the operation of the prosthesis. Patients may be dependent on a prosthesis, but they may also despise the experience of wearing and using one.

Actions/Interventions	**Rationales**
■ Note the patient's behavior regarding the actual or perceived changed body part or function. Assess the patient's ability to use effective coping mechanisms.	There is a broad range of behaviors associated with body image disturbance, ranging from totally ignoring the altered structure or function to preoccupation with it. At the heart of the adaptive process for the patient with an amputation is the need to accept the loss of the limb and to realize that the loss is permanent. Patients will express a wide range of feelings in response to their loss, including anger, rage, sadness, helplessness, and hopelessness. Patients will be likely to fall back on known coping skills, including humor, denial, distraction, and expression of thoughts and feelings in talk and writing. Previously successful coping skills may not be effective in the present situation.
■ Assess the patient's perception of the impact of the amputation on his or her ability to perform self-care measures and on his or her social behavior, personal relationships, and occupational activities.	For some patients who have undergone an amputation, the psychological and social aspects of amputation are experienced as far greater consequences of the surgical procedure.
■ Note the frequency of the patient's self-critical remarks.	Negative statements about the affected body part indicate limited ability to integrate the change into the patient's self-concept.
■ Assess the need for a support group.	Support groups are usually a component of most formal rehabilitation programs; however, patients may require this kind of intervention earlier, in the immediate postoperative period.

Therapeutic Interventions

Actions/Interventions	**Rationales**
■ Encourage verbalization of feelings.	Loss of a limb requires significant psychological adjustment. It is worthwhile to encourage the patient to separate feelings about changes in body structure and/or function from feelings about self-worth. Expression of feelings can enhance the person's coping strategies.
■ Allow the patient time to work through grief stages.	Working through stages of grief over loss of a body part or function is normal and typically involves a period of denial, the length of which varies between individuals. Patients will do this at their own pace and in their own way. Accommodation to amputation is a lifetime process for some patients.
■ Listen and support verbalized feelings about body and lifestyle changes.	These changes will be massive. There is no way to prepare patients for the impact this will have on their lives. It is important that the health care provider not minimize or negate the patient's experiences.
■ Encourage the patient to participate fully in design of the therapeutic regimen.	This fosters a sense of still being in control of one's own life.
■ Encourage family members to support the patient and allow independence.	A grieving family may have a need to take care of the patient, but this response may feed into an unhealthy dependence, setting a precedent that is difficult to disrupt later in the recovery period and that communicates the concept of the patient as damaged.
■ Encourage the patient to participate in the care of the residual limb when able.	Such activity promotes independence and helps the patient's adjustment to a new body image.
■ Allow the patient sufficient time to perform ADLs.	Amputees experience an overall increase in fatigue as they perform even normal activities. In addition to this, conscious attention must be paid to functions that one carried out on a fairly autonomic level when the neuromuscular system was intact. Attention to this level of detail is exhausting and limits the number of activities that can be carried out at the same time.

■ = Independent   ▲ = Collaborative

Actions/Interventions	Rationales
■ Encourage use of clothing to enhance appearance.	Amputation is a very public disability. It may be the first thing people notice about an individual. Shock and embarrassment are often initial responses of the public to seeing an individual with an amputation. Attractive clothing can enhance a patient's self-image and confidence.
■ Discuss use of a prosthesis for both cosmetic and functional purposes.	Both are equally acceptable reasons to use a prosthesis. Some people have more than one device, one for cosmetic use and one for functional use.
▲ Consult social services for support groups.	Persons who have themselves experienced an amputation can offer a unique type of support that is perceived as helpful by patients. It is often possible to match up individuals by age, sex, and education; in some situations, career matches can be made. Opportunities for positive feedback and success in social situations may hasten adaptation.

 NANDA-I NDx **Acute Pain and Chronic Pain**

Common Related Factors

Phantom sensation
Phantom pain
Surgical procedure
Decreased mobility
Prosthesis fit

Defining Characteristics

Verbal complaints
Nonverbal signs of pain
Facial expressions of discomfort
Protection of residual limb
Refusal to be mobile
Refusal to participate in rehabilitation
Crying, moaning
Restlessness
Withdrawal, irritability

Common Expected Outcomes

Patient reports pain at a level less than 3 to 4 on a 0 to 10 rating scale.
Patient implements a pain management plan that includes pharmacological and nonpharmacological strategies.
Patient verbalizes understanding of phantom limb sensation.
Patient verbalizes that phantom pain is adequately relieved.

NOC Outcomes
Pain Control; Medication Response
NIC Interventions
Analgesic Administration; Pain Management

Ongoing Assessment

Actions/Interventions	Rationales
■ Assess the patient's description of pain. Have the patient rate the pain on the pain scale.	Thorough assessment of pain characteristics will assist the nurse in differentiating phantom limb sensation from incision pain. The nurse needs to understand the type of pain the patient is experiencing in order to select appropriate pain management interventions. Pain is what the patient states it is. Early detection and intervention promote patient comfort.
■ Assess for nonverbal signs of pain. Observe for tense posture, tightening fists, diaphoresis, and increased pulse rate.	Behavioral pain responses may be the only indication of acute pain.

Actions/Interventions	Rationales
■ Assess the patient's understanding of the occurrence and management of phantom limb sensations.	Phantom limb sensations are the painless awareness of the presence of the amputated part and are often experienced as a tingling sensation caused by nerve stimulation proximal to the level of amputation but perceived as coming from the amputated limb. These sensations are frequently experienced as incomplete. In a lower limb amputation, sensations in the foot will be experienced more strongly than the leg and the great toe more strongly than the other toes.
■ Assess understanding of phantom pain.	When phantom limb sensations become disagreeable and painful, they are called *phantom pain*. Phantom limb pain may be continuous or occasional, with a wide range in the intensity experienced by the patient. Patients may experience the pain as a cramping or squeezing sensation; a burning sensation; or a sharp, shooting pain. Phantom limb pain tends to disappear over time, but phantom limb sensation tends to remain indefinitely.
■ Assess the fit of the prosthesis to determine whether the fit is resulting in the development of pressure points.	A properly fitting prosthetic device is almost always experienced as uncomfortable by the patient. Furthermore, prosthetic devices are fitted over tissues that would not normally bear weight. Patients will experience significant discomfort until these tissues become adjusted. Assessments as to the fit of the device should be made by the device maker.

Therapeutic Interventions

Actions/Interventions	Rationales
▲ Provide medications as prescribed for surgical pain relief; evaluate effectiveness and modify doses as needed.	Patients have a right to adequate pain relief. Bone surgery is extremely painful and generally requires higher levels of narcotic relief. Phantom limb pain is real pain, and the patient requires appropriate analgesics as part of a total pain management program. Patients receiving oral analgesics or intramuscular injections could benefit from analgesics delivered via the epidural route or through intravenous patient-controlled analgesia.
▲ Use additional comfort measures as appropriate to relieve phantom sensations: diversional activities; relaxation techniques; position change, exercise; ROM of residual limb; application of pressure to residual limb; and transcutaneous electrical nerve stimulation.	Long-term management of phantom limb sensations includes the use of nonpharmacological measures. Current research indicates that these measures are effective.

Deficient Knowledge

Common Related Factor	Defining Characteristics
New condition	Expressed concerns about home management Questions about treatment Questions about rehabilitation/prosthesis management

■ = Independent ▲ = Collaborative

Common Expected Outcomes

Patient verbalizes understanding of residual limb care.
Patient verbalizes understanding of the rehabilitation program.
Patient describes course of prosthetic fitting.

NOC Outcomes
Knowledge: Disease Process; Knowledge: Treatment Regimen

NIC Interventions
Teaching: Disease Process; Teaching: Psycho-motor Skills

Ongoing Assessment

Actions/Interventions	Rationales
■ Assess knowledge of the following: care of residual limb, phantom limb pain management, signs and symptoms of circulatory problems, prosthetic care, follow-up appointments, and community resources.	Accurate understanding of self-care issues facilitates smooth transition from hospital to home.

Therapeutic Interventions

Actions/Interventions	Rationales
■ Inform of discharge medications, exercises, and follow-up appointments.	This information promotes effective self-care by the patient.
■ Reinforce teaching for care of residual limb (e.g., wrapping the residual limb, skin care, and weight-bearing limitations).	Accurate self-care measures promote optimal rehabilitation. The patient may need to continue wrapping the residual limb to promote effective shaping and successful fit of a prosthesis.
■ Provide information for phantom limb pain or sensation management.	Phantom limb sensations may continue for several months or longer.
■ Discuss signs and symptoms of circulatory problems. Reinforce the need for the patient to protect the residual limb from infection and circulatory compromise or damage.	Signs of infection, circulatory compromise, or skin breakdown should be reported to the physician immediately.
■ Reinforce teaching about care of prosthesis if applicable.	Some patients may go home with a temporary prosthesis. The patient needs to understand how to maintain the prosthesis in proper working order.
▲ Coordinate social services, physical therapy, and occupational therapy.	Such services enhance adequate discharge planning and home treatments after discharge.
▲ Contact social services for information about community resources and support groups (e.g., home care nurses, homemakers, outpatient therapy).	Special assistance may be necessary to help the patient accept and adapt to the amputation.

Related Care Plans

Ineffective coping, p. 49
Risks for falls, p. 60
Risk for infection, p. 114
Ineffective tissue perfusion, p. 199

Arthritis, Rheumatoid

Rheumatoid arthritis (RA) is a chronic, systemic, inflammatory disease. RA is classified as an autoimmune disorder that develops as a result of interactions between autoantibodies and immunoglobulins. Rheumatoid factor (RF) is the primary autoantibody that acts against immunoglobulin G (IgG). The disorder usually presents as symmetrical synovitis primarily of the small joints of the body. The diagnosis of RA is based on the presence of criteria established by the American Rheumatism Association. These criteria include morning joint stiffness lasting at least 1 hour, soft tissue swelling of three or more joint areas, simultaneous symmetrical joint swelling, subcutaneous rheumatoid nodules, presence of rheumatoid factor, and radiographic evidence of joint erosion or periarticular osteopenia. Synovial fluid analysis may be done to confirm the diagnosis of RA. Extraarticular manifestations may include rheumatoid nodules, pericarditis, scleritis, and arteritis. RA is characterized by periods of remission and prolonged exacerbation of the disease, during which the joints can become damaged. In the initial phase of RA, the synovial membrane becomes inflamed and thickens, associated with an increased production of synovial fluid. As this tissue develops, it causes erosion and destruction of the joint capsule and subchondral bone. These processes result in decreased joint motion, deformity, and finally ankylosis, or joint immobilization. Anyone can develop RA, including children and older adults, but it usually strikes people in the young to middle years. RA strikes women at a 3:1 ratio compared with men and occurs in all ethnic groups worldwide. The specific cause of RA is unknown, but the tendency to develop it may be inherited. The gene that seems to control RA is one of the genes that control the immune system, but not everyone who has this gene goes on to develop RA. The disease behaves differently in each person who contracts it. In some people the joint inflammation that marks RA will be mild with long periods of remission between "exacerbations," or increased periods of disease activity. For others the activity of the disease may seem continuous and worsening as time passes. The goals of treatment are to relieve pain and inflammation and to reduce joint damage. The long-term goal of treatment is to maintain or restore use in the joints damaged by RA. This care plan focuses on the outpatient management of patients who are affected by RA.

NANDA-I
NDx **Deficient Knowledge**

Common Related Factors

New disease/procedures
Unfamiliarity with treatment regimen
Lack of interest/denial

Defining Characteristics

Multiple questions
Lack of questions
Verbalized misconceptions
Verbalized lack of knowledge
Inaccurate follow-through of previous instructions

Common Expected Outcome

Patient verbalizes understanding of RA and treatment.

NOC Outcomes
Knowledge: Disease Process; Knowledge:
   Medication; Knowledge: Treatment Regimen
NIC Interventions
Teaching: Disease Process; Teaching:
   Prescribed Medications

■ = Independent   ▲ = Collaborative

Ongoing Assessment

Actions/Interventions	Rationales
■ Assess the patient's level of knowledge of RA and its treatment.	Patients will be responsible for evaluating their condition on a daily basis to make determinations about exercise, the use of analgesics, and seeking medical intervention.

Therapeutic Interventions

Actions/Interventions	Rationales
■ Introduce or reinforce disease process information: unknown cause, chronicity of RA, process of inflammation, joint and other organ involvement, remissions and exacerbations, and control versus cure.	Patients must have a comprehensive understanding of the disease to actively participate in their own care.
Initial Presentation With Symptoms of Joint Inflammation	Simultaneous, symmetrical joint inflammation differentiates RA from other forms of arthritis. This inflammatory process is not limited to the joints; progressive changes occur in the heart, with pericarditis, congestive heart failure, and cardiomyopathies developing; in the skin; in the kidneys, with chronic renal failure developing; and in the lungs, with chronic restrictive pulmonary disease and repeated infections occurring.
• Patients may feel systemically ill with additional symptoms of fever, chills, loss of appetite, decreased energy, and weight loss.	
• The synovial lining of the joints and tendons becomes inflamed, with a progressive proliferation of the synovium within and outside of the joint capsule itself (pannus formation).	
• Joint inflammation may affect more than one joint at a time, and usually the inflammation affects the same joint bilaterally.	
• Cartilage eventually becomes involved; the inflammatory process erodes the surface between the bone ends, leaving the surfaces exposed.	
• Further inflammation results in the development of bone fissures, cysts on the bones, spurs, fibrosis, and shortening of the tendons.	
Diagnosis	
• Laboratory tests:	
• Anti–cyclic citrullinated peptide antibodies (anti-CCP)	Anti-CCP is a predictive diagnostic marker for development of RA.
• Rheumatoid factor (or the RA antibody)	It is important to note that not all people with RA will have a positive antibody titer. No single laboratory test is capable of ruling out RA.
• Hemoglobin and hematocrit	Patients with RA may develop normocytic, hypochromic anemia. Iron deficiency anemia may be present.
• Serum complement	This laboratory value is decreased during periods of exacerbation.
• Erythrocyte sedimentation rate (ESR) • C-reactive protein	Laboratory tests should include acute phase reactors (ESR and C-reactive protein). These two tests are good indicators of the inflammatory activity of the disease.
• Liver function tests and kidney function tests	These tests help facilitate rheumatoid arthritis monitoring, early detection of disease complications, and side effects of treatments.
• X-ray films of the hands, feet, and chest are recommended initially, and x-ray films of the feet and hands should be repeated annually for the first 3 years of the disease.	X-ray films should be examined for the presence of bony erosions, which are more frequent at the beginning of the disease process. Erosions of the hands or feet develop in about 70% of patients by the end of the first 2 to 3 years. Their presence and the speed of onset are associated with poorer outcomes. A chest x-ray film is recommended for initial evaluation and to identify the appearance of possible problems during the course of the disease and its treatment.

Actions/Interventions	Rationales
• Joint arthroscopy	Arthroscopic examinations are used to evaluate for characteristic changes in synovial fluid. Cartilage destruction and pannus formation may be identified.

General Treatment/Management Guidelines

Actions/Interventions	Rationales
• Adequate sleep, at least 8 to 10 hours each night with periods of rest during the day	Sleep enhances immune system function to reduce inflammation. Fatigue contributes to increased joint pain.
• Rest of the affected joints with splinting	Splinting is sometimes helpful in protecting joints, which can become overused during the course of daily activities.
• Application of hot or cold packs on painful, inflamed joints	Alternating use of hot and cold is sometimes helpful in reducing the local inflammatory process in the joints. Individual patients may prefer heat over cold or vice versa.
• Physical therapy especially designed for the individual patient	This therapy provides a balance between maintaining function in a threatened joint while respecting the inflammatory nature of the disease.
• Relearning how to perform activities of daily living (ADLs) and professional roles within the limitations of the disease (may require the help of an occupational therapist)	As joint deformity progresses and joint mobility decreases, the patient may benefit from using assistive devices to complete ADLs, such as using long-handled eating utensils. The occupational therapist can evaluate the patient's needs and provide devices that can be adjusted to fit the individual patient.
• Prescribed medications	Single drug therapy is rarely effective. Patients may be taking many drugs and need to understand the different methods of administration and the potential side effects. Patients usually benefit from a combination drug plan that includes a nonsteroidal antiinflammatory drug (NSAID) and a disease-modifying antirheumatic drug (DMARD) or a biological response modifier (BRM). Short-term therapy with corticosteroids may be included during exacerbations.
• Acetaminophen	Simple analgesics such as acetaminophen may be used first. They relieve pain but have no effect on inflammation.
• Salicylates: aspirin, salsalate, magnesium salicylate, choline salicylate, and combination salicylate	These drugs relieve pain in the mild to moderate range and have an antiinflammatory effect. Side effects include gastrointestinal (GI) disturbances, increased risk for bleeding, and tinnitus.
• NSAIDs: phenylacetic acid, oxicam, indole, propionic acid, and pyrazolone derivatives	NSAIDs are recommended at disease onset, when a new DMARD is introduced, and when uncontrolled isolated symptoms persist despite good response to antirheumatic drugs. Patients should be aware of the risks and benefits of using NSAIDs. Potential complications include GI and cardiovascular risks. NSAIDs relieve pain and reduce minor inflammation, but they are not strong enough to alter the long-term damaging effects of rheumatoid arthritis on the joints.
• Selective NSAIDs, cyclooxygenase-2 (COX-2) inhibitors (celecoxib)	These drugs act by reducing prostaglandin synthesis via inhibition of cyclooxygenase-2. People who have a history of coronary artery disease, angina, a stroke, or are at a higher-than-average-risk for these diseases and who are not taking aspirin may want to avoid the COX-2 inhibitors until more information is available on the safety of this class of drugs.

Actions/Interventions	Rationales
• Corticosteroids: cortisone, hydrocortisone, prednisone, triamcinolone, methylprednisolone, dexamethasone, and betamethasone	Corticosteroids are used when NSAIDs are contraindicated or have a high risk for adverse side effects, as bridge therapy until the onset of disease-modifying antirheumatic drug therapy, or when NSAIDs do not adequately control inflammation. Steroids have strong antiinflammatory effects. Steroids may be taken orally, be administered intravenously, or be injected directly into a joint. Steroids promptly improve symptoms of RA such as pain and stiffness, and they decrease joint tenderness and swelling. However, if used alone, steroids have only a modest effect on decreasing arthritis damage.
• DMARDs: hydroxychloroquine (Plaquenil), methotrexate (Rheumatrex), gold salts (Ridaura, Solganal), sulfasalazine (Azulfidine), azathioprine (Imuran), leflunomide (Arava), and cyclosporine (Sandimmune, Neoral)	These drugs substantially reduce inflammation of rheumatoid arthritis, although DMARDs act slowly when compared with steroids. Studies suggest that DMARDs can reduce or prevent joint damage, preserve structure and function, and enable a person to continue his or her daily activities. Several weeks to months of treatment are often necessary before the effects of DMARDs become evident.
	Because of its efficacy and toxicity profile, methotrexate is the recommended initial treatment in all patients who have not previously received DMARDs.
• Biological response modifiers (BRM): etanercept (Enbrel), adalimumab (Humira), infliximab (Remicade), anakinra (Kineret), abatacipt (Orencia)	This class of drugs treats RA by interfering with signaling pathways involved in inflammation. The onset of action of these medications is more rapid than that of DMARDs. Because of the cost of these medications and uncertainty about their long-term effects, they are often reserved for people who have not responded fully to DMARDs and for people who cannot tolerate DMARDs in doses large enough to control inflammation.
	These drugs interfere with the ability to fight infection; these should not be used in people with serious infections such as kidney infection or pneumonia.
■ Stress the importance of long-term follow-up.	Patients with RA should be monitored for an indefinite period of time. Patients in complete remission should be seen every 6 months or yearly; patients with recent disease onset, frequent exacerbations, or persistent activity should be seen on demand (in general every 1 to 2 months) depending on the treatment used and disease activity until control is achieved. Aging may alter hepatic function, thus decreasing the metabolization of drugs that are broken down in the liver. The possibility of adverse effects and drug interactions should be monitored in older patients.
■ Encourage the patient to discuss new or over-the-counter treatments with health care workers.	The patient may be vulnerable to fads or advertisements claiming curative effects of high-dose vitamins, special health foods, or copper bracelets.
■ Inform the patient of resources such as the Arthritis Foundation.	This is a comprehensive resource center for patients suffering with RA.
▲ Suggest referral to an arthritis specialist for optimal treatment.	This practitioner may be in the best position to understand the nuances of an individual's disease, because so much of it is seen within the practice. In addition, the rheumatologist will be aware of the latest treatment regimens.

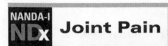

NANDA-I NDx Joint Pain

Common Related Factors

Inflammation associated with increased disease activity
Degenerative changes secondary to longstanding inflammation

Defining Characteristics

Patient report of pain
Guarding on motion of affected joints
Facial mask of pain
Moaning or other sounds associated with pain and movement

Common Expected Outcomes

Patient reports pain at a level less than 3 to 4 on a 0 to 10 rating scale.
Patient implements a pain management plan that includes pharmacological and nonpharmacological strategies.
Patient engages in desired activities without an increase in pain level.

NOC Outcomes

Pain Control; Medication Response

NIC Interventions

Pain Management; Analgesic Administration

Ongoing Assessment

Actions/Interventions	Rationales
■ Assess for signs of joint inflammation (redness, warmth, swelling, decreased motion).	Local signs of inflammation may be the first to manifest. Joint swelling usually accompanies joint pain.
■ Evaluate location and description of pain.	Pain occurs primarily in small joints, such as hands, wrists, fingers, and ankles. Assessment includes a "joint count" of the number of joints affected by pain and swelling.
■ Assess interference with lifestyle.	Joint pain and decreased range of motion (ROM) can limit the fine motor and gross motor movements required for completing ADLs.

Therapeutic Interventions

Actions/Interventions	Rationales
■ Instruct the patient to take antiinflammatory medication as prescribed.	Antiinflammatory drugs should not be taken on an empty stomach (they can irritate the stomach lining and lead to ulcer disease).
■ Encourage the patient to continue with DMARD/BRM therapy.	Drug therapy to manage the autoimmune basis of RA can reduce episodes of joint pain and swelling. Some drugs may take weeks or months for a full therapeutic effect to be evident.
▲ Suggest the use of nonnarcotic analgesic as necessary.	Central-acting analgesics such as narcotics are not as effective in relieving inflammatory pain.
■ Encourage the patient to monitor position and to always maintain anatomically correct alignment of the body.	Muscle spasms can result from nonfunctional body alignment and result in pain and predispose to deformity formation.
■ Instruct to:	
• Not use knee gatch or pillows to prop knees.	Prolonged knee flexion can lead to decreased ROM and increased pain.
• Use small flat pillow under head.	It is important not to increase the flexion of the neck, which could lead to further deformity and neck strain.
• Wear splints as prescribed.	Splints provide rest to inflamed joints and may reduce muscle spasm.
■ Recommend use of hot (e.g., heating pad) or cold packs on painful, inflamed joints.	Alternating use of hot and cold is sometimes helpful in reducing the inflammatory response in the joints. Individual patients may prefer heat over cold or vice versa.

■ = Independent   ▲ = Collaborative

Actions/Interventions

- Encourage use of ambulation aids when pain is related to weight bearing.

- Suggest that the patient apply a bed cradle.

- Encourage use of alternative methods of pain control such as relaxation, guided imagery, or distraction.

Rationales

Some of the weight normally transferred to the affected extremity can be shifted to the ambulation device; the device may also improve balance.

Protective devices keep pressure of bed covers off inflamed lower extremities and prevent the development of contractures.

These measures may augment other medications to diminish pain.

NDx Joint Stiffness

Common Related Factors

Inflammation associated with increased disease activity
Degenerative changes secondary to longstanding inflammation

Common Expected Outcomes

Patient verbalizes decrease in stiffness.
Patient is able to participate in self-care activities.

Defining Characteristics

Patient's complaint of joint stiffness
Guarding on motion of affected joints
Refusal to participate in usual self-care activities
Decreased functional ability

NOC Outcomes
Pain Control; Coordinated Movement
NIC Interventions
Pain Management; Heat Therapy

Ongoing Assessment

Actions/Interventions

- Assess the patient's description of stiffness:
  - Location: What specific joints are affected?
  - Timing (morning, night, all day)
  - Length of time the stiffness persists

  - Relationship to activities (aggravate or alleviate stiffness)

  - Measures used to alleviate stiffness

- Assess how stiffness interferes with lifestyle.

Rationales

Stiffness may rotate among various joints involved in RA.
Stiffness characteristically occurs on awaking in the morning.
Stiffness usually lasts 30 minutes; it may last longer as the disease progresses.
Stiffness is usually aggravated by prolonged inactivity; it may be precipitated by joint motion.
Most patients will have rituals that they perform to reduce pain (e.g., taking a warm bath, foot soaks).
RA is a chronic disease with periods of remission and exacerbation.

Therapeutic Interventions

Actions/Interventions

- Encourage the patient to take a 15-minute warm shower or bath on arising. Localized heat (hand soaking) is also useful. Encourage the patient to perform ROM exercises after the shower or bath, two repetitions per joint.
- Suggest that the patient plan sufficient time for performing activities and avoid scheduling tasks or therapy when stiffness is present.

Rationales

Warm water reduces stiffness and relieves pain and muscle spasms. ROM is important to maintain joint mobility.

Performing tasks while joints are stiff depletes energy, because the functional capacity of the joints may be reduced. Performing simple tasks may take longer. Excessive movement at these times may increase the inflammatory response.

Actions/Interventions

- Instruct the patient to take antiinflammatory medications in the morning. Remind the patient that antiinflammatory drugs should not be taken on an empty stomach.

- Suggest use of elastic gloves (e.g., Isotoner) at night.
- Remind the patient to avoid prolonged periods of inactivity.

Rationales

The first dose of the day should be taken as early in the morning as possible, with a small snack. The sooner the patient takes the medication, the sooner stiffness will abate. Antiinflammatory agents are caustic to the gastric mucosa.
Supportive gloves may decrease hand stiffness.
Muscle activity must be balanced with rest, or the joint will become frozen and muscles will atrophy.

 NANDA-I NDx

Impaired Physical Mobility

Common Related Factors

Pain
Stiffness
Fatigue
Psychosocial factors
Altered joint function
Muscle weakness

Common Expected Outcomes

Patient performs physical activity independently within limits of RA.
Patient demonstrates use of adaptive techniques that promote ambulation and transfer.

Defining Characteristics

Patient's description of difficulty with purposeful movement
Decreased ability to transfer and ambulate
Reluctance to attempt movement
Decreased muscle strength
Decreased ROM

NOC Outcomes
Ambulation; Self-Care: ADLs
NIC Interventions
Exercise Therapy: Ambulation; Self-Care Assistance

Ongoing Assessment

Actions/Interventions

- Assess the patient's description of what type of movement aggravates or alleviates the condition and to what degree these things interfere with lifestyle.
- Observe the patient's ability to ambulate and to move all joints functionally.
- Assess the need for analgesics before activity.
- Observe the patient's ability to bathe, carry out personal hygiene, dress, toilet, and eat.
- Assess the impact of self-care deficit on lifestyle.

- Determine the need for assistive or adaptive devices to use in self-care activities.
- Assess the need for home care during exacerbations.

Rationales

Symptoms will change as the disease progresses.

Pain and fatigue may cause progressive loss of function.

Pain may be dealt with effectively by preventing or reducing it.
Joint pain and stiffness interfere with performing ADLs.

Some patients have successfully adjusted their routines and complete required tasks. Other patients may be unable to care for themselves.
The patient may not have knowledge of newly available assistive devices.
Home care services can help the patient remain in the home setting as the disease progresses.

Therapeutic Interventions

Actions/Interventions

- Reinforce the need for adequate time to perform activities.

- Reinforce proper use of ambulation devices as taught by the physical therapist.

Rationales

The patient may need more time than others to complete same tasks.
Proper use conserves energy and provides more protection and support to the patient. It also reduces the load on joints.

■ = Independent   ▲ = Collaborative

Actions/Interventions

- Encourage the patient to wear proper footwear (properly fitting, with good support and nonskid bottoms) when ambulating, and to avoid wearing house slippers.
- Assist with ambulation as necessary.

- Reinforce techniques of therapeutic exercise taught by the physical therapist.

- Instruct the patient to avoid excessive exercise during acute inflammatory exacerbations.
- Reinforce principles of joint protection taught by the occupational therapist.
- Reinforce proper body alignment when sitting, standing, walking, and lying down.
- Encourage family members to promote independence by:
  - Assisting the patient only as necessary

  - Providing necessary adaptive equipment (e.g., raised toilet seat, dressing aids, eating aids)
  - Providing enough time for the patient to complete tasks

Rationales

Patients may select floppy shoes because of pain or because of deformities in the foot. It is important for the patient's safety that footwear fit correctly and be properly supportive.

The first few minutes of weight bearing may be difficult on a joint; support to the standing or sitting position may be helpful to the patient.

ROM, muscle strengthening, and endurance exercise within a prescribed regimen promote joint function and increase physical stamina.

Exercise during this time may exaggerate the inflammatory process.

Joint protection preserves joint mobility and prevents injury that increases inflammation.

Improper body alignment can lead to unnecessary pain and contracture.

During times of exacerbations, patients need more assistance than at other times; the family needs to be sensitive to this.

Such aids promote independence and may enhance safety.

The patient's self-image improves when he or she can perform personal care independently.

Related Care Plans

Chronic pain, p. 155
Fatigue, 66
Self-care deficit, 170
Risk for infection, 114

Arthroscopy

Arthroscopy is the direct visualization of a joint interior using a rigid fiberoptic endoscope. The procedure can be done for diagnostic evaluation and/or surgical repair of a joint. Arthroscopy is used when joint problems cannot be identified by noninvasive techniques such as x-ray examination. The procedure has wide application in the diagnosis and management of joint problems associated with sports injuries, degenerative disorders, and acute or chronic inflammatory disorders. Most arthroscopic procedures are done to evaluate and correct injuries to the knee. Problems related to the meniscus, cartilage, and ligaments of the knee can be repaired with arthroscopy. There is increasing use of the technique with other joints in the body such as rotator cuff injuries of the shoulder. Joint arthroscopy may be used in patients with rheumatoid arthritis to remove joint debris and thereby reduce joint pain. Advantages of this procedure for the patient include decreased surgical risks and fewer complications because it can be done using smaller incisions and usually with local or regional anesthesia. Complications of arthroscopy are not common but include infection, neurovascular damage, hemarthrosis (bleeding into the joint), and joint injury. The majority of arthroscopic procedures are done on an outpatient basis.

Deficient Knowledge

Common Related Factor
Unfamiliarity with procedure

Common Expected Outcome
Patient verbalizes understanding of the procedure and postprocedure home care.

Defining Characteristics
Multiple questions about procedure and follow-up care
Verbalized lack of knowledge about procedure

NOC Outcome
Knowledge: Treatment Procedure
NIC Interventions
Teaching: Preoperative; Teaching: Procedure/ Treatment

Ongoing Assessment

Actions/Interventions	Rationales
■ Assess the patient's understanding of arthroscopy.	Patients' anxiety level may be decreased if they know what to expect. Patients will be able to cooperate during the procedure if they understand what is going to occur.
■ Assess the patient's level of knowledge about home care after the procedure.	Patients will be responsible for monitoring their status after the procedure and implementing care to prevent complications.

Therapeutic Interventions

Actions/Interventions

■ Introduce or reinforce information about the arthroscopic procedure.

• The patient may need to be NPO (nothing by mouth) for at least 6 to 8 hours before the procedure.

• The hair around the joint will be shaved before the procedure.

• An intravenous infusion will be started to facilitate administration of sedatives and other medications for anesthesia during the procedure.

• The procedure will be started after an appropriate level of anesthesia has been achieved.

• The patient may experience transient sensations of joint pressure during the procedure when local or regional anesthesia is used.

• A tourniquet or compression bandage may be applied to the affected extremity.

Rationales

Restriction of food and fluids before the procedure will depend on the type of anesthesia. For patients receiving general anesthesia, fasting from solid foods before the procedure reduces the risk for vomiting and respiratory aspiration. Some patients may be allowed clear liquids up to 2 hours before the procedure to maintain hydration. Patients may be able to take certain prescription medications with small sips of water before the procedure.

Hair is usually removed in an area 6 inches above and below the affected joint. Hair removal reduces the risk for wound contamination during the procedure.

Drugs for anesthesia have a faster onset of action when administered intravenously. The surgeon and anesthesia care provider will determine the type of anesthesia required for the procedure. The choice of local or general anesthesia will be based on the extent of the procedure.

Patients need to be assured that they will not feel pain during the procedure, if they are to be awake and a local or regional anesthesia is used.

Informing patients about sensory experiences during the procedure may reduce their anxiety.

These measures are used to control bleeding during the procedure.

■ = Independent   ▲ = Collaborative

Actions/Interventions

- Introduce or reinforce information concerning home care after the procedure.
  - Pain management
  - Use of joint immobilizers
  - Activity and weight bearing
  - Care of incisions
  - Signs and symptoms to report to the physician

Rationales

Patients may be discharged with prescription for NSAIDS alone or combined with opiod analgesics for pain management. Joint immobilizers are applied to reduce pain and prevent further joint injury. Activity and weight bearing limitations will depend on the reason for the procedure. The patient may have more restrictions if joint repair was done during the procedure. The patient should be alert for signs of infection such as fever, joint swelling and increased pain, redness, warmth, or drainage from the incision. These signs should be reported to the physician as soon as possible. If Steri-Strips are used for wound closure, the patient may be instructed to leave them in place until they fall off on their own. Adhesive bandages may be used to cover wounds and prevent irritation from joint immobilizers. Skin sutures are usually removed in 7 days.

 NANDA-I NDx **Acute Pain**

Common Related Factors

Bone and soft tissue trauma caused by the procedure
Swelling of affected joint

Defining Characteristics

Verbal report of pain
Irritability
Restlessness
Protective behavior of joint
Positioning of joint to avoid pain

Common Expected Outcomes

Patient reports satisfactory pain control at a level less than 3 to 4 on a 0 to 10 rating scale.
Patient uses pharmacological and nonpharmacological pain relief strategies.
Patient exhibits increased comfort such as baseline levels for pulse, blood pressure, respirations, and relaxed muscle tone or body posture.

NOC Outcomes
Pain Control; Pain Level
NIC Interventions
Analgesic Administration; Pain Management

Ongoing Assessment

Actions/Interventions

- Assess the patient's description of pain.

- Assess the patient's expectations and goals for pain relief.

Rationales

The first step in effective pain management is assessing the location, severity, and quantity of pain experienced by the patient. Postprocedure pain is usually restricted to the affected joint. The patient may describe the pain as acute, sharp, or throbbing. The pain should decrease in intensity during the first 5 to 7 days after the procedure. Pain levels that persist or increase after 5 days may be indications of infection or joint injury.

Pain management is not effective until the patient is satisfied with the level of comfort achieved.

Therapeutic Interventions

Actions/Interventions	Rationales
■ Teach the patient about using analgesic medications.	The patient will be responsible for pain management and needs information to support decision making. After arthroscopy, most patients require mild analgesics for effective pain relief. Acetaminophen, nonsteroidal anti-inflammatory drugs (NSAIDs), or oral opioids may be prescribed for pain management.
• Take medications before the pain becomes severe.	If the patient waits until the pain is severe before taking analgesics, it takes longer to obtain effective relief.
• Take medications at regular intervals.	Regular dosing with analgesics achieves stable serum drug levels that provide effective pain management.
■ Apply ice packs to the affected joint.	Cold therapy produces vasoconstriction and reduces swelling. Release of pain-causing chemicals and conduction of pain impulses are decreased with cold therapy.
■ Maintain joint immobilizers applied after the procedure.	Immobilization of the joint after arthroscopy reduces unnecessary movement that causes pain and further joint injury.

NANDA-I NDx

Impaired Physical Mobility

Common Related Factors
Prescribed activity restrictions for joint movement and weight bearing
Pain

Defining Characteristics
Limited range of motion (ROM) of affected joint
Reluctance to move
Presence of joint immobilizer

Common Expected Outcomes
Patient maintains mobility level within limits of prescribed restrictions.
Patient uses assistive devices for mobility.

NOC Outcomes
Mobility Level; Coordinated Movement; Knowledge: Prescribed Activity
NIC Interventions
Teaching: Prescribed Activity/Exercise; Exercise Therapy: Joint Mobility

---

Ongoing Assessment

Actions/Interventions	Rationales
■ Assess ROM in unaffected and affected joints.	After arthroscopy, the affected joint may be immobilized with slings, splints, or commercially made immobilizers. The type of immobilizer used and the length of time the joint will be immobilized depend on the extent of the procedure.
■ Assess muscle strength, coordination, and ability to use mobility aids.	The patient's overall strength and coordination will determine the type of mobility aids needed after arthroscopy.

Therapeutic Interventions

Actions/Interventions	Rationales
■ Instruct the patient in proper application and use of the prescribed immobilizer.	The immobilizer maintains the joint in anatomical alignment and protects the joint from unnecessary movement during the healing process. Such movements can lead to increased pain and joint injury.

■ = Independent ▲ = Collaborative

Actions/Interventions

- Teach the patient about activity and weight-bearing restrictions.

- Instruct the patient in use of mobility aids.

- ▲ Refer to physical therapist.

Rationales

The degree of mobility restrictions depends on the extent of the procedure. Most patients with diagnostic arthroscopy can resume weight bearing. Activity and excessive use of the joint may be limited for several days after the procedure.

Crutches, canes, or walkers may be provided to assist the patient with mobility until activity restrictions are no longer needed.

The patient is often referred to a physical therapist for progressive ROM and joint-strengthening exercises. The physical therapist will educate the patient on proper techniques for using mobility aids.

Fibromyalgia

Fibromyalgia Syndrome; Fibromyositis; Fibrositis

Fibromyalgia is a common, complex pain syndrome that affects an estimated 10 million Americans. The syndrome can be extremely debilitating for patients with severe symptoms, interfering with performance of basic activities of daily living. It is characterized by chronic, widespread pain and abnormal pain processing; multiple tender points; sleep disturbances and fatigue; and frequent psychological distress. The pain frequently has been described as stabbing or shooting, or as a deep muscle ache or twitch. Numbness, tingling, and burning often add to the patient's discomfort. The fatigue of fibromyalgia is marked by profound exhaustion and poor stamina. Sleep problems include documented abnormalities in Stage 4 deep sleep that prevent patients from getting adequate rest. Additional symptoms may include irritable bowel and bladder, headaches and migraines, restless legs syndrome, impaired memory and concentration, Raynaud's syndrome, anxiety, and depression. Fibromyalgia has no known cause, but most researchers agree it results from a disorder of central processing with neuroendocrine/neurotransmitter dysregulation. Recent research also suggests a genetic component because the syndrome is seen in families, among siblings, or in mothers and their children. No laboratory tests or radiological studies are available for diagnosing fibromyalgia. The health care provider instead relies on patient history, a physical examination, and accurate manual tender point examination; multiple tender points at characteristic locations are typical in fibromyalgia. Because laboratory tests often are negative and symptoms overlap with other disorders, accurate diagnosis of fibromyalgia can take an average of 5 years. Diagnosis usually is made in persons ages 20 to 50, but incidence rises with age. Fibromyalgia occurs more often in women, although it also affects men and children. It occurs in all ethnic groups. No cure exists for the syndrome, but clinical advances in the last decade have allowed patients to reduce their symptoms with a variety of treatments. Because one of the most important factors in improving the symptoms of fibromyalgia is lifestyle adaptation, this care plan focuses on patient education regarding self-care needs.

Deficient Knowledge

Common Related Factor

Unfamiliarity with disease process and management

Defining Characteristics

Lack of questions
Multiple questions
Misconceptions

Common Expected Outcome

Patient and family verbalize knowledge of chronic nature of fibromyalgia, self-care and need for lifestyle modification, and available community resources.

NOC Outcome

Knowledge: Disease Process, Knowledge: Medication

NIC Intervention

Teaching: Disease Process, Teaching: Prescribed Medication

Ongoing Assessment

Actions/Interventions	Rationales
■ Assess the patient's level of knowledge regarding fibromyalgia and its management.	Patients will be responsible for evaluating their condition on a daily basis to determine their need for exercise, analgesics, and other interventions.
■ Evaluate knowledge or awareness of community support groups.	Awareness of other resources may improve patients' coping abilities.

Therapeutic Interventions

Actions/Interventions	Rationales
■ Introduce or reinforce information about disease process, diagnosis, and management: chronic pain syndrome of unknown cause characterized by multiple tender points, sleep disturbances, and fatigue.	Patients and families need to understand the disease process and diagnosis in order to manage fibromyalgia successfully. Patients with fibromyalgia tend to look well and have normal results for conventional tests. Awareness of the extent of their symptoms will allow them to dialogue appropriately with a knowledgeable health care provider.
Initial Presentation With Pain and Tender Points	
• Extent and severity of pain	Patients' pain may be widespread, migrating to all areas of the body. Pain severity and stiffness are often worse in the morning; other aggravating factors include cold/humid weather, nonrestorative sleep, physical and mental fatigue, excessive physical activity, inactivity, anxiety, and stress.
• Related systemic symptoms	Patients and family members need to understand that fibromyalgia is associated with symptoms other than pain. Additional symptoms may include sleep disorders and severe fatigue, problems with cognitive function, irritable bowel syndrome (IBS), anxiety and depression, and environmental sensitivities.
Diagnosis	
• Diagnosis by history and examination based on American College of Rheumatology diagnostic criteria and palpation of multiple tender points.	No laboratory or radiological tests can aid in diagnosis of fibromyalgia. Patients need to be able to describe their specific symptoms in order to aid the health care provider in diagnosis. Patient must have widespread pain in all body quadrants for a minimum of 3 months; tenderness or pain in at least 11 of 18 specified tender points when pressure is applied.

■ = Independent ▲ = Collaborative

Actions/Interventions

General Treatment/Management Guidelines

- Medications to treat fibromyalgia pain include pregabalin, duloxetine, and milnacipran, nonopiates such as tramadol or nonsteroidal antiinflammatory drugs, muscle relaxants, and Lidocaine injections into tender spots.

- A regular program of gentle exercise should be performed daily. A physical therapy referral may be beneficial to structure this program.
- Regular sleep regimen

- Diet modification

- Complementary therapies may include therapeutic massage, acupuncture and acupressure, yoga, aromatherapy, biofeedback, herbs/nutritional supplements, and chiropractic manipulation.

- Provide information on fibromyalgia support groups:
  National Fibromyalgia Association
  2121 S. Towne Centre Place, Suite 300
  Anaheim, CA 92806
  (714) 921-0150
  www.fmaware.org

Rationales

Pain is the hallmark symptom of fibromyalgia. Its management contributes to patients' ability to cope effectively with the syndrome. Pregabalin is an anticonvulsant drug that is effective in relieving pain and improving the quality of sleep for the patient with fibromyalgia. Selective serotonin/norepinephrine reuptake inhibitors such as duloxetine and milnacipran produce improvement in fibromyalgia pain, physical functioning, and the patient's overall sense of well-being. NSAIDS and nonopiate analgesics reduce pain especially when used in combination with other drugs for fibromyalgia. Muscles relaxants have been found to reduce fibromyalgia pain but do relieve muscle spasms in these patients. Injections of anesthetics such as Lidocaine directly into tender points improve muscle stretching with decreased pain. The injections may need to be repeated one or more times over several weeks to achieve full effectiveness.

Exercise and stretching maintain muscle tone, and reduce pain and stiffness. Water-based exercises may be especially beneficial for patients with fibromyalgia.

Adequate rest contributes to improved overall symptom management. Specific activities to improve sleep include going to bed and getting up at the same time each day; ensuring the sleep environment is conducive to rest (i.e., quiet, free of distractions; comfortable room temperature; supportive bed); avoiding caffeine, sugar, and alcohol before bedtime; avoiding eating before bedtime; practicing relaxation exercises at bedtime.

Diet modification may lead to increased energy and decreased pain for patients with fibromyalgia. Specific dietary changes may include limiting high-fat foods, sweets, large amounts of grains and legumes, excessive raw fruits or vegetables, and alcohol. Consultation with a nutritionist or practitioner of Chinese medicine may be indicated.

The benefits of various complementary therapies for fibromyalgia remain unclear; well-designed controlled trials are needed to identify their potential role in syndrome management. However, because studies have not reported safety issues for patients with fibromyalgia, complementary therapies may be considered for those who are unresponsive or resistant to medications and self-management approaches. Discussion with their health care providers may help patients avoid fads or products that claim curative effects.

Living with a chronic condition can challenge patients emotionally. Group membership and counseling supports patients' efforts to understand and live successfully with fibromyalgia. This organization provides patients and families with information and links them with appropriate resources to support quality of life.

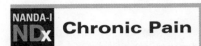
Chronic Pain

Common Related Factor

Diffuse body pain and tenderness at specified points

Defining Characteristics

Patient report of pain
Facial mask of pain
Moaning or other sounds associated with pain and movement

Common Expected Outcomes

Patient reports pain at a level less than 3 to 4 on a 0 to 10 rating scale.
Patient implements a pain management plan that includes pharmacological and nonpharmacological strategies.
Patient engages in desired activities without an increase in pain level.

NOC Outcomes
Pain Control; Quality of Life
NIC Interventions
Pain Management; Analgesic Administration; Acupressure; Heat/Cold Application; Simple Massage

---

Ongoing Assessment

Actions/Interventions	Rationales
■ Assess severity and location of patient's pain.	Pain typically is diffuse, with multiple tender points.
■ Assess interference with lifestyle.	Severe pain may affect patients' ability to participate in activities of daily living.
■ Assess patient's perception of the effectiveness of all pain management strategies.	Evaluation of the treatment regimen allows patients and health care providers to determine appropriate changes.
■ Assess patient's ability to complete customary activities.	Chronic pain, as well as any associated depression or anxiety, can limit patients' ability to complete self-care activities and activities of daily living.

Therapeutic Interventions

Actions/Interventions	Rationales
■ Instruct the patient to take medications as prescribed.	To avoid stomach irritation or ulcer disease, patients should not take antiinflammatory drugs on an empty stomach. Because of potential interactions, patients who are taking pregabalin should avoid alcohol and inform their health care providers if they also take diabetes medications, phenothiazines, or antidepressants.
■ Suggest the use of nonpharmacological treatments for pain.	Medications may be of limited use in the treatment of fibromyalgia pain. Nonpharmacological strategies have little risk and may be helpful as part of a comprehensive treatment plan.
• Pacing activities	Keeping activity levels within the limits imposed by the syndrome can reduce pain. For example, spread chores over a day instead of trying to do them all in the morning.
• Relaxation	Pain often triggers tension and anxiety, which in turn can intensify the experience of pain. In addition to decreasing tension and stress, relaxation also offers a distraction from pain and can improve sleep. Strategies include breathing exercises, baths and hot tubs, massage, rest, and listening to CDs.
• Problem solving	Identifying situations that trigger pain helps the patient alter those situations.

■ = Independent ▲ = Collaborative

Actions/Interventions

- Exercise and movement

- Heat, cold, and massage

Rationales

A comprehensive exercise program that includes flexibility, strengthening, and endurance activities may lessen both pain and fatigue by increasing stamina.

Heat may be effective for pain that results from muscle tension or inactivity; warm baths may provide overall relief, whereas heating pads or hot packs may improve localized pain. Massage serves the same purpose. Cold therapy reduces blood flow to an area and may provide some anesthetic effect. Both heat and cold should be used no more than 15 to 20 minutes at a time.

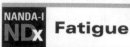 **Fatigue**

Common Related Factors

Increased pain
Poor sleep pattern

Defining Characteristics

Patient describes lack of energy, exhaustion, listlessness
Decreased attention span
Facial expressions: yawning, sadness
Decreased functional capacity

Common Expected Outcomes

Patient verbalizes reduction of fatigue as evidenced by reports of increased energy and ability to perform desired activities.
Patient demonstrates use of energy-conservation principles.

NOC Outcomes

Activity Tolerance; Endurance; Energy Conservation

NIC Interventions

Energy Management; Sleep Enhancement

Ongoing Assessment

Actions/Interventions

■ Assess the patient's description of fatigue: timing (continuous or at the end of the day), aggravating and alleviating factors.

■ Assess the patient's emotional response to fatigue.

■ Determine the patient's nighttime sleep pattern.

Rationales

Patients' descriptions of fatigue contribute to the development of an individualized approach to care.

Anxiety and depression can result from fatigue and also contribute to its continuation. Additional treatment for these emotional disorders may be needed.

Chronic pain and dysfunctional pain processing associated with fibromyalgia may interfere with patients' restful sleep.

Therapeutic Interventions

Actions/Interventions

■ Encourage the patient to keep a 24-hour fatigue/activity log for at least 1 week.

■ Help the patient develop a daily schedule that balances rest and activity.

Rationales

Logs allow patients to correlate specific activities with their levels of fatigue. Information can help patients determine how to arrange activities to minimize fatigue.

A plan can help patients complete desired activities without increasing their fatigue.

Actions/Interventions

- As part of an energy conservation plan, encourage the patient to identify tasks that can be delegated to others.
- Encourage patient to maintain nutritional intake for adequate caloric requirements.
- Encourage good sleep hygiene to maximize rest (see Deficient Knowledge).

Rationales

Delegation can help patients conserve energy.

An appropriate diet provides adequate energy resources.

Adequate rest minimizes fatigue and other symptoms of fibromyalgia.

Related Care Plans

Activity intolerance, p. 8
Hopelessness, p. 98
Ineffective coping, p. 49
Ineffective therapeutic regimen management, p. 194
Insomnia, p. 117

Fractures: Extremity and Pelvic

Closed Reduction; Open Reduction; Internal Fixation; External Fixation

A fracture is a break or disruption in the continuity of a bone. Fractures occur when a bone is subjected to more stress than it can absorb. Fractures are treated by one or a combination of the following: closed reduction—alignment of bone fragments by manual manipulation without surgery; open reduction—alignment of bone fragments by surgery; internal fixation—immobilization of fracture site during surgery with rods, pins, plates, screws, wires, or other hardware or immobilization through use of casts, splints, traction, or posterior molds; external fixation—immobilization of bone fragments with the use of rods and pins that extend from the incision externally and are fixed. This care plan covers the management of patients with fractures and cast immobilization and contains occasional references to more complicated fractures.

 Acute Pain

Common Related Factors	Defining Characteristics
Fracture	Complaints of pain or discomfort
Soft tissue injury	Guarding behavior
	Increased muscle spasm
	Increased pulse rate
	Increased blood pressure (BP)
	Crying, moaning
	Grimacing
	Anxiety
	Restlessness
	Withdrawal
	Irritability

■ = Independent   ▲ = Collaborative

Common Expected Outcomes

Patient reports satisfactory pain control at a level less than 3 to 4 on a 0 to 10 rating scale.

Patient uses pharmacological and nonpharmacological pain relief strategies.

Patient exhibits increased comfort such as baseline levels for pulse, blood pressure, respirations, and relaxed muscle tone or body posture.

NOC Outcomes
Pain Control; Medication Response

NIC Interventions
Pain Management; Analgesic Administration

Ongoing Assessment

Actions/Interventions	Rationales
■ Assess for pain or discomfort.	Immediately after the fracture, there may be a period of 15 to 20 minutes in which no pain is apparent. This period of transient anesthesia may be related to the immediate response of nerves that are damaged by the trauma of the fracture. Eventually, sensation is returned and the traumatized area becomes painful enough for the patient to guard the affected area. Subsequent pain from a fracture is associated with muscle spasms and soft tissue injury. The pain may be aggravated by movement of the affected area.
■ Assess the patient's description of pain.	Patients with pelvic fractures may have intense pain from secondary injuries associated with the fracture. These injuries include trauma to pelvic blood vessels, the intestines, or the urinary bladder. Intense pain that persists or pain that returns to previous levels of intensity may indicate a developing complication such as infection or compartment syndrome.
■ Assess effectiveness of pain-relieving interventions.	Patients have a right to effective pain relief. Pain relief is not determined to be effective until the patient indicates that it is acceptable.

Therapeutic Interventions

Actions/Interventions	Rationales
■ Explain analgesic therapy, including medication and schedule; instruct the patient to take pain medications as needed. Instruct the patient to request pain medication before the pain becomes severe.	Discomfort will be directly related to the type of fracture and the amount of soft tissue damage. Pain with simple fractures may be effectively managed with ibuprofen or aspirin. Pain related to more serious fractures with complicated types of tissue damage and need for surgical reduction requires opioid analgesics. Care providers often assume that the patient will request pain medication when needed. The patient may think it is his or her duty or responsibility to tolerate pain until it can no longer be tolerated and may be waiting for the nurse to offer pain medication when it is available. If pain is too severe before analgesics or therapy is instituted, relief takes longer.
■ If the patient is a candidate for intravenous PCA (inpatients only), explain its concept and use.	PCA refers to a method that allows the patient to control pain by using an intravenous drug delivery system. This method allows the patient to self-administer a prescribed narcotic analgesic in controlled doses at a frequency necessary to effectively manage the pain. Successful use of PCA requires the patient to have knowledge of its use and the manual dexterity to operate it.

Actions/Interventions

▲ Administer narcotic analgesics every 3 to 4 hours around the clock for the first 24 hours after surgical reduction or pin placement.

■ Encourage use of analgesics 30 to 45 minutes before physical therapy.

■ Encourage the patient to change position every 2 hours or more often for comfort.

■ Maintain immobilization and support of affected part. Elevate the affected extremity.

■ Reposition and support the unaffected parts as permitted.

■ Apply ice packs for 20 to 30 minutes every 1 to 2 hours.

■ Teach relaxation techniques.

▲ Administer muscle relaxants as necessary.

Rationales

Manipulation, nerve trauma, and tissue damage result from the fracture and the surgical procedure. Assume that the patient requires analgesia. The patient's ability to fall asleep between pain assessments is not a good indicator of the patient's level of comfort. Adjusting to pain depletes the patient's energy levels and leads to fatigue.

Unrelieved pain hinders rehabilitative progress.

Repositioning reduces pressure and pain on bony prominences.

Immobility prevents further tissue damage and muscle spasm. Elevation decreases vasocongestion and edema.

These techniques promote general comfort and maintain good body alignment.

Cold therapy decreases swelling (first 24 to 48 hours).

Complementary therapies can enhance the effects of analgesic agents.

These medications prevent muscle spasms, which may be painful.

 Impaired Physical Mobility

Common Related Factors

Cast
Fixation device
Immobilizer device
Pain
Surgical procedure

Defining Characteristics

Reluctance to attempt movement
Limited range of motion (ROM)
Mechanical restriction of movement
Decreased muscle strength and/or control
Impaired coordination
Inability to move purposefully within physical environment (bed, mobility, transfer, ambulation)

Common Expected Outcomes

Patient performs physical activity independently or within limits of activity restrictions.

Patient demonstrates use of adaptive techniques that promote ambulation and transferring.

Patient is free of complications of immobility, as evidenced by intact skin, absence of thrombophlebitis, normal bowel pattern, and clear breath sounds.

NOC Outcomes

Ambulation; Mobility; Balance; Bone Healing

NIC Interventions

Exercise Therapy: Joint Mobility; Exercise: Ambulation

Ongoing Assessment

Actions/Interventions

■ Assess ROM of unaffected joints proximal and distal to the immobilization device.

■ Determine the type of assistive devices the patient will require for ambulation in anticipation of discharge.

Rationales

Patients with casts, external fixators, or other immobilizer devices will experience some degree of limited ROM to the affected area. Optimal ROM is critical for movement and necessary for rehabilitation.

Patients may require a cane, walker, or crutches to enhance ambulation.

■ = Independent   ▲ = Collaborative

Actions/Interventions

■ Assess muscle strength in all extremities.

Rationales

The rehabilitation program will be geared toward maximizing strength in the unaffected extremities and maintaining as much strength as possible in the affected or immobilized extremity.

Therapeutic Interventions

Actions/Interventions

■ Encourage isometric, active, and resistive ROM exercises to all unaffected joints on a schedule consistent with the rehabilitation program and as tolerated.

■ Perform flexion and extension exercises to proximal and distal joints of the affected extremity, when indicated.

■ Assist the patient up to chair when ordered; teach transfer technique. Lift extremity by external fixation frame if stable; avoid handling of injured soft tissue.

▲ Reinforce crutch ambulation taught by physical therapist, using appropriate weight-bearing techniques as prescribed.

Rationales

Exercise prevents muscle atrophy and maintains adequate muscle strength required for mobility.

These exercises serve to maintain mobility.

Early mobility reduces the complication of immobility. Learning the correct way to transfer is important to maintain optimal mobility and patient safety.

Some patients will have limited or no weight bearing on the affected extremity to allow the fracture adequate time to begin healing.

NANDA-I NDx Risk for Ineffective Tissue Perfusion

Common Risk Factors

Cast
Fracture
Manipulation
Inflammatory process and edema
Mobilization of a fat embolism
Immobility

Common Expected Outcome

Patient maintains optimal tissue perfusion, as evidenced by warm extremities, good color, good capillary refill (less than or equal to 2 seconds), absence of pain and numbness, and bilaterally strong, palpable pulses.

NOC Outcomes
Tissue Perfusion: Peripheral; Risk Control; Risk Detection
NIC Interventions
Circulatory Care; Circulatory Precautions

Ongoing Assessment

Actions/Interventions

■ Assess and compare neurovascular status of all extremities before and after the application of a cast or surgical reduction of a fracture.

■ Assess the affected extremity every 1 to 2 hours for signs of neurovascular compromise and damage:
  • Skin temperature

Rationales

Changes in neurovascular assessment findings may indicate the onset of compartment syndrome. Assessment must include unaffected and affected extremity to establish baseline and monitor for change in neurovascular status.

Injured tissues are usually cooler than those on the nonaffected side. Normal temperature indicates adequate perfusion.

Actions/Interventions	**Rationales**
• Capillary refill of nail beds	Normal refill is 2 to 4 seconds. In the first hours after injury, capillary refill may be sluggish, but refill that exceeds 4 to 6 seconds should be reported to the physician.
• Skin color	Color should be pink, not pale or white. The affected area may be paler than the unaffected area.
• Peripheral pulses	All peripheral pulses will be felt; however, the posterior tibialis and the dorsalis pedis in the lower extremities and the radial and ulnar pulses in the upper extremities may be weaker than in the unaffected area.
• Paresthesias	Complaints of numbness, tingling, or "pins and needles" feeling may indicate pressure on nerves and should be investigated.
• ROM	ROM indicates the amount and degree of limitation. Injured tissues will have decreased ROM. Opposite side should have normal ROM. Decreased ability to wiggle fingers or toes occurs with nerve damage from compartment syndrome.
• Pain	Pain indicates injury, trauma, or pressure. The surgical site will normally be painful. Monitor and report excessive complaints of pain as a possible harbinger of compartment syndrome.
▲ Monitor results of lung scans, chest films, and films of extremity fracture.	These tests may be used to identify a nonhealing fracture or respiratory complications, such as a pulmonary embolus or a fat embolus.
■ Assess for symptoms of fat embolism.	The patient may experience a sense of impending doom; chest pain; and signs and symptoms of shock, including tachypnea, tachycardia, hypoxia confusion, or disorientation. The patient may manifest a rash over the chest from below the nipple line up to the neck (may also include the conjunctivae).

Therapeutic Interventions

Actions/Interventions	**Rationales**
■ Notify the physician immediately if signs of altered circulation are noted.	Venous pressures in the interstitial area surrounding an operative site can be measured through a small catheter inserted into the compartment. A surgical fasciotomy can be performed, which would release constriction and increase arterial inflow, restoring adequate circulation. The best indicators of developing compartment syndrome are patient complaints of excessive pain, peripheral pulses becoming weaker or absent, and an increase in pain on passive movement of the distal part.
■ Elevate extremity, and apply ice packs after surgical reduction (ORIF) or cast application.	These measures reduce edema formation and decrease the risk for compartment syndrome.
▲ Administer anticoagulants as ordered	These drugs may be given prophylactically to reduce threat of deep vein thrombosis.
▲ Apply antiembolic hose or sequential compression devices as indicated.	These devices decrease venous pooling and may enhance venous return, thereby reducing the risk for thrombus formation.
▲ Split or bivalve cast as needed.	This technique may be done on an emergency basis to reduce restriction and improve impaired circulation resulting from compression and edema of the injured extremity.

■ = Independent   ▲ = Collaborative

Actions/Interventions

■ Instruct the patient in the symptoms of fat embolism.

▲ Implement emergency measures in the presence of symptoms of fat embolism:
- Administer oxygen to keep saturation level greater than 90%.

- Titrate intravenous fluids closely.
- Transfer patient to intensive care unit.

Rationales

This complication occurs most often within 2 to 4 days after long bone or pelvic fractures. It may occur because fat molecules are mobilized into general circulation from the bone marrow during a fracture. Fat emboli represent a fatal risk to patients as much as 40% of the time and must be regarded as a potential life-threatening risk.

Impaired gas exchange is a priority concern. Supplemental oxygen will improve gas exchange and promote effective breathing.
Fluid overload can lead to pulmonary edema.
Significantly compromised or unstable patients require critical care management.

NANDA-I NDx Deficient Knowledge

Common Related Factors

New procedures or treatment
New condition
Home care needs

Defining Characteristics

Verbalizes inadequate knowledge of care or use of immobilization device, mobility limitations, complications, and follow-up care
Expresses concerns about ability to manage independently at home
Confusion; asking multiple questions
Lack of questions
Inaccurate follow-through of instruction

Common Expected Outcome

Patient or caregiver verbalizes understanding of treatment, possible complications, and follow-up care.

NOC Outcomes
Knowledge: Treatment Regimen; Safety Behavior: Home Physical Environment
NIC Interventions
Cast Care: Maintenance; Teaching: Psychomotor Skill; Teaching: Prescribed Activity/Exercise

---

Ongoing Assessment

Actions/Interventions

■ Assess the patient's understanding of the factors that facilitate bone healing:
- The bone ends and/or fragments must be brought into anatomical alignment.
- Fracture site is immobilized.
- Weight bearing is reduced or prohibited.
- Joints above and below the injury may be immobilized to prevent movement that might dislodge bone ends.

Rationales

Knowledge about fractures and the treatment procedures can help the patient be an active participant in making decisions about his or her care. The patient needs to understand that limited weight bearing on the affected extremity is a necessary component of the healing process for a fracture.

Actions/Interventions

■ Assess current understanding of treatment, follow-up care, and readiness and ability to assume self-care and activities of daily living (ADLs).

■ Determine the patient's recognition of hazards in the home that will compromise the patient's ability to be effectively mobile at home.

■ Assess the availability of people on whom the patient may rely for support and assistance while mobility is impaired.

Rationales

Effective discharge planning is based on a clear understanding of the needs of the patient and family members who will assume caregiver roles. Referral to a home care agency may be necessary to support a safe transition from hospital to home for the patient and family caregivers.

Stairs, areas rugs, and so on can limit the patient's progressive mobility and increase the risk for falls.

A social support network can help the patient cooperate with mobility restrictions during the healing process.

Therapeutic Interventions

Actions/Interventions

■ Instruct patient/caregiver to:
  • Perform prescribed exercises several times a day.

  • Use appropriate assistive device (walker, crutches), and maintain prescribed weight-bearing status.
  • Identify and report to the physician signs of neurovascular compromise of the extremity: pain, numbness, tingling, burning, swelling, or discoloration.
  • Use pain relief measures as ordered.

  • Obtain proper nutrition.

  • Keep all follow-up and physical therapy appointments.

■ Instruct the patient in cast care:
  • To keep the cast clean and dry; tub bathe only if the cast is protected, not immersed
  • To inspect skin around cast edges for irritation

  • Not to put anything under the cast, poke under the cast, or put powder or lotion under the cast
  • To notify the physician if the cast cracks or breaks, of foul odor under the cast, of fresh drainage through the cast, if anything gets inside the cast, of areas of skin breakdown around the cast, of pain or burning inside the cast, or of warm areas on the cast
■ Instruct the patient with a surgical incision to observe for signs of infection and to notify the physician if they develop.
■ Instruct the patient with an external fixation device to perform pin care, perform wound care, and observe for loosening of pins.
■ Involve the patient or caregiver in procedures. Supervise those performing procedures, and teach proper technique.

■ Provide the patient with medical supplies and assistive devices as needed.

Rationales

Regular exercise is necessary to maintain muscle tone and promote bone healing.
Assistive devices help the patient maintain mobility.

Early assessment reduces the risk for injury or complications.

Knowledge helps the patient make decisions about measures to achieve effective pain management.
A diet with sufficient protein, vitamin D, calcium, and fiber promotes bone and wound healing and prevents constipation.
The rehabilitation program will be modified regularly as the fracture heals.

Moisture can break down the cast and limits the cast's ability to stabilize the fracture during healing.
Rough edges of the cast can lead to skin irritation and breakdown.
These actions may abrade skin and cause infection.

The cast may need to be removed and reapplied if infection or skin breakdown occurs.

Prompt treatment of infection is necessary to prevent osteomyelitis.

A strong knowledge base optimizes the patient's sense of independence and sense of mastery over the ability to perform self-care.
Ability to perform self-care procedures decreases risk for infection and optimizes therapeutic effect in the home care environment.
Efforts to enhance self-care abilities promote successful transition and accommodation to home environment.

■ = Independent   ▲ = Collaborative

NANDA-I NDx **Risk for Impaired Urinary Elimination**

Common Risk Factors

Urinary tract injuries (e.g., urethral tear secondary to high-velocity trauma)
Bladder rupture secondary to punctures from bony fragments
Immobility
Presence of catheter
Infection

Common Expected Outcome

Patient maintains urine output greater than 30 mL/hr with normal color.

NOC Outcome
Urinary Elimination
NIC Interventions
Urinary Retention Care; Urinary Catheterization

Ongoing Assessment

Actions/Interventions	Rationales
■ Assess frequency, amount, and character of urine and for any signs of incontinence.	Bladder trauma may occur with pelvic fractures and result in changes in urinary elimination.
■ Observe for gross hematuria, pelvic hematoma, and edematous and ecchymotic scrotum.	Blood-tinged urine may reflect trauma or damage of the urinary tract system. Excessive bruising or hematoma formation in the pelvic or perineal area may indicate bladder trauma has occurred.
■ Record intake and output.	This information enables the care provider to determine adequate fluid balance. Hourly output should not fall below 30 mL/hr. A Foley catheter may be required to assess output.
■ Palpate suprapubic area of abdomen for bladder distention or suprapubic pain.	Urinary retention may indicate edema or nerve damage secondary to the trauma. Pelvic injuries frequently cause internal injury to the urinary tract; intravenous pyelogram, cystogram, and a kidney and ureter bladder examination may be required for diagnosis.
■ Assess for signs and symptoms of urinary tract infection: frequency, burning on urination, elevated temperature, and elevated white blood cell count.	Urinary tract infection may be a complication of bladder trauma.

Therapeutic Interventions

Actions/Interventions	Rationales
■ Encourage oral fluids.	If the urine is kept dilute, calcium particles are less likely to precipitate and stasis with resultant infection is less likely.
▲ Insert Foley catheter, or institute intermittent catheterization using aseptic technique, as prescribed.	Catheterization prevents bladder distention and further trauma to bladder.
▲ Administer antibiotics, as prescribed.	Antibiotics may be given to reduce the risk for urinary tract infection from bladder trauma.
■ Notify the physician immediately of any abnormalities in the urine or the process of voiding.	Bladder trauma may not be immediately apparent after pelvic fracture.

Risk for Injury

Common Risk Factors

Improper positioning of immobilization device—sling, external fixator
If cast is in place, loss of continuity of cast
Pelvic fracture

Common Expected Outcomes

Patient maintains correct body position and alignment.
Patient maintains intact cast.

NOC Outcomes
Risk Control; Risk Detection; Bone Healing
NIC Interventions
Cast Care: Wet; Cast Care: Maintenance; Traction/Immobilization Care

---

Ongoing Assessment

Actions/Interventions	Rationales
■ Assess stabilization device for pelvic fracture.	Application of an external compression device is indicated for unstable pelvic fracture. For pelvic stabilization to be effective, the device must be properly applied. The patient's own movement may result in subtle changes in the apparatus, which can result in malalignment. This would result in patient discomfort and poor healing of the fracture.
■ Assess the patient's position in the immobilization apparatus.	The patient should be in an anatomically correct body alignment. If not, painful muscle spasms, muscle fatigue, and malalignment of the healing pelvic bones can occur.
■ Assess the cast for cracks; weakened, softened, or wet areas; indentations; or odors.	A weakened cast cannot adequately hold the patient's limbs in the positions necessary for correct healing. It may also indicate that there is bleeding or an infective process going on within the cast.

Therapeutic Interventions

Actions/Interventions	Rationales
Pelvic Stabilization	
■ Maintain proper alignment of the pelvis and of the affected extremity.	Only in this position will it be possible for the fracture to be reduced (the edge of the fracture will be properly aligned and juxtaposed).
▲ Verify with the physician how much lifting and turning the patient is allowed.	Activity limitations are necessary to enhance healing and recovery.
Cast:	
■ Leave the cast open to air until completely dry. Do not cover with blankets or sheets or balance on the edge of a hard surface.	Coverings may retain moisture and prevent the proper drying of the cast. Resting the cast on the edge of a hard surface will cause indentation.
■ Prevent indenting of the wet cast by moving and supporting it with the palms of your hands.	Indentations will contribute to skin irritation under the cast.
■ Reposition the patient in a cast every 2 hours.	Changing position allows for complete drying.

■ = Independent   ▲ = Collaborative

Actions/Interventions

- Instruct the patient not to insert anything into the cast (such as an object that might be used to scratch an itch).

- Petal the edges of the cast with tape.

Rationales

Objects may damage the underlying tissue and result in infection or may become trapped within the cast and cause constriction and nerve damage.

This procedure reduces or prevents tissue trauma to the skin underlying the edges of the cast.

Related Care Plans

Deficient fluid volume, p. 72
Disturbed body image, p. 24
Risk for impaired skin integrity, p. 185

Joint Arthroplasty/Replacement: Total Hip, Knee, Shoulder

Total hip arthroplasty/replacement is a total joint replacement by surgical removal of the diseased hip joint, including the femoral neck and head, as well as the acetabulum. The femoral canal is reamed to accept a metal component placed into the femoral shaft, which replaces the femoral head and neck. A polyethylene cup replaces the reamed acetabulum. The prosthesis is either cemented into place or a porous coated prosthesis is used, which allows bio-ingrowth, resulting in retention and stability of the joint. Some arthroplasty procedures are done using a minimally invasive approach. These techniques use multiple small incisions compared to the more traditional approach that uses a single, long incision. A less invasive surgical technique for joint arthroplasty is associated with earlier ambulation, decreased incidence of joint dislocation, and shorter length of stay postoperatively.

Knee hemiarthroplasty is replacement of deteriorated femoral, tibial, and patellar articular surfaces with prosthetic metal and plastic components. The prosthetic devices are held in place through the use of cement or the device is porous, allowing for bio-ingrowth, which eventually secures the replacement. Total knee replacement is the preferred treatment for the older patient with advanced osteoarthritis and for the young and elderly with rheumatoid arthritis. Although knee implants are thought to be durable over time and result in a degree of predictable pain relief, which makes them desirable for all patients, younger patients will almost certainly require revision at some point after the device becomes worn. The hospitalization for total knee replacement rarely exceeds 5 days, with rehabilitation and recovery expected to take from 6 weeks to 3 months. Elderly patients may require additional care in a rehabilitation setting.

Shoulder hemiarthroplasty is the surgical removal of the head of the humerus with replacement by a prosthesis. Total shoulder arthroplasty is the surgical removal of the head of the humerus and the glenoid cavity of the scapula, with replacement by an articulating prosthesis. A metallic humerus is inserted into the shaft, and a high-density polyethylene cup is cemented into place. Patients most likely to undergo this procedure (many of whom are older) have experienced joint damage and functional limitations secondary to osteoarthritis or rheumatoid arthritis. Many arthropathies are bilateral, necessitating the eventual replacement of both shoulder joints. Full recovery takes 3 to 6 months for optimal movement (70 to 90 degrees of abduction is usual, but the quality of postsurgical joint function is directly linked to the strength of the muscles that will move the implant).

Acute Pain

Common Related Factors

Bones and soft tissue trauma caused by surgery
Intense physical therapy or rehabilitation program
Restricted mobility

Defining Characteristics

Complaint of pain
Facial grimaces, guarding behavior, crying
Withdrawal, restlessness, irritability
Altered vital signs
Refusal to participate in a physical therapy or rehabilitation
  program

Common Expected Outcomes

Patient reports satisfactory pain control at a level less than
  3 to 4 on a 0 to 10 rating scale.
Patient uses pharmacological and nonpharmacological
  pain relief strategies.
Patient exhibits increased comfort such as baseline levels
  for pulse, blood pressure, respirations, and relaxed
  muscle tone or body posture.

NOC Outcomes
Pain Control; Medication Response; Self-Care:
  Parenteral Medication
NIC Interventions
Pain Management; Analgesic Management;
  Patient-Controlled Analgesia

Ongoing Assessment

Actions/Interventions	Rationales
■ Assess the patient's description of pain.	The first step in alleviating pain is assessing location, severity, and degree of both physical and emotional pain. Postoperative pain is usually localized to the affected joint. It will be acute and sharp. The pain should decrease in intensity over the 5 days after surgery. Intense pain that persists or pain that returns to previous levels of intensity may indicate a developing complication such as infection or compartment syndrome. Compartment syndrome is a condition that results from the unyielding nature of fascial coverings over muscles. The inflammatory process, which is the result of injured tissues (tissues traumatized by surgery), increases venous pressure, reduces venous return, and subsequently decreases arterial inflow. If tissue ischemia persists for longer than 6 hours, permanent tissue damage may result.
■ Assess effectiveness of pain-relieving interventions.	Patients have a right to effective pain relief. Pain relief is not determined to be effective until the patient indicates that it is acceptable.

Therapeutic Interventions

Actions/Interventions	Rationales
■ Explain analgesic therapy, including medication and schedule. If the patient is a candidate for PCA, explain the concept and routine. Instruct the patient to request pain medication before the pain becomes severe.	Care providers often assume that the patient will request pain medication when needed. The patient may be waiting for the nurse to offer it when it is available and may think it is his or her duty or responsibility to tolerate pain until it can no longer be tolerated. Successful use of PCA requires the patient to have knowledge of its use and the manual dexterity to operate it. If pain is too severe before analgesics or therapy is instituted, relief takes longer.

■ = Independent ▲ = Collaborative

Musculoskeletal Care Plans

Actions/Interventions

▲ Administer narcotic analgesics every 3 to 4 hours around-the-clock for the first 24 hours.

■ Encourage use of analgesics 30 to 45 minutes before physical therapy.

■ Change position (within hip precautions) every 2 hours or more often for comfort.

▲ Apply ice packs as ordered.

■ Provide comfort measures (frequent repositioning, back rubs, diversional activities). Encourage stress management techniques (guided imagery, progressive relaxation).

■ Maintain proper position of the operated extremity.

■ Investigate reports of sudden severe joint pain with muscle spasms and changes in joint mobility, and of sudden severe chest pain with dyspnea and restlessness.

Rationales

There is a massive amount of manipulation, nerve trauma, and tissue damage done during the surgical procedure. Assume that the patient requires analgesia. The patient's ability to fall asleep between pain assessments is not a good indicator of the patient's level of comfort. Coping with unrelieved pain depletes energy reserves and contributes to fatigue. The patient may sleep and still be in pain.

Unrelieved pain hinders the rehabilitative progress. Adequate pain relief will enhance the patient's level of participation in physical therapy activities.

The patient's inability to move freely and independently may result in pressure and pain on bony prominences.

Cold therapy may decrease edema and enhance comfort.

These measures reduce muscle tension, refocus attention, promote a sense of control, and may enhance coping abilities in relation to pain.

This reduces muscle spasm and undue tension on the new prosthesis and surrounding tissue.

Early recognition of developing problems such as dislocation of prosthesis or pulmonary emboli provides for prompt intervention and treatment of more serious complications.

NANDA-I NDx **Impaired Physical Mobility**

Common Related Factors

Surgical procedure
Discomfort
Pain

Defining Characteristic

Limited ability to ambulate or move in bed
Reluctance to attempt movement
Limited range of motion
Inability to perform action as desired

Common Expected Outcomes

Patient performs physical activity within limitations of prescribed mobility restrictions.
Patient demonstrates use of adaptive techniques that promote ambulation and transferring.

NOC Outcomes

Bone Healing; Ambulation; Coordinated Movement

NIC Interventions

Positioning; Exercise Therapy: Joint Mobility; Exercise Therapy: Ambulation

---

Ongoing Assessment

Actions/Interventions

■ Assess fear and anxiety about transferring or ambulating.

■ Assess the level of understanding of postoperative restriction.

Rationales

The patient may be fearful of injuring the joint replacement. Allaying anxiety or fear will allow the patient to concentrate on correct techniques.

Postoperative mobility restrictions must be maintained at all times to prevent dislocation.

Actions/Interventions	**Rationales**
■ Assess postoperative range of motion (ROM); document improvement and failure to progress compared with preoperative status.	ROM of joints must be maintained during periods of decreased activity. Arthritic joints lose function more rapidly when activity is restricted.

Therapeutic Interventions

Actions/Interventions:

Hip

Rationales

■ Encourage active ROM with all unaffected extremities.

Decreased mobility results in the loss of muscle tone in all muscle groups. Active ROM promotes muscle tone.

■ Encourage exercise as prescribed to affected joint.

Such exercise aids in increasing muscle strength and tone in the affected extremity.

■ Encourage use of analgesic before position changes.

Decreased or controlled pain allows better performance during therapy.

■ Use trapeze bar in bed to assist in mobility.

This device facilitates movement in bed.

■ Instruct the patient in maintaining total hip arthroplasty precautions during position changes.

These precautions prevent hip dislocation. These precautions may include use of an abductor wedge while in bed, no hip flexion greater than 90 degrees, and no bending from the waist.

▲ Maintain weight-bearing status on the affected extremity as prescribed.

Excessive weight bearing on the new hip increases risk for dislocation until healing occurs. Patients will begin physical therapy within 24 hours postoperatively.

Knee

▲ If prescribed, apply continuous passive motion (CPM) machine to affected leg at prescribed degrees.

CPM facilitates joint ROM, promotes wound healing, maintains mobility of knee, and prevents formation of adhesions to operative knee.

▲ Maintain proper position in CPM: maintain leg in neutral position; adjust CPM so knee joint corresponds to bend in CPM machine; adjust foot plate so foot is in a neutral position in the boot; instruct patient to keep opposite leg away from machine.

Proper positioning is imperative to prevent injury from moving parts.

■ Assist and encourage the patient to perform quad sets, gluteal sets, and ROM to both legs.

These exercises increase muscle strength and tone. Maintenance of optimal function in all unaffected joints is critical to overall recovery, because collateral extremities will be performing all activities of daily living (ADLs) until recovery is completed.

▲ Reinforce muscle-strengthening exercises taught by the physical therapist.

These exercises optimize return of full knee extension.

■ Elevate leg on a pillow when not in CPM. Place pillow under calf.

This position promotes full leg extension.

■ Encourage and assist the patient with sitting in a chair on first and second postoperative days. Instruct to sit with legs dependent several times a day. Initiate weight bearing as prescribed.

Patients will progress from a walker to crutches and finally to a cane. Weight bearing progresses with each advancement.

■ Encourage ambulation with walker or canes after initiated by the physical therapist.

Progressive daily ambulation promotes the patient's return to increased physical activity and self-care.

Shoulder

■ Maintain arm in shoulder immobilizer for 1 to 2 days or as prescribed. After the immobilizer is removed, maintain the patient's arm in a sling.

The immobilizer may consist of a sling or a sling and a strap that is applied around the body to restrain the arm and maintain proper body alignment.

■ Encourage and assist the patient in performing basic ADLs: self-feeding, brushing teeth, and combing hair. Provide extra time for the performance of these activities.

The patient may be performing ADLs using the nondominant arm, if the surgical site is located in the dominant arm.

■ = Independent ▲ = Collaborative

NANDA-I NDx Risk for Ineffective Tissue Perfusion

Common Risk Factors

Surgical procedure
Immobility

Common Expected Outcomes

Patient maintains adequate tissue perfusion, as evidenced by warm extremities, good color, good capillary refill, absence of pain and numbness, and bilaterally equal pulses.

Patient is free of signs and symptoms of deep vein thrombosis (DVT), pulmonary embolus (PE), and fat embolism, as evidenced by negative Homans' sign, normal respiratory status, stable vital signs, and normal arterial blood gases (ABGs).

NOC Outcome
Tissue Perfusion: Peripheral
NIC Interventions
Circulatory Care; Circulatory Precautions

Ongoing Assessment

Actions/Interventions	Rationales
■ Assess and compare neurovascular status of affected limb preoperatively and postoperatively.	Assessment must include unaffected and affected extremity to establish baseline and monitor for change in neurovascular status. Changes in neurovascular assessment findings may indicate the onset of compartment syndrome, peripheral arterial embolism, or DVT.
■ Assess affected extremity every 1 to 2 hours for signs of neurovascular compromise and damage:	
• Skin temperature	Injured tissues are usually cooler than on the nonoperative side. Normal temperature indicates adequate perfusion.
• Capillary refill of nail beds	Normal refill is 2 to 4 seconds. In the first hours after surgery, capillary refill may be sluggish, but refill that exceeds 4 to 6 seconds should be reported to the physician.
• Skin color	Color should be pink, not pale or white. The affected extremity may be paler than the unaffected extremity.
• Peripheral pulses	All peripheral pulses will be felt; however, the posterior tibialis and the dorsalis pedis in the lower extremities and the radial and ulnar pulses in the upper extremities may be weaker than in the unaffected area.
• Paresthesias	Complaints of numbness, tingling, or "pins and needles" feeling may indicate pressure on nerves.
• ROM	This evaluation indicates the amount and degree of limitations. Injured tissues will have decreased ROM. Decreased ability to wiggle findgers or toes occurs with nerve damage from compartment syndrome.
• Pain	Pain indicates injury, trauma, or pressure. Surgical site will normally be painful. Monitor and report excessive complaints of pain as a possible harbinger of compartment syndrome.
▲ Check sequential compression device and thromboembolic disease support (TED) stocking for extreme tightness.	Excessive compression may result in neurovascular compromise.
■ Assess for signs and symptoms of DVT:	DVT is a serious complication after joint replacement surgery.
• Positive Homans' sign	The examiner dorsiflexes the patient's foot toward the tibia, and the patient experiences pain in the calf muscles. Homans' sign may be absent with a DVT.

Actions/Interventions

- Swelling, tenderness, redness in calf; palpable cords

- Abnormal blood flow study findings (if prescribed)
■ Assess for signs and symptoms of PE: tachypnea, chest pain, dyspnea, tachycardia, hemoptysis, cyanosis, anxiety, abnormal ABGs, and abnormal ventilation-perfusion scan result.
■ Assess for signs and symptoms of fat embolism: pulmonary (dyspnea, tachypnea, cyanosis); cerebral (headache, irritability, delirium, coma); cardiac (tachycardia, decreased blood pressure, petechial hemorrhage of upper chest, axillae, and conjunctivae); fat globules in urine.

Rationales

Redness, swelling, and tenderness in the calf region may be indicative of a DVT. Further studies are indicated.
A Doppler ultrasound may be performed to diagnose a DVT.
Onset of symptoms can be sudden and overwhelming and can constitute an immediate threat to the life of the patient.
Fat embolism is usually seen the second day after surgery. Symptoms may be sudden and precipitous and represent an immediate threat to the patient's life.

Therapeutic Interventions

Actions/Interventions

▲ Notify the physician immediately if signs of compartment syndrome are noted.

■ Encourage leg exercises, including quad sets, gluteal sets, and active ankle ROM.
▲ Institute antiembolic devices as prescribed (sequential compression device or TED hose).

▲ Administer anticoagulant agents as ordered.

■ Encourage the patient to be out of bed as soon as prescribed.

Rationales

Venous pressures in the interstitial area surrounding an operative site can be measured through a small catheter inserted into the compartment. A surgical fasciotomy can be performed, which would release constriction and increase arterial inflow, restoring adequate circulation. The best indicators of developing compartment syndrome are patient complaint of excessive pain, peripheral pulses becoming weaker or absent, and an increase in pain on passive movement of the distal part to the surgery.
Venous stasis may predispose the patient to circulatory compromise.
Antiembolic devices increase venous blood flow to the heart and decrease venous stasis, thereby decreasing the risk of DVT and PE.
Prophylactic anticoagulants reduce the risk of thrombophlebitis or thromboembolism. The patient must be monitored closely because these medications may cause bleeding.
Mobility restores normal circulatory function and decreases the risk of venous stasis.

 NANDA-I NDx Deficient Knowledge

Common Related Factors

New condition
Unfamiliarity with discharge and rehabilitation plan

Defining Characteristics

Lack of or multitude of questions
Expressed confusion about arthroplasty precautions
Inability to follow mobility instructions

Common Expected Outcome

Patient verbalizes understanding of discharge instructions and follow-up rehabilitation regimen.

NOC Outcomes
Knowledge: Disease Process; Knowledge: Treatment Regimen; Knowledge: Prescribed Activity

NIC Interventions
Teaching: Disease Process; Teaching: Prescribed Activity/Exercise

■ = Independent   ▲ = Collaborative

Ongoing Assessment

Actions/Interventions	Rationales
■ Assess understanding of discharge instructions and follow-up regimen.	An individualized teaching plan is based on the patient's understanding of the treatment plan.
■ Assess home and support systems.	These assessments ensure that the environment is safe and supportive to the recovering patient.

Therapeutic Interventions

Actions/Interventions	Rationales
■ Review total hip arthroplasty precautions:	
• Maintain abduction with abductor device when at rest.	The patient needs to understand how to prevent hip dislocation. Extremes of joint flexion and adduction during the healing process increase the risk of dislocation.
• Always keep legs externally or neutrally rotated.	
• Avoid hip flexion of greater than 90 degrees.	Bending causes hip flexion of greater than 90 degrees.
• Avoid bending from waist.	This position causes adduction, which can lead to dislocation.
• Do not cross legs.	
• Ambulate (weight bearing as instructed) with assistive device (walker or crutches).	Protected ambulation promotes healing of the affected hip.
• Call the physician immediately if sharp pain or "popping" is felt in the affected extremity or if there is a feeling of the hip being "out of socket."	Dislocation of the prosthesis requires immediate attention and possible surgical intervention.
• Instruct the patient not to drive until directed by physician.	Muscle contraction and joint movement associated with operating the accelerator and brake pedals puts stress on the healing prosthetic joint.
■ Review knee arthroplasty precautions:	
• Use walker or crutches to ambulate with prescribed weight bearing on the operative knee.	Assistive devices reduce stress on the affected joint during the healing process.
• Do not participate in sports until the physician indicates that it is permissible.	The patient needs to limit activities that put stress on the affected joint during healing.
• Notify the physician of knee pain that returns to a previous level of discomfort, excessive swelling, leaking of fluid from incision, chest pain, shortness of breath, or pain and swelling in the calf of either leg.	These symptoms indicate complications of joint replacement and require immediate attention.
■ Review shoulder arthroplasty precautions:	
• Initially, perform only passive ROM exercises, gradually adding active exercises as instructed.	Gradual increase in ROM and weight bearing as necessary allows healing of the affected joint and prevents dislocation of the prosthesis.
• Avoid using affected arm for heavy lifting (greater than 5 pounds), pulling, or pushing. Follow weight-bearing precautions as instructed.	
• Avoid activities that involve exaggerated external rotation and abduction of the affected shoulder.	
■ Reinforce the need to continue prescribed ROM exercises. This may require home physical therapy.	Physical therapy at home helps the patient gain strength in muscle groups to support the integrity of the prosthetic joint.
■ Emphasize importance of removing environmental hazards (e.g., throw rugs, low tables, pets, electrical cords, toys).	The patient needs to understand how to maintain a safe home environment to promote progressive ambulation and prevent falls.

Osteoarthritis

Osteoarthritis (OA) is the most common kind of arthritis and generally is a disease of older adults. This disorder was formerly known as degenerative joint disease (DJD). Idiopathic (primary) OA is more likely to affect women over age 65. People with this type of OA usually have a family history of the disorder but no direct history of joint disease or injury. Weight-bearing joints and the spine are affected most often. Secondary OA occurs more often in men. People with this type of OA are likely to have a history of joint trauma or repetitive joint injury related to the person's occupation or sports activity. OA is characterized by a progressive degeneration of the cartilage in a joint. The changes in articular cartilage represent an imbalance between lysosomal enzyme destruction of and chrondrocyte production of cartilage matrix. This imbalance leads to an inability of the cartilage to withstand the normal weight-bearing stress in the joint. Cartilage becomes thin, rough, and uneven with areas that soften, eventually allowing bone ends to come closer together. Microfragments of the cartilage may float about freely within the joint space, and as a result inflammation occurs. True to the progressive nature of the disease, the cartilage continues to degenerate, and bone spurs called osteophytes develop at the joint margins and at the attachment sites of the tendons and ligaments. Over time these changes have an effect on the mobility and size of the joint. As joint cartilage becomes fissured, synovial fluid leaks out of the subchondral bone and cysts develop on the bone. Treatment is aimed at relieving pain, maintaining optimal joint function, and preventing progressive disability. This care plan focuses on the outpatient nursing management for this group of patients.

 ## Acute Pain/Chronic Pain

Common Related Factors

Joint degeneration
Muscle spasm
Physical activity
Bone deformities

Defining Characteristics

Reports of pain, spasm, tingling, numbness
Reports of a decreased ability to perform activities of daily living because of discomfort
Facial grimaces
Crying
Protective, guarded behavior
Restlessness
Withdrawal
Irritability
Refusal or inability to participate in ongoing exercise or rehabilitation program

Common Expected Outcomes

Patient reports satisfactory pain control at a level less than 3 to 4 on a 0 to 10 rating scale.
Patient uses pharmacological and nonpharmacological pain relief strategies.
Patient exhibits increased comfort such as baseline levels for pulse, blood pressure, respirations, and relaxed muscle tone or body posture.
Patient engages in desired activities without an increase in pain level.

NOC Outcomes

Pain Control; Medication Response

NIC Interventions

Medication Administration; Analgesic Administration

■ = Independent ▲ = Collaborative

Ongoing Assessment

Actions/Interventions

- Assess the patient's description of pain:
  - Pain is usually provoked by activity and relieved by rest; joint pain and aching may also be present when the patient is at rest.
  - Pain may manifest as an ache, progressing to sharp pain when the affected area is brought to full weight bearing or full range of motion (ROM).
  - Sharp, painful muscle spasms may be present.
  - Tingling or numbness may be present.
- Identify factors or activities that seem to precipitate acute episodes or aggravate a chronic condition.
- Assess previous experiences with pain and pain relief.

- Determine the patient's emotional reaction to chronic pain.
- Determine whether the patient is reporting all of the pain he or she is experiencing.

Rationales

The patient may manifest any part of the defining characteristics, so focused assessment is important. The patient may report pain in fingers, hips, knees, lower lumbar spine, and cervical vertebrae.

Pain may be associated with specific movements, especially repetitive movements.

The patient may have a tried-and-true plan to implement when OA becomes exacerbated. Consideration should be given to implementing this plan, with modifications if necessary, when pain becomes acute.

The patient may find coping with a progressive, debilitating disease difficult.

Patients who have become accustomed to living with chronic pain may learn to tolerate basal levels of discomfort and only report those discomforts that exceed these "normal levels." The care provider is not getting an accurate picture of patient status if this pain is not reported. The nurse may need to be sensitive to nonverbal cues that pain is present.

Therapeutic Interventions

Actions/Interventions

- Develop a pain relief regimen based on the patient's identified aggravating and relieving factors. Instruct the patient to do the following:
  - Change positions frequently while maintaining functional alignment.
  - Support joints in slightly flexed position through the use of pillows, rolls, and towels.
  - Apply hot or cold pack.

  - Provide for adequate rest periods.
  - Use adaptive equipment (e.g., cane, walker), as necessary.
  - Medicate for pain before activity and exercise therapy.

  - Eliminate additional stressors.

- Take prescribed analgesics and/or antiinflammatory medication. Provide instruction in important side effects.
  - Acetaminophen

Rationales

Muscle spasms may result from poor body alignment, resulting in increased discomfort.

Flexion of the joint may reduce muscle spasms and other discomforts.

Some patients prefer hot therapy over cold therapy to provide comfort.

Fatigue impairs ability to cope with discomfort.

These aids assist in ambulation and reduce joint stress.

Exercise is necessary to maintain joint mobility, but patients may be reluctant to participate in exercise if they are in too much pain.

Chronic pain takes an enormous emotional toll on its victims. Reducing other factors that cause stress may make it possible for the patient to have greater reserves of emotional energy for effective coping.

Simple analgesics such as acetaminophen should be used first. They relieve pain but have no effect on inflammation. This drug has fewer gastrointestinal (GI) side effects than nonsteroidal antiinflammatory drugs (NSAIDs).

Actions/Interventions

- Salicylates

- Non-selective NSAIDs

- Selective NSAIDs

- Corticosteroids

- Muscle relaxants

Rationales

These drugs relieve pain in the mild to moderate range and have an antiinflammatory effect. Side effects include GI disturbances, risk for bleeding, and tinnitus.

These drugs are antiinflammatory, antipyretic, and analgesic agents. They are usually used for their antiinflammatory action to relieve mild to moderate pain. Side effects include mild GI disturbances and fluid retention.

This class of drugs acts by reducing prostaglandin synthesis via inhibition of cyclooxygenase-2 (COX-2). These drugs are used with caution in people with a history of gastric ulcers, liver disease, stroke, or cardiovascular disease.

These drugs are antiinflammatory and usually used over a short period of time for the treatment of acute episodes of musculoskeletal pain disorders. In long-term therapy (exceeding 1 week), a vast array of symptoms may be seen, including sodium retention and edema, weight gain, glaucoma, psychosis, Cushing-like syndrome, and altered adrenal function.

These drugs may relax painful muscle spasms. They may cause drowsiness and may exaggerate the central nervous system depressive effects of alcohol and other drugs.

NANDA-I NDx **Impaired Physical Mobility**

Common Related Factors

Pain
Stiffness
Fatigue
Restricted joint movement
Muscle weakness

Defining Characteristics

Reluctance to move
Limited ROM
Decreased muscle strength
Decreased ability/refusal to transfer and ambulate or perform activities of daily living (ADLs)

Common Expected Outcomes

Patient performs physical activity independently or within limits of activity restrictions.
Patient demonstrates use of adaptive techniques that promote ambulation and transferring.
Patient is free of complications of immobility, as evidenced by intact skin, absence of thrombophlebitis, normal bowel pattern, and clear breath sounds.

NOC Outcomes

Ambulation; Knowledge: Prescribed Activity

NIC Interventions

Exercise Therapy: Joint Mobility; Exercise Therapy: Ambulation; Teaching: Prescribed Activity/Exercise

---

Ongoing Assessment

Actions/Interventions

■ Assess ROM in all joints. Assess the patient's range, comparing passive and active ROM in all joints.
■ Assess posture and gait.

Rationales

Pain or joint deformity may cause progressive loss of range of motion.
It is important to assess for indicators of decreased ability to ambulate and move purposefully: shorter steps, making gait appear unstable; uneven weight bearing; an observable limp; or a rounding of the back or hunching of the shoulders.

■ = Independent   ▲ = Collaborative

Actions/Interventions

- Assess ability to perform ADLs. Determine what adaptive measures the patient has already taken to be able to perform self-care measures.

- Assess the patient's comfort with and knowledge of how to use assistive devices.

- Assess weight.
- Assess the patient's vital signs after physical activity.

Rationales

Spouse may assist in buttoning clothes or picking up dropped objects. The patient may have had assistive devices installed in the shower or near the toilet (e.g., handlebars, raised toilet seat). Knowing this gives the nurse a sense of the measures the patient has had to take to remain functional.

Correct use of assistive devices for ambulation can improve mobility and reduce risk for falls. Some patients refuse to use assistive devices because they attract attention to their disability.

Excessive weight may be additionally stressing painful joints.

Elevations in heart rate, respiratory rate, and blood pressure may be a function of increased effort and discomfort during the performance of tasks.

Therapeutic Interventions

Actions/Interventions

- Instruct the patient in how to perform isometric, and active and passive ROM exercises to all extremities.

- Encourage the patient to increase activity as indicated.

- ▲ Consult physical therapy staff to prescribe an exercise program.
- Encourage the patient to ambulate with assistive devices (e.g., crutches, walker, cane).
- Encourage sitting in a chair with a raised seat and firm support.
- Encourage the patient to rest between activities that are tiring. Suggest strategies for getting out of bed, rising from chairs, and picking up objects from the floor to conserve energy.
- Stress the importance of the patient taking adequate time for activities.

- Discuss environmental barriers to mobility.

- Provide the patient with access to and support during weight-reduction programs.
- Suggest referral to community resources such as the Arthritis Foundation.

Rationales

Muscular exertion through exercise promotes circulation and free joint mobility, strengthens muscle tone, develops coordination, and prevents nonfunctional contracture.

Increasing activity at home can be effective in maintaining joint function and independence. A balance must exist between the patient performing enough activity to keep joints mobile and not taxing the joint too much.

The physical therapist can evaluate the patient's need for an individualized program.

Using mobility aids reduces the load on the joint and promotes safety.

This adaptive technique facilitates getting in and out of a chair.

Rest periods are necessary to conserve energy. The patient must learn to respect the limitations of his or her joints; pushing beyond the point of pain will only increase the stress on the joint.

The patient will need to recognize and accept the limitations of his or her joints. Rushing is likely to be frustrating and self-defeating and may result in unsafe conditions for the patient.

It may no longer be reasonable for the patient to continue to live in a home or apartment with multiple flights of stairs or to continue to try to take care of a large home. If the patient is using a cane or walker, carpets must be tacked down or removed. Items that are used often should be kept within reach.

Weight reduction results in decreased trauma to bones, muscles, and joints.

Community resources can provide the patient with peer support and additional information about resources (e.g., assistive devices).

Related Care Plans

Osteomyelitis

Bone Infection

Osteomyelitis is an infection of the bone that occurs as a result of direct or indirect invasion of an infective agent. Direct entry of the infective agent occurs after fracture or surgical intervention. Indirect entry (also called hematogenous infection) occurs as a result of a blood-borne infection with seeding of the infective organism, usually in the metaphysis of the bone. The most common site for the infection is in the long bones of the leg, although any bone can be affected. Older adults who are at greatest risk for developing osteomyelitis via the indirect route commonly have a debilitating disease such as diabetes, sickle cell disease, peripheral vascular disease, or trauma to the specific bone. The most common infective agent is *Staphylococcus aureus,* which accounts for more than 90% of osteomyelitis infections; other organisms identified include group B streptococci and gram negative bacteria. Osteomyelitis may be acute (less than 1 month's duration) or chronic (greater than 1 month's duration or unresponsive to one course of adequate antibiotic treatment). The bone infection is stabilized with intravenous (IV) antibiotics. Surgical debridement may be performed to infective areas on the bone. Patients are often discharged with IV access devices that allow them to continue aggressive antibiotic therapy at home, and home care nurses monitor patients' progress and coordinate the activities of other agencies, including social services and physical therapy. Complications of this disease include pathological fracture and the development of a systemic infection, which can be fatal.

NDx Infection

Common Related Factors

Infection of a bone resulting from an infective organism that enters through an open wound
Infection that has migrated to bone tissue from another source

Common Expected Outcome

Patient responds to antibiotic therapy, as evidenced by absence of fever, normal white blood cell (WBC) count, and negative wound culture findings.

Defining Characteristics

Local inflammation over the site of the involved bone characterized by edema, tenderness, redness, and warmth with or without a palpable mass over the site
Wound drainage

NOC Outcomes

Medication Response; Knowledge: Infection Control; Wound Healing: Primary Intention; Wound Healing: Secondary Intention

NIC Interventions

Infection Precautions; Wound Care; Medication Administration: Parenteral

Ongoing Assessment

Actions/Interventions	Rationales
■ Assess affected area for signs and symptoms of infection. Monitor temperature.	Symptoms of inflammation such as redness, warmth, or edema may be noted. Other symptoms might include malaise, chills, fever, diaphoresis, headache, and nausea.
▲ Assess laboratory values, especially WBC count.	WBC values will be extremely elevated; they may exceed 30,000/mm³.

■ = Independent   ▲ = Collaborative

Actions/Interventions

▲ Assess X-ray film and bone scan findings.

▲ Obtain appropriate culture and sensitivity specimens.

Rationales

Early x-ray films may be negative for as long as 2 weeks. Later, bone in the infected area will show destruction and decalcification. Later still, the bone will appear moth-eaten, and the dead bone may be surrounded by an area of sequestration where the infection has been sealed off and is impervious to the effects of antibiotics. Eventually new areas of infection will be apparent proximal to the original infection. Computed tomography (CT) scans may be more useful in the early days of the infection, because they can reflect more subtle changes. CT scans can also reveal the spread of the infection to soft tissues.

Aspirate from the affected bone will reflect the causative organism. Blood cultures will rule out bacteremia or septicemia. Blood cultures may reveal infecting organisms when the infection has become systemic.

Therapeutic Interventions

Actions/Interventions

▲ Administer IV antibiotics as ordered.

▲ Administer antipyretics, and provide fluids.

■ Use specialized cooling blankets or mattresses.
■ Provide nutritional supplementation, increased levels of protein, and vitamins A, B, and C.
▲ For patients with chronic osteomyelitis, prepare for surgical debridement.

Rationales

Aggressive antibiotic treatment is the primary therapy. Type and dosage of the medications ordered are specific for the patient with consideration of the patient's age and weight and the identified organism.

Drug therapy and fluid replacement prevent dehydration while the patient is in a febrile state. Temperatures may reach as high as 40° C (104° F).

These devices are used to reduce fever.

Adequate nutrition enhances cellular healing.

Surgery may be necessary to remove infected tissue and bone. Anticipate constant wound irrigation with antibiotics. Sepsis and unsuccessful antibiotic therapy are major complications.

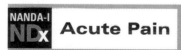

Acute Pain

Common Related Factors

Fractured limb
Muscle spasms
Bone and soft tissue trauma caused by surgery or infection
Restricted mobility

Defining Characteristics

Verbalized pain
Irritability
Restlessness
Crying, moaning
Facial grimaces
Altered vital signs; increased pulse, increased blood pressure, increased respirations
Withdrawal
Unwillingness to change position
Inability to sleep

Common Expected Outcomes

Patient reports satisfactory pain control at a level less than 3 to 4 on a 0 to 10 rating scale.

Patient uses pharmacological and nonpharmacological pain relief strategies.

Patient exhibits increased comfort such as baseline levels for pulse, blood pressure, respirations, and relaxed muscle tone or body posture.

NOC Outcomes
Pain Control; Medication Response; Self-Care: Parenteral Medication

NIC Interventions
Pain Management; Analgesic Management; Patient-Controlled Analgesia; Positioning; Splinting

Ongoing Assessment

Actions/Interventions	Rationales
■ Assess the patient's description of pain.	A careful analysis of the pain is essential to adequately treat it. Postoperative pain is usually localized to the surgical area. It will be acute and sharp. The pain should decrease in intensity over the 5 days after surgery. Intense pain that persists or pain that returns to previous levels of intensity may indicate a developing complication such as infection or compartment syndrome. Pain related to the infective process and the muscle spasms caused by osteomyelitis may be acute in the infective area until antibiotics sufficiently diminish the infective process.
■ Assess for correct positioning and alignment of affected extremity.	Incorrect positioning and malalignment can result in muscle spasms, which may be painful.
■ Identify the types of activity or positions that increase pain.	Measures may be taken to avoid precipitating factors.
■ Assess effectiveness of present pain relief measures.	Patients may know that their pain is effectively managed by a specific medication and dosage. This knowledge should be integrated into the nursing plan for pain management.

Therapeutic Interventions

Actions/Interventions	Rationales
■ Elevate and support the affected extremity.	Elevation of the affected extremity promotes venous return to reduce inflammatory edema. Supportive positioning protects against muscle strain and spasm.
■ Explain analgesic therapy, including medication and schedule. If the patient is a candidate for PCA, explain its concept and routine.	Care providers often assume that the patient will request pain medication when needed. The patient may think it is his or her duty or responsibility to tolerate pain until it can no longer be tolerated and may be waiting for the nurse to offer it when it is available.
▲ Administer narcotic analgesics and nonsteroidal antiinflammatory drugs as ordered, and carefully monitor their effectiveness. Monitor for adverse side effects.	There is a massive amount of manipulation, nerve trauma, and tissue damage as a result of the infective process. Assume that the patient requires analgesia. The patient's ability to fall asleep between pain assessments is not a good indicator of the patient's level of comfort.
■ Instruct the patient to request pain medication before the pain becomes severe.	If pain is too severe before analgesics or therapy is instituted, relief takes longer.
■ Encourage use of analgesics 30 to 45 minutes before physical therapy.	Unrelieved pain hinders the patient's ability to participate in the rehabilitative progress.
■ Change or assist the patient in changing position every 2 hours or more often for comfort.	The patient's inability to move freely and independently may result in pressure and pain on bony prominences.

■ = Independent ▲ = Collaborative

Actions/Interventions

- Eliminate additional stressors or sources of pain and discomfort by providing comfort measures: relaxation techniques, diversionary activity (e.g., books, games, television, sewing, radio), heat or cold application, position changes, and touch (e.g., back rubs).
- If indicated, explain that immobilization devices such as splints and external fixation devices may decrease muscle spasms and abrupt movement of the affected extremity, thereby helping to reduce pain.

Rationales

Directing attention away from pain or to other body areas decreases perception of pain.

Information about the purpose of immobilization devices can reduce the patient's anxiety, which may aggravate pain.

Related Care Plans

Ineffective coping, p. 49
Self-care deficit, p. 170

Osteoporosis

Brittle Bone

Osteoporosis is a metabolic bone disease characterized by a decrease in bone mass, resulting in porosity and brittleness. Bone resorption occurs at a rate that is faster than the process of bone deposition. Primary causes are a decrease in dietary intake of calcium or a decrease in calcium absorption and estrogen deficiency. Secondary causes may include steroid use, tobacco and alcohol use, and endocrine and liver diseases. Osteoporosis occurs most commonly in women who are menopausal, although it may also be present in women who exercise to such an extent that menstruation and resultant estrogen production are suppressed. Estrogen has been demonstrated to have a protective effect against the development and progression of bone changes that result in osteoporosis. Men and African American women have denser bones than white women. Men develop osteoporosis much later in life than women. These factors together with a decrease in physical activity and weight-bearing activities result in bones that are brittle and fragile. Even normal physical activity can result in fracture. Common fractures include compression fractures of the vertebrae and fractures of the femur, hip, and forearm. Vertebral compression fractures result in a progressive decrease in height and development of kyphosis. Osteoporosis combined with an increased incidence of falls in the elderly puts the older adult at higher risk for fractures. Adequate calcium and vitamin D intake are fundamental to all prevention and treatment programs for osteoporosis. Bisphosphonates (Fosamax, Actonel), salmon calcitonin, and raloxifene are medications used to prevent and treat osteoporosis. They act by reducing bone resorption. A program of moderate exercise has been demonstrated to arrest the progression of osteoporosis and reverse some of the effects of the disease. This care plan focuses on early identification and prevention of the disease.

 NANDA-I NDx ## Deficient Knowledge

Common Related Factors

Lack of information about dietary intake and bone density
Lack of information about prevention
Newly diagnosed with osteoporosis
Unfamiliarity with treatment regimen
Lifestyle places patient at risk for osteoporosis

Defining Characteristics

Multiple questions
Verbalized misconceptions
Request for help

Common Expected Outcomes

Patient verbalizes an understanding of prevention measures. Patient verbalizes understanding of the disease and treatment.

NOC Outcomes

Knowledge: Disease Process; Knowledge: Medication; Knowledge: Diet; Safety Behavior: Fall Prevention

NIC Interventions

Teaching: Disease Process; Teaching: Prescribed Diet; Teaching: Prescribed Medication

---

Ongoing Assessment

Actions/Interventions	Rationales
■ Assess the patient's knowledge of osteoporosis and treatment.	As people live longer, the risk for osteoporosis increases. However, many people do not believe that they are susceptible to it, do not understand the life-threatening injuries that may occur secondary to it, and do not realize that it can be prevented. Men may believe that only women develop osteoporosis.
■ Assess the patient's dietary intake of calcium and use of calcium supplementation.	Daily dietary intake of 1000 to 1200 mg of calcium is necessary. Calcium supplements are necessary if dietary intake is inadequate. Some people stop taking calcium supplements because of gastrointestinal (GI) upset, constipation, or cost.
■ Assess whether the patient is postmenopausal or has had hysterectomy with bilateral oophorectomy.	Resorption of bone is accelerated with natural or surgically induced menopause.
■ Assess tobacco, alcohol, exercise history, and if the patient is taking medications that decrease calcium absorption.	Smoking, drinking alcohol, and having only minimal weight-bearing exercise are risk factors for the development of osteoporosis. Medication such as cortisone, antacids, tetracycline, and laxatives may inhibit calcium absorption.
▲ Monitor calcium levels.	Elevated calcium levels indicate calcium malabsorption. This may indicate the need for vitamin D supplementation to aid in calcium absorption. The usual dose is 200 to 400 international units daily.

Therapeutic Interventions

Actions/Interventions	Rationales
■ Instruct or reinforce regarding risk factors for osteoporosis: 　• Risk factors are an inadequate dietary calcium intake, family history, and an inactive lifestyle. Also at risk are people who use cigarettes, caffeine, and alcohol and are older than 45 years, with or without endocrine disease. Estrogen deficiency is the primary risk factor for women.	This knowledge allows the patient to make decisions about lifestyle modifications to delay development of osteoporosis.
■ Describe diagnostic tests available: 　• Dual-energy x-ray absorptiometry (DEXA)	This test is used for early detection of the disease. Dual photons are used to measure bone density. This type of screening can be done for the hip, wrist, or spinal column. Patients at risk for osteoporosis should begin bone density screening in their 40s.
• Quantitative computed tomography (QCT)	QCT measures the density of bone.
• Ultrasound	Ultrasound measures of bone density of the heel have been found to reliably detect osteoporosis and risk for subsequent fractures of the hip.

■ = Independent   ▲ = Collaborative

Actions/Interventions

- Biochemical assessment

■ Reinforce dietary teaching about increased calcium intake. Encourage increased intake of calcium-rich foods: skim milk, cheeses, yogurt, ice cream; whole-grain cereals; green leafy vegetables; almonds and hazelnuts.

▲ Consult a dietitian when appropriate. Reinforce meal planning taught by the dietitian.

▲ Instruct the patient in taking calcium supplementation therapy as ordered.

■ Introduce or reinforce self-management techniques:
- Physical activity, at least 30 minutes most days of the week

- Use of assistive devices (e.g., canes, walkers)

- Protection from injury and falls

■ Introduce or reinforce information on medications:
- Bisphosphonates given in conjunction with calcitonin

- Calcitonin injection or nasal spray

- Selective estrogen receptor modulators (SERMs)

Rationales

Tests such as serum osteocalcin provide information on osteoblastic activity. Low levels of alkaline phosphatase are present in patients with osteoporosis.

Natural sources of calcium may provide more elemental or useful forms.

A registered dietitian can provide specific dietary guidelines for calcium and vitamin D intake based on analysis of the patient's dietary history.

The patient needs to understand that calcium supplements are available as calcium compounds. Calcium carbonate has the highest concentration of elemental calcium. This compound is often the least expensive. The patient should read labels and look for the word "purified" or "USP" (United States Pharmacopeia). Supplements without these words may be less reliable and may contain high levels of lead. Calcium supplements are better absorbed when taken with meals. If flatulence or constipation occurs with taking calcium supplements, the patient can increase his or her fluid and dietary fiber intake. However, eating large amounts of dietary fiber can interfere with calcium absorption. Foods high in oxalates such as spinach may also interfere with calcium absorption.

Weight-bearing exercise at a moderate level, such as walking, running, dancing, skipping rope, or circuit-resistance training, aids in development and maintenance of bone mass.

These devices assist in balance and take up partial weight bearing. They can help prevent falls and associated fractures in the patient with osteoporosis.

Until bone density is enhanced and stabilized, falls will constitute a grave risk to the patient manifesting symptoms of osteoporosis. Severe hip fractures can be fatal in certain debilitated populations.

These compounds inhibit bone breakdown and slow bone removal. Bisphosphonates increase bone density and decrease the risk for fractures. Patients taking oral bisphosphonates need to learn the correct method of administration. These drugs are best taken in the morning, 30 to 60 minutes before breakfast. The patient needs to remain upright during this time to reduce the risk of esophageal reflux. Intravenous (IV) forms of these drugs are available for patients who do not tolerate the oral preparations. The IV bisphosphonates are administered once a year to four times a year, depending on the specific drug.

Calcitonin is a naturally occurring hormone involved in calcium regulation and bone metabolism. Calcitonin prevents further bone loss by slowing the removal of bone and may be helpful in relieving the pain associated with osteoporosis.

SERMs activate estrogen receptors in target organs to produce effects on estrogen-responsive tissues. Raloxifene (Evista) is given for prevention and treatment of postmenopausal osteoporosis.

Actions/Interventions

- Teriparatide

Rationales

Teriparatide is a recombinant human parathyroid hormone used for the treatment of postmenopausal osteoporosis and in men with idiopathic or hypogonadal osteoporosis who are at high risk for fractures or who failed or are intolerant to prior osteoporosis therapy.

 Risk for Falls

Common Risk Factors

Impaired balance
Pain

Common Expected Outcome

Patient will not sustain a fall.

NOC Outcome
Fall Prevention Behavior
NIC Interventions
Fall Prevention; Environmental Management

Ongoing Assessment

Actions/Interventions

- Observe the patient's ability to ambulate and to move all body parts functionally.

- Assess the environment for safety.

Rationales

Walking or getting up from a chair or bed may present difficulty to the patient because of pain, balance, or gait problems. Because fractures can occur spontaneously with normal activity, protective measures must be taken until bone density has increased sufficiently to tolerate exercise.
A safe environment reduces the risk for falls and potential fractures.

Therapeutic Interventions

Actions/Interventions

- Promote mobility through physical therapy and exercise. Suggest moderate weight-bearing exercise (e.g., walking, bicycling, dancing) for 30 minutes three times a week. Reinforce techniques of therapeutic exercise (range of motion and muscle strengthening) taught by a physical therapist.
- Encourage the patient to request assistance with ambulation as necessary. Recommend low, comfortable shoes for walking. Provide adaptive equipment (e.g., cane, walker) as necessary.
- Teach the patient to create a safe environment at home: remove or tack down throw rugs, wear firm-soled shoes, install grab bars in bathroom, do not carry heavy objects.
- If a patient is hospitalized, provide a safe environment: bed rails up, bed in down position, necessary items (e.g., telephone, call light, walker, cane) within reach, adequate lighting, grab bars in bathroom (if available).

Rationales

Weight bearing stimulates osteoblastic activity and new bone growth. An exercise program will require modification on an ongoing basis as the patient's condition improves and bone strength is enhanced.

Pathological fractures are a complication of falls. Safety is a priority with activity. Assistive devices promote safety with ambulation.

A safe home environment is necessary to prevent falls and potential fractures.

These measures may decrease the risk for falls.

■ = Independent   ▲ = Collaborative

Disturbed Body Image

Common Related Factors
Deformities
Use of assistive devices

Defining Characteristics
Verbalization of negative feelings about kyphosis or decreased height
Refusal to use assistive devices

Common Expected Outcome
Patient demonstrates enhanced body image and self-esteem, as evidenced by ability to look at, touch, talk about, and care for actual or perceived change in posture and height.

NOC Outcomes
Body Image; Acceptance: Health Status
NIC Interventions
Body Image Enhancement; Self-Awareness Enhancement; Support Group

Ongoing Assessment

Actions/Interventions	Rationales
■ Assess perception of change in posture and height.	Bone loss causes loss of height and appearance of humped back (dowager's hump). Kyphosis and lordosis are deformities often found in osteoporosis.
■ Assess perception of how physical changes associated with osteoporosis change the patient's ability to perform activities of daily living, interact with others, and continue to be involved in occupational and diversional activities.	The patient may isolate self for fear of falling, difficulty in getting around, or self-consciousness about changed appearance.

Therapeutic Interventions

Actions/Interventions	Rationales
■ Acknowledge the emotional response to actual or perceived change in posture or height.	Once these changes have been acknowledged, ways can be found to reenter social life, interpersonal relationships, and occupational activities while still respecting actual limitations.
■ Encourage a positive attitude that some of the physical disabilities experienced will respond to adequate treatment and be abolished, reduced, or controlled.	The therapeutic regimen can be effective in reversing some of the early changes of osteoporosis.
■ Remind the patient to allow adequate time for self-care activities.	The patient's self-image improves when he or she can perform personal care independently.
▲ Reinforce self-care techniques taught by an occupational therapist.	Patients can learn new ways to perform self-care activities; this increases their sense of independence.
■ Provide the patient with community resources that can be helpful in supporting special needs in the home.	Such resources can increase independence and foster enhanced self-image.
■ Encourage participation in support groups.	This allows for open, nonthreatening discussion of feelings with others with similar experiences. Groups can give a realistic picture of the condition and suggestions for problem solving and coping.

Hematolymphatic, Immunological, and Oncological Care Plans

Anemia

Iron Deficiency; Cobalamin (B₁₂) Deficiency; Aplastic Anemia; Pernicious Anemia

Anemia is a general diagnostic term referring to a decrease in number or derangement in function of erythrocytes (red blood cells [RBCs]), and is the most common hematological disorder. Classification of the type of anemia begins with the complete blood count, with subsequent stepwise testing providing the actual diagnosis that guides treatment and prognosis. Three anemia classification strategies exist: cytometric, which measures the RBC mass and hemoglobin concentration; erythrokinetic, which measures RBC destruction and production; and biochemical, which looks at DNA. Cytometric measurements are easily measured and begin with evaluation of the mean corpuscular hemoglobin concentration (MCHC) and mean corpuscular volume (MCV). MCHC may be normocytic or hypochromic. MCV may be normocytic, macrocytic, or microcytic. The pattern of combination of these indexes classifies the anemia, directing the next sequence of blood work to assist in diagnosis and etiology of the anemia.

Normochromic/normocytic anemia (normal MCHC, normal MCV)	Anemia of chronic disease Acute hemorrhage Hemolytic ancmias Aplastic anemia
Hypochromic/microcytic anemia (low MCHC, low MCV)	Iron deficiency anemia Thalassemia major and minor
Normochromic/macrocytic anemia (normal MCHC, high MCV)	B₁₂ deficiency Folate deficiency

Iron deficiency anemia is a hypochromic, microcytic anemia usually occurring over time, resulting from dietary deficiencies, poor absorption, chronic blood loss as seen in younger women with heavy menses or older persons with gastrointestinal (GI) loss from ulcer, use of nonsteroidal medications, or GI malignancy. Cobalamin or B₁₂ deficiency and pernicious anemia arc both caused by deficiency of B₁₂. Pernicious anemia impedes B₁₂ absorption by lack of intrinsic factor in the stomach. Poor diet intake, certain medications, alcoholism, and some bowel disorders can cause cobalamin deficiency, resulting in this macrocytic anemia.

Aplastic anemia is a disease of diverse causes characterized by a decrease in precursor cells in the bone marrow and replacement of the marrow with fat. Aplastic anemia is characterized by pancytopenia, depression of all blood elements: white blood cells (WBCs) (leukopenia), RBCs (anemia), and platelets (thrombocytopenia). The underlying cause of aplastic anemia remains unknown. Possible pathophysiological mechanisms include certain infections, toxic dosages of chemicals and drugs, radiation damage, and impairment of cellular interactions necessary to sustain hematopoiesis. Advances in bone marrow transplantation and immunosuppressive therapy have significantly improved outcomes. This care plan focuses on ongoing care in the ambulatory care setting.

 NANDA-I NDx ## Deficient Knowledge

Common Related Factors
Unfamiliarity with disease
Lack of resources
Lack of recall
New condition or treatment
Complexity of treatment

Defining Characteristics
Questioning members of health care team
Verbalized inaccurate information
Inaccurate follow-through of instructions

Common Expected Outcome
Patient verbalizes understanding of own disease and treatment plan.

NOC Outcomes
Knowledge: Disease Process; Knowledge: Treatment Procedures

NIC Interventions
Teaching: Disease Process; Teaching: Procedure/Treatment

Ongoing Assessment

Actions/Interventions	Rationales
■ Assess the patient and family's understanding of new medical vocabulary.	Most persons have little exposure to hematological diseases and therefore have not heard or do not understand terms commonly used by health professionals.
■ Assess current knowledge of diagnosis, possible causative factors, disease process, and treatment.	Appropriate and individualized teaching can begin only after the patient's current knowledge and perceptions are determined. Patients may have a general understanding of anemia related to iron deficiency but lack knowledge of other types of anemia.

Therapeutic Interventions

Actions/Interventions	Rationales
■ Explain hematological vocabulary and functions of blood elements, such as RBCs, WBCs, and platelets.	Patients commonly have only a basic understanding of the hematological system.
■ Instruct the patient to avoid causative factor if known (e.g., certain chemicals).	A range of etiologies are possible including dietary deficiencies, medication side effects, alcohoism, and a variety of toxic chemicals. The anemia may be acute or chronic, depending on the etiology.
■ Explain the necessity for diagnostic procedures, including possible referral to hematology specialist and bone marrow aspiration.	Diagnosis of anemia is based on characteristic changes in RBC indexes and bone marrow. Often, stepwise testing is necessary to make the diagnosis.

Actions/Interventions

For nutritional deficiency anemias:

■ Explain the use of diet therapy and medications.
- Teach the patient and family about food sources of iron, folic acid, and vitamin B_{12}.

- Teach the patient and family about replacement therapy with iron and folic acid.

- Explain the need for vitamin B_{12} replacement.

For blood loss anemia:

■ Instruct the patient regarding medications that may stimulate RBC production in the bone marrow.

■ Explain that a transfusion of packed RBCs may be needed.

For aplastic anemia:

■ Explain the need for rapid human leukocyte antigen (HLA) typing.
■ Explain that allogeneic bone marrow transplantation is the recommended treatment for patients younger than 40 years of age who have HLA-identical related donors.
■ Explain that blood transfusions from prospective marrow donors should be avoided.
■ Explain that immunosuppressive therapy is the treatment of choice in patients without HLA-matched donors and/or older than 40 years of age.
- Immunosuppressive therapy includes antithymocyte globulin, cyclophosphamide, antilymphocyte globulin, granulocyte-macrophage colony-stimulating factor, and cyclosporine.

- Drug administration requires continuous monitoring of heart rate and blood pressure. Emergency resuscitation equipment must be immediately available.

Rationales

A balanced diet that includes a variety of foods from each food group usually contains adequate nutrients to support RBC formation. In particular, patients need to have adequate intake of dark-green, leafy vegetables; meat; eggs; and whole grain, enriched, and fortified breads and cereals.

Dietary replacement may not be sufficient to correct nutritional deficiency anemia. Supplementation is often necessary to support the formation of normal RBCs. The dosage and frequency of administration will depend on the severity of the anemia. Folic acid is given orally. Iron supplements may be given orally with meals to reduce gastric irritation. Stool discoloration is common with oral supplementation. Feces may have a dark greenish or black color and a tarry consistency. Intramuscular injections of iron may be given using the Z-track method to prevent leakage of the solution into subcutaneous tissue along the needle track.

Vitamin B_{12} injections are the primary therapy for this vitamin deficiency. These injections may need to be given monthly for the remainder of the patient's life. High doses of oral vitamin B_{12} have been shown to be effective in overcoming impaired vitamin absorption resulting from a lack of intrinsic factor.

Recombinant human erythropoietin, a hematological growth factor, increases hemoglobin and decreases the need for RBC transfusions.

Packed RBCs can be transfused to increase the amount of hemoglobin in the blood that can carry oxygen. One unit of PRBC typically will raise the hemoglobin concentration by 1g/dL.

This typing is performed to identify possible marrow donors.

Bone marrow transplantation has a very high success rate.

Histocompatibility antigens could lead to rejection of donor marrow.

Immunosuppressive therapy has become standard therapy for patients who do not have an HLA-identical donor. Autologous transplantation is not an option, because the patient's own marrow is defective. Marrow must be transferred from an identically matched donor who is healthy (i.e., allogeneic transplantation with identical HLA-matched donor).

These medications are not without significant side effects. Because of the risk for severe anaphylaxis, some centers admit patients to the critical care unit for drug administration. Patient safety is a priority.

■ = Independent   ▲ = Collaborative

Actions/Interventions	Rationales
• Complications:	
• Rejection of donor marrow	Rejection results from sensitization to histocompatibility antigens acquired during previous blood transfusions and carries a high mortality rate. Conditioning regimens using cyclophosphamide (Cytoxan) and total lymphoid irradiation show a reduction in the risk for graft failure.
• Acute graft-versus-host disease (GVHD)	A red maculopapular rash within 3 months after transplantation signals acute GVHD and carries a 20% to 40% mortality rate.
• Chronic GVHD	This can be manifested by many symptoms. Mucosal degeneration leading to guaiac-positive diarrhea, vomiting, and malnutrition is one manifestation.

NANDA-I NDx Fatigue

Common Related Factor

Reduced oxygen-carrying capacity of blood from decreased number of RBCs

Defining Characteristics

Report of fatigue and lack of energy
Exertional discomfort or dyspnea
Inability to maintain usual level of physical activity
Increased rest requirements

Common Expected Outcomes

Patient verbalizes reduction in fatigue, as evidenced by reports of increased energy and ability to perform desired activities.
Patient verbalizes use of energy-conservation principles.

NOC Outcomes

Endurance Energy Conservation; Activity Tolerance

NIC Intervention

Energy Management

Ongoing Assessment

Actions/Interventions	Rationales
■ Assess ability to perform activities of daily living (ADL), instrumental ADL and demands of daily living.	Fatigue can limit the person's ability to participate in self-care and perform his or her role responsibilities in family and society, such as working outside the home.
■ Assess specific cause of fatigue.	Besides tissue hypoxia from normocytic anemia, the patient may have associated depression or related medical problems that can compromise activity tolerance.
▲ Monitor hemoglobin, hematocrit, RBC counts, and reticulocyte counts.	Decreased RBC indexes are associated with decreased oxygen-carrying capacity of the blood. It is critical to compare serial laboratory values to evaluate progression or deterioration in the patient and to identify changes before they become potentially life-threatening.

Therapeutic Interventions

Actions/Interventions	Rationales
■ Teach energy-conservation techniques.	Patients and caregivers may need to learn skills for delegating tasks to others, setting priorities, and clustering care to use available energy to complete desired activities. Organization and time management can help the patient conserve energy and reduce fatigue.
■ Assist the patient in planning activities of daily living (ADLs). Guide in prioritizing activities for the day.	Setting priorities is one example of an energy-conservation technique that allows the patient to use available energy to accomplish important activities. Not all self-care and hygiene activities need to be completed in the morning. Likewise, not all housework needs to be completed in 1 day.
■ Assist the patient in developing a schedule for daily activity and rest. Stress the importance of frequent rest periods.	Energy reserves may be depleted unless the patient respects the body's need for increased rest. A plan that balances periods of activity with periods of rest can help the patient complete desired activities without adding to levels of fatigue.
▲ Refer the patient and family to an occupational therapist.	The occupational therapist can teach the patient about using assistive devices. The therapist also can help the patient and family evaluate the need for additional energy-conservation measures in the home setting.
■ Instruct regarding medications that may stimulate RBC production in the bone marrow.	Recombinant human erythropoietin, a hematological growth factor, increases hemoglobin and decreases the need for RBC transfusions.
▲ Anticipate the need for transfusion of packed RBCs.	Packed RBCs increase oxygen-carrying capacity of the blood.
▲ Institute supplemental oxygen therapy, as needed.	Oxygen saturation should be kept at 90% or greater.

Risk for Bleeding

NANDA-I NDx

Common Risk Factors

Bone marrow malfunction
Marrow replacement with fat in aplastic anemia

Common Expected Outcome

Patient has reduced risk for bleeding, as evidenced by normal or adequate platelet levels and absence of bruises and petechiae.

NOC Outcome
Blood Coagulation

NIC Intervention
Bleeding Reduction; Bleeding Precautions

Ongoing Assessment

Actions/Interventions	Rationales
▲ Monitor platelet count.	Thrombocytopenia, or low platelet count, is due to bone marrow malfunction caused by nutritional deficiencies, drugs, certain viral etiologies, or aplastic anemia. Some causes may result in temporary platelet abnormalities, whereas others are permanent. Risk for bleeding is increased as platelet counts are decreased.

■ = Independent   ▲ = Collaborative

Actions/Interventions

■ Assess skin for evidence of petechiae or bruising.

■ Assess for frank bleeding from nose, gums, vagina, or urinary or gastrointestinal tract.

■ Monitor stool (guaiac) and urine (Hemastix) for occult blood.

Rationales

Petechiae or bruising is usually seen when platelet count falls below 20,000/mm³.

Early assessment facilitates prompt treatment. These sites are most common for spontaneous bleeding.

These tests help identify the site of bleeding.

Therapeutic Interventions

Actions/Interventions

■ Consolidate laboratory blood sampling tests.

■ Instruct the patient regarding bleeding precautions, also known as platelet precautions:
  • Avoid rectal procedures such as enemas, suppositories, and temperature readings. Also avoid douching, vaginal suppositories, and tampons. During sexual intercourse the patient and his or her partner should avoid vigorous thrusting and use water-based lubricant to reduce friction and potential tissue tearing.
  • Instruct the patient to shave with an electric razor and to use a soft toothbrush.

■ Instruct in dietary modifications to reduce constipation.

▲ If platelet counts are very low, anticipate the need for platelet transfusions and premedication with antipyretics and antihistamines.

Rationales

Frequent blood sampling over time can contribute to anemia. Consolidation reduces the number of venipunctures and optimizes blood volume.

Precautions are necessary when platelet count falls below 50,000/mm³.

These activities can stimulate bleeding.

Trauma should be avoided to reduce risk for bleeding.

Constipation results in the passage of hard stools that can irritate the rectal mucosa and stimulate bleeding. Modifications include increased water intake to soften stool and avoiding rough foods. Stool softeners may be needed.

Platelet replacement may be required to reduce risk of bleeding. Premedication may reduce transfusion reaction effects.

Risk for Infection

Common Risk Factors

Bone marrow malfunction
Marrow replacement with fat in aplastic anemia

Common Expected Outcome

Patient has reduced risk for infection, as evidenced by normal WBC count, absence of fever, and implementation of preventive measures.

NOC Outcome
Immune Status

NIC Intervention
Infection Protection

Ongoing Assessment

Actions/Interventions

▲ Monitor trends in WBC lab values.

■ Assess for local or systemic signs of infection, such as fever, chills, malaise, swelling, and pain.

Rationales

A low WBC count, or leukopenia, is a decrease in disease-fighting cells circulating in the body. A low WBC count in adults is generally fewer than 3500/mm³.

Opportunistic infections can easily develop, especially in immunosuppressed patients.

Therapeutic Interventions

Actions/Interventions

Rationales

■ Stress the importance of thorough hand washing by the patient, caregiver, and visitors.

Meticulous hand washing is a priority in both the hospital and the outpatient or home setting to prevent transmission of pathogens.

■ Reinforce the need for daily hygiene, mouth care, and perineal care.

These measures prevent skin breakdown and reduce the risk for infection.

■ Instruct the patient to avoid contact with persons with colds or infections.

These are sources of infection for the compromised patient. Children 12 years of age or younger put the patient at particular risk because they can be "carriers" of infection, especially upper respiratory infections.

■ Instruct the patient to avoid eating raw fruits and vegetables and uncooked meat.

These foods can harbor bacteria. A low-bacterial diet protects the patient from exposure to pathogens.

▲ Administer WBC growth factor to stimulate production of neutrophils.

Granulocyte colony-stimulating factor (G-CSF), granulocyte-macrophage colony-stimulating factor (GM-CSF), filgrastim, and long-acting pegfilgrastim are effective as mobilizers of peripheral blood progenitor cells.

■ Instruct the patient to report signs and symptoms of infection immediately.

Any fever is significant. Antibiotics may be indicated.

▲ Anticipate the need for antibiotic, antifungal, and antiviral intravenous agents.

These agents counteract opportunistic infections.

■ If the patient is hospitalized, provide a private room for protective isolation.

Environmental changes may be necessary if absolute neutrophil count is less than 500/mm^3. Protective isolation precautions may include placing the patient in private room, limiting visitors, and having all people who come in contact with patient use masks, gloves, and gowns. These patients are at significant risk for infection.

Related Care Plan

Hematopoietic stem cell transplantation, p. 703

Cancer Chemotherapy

Cancer chemotherapy is the administration of cytotoxic drugs by various routes for the purpose of destroying malignant cells. Chemotherapeutic drugs are commonly classified according to their antineoplastic action: alkylating agents, antitumor antibiotics, antimetabolites, vinca alkaloids, and hormonal agents. Another way of classifying cancer chemotherapeutic agents is based on where in the cancer cell's life cycle the drug has its effect. Cell cycle–specific drugs exert their cytotoxic effect at a specific point in the cell cycle. Drugs that affect the cancer cell at any point in its cycle are called cell cycle–nonspecific drugs. These drugs are dose dependent in their therapeutic effect. Typically a combination of chemotherapeutic agents is administered to destroy the greatest number of tumor cells at different stages of cell replication. Cancer chemotherapy may be administered in the hospital, ambulatory care, or even home setting. It is recommended by the Oncology Nursing Society (ONS) that chemotherapy, biotherapy, and targeted therapies be administered by a qualified chemotherapy-competent nurse. Depending upon the specific cancer, cell type, cellular mutations, and stage of disease, newer targeted therapies and/or biotherapies may be administered along with chemotherapy. The goal of systemic treatment is cure, control, or symptom

■ = Independent ▲ = Collaborative

relief. It is often used as an adjunct to surgery and radiation. Because chemotherapy drugs are highly toxic and are given systemically, they affect normal cells as well as cancer cells. Most of the side effects of cancer chemotherapy are the result of the drugs' effects on rapidly dividing normal cells in the hair follicles, the gastrointestinal tract, and the bone marrow. The Oncology Nursing Society has developed evidence-based resources for patients experiencing chemotherapy-related side effects.

NANDA-I NDx Deficient Knowledge

Common Related Factors

Complex treatment
Unfamiliarity with proposed treatment plan and procedures
Misinterpretations of information
Unfamiliarity with discharge and follow-up care

Common Expected Outcome

Patient or caregiver verbalizes understanding of chemotherapy treatment, including rationale for treatment, self-management of interventions to prevent or control side effects, and follow-up care.

Defining Characteristics

Verbalized lack of knowledge
Expressed need for information
Questions to health care team
Verbalized misconceptions
Verbalized confusion over events

NOC Outcome
Knowledge: Treatment Procedure
NIC Interventions
Teaching: Procedure/Treatment; Chemotherapy Management

Ongoing Assessment

Actions/Interventions	Rationales
■ Assess patient and family's prior experiences with chemotherapy.	An individual's beliefs and expectations regarding treatment may be influenced by past experiences and hearsay.
■ Assess understanding of rationale for chemotherapy and type and goal of treatment.	The patient and family need information based on their understanding of the treatment plan using chemotherapeutic agents. A successful treatment plan requires the cooperation of the patient and support of the patient's family members.

Therapeutic Interventions

Actions/Interventions	Rationales
■ Instruct the patient and caregiver as needed:	
Treatment plan:	
• Need and schedule for laboratory tests before and during treatment	Regular laboratory tests are done to assess for electrolyte and metabolic changes; cardiac, pulmonary, and renal alterations; bone marrow function; the need for blood component transfusions; and the presence of infection.
• Chemotherapy agents to be used	Single agents are rarely used. Instead, combination therapies are used for their synergistic effects and to capitalize on their different mechanisms of action and side effect profiles. Many chemotherapy agents in combination with targeted therapies or monoclonal antibody regimens are approved and are in wide use.

Actions/Interventions	Rationales
• Method of administration	Oral and intravenous (IV) routes are most common, although regional delivery directly to the tumor site may be selected.
• Schedule of administration	Each drug protocol has a preferred time for administration followed by a rest period. Therapy is usually given in cycles.
• Setting for administration	Although therapy may be initially started in the hospital setting, the vast majority of systemic treatment is given in the outpatient setting.

Chemotherapy side effects:

• Potential short- and long-term side effects and toxicities	A variety of serious and distressing side effects occur with aggressive chemotherapy. These may include nausea, vomiting, constipation, fatigue, mucositis, alopecia and peripheral neuropathy.
• Period of anticipated side effects and toxicities	Patients need to be informed of the side effect profile for their specific agents.
• Preventive measures to minimize or alleviate potential side effects and toxicities	Patients need to be informed that most side effects can be managed to some degree.

Discharge planning and teaching:

• Catheter care (central venous, arterial, intraperitoneal catheters and devices)	Ongoing care is an important responsibility. Refer to the care plan for Central Venous Access Devices on the **Evolve** website.
• Signs and symptoms to report to health care professionals (e.g., bleeding, fever, acute pain, shortness of breath, intractable nausea and vomiting, inability to eat or drink, diarrhea)	Patients and family caregivers need to be able to recognize early indications of drug side effects. Early interventions to control side effects can minimize the impact on the patient's daily routines.
• Measures to prevent infection	The patient's immune function is usually impaired by chemotherapy-induced bone marrow suppression. Patient must understand strategies and measures by which they can protect themselves during times of compromised defense. Measures include following a low-bacterial diet, avoiding exposure to anyone with an infection, maintaining meticulous oral hygiene.
• Importance of balanced diet and adequate fluid intake	The patient and family caregivers need to understand how adequate nutrition can promote improvement in the patient's quality of life, but patients should not be forced to eat.
• Medications after discharge	Patients will be assuming responsibility for care.
• Activities of daily living (ADLs)	Fatigue, neutropenia, and other side effects will determine the patient's rate of return to activities of daily living.
• Follow-up care	Periodic evaluation of the patient's response to therapy will need to be closely monitored.
• Community resources and support systems	Advocates are available for information, support, and even caregiving.

■ = Independent   ▲ = Collaborative

NANDA-I NDx **Nausea**

Common Related Factors

Treatment related:
- Side effects of chemotherapy (inability to taste and smell foods, loss of appetite, nausea, vomiting, mucositis, dry mouth, diarrhea)
- Medications (e.g., narcotics, antibiotics, vitamins)

Disease effects:
- Primary malignancy or metastasis

Psychogenic effects:
- Conditioning to adverse stimuli (e.g., anticipatory nausea and vomiting; tension, anxiety, stress)
- Depression

Defining Characteristics

Reports "nausea" or "sick to stomach"
Increased salivation
Increased swallowing
Gagging sensation
Sour taste in mouth
Aversion to food

Common Expected Outcome

Patient reports diminished severity or elimination of nausea.

NOC Outcomes

Medication Response; Nutritional Status; Food and Fluid Intake; Comfort Level; Symptom Severity

NIC Interventions

Chemotherapy Management; Nutrition Therapy; Oral Health Maintenance; Medication Administration

Ongoing Assessment

Actions/Interventions

- Obtain history of previous patterns of nausea and vomiting and any treatment measures effective in the past.

- Assess the patient's description of nausea and vomiting pattern prior to each cycle of chemotherapy.

- Evaluate the effectiveness of the antiemetic and comfort measure regimens.
- Observe the patient for potential complications of prolonged nausea and vomiting.

Rationales

Chemotherapeutic drugs produce nausea and vomiting as a side effect by stimulating central receptors in the chemoreceptor trigger zone in the medulla or in the cerebral cortex. Some of the drugs stimulate peripheral receptors in the GI tract to cause nausea and vomiting. Nausea and vomiting are the most distressing side effects for patients and families and can significantly affect the quality of one's life. However, newer antiemetic medications have improved this condition for many patients.

Patient responses are individualized, depending on type and dosage of chemotherapy. Nausea and vomiting may be acute, delayed, and for some patients even prior to ("anticipatory") the chemotherapy treatment.

Patient responses to antiemetic medications are highly variable and must be explored with each patient.

Nausea and vomiting can alter a patient's hydration status because of fluid loss and effect electrolyte imbalance (hypokalemia; decreased sodium and chloride). Persistent vomiting and reduced nutritional intake can result in weight losss, decreased activity level, and lethargy.

Actions/Interventions

- Weigh the patient weekly or twice weekly at the same time and with the same scale. If the patient is at home, stress the importance of maintaining a log.
- Encourage the patient to record any food intake using a daily log.

Rationales

Consistent weighing ensures accuracy. Without monitoring, the patient may be unaware of actual weight loss due to imbalanced nutrition.

Determination of type, amount, and pattern of food intake (if any) is facilitated by accurate documentation, which provides data as to whether oral intake meets daily nutritional requirements.

Therapeutic Interventions

Actions/Interventions

▲ Administer antiemetics according to protocol.

- Explain that the selection of antiemetic agents should be based upon the emetic risk of the therapy and risk factors in the patient.

▲ Administer antiemetic around-the-clock rather than as needed during periods of high incidence of nausea and vomiting.

- Institute or teach measures to reduce or prevent nausea and vomiting:

  • Small dietary intake before treatments

  • Foods with low potential to cause nausea and vomiting (e.g., dry toast, crackers, ginger ale, cola, Popsicles, gelatin, baked or boiled potatoes, fresh and canned fruit, bland foods).

Rationales

Newer agents are much more effective in reducing the incidence and severity of emesis. Treatment protocols using a combination of antiemetic medications are most effective in controlling the nausea and vomiting associated with chemotherapy. This approach uses drugs that block nausea receptors at different sites and through different mechanisms of action. Antiemetic regimens are more effective in treating vomiting than nausea. A typical combination protocol may include administration of a 5HT3 (serotonin) receptor antagonist such as ondansetron and dexamethasone before chemotherapy. For delayed nausea, the protocol may include administration of dexamethasone and metoclopramide. New agents currently approved for acute and delayed nausea and vomiting include aprepitant and palonosetron. Other classes of drugs used to control nausea and vomiting include phenothiazines, butyrophenones, cannabinoids, and benzodiazepines.

The Oncology Nursing Society provides resources for recommended antiemetic regimens for high, moderately high, low, and minimal emetogenic chemotherapy. Administration of optimal antiemetic therapy during every cycle of chemotherapy will reduce the risk for development of anticipatory nausea and vomiting.

Effectiveness of antiemetic therapy is increased when adequate plasma levels are maintained.

Behavioral and dietary interventions seem to be most effective in the management of anticipatory nausea and vomiting. This pattern of nausea and vomiting is related to classical conditioning. The patient develops nausea and vomiting in response to stimuli associated with administration of chemotherapeutic drugs. Patients may try a variety of interventions to find those that best control this type of nausea and vomiting before drug administration. Antiemetic medications are less effective in the management of anticipatory nausea and vomiting. However, antianxiety medications such as lorazepam may be effective.

Having some food in the stomach prior to chemotherapy may reduce emesis. Easting small amounts reduces gastric overstimulation, thus reducing vomiting risk.

These foods are easily digested and provide a measure of success to augment nutrition.

■ = Independent   ▲ = Collaborative

Actions/Interventions	Rationales
• Avoidance of spices, gravy, greasy fried foods, and foods with strong odors	Fats are difficult to digest and may exacerbate nausea and can stimulate gastric motility.
• Meals at room temperature. Serve foods cold if odors cause aversions	The smell of cooking foods may aggravate feelings of nausea. Hot foods can stimulate peristalsis.
• Avoidance of coaxing, bribing, or threatening in relation to intake (help family to avoid being "food pushers")	Such behaviors tend to only aggravate the situation.
• Sucking on hard candy (e.g., peppermint) while receiving chemotherapeutic drugs with "metallic taste" (e.g., Cytoxan, dacarbazine [DTIC], cisplatin, oxaliplatin, actinomycin D, Mustargen, methotrexate)	Hard candies can reduce metallic or bitter taste.
• Drinking fluids at a different time than when eating solid snacks or meals	Separating fluids from solids will help not "filling" the stomach quickly. This may help prevent nausea as well.
• Minimal physical activity and no sudden rapid movement during times of increased nausea	Activity or sudden movement may potentiate nausea and vomiting.
• Relaxation and distraction techniques, guided imagery	These techniques, especially guided imagery, are useful adjuncts to antiemetic drug therapy. They can be helpful if used before nausea occurs or increases.
• Antiemetic half an hour before meals as prescribed	Appropriate timing of meds can reduce onset/severity of nausea.
• Use of acupuncture or acupressure.	Several small studies report acupuncture and acupressure to be useful measures in reducing nausea/vomiting risk.
• Offering meat dishes in the morning.	Aversions tend to increase during the day; chicken, cheese, and eggs are usually well-tolerated protein sources.

NDx Cancer-Related Fatigue

Common Related Factors

Tumor and metastatic disease
Chemotherapy/targeted therapy
Radiation
Pain
Distress (spiritual or emotional)
Anxiety/fear
Malnutrition
Anemia

Defining Characteristics

A sense of physical or emotional tiredness that is not proportional to recent activity or treatment and interferes with the individual's daily functioning.
Inability to restore energy, even after sleep
Verbalization of an overwhelming lack of energy

Common Expected Outcomes

Patient reports reduction in fatigue, as evidenced by reports of increased energy and ability to perform desired activities.
Patient reports use of energy-conservation principles.

NOC Outcomes

Activity Tolerance; Endurance; Energy Conservation; Self-Care: Activities

NIC Interventions

Energy Management; Nutrition Management; Sleep Enhancement; Exercise Promotion

Ongoing Assessment

Actions/Interventions	Rationales
■ Assess for fatigue regularly using 0 to 10 scale and defining characteristics.	Fatigue has become the most common and distressing complaint for cancer patients, especially during treatment. Regular assessment allows the nurse to evaluate the fatigue and response to interventions and to develop and alter the plan accordingly.
■ Refer to Fatigue (p. 66).	

Interventions

Actions/Interventions	Rationales

In addition to the interventions in the Fatigue care plan, consider the following:

■ Educate patient regarding these treatments:

• Assigning priorities to activities to accommodate energy levels	Setting priorities while conserving energy will allow the patient to achieve most desired goals and feel a sense of accomplishment.
• Energy-conservation strategies, such as:	Energy conservation techniques reduce oxygen consumption, allowing more prolonged activity.
• Sitting to do tasks	
• Pushing rather than pulling	
• Working at an even pace	
• Placing frequently used items within easy reach	
• Using wheeled carts for laundry, shopping, cleaning needs (see Fatigue, p. 66)	
• Limiting naps to 20 to 30 minutes	Limiting the amount of sleep during naps will help the individual to sleep at night.
• Use of psychostimulants after ruling out other causes	These medications have been used cautiously and demonstrate improved symptoms of fatigue in some patients.
• Treatment for anemia as indicated	Cancer patients' anemia results from the disease itself and treatment. Correcting the anemia may improve the patient's energy level.
• Cognitive behavioral therapy (CBT)	This type of psychotherapy facilitates psychological adjustment to cancer experience by helping certain patients recognize and change maladaptive thoughts.
• Nutrition consultation	Dietitian can counsel patient and family on how to maximize the patient's intake during treatment for optimal nutritional needs.

NANDA-I NDx Risk for Bleeding

Common Risk Factors

Bone marrow toxicity of chemotherapy
Disease of bone marrow
Invasion of bone marrow by malignant cells
Genetically transmitted platelet deficiency coagulopathies
   (tumor related or other)
Abnormal hepatic or renal function
Exposure to toxic substances (e.g., benzene, antibiotics)

■ = Independent   ▲ = Collaborative

Common Expected Outcomes

Patient has reduced risk for bleeding, as evidenced by platelets within acceptable limits, coagulation and fibrinogen within acceptable limits, and absence of overt and occult bleeding.

Patient is free of anemia, as evidenced by heart rate and blood pressure (BP) within normal limits, hemoglobin (Hgb) and hematocrit (Hct) within normal limits, and ability to perform ADLs.

NOC Outcome
Blood Coagulation
NIC Interventions
Bleeding Precautions; Chemotherapy Management; Blood Product Administration

Ongoing Assessment

Actions/Interventions	Rationales
▲ Monitor platelets daily. Anticipate platelet count nadir.	Risk for bleeding increases as platelet count drops: Nadir is when platelets are at lowest point. • Less than 20,000/mm³ = Severe risk • 20,000 to 50,000/mm³ = Moderate risk; may note prolonged bleeding at invasive sites • 50,000 to 100,000/mm³ = Mild risk; does not usually require treatment • Greater than 100,000/mm³ = No significant risk
▲ Monitor coagulation parameters (fibrinogen, thrombin time, bleeding time, fibrin degradation products) if indicated.	The blood clotting cascade is an integrated system requiring intrinsic and extrinsic factors. Derangements in any factors can affect clotting ability. These lab tests provide important information on clotting ability and bleeding potential.
■ Evaluate for any medications that can interfere with hemostasis (e.g., salicylates, anticoagulants, nonsteroidal antiinflammatory drugs).	Drugs that interfere with clotting mechanisms or platelet activity increase risk for bleeding.
■ Assess patient regularly for evidence of the following: • Spontaneous petechiae (all skin surfaces, including oral mucosa) • Prolonged bleeding or new areas of ecchymoses or hematoma from invasive procedures (venipuncture, injection, and bone marrow sites) • Oozing of blood from nose or gums • Rectal bleeding, vaginal bleeding, and/or increased menstruation • Neurological status	Changes in coagulation profile may be marked by ecchymosis, hematomas, petechiae, blood in body excretions, bleeding from body orifices, and change in neurological status (including headache, visual disturbances, or change in level of consciousness).
▲ If any significant bleeding occurs, monitor vital signs closely until bleeding is controlled.	Sinus tachycardia and increased arterial BP are seen in early stages to maintain an adequate CO. BP drops as condition deteriorates.
For risk for anemia: ■ Assess for signs of anemia secondary to bone marrow toxicity of chemotherapy or radiation therapy: tiredness, weakness, fatigue; pallor; dyspnea on exertion, palpitations or chest pain on exertion; dizziness; tachycardia; hypotension.	Although anemia may not signify a life-threatening problem such as infection or bleeding, it can significantly impact the quality of one's life.
▲ Monitor Hgb/Hct regularly based upon condition.	Low hemoglobin affects the oxygen-carrying capacity of the blood.
■ Assess for orthostatic changes secondary to reduced blood volume.	Postural hypotension is a common manifestation of fluid loss with active bleeding. Assessment may be more significant in older patients.
■ Determine nadir and anticipated recovery of bone marrow after chemotherapy administration.	This information helps in planning nursing measures.

Therapeutic Interventions

Actions/Interventions	Rationales

■ Instruct patient or significant others of relationship between platelets and bleeding:
- Platelet function
- Normal platelet count
- Effects of chemotherapy on bone marrow function and platelet count

A successful treatment plan requires the knowledge and cooperation of the patient and family members.

■ Implement bleeding precautions for a platelet count of less than 50,000/mm^3.

Understanding of precautionary measures reduces risk of bleeding. At platelet counts less than 50,000/mm^3 spontaneous bleeding can occur.

■ Avoid nonessential invasive procedures, punctures, and injections.

This practice reduces bleeding at vascular access sites.

■ Avoid rectal thermometers, suppositories, and enemas.

Use increases the chance of rectal bleeding.

▲ Communicate the anticipated need for platelet support to a transfusion center. Transfuse single or random donor platelets, as ordered.

It is important to have platelets available when needed (e.g., when platelets are less than 10,000/mm^3 or in the presence of active bleeding). Platelet thresholds need to be individualized. Prophylactic platelet transfusions may be administered.

▲ Administer fresh frozen plasma or coagulation factors, as prescribed.

These therapies provide all the needed clotting factors, except platelets.

■ See additional bleeding precautions and nursing interventions, in Leukemia, p. 724.

For risk for anemia:

■ Estimate energy expenditures of ADLs; prioritize activities accordingly. Plan or promote rest periods.

A plan that balances periods of activity with periods of rest can help the patient complete desired activities without increased fatigue. Rest lowers the body's oxygen requirement and decreases cardiopulmonary strain.

■ Instruct the patient to change position slowly.

This method allows for circulatory compensation to prevent dizziness and possible injury.

▲ Administer erythropoietin agent as ordered (e.g., epoetin alfa, darbepoetin alfa).

These agents correct anemia by stimulating production of RBCs in the same way as endogenous human erythropoietin.

▲ Maintain a current blood sample for "type and screen" in the transfusion center. Transfuse packed red blood cells (RBCs), as ordered.

This practice ensures availability and readiness of packed RBCs when needed. Transfusion may be required to restore Hgb/Hct to levels at which the patient experiences minimal symptoms.

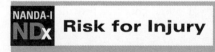

NANDA-I NDx Risk for Injury

Common Risk Factors

Hypersensitivity to drugs
Potential side effects and toxicities of drugs
Extravasation
Infiltration of drug from vein

■ = Independent   ▲ = Collaborative

Common Expected Outcome

Patient has reduced risk for injury from drug therapy, as evidenced by normal vital signs, absence of reaction, no pain at infusion site, adequate blood return from IV catheter, and prompt reporting of adverse signs and symptoms.

NOC Outcomes
Blood Circulation; Medication Response; Risk Control; Risk Detection

NIC Interventions
Allergy Management; Medication Administration; Emergency Care; IV Therapy; Venous Access Device Management

Ongoing Assessment

Actions/Interventions	Rationales
■ Note allergy history.	Drug hypersensitivity is an immune-mediated reaction to a drug. Symptoms range from mild to severe. This information guides selection of prescribed meds. Patient safety is a priority.
■ Monitor for potential hypersensitivity, side effects, or toxicities to chemotherapeutic drugs.	Patients, family, and staff need to be vigilant when the patient is starting any new agent, as well as monitoring effects for prolonged periods. A variety of responses to chemotherapy are possible. These can include restlessness, facial edema and flushing, wheezes, bronchospasms, tachycardia, hypotension or hypertension, diaphoresis, fever, increased uric acid levels, runny nose, skin rash, temporomandibular joint pain, frontal sinusitis, ileus, diarrhea.
■ Monitor for hypersensitivity, side effects, or toxicities to common antiemetic drugs.	Antiemetic medications meant to be helpful also exhibit their own side effects. These can include agitation and restlessness, hypotension, tachycardia, irritability, facial flushing, extrapyramidal reactions, dry mouth, sedation, blurred vision, drowsiness, dizziness, headache, diarrhea, urine retention.
▲ Monitor relevant laboratory data.	Complete blood count, differential, platelets, metabolic panel, and electrocardiogram provide baseline and response data.
■ Assess IV insertion site at frequent intervals according to established hospital policy and procedure: blood return, patency of vein and catheter, signs of infiltration.	Defective or malpositioned indwelling central venous catheter or access device can cause extravasation into local subcutaneous tissue surrounding the administration site.
■ Determine whether the chemotherapeutic agent has vesicant properties. Observe injection or infusion site closely during chemotherapy administration.	Chemotherapy can cause tissue damage if it leaks outside the vein; however, not all agents have the same likelihood of causing tissue damage if infiltrated. Refer to hospital policy and procedure manual for guidelines.

Therapeutic Interventions

Actions/Interventions	Rationales
■ Insure that two chemotherapy-competent RNs perform independent double check of written order for each agent for specific drug name, dose, route, time, and frequency of antiemetic or chemotherapy drugs to be administered, based upon patient's body surface area and treatment regimen.	Patient safety is a priority. Double-checking provides a measure of safety.
■ Know immediate and delayed side effects of drugs to be administered.	Each nurse has a responsibility to be familiar with potential side effects or complications associated with each agent being administered, whether a standard or experimental drug treatment.

Actions/Interventions

- Inform the patient or significant others to report adverse effects. Delineate which changes indicate emergencies that must be reported immediately.
- Maintain or restore adequate fluid balance.

▲ For drugs associated with a high risk for anaphylaxis:
  - Administer the first dose in a hospital setting. Stay with the patient while the drug is being administered.
▲ When an adverse drug reaction is suspected, stop infusion; administer emergency drugs as prescribed; notify physician; take and record vital signs; maintain patent IV with normal saline solution; reassure patient.
- Select veins most suitable for administration of chemotherapeutic agents.

- Avoid veins in the antecubital fossa, near the wrist, or on the dorsal surface of the hand.
- Instruct the patient to report tenderness, stinging, burning, or other unusual sensation at the IV site immediately. Evaluate patient complaints of "painful infusion."

▲ Keep extravasation kit and chemotherapy spill kits available.

▲ When drug extravasation is suspected, stop infusion, initiate extravasation management appropriate for the chemotherapeutic drug being infiltrated, notify the physician, reassure the patient, and document the incident according to institutional policy and procedure.

Rationales

Changes that a patient perceives as "minor" may be highly significant.

Fluid therapy reduces potential drug toxicity in that fluids help clear the body of accumulated metabolic by-products. Older patients with reduced blood volumes and functional deterioration are especially at risk.

Patient safety is a priority. Prompt treatment reduces further injury.
Prompt treatment reduces complications and provides reassurance to the patient.

These are the cephalic, median brachial, and basilic veins in the mid-forearm area. Venous access devices may also be used. NOTE: Only specially trained and competencied nurses can administer chemotherapy.
Damage to underlying tendons and nerves may occur in the event of drug extravasation of a vesicant.
Infiltration of chemicals (vesicants) causes tissue damage on direct contact, with pain as the most frequent complaint. Accurate assessment guides treatment. It is important to rule out the source of extravasation versus other causes of pain (which may include chemical composition of drug, venous spasm, phlebitis, and/or psychogenic factors).
Contents vary according to hospital policy. Kits and procedures for treating extravasation must also be available in the home if chemotherapy is being administered in that setting. Chemotherapy spill kits should also be available in the home.
Management of the site after extravasation remains a controversial issue in chemotherapy administration. However, most hospitals and agencies have developed care standards in management of extravasation of drugs classified as "vesicants." These agents potentially cause cellular damage, ulceration, and tissue necrosis. A plastic surgeon may be consulted for debridement or skin grafting, depending on the extent of injury.

NANDA-I NDx
Disturbed Body Image

Common Related Factors

Loss of hair (scalp, eyebrows, eyelashes, pubic and body hair)
Discoloration of fingernails, veins
Breakage or loss of fingernails
Changes in skin color and texture
Generalized "wasting"
Presence of externalized or implanted venous access device
Concurrent surgical changes (mastectomy, colostomy)

Defining Characteristics

Self-deprecating remarks
Verbal preoccupation with changed body parts
Refusal to look at self in mirror
Crying
Anger
Decreased attention to grooming
Compensatory use of makeup, concealing makeup, clothing, devices
Decreased social interaction

■ = Independent ▲ = Collaborative

Common Expected Outcomes

Patient demonstrates enhanced body image as evidenced by ability to look at, touch, talk about, and care for altered body part.

Patient verbalizes understanding of temporary nature of side effects.

Patient engages in meaningful social interactions.

NOC Outcomes
Body Image; Self Esteem

NIC Interventions
Body Image Enhancement; Hope Installation; Coping Enhancement

Ongoing Assessment

Actions/Interventions	Rationales
■ Assess perception of change in structure or function of body part.	The extent of the response is more related to the value or importance the patient places on the part than the actual value.
■ Note the frequency of the patient's self-critical remarks.	Negative statements about the affected body part indicate limited ability to integrate the change into the patient's self-concept.
■ Note the patient's behavior regarding the actual or perceived changed body part.	There is a broad range of behaviors associated with body image disturbance, ranging from totally ignoring the altered structure or function to preoccupation with it.

Therapeutic Interventions

Actions/Interventions	Rationales
■ Acknowledge normalcy of emotional response to the actual or perceived changes in physical appearance.	For some patients, the fear of treatment side effects can feel worse than the disease.
■ Encourage verbalization of feelings; listen to concerns.	This may open lines of communication and help relieve anxiety. Expression of feelings can enhance the person's coping strategies.
■ Convey feelings of acceptance and understanding.	The nurse is in an ideal position to promote acceptance of the situation.
■ Provide anticipatory guidance on hair alternatives for alopecia (e.g., suggest purchase of a wig or turbans before chemotherapy), on makeup and skin care for changes in skin color and texture, and on clothing to camouflage venous access device.	Adaptive behaviors can compensate for the changed body structure and function. Patients need to understand that hair loss may occur over a short period of time. Some patients begin wearing wigs, scarves, or other types of head coverings before the hair loss occurs. This approach decreases the dramatic changes in their appearance.
■ Offer realistic assurance of temporary nature of some physical changes.	It is important that the patient understand that hair and nails will begin to regrow, usually within 1 to 2 months after chemotherapy is completed, and that external or implanted venous access devices will eventually be removed.
■ Refer to support group composted of individuals with similar alterations.	Groups that come together for mutual support and information can be a valuable resource. Although family and friends can be great allies, often a formal support group or communication with a cancer survivor is most helpful.

NANDA-I NDx **Risk for Injury**

Common Risk Factor

Improper handling or disposal of waste material in the home

Common Expected Outcome

Nurse, patient, or caregiver maintains safe handling and disposal of waste material according to institutional procedures and policies.

NOC Outcome
Safe Home Environment

NIC Interventions

Surveillance: Safety; Home Maintenance Assistance

Ongoing Assessment

Actions/Interventions	**Rationales**
If chemotherapy is administered in the home:	Safety is a priority. Special heavy duty plastic bags are used that are leak resistant when being transported. Bags should include a chemotherapy bio-hazard warning.
■ Determine that chemotherapy medications are clearly labeled and safely transported to the home.	
■ Determine that an adequate area is available for the safe preparation of the medication.	This area should be at a bathroom or kitchen counter but away from food items that could become contaminated.
■ Ensure that waste materials are disposed of in accordance with established policies (e.g., not flushing unused medication or fluids down the toilet; always placing contaminated needles, tubing, and syringes in biohazard containers).	Waste materials are usually returned to the health care facility for appropriate disposal.

Therapeutic Interventions

Actions/Interventions	**Rationales**
■ Instruct the family and caregiver to avoid contact with the patient's excreta.	The patient may need to use a private bathroom. Contaminated linen should be cared for according to established procedure.
■ If a spill occurs, institute safety precautions according to established procedures (e.g., use of gloves, gown, goggles, plastic disposal bags).	These measures should be rehearsed in the home environment so patient and caregivers are prepared to act.

Related Care Plans

Anxiety, p. 18
Deficient fluid volume, p. 72
Diarrhea, p. 54
Fatigue, p. 66
Fear, p. 69
Hematopoietic stem cell collection (see the **Evolve** website)
Imbalanced nutrition: less than body requirements, p. 142
Neutropenia, p. 753
Risk for infection, p. 114

■ = Independent   ▲ = Collaborative

Hematolymphatic, Immunological and Oncological Care Plans

Cancer Radiation Therapy

External Beam; Brachytherapy; Teletherapy

Radiation therapy is the use of ionizing radiation delivered in prescribed doses to a malignancy. Ionizing radiation interacts with the atoms and molecules of malignant cells, interfering with mitotic activity, thereby causing DNA damage. This damage interferes with the malignant cell's ability to reproduce. Adjacent healthy cells experience the same detrimental effects, however, resulting in untoward side effects to radiation therapy. Radiation therapy may be curative of some cancers, or it may be used as a palliative treatment to reduce the pain and pressure from large tumors. Radiation may be used alone or in combination with other treatment modalities such as surgery, chemotherapy, and/or biotherapy.

Radiation therapy can be divided into two broad categories: external radiation, also known as *teletherapy,* and internal radiation, commonly known as *brachytherapy.* Teletherapy administers a prescribed dosage of radiation at a distance from the patient using a machine, such as a linear accelerator. Brachytherapy is the implantation of either sealed (solid) or unsealed (fluid) radioactive sources. The sealed radioactive implant may be contained within an applicator, needle, or seed, and is placed in or near the malignancy. The unsealed radioactive isotope can be administered through the intravenous or oral route or by instillation into a specific body cavity.

The radiation oncologist prescribes the treatment modality and amount of treatment necessary. This treatment plan is based on the location, size, and biological characteristics of the malignancy. The patient's health history, current health status, and previous cancer treatments are taken into consideration in treatment planning. All health care providers need to implement principles of radiation safety when caring for patients undergoing radiation therapy.

NANDA-I NDx Deficient Knowledge

Common Related Factors
Unfamiliarity with treatment protocols
Misinformation about radiation therapy

Defining Characteristics
Verbalizes anxiety about therapy
Asks many questions about treatment
Lack of questions about treatment

Common Expected Outcome
Patient verbalizes accurate knowledge about radiation therapy.

NOC Outcomes
Knowledge: Treatment Procedure; Anxiety Self-Control

NIC Interventions
Teaching: Procedure/Treatment; Radiation Therapy Management; Anxiety Reduction

---

Ongoing Assessment

Actions/Interventions	Rationales
■ Assess the patient's knowledge of and previous experience with radiation therapy.	Appropriate and individualized teaching is based on the patient's current knowledge and perceptions.
■ Assess any fears, myths, or misconceptions that the patient has about radiation therapy.	Patients and families may have anxiety and fear about the radioactivity of the patient during therapy. These misconceptions need to be clarified and corrected to promote the patient's cooperation with the treatment plan.

Therapeutic Interventions

Actions/Interventions	Rationales
■ Explain the purpose of radiation therapy.	The patient and family need to understand the role that radiation therapy has in the treatment of the patient's cancer. They need to understand whether the treatment goal is curative or palliative and how it may work with other treatment procedures.
■ Teach the patient and family what to expect during the treatment procedure: • Planning simulation • External beam treatment • Insertion of internal radiation	The process of preparation for therapy can be more anxiety producing than the actual procedure itself. Patients having external beam therapy will undergo an extensive and time-consuming planning process that includes a simulation of the treatment. During this simulation, the treatment area is located and marked on the skin. Adjacent tissue areas that will be shielded or blocked during therapy are identified. The procedure for implanting internal radiation will depend on the location of the malignancy.
■ Explain all site-specific care to the patient and family.	For the patient with external beam therapy, maintaining skin integrity and reporting side effects will facilitate prompt intervention and reduce complications. The generalized side effects associated with radiation therapy are fatigue and anorexia.
■ Correct any misconceptions the patient and family have about radioactivity.	The patient undergoing external beam therapy is never radioactive. The patient and family do not need to take any special safety precautions. The patient with a temporary implant emits radioactivity during the time the implant is in place. These patients are usually hospitalized, and specific precautions are taken to reduce radiation exposure to staff and visitors. The patient with a permanent sealed implant has a low level of radiation outside the body and the risk to others is minimal. The patient and family will be taught specific precautions to be taken at home depending on the location of the implant and the half-life of the isotope.
■ Provide information about common side effects.	Side effects depend on the treatment dose and the part of the body that is treated. Fatigue and skin reactions are commonly experienced during radiation to any site. Fatigue can be debilitating. Site-specific side effects may include dry mouth, difficulty swallowing, and bone changes. Anorexia is likewise commonly experienced.

 NANDA-I NDx **Risk for Impaired Skin Integrity**

Common Risk Factor

External beam radiation

Common Expected Outcome

The patient's skin will remain intact and free of irritation or breakdown.

NOC Outcome
Tissue Integrity: Skin and Mucous Membranes
NIC Interventions
Skin Surveillance; Radiation Therapy Management; Skin Care: Topical Treatments

---

■ = Independent   ▲ = Collaborative

Ongoing Assessment

Actions/Interventions	Rationales
■ Assess the patient's skin in the treatment area for signs of radiation effects.	Every effort is made in planning external beam treatment to implement skin-sparing approaches to minimize the effect on healthy skin.
• Erythema and darkening	Redness of skin may develop within the first 24 hours after the first treatment. As the melanocytes in the skin are stimulated during treatment, the skin may appear darker.
• Dry desquamation	When basal cells of the epidermis are affected by radiation, they begin to shed from the skin and allow new cells to develop.
• Wet desquamation	If the rate of epidermal cell sloughing exceeds the rate of new cell replacement, the skin becomes moist and begins to break down.
■ Assess the skin for long-term effects of radiation therapy.	Long-term changes in the skin are related to the total amount of radiation the patient received during therapy. The epidermis may be thinner, with less hair and fewer sweat glands in the treatment area. The skin will be less resistant to trauma and may take longer to heal. Fibrosis of the dermis and hyperplasia of the blood vessels may lead to development of telangiectasia and spider veins.

Therapeutic Interventions

Actions/Interventions	Rationales
■ Clean the skin in the treatment area with a mild, nonperfumed soap and tepid water. Use a soft cloth, and avoid rubbing the skin. Dry thoroughly. Do not apply any skin care products within 4 hours before treatment.	Any markings used as treatment guidelines should not be removed from the skin until therapy is completed. Keeping the skin clean, dry, and free of irritants will promote skin integrity and reduce the risk for wet desquamation.
■ Apply lubricating lotions or creams that do not contain metals, alcohol, fragrances, or additives that irritate the skin. This includes antiperspirants containing aluminum.	Intervention protocols may vary among treatment centers. The radiation oncologist may recommend particular brands of moisturizers to relieve dry skin.
■ Teach the patient to avoid scratching dry, itchy skin.	Scratching increases skin trauma in the treatment area. Cornstarch, sprinkled on the skin, may provide some relief from itching.
■ Teach the patient to avoid exposing the skin to pressure, sunlight, rough clothing, shaving, and extremes of temperature. Avoid tape or other products that may cause tearing or scratching of the skin.	Pressure from tight or irritating clothing will increase skin irritation and the risk for skin breakdown in the treatment area. Lightweight cotton clothing is best. The skin in the treatment area is more vulnerable to the effects of heat, cold, and ultraviolet light from sunlight or artificial sources such as tanning lamps. Use of protective clothing and sunscreens is recommended for the treatment area even after therapy is completed.
▲ Implement skin care protocol for wet desquamation.	Treatment of wet desquamation varies among treatment centers. A standard treatment protocol may include irrigation of the area with a solution of one part hydrogen peroxide with three parts normal saline. Consult with radiation oncologist or wound care specialist for recommendations. Dry the area thoroughly, and leave open to air. If drainage is present or if the area comes in contact with clothing, a nonadherent dressing may be applied. Use nontape methods to secure the dressing.

Risk for Injury (Radiation Exposure)

Common Risk Factors

Internal radiation
Dislodged radiation implant
Lack of knowledge of radiation safety principles

Common Expected Outcome

Health care providers and visitors will have minimal radiation exposure.

NOC Outcomes
Knowledge: Personal Safety; Risk Control; Risk Detection

NIC Interventions
Radiation Therapy Management; Environment Management; Worker Safety

Ongoing Assessment

Actions/Interventions	Rationales
■ Review the radiation treatment plan: • Type of radiation • Isotope half-life • Method of delivery • Duration of treatment	Implementation of radiation safety precautions will depend on the amount of energy emitted by the isotope, the half-life of the isotope, and the method used to deliver the radiation. With a sealed implant, the patient's excreta are not radioactive, but the actual implant is. If a systemic unsealed delivery method is used, the patient's secretions and excretions will be radioactive for a time based on the isotope's half-life.

Therapeutic Interventions

Actions/Interventions	Rationales
■ Provide the patient with a private room and a private bathroom.	This type of room placement reduces the risk for radiation exposure to other patients.
▲ Consult with the hospital's radiation safety officer about appropriate radiation safety protocols.	The radiation safety officer will provide appropriate safety guidelines based on the type of internal radiation to be used.
■ Post signs outside the patient's room. Many hospitals have specialized rooms or units designated for this purpose.	Health care providers and visitors at risk for the effects of radiation need to be warned before entering the patient's room. The signs should indicate precautions to be used when entering the patient's room. Women who are pregnant should avoid all direct contact with the patient until radiation treatment is completed.
■ Provide film badges to staff members who are responsible for direct care of the patient.	Film badges record the amount of exposure to a radiation source. The badge should be worn outside the clothing during all direct contact activities with the patient. The radiation safety officer will periodically review all film badges and quantify the staff member's amount of radiation exposure.
■ For patients with encapsulated forms of internal radiation, keep appropriate lead-lined containers in the patient's room.	When an implanted radiation source becomes dislodged, most institutions require nurses not to touch the source but to call a radiation safety officer to handle the source. The nurse should never pick up a radiation source with bare hands.

■ = Independent   ▲ = Collaborative

Hematolymphatic, Immunological and Oncological Care Plans

Actions/Interventions

■ Implement all direct patient care activities using principles of time and distance.
  • Organize care activities to minimize the amount of time at the patient's bedside.
  • Provide only essential care to promote patient comfort.
  • Prepare meal trays outside the room.
  • Keep bedside tables, call lights, and personal care items within easy reach of the patient at all times to reduce return trips to the bedside.

Rationales

Radiation exposure is based on the law of inverse squares. The amount of radiation exposure is inversely related to the square of the distance from the radiation source. A nurse standing 2 feet from the patient has one-quarter the exposure of someone standing next to the patient ($2^2 = 4$; the inverse of 4 is ¼).

Related Care Plan

Fatigue, p. 66

Disseminated Intravascular Coagulation (DIC)

Coagulopathy; Defibrination Syndrome

Disseminated intravascular coagulation (DIC) is a coagulation disorder that prompts over-stimulation of the normal clotting cascade and results in simultaneous thrombosis and hemorrhage. The formation of microclots affects tissue perfusion in the major organs, causing hypoxia, ischemia, and tissue damage. Coagulation occurs in two different pathways: intrinsic and extrinsic. These pathways are responsible for formation of fibrin clots and blood clotting, which maintains hemostasis. In the intrinsic pathway, endothelial cell damage commonly occurs because of sepsis or infection. The extrinsic pathway is initiated by tissue injury such as from malignancy, trauma, or obstetrical complications. DIC may present as an acute or chronic condition. The medical management of DIC is primarily aimed at (1) treating the underlying cause, (2) managing complications from both primary and secondary causes, (3) supporting organ function, and (4) stopping abnormal coagulation and controlling bleeding. Morbidity and mortality depend on underlying cause and severity of the coagulopathy.

NANDA-I NDx **Risk for Bleeding**

Common Risk Factors

Abnormal blood profiles (depleted coagulation factors)
Drug therapy (adverse effects of heparin)

Defining Characteristics

Active bleeding
Abnormal clotting times
Blood clots

Common Expected Outcomes

Patient experiences reduced episodes of bleeding and hematomas.
Patient maintains therapeutic levels of coagulation lab profiles (PPT, PT, fibrinogen, fibrin split products, bleeding time).
Patient's side effects of medication therapy are reduced through ongoing assessment and early intervention.

NOC Outcomes
Blood Coagulation; Circulation Status
NIC Interventions
Bleeding Precautions; Bleeding Reduction; Blood Product Administration; Medication Administration

Ongoing Assessment

Actions/Interventions	Rationales
■ Assess for underlying cause of DIC.	DIC is not a primary disease but occurs in response to a precipitating factor such as infection or tumor. Successful treatment of DIC includes management of the underlying disorder.
▲ Monitor serial coagulation profiles.	Initially, accelerated clotting is noted. As the clotting then stimulates the fibrinolytic system, clotting factors become depleted and large quantities of proteins are produced as part of the fibrin degradation process. Common laboratory values in DIC are prothrombin time (PT) greater than 15 seconds, partial thromboplastin time (PTT) greater than 60 to 90 seconds, hypofibrinogenemia, thrombocytopenia, elevated fibrin split products (FSPs), elevated D-dimers (a type of FSP), and prolonged bleeding time. All put the patient at risk for increased bleeding. Specific deficiencies guide treatment therapy.
▲ Monitor hematocrit (Hct) and hemoglobin (Hgb).	Decreased Hgb and Hct levels are associated with bleeding from DIC.
■ Examine skin surface for signs of bleeding. Note petechiae; purpura; hematomas; oozing of blood from intravenous (IV) sites, drains, and wounds; and bleeding from mucous membranes.	Prolonged oozing of blood from injection sites or venipuncture sites could be the first indication of DIC.
■ Observe for signs of external bleeding from gastrointestinal (GI) and genitourinary (GU) tracts.	One of the diagnostic hallmarks of acute DIC can be manifested as bleeding simultaneously from at least three unrelated sites associated with shock, respiratory failure, or renal failure. For example, the patient may have increased skin bruising, hemoptysis, and hematuria.
■ Note any hemoptysis or blood obtained during suctioning.	These are common manifestations of acute DIC.
■ Observe for signs of internal bleeding, such as pain or changes in level of consciousness. Institute neurological checklist.	Changes in level of consciousness may occur with the decreased fluid volume or with decreasing Hgb.
■ Monitor heart rate and BP. Observe for signs of orthostatic hypotension.	Tachycardia and hypotension are signs of decreased cardiac output. Orthostasis (a drop of more than 15 mm Hg when changing from supine to sitting position) indicates reduced circulating fluids.
■ If heparin therapy is initiated, observe for: • Any increase in bleeding from IV sites, GI/GU tracts, respiratory tract, or wounds • New purpura, petechiae, or hematomas	Heparin is used for milder cases when clotting is more of a problem than bleeding. It aborts clotting process by blocking thrombin production.

Therapeutic Interventions

Actions/Interventions	Rationales
■ Institute precautionary measures: • Avoid unnecessary venipunctures; draw all laboratory specimens through an existing line: arterial line or venous heparin lock line. • Use only compressible vessels for IV sites. • Apply pressure to any oozing site. • Avoid intramuscular injections. • Prevent trauma to the catheters and tubes by proper taping; minimize pulling. • Minimize number of cuff BPs. • Use gentle suctioning.	Nursing interventions should be planned and implemented to eliminate potential sources of bleeding and to control the amount of potential bleeding and tissue injury.

■ = Independent ▲ = Collaborative

Hematolymphatic, Immunological and Oncological Care Plans

Actions/Interventions

- Use gentle chest physiotherapy, such as turning, repositioning, coughing, deep breathing, percussion, and vibration.
- Provide gentle oral care, using saline and water rinses instead of toothbrushes.
- Use electric rather than safety razor for shaving.
- If the patient is confused or agitated, pad the side rails.

▲ Administer blood products as prescribed: red blood cells (RBCs), fresh frozen plasma (FFP), cryoprecipitate, and platelets.

▲ Administer heparin therapy as prescribed. Dose may be titrated based on laboratory values and clinical situation. If bleeding is increased, notify the physician of the possible need to decrease the IV drip.

▲ Administer parenteral fluids as prescribed. Anticipate the need for an IV fluid challenge with immediate infusion of fluids for patients with hypotension.

▲ Administer additional medications or investigational drugs as ordered:

- Antithrombin III concentration

- Recombinant human activated protein C
- Amicar (epsilon aminocaproic acid)

- Hirudin

Rationales

Blood/plasma transfusions replace blood clotting factors. RBCs increase oxygen-carrying capacity; FFP replaces clotting factors and inhibitors; platelets and cryoprecipitate provide proteins for coagulation.

Heparin is used for milder cases when clotting is more of a problem than bleeding. Heparin augments antithrombin III activity that interrupts the clotting cycle and conversion of fibrinogen to fibrin. It also blocks the intrinsic and extrinsic pathways by inhibiting factor X, which slows clot formation. As the clinical situation improves, the need for heparin decreases. The challenge lies in differentiating the blood loss as an untoward effect of heparin therapy from a worsening of DIC.

Maintenance of an adequate blood volume is vital for maintaining cardiac output and systemic perfusion.

A hematologist can guide medical treatment.

This is a cofactor of heparin used for more severe cases. The antiinflammatory properties may be of benefit when sepsis is the causative factor.

This inhibits factors Va and VIIIa of the coagulation cascade.

This antifibrinolytic agent is reserved for when other measures have failed. Its use can lead to organ failure from large vessel thrombosis, and thus its use is controversial.

This is a thrombin inhibitor and neutralizer; there is limited clinical experience with this drug.

NANDA-I NDx Impaired Gas Exchange

Common Related Factor	Defining Characteristics
Altered oxygen-carrying capacity of blood	Confusion Somnolence Restlessness Irritability Hypercapnia Hypoxia/hypoxemia Abnormal breathing (rate, rhythm, depth) Dyspnea Abnormal arterial blood gases

Common Expected Outcome

Patient maintains optimal gas exchange, as evidenced by arterial blood gases (ABGs) within patient's usual range; oxygen saturation of 90% or greater; alert, responsive mentation or no further reduction in level of consciousness; and relaxed breathing and baseline HR for patient.

NOC Outcome
Respiratory Status: Gas Exchange

NIC Interventions
Respiratory Monitoring; Oxygen Therapy; Ventilation Assistance

Ongoing Assessment

Actions/Interventions

- Assess respiratory rate, rhythm, and depth.

- Assess for tachycardia, shortness of breath, use of accessory muscles.

- Assess breath sounds. Assess cough for signs of bloody sputum.

- Assess for changes in level of consciousness.

- ▲ Use pulse oximeter to monitor oxygen saturation; assess ABGs.

Rationales

Patient will adapt breathing pattern over time to facilitate gas exchange. Rapid, shallow respirations may result from hypoxia or from the acidosis with the shock state. Development of hypoventilation indicates that immediate ventilator support is needed.

These signify an increased work of breathing. With initial hypoxia, HR increases,. Use of accessory muscles increases chest excursion to facilitate effective breathing.

Changes in breath sounds reveal etiology of impaired gas exchange. Hemoptysis is an indication of bleeding in the respiratory tract.

Early signs of cerebral hypoxia are restlessness and anxiety; later signs are agitation, lethargy and confusion.

Pulse oximetry is a useful tool to detect early changes in oxygen saturation. O_2 saturation should be kept at 90% or greater. However, for CO_2 levels, ABGs need to be obtained.

Therapeutic Interventions

Actions/Interventions

- Position the patient in high-Fowler's position (if hemodynamically stable).
- Change the patient's position every 2 hours, and perform chest physiotherapy.
- Suction as needed.

- Provide reassurance and allay anxiety by staying with the patient during acute episodes of respiratory distress.
- ▲ Maintain oxygen delivery system.

- ▲ Anticipate the need for intubation and mechanical ventilation.

Rationales

A sitting position allows for adequate diaphramatic and lung excursion and promotes optimal lung expansion.

These maneuvers facilitate movement and drainage of secretions.

Productive coughing is the most effective way to remove most secretions. If patient is unable to perform independently, suctioning may be needed to promote airway patency and reduce work of breathing.

Anxiety increases dyspnea, work of breathing, and respiratory rate.

The appropriate amount of oxygen must be delivered continuously so that the patient maintains an oxygen saturation of 90% or greater.

Early intubation and mechanical ventilation are recommended to prevent full decompensation of the patient.

■ = Independent   ▲ = Collaborative

NANDA-I NDx Deficient Knowledge

Common Related Factors
New condition/treatment
Complexity of treatment
Emotional state affecting learning
Unfamiliar environment

Defining Characteristics
Questioning health care team
Verbalizing inaccurate information

Common Expected Outcome
Patient/significant others verbalize basic understanding of DIC and its management.

NOC Outcomes
Knowledge: Disease Process; Knowledge: Treatment Procedures

NIC Interventions
Teaching: Disease Process; Bleeding Precautions

Ongoing Assessment

Actions/Interventions	Rationales
■ Assess knowledge of DIC.	DIC usually occurs acutely, so the patient and family have no prior knowledge of it. Assessment provides baseline for teaching.

Therapeutic Interventions

Actions/Interventions	Rationales
■ Carefully explain the underlying etiology that precipitated DIC.	Patients are better able to ask questions when they have basic information about what to expect.
■ Instruct the patient or significant others to notify the nurse of new bleeding from wounds or IV sites.	This notification can aid in achieving early intervention at bleeding sites. However, any new episodes of bleeding may have a traumatic impact on the patient and family.
■ Explain the purpose of drug and transfusion therapy.	The controversial nature of treatment may be difficult for the patient or significant others to understand in the acute setting. In addition, frequent use of blood components may cause fear regarding transmission of infectious diseases such as hepatitis or human immunodeficiency virus.

Related Care Plans

Acute pain, p. 151
Anxiety, p. 18
Deficient fluid volume, p. 72
Mechanical ventilation, p. 418
Acute respiratory distress syndrome, p. 358
Ineffective tissue perfusion, p. 199

Hematopoietic Stem Cell Transplantation (HSCT)

Bone Marrow Transplant; Peripheral Blood Stem Cell Transplant

Bone marrow transplantation (BMT) and peripheral blood stem cell transplantation (PBSCT) are terms that now more commonly fall under the umbrella term of *hematopoietic stem cell transplantation (HSCT)*. The indications for HSCT are expanding; it is used as both a curative and investigational treatment for both malignant and nonmalignant conditions. HSCT should not be confused with the controversial field of embryonic stem cells. Embryonic stem cells, derived from fertilized embryos, are undifferentiated cells that have the ability to form any adult cell. Hematopoietic stem cells are the "mother" cells that differentiate only into the cells of the blood system (e.g., white blood cells [WBCs], red blood cells [RBCs], platelets).

HSCT is used to replace diseased bone marrow, as a hematopoietic rescue after high-dose therapy (radiation and/or chemotherapy), as a form of immunotherapy, and as a vehicle for gene therapy.

There are three major types of transplants:

- *Autologous:* self
- *Syngeneic:* donor from an identical twin
- *Allogeneic:* can be related (from a matched sibling), or unrelated (from a volunteer in the Be The Match Registry). This is also referred to as a MUD (matched unrelated donor) transplant.

There are three sources of hematopoietic stem cells:

- *Bone marrow:* These cells are collected from the pelvic bones through a series of aspirations. Bone marrow harvesting is a surgical procedure done under general anesthesia.
- *Peripheral blood:* The stem cells that normally reside in the bone marrow can be moved or mobilized into the bloodstream (peripheral circulation) and collected in an outpatient procedure via a cell separator or apheresis machine. This procedure does not require anesthesia. The majority of all transplants performed today (greater than 95%) use peripheral blood stem cells rather than bone marrow stem cells.
- *Umbilical cord, placental:* This is a rich source of stem cells that are collected at the time of delivery from tissue that is normally discarded.

There is one other classification of transplant based on the amount and type of pretransplant therapy that is administered. Standard transplants use strong treatment (chemotherapy and/or radiation therapy) administered before transplantation to destroy the host's diseased cells and suppress the host's immune system. This therapy is referred to as *ablative therapy,* because it eliminates all host blood and immune cells. Reduced-intensity transplants—also called *nonmyeloablative transplants* or *minitransplants*—are transplants that use less intense treatment to prepare for transplantation than a standard transplant does. Thus the doses of chemotherapy given before transplantation are much lower and do not necessarily eliminate all diseased cells. This type of transplant is only used in the allogeneic setting, because this method relies on the donor's immune cells to fight disease. This care plan focuses on inpatient care. Emotional issues related to HSCT are not addressed here.

Deficient Knowledge

Common Related Factors

New condition, procedure, or treatment
Complexity of treatment
Misinterpretation of information
Emotional state affecting learning
Unfamiliarity with information resources
Lack of recall

Defining Characteristics

Verbalized inaccurate information
Expressed need for information
Questioning members of health care team

■ = Independent   ▲ = Collaborative

Common Expected Outcome

Patient or significant others verbalize understanding of procedures, treatments, possible complications, and follow-up care.

NOC Outcomes
Knowledge: Disease Process; Knowledge: Treatment Procedure

NIC Interventions
Teaching: Disease Process; Teaching: Preoperative; Teaching: Prescribed Medications; Teaching: Procedure/Treatment

Ongoing Assessment

Actions/Interventions	Rationales
■ Assess the patient's and significant others' understanding of procedures, treatment protocol, potential side effects and complications, schedule of overall treatment plan, and follow-up care after discharge.	The patient and family need information based on their understanding of the treatment care plan. A successful treatment plan requires the cooperation of the patient and support of the patient's family.

Therapeutic Interventions

Actions/Interventions	Rationales
■ Share with the patient a written calendar or schedule of the overall treatment plan.	This schedule helps the patient process the timeline for treatment. The transplantation process includes several phases (i.e., mobilization, collection of HSC, conditioning, reinfusion, engraftment) depending on the type of transplant.
■ Instruct the patient (significant others as needed) about central venous access device if not already in place.	Accurate information provides rationale for treatment. The device is used for administration of chemotherapy, collection of peripheral blood stem cells, stem cell infusion, antibiotic treatment, blood draws, blood component replacement, and total parenteral nutrition (TPN) as appropriate. These catheters may remain in place for several months or longer.
■ Explain bone marrow or peripheral stem cell collection, storage, and potential complications.	If bone marrow is used, the patient will require preoperative and postoperative teaching. If peripheral blood stem cells are used, the patient will require mobilization therapy with chemotherapy and/or growth factors, and/or a CXCR4 chemokine receptor antagonist and collection of peripheral blood stem cells via apheresis (see Hematopoietic Stem Cell Collection care plan on the **Evolve** website).
■ Discuss preparative or conditioning regimen, potential short- and long-term side effects, and preventive measures to minimize or alleviate toxicities (e.g., antiemetic, oral regimens, pain control).	The conditioning regimen can be ablative (high-dose) or nonmyeloablative (reduced-intensity). Potential side effects will vary (e.g., nausea and vomiting and loss of appetite are generally less with the nonmyeloablative conditioning protocols).
■ Discuss the HSCT procedure for peripheral stem cell infusion and potential complications.	The procedure and potential complications for stem cell infusion depend on whether the stem cell product is fresh or frozen. Allogeneic transplants generally mean that the stem cell product is collected from the donor and infused to the recipient on the same day (i.e., "fresh"). In this case, the stem cell infusion is similar to a blood transfusion. Autologous transplants use frozen stem cells, in that stem cells from the donor (i.e., the patient) have been collected and stored ahead of time. Infusion of frozen or cryopreserved stem cells is more involved, with more potential complications related to infusion of the cryopreservative (DMSO), which can cause side effects in the recipient.

Actions/Interventions	Rationales
■ Discuss the time frame for marrow engraftment.	After infusion, stem cells travel to the bone marrow and stimulate production of new blood cells (RBCs, WBCs, and platelets). This process is referred to as *engraftment*. The time after transplantation until engraftment depends upon the source of cells: for peripheral blood stem cells, engraftment occurs as early as 7 to 10 days but can take up to 21 days. Cord blood transplants take longer to engraft (21 to 35 days). Full recovery of function may take up to several months or longer (1 to 2 years) depending on the type of transplant.
■ Discuss administration of neutrophil growth factors (i.e., granulocyte colony-stimulating factor [G-CSF]).	Growth factors are sometimes administered after stem cell infusion to accelerate engraftment.
■ Discuss blood component transfusions (i.e., packed RBCs and platelets). Encourage the patient and significant others to participate in blood component donor accrual to fulfill transfusion requirements as needed.	These transfusions constitute adjunct management of anemia and thrombocytopenia. The widespread adoption of peripheral blood as the stem cell source has resulted in a reduced period of pancytopenia and a subsequent reduced need for transfusion support. Many patients get through the peritransplant phase without ever needing an RBC or platelet transfusion. However, families can still be encouraged to donate blood products, although this is not required specifically for family members.
■ Discuss the need to maintain a protective environment (e.g., private room, laminar airflow room). Provide information about isolation techniques and procedures.	Environmental changes protect the patient from contagions during the myelosuppression period.
■ Discuss antibacterial, antifungal, and antiviral therapy to prevent and treat infections.	Infections can be caused by bacteria, viruses, or fungi. Patients are given drugs to prevent infection even if they do not have any signs of such.
■ Discuss dietary modifications, which may include a low-bacterial diet (no fresh fruits or vegetables; "well-cooked" food items).	This diet decreases bacterial contamination of the alimentary tract.
■ Explain the need for frequent blood sampling.	Sampling is indicated to assess for electrolyte and metabolic changes; cardiac, pulmonary, and renal alterations; bone marrow function; the need for blood component transfusions; and the presence of infection. Cultures provide data on which microorganisms are causing infection and antibiotic drug sensitivity.
■ Explain the need for frequent inspection and culturing of all orifices and potential infection sites.	This assessment is required for surveillance of opportunistic microorganisms, early detection, and prompt treatment of infection.
■ Discuss discharge planning and teaching: • Timing of discharge	Timing depends on type of transplant and course of postengraftment period. Length of stay averages 14 to 21 days. Discharge criteria include absolute granulocyte count above 500 to 1000/mm^3, oral intake of at least 1000 kcal/day, no evidence of infection or bleeding, adequate oral hydration of at least 2 liters, and psychological readiness to return home.
• Importance of follow-up visits for blood studies and monitoring for potential complications	Information aids the patient in assuming responsibility for ongoing care.
• Activities of daily living	The patient should gradually resume activities, because fatigue and reduced endurance will be a problem.
• Medications after discharge	Patients are better able to ask questions and seek assistance when they know basic information about all medications prescribed.
• Importance of balanced diet/adequate fluid intake	Information provides rationale for therapy.

■ = Independent   ▲ = Collaborative

Actions/Interventions

- Central venous catheter care (e.g., Hickman, Permcath)

- Measures to prevent infection (e.g., avoiding children with infections or who have recently been immunized, avoiding crowds)

- Recognition and reporting of signs and symptoms of bleeding, low RBC count, and infection
- Sexual relations and contraception

- Return to work or school

Rationales

Risk for complications is associated with long-term use. Aseptic techniques need to be taught.

The patient's immune function is not fully restored until about 6 to 12 months after transplantation; many patients are fearful of leaving the hospital's "protective isolation" environment, and thus need information to optimize their self-care regimen.

Early assessment facilitates prompt treatment.

Libido may be decreased. Women may need vaginal lubrication. Men may need medical management for erectile dysfunction.

Timing for return is related to risk for infection and performance status.

NANDA-I NDx Risk for Infection

Common Risk Factors

Immunosuppression secondary to high-dose chemotherapy or radiation therapy
Antimicrobial therapy (i.e., superimposed infection)
Prolonged bone marrow regeneration
Failure of bone marrow graft
Cytomegalovirus (CMV)/herpes simplex virus seropositivity

Common Expected Outcome

Patient is at reduced risk for local and systemic infection, as evidenced by negative blood surveillance culture findings, compliance with preventive measures, normal chest radiograph, intact mucous membranes and skin, and prompt reporting of early signs of infection.

NOC Outcomes
Infection Status; Medication Response
NIC Interventions
Infection Protection; Chemotherapy Management; Medication Administration; Teaching: Individual

---

Ongoing Assessment

Actions/Interventions

- Inspect body sites with high potential for infection (mouth, throat, axilla, perineum, rectum).

- Inspect peripheral intravenous and/or catheter sites for redness and tenderness.

Rationales

Opportunist infections are often the first type of infection to develop in immunosuppressed patients. Early detection facilitates prompt treatment.

These are frequent sites of infection.

Actions/Interventions

■ Observe closely for fever and chills.

■ Auscultate lung field for crackles, rhonchi, and breath sounds.
■ Assess risk factors predisposing to CMV infection.

▲ Monitor WBC count with differential and absolute neutrophil count daily for evidence of rising or falling counts.

▲ Monitor cultures and sensitivities and CMV titers of blood, sputum, and urine.

Rationales

A temperature greater than 37° C (98.6° F) may indicate systemic infection. This may be the initial presentation of infection because, in the absence of granulocytes, the locus of infection may develop without characteristic inflammation or pus formation at the site.

Pneumonia infections are common and can be fatal in this population.

Infections are common post transplant, especially to cytomegalovirus (CMV). Specific risk factors in this population include: allogenic transplants, CMV seropositivity, total body irradiation, and acute graft-versus-host disease (GVHD).

Neutropenia puts patients at increased risk, especially before engraftment. Even a slight rise in WBC count may signal an infection because of the patient's impaired immune system.

Cultures provide data on which microorganisms are causing infection and antibiotic drug sensitivity.

Therapeutic Interventions

Actions/Interventions

▲ Place the patient in protective isolation according to transplant protocol.

■ Ensure thorough hand washing (using vigorous friction) by the staff and visitors before physical contact with the patient.
■ Teach or provide meticulous total body hygiene with special attention to frequent sites of infection (e.g., anal area, groin, breast folds, skin folds).
■ Implement a meticulous oral hygiene regimen.

▲ Institute a low-bacterial diet.

▲ Administer antiinfective drugs for prophylaxis or treatment, as prescribed.

■ Explain the effects of chemotherapy and radiation therapy on the immune system.

Rationales

Protective isolation precautions may include placing the patient in a private room, limiting visitors, and having all people who come in contact with the patient use masks, gloves, and gowns. Some hospitals may place patients in special sterile laminar airflow rooms. These precautions reduce the risk for patient exposure to opportunistic infections.

Hand washing removes transient and resident bacteria from hands, thus minimizing or preventing transmission to the patient.

The perineal area is a source of many pathogens and frequent portal of entry for microorganisms. Skin fold areas can also harbor pathogens.

Oral hygiene is important in prevention of periodontal disease as a locus of infection.

This diet protects the patient from exposure to pathogens from foods at a time when host defenses are greatly compromised.

Medications may be given before and after transplant for prophylactic, empiric, or actual treatment. Prophylactic antiinfective administration is given to prevent viral, fungal, and bacterial infections through immune reconstitution.

Information provides basis for ongoing education.

■ = Independent   ▲ = Collaborative

Actions/Interventions

■ Explain to the patient or significant others the role of WBCs in infection prevention:
- Normal range of WBCs
- Function of leukocytes and neutrophils
- Meaning or importance of absolute neutrophil count (ANC):
  - Greater than 2000/mm^3 = No risk
  - 1500 to 2000/mm^3 = Mild risk
  - 1000 to 1499/mm^3 = Moderate risk
  - 500 to 999/mm^3 = High risk
  - Less than 500/mm^3 = Life-threatening risk

■ Teach the patient or significant others measures to prevent infection after discharge until immune function is fully restored (about 9 to 12 months after transplantation):
- Avoid crowds or contact with persons with known infections.
- Avoid contact with cat litter boxes, fish tanks, bird cages, and dog and human excreta.
- Avoid swimming in private or public pools for at least a year.
- Avoid construction sites and home remodeling.
- Avoid sweeping and vacuuming.
- Practice meticulous oral and body hygiene, including frequent hand washing, especially before handling food.
- Use aseptic technique when caring for a central venous catheter.
- Maintain a balanced diet with sufficient protein, calories, vitamins, minerals, and fluids.

Rationales

Patients need to be comanagers of their treatment plan. Adequate knowledge is necessary for ongoing monitoring of potential complications. Patients may be unaware of the many medical terms used to guide therapy.

Patients and family members are more likely to implement infection control measures at home when they understand the risks and benefits to the patient. Animal excreta, soil, and people with known infections are sources of opportunistic infections for the immune-compromised patient after transplantation.

NANDA-I NDx **Ineffective Protection**

Common Related Factors

Bone marrow suppression secondary to chemotherapy and radiation therapy
Prolonged bone marrow regeneration
Failure of bone marrow graft
Invasion of bone marrow by malignant cells
Sinusoidal occlusive disease (SOD)
GVHD
Drug injury (chemotherapy or antimicrobial therapy)
Hepatic malignancy
Immunosuppressive therapy (e.g., cyclosporine, tacrolimus, sirolimus, methotrexate, steroids, antithymocyte globulins)
Drug or transfusion reactions

Defining Characteristics

Pancytopenia: reduced platelets, reduced RBCs, reduced WBCs
Liver dysfunction or failure
Renal dysfunction
Facial edema and flushing
Wheezing
Skin rashes

Common Expected Outcomes

Patient maintains reduced risk for bleeding, as evidenced by normal platelet count, absence of signs of bleeding, and early report of any signs of bleeding.

Patient maintains optimal liver function, as evidenced by serum and urine laboratory values within normal limits, absence of ascites, balanced intake and output (I&O), and normal weight for patient.

Patient maintains optimal renal function, as evidenced by balanced I&O, weight within normal limits, normal vital signs, and normal level of consciousness.

Patient maintains optimal skin integrity.

Patient is free of injury from drug or blood therapy as evidenced by normal vital signs, absence of pain, and absence of nausea and vomiting.

NOC Outcomes
Circulation Status; Blood Coagulation; Vital Signs

NIC Interventions
Chemotherapy Management; Bleeding Precautions; Hemodynamic Regulation; Vital Sign Monitoring

Ongoing Assessment

Actions/Interventions

For risk for bleeding:

■ Assess for any signs of bleeding. Signs may be obvious (e.g., epistaxis, bleeding gums, petechiae, bruising, hematomas, hematemesis, hemoptysis, retinal hemorrhages, melena, hematuria, vaginal bleeding) or occult (e.g., neurological changes, dizziness).

■ Monitor vital signs as needed.

▲ Monitor platelets, RBCs, hemoglobin (Hgb), and hematocrit (Hct).

For risk for liver dysfunction:

■ Assess for risk factors predisposing to development of sinusoidal occlusive disease (SOD), previously called venoocclusive disease:
  • Intense toxic conditioning regimen
  • Total body irradiation
  • Liver abnormalities before transplantation (hepatitis)
  • Allogeneic stem cell transplant or HSCT
  • Patients with malignant diseases (leukemia, lymphoma, solid tumors)
  • Second stem cell transplant or HSCT

■ Assess for signs of liver dysfunction: sudden weight gain, enlarged liver, right upper quadrant pain, ascites, jaundice, tea-colored urine, labored and shallow respirations, dyspnea, confusion, and lethargy and fatigue.

Rationales

Early assessment facilitates prompt treatment and reduced risk for complications. Signs of bleeding are most commonly seen during the first 4 weeks after transplant.

Increased heart rate and orthostatic blood pressure changes accompany bleeding.

After entering the blood stream, the stem cells travel to the bone marrow where they begin to produce new red blood cells, platelets and white blood cells in a process known as engraftment. Engraftment begins in 1 to 2 weeks, though time can vary depending on the type of stem cell transplant. Normal values from successful engraftment may be seen in 2 to 3 months.

Chemotherapy or radiation therapy can cause deposits of fibrous materials to form in the small veins of the liver, obstructing blood flow from it. SOD is the occlusion of these vessels. There is no proven preventive therapy for SOD.

Classic signs of SOD include weight gain, ascites, hepatomegaly. Typically, symptoms develop 1 to 4 weeks after transplantation. Patients usually present with some but not all of these symptoms.

■ = Independent   ▲ = Collaborative

Actions/Interventions	Rationales
▲ Monitor laboratory values daily for: • Increased alkaline phosphatase, bilirubin, serum aspartate aminotransferase, alanine aminotransferase, lactic dehydrogenase, and ammonia levels • Decreased serum albumin level • Electrolyte imbalance • Abnormal coagulation profile	These lab tests provide data on liver function. Specific deficiencies guide treatment.
For risk for renal dysfunction: ■ Monitor urine output.	Decreased urine volume less than 30 mL/hr suggests renal insufficiency.
▲ Monitor laboratory data: sodium, potassium, blood urea nitrogen (BUN), creatinine, osmolality.	Increased potassium, BUN, and creatinine are associated with decreased renal function. Chemotherapy, radiation therapy, antibiotics, and immunosuppressive drugs may cause renal failure.
■ Monitor fluid balance (at minimum, I&O every 8 hours and daily weight).	Close monitoring of fluid balance is necessary to determine adequate replacement needs and to prevent excessive administration of oral or IV fluids during decreased renal function. Body weight is a more sensitive indicator of fluid retention than intake and output.
■ Observe for presence of peripheral and/or dependent edema.	Edema occurs when fluid accumulates in the extravascular spaces. These changes reflect fluid imbalance.
■ Monitor for changes in level of consciousness.	BUN and other waste products can build up in the blood and can cause uremic encephalopathy.
■ Monitor drug profile for medications potentially contributing to renal insufficiency and/or changes in level of consciousness.	Drug dosage adjustment or discontinuation may be necessary to prevent toxic side effects of poorly excreted drugs.
For risk for drug or transfusion reactions: ■ Assess for reaction from chemotherapeutic drugs: restlessness, facial edema and flushing, wheezing, skin rash, tachycardia, hypotension, hematuria (Cytoxan), and increased uric acid levels.	Careful monitoring for potential adverse effects is required both during and after administration.
■ Test urine for blood.	Hematuria may be caused by irritation of the bladder lining secondary to the conditioning regimen or infection. High urine flow, alkalinization of urine, and frequent voiding help prevent concentration of metabolites in the bladder, thus reducing risk for hemorrhagic cystitis.
■ Assess for reactions from immunoglobulins: urticaria, pain (local crythema), headache, muscle stiffness, fever and malaise, nephrotic syndrome, angioedema, and anaphylaxis.	Reactions can be serious and even life threatening.
■ Assess for reactions to immunosuppressive therapy: mucositis, nausea and vomiting, bone marrow suppression, fluid retention, hypertension, headache, hypomagnesemia, renal toxicity, tingling in extremities, tremors, and anaphylaxis-like reactions.	A variety of reactions may occur, depending on the agent administered.
For risk for GVHD: ■ Assess risk factors predisposing to development of GVHD: older age, sex-mismatched donor, human leukocyte antigen–mismatched donor.	GVHD is one of the most serious complications of allogeneic HSCT. It occurs when T cells from the donated marrow (the "graft") identify the recipient body (the "host") as foreign and attack it. However, the presence of some level of GVHD does indicate adequate or successful engraftment.
■ Assess for signs of acute GVHD: skin rash or scaling, elevated bilirubin levels, gastrointestinal (GI) changes (diarrhea, abdominal cramps).	GVHD can affect skin, GI tract, and liver. Inflammation and sensitivity on the palms of the hands and plantar surfaces of the feet are early signs of GVHD.

Therapeutic Interventions

Actions/Interventions	Rationales
For risk for bleeding:	
▲ Implement bleeding precautions for platelet count less than 50,000/mm³:	Understanding of importance of precautionary measures reduces risk for bleeding. At this level, spontaneous bleeding can occur.
	This precaution reduces bleeding at vascular access sites.
• Avoid nonessential invasive procedures, punctures, and injections.	
• Avoid rectal thermometers, suppositories, and enemas.	This reduces mucosal injury.
• Maintain appropriate fall precautions.	Safety measures reduce risk for trauma.
▲ Communicate anticipated need for platelet support to transfusion center. Transfuse platelets as prescribed.	This measure ensures availability and readiness of platelets when needed to prevent spontaneous or excessive bleeding. Platelet transfusion is indicated for counts less than or equal to 10,000/mm³ unless the patient is actively bleeding; this decreases the risk for the patient becoming refractory to platelet transfusions.
▲ Maintain a current blood sample for "type and screen" in the transfusion center. If a significant drop in Hgb and Hct is noted, transfuse packed RBCs as prescribed.	This ensures availability and readiness of packed RBCs. Packed RBCs are used to restore Hgb and Hct to levels where the patient experiences minimal symptoms. All products transfused should be leukocyte-reduced, CMV-negative, and irradiated products.
For risk for liver dysfunction:	
▲ Restrict fluids and sodium as prescribed.	Restrictions reduce fluid buildup. Fluid management is key.
▲ Consult a dietitian about dietary modifications in enteral or parenteral nutrition.	Oral protein may need to be restricted; TPN solutions may need to be concentrated.
▲ Administer Actigall as ordered.	This medication is used routinely for patients at high risk for SOD or those exhibiting signs and symptoms of potential SOD.
▲ Administer IV medications with minimal amount of solution. Consult a pharmacist.	This measure decreases unnecessary fluids.
▲ Administer diuretics as prescribed.	Diuretics decrease the amount of ascites and help maintain adequate renal perfusion.
▲ Transfuse packed RBCs as prescribed.	Packed RBCs maintain intravascular fluid volume. The goal of hypertransfusion of packed RBCs is to attain a Hct of 40 or greater, which helps maintain high osmotic pressure within the vascular space. This in turn draws extravascular interstitial fluid back into the vessels.
▲ Administer analgesics as prescribed.	Analgesics are used to reduce patient discomfort with ascites and related problems. Narcotics and sedatives with shorter half-lives and fewer metabolites given in reduced doses should be considered to prevent compounding of hepatic encephalopathy.
For risk for renal dysfunction:	
▲ Administer IV fluids and diuretics as prescribed.	These therapies are used to correct vascular volume disequilibrium.
▲ Administer electrolytes in IV fluids.	Replacement is necessary to match calculated loss and correct any deficit.
▲ Administer low-dose ("renal dose") dopamine.	This medication is indicated to maintain urine flow. However, it does not offer reno-protective effects.
▲ Consult a dietitian about dietary modifications in enteral or parenteral nutrition.	Specialty expertise may be needed to balance fluid and nutritional needs.
For risk for drug or blood reactions:	
▲ Keep emergency drugs (IV Benadryl, hydrocortisone, epinephrine 1:1000) readily available.	Patient safety is a priority. Being prepared reduces complications.

■ = Independent   ▲ = Collaborative

Hematolymphatic, Immunological and Oncological Care Plans

Actions/Interventions

▲ Administer IV fluids and diuretics before, during, and after conditioning regimen, as prescribed.

▲ Premedicate patient with antiemetic and antihistamine as prescribed before infusion.

■ Provide warm blankets if chills occur during reinfusion.

▲ Do the following when drug or transfusion reaction is suspected: stop infusion, notify physician, administer emergency drugs as prescribed, and reassure the patient.

For GVHD:

▲ Administer immunosuppressive drugs as prescribed.

▲ Implement the following once signs of GVHD skin changes are present:
- Use mild soap and oatmeal bath preparation daily.
- Administer antipruritic medications (i.e., antihistamines).
- Trim the patient's nails, and discourage him or her from scratching; consider use of mittens.
- Lubricate skin well with frequent applications of a mixture of half-and-half mineral oil and ointment.

Rationales

These are used to maintain good urine output and counteract antidiuretic effect of medications. As chemotherapy destroys tumor cells, uric acid is liberated and accumulates in blood. High urine flow prevents uric acid deposits in kidneys.

These medications are used to reduce incidence of nausea and vomiting and of allergic reactions. Allergic reactions, including shortness of breath, are possibly the result of liberation of histamines from broken marrow cells.

Chills usually are secondary to cool temperature of thawed marrow or peripheral stem cell concentrate.

Rapid, efficient intervention is critical to saving life.

These drugs are used to prevent or treat acute GVHD (drugs include cyclosporine, tacrolimus, methotrexate, steroids, immunoglobulins). GVHD results when the T lymphocytes in the transplanted donor bone marrow recognize the marrow recipient as "foreign" and mount an immunological "attack" against the "host." GVHD generally is seen in patients receiving allogeneic HSCT. It remains one of the major causes of transplantation-related mortality.

These soothe dry, flaky, irritated skin.

Systemic agents can be effective in relieving itching and promoting comfort.

This measure reduces skin trauma.

Lubrication provides relief to skin.

NANDA-I NDx   Diarrhea

Common Related Factors
Intestinal GVHD
Side effects of high-dose chemotherapy or radiation therapy
Oral magnesium
Medication use: antacids, antibiotic therapy
Infection

Defining Characteristics
Abdominal pain
Cramping
Frequency of stools
Loose or liquid stools
Urgency
Hyperactive bowel sounds and sensations

Common Expected Outcome
Patient passes soft, formed stool no more than three times per day.
Patient has negative stool cultures.

NOC Outcomes
Bowel Elimination; Fluid Balance; Medication Response

NIC Interventions
Diarrhea Management; Nutrition Therapy; Medication Administration; Perineal Care

Ongoing Assessment

Actions/Interventions	Rationales
■ Check bowel sounds; observe for abdominal distention, rigidity, and discomfort.	Hyperactive bowel sounds and abdominal pain and cramping are associated with diarrhea.
■ Monitor stool pattern; record frequency, character, and volume.	Diarrhea can be the first manifestation of GVHD; it is usually high volume (500 to 1500 mL/day) and watery green and contains mucous strands, protein, and cellular debris.
▲ Obtain stool specimen for culture and sensitivity, as prescribed.	Specimen provides evidence of causative organism, such as *Clostridium difficile*.
■ Hematest all watery stools.	Hematest aids in detecting possible GI mucosal sloughing caused by chemotherapy or radiation therapy or by GVHD-related mucosal injury.

Therapeutic Interventions

Actions/Interventions	Rationales
▲ Administer antidiarrheal, and antispasmodic medications as prescribed; document effectiveness.	Most antidiarrheal drugs suppress GI motility, thus allowing for more fluid absorption. Antispasmotics drugs relieve cramps or spasms of the stomach or intestines.
▲ Administer IV analgesics.	These medications may be needed to relieve abdominal pain and cramping.
■ Implement meticulous perianal care regimen.	Perianal care prevents mucosal irritation/breakdown.
▲ Administer parenteral nutrition as prescribed.	Optimal nutritional support is important in view of inadequate oral intake and decreased absorption secondary to diarrhea and intestinal GVHD.
▲ Consult a dietitian for diet specifications.	Specialist may be able to tailor an optimal meal plan for the patient.

 Risk for Imbalanced Nutrition: Less Than Body Requirements

Common Risk Factors

Side effects of chemotherapy or radiation therapy (inability to taste and smell foods, loss of appetite, nausea and vomiting, mucositis, mouth and throat lesions, xerostomia, diarrhea)

Intestinal GVHD: abdominal cramping, diarrhea, and malabsorption of nutrients

Increased metabolic rate secondary to fever or infection and other metabolic alterations

Common Expected Outcome

Patient maintains optimal nutritional status and protein stores as evidenced by caloric intake adequate to meet body requirements, balanced intake and output, and absence of nausea and vomiting or other GI symptoms.

NOC Outcomes
Nutritional Status: Food and Fluid Intake;
  Nutritional Status: Nutrient Intake

NIC Interventions
Nutrition Therapy; Total Parenteral Nutrition;
  Chemotherapy Management

■ = Independent   ▲ = Collaborative

Ongoing Assessment

Actions/Interventions	Rationales
■ Determine specific cause or causes for imbalanced nutrition.	Specific cause guides treatment plan. These may include side effects of chemotherapy or radiation therapy, GVHD, and infection.
■ Obtain history of side effects of previous chemotherapy or radiation therapy and treatment measures used in the past.	Patients may have had adverse side effects in the past. However, newer antiemetic agents have improved the management of nausea and vomiting for many patients.
■ Review the patient's description of current nausea and vomiting pattern, if present.	Pattern may guide treatment because not all patients experience the same response.
■ Evaluate the effectiveness of the current antiemetic regimen.	Ongoing nausea and vomiting can significantly affect the quality of one's life. Patient response to antiemetic and comfort medications is highly variable and must be explored with each patient. Newer antiemetics may be effective.
■ Monitor daily calorie counts and I&O.	These assessments are important to determine whether the patient's oral intake meets daily nutritional requirements.
■ Weigh the patient daily on the same scale and at the same time.	Consistent weighing is important to ensure accuracy of weight. Without monitoring, the patient may be unaware of small weight changes.
▲ Monitor laboratory values: red and white blood cell counts; serum electrolytes; transferrin, and serum albumin.	Laboratory values provide information on nutrition and electrolyte status. Albumen indicates degree of protein depletion; transferrin is important for iron transfer and typically decreases as serum protein decreases. Anemia and leukopenia occur in malnutrition. Potassium typically increases, and sodium is typically decreased in malabsorption.
■ If on TPN, monitor closely for tolerance to TPN solution and for any potential adverse complications.	Common problems include hyperglycemia or hypoglycemia, hypophosphatemia, electrolyte disorders, hyperosmolarity, dislodgment of catheter or infiltration, and catheter sepsis.

Therapeutic Interventions

Actions/Interventions	Rationales
■ Identify and provide favorite foods; avoid serving them during periods of nausea and vomiting.	The patient may develop an aversion to specific foods as a result of drug side effects.
▲ Administer supplemental feedings or fluids, as prescribed.	Such supplements can be used to increase calories and protein.
■ Implement appropriate GVHD diet or NPO (nothing by mouth) status ("gut rest") in the presence of abdominal cramps, pain, or diarrhea.	These symptoms generally indicate injury to intestinal mucosal surfaces, resulting in nutrient malabsorption. TPN support may be necessary to maintain balanced nutrition.
■ Teach methods to minimize or prevent nausea and vomiting and maintain adequate nutritional intake:	Modifications in dietary intake may reduce the stimulus for nausea and vomiting. Interventions to stimulate appetite and reduce noxious environmental stimuli may enhance nutrient intake.
• Small dietary intake before treatments	Limited intake reduces gastric overdistention. Having some food in the stomach prior to treatment may reduce emesis.
• Foods with low potential for nausea (e.g., dry toast, crackers, ginger ale, cola, Popsicles, gelatin, baked or boiled potatoes)	These foods are easily digested and provide a measure of success to augment nutrition.
• Avoidance of spices, gravy, greasy foods, and foods with strong odors	Fats are difficult to digest and may exacerbate nausea, and can stimulate gastric motility.
• Modification of food consistency or type, as needed	Bland foods may be better tolerated.
• Oral hygiene measures before, after, and between meals	Nausea is often associated with anorexia and increased salivation. Oral hygiene will help promote comfort.

Actions/Interventions

- Antiemetic half an hour before meals, as prescribed

- Relaxation therapy, guided imagery

▲ Administer antiemetic around-the-clock rather than as needed. Schedule before, during, and after chemotherapy or radiation therapy.

Rationales

Antiemetics relieve nausea and vomiting. Selection of antiemetic agents should be based on the risk factors of the patient for nausea/vomiting.

These techniques can be helpful if used before nausea occurs or increases.

Effectiveness of therapy is increased when adequate plasma levels are maintained.

Related Care Plans

Central venous access devices (see the **Evolve** website)
Leukemia, p. 724
Neutropenia, p. 753

Human Immunodeficiency Virus (HIV)

Acquired Immunodeficiency Syndrome (AIDS)

Human immunodeficiency virus (HIV) causes acquired immunodeficiency syndrome (AIDS). Transmission of HIV occurs in situations that allow contact with body fluids that are infected with the virus. The primary body fluids associated with transmission are blood, vaginal secretions, semen, and breast milk. Transmission of HIV can occur during sexual intercourse with an infected partner. Transmission through blood and blood product administration occurred early in the history of HIV in the United States. With current methods for screening blood donors and testing donated blood before transfusion, this is no longer considered a route of infection transmission. However, contact with infected blood through shared intravenous equipment and accidental needle sticks is still possible. Perinatal transmission of the virus from mother to baby is thought to occur during pregnancy, during delivery, or through breast-feeding. Most of the early victims of the syndrome were homosexual men; however, in many cities today, infected intravenous (IV) drug users, their sexual partners, and their children outnumber infected homosexual men. Despite efforts to increase routine voluntary testing and counseling for HIV, many patients first learn that they are infected after their disease is advanced.

The first signs of HIV infection occur when the body produces HIV antibodies. Flulike signs and symptoms that may last 1 to 2 weeks characterize this stage of the infection. After this stage, the patient may be asymptomatic for acute infection, depending on his or her general state of health. This asymptomatic stage can last 10 years or longer. When the immune system begins to fail, the patient exhibits signs of immune system incompetence. The patient begins to develop clinical conditions such as cancers and opportunistic infections. When the patient's CD4 lymphocyte count falls below 200, AIDS is diagnosed. Patients present at various stages of the disease. Treatment regimens are changing rapidly. Patients are treated in hospital, ambulatory care, and home care settings. People may receive prophylactic antiretroviral therapy following high-risk, unprotected sex or injection drug exposures. The nursing diagnosis list of problems for various stages of HIV/AIDS is extensive. Some are highlighted here.

NANDA-I NDx Deficient Knowledge: Disease and Transmission

Common Related Factors

New condition and treatment regimen
Decreased motivation to learn
Emotional state affecting learning (e.g., fear of AIDS)
Unfamiliarity with information resources
Complexity of treatment
Misinterpretation of information

Defining Characteristics

Questioning members of health care team
Verbalizing inaccurate information
Inaccurate follow-through of instruction

Common Expected Outcome

Patient verbalizes understanding of desired content and/or performs desired skills.

NOC Outcomes

Knowledge: Disease Process; Knowledge: Infection Control; Knowledge: Sexual Functioning

NIC Interventions

Teaching: Disease Process; Teaching: Prescribed Medications; Teaching: Safe Sex; Teaching: Individual; Infection Protection

---

Ongoing Assessment

Actions/Interventions	Rationales
■ Assess the patient's knowledge of the disease process, routes of transmission, complications, and treatment modalities.	Because of the chronic nature of HIV infection, the patient needs information about the disease and its treatment to make appropriate decisions about his or her health behaviors.
■ Determine the patient's or significant others' concerns about HIV infection.	Patients, family members, and significant others may have fear of rejection or retaliation when disclosing a patient's HIV infection. Lack of accurate information about the disease and its transmission may interfere with interpersonal relationships and social support for the patient.
■ Determine at-risk behaviors, including sexual activities and IV drug use.	HIV is spread primarily through unprotected sexual activity and by sharing contaminated needles and syringes for IV drug use.

Therapeutic Interventions

Actions/Interventions	Rationales
■ Instruct the patient about a schedule of appointments and treatments.	Patients are better able to ask questions when they have basic information about what to expect. Accurate, clear information provides rationale for treatment and aids the patient in assuming responsibility for care.
■ Instruct the patient in the signs and symptoms of disease, opportunistic infections, and neoplasms, as well as the person to whom information should be reported.	Collaborative management of this disease focuses on monitoring for progression of disease, effectiveness of drug therapy, side effects experienced, and occurrence of complications. This requires an ongoing relationship with the health care provider.
■ Instruct the patient regarding interventions to prevent opportunistic infections:	Appropriate prophylaxis can reduce morbidity and mortality.

Actions/Interventions	Rationales
• Vaccines	Vaccines may include hepatitis B virus (HBV) vaccine, as well as annual influenza and pneumococcal vaccines.
• Medications	Patients with a lymphocyte count of less than 200 CD4 cells need medications to prevent *Pneumocystis carinii* pneumonia (PCP). Patients with a lymphocyte count of less than 100 CD4 cells who are infected with *Toxoplasma gondii* need medication to prevent reactivation. Patients with a lymphocyte count of less than 50 CD4 cells need medication to prevent *Mycobacterium avium* complex (MAC) infection. Patients with a history of cryptococcal meningitis or end-organ cytomegalovirus disease need ongoing medication to prevent recurrence. Patients with tuberculosis (TB) skin test results that indicate latent TB infection need treatment to prevent progression to TB.
• Other • Avoid raw vegetables, raw fish, milk, and raw meat.	These foods harbor bacteria and protozoa that may cause infection in severely compromised people.
• Avoid changing the cat's litter box.	*T. gondii* may be transmitted from the stool of an infected cat.
■ Instruct the patient in methods of preventing HIV transmission sexually: • Safe sex: kissing, touching, mutual masturbation • Probably safe: vaginal or anal intercourse with latex condom and spermicidal lubricant • Possibly safe: oral intercourse between man and woman, two men, or two women • Unsafe: vaginal or anal intercourse without condom; sexual activities that cause bleeding	Activities in which there is no contact with a partner's blood, semen, or vaginal secretions are safe. When properly used, latex condoms reduce the risk for HIV transmission for both partners. Both male and female condoms are available.
■ Explore ways to express physical intimacy that do not lead to infection.	Patients need to have open communication with their sexual partners to negotiate risk-reduction methods.
■ Explore the patient's sexual partner's perception of personal risk for HIV infection.	It is important to assess knowledge rather than make assumptions.
■ Role-play to practice new behaviors (e.g., saying "no" or negotiating condom use) in situations that may lead to transmission.	Practice instills confidence to perform desired behavior. Older adults may be reluctant to use condoms because they are past childbearing age.
■ Explore the benefits and drawbacks of HIV testing of sexual partners and needle-sharing partners.	If the test is positive, benefits include initiation of antiviral therapy; drawbacks include possible discrimination and emotional depression.
■ Instruct the patient and partners to prevent pregnancy. Instruct in birth control methods, including condom use.	Without treatment, approximately 15% to 50% of infants of HIV-infected mothers are infected. Antiretroviral medication administered to the mother during pregnancy and to the infant after birth reduces the infant's risk for becoming infected with HIV.
■ Counsel pregnant women at high risk for HIV infection to be tested for HIV.	Only through early diagnosis can both mother and baby reduce their risk.
■ Encourage use of clean IV equipment when recreational drugs are used. Refer patients to drug rehabilitation programs as appropriate.	HIV is quickly killed by 10% hypochlorite solution. Flush syringe and needles with household bleach diluted ninefold with water; rinse with tap water.
■ Explain the importance of the following: • Refraining from donating blood, semen, or organs	These are established modes of transmission.
• Cleaning blood or excreta containing blood with 10% hypochlorite solution	This solution should be used on blood and stool (carriers of HIV) but it is not necessary to use bleach to wash the patient's dishes, clothes, or personal items.

■ = Independent   ▲ = Collaborative

Actions/Interventions

■ Instruct the patient to avoid exposure to infectious diseases:
  • Avoid sexual practice that leads to sexually transmitted infections (STIs).
  • Avoid contact with people who have infectious diseases.

Rationales

Immunocompromised people are especially vulnerable to viral infections (e.g., herpes or genital warts). Syphilis is more difficult to diagnose and treat in HIV-infected persons and progresses more rapidly. Normally nonpathogenic intestinal flora may cause disease in HIV-infected persons; therefore, such persons should refrain from anal-oral sexual activities. Used properly, condoms can help prevent STIs spread during vaginal or anal intercourse.

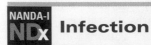 **Infection**

Common Related Factor	**Defining Characteristics**
HIV infection	Decreased number of CD4 cells Positive HIV antibody with confirmatory Western blot Detectable HIV viral load (HIV-1 RNA)

Common Expected Outcomes

Patient does not experience opportunistic infections.
The number of CD4 cells stabilizes or increases.
HIV-1 RNA level drops below limits of assay detection.

NOC Outcomes
Medication Response; Infection Status
NIC Interventions
Infection Protection; Medication Administration

Ongoing Assessment

Actions/Interventions

■ Monitor CD4 level and viral load.

Rationales

Patients need to have regular laboratory testing of CD4 levels and viral load to monitor the status of HIV. Decreasing CD4 levels and increasing viral load indicate progression of the infection and increasing risk for opportunistic infections.

Therapeutic Interventions

Actions/Interventions

■ Instruct in the terminology commonly used in treatments.
  • CD4 cell count
  • Viral load
  • Antiretroviral

■ Instruct about when to start treatment.

Rationales

CD4 cells (T cells) are white blood cells that fight infection.
Viral load is the amount of HIV in a sample of blood.
Antiretrovirals are medications that interfere with the replication of retroviruses such as HIV.
Treatment with antiretroviral medications may begin at any CD4 cell count when the patient is ready to accept treatment and any of the following conditions exist:
  • High plasma viral load of HIV
  • Rapid decline in CD4 cell count (greater than 100 µL per year)
  • High risk of cardiovascular disease (hypertension, hyperlipidemia, diabetes, or tobacco use)
  • HIV-associated nephropathy
  • Active co-infection with HBV or hepatitis C (HCV)
  • Symptoms of HIV disease

Actions/Interventions	Rationales
	• Otherwise, treatment begins when the CD4 cell count drops below 350 μL.
	• See current guidelines for treating pregnant women, newborns, and children.
■ Complete medication reconciliation.	At admission, transfer, and discharge, as well as at every home health or outpatient encounter, a complete medication profile should be completed, including over-the-counter medications and herbal remedies, to reduce medication errors, to minimize the risk for adverse drug reactions, and to guide patient teaching.
	Doses of many antiretrovirals are adjusted for patients with preexisting kidney or liver damage.
■ Instruct about antiretroviral medications and potential therapeutic effects and side effects to monitor.	Antiretrovirals are usually used in combinations; however, each regimen is tailored to the individual patient. Regimens may include fixed-dose combinations of medication. Additional experimental medications may be available through clinical trials. Choice of medications may also depend on chronic conditions, such as renal failure, hepatic dysfunction, diabetes, TB, or cardiovascular disease. Review recent laboratory values to evaluate renal and hepatic functions.
A. Treatment effects	Successful treatment usually results in at least a 10-fold reduction in HIV-1 RNA copies/mL during the first month and a further drop to 50 copies/mL by 6 months, depending on the baseline value of viral load. To evaluate treatment, viral load tests are usually repeated every 3 or 4 months.
	Rising viral loads (HIV-1 RNA greater than 500 to 1000 copies/mL) indicate treatment failure, and antiretroviral drug-resistance testing should be performed while the patient still takes the failing regimen.
B. Indications for special drug monitoring	Therapeutic drug monitoring by quality-assured laboratories of certain antiretrovirals may be considered for the following patients:
	• Pregnant women
	• Children
	• Patients with liver or kidney failure
	• Patients with complex drug-drug interactions
	• Patients whose viral loads continue to rise despite adherence to treatment and the absence of antiretroviral drug resistance
C. Drug-specific actions/interactions	Before instructing a patient, review the current medication profile with a clinical pharmacist to clarify:
	• Preferred formulation and release formulation
	• Whether formulation can be opened, crushed, or chewed
	• Potential drug-drug interactions that may result in dosage alterations or changes in administration times or frequencies
	• Potential drug–oral contraceptive interactions that may require alternative methods of birth control
	• Potential drug-alcohol interactions
	• Potential drug-methadone interactions
	• Potential food-drug interactions
	• Potential dosage alterations because of renal or hepatic functions
	• When to repeat monitoring
	• How to store medication

■ = Independent   ▲ = Collaborative

Actions/Interventions	Rationales
Nucleoside reverse transcriptase inhibitors (NRTIs):	NRTIs block reverse transcriptase, an enzyme that HIV needs to make more copies of itself.
• Emtricitabine (Emtriva, FTC): Monitor for nausea, vomiting, abdominal pain, lack of appetite, weight loss, difficulty breathing, and fatigue.	This drug may also cause headache, diarrhea, rash, and skin discoloration.
• Lamivudine (Epivir, 3TC): Monitor for severe abdominal pain, as well as pain, numbness, tingling, and burning in the extremities.	This drug may also cause nausea, vomiting, mouth sores, ear discharge, ear swelling, rash, and warm skin.
• Zalcitabine, dideoxycytidine (Hivid, ddC): Monitor liver function (especially among patients with preexisting liver damage). Monitor for severe pancreatitis, peripheral neuropathy, and lactic acidosis with hepatomegaly with steatosis.	Peripheral neuropathy occurs in up to one-third of patients with advanced HIV disease treated with this drug. May also cause stomatitis or aphthous ulcers.
• Zidovudine, azidothymidine (Retrovir, AZT, ZDV): Monitor complete blood count (CBC) for neutropenia and anemia.	This drug may cause fever, chills, sore throat, headache, sleep disturbances, muscle soreness, and nausea.
• Didanosine enteric coated (Videx, Videx EC, ddI): Monitor renal function, hepatic function, for signs of severe pancreatitis, for signs of lactic acidosis, peripheral neuropathy, cardiac dysrhythmias, and vision disturbances.	This drug may also cause diarrhea, nausea, vomiting, headache, dizziness, anxiety, sleep disturbances, and rash.
• Tenofovir disoproxil fumarate (Viread, TDF): Monitor renal function, hepatic function, and for signs of severe pancreatitis. Monitor for signs of lactic acidosis and hepatic steatosis. Monitor for signs of exacerbation of chronic HBV after discontinuation of medication among people co-infected with HBV and HIV.	This drug may also cause diarrhea, dizziness, abdominal pain, flatulence, headache, and rash.
• Stavudine (Zerit [IR immediate release or XR extended release], d4T): Monitor liver function, for symptoms of pancreatitis, and for symptoms of peripheral neuropathy.	This drug may also cause nausea, fever, rash, vomiting, stomach pain, and joint or muscle pain.
• Abacavir sulfate (Ziagen, ABC): Before use, screen patients for HLA-B 5701 genotype. Monitor for skin rash (potentially fatal hypersensitivity reaction) and lactic acidosis with hepatic steatosis (rare but life-threatening).	Risk for hypersensitivity reaction greater for positive HLA-B 5701 genotype. Hypersensitivity usually occurs within the first 6 weeks of treatment. Report rash, fever, and GI upset immediately. This drug may also cause changes in body fat, elevated blood glucose, and liver damage.
Nonnucleoside reverse transcriptase inhibitors (NNRTIs):	NNRTIs block reverse transcriptase, an enzyme that HIV needs to make more copies of itself.
• Etravirine (Intelence, TMC125): Monitor blood pressure (BP) and for severe rash.	Mild-to-moderate rash may occur during the first weeks of treatment and often resolves after a few weeks of continued therapy. This drug may also cause nausea, diarrhea, abdominal pain, vomiting, fatigue, headache, and peripheral neuropathy.
• Delavirdine (Rescriptor, DLV): Monitor for anemia, liver function, and kidney function. Also monitor for severe rash, muscle, and joint pain.	This drug may also cause diarrhea, nausea, vomiting, fatigue, and headache. Many people develop a rash on their upper bodies and arms during the first weeks of treatment, which usually resolves within weeks.
• Efavirenz (Sustiva, EFV): Monitor for disturbed thinking, hallucinations, nightmares, depression, memory loss, and thoughts of suicide. Monitor liver function.	This drug may also cause nausea, diarrhea, sleep problems, abnormal dreams, dizziness, headache, and impaired concentration. Laboratory screens may be falsely positive for marijuana.
• Nevirapine (Viramune, NVP): Monitor liver function and signs of liver disease, including severe skin rash, fever, sore throat, and flulike symptoms.	This drug may also cause stomach pain, nausea, diarrhea, fatigue, and headache.

Actions/Interventions

Protease inhibitors (PIs):

- Tipranavir (Aptivus, TPV): Must be boosted with low-dose ritonavir. Monitor for liver toxicity, intracranial hemorrhage, rash, and elevated lipids.

- Indinavir (Crixivan, IDV): Monitor for signs of kidney stones—flank pain and hematuria; advise all patients to maintain good hydration. Monitor glucose and lipids. Monitor for signs of increased bleeding in patients with hemophilia.

- Saquinavir mesylate (Invirase, SQV): Must be boosted with ritonavir. Monitor glucose and lipids. Monitor for signs of increased bleeding in patients with hemophilia.

- Lopinavir and ritonavir (Kaletra, LPV/RTV): The ritonavir portion of this medication functions as a metabolic booster. Monitor glucose, lipids, and liver function. Monitor for pancreatitis. Monitor for signs of increased bleeding in patients with hemophilia.

- Fosamprenavir calcium (Lexiva, FOS-APV): This is a prodrug that is converted by the body to amprenavir. It may be boosted with low-dose ritonavir. Dosages depend on how much ritonavir is used to boost and whether there is liver damage. Monitor glucose, liver function, severe rash, lipids, and increased bleeding in patients with hemophilia.

- Ritonavir (Norvir, RTV): Monitor glucose, lipids, liver function, and signs of pancreatitis. Monitor for increased bleeding in patients with hemophilia. Monitor for cardiac dysrhythmias, including symptoms of dizziness, light-headedness, and fainting.

- Darunavir (Prezista): Must be boosted with low-dose ritonavir. Monitor liver function, lipids, glucose, and for severe rash. Monitor for rhabdomyolysis and hypersensitivity with facial swelling (rare).

- Atazanavir sulfate (Reyataz, ATV): Monitor glucose, BP, lipids, bilirubin, liver function, hematuria, and cardiac dysrhythmias.
- Nelfinavir mesylate (Viracept, NFV): Monitor lipids, glucose, and liver function. Monitor for signs of increased bleeding in patients with hemophilia.

Entry inhibitors CCR5 coreceptor antagonists:

Rationales

Protease inhibitors block protease, an enzyme that HIV needs to make more copies of itself.

Patients with advanced HIV disease, preexisting liver damage, or co-infected with HBV or HCV require careful monitoring. This drug may also cause diarrhea, nausea, vomiting, and unusual fatigue. Women taking oral contraceptives are more likely to develop a rash. Report signs of liver damage or intracranial hemorrhage immediately.

This drug may also cause changes in sense of taste, diarrhea, nausea, vomiting, weakness, headache, stomach pain, sleep disturbances. Hydration may help prevent kidney stones.

This drug may also cause anxiety, changes in sense of taste, constipation, depression, diarrhea, dizziness, eczema, flatulence, weakness, headache, mouth sores, nausea, vomiting, sleep disturbances, and peripheral neuropathy.

This drug may also cause diarrhea, headache, nausea, rash, trouble sleeping, vomiting, and weakness.

This drug may also cause depression, diarrhea, rash, nausea, numbness, mood changes, vomiting, stomach pain, fatigue, and unusual sense of taste. Report a severe rash immediately.

Because ritonavir inhibits metabolism of other PIs, it is often used to "boost" and maintain the plasma concentrations of other PIs for longer periods of time. Ritonavir-boost regimens alter the dose and frequency of other medications. This drug may also cause weakness, peripheral neuropathy, stomach pain, diarrhea, vomiting, flatulence, indigestion, constipation, loss of appetite, fever, throat irritation, rash, sweating, and disturbed sleep.

Patients with preexisting liver damage or co-infected with HBV or HCV require careful monitoring during the first months of treatment. This drug may also cause diarrhea, nausea, headache, runny nose, and sore throat. Report signs of liver damage immediately.

This drug may also cause headache, rash, stomach pain, vomiting, depression, cough, sleep disturbances, fatigue, back and joint pain, and peripheral neuropathy.

This drug may cause diarrhea, nausea, and rash.

Chemokine receptor 5 (CCR5) antagonists work by blocking one of the receptors needed by HIV to enter cells. They are effective only for patients with CCR5-tropic variants of HIV-1. Over time HIV-1 may adapt to use an alternative CXCR4 receptor, which renders this drug class ineffective.

Hematolymphatic, Immunological and Oncological Care Plans

■ = Independent ▲ = Collaborative

Actions/Interventions	Rationales
• Maraviroc (Selzentry): Before use, patients must be screened for CCR5 tropism. Monitor for cardiovascular disease, including myocardial ischemia or infarction (rare).	This drug may also cause cough, fever, dizziness, headache, low blood pressure, nausea, and bladder irritation. Report chest pain immediately.
HIV integrase strand transfer inhibitors:	Integrase inhibitors block integrase, a protein that HIV needs to put its genetic material in the genetic material of an infected cell.
• Raltegravir (Isentress): Used by patients with advanced HIV disease inadequately controlled by other medications.	This drug may cause diarrhea, nausea, headache, and fever.
Fusion inhibitors:	Fusion inhibitors block HIV from entering cells.
• Enfuvirtide (Fuzeon, T-20): Used by patients with advanced HIV disease inadequately controlled by other medications. Monitor for signs of injection-site reaction and signs of serious hypersensitivity reactions.	Administer subcutaneously following the manufacturer's instructions at sites without large nerves that are close to the skin. This drug usually causes mild-to-moderate injection-site reactions. Report infection or nerve pain at injection site, as well as signs of pneumonia. This drug may also cause bad taste in the mouth, constipation, cough, depression, diarrhea, rash, fatigue, flulike illness, muscle pain, weakness, nervousness, trouble sleeping, nausea, loss of appetite, and pain and tingling in the extremities.
Fixed-dose combination products: • Atripla contains efavirenz, emtricitabine, and tenofovir disoproxil fumarate. • Combivir contains lamivudine and zidovudine. • Epzicom contains abacavir and lamivudine. • Trizivir contains abacavir, zidovudine, and lamivudine. • Truvada contains emtricitabine and tenofovir disoproxil fumarate.	
■ Encourage adherence to therapy, and avoid interruptions of therapy.	Strict adherence is needed to stall the emergence of drug-resistant HIV. Antiretrovirals are taken throughout the course of infection unless the toxicities outweigh the potential benefits.
▲ Follow local regulations for obtaining a separate consent to be tested for HIV and for reporting results to the health department.	Pregnant women may be required to be tested because of local or state regulations.

Imbalanced Nutrition: Less Than Body Requirements

Common Related Factors	Defining Characteristics
Loss of appetite Fatigue Oral or esophageal candidiasis Cryptosporidiosis Enteric cytomegalovirus disease MAC (cultured from blood, bone marrow, or lymph node biopsy specimen) Increased nutritional needs Nausea and vomiting Malabsorption	Loss of weight Caloric intake inadequate to meet metabolic requirements Loss of fat and muscle Decreased body mass index (BMI)

Common Expected Outcomes

Patient regains weight or does not lose additional weight. Patient verbalizes understanding of necessary caloric intake to achieve a cessation of weight loss.

NOC Outcomes

Nutritional Status: Food and Fluid Intake; Nutrient Intake

NIC Interventions

Nutrition Monitoring: Nutrition Therapy; Medication Administration; Total Parenteral Nutrition; Oral Health Restoration

Ongoing Assessment

Actions/Interventions	Rationales
■ Assess changes in weight.	HIV wasting syndrome is one of the clinical conditions that occur with AIDS. This condition is defined as an involuntary loss of more than 10% of total body weight. Persistent diarrhea and recurrent fevers are associated with the syndrome. Other factors contributing to weight loss in the patient with HIV infection include reduced food intake from anorexia, oral or esophageal lesions from candidiasis, and drug side effects. Inflammatory bowel disease from HIV may lead to malabsorption syndromes. Chronic HIV infection increases metabolic demands.
▲ Obtain nutritional history: intake, difficulty in swallowing, weight loss. Consult with dietician.	Attention to individual factors helps in designing an appropriate plan. Routine evaluations of changes in weight and caloric intake are useful to prevent weight loss and malnutrition.
▲ Inspect mouth for candidal infection.	This infection causes difficulty in swallowing.
■ Evaluate for possible adverse reactions to medications.	Many drugs used to treat HIV can cause anorexia, nausea and vomiting, and weight loss.
▲ If the patient receives total parenteral nutrition (TPN), monitor serum glucose and electrolyte levels.	The high glucose content of TPN solutions can cause short-term hyperglycemia that may require insulin administration.

Therapeutic Interventions

Actions/Interventions	Rationales
■ Provide dietary planning to encourage intake of high-calorie, high-protein foods and dietary supplements.	Patients may not easily understand what is involved in a special dietary plan.
▲ Provide antiemetics before meals.	Antiemetics can reduce nausea and improve intake.
■ Assist with meals as needed.	Fatigue and weakness may prevent the patient from eating.
■ Encourage exercise as tolerated.	Metabolism and utilization of nutrients are enhanced by activity.
▲ Administer dietary supplements or TPN, as ordered.	HIV may cause wasting syndrome. Oral nutritional supplements should be tried first. Parenteral nutrition should be reserved for severe intestinal dysfunction.
▲ Administer antimonilial medication, as prescribed.	Oral and esophageal candidiasis can cause sore throat, which may cause lack of appetite.
▲ Administer megestrol acetate (Megace), as prescribed.	This is a synthetic progestational drug that increases body weight by increasing appetite. Dose will be individualized to degree of wasting and patient's response. Side effects include carpal tunnel syndrome, thrombophlebitis, alopecia, reduced sex drive, and impotence.

■ = Independent   ▲ = Collaborative

Actions/Interventions

▲ Administer anabolic steroids or testosterone supplements, as ordered.

▲ Administer human growth hormones, as ordered. Monitor for hyperglycemia and hypertriglyceridemia.

▲ Administer dronabinol (THC, Marinol) as ordered.

▲ Administer medications for opportunistic pathogens affecting the gastrointestinal (GI) tract.

▲ Administer clarithromycin (Biaxin), rifabutin (Mycobutin), or azithromycin (Zithromax).

Rationales

These can enhance appetite but are not without their own side effects. Monitor for edema and jaundice.

Human growth hormone has been found to increase weight and lean body mass in people with AIDS wasting. Hormones may cause arthralgia, joint stiffness, or carpal tunnel syndrome.

Dronabinol is a synthetic derivative of marijuana and is associated with increased appetite and control of weight loss. It may cause restlessness, insomnia, dizziness, loss of coordination, and clouded sensorium or euphoria.

Bowel inflammation from opportunistic infections causes malabsorption of nutrients.

These help prevent MAC in patients with advanced disease.

Related Care Plans

Diabetes mellitus, p. 911
Diarrhea, p. 54
Disturbed body image, p. 24
Fatigue, p. 66
Hepatitis, p. 593
Ineffective coping, p. 49
Ineffective therapeutic regimen management, p. 194
Pancreatitis, p. 607
Renal failure, chronic/end-stage renal disease, p. 818
Spiritual distress, p. 189

Leukemia

Acute Lymphocytic Leukemia; Acute Myelocytic Leukemia; Chronic Lymphocytic Leukemia; Lymphocytic Leukemia; Chronic Myelocytic Leukemia; Nonlymphocytic Leukemia; Myelogenous Leukemia; Granulocytic Leukemia

Leukemia is a malignant disorder of the blood-forming system, including the bone marrow and spleen. The proliferation of immature white blood cells (WBCs) interferes with the production and function of the red blood cells (RBCs) and platelets. Leukemia can be characterized by identification of the type of leukocyte involved: myelogenous or lymphocytic. In acute lymphocytic leukemia there is a proliferation of lymphoblasts (most commonly seen in children); in acute myelocytic leukemia (most common after 60 years of age), there is a proliferation of myeloblasts. In chronic lymphocytic leukemia, there are increased lymphocytes (more common in men, especially after 50 years of age); in chronic myelocytic leukemia, granulocytes are increased (common in middle age).

Depending on the type of leukemia, therapeutic management may consist of combined chemotherapeutic agents, radiation therapy, and/or stem cell transplantation. Chemotherapeutic treatment consists of several stages: induction therapy, intensification, consolidation therapy, and maintenance therapy. The goals of nursing care are to prevent complications and to provide educational and emotional support. This care plan addresses ongoing care of a patient in an ambulatory setting receiving maintenance therapy.

NANDA-I NDx **Deficient Knowledge**

Common Related Factors

New disease/procedure/treatment
Lack of information resources
Complexity of treatment
Misinterpretation of information
Emotional state affecting learning
Lack of recall

Defining Characteristics

Questioning health care team
Verbalizing inaccurate information
Inaccurate follow-through of instruction

Common Expected Outcome

Patient verbalizes understanding of diagnosis, treatment strategies, and prognosis.

NOC Outcomes

Knowledge: Disease Process; Knowledge: Treatment Procedures

NIC Intervention

Teaching: Disease Process

Ongoing Assessment

Actions/Interventions	Rationales
■ Assess knowledge of disease, treatment strategies, and prognosis.	Several types of leukemia occur, which can be confusing. Each has its own treatment approach and prognosis.

Therapeutic Interventions

Actions/Interventions	Rationales
■ Describe the etiology of leukemia: • Not well understood; probably multifactorial • May be related to exposure to radiation or chemical agents, genetic factors, congenital abnormalities, viruses, immunological deficiencies, or antineoplastic drugs	The exact cause of leukemia is unknown. Many causative factors seem to play a role in the development of both the acute and chronic forms of the disease. A group of preleukemic or myelodysplastic syndromes has been identified as significant in the development of leukemia in older adults.
■ Explain the blood-forming changes that occur with all types of leukemia: • Bone marrow failure; leukemic infiltrates • Granulocytopenia from reduced number of WBCs • Anemia from reduced RBC production • Thrombocytopenia from decreased platelet production	Most people are unfamiliar with the various components of normal blood and marrow and the respective functions of the different blood cells.
■ Clarify the difference between acute and chronic leukemia: • Acute leukemia is abnormal proliferation of *immature* leukocytes or blasts with rapid onset of symptoms. • Chronic leukemia is characterized by disease of *mature* WBCs with a progressive, gradual onset of symptoms.	Knowing type will guide treatment. Acute leukemia is treated immediately, whereas in chronic leukemia symptoms may be "watched" until they worsen. Leukemias may be further classified as lymphocytic or myelocytic according to the type of WBC that is involved in the disease.
■ Describe the patient's specific type of leukemia.	Four major types of leukemia are known, as described in the introductory paragraph. Distinguishing specific subtypes is important to guide appropriate therapy.
■ Explain the diagnostic process: • Peripheral blood analysis • Bone marrow examination/biopsy • Lumbar puncture and computed tomography scan	Analysis is necessary to detect immature blood cells. This is the key diagnostic tool and assists in staging of disease. These tests are done to determine the presence of leukemic cells throughout the body.

■ = Independent   ▲ = Collaborative

Actions/Interventions	Rationales
■ Describe common approaches to treatment:	Treatment is guided by current research findings and definitive protocols for specific types of leukemia. Initial chemotherapy doses may be given in the hospital. However, follow-up courses may be administered in an outpatient or even in a home setting.
• Combination chemotherapy	Chemotherapy is the primary treatment. It has reduced side effects and improved response. A variety of drugs are available depending on leukemia type.
• Targeted therapy	Targeted therapy blocks cancer cells but not normal cells. For example, Gleevec is used for chronic myeloid leukemia.
• Radiation therapy	Radiation therapy may be used as an adjunct to chemotherapy to keep acute leukemia from spreading, or to relieve pain in chronic leukemia.
• Stem cell transplantation, especially with acute myelocytic leukemia	Transplantation is a standard treatment for leukemia.
• Biological therapies	Several types of biological therapies can treat leukemia. This type of therapy improves the body's natural defenses against cancer. Examples include monoclonal antibody for chronic lymphocytic leukemia and interferon for chronic myelocytic leukemia.
• Clinical trials	Ongoing research continues to explore improved treatments. Some are indicated for patients *before* any treatment, others for patients with refractory disease.
■ Explain common complications of therapy.	Complications include pancytopenia from radiation and chemotherapy (anemia, bleeding, infection); nausea and vomiting from chemotherapy; fatigue and weakness.
■ Discuss prognosis: • The prognosis is hopeful, with the treatment goal being a curative attempt, although at times the treatment may only result in prolonged remission. • Patients may be in remission for a long time, especially with chronic leukemia.	The patient's adjustment to any form of leukemia and its treatment requires understanding of the expected course of exacerbations and remissions.

NANDA-I NDx   Risk for Ineffective Coping

Common Risk Factors

Situational crisis
Inadequate support system
Inadequate coping methods

Common Expected Outcomes

Patient demonstrates positive coping strategies.
Patient uses available resources and support systems.
Patient verbalizes realistic goal setting for future.

NOC Outcomes
Coping; Social Support; Family Coping

NIC Interventions
Coping Enhancement; Hope Instillation; Grief Work Facilitation; Support System Enhancement

Ongoing Assessment

Actions/Interventions	Rationales
■ Assess the patient's knowledge of disease and treatment plan.	Because leukemia is cancer, patients may expect to die. Realistic but positive information may be indicated.
■ Assess for coping mechanisms used in previous illnesses and hospitalization experiences.	Successful coping is influenced by previous success. Patients with a history of maladaptive coping may require additional resources. Likewise, previously successful coping skills may be inadequate in the present situation.
■ Evaluate resources and support systems available to the patient in the home and community.	Leukemia treatment may include months and years of ongoing chemotherapy, depending on the length of remission. The demands of managing therapy and preventing complications in the home setting can disrupt the lives of both the patient and the family members. Availability of support systems may change over time.
■ Assess financial resources required for expensive long-term therapy.	The financial aspects of acute care and long-term follow-up can be overwhelming, especially when the patient is dealing with a new diagnosis.

Therapeutic Interventions

Actions/Interventions	Rationales
■ Establish open lines of communication; establish a working relationship with the patient through continuity of care.	The nurse may be the first source of support for the patient and family. An ongoing relationship establishes trust, reduces the feeling of isolation, and may facilitate coping.
■ Provide opportunities for the patient and significant others to openly express feelings, fears, and concerns. Provide hope but avoid false reassurances.	Verbalization of actual or perceived threats can help reduce anxiety and open doors for ongoing communication. An honest relationship facilitates problem solving and successful coping. False reassurances are never helpful to the patient and only serve to relieve the discomfort of care provider.
■ Assist the patient and significant others in redefining hopes and components of individuality (e.g., roles, values, and attitudes).	Emphasizing the patient's intrinsic worth and viewing the immediate situation as manageable in time may provide support.
■ Encourage the patient to seek information that will improve coping skills.	Patients who are not coping well may need more guidance initially.
■ Introduce new information about disease treatment as available.	Chronic leukemia is seldom cured. However, remission is possible, and long-term survival is feasible. Acute leukemia is treated to remission stage, with maintenance therapy given to prevent relapse.
■ Assist the patient in becoming involved as a comanager of the treatment plan.	Involvement helps the patient regain control over the situation. Many patients become educated about their chemotherapeutic agents, using abbreviations fluently (e.g., MOPP, COAP). Others become knowledgeable about blood components and vigilantly record daily or weekly laboratory results.
■ Describe community resources available to meet the unique demands of leukemia, its treatment, and survival (e.g., Leukemia and Lymphoma Society, American Cancer Society, National Coalition for Cancer Survivorship).	It is helpful for patients to have more than one resource for helping them in this process. Reliable websites may likewise offer information and support.
▲ Refer to a social worker for financial assistance, as indicated.	The social worker can assist the patient and family with decisions about finances, living arrangements, wills, advance directives, and power of attorney.

■ = Independent   ▲ = Collaborative

Hematolymphatic, Immunological and Oncological Care Plans

Actions/Interventions

- Assist in the development of an alternative support system, as indicated. Encourage participation in self-help groups as available.

- Assist the patient in grieving and working through the losses from life-threatening illness and change in body function.

Rationales

Relationships with persons with common interests and goals can be beneficial. Participation in support groups may allow the individual to realize that others have the same problem, and they may use this as an aid for coping.

Grief is a universal experience; people who have successfully undergone grief over loss can be enormously helpful to others undergoing the same feelings.

NANDA-I NDx Risk for Infection

Common Risk Factors

Cancer, resulting in altered immunological responses
Immunosuppression secondary to chemotherapy or radiation therapy

Common Expected Outcome

Patient is at reduced risk for local or systemic infection, as evidenced by afebrile state, normal vital signs, chest x-ray film results within normal limits, negative results of blood and surveillance cultures, compliance with preventive measures, and prompt reporting of early signs of infection.

NOC Outcomes

Immune Status; Knowledge: Infection Control; Tissue Integrity: Skin and Mucous Membranes

NIC Interventions

Infection Protection; Teaching: Disease Process; Oral Health Maintenance

---

Ongoing Assessment

Actions/Interventions

- Auscultate lung fields for crackles, rhonchi, and decreased breath sounds.
- Observe the patient for coughing spells and character of sputum.

- Inspect body sites with high infection potential (mouth, throat, axilla, perineum, rectum).

- Inspect intravenous or central catheter site for redness, tenderness, pain, and itching.
- Observe for changes in color, character, and frequency of urine and stool.
- Monitor temperature as indicated. Report temperature higher than 38° C (100.4° F).
- ▲ Obtain cultures as indicated.

Rationales

Pulmonary infections are common, especially in immunosuppressed patients.

Increased sputum production and change in color from clear or white to yellow or green may indicate respiratory infection.

Many infections that occur in patients with leukemia are opportunistic because of the patients' immunocompromised status. Opportunistic infections of the mucous membrane surfaces of the body are often the first type of infection to develop in immunosuppressed patients.

In the absence of granulocytes, site of infection may develop without characteristic pus formation.

These observations provides data on possible urinary tract infection or intestinal infection.

Fever may be the only sign of infection. Patients need to be instructed to record serial temperatures at home.

Cultures are required to determine the organism causing the infection and antibiotic sensitivity.

Therapeutic Interventions

Actions/Interventions	Rationales

■ Explain the cause and effects of leukopenia.

Leukemic cells replace normal cells. Also, chemotherapy causes bone marrow suppression and reduced number of neutrophils needed to fight infection.

■ Instruct the patient to maintain personal hygiene, especially at home:
- To bathe with chlorhexidine (Hibiclens)
- To wash hands well before eating and after using bathroom
- To wipe perineal area from front to back

Hand washing removes transient and residual bacteria from hands. The perineal area is a source of pathogens and a frequent entry port for microorganisms.

■ Instruct the patient to brush teeth with a soft toothbrush four times a day and as necessary, to remove dentures at night, and to rinse mouth after each emesis or when expectorating phlegm.

Keeping oral mucous membranes intact reduces a possible site for opportunistic infection to develop. Periodontal disease is a locus of infection.

■ Teach the patient to inspect the oropharyngeal area daily for white patches in the mouth, coated or encrusted oral ulcerations, swollen and erythematous tongue with white or brown coating, infected throat and pain on swallowing, debris on teeth, ill-fitting dentures.

The oral cavity and upper respiratory tract are common infection sites in patients with leukemia and neutropenia. Candidiasis is a common opportunistic infection in the immunocompromised patient.

■ Teach the patient to avoid mouthwashes that contain alcohol and to avoid irritating foods and acidic drinks.

Alcohol has a drying effect on mucous membranes which can impair their integrity.

■ Teach the patient to use prescribed topical medications (e.g., nystatin [Nilstat] and lidocaine [Xylocaine]).

These agents may require specific instruction.

■ Instruct the patient and caregiver to maintain strict aseptic technique when changing dressings and to avoid wetting central catheter dressings.

These measures help prevent bacterial growth.

■ Instruct the patient to observe for fever spikes and flulike symptoms (e.g., malaise, weakness, myalgia) and to notify the nurse or physician if they occur.

Early assessment facilitates prompt treatment.

■ Instruct the patient and caregiver regarding the importance of eliminating potential sources of infection at home (especially when neutrophil counts are low):
- Avoidance of contact with visitors and family, especially children with colds or infections
- Avoidance of shared drinking and eating utensils
- Avoidance of contact with cat litter boxes, fish tanks, and human or animal excreta
- Avoidance of swimming in private or public pools
- Restricting contact with live plants

Patients must understand strategies and measures by which they can protect themselves during times of compromised defense. Animal excreta, soil, and people with known infections are sources of opportunistic infection for the immunocompromised patient.

■ Instruct the patient regarding "protective isolation" if laboratory results indicate neutropenia (absolute neutrophil count [ANC] less than 500 to 1000/mm^3):
- Implement thorough hand washing for staff and visitors before physical contact with the patient.

Institutional protocols may vary.

Hand washing removes transient and resident bacteria from hands, thus minimizing or preventing transmission to patient.

■ Instruct the patient to take prescribed antibiotic, antifungal, or antiviral drugs on time.

A regular schedule is needed to maintain therapeutic drug levels.

▲ Refer the patient to a dietitian for instructions on maintenance of a well-balanced diet.

A specialist may provide additional help. This diet is for maintenance of optimal health status, which promotes improvement of host resistance and bone marrow recovery.

■ = Independent   ▲ = Collaborative

Risk for Bleeding

Common Risk Factors

Bone marrow depression secondary to chemotherapy
Proliferation of leukemic cells

Common Expected Outcome

Patient's risk for bleeding is reduced, as evidenced by platelet count within acceptable limits, compliance with preventive measures, and prompt reporting of early signs and symptoms.

NOC Outcomes

Blood Coagulation; Knowledge: Treatment Regimen

NIC Interventions

Bleeding Precautions; Teaching: Disease Process

Ongoing Assessment

Actions/Interventions	Rationales
▲ Monitor platelet count.	Risk for bleeding increases as platelet count drops: • Mild thrombocytopenia: platelets 50,000 to 100,000/mm^3 • Moderate risk: platelets 20,000 to 50,000/mm^3 • Severe: platelets 20,000/mm^3 or less • Transfusion threshold: platelet count less than 10,000/mm^3 or signs of active bleeding
■ Assess for signs and symptoms of bleeding. These may include petechiae and bruising; hemoptysis; epistaxis; bleeding in oral mucosa; hematemesis; hematochezia; melena; vaginal bleeding; dizziness; orthostatic changes; decreased blood pressure (BP); headaches; changes in mental and visual acuity; and increased pulse rate.	Early assessment facilitates prompt treatment and reduced risk for complications.
■ Note bleeding from any recent puncture site (e.g., venipuncture, bone marrow aspiration site).	Prolonged oozing of blood from puncture sites may be the first sign of a coagulation problem.

Therapeutic Interventions

Actions/Interventions	Rationales
■ Explain to the patient and significant others the symptoms of thrombocytopenia and the functions of platelets: • Normal range of platelet count • Effects of thrombocytopenia • Rationale of bleeding precautions	Most individuals are not familiar with the complexities of the hematological system. A successful plan requires the knowledge and cooperation of the patient and family members.
■ Instruct the patient in precautionary measures. Initiate bleeding precautions for platelet count less than 50,000/mm^3: • Use soft toothbrush and nonabrasive toothpaste. • Inspect gums for oozing. • Avoid use of toothpicks and dental floss. • Avoid rectal suppositories, thermometers, enemas, vaginal douches, and tampons. • Avoid aspirin or aspirin-containing products, nonsteroidal antiinflammatory drugs (NSAIDs), and anticoagulants.	Understanding of precautionary measures reduces risk for bleeding. At this level, spontaneous bleeding can occur. This method reduces risk for bleeding. Oozing can be an early sign of bleeding. It is important to reduce mucosal trauma. This measure reduces mucosal trauma. These medications interfere with platelet function.

Actions/Interventions

- Avoid straining with bowel movements, forceful nose blowing, coughing, or sneezing.
- Count used sanitary pads during menstruation. Report menstrual cycle changes.
- Avoid sharp objects such as scissors and knives. Use electric razor for shaving (not razor blades).

- Lubricate nostrils with saline solution drops as necessary and lips with petroleum jelly as needed.
- Practice gentle sex; use water-based lubricant before sexual intercourse.
- Protect self from injury and trauma (e.g., falls, bumps, strenuous exercise, contact sports).

In the health care setting:

- Avoid finger sticks if possible. Coordinate laboratory work so all tests are done at one time.
- Avoid intramuscular and subcutaneous injections. If necessary, use small-bore needles for injections and apply ice to the injection site for 5 minutes. Observe the site for oozing.
- Apply pressure, dressing, or sandbag to the bone marrow aspiration site.

- Give the patient and family at least two telephone numbers to call in case of bleeding.
- ▲ Apply ice or topical thrombin promptly as prescribed for bleeding mucous membranes.
- Instruct the patient to take antacids as prescribed when taking steroids, NSAIDs, and/or aspirin.
- Discuss the possibility of platelet transfusions. Teach the patient the purpose and possible reactions to transfusions.

- ▲ Ensure availability and readiness of platelets for transfusion.

Rationales

This measure reduces the risk for bleeding.

This measure provides data on bleeding status.

It is important to prevent cuts, which would not only bleed but also become portals of entry for microorganisms, leading to infection in the presence of neutropenia.
Lubrication prevents drying and cracking.

These measures prevent mucosal trauma.

Patient safety is a priority.

This precaution reduces bleeding potential.

These measures reduce bleeding potential at the injection sites.

This procedure prevents excessive pressure when compressing soft tissues and deeper structures of the arm, because this may lead to bruising or hematomas.
Prearranged contact information facilitates early treatment.

Thrombin promotes clot formation.

Antacids reduce gastric irritation which can lead to bleeding.

Knowledge reduces anxiety. Transfusions may be needed to maintain adequate platelet count to prevent spontaneous or excessive bleeding.
It is important to have platelets available when needed to prevent spontaneous or excessive bleeding (generally for platelet count less than 10,000/mm³, unless active bleeding is present, or according to institutional protocol).

NDx Cancer-Related Fatigue

Common Related Factors

Tumor and metastatic disease
Chemotherapy/targeted therapy
Radiation
Pain
Distress (spiritual or emotional)
Anxiety/fear
Malnutrition
Anemia

Defining Characteristics

A sense of physical or emotional tiredness that is not proportional to recent activity or treatment and interferes with the individual's daily functioning.
Inability to restore energy, even after sleep
Verbalization of an overwhelming lack of energy

■ = Independent   ▲ = Collaborative

Common Expected Outcomes

Patient reports reduction in fatigue, as evidenced by reports of increased energy and ability to perform desired activities.

Patient reports use of energy-conservation principles.

NOC Outcomes

Activity Tolerance; Endurance; Energy Conservation; Self-Care: Activities

NIC Interventions

Energy Management; Nutrition Management; Sleep Enhancement; Exercise Promotion

Ongoing Assessment

Actions/Interventions	Rationales
■ Assess for fatigue regularly using 0 to 10 scale and defining characteristics.	Fatigue has become the most common and distressing complaint for cancer patients, especially during treatment. Regular assessment allows the nurse to evaluate the fatigue and response to interventions and to develop and alter the plan accordingly.
■ Refer to Fatigue (p. 66)	

Interventions

Actions/Interventions	Rationales
In addition to the Fatigue care plan, consider interventions in the following:	
■ Educate patient regarding these treatments:	
• Assigning priorities to activities to accommodate energy levels	Setting priorities while conserving energy will allow the patient to achieve most desired goals and feel a sense of accomplishment.
• Energy-conservation strategies, such as:	Energy-conservation techniques reduce oxygen consumption, allowing more prolonged activity.
• Sitting to do tasks	
• Pushing rather than pulling	
• Working at an even pace	
• Placing frequently used items within easy reach	
• Using wheeled carts for laundry, shopping, cleaning needs (see Fatigue, p. 66)	
• Limiting naps to 20 to 30 minutes	Limiting the amount of sleep during naps will help the individual to sleep at night.
• Use of psychostimulants after ruling out other causes	These medications have been used cautiously and demonstrate improved symptoms of fatigue in some patients.
• Treatment for anemia as indicated	Cancer patients' anemia results from the disease itself and treatment. Correcting the anemia may improve the patient's energy level.
• Cognitive behavioral therapy (CBT)	This type of psychotherapy facilitates psychological adjustment to the cancer experience by helping certain patients recognize and change maladaptive thoughts.
• Nutrition consultation	Dietitian can counsel patient and family on how to maximize the patient's intake during treatment for optimal nutritional needs.

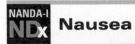

Nausea

Common Related Factors

Treatment effects:
- Side effects of chemotherapy (inability to taste and smell foods, loss of appetite, nausea, vomiting, mucositis, dry mouth, diarrhea)
- Medications (e.g., narcotics, antibiotics, vitamins)

Disease effects:
- Primary malignancy or metastasis
- Tumor waste products

Psychogenic effects:
- Conditioning to adverse stimuli (e.g., anticipatory nausea and vomiting, tension, anxiety, stress)
- Depression

Defining Characteristics

Reports "nausea" or "sick to stomach"
Increased salivation
Increased swallowing
Gagging sensation
Sour taste in mouth
Aversion to food

Common Expected Outcome

Patient maintains optimal nutritional status, as evidenced by caloric intake adequate to meet body requirements, balanced intake and output, weight gain or reduced loss, absence of nausea and vomiting, and good skin turgor.

NOC Outcomes

Nutritional Status: Food and Fluid Intake; Nutritional Status: Comfort Level; Symptom Severity

NIC Interventions

Chemotherapy Management; Nutrition Therapy; Oral Health Maintenance; Medication Administration

Ongoing Assessment

Actions/Interventions	Rationales
■ Obtain history of previous patterns of nausea and vomiting and treatment measures effective in the past.	Chemotherapeutic drugs produce nausea and vomiting as a side effect by stimulating central receptors in the chemoreceptor trigger zone in the medulla or in the cerebral cortex. Some of the drugs stimulate peripheral receptors in the gastrointestinal tract to cause nausea and vomiting. Nausea and vomiting are the most distressing side effects for patients and families and can significantly affect the quality of one's life. . However, newer antiemetic medications have improved this condition for many patients.
■ Assess the patient's description of nausea and vomiting pattern prior to each cycle of chemotherapy.	Patient responses are individualized, depending on type and dosage of chemotherapy. Ongoing assessment is important so that treatment plans can be revised as needed. Assessment data should include the number of episodes of nausea/vomiting, timing of nausea and vomiting, ability to eat after chemo, antiemetics taken, and other related symptoms.

■ = Independent   ▲ = Collaborative

Actions/Interventions

- Evaluate the effectiveness of the antiemetic and comfort measures regimens.
- Weigh the patient daily at the same time and with the same scale. If the patient is at home, stress the importance of maintaining a daily log.
- Encourage the patient to record any food intake using a daily log.

Rationales

Patient response to antiemetic and comfort medications is highly variable and must be explored with each patient.

Consistent weighing is important to ensure accuracy. Without monitoring, the patient may be unaware of small changes in weight due to imbalanced nutrition.

Determination of type, amount, and pattern of food intake (if any) is facilitated by accurate documentation, which provides information as to whether oral intake meets daily nutritional requirements.

Therapeutic Interventions

Actions/Interventions

▲ Administer antiemetics according to protocol.

- Explain that the selection of antiemetic agents should be based upon the emetic risk of the therapy and risk factors in the patient.

▲ Administer antiemetic around-the-clock rather than as needed during periods of high incidence of nausea and vomiting.

- Institute or teach measures to reduce or prevent nausea and vomiting:

Rationales

Newer agents are much more affective in reducing the incidence and severity of emesis. Treatment protocols using a combination of antiemetic medications are most effective in controlling nausea and vomiting associated with chemotherapy. This approach uses drugs that block nausea receptors at different sites and through different mechanisms of action. A typical combination protocol may include administration of a 5HT3 (serotonin) receptor antagonist such as ondansetron and dexamethasone before chemotherapy. For delayed nausea, the protocol may include administration of dexamethasone and metoclopramide. Other classes of drugs used to control nausea and vomiting include phenothiazines, butyrophenones, cannabinoids, and benzodiazepines.

The Oncology Nursing Society provides resources for recommended antiemetic regimen for high, moderately high, low and minimal emetogenic chemotherapy. Administration of optimal antiemetic therapy during every cycle of chemotherapy will reduce development of anticipatory nausea and vomiting.

Effectiveness of antiemetic therapy is increased when adequate plasma levels are maintained.

Behavioral and dietary interventions seem to be most effective in the management of anticipatory nausea and vomiting. This pattern of nausea and vomiting is related to classic conditioning. The patient develops nausea and vomiting in response to stimuli associated with administration of chemotherapeutic drugs. Patients may try a variety of interventions to find those that best control this type of nausea and vomiting before drug administration. Antiemetic medications have been found to be less effective in managing anticipatory nausea and vomiting. However, antianxiety medications such as lorazepam may be effective.

Actions/Interventions

- Small dietary intake before treatment

- Foods with low potential to cause nausea and vomiting (e.g., dry toast, crackers, ginger ale, cola, Popsicles, gelatin, baked or boiled potatoes, fresh or canned fruit)
- Avoidance of spices, gravy, greasy fried foods, and foods with strong odors
- Meals at room temperature. Serve foods cold if odors cause aversions.
- Avoidance of coaxing, bribing, or threatening in relation to intake (help family avoid being "food pushers")
- Sucking on hard candy (e.g., peppermint) while receiving chemotherapeutic drugs with "metallic taste"
- Drinking fluids at a different time than when eating solid snacks or meals
- Minimal physical activity and no sudden rapid movement during times of increased nausea
- Relaxation and distraction techniques; guided imagery

- Antiemetic half an hour before meals as prescribed

- Use of acupressure or acupuncture

- Offering meat dishes in the morning.

Rationales

Eating small amounts reduces gastric overstimulation, thus reducing vomiting risk.
These foods are easily digested and provide a measure of success to augment nutrition.

Fats are difficult to digest and may exacerbate nausea, and stimulate gastric motility.
Hot foods can stimulate peristalsis. The smell of cooking food may aggravate feelings of nausea.
Such behaviors tend to only aggravate the situation.

Hard candies can reduce metallic or bitter taste.

Separating fluids from solids will help not "filling" the stomach quickly. This may help prevent nausea as well.
Activity or sudden movement may potentiate nausea and vomiting.
These techniques especially guided imagery, are useful adjuncts to antiemetic drug therapy. They can be helpful if used before nausea occurs or increases.
Appropriate timing of meds can reduce onset/severity of nausea.
Several small studies report acupressure and acupuncture to be useful measures in reducing nausea/vomiting risk.
Aversions tend to increase during the day: chicken, cheese, eggs, and fish are usually well-tolerated protein sources.

Related Care Plans

■ = Independent   ▲ = Collaborative

Lymphoma: Hodgkin Lymphoma (HL); Non-Hodgkin Lymphoma (NHL)

Lymphoma is a malignant disorder of the lymph nodes, spleen, and other lymphoid tissue. Lymphomas include a number of related diseases with a variety of symptoms, treatment options, and outcomes depending on the lymphocyte type and stage of disease. Lymphomas are classified as either Hodgkin lymphoma or non-Hodgkin lymphoma. A specific etiology has not been identified, although associations with viral disease such as Epstein-Barr and mononucleosis and environmental exposure to toxins have been noted. The Centers for Disease Control and Prevention has included lymphoma in the list of clinical conditions that are part of the case definition for acquired immunodeficiency syndrome (AIDS).

Hodgkin lymphoma is a disorder of the lymph nodes, usually presenting with node enlargement. It is seen more frequently in men than women, first between the ages of 20 and 40, and then again after 55 years of age. Non-Hodgkin lymphoma is a disorder of the lymphocytes that involves many different histological variations. It is seen more frequently in middle-age men.

Depending on the type of lymphoma, therapeutic management may consist of combination chemotherapy, radiation therapy, and/or stem cell transplantation. The prognosis is usually poorer for non-Hodgkin lymphoma because of its later stage at diagnosis.

The goals of nursing care are to provide educational and emotional support and to prevent complications. This care plan addresses ongoing care of a patient in an ambulatory setting receiving maintenance therapy.

NANDA-I NDx Deficient Knowledge

Common Related Factors

New disease/procedure/treatment
Lack of information resources
Complexity of treatment
Misinterpretation of information
Emotional state affecting learning
Lack of recall

Defining Characteristics

Questioning members of health care team
Inaccurate follow-through of instruction
Verbalizing inaccurate information

Common Expected Outcome

Patient verbalizes understanding of diagnosis, treatment strategies, and prognosis.

NOC Outcomes

Knowledge: Disease Process; Knowledge: Treatment Procedures

NIC Interventions

Teaching: Disease Process; Teaching: Procedures/Treatment

Ongoing Assessment

Actions/Interventions	Rationales
■ Assess knowledge of disease, treatment strategies, and prognosis.	Several types of lymphoma occur, each with its own treatment approach and prognosis; this can be confusing.

Therapeutic Interventions

Actions/Interventions	Rationales
■ Describe the function of the lymphatic system and the abnormalities associated with lymphoma.	Most individuals are not familiar with the complexities of the hematological system unless an illness strikes.
■ Clarify the diagnostic process:	
• Peripheral blood analysis	Analysis may reveal a microcytic hypochromic anemia, lymphopenia (neutrophilic leukocytosis), and elevated platelet count.
• Lymph node biopsy	Lymph node biopsy provides tissue for histological examination that is needed in diagnosing cell type and staging the disease. Knowing the stage of the disease determines treatment and aids in estimation of prognosis. Biopsy may be performed either as open biopsy (in operating room) or a closed needle biopsy (at bedside or as outpatient).
• Bone marrow biopsy	Bone marrow biopsy can assist with staging of disease.
• Computed tomography scan/magnetic resonance imaging (MRI)	These scans are used to assess abdominal lymph nodes and liver, spleen, bone, and brain infiltrates.
• X-ray study	X-ray study is used to detect lymphoma in the chest area as well as additional sites of disease.
• Positron emission tomography (PET) scan	PET scan provides information on site of tumor using increased metabolic activity as a marker.
■ Clarify the similarities and differences between Hodgkin lymphoma and non-Hodgkin lymphoma.	Although both have similar presenting symptoms and treatment approaches, significant differences in actual treatment therapies and response to therapy do exist. Non-Hodgkin lymphoma has a poorer prognosis because of its later stage at diagnosis.
• Common presenting symptoms include fever, weight loss, night sweats, pruritus, nontender enlarged lymph nodes, and possibly enlarged spleen and liver.	
■ Discuss common treatment approaches:	
• Radiation therapy	Radiation therapy is indicated for stages 1 and 2 in Hodgkin lymphoma and for localized non-Hodgkin lymphoma.
• Combined chemotherapy	Combined chemotherapy is common for stages 3 and 4 in Hodgkin lymphoma. Chemotherapy is also indicated for generalized non-Hodgkin lymphoma. Many protocols exist depending on the type of lymphoma. NOTE: Older patients have significant problems dealing with the adverse side effects of these aggressive treatments. Initial chemotherapy is performed in the hospital. However, follow-up courses may be administered in an outpatient or sometimes a home setting.
• Biological therapy (immunotherapy)	Investigational and clinical trials for biological therapy include the use of cytokines such as interferon, interleukin, and colony-stimulating factors, and monoclonal antibodies that bind to the lymphoma cells and allow the patient's own immune system to recognize and destroy malignant cells.
• Stem cell transplantation	Transplantation is indicated when patients have not shown remission with radiation and/or chemotherapy or have relapsed after chemotherapy. Autologous (patient is donor) transplantations are most frequently used. Allogenic (matched donor) transplantation is used if the disease has spread to the bone marrow.
• Participating in a clinical trial	Clinical trials may be an option for patients before starting standard treatment or for those nonresponsive to treatment.
■ Explain common complications of the therapy.	Complications include pancytopenia from radiation and chemotherapy (anemia, bleeding, infection); nausea and vomiting from chemotherapy; fatigue and weakness.

■ = Independent   ▲ = Collaborative

Actions/Interventions

- Discuss prognosis.

Rationales

Prognosis depends on type of disease, stage at which diagnosis was made, and response to treatment plan. Generally complete remissions are possible in about 80% of patients with Hodgkin lymphoma. Patients with non-Hodgkin lymphoma usually have a poorer prognosis because of later stage at diagnosis.

NDx Cancer-Related Fatigue

Common Related Factors

Tumor and metastatic disease
Chemotherapy/targeted therapy
Radiation
Pain
Distress (spiritual or emotional)
Anxiety/fear
Malnutrition
Anemia

Defining Characteristics

A sense of physical or emotional tiredness that is not proportional to recent activity or treatment and interferes with the individual's daily functioning.
Inability to restore energy, even after sleep
Verbalization of an overwhelming lack of energy

Common Expected Outcomes

Patient reports reduction in fatigue, as evidenced by reports of increased energy and ability to perform desired activities.
Patient reports use of energy-conservation principles.

NOC Outcomes

Activity Tolerance; Endurance; Energy Conservation; Self-Care: Activities

NIC Interventions

Energy Management; Nutrition Management; Sleep Enhancement; Exercise Promotion

---

Ongoing Assessment

Actions/Interventions

- Assess for fatigue regularly using 0 to 10 scale and defining characteristics.

- Refer to Fatigue (p. 66)

Rationales

Fatigue has become the most common and distressing complaint for cancer patients, especially during treatment. Regular assessment allows the nurse to evaluate the fatigue and response to interventions and to develop and alter the plan accordingly.

Therapeutic Interventions

Actions/Interventions

In addition to the interventions in the Fatigue care plan, consider the following:

- Educate patient regarding these treatments:
  - Assigning priorities to activities to accommodate energy levels

  - Energy-conservation strategies, such as:
    - Sitting to do tasks
    - Pushing rather than pulling
    - Working at an even pace
    - Placing frequently used items within easy reach
    - Using wheeled carts for laundry, shopping, cleaning needs

Rationales

Setting priorities while conserving energy will allow the patient to achieve most desired goals and feel a sense of accomplishment.
Energy-conservation techniques reduce oxygen consumption, allowing more prolonged activity

Actions/Interventions	Rationales
• Limiting naps to 20 to 30 minutes	Limiting the amount of sleep during naps will help the individual to sleep at night.
• Use of psychostimulants after ruling out other causes	These medications have been used cautiously and demonstrate improved symptoms of fatigue in some patients.
• Treatment for anemia as indicated	Cancer patients' anemia results from the disease itself and treatment. Correcting the anemia may improve the patient's energy level.
• Cognitive behavioral therapy	This type of psychotherapy facilitates psychological adjustment to cancer experience by helping certain patients recognize and change maladaptive thoughts.
• Nutrition consultation	Dietitian can counsel patient and family on how to maximize the patient's intake during treatment for optimal nutritional needs.

NANDA-I NDx   Risk for Ineffective Coping

Common Risk Factors

Situational crisis
Inadequate support system
Inadequate coping methods

Common Expected Outcome

Patient demonstrates positive coping strategies, as evidenced by expression of feelings and hopes, realistic goal setting for future, and use of available resources and support systems.

NOC Outcomes
Coping; Social Support; Family Coping
NIC Interventions
Coping Enhancement; Hope Instillation; Grief Work Facilitation; Support System Enhancement

---

Ongoing Assessment

Actions/Interventions	Rationales
■ Assess patient's knowledge of disease and treatment plan.	Because lymphoma is a cancer, the patient may expect to die. Realistic but positive information may be indicated.
■ Assess for coping mechanisms used in previous illnesses or prior hospitalizations.	Successful coping is influenced by previous successes. Patients with a history of maladaptive coping may require additional resources. Likewise, previously successful coping skills may be inadequate in the present situation.
■ Evaluate resources and support systems available to the patient at home and in the community.	Lymphoma treatment may require months and years of ongoing chemotherapy, depending on length of remission. Available support systems may change over time.
■ Assess financial resources required for extensive long-term therapy.	The financial aspects of acute care and long-term follow-up can be overwhelming, especially when the patient is dealing with a new diagnosis.

■ = Independent   ▲ = Collaborative

Hematolymphatic, Immunological and Oncological Care Plans

Therapeutic Interventions

Actions/Interventions	Rationales
■ Establish open lines of communication; establish a working relationship with the patient through continuity of care.	The nurse may be the first person the patient and family turn to as a source of support. An ongoing relationship establishes trust, reduces the feeling of isolation, and may facilitate coping.
■ Provide opportunities for the patient and significant others to openly express feelings, fears, and concerns. Provide hope but avoid false reassurances.	Verbalization of actual or perceived threats can help reduce anxiety and open doors for ongoing communication. An honest relationship facilitates problem solving and successful coping. False reassurances are never helpful to the patient and only serve to relieve the discomfort of care providers.
■ Assist the patient in grieving and working through the losses associated with life-threatening illness, if appropriate.	Grief is a universal experience; people who have successfully undergone grief over a loss can be enormously helpful to others undergoing the same feelings.
■ Assist the patient and significant others in redefining hopes and components of individuality (e.g., roles, values, and attitudes).	Emphasizing the patient's intrinsic worth and viewing the immediate situation as manageable in time may provide support.
■ Introduce new information about disease treatment, as available.	Chemotherapy agents may change. The patient may become a candidate for stem cell transplantation. Clinical trials are also available for these patients.
■ Assist the patient in becoming involved as a comanager of the treatment plan.	This helps the patient regain control over the situation. Many patients become educated about their chemotherapeutic agents and possible side effects.
■ Assist in the development of an alternative support system. Encourage participation in self-help groups as available.	Relationships with persons with common interests and goals can be beneficial. Participation in support groups may allow the individual to realize that others have the same problem, and they may use this as an aid for coping.
■ Describe community resources available to meet unique demands of lymphoma, its treatment, and survival.	It is helpful for patients to have more than one resource for assisting them in this process. Reliable websites may likewise offer information and support.
▲ Refer to a social worker for financial assistance as indicated.	The social worker can assist the patient and family with decisions about finances, living arrangements, wills, advance directives, and power of attorney.

NANDA-I NDx   Risk for Infection

Common Risk Factors

Cancer resulting in altered immunological responses
Immunosuppression secondary to chemotherapy and radiation therapy

Common Expected Outcome

Patient is at reduced risk for local or systemic infection, as evidenced by afebrile state, normal vital signs, chest x-ray film results within normal limits, negative results of blood and surveillance cultures, compliance with preventive measures, and prompt reporting of early signs of infection.

NOC Outcomes
Immune Status; Knowledge: Infection Control; Tissue Integrity: Skin and Mucous Membranes

NIC Interventions
Infection Protection; Teaching: Disease Process; Oral Health Maintenance

Ongoing Assessment

Actions/Interventions	Rationales
■ Auscultate lung fields for crackles, rhonchi, and decreased breath sounds.	Pulmonary infections are common in immunocompromised patients.
■ Observe patient for coughing spells and character of sputum.	Increase in the amount of sputum and changes in color from clear or white to yellow or green may indicate a respiratory infection.
■ Inspect body sites with high infection potential (mouth, throat, axilla, perineum, rectum).	Opportunistic infections of the mucous membrane surfaces of the body are often the first type of infection to develop in the immunocompromised patient.
■ Inspect intravenous central catheter sites for redness, tenderness, pain, and itching.	In the absence of granulocytes, site of infection may develop without characteristic pus formation.
■ Observe for changes in color, character, and frequency of urine and stool.	These observations provide data on possible urinary tract infection or intestinal infection.
■ Monitor temperature as indicated. Report if higher than 38° C (100.4° F).	Fever may be the only sign of infection. Patients need to be instructed to record serial temperatures at home.
▲ Obtain cultures as indicated.	Cultures are required to determine the organism causing the infection and antibiotic sensitivity.

Therapeutic Interventions

Actions/Interventions	Rationales
■ Explain the cause and effects of leukopenia.	Leukopenic cells replace normal cells. Also, chemotherapy causes bone marrow suppression and reduced number of neutrophils needed to fight infection.
■ Instruct the patient to maintain personal hygiene, especially at home: • To bathe with a mild antiseptic soap • To wash hands well before eating and after using bathroom • To wipe perineal area from front to back	Hand washing removes transient and residual bacteria from hands. The perineal area is a source of pathogens and a frequent entry port for microorganisms.
■ Instruct the patient to brush teeth with a soft toothbrush four times a day and as necessary, to remove dentures at night, and to rinse mouth after each emesis or when expectorating phlegm.	Intact oral mucous membranes are the first line of defense in controlling development of oral infections. Periodontal disease is a locus of infection.
■ Teach the patient to inspect the oropharyngeal area daily for white patches in the mouth, coated or encrusted oral ulcerations, swollen and erythematous tongue with white or brown coating, infected throat and pain on swallowing, debris on teeth, ill-fitting dentures, and amount and viscosity of saliva.	The oral cavity and upper respiratory tract are common infection sites in patients with lymphoma and neutropenia. Candidiasis is a common opportunistic infection of the oral and esophageal mucous membranes.
■ Teach the patient to avoid mouthwashes that contain alcohol and to avoid irritating foods and acidic drinks.	Alcohol has a drying effect on mucous membranes.
■ Teach the patient to use prescribed topical medications (e.g., nystatin [Nilstat] and lidocaine [Xylocaine]).	These agents may require specific instructions.
■ Instruct the patient and caregiver to maintain strict aseptic technique when changing dressings and to avoid wetting central catheter dressings.	These measures help prevent bacterial growth.
■ Instruct the patient to observe for fever spikes and flulike symptoms (e.g., malaise, weakness, myalgia) and to notify the nurse or physician if they occur.	Early assessment facilitates prompt treatment.

■ = Independent   ▲ = Collaborative

Actions/Interventions

- Instruct the patient and caregiver regarding the importance of eliminating potential sources of infection at home (especially when neutrophil counts are low):
  - Avoid contact with visitors or family, especially children with colds or infections and/or who attend daycare, preschool, or elementary school.
  - Avoid shared drinking and eating utensils.
  - Avoid contact with cat litter boxes, fish tanks, and human or animal excreta.
  - Avoid swimming in private or public pools.
  - Restrict contact with live plants.
- Instruct the patient regarding "protective isolation" if laboratory results indicate neutropenia (absolute neutrophil count [ANC] less than 500 to 1000/mm^3).
  - Implement thorough hand washing for staff and visitors before physical contact with the patient.

- Instruct the patient to take prescribed antibiotic, antifungal, or antiviral drugs on time.
- ▲ Refer the patient to a dietitian for instructions on maintenance of a well-balanced diet.

Rationales

Patients must understand strategies/measures by which they can protect themselves during times of compromised defense. Animal excreta, soil, and people with known infections are sources of opportunistic infection for the immunocompromised patient.

Institutional protocols may vary.

Hand washing removes transient and resident bacteria from hands, thus minimizing or preventing transmission to the patient.

A regular schedule is needed to maintain therapeutic drug levels.

A specialist may provide additional help. This diet is for maintenance of optimal health status, which promotes improvement of host resistance and bone marrow recovery.

NANDA-I NDx **Risk for Bleeding**

Common Risk Factor
Bone marrow depression secondary to chemotherapy or radiation therapy

Common Expected Outcome
Patient's risk for bleeding is reduced, as evidenced by platelet count within acceptable limits, compliance with preventive measures, and prompt reporting of early signs and symptoms.

NOC Outcomes
Blood Coagulation; Knowledge: Disease Process
NIC Interventions
Bleeding Precautions; Teaching: Disease Process

Ongoing Assessment

Actions/Interventions

▲ Monitor platelet count.

Rationales

Risk for bleeding increases as platelet count drops:
- Mild thrombocytopenia: platelets 50,000 to 100,000/mm^3
- Moderate risk: platelets 20,000 to 50,000/mm^3
- Severe: platelets 20,000/mm^3 or less
- Transfusion threshold: platelet count less than 10,000/mm^3 or signs of active bleeding

Actions/Interventions

- Assess for signs and symptoms of bleeding. These may include petechiae and bruising, hemoptysis, epistaxis, bleeding in oral mucosa, hematemesis, hematochezia, melena, vaginal bleeding, dizziness, orthostatic changes, decreased blood pressure (BP), headaches, changes in mental and visual acuity, and increased pulse rate.
- Note bleeding from any recent puncture site (e.g., venipuncture, bone marrow aspiration site).

Rationales

Early assessment facilitates prompt treatment and reduced risk for complications.

Prolonged oozing from puncture sites may be the first sign of bleeding problems.

Therapeutic Interventions

Actions/Interventions

- Explain to the patient and significant others the symptoms of thrombocytopenia and the functions of platelets:
  - Normal range of platelet count
  - Effects of thrombocytopenia
  - Rationale of bleeding precautions
- Instruct the patient in precautionary measures. Initiate bleeding precautions for platelet count less than 50,000/mm³:
  - Use soft toothbrush and nonabrasive toothpaste.
  - Inspect gums for oozing.
  - Avoid use of toothpicks and dental floss.
  - Avoid rectal suppositories, thermometers, enemas, vaginal douches, and tampons.
  - Avoid aspirin or aspirin-containing products, nonsteroidal antiinflammatory drugs (NSAIDs), and anticoagulants.
  - Avoid straining with bowel movements, forceful nose blowing, coughing, or sneezing.
  - Count used sanitary pads during menstruation. Report menstrual cycle changes.
  - Avoid sharp objects such as scissors and knives. Use electric razor for shaving (not razor blades).

  - Lubricate nostrils with saline solution drops as necessary, and lips with petroleum jelly as needed.
  - Practice gentle sex; use water-based lubricant before sexual intercourse.
  - Protect self from injury and trauma (e.g., falls, bumps, strenuous exercise, contact sports).

In the health care setting:
- Avoid finger-sticks if possible. Coordinate laboratory work so all tests are done at one time.
- Avoid intramuscular and subcutaneous injections. If necessary, use small-bore needles for injections and apply ice to the injection site for 5 minutes. Observe the site for oozing.
- Apply pressure, dressing, or sandbag to the bone marrow aspiration site.

- Give the patient and family at least two telephone numbers to call in case of bleeding.
- ▲ Apply ice or topical thrombin promptly as prescribed for bleeding mucous membranes.
- Instruct the patient to take antacids as prescribed when taking steroids, NSAIDs, and/or aspirin.

Rationales

Most individuals are not familiar with the complexities of the hematological system. A successful plan requires the knowledge and cooperation of the patient and family members.

Understanding of precautionary measures reduces risk for bleeding. At this level, spontaneous bleeding can occur.
This method reduces risk for bleeding.
Oozing can be an early sign of bleeding.
These items stimulate bleeding.
This measure reduces mucosal trauma.

These medications interfere with platelet function.

This measure reduces the risk for bleeding.

This measure provides data on bleeding status.

It is important to prevent cuts, which would not only bleed but also become portals of entry for microorganisms, leading to infection in the presence of neutropenia.
Lubrication prevents drying and cracking.

These measures prevent mucosal trauma.

Patient safety is a priority.

This precaution reduces bleeding risk.

These measures reduce bleeding potential at the injection site.

This procedure prevents excessive pressure when compressing soft tissues and deeper structures of the arm, because this may lead to bruising or hematomas.
Prearranged contact information facilitates early treatment.

Thrombin promotes clot formation.

Antacids reduce gastric irritation.

■ = Independent   ▲ = Collaborative

Actions/Interventions

■ Discuss the possibility of platelet transfusions. Teach the patient the purpose and possible reactions to transfusions.

▲ Ensure availability and readiness of platelets for transfusion.

Rationales

Knowledge reduces anxiety. Transfusions may be needed to maintain adequate platelet count to prevent spontaneous or excessive bleeding.

It is important to have platelets available when needed to prevent spontaneous or excessive bleeding (generally for platelet count less than 20,000/mm³, or according to institutional protocol).

NANDA-I NDx Nausea

Common Related Factors

Treatment effects:
- Side effects of chemotherapy (inability to taste and smell foods, loss of appetite, nausea, vomiting, mucositis, dry mouth, diarrhea)
- Medications (e.g., narcotics, antibiotics, vitamins)

Disease effects:
- Primary malignancy or metastasis
- Tumor waste products

Psychogenic effects:
- Conditioning to adverse stimuli (e.g., anticipatory nausea and vomiting, tension, anxiety, stress)
- Depression

Defining Characteristics

Reports "nausea" or "sick to stomach"
Increased salivation
Increased swallowing
Gagging sensation
Sour taste in mouth
Aversion to food

Common Expected Outcome

Patient reports diminished severity or elimination of nausea.

NOC Outcomes

Nutritional Status: Food and Fluid Intake; Comfort Level; Symptom Severity

NIC Interventions

Chemotherapy Management; Nutrition Therapy; Oral Health Maintenance; Medication Administration

Ongoing Assessment

Actions/Interventions

■ Obtain history of previous patterns of nausea and vomiting and treatment measures effective in the past.

Rationales

Chemotherapeutic drugs produce nausea and vomiting as a side effect by stimulating central receptors in the chemoreceptor trigger zone in the medulla or in the cerebral cortex. Some of the drugs stimulate peripheral receptors in the gastrointestinal tract to cause nausea and vomiting. Nausea and vomiting are the most distressing side effects for patients and families. However, newer antiemetic medications have improved this condition for many patients. Nausea and vomiting are the most distressing side effects for patients and families and can significantly affect the quality of one's life.

Actions/Interventions

■ Assess the patient's description of nausea and vomiting pattern prior to each cycle of chemotherapy.

■ Evaluate the effectiveness of the antiemetic and comfort measure regimens.

■ Observe the patient for potential complications of prolonged nausea and vomiting.

■ Weigh the patient daily at the same time and with the same scale. If the patient is at home, stress the importance of maintaining a daily log.

■ Encourage the patient to record any food intake using a daily log.

Rationales

Patient responses are individualized, depending on type and dosage of chemotherapy. Ongoing assessment is important so that treatment plans can be revised as needed. Assessment data should include the number of episodes of nausea/vomiting after therapy; timing of nausea/vomiting; ability to eat after therapy; antiemetics taken; and other related symptoms. Nausea and vomiting may be acute, delayed, and for some patients even before ("anticipatory") the chemotherapy treatment.

Patient response to antiemetic and comfort medications is highly variable and must be explored with each patient. Anticipatory nausea can be difficult to overcome.

Nausea and vomiting can alter a patient's hydration status because of fluid loss and effect electrolyte imbalance (hypokalemia; decreased sodium and chloride). Persistent vomiting and reduced nutritional intake can result in weight loss, decreased activity level and lethargy.

Consistent weighing is important to ensure accuracy. Without monitoring, the patient may be unaware of small changes in weight.

Determination of type, amount, and pattern of food intake (if any) is facilitated by accurate documentation, which provides information as to whether oral intake meets daily nutritional requirements.

Therapeutic Interventions

Actions/Interventions

▲ Administer antiemetics according to protocol.

■ Explain that the selection of antiemetic agents should be based upon the emetic risk of the therapy and risk factors in the patient.

▲ Administer antiemetic around-the-clock rather than as needed during periods of high incidence of nausea and vomiting.

Rationales

Newer agents are much more effective in reducing the incidence and severity of emesis. Treatment protocols using a combination of antiemetic medications are most effective in controlling nausea and vomiting associated with chemotherapy. This approach uses drugs that block nausea receptors at different sites and through different mechanisms of action. Antiemetic regimens are more effective in treating vomiting than nausea. A typical combination protocol may include administration of a 5HT3 (serotonin) receptor antagonist such as ondansetron and dexamethasone before chemotherapy. For delayed nausea, the protocol may include administration of dexamethasone and metoclopramide. Other classes of drugs used to control nausea and vomiting include phenothiazines, butyrophenones, cannabinoids, and benzodiazepines.

The Oncology Nursing Society provides resources for recommended antiemetic regimens for high, moderately high, low and minimal emetogenic chemotherapy. Administration of optimal antiemetic therapy during every cycle of chemotherapy will reduce development of anticipatory nausea and vomiting.

Effectiveness of antiemetic therapy is increased when adequate plasma levels are maintained.

■ = Independent   ▲ = Collaborative

Actions/Interventions

■ Institute or teach measures to reduce or prevent nausea and vomiting:

- Small dietary intake before treatment

- Foods with low potential to cause nausea and vomiting (e.g., dry toast, crackers, ginger ale, cola, Popsicles, gelatin, baked or boiled potatoes, fresh or canned fruit, bland foods).
- Avoidance of spices, gravy, greasy fried foods, and foods with strong odors
- Meals at room temperature. Serve foods cold if odors cause aversions.
- Avoidance of coaxing, bribing, or threatening in relation to intake (help family avoid being "food pushers")
- Sucking on hard candy (e.g., peppermint) while receiving chemotherapeutic drugs with "metallic taste"
- Drinking fluids at a different time than when eating solid snacks or meals
- Minimal physical activity and no sudden rapid movement during times of increased nausea
- Relaxation and distraction techniques; guided imagery

- Antiemetic half an hour before meals as prescribed

- Use of acupuncture or acupressure.

- Offering meat dishes in the morning.

Rationales

Behavioral and dietary interventions seem to be most effective in the management of anticipatory nausea and vomiting. This pattern of nausea and vomiting is related to classical conditioning. The patient develops nausea and vomiting in response to stimuli associated with administration of chemotherapeutic drugs. Patients may try a variety of interventions to find those that best control this type of nausea and vomiting before drug administration. Antiemetic medications have been found to be less effective in the management of anticipatory nausea and vomiting. However, antianxiety medications such as lorazepam may be effective.

Eating small amounts reduces gastric overstimulation, thus reducing vomiting risk

These foods are easily digested and provide a measure of success to augment nutrition.

Fats are difficult to digest and may exacerbate nausea and can stimulate gastric motility.

Hot foods can stimulate peristalsis. The smell of cooking foods may aggravate feelings of nausea.

Such behaviors tend to only aggravate the situation.

Hard candies can reduce metallic or bitter taste.

Separating fluids from solids will help not "filling" the stomach quickly. This may help prevent nausea as well.

Activity or sudden movement may potentiate nausea and vomiting.

These techniques, especially guided imagery, are useful adjuncts to antiemetic drug therapy. They can be helpful if used before nausea occurs or increases.

Antiemetics relieve nausea and vomiting. Appropriate timing of meds can reduce onset/severity of nausea.

Several small studies report acupuncture and acupressure to be useful measures in reducing nausea/vomiting risk.

Aversions tend to increase during the day: chicken, cheese, eggs, and fish are usually well-tolerated protein sources.

Related Care Plans

Cancer chemotherapy, p. 681
Cancer radiation therapy, p. 694
Caregiver role strain, p. 36
Deficient fluid volume, p. 72
Disturbed body image, p. 24
Fear, p. 69
Hematopoietic stem cell transplantation, p. 703

Multiple Myeloma

Plasmacytoma; Myelomatosis; Plasma Cell Myeloma

Multiple myeloma is the second most common hematological malignancy. It is a plasma B-cell malignancy that is characterized by the overproduction of immunoglobulins. This pathophysiology results in disruption of normal red blood cells, leukocytes, and platelets, resulting in anemia, infection, and bleeding problems. The cause of multiple myeloma is unknown with no clear risk factors identified beyond age. There are no specific symptoms with multiple myeloma. Clinically, it may present itself as destruction of bone, infiltration of bone marrow, the presence of immunoglobulins in the urine or serum, recurrent infections, pain, fatigue, or symptoms of renal failure. This disease affects older adults, with a median age at diagnosis of 62 years. It is more common in African Americans than in whites, and in men than in women.

NANDA-I NDx Deficient Knowledge

Common Related Factors

New diagnosis
Unfamiliarity with disease process, treatment, and discharge and follow-up care
Complexity of treatment
Misinterpretation of information
Emotional state affecting learning
Unfamiliarity with information resources

Defining Characteristics

Questions to health care team
Verbalizing inaccurate information

Common Expected Outcome

Patient and significant others verbalize understanding of diagnosis and treatment plan, side effects of medications, and follow-up care.

NOC Outcomes

Knowledge: Disease Process; Knowledge: Treatment Procedures

NIC Interventions

Teaching: Disease Process; Support System Enhancement

Ongoing Assessment

Actions/Interventions	Rationales
■ Assess knowledge of disease, treatment plan, and prognosis.	This type of cancer is less publicized in the media than lung, breast, and colon cancers, with which patients may be quite familiar.

Therapeutic Interventions

Actions/Interventions	Rationales
■ Provide information on the following:	
• Nature of disease	Malignant plasma cells infiltrate the bone marrow and disrupt blood cells.
• Diagnosis	Diagnosis of multiple myeloma requires consideration of a number of factors: physical examination, laboratory tests, and symptoms

■ = Independent   ▲ = Collaborative

Actions/Interventions	Rationales
• Bone marrow analysis	Large numbers of immature plasma cells are noted with this diagnosis.
• Computed tomography bone scans and skeletal survey	This test shows degree of demineralization and osteoporosis.
• Laboratory studies (chemistry, complete blood count, serum protein electrophoresis, C-reactive protein [CRP], monoclonal immunoglobulin levels)	An abnormal globulin (Bence Jones protein) is seen in serum and urine; increased serum calcium is noted. Because of the increased number of plasma cells producing immuno-globulins, plasma electrophoresis is performed to quanti-tate amounts.
• Twenty-four–hour urine protein and urine protein electrophoresis	These tests show the presence of myeloma protein in the urine and help stage the disease.
• Treatment plan—medical treatment of signs and symp-toms: calcitonin to reduce hypercalcemia; alkylating chemotherapeutic agents; newer therapies such as pro-teasome inhibitors and thalidomide; corticosteroids; high-dose chemotherapy; palliative radiation therapy to treat bone pain; or stem cell transplantation	Treatment is focused on managing both disease and its symp-toms. Many combinations are available depending on type of myeloma and stage of disease.
• Pain management strategies	Analgesic combination is often required for relief.
• Diet and fluid therapy	Therapy is required to prevent or treat hypercalcemia, hyper-uricemia, and renal impairment.
• Importance of mobility	Weight bearing prevents further bone demineralization.
• Safety precautions	Great care must be taken to prevent falls and pathological fractures in this high-risk population.
■ Refer to the U.S. Department of Health and Human Ser-vices (for information on multiple myeloma) and the American Cancer Society.	New treatments continue to be studied.
■ Involve the family and caregivers so they can effectively provide support in the home environment.	Because more patients are older, a variety of support services may be required.

NANDA-I NDx Acute Pain

Common Related Factors

Pain resulting from medical problem (invasion of marrow and bone by plasma cells)
Pathological fractures

Defining Characteristics

Patient reports pain:
- Constant, severe bone pain on movement
- Low back pain
- Abdominal pain

Swelling, tenderness
Guarding behavior
Relief or distraction behavior:
- Moaning, crying
- Pacing, restlessness, irritability

Common Expected Outcomes

Patient reports satisfactory pain control at a level less than 3 to 4 on a 0 to 10 rating scale.
Patient uses pharmacological and nonpharmacological pain relief measures.
Patient exhibits increased comfort such as baseline levels for BP, pulse, respirations, and relaxed muscle tone or body posture.

NOC Outcomes

Pain Control; Comfort Status; Medication Response

NIC Interventions

Pain Management; Analgesic Administration; Distraction

Ongoing Assessment

Actions/Interventions	Rationales
■ Assess pain characteristics.	Assessment of the pain experience is the first step in planning pain management strategies. Skeletal pain, especially in the lower back and ribs, occurs most commonly and is often the presenting symptom.
■ Assess effectiveness of relief measures.	It is important to help patients express as factually as possible the effect of pain relief measures. During terminal stages, pain management is extremely challenging.

Therapeutic Interventions

Actions/Interventions	Rationales
▲ Provide analgesics in dosage, route, and frequency best suited to the individual patient. Consider around-the-clock schedule, continuous infusion, fentanyl (Duragesic) patch, or patient-controlled analgesia. Consider combination analgesics.	The patient with multiple myeloma responds to a combination of interventions for effective pain management. Drug therapy that combines nonsteroidal antiinflammatory drugs with low doses of opioid analgesics is often more effective in decreasing bone pain.
■ Instruct the patient to take analgesics early and regularly to prevent severe pain. Schedule pain-inducing procedures and activities during peak analgesic effect.	Timing of administration is crucial to prevent peak pain periods. Unless contraindicated, all patients with acute pain should receive around-the-clock analgesics. Each patient must be evaluated individually as to the optimal regimen.
■ Suggest nonpharmacological measures for comfort: decreased noise and activity, relaxation and distraction techniques, good body alignment, additional rest and sleep periods, and ambulation unless contraindicated (e.g., because of spinal lesions).	Patients may not be aware of the effectiveness of nonpharmacological therapies. A trial-and-error period may be required to match therapy to patient preference. Immobilization of painful areas with braces and splints may enhance pain relief.
▲ Notify the physician if pain medications are ineffective.	Pain service may need to be consulted. Radiation therapy may be required to decrease the size of lesions causing pain.

NANDA-I NDx **Impaired Physical Mobility**

Common Related Factors

Bone weakness and osteoporosis
Generalized weakness caused by chemotherapy
Pain or discomfort
Depression
Deconditioning
Decreased endurance
Decreased muscle strength or control
Restricted movement and impaired coordination

Defining Characteristics

Inability to move purposefully within physical environment
Decrease in activities of daily living (ADLs)
Reluctance to attempt movement
Limited range of motion (ROM)

Common Expected Outcomes

Patient performs physical activity independently or within limits of disease.
Patient demonstrates adaptive techniques that promote ambulation and transfer.

NOC Outcomes

Ambulation; Mobility Level

NIC Interventions

Exercise Therapy: Joint Mobility; Exercise Therapy: Muscle Control; Exercise Therapy: Ambulation

---

■ = Independent   ▲ = Collaborative

Ongoing Assessment

Actions/Interventions	**Rationales**
■ Assess ability to carry out ADLs effectively and safely.	Osteoporosis, progressive weakness, skeletal muscle pain, and malaise are common symptoms of this disease and reduce mobility.
■ Assess ability to perform ROM and the level of muscle strength.	Assessment provides data on extent of physical problems. Decreases in ROM and muscle strength occur as a result of decreased mobility.

Therapeutic Interventions

Actions/Interventions	**Rationales**
■ Instruct regarding the importance of ambulation.	Weight bearing stimulates reabsorption and helps prevent further bone demineralization.
■ Stress the importance of maintaining an uncluttered environment.	This prevents falls and bumping into objects. Bone weakening can readily result in fractures.
■ Encourage the patient to perform ROM exercises.	Exercises promote increased venous return, prevent stiffness, and maintain muscle strength and endurance. To be most effective, all joints should be exercised to prevent contractures.
■ Instruct the patient to change position every 1 to 2 hours and to get up in a chair as tolerated.	Position changes optimize circulation to all tissues and relieve pressure. Activity and movement reduce risk for pneumonia, a complication of immobility, especially in older patients.
■ Encourage caregivers to assist the patient with ADLs as indicated.	Help may be required for safety and comfort, but it needs to be balanced with not making the patient unnecessarily dependent.
■ Provide assistive devices (e.g., walker, cane, back brace) as needed.	These devices assist the patient with mobility and enhance patient safety.
■ Teach energy-saving techniques, and stress the importance of rest periods after ambulation.	Rest periods are necessary to conserve energy. The patient must learn to respect the limits of his or her restrictions.

 NANDA-I NDx **Risk for Impaired Urinary Elimination**

Common Risk Factors

Immunoglobulin precipitates
Hypercalcemia, hypercalciuria
Hyperuricemia
Pyelonephritis
Myeloma kidney/renal failure
Renal vein thrombosis
Spinal cord compression

Common Expected Outcome

Patient maintains optimal renal function, as evidenced by serum and urine laboratory values within normal limits, balanced intake and output, and normal blood pressure.

NOC Outcome
Electrolyte and Acid-Base Balance
NIC Interventions
Electrolyte Management: Hypercalcemia; Fluid Management

Ongoing Assessment

Actions/Interventions	Rationales
▲ Monitor serum laboratory values.	Hypercalcemia and increased uric acid levels occur from bone destruction. Crystallization leads to renal impairment as seen by increased blood urea nitrogen and creatinine levels.
■ Assess for signs of hypercalcemia: nausea, vomiting, anorexia, confusion, weakness, constipation, ileus, or abdominal pain.	Gastrointestinal and neurological changes are common manifestations.
■ Monitor for signs of decreased urine output related to impaired renal function.	Hyperuricemia may cause renal tubular obstruction and interstitial nephritis from uric acid buildup.
■ Assess for signs of fluid overload: dyspnea, tachycardia, crackles, distended neck veins, and peripheral edema.	Hydration is used to counterbalance effects of calcium and protein buildup. Overhydration needs to be prevented.
■ Monitor urine for specific gravity, pH, color, odor, and blood.	These tests provide data on fluid balance, as well as evidence of bleeding.
■ Palpate abdomen for bladder distention.	Bladder distention may indicate spinal cord compression from bone damage.

Therapeutic Interventions

Actions/Interventions	Rationales
■ Promote calcium excretion; prevent dehydration.	The effects of hypercalcemia are reduced when urine output is maintained at a level of 1.5 to 2 liters per 24 hours.
▲ If hypercalcemia is present, increase fluids to 2500 to 3000 mL/day as prescribed.	Hydration dilutes calcium and prevents renal tubular obstruction from protein buildup.
▲ Provide low-calcium, low-purine diet, if prescribed.	Hypercalcemia is a clinical manifestation of multiple myeloma.
▲ Administer medications as ordered: Didronel, Aredia, Mithracin, calcitonin, Ganite.	These may be used for hypercalcemia to inhibit resorption of bone. NOTE: Some arc given intravenously and require aggressive intravenous hydration with 0.9% normal saline; allopurinol is given for hyperuricemia; oral phosphates are given for hypophosphatemia.
■ If the patient is confused secondary to increased calcium, provide a safe environment.	Safety is a priority.
▲ Prepare for dialysis or plasmapheresis for ongoing renal problems.	These therapies may be indicated to prevent or treat impending renal failure.

Ineffective Protection

Common Related Factors	Defining Characteristics
Bone marrow depression or failure	Bleeding
Replacement or invasion of bone marrow by neoplastic plasma cells	Thrombocytopenia
Decrease in synthesis of immunoglobulin by plasma cells secondary to decrease in normal circulating antibodies	Anemia
Decreased autoimmune response	Infection
Chemotherapy	
Bone marrow transplantation	

■ = Independent   ▲ = Collaborative

Common Expected Outcomes

Patient maintains hemoglobin (Hgb), hematocrit (Hct), and platelets within normal limits.

Patient's risk for infection is reduced or prevented, as evidenced by normal temperature and absence of active infection.

NOC Outcomes
Immune Status; Blood Coagulation; Infection Status

NIC Interventions
Chemotherapy Management; Bleeding Precautions; Infection Protection

Ongoing Assessment

Actions/Interventions	Rationales
▲ Monitor Hgb, Hct, red blood cells, and platelet count.	Impaired bone marrow function caused by infiltration by plasma cells can predispose the patient to bleeding.
■ If on chemotherapy, evaluate regimens for potential myelosuppression.	Chemotherapy may aggravate an already existing problem.
■ If the patient is a candidate for stem cell transplant, monitor closely for signs of anemia, bleeding, and infection.	Pretreatment with high-dose chemotherapy to eradicate disease may cause significant problems.
■ Observe for signs and symptoms of bleeding.	Abnormal platelet production increases risk for bleeding.
■ Monitor for signs of infection.	Infection is a frequent complication secondary to deficient antibody production and reduced granulocytes from bone marrow depression.
■ Observe for coughing (productive and nonproductive) and changes in color and odor of sputum.	Bronchopneumonia is a common complication, especially in immunocompromised patients.
■ Review medications.	The patient taking steroids may not have overt infection symptoms.
▲ Obtain urine, sputum, and blood for culture and sensitivity testing and x-ray study if temperature exceeds 37.7° C (100° F).	Culture and sensitivity results guide antibiotic therapy.

Therapeutic Interventions

Actions/Interventions	Rationales
■ Instruct the patient to avoid unnecessary trauma.	Platelet abnormalities increase risk for bleeding.
▲ Avoid unnecessary intravenous or intramuscular (IM) injections; if necessary, use smallest needle possible; apply direct pressure for 3 to 5 minutes after IM injection, venipuncture, and bone marrow aspiration.	This measure reduces the potential for bleeding from injection sites.
■ Instruct the patient to: • Prevent constipation by increasing oral fluid, increasing fiber intake, and using stool softeners, as prescribed. • Use soft toothbrushes. • Use electric razor, not blades. • Avoid rectal temperatures and enemas.	Precautions reduce risk for trauma. Straining causes breakage of small blood vessels around the anus. Rectal procedures can traumatize the intestinal mucosa.
■ Instruct the patient to avoid aspirin and aspirin-containing compounds.	These drugs interfere with hemostatic platelet function.
▲ Administer hormones (steroids and androgens) and erythropoietin agents as ordered (e.g., epoetin alfa).	These agents stimulate red blood cell production.
▲ Consider platelet and packed red blood cell transfusion for platelet count below 20,000/mm³, Hgb below 10 g/dL, or Hct below 30%.	Replacement therapy is indicated to correct deficiencies.
■ Discourage exposure to visitors and friends with current or recent infection (e.g., a family member with an upper respiratory infection should wear a mask).	Multiple myeloma weakens the immune system.

Actions/Interventions

▲ If granulocyte counts are low, institute low-bacteria, no-fresh-fruit diet. Avoid contact with living plants.

▲ Maintain normal or near-normal body temperature with medications as prescribed, tepid bath, cooling blanket, and ice packs.

Rationales

These measures reduce exposure to microbes in food and the environment, which could colonize and increase risk for infection.

Normothermia prevents stress on the body and promotes comfort.

Related Care Plans

Grieving, p. 82
Cancer chemotherapy, p. 681
Ineffective coping, p. 49
Neutropenia, p. 753
Risk for falls, p. 60

Neutropenia

Granulocytopenia

Neutropenia is a deficiency in granulocytes, a type of white blood cell (WBC). There are three types of granulocytes: basophils, eosinophils, and neutrophils. Neutropenia and its complications center around the neutrophilic granulocyte. Neutropenia is a below-normal number of circulating neutrophils that may result in overwhelming, potentially life-threatening infection. Neutrophils constitute 45% to 75% of all WBCs. Their primary function is phagocytosis, the digestion and subsequent destruction of microorganisms; as such, they are one of the body's most powerful first lines of defense against infection. The chance of developing a serious infection is related not only to the absolute level of circulating neutrophils but also to the length of time the patient is neutropenic. Prolonged duration predisposes the patient to a higher risk for infection. Neutropenia not only predisposes one to infection but also causes it to be more severe when an infection occurs. Neutropenia is usually associated with another medical condition being treated. It can be acute or chronic. Primary diagnosis is by complete blood cell count and bone marrow aspiration. Treatment depends on cause and severity. This care plan focuses on outpatient management.

Risk for Infection

Common Risk Factors

Neutropenia, secondary to:
- Cancer or similar diseases that destroy bone marrow
- Radiation therapy that damages bone marrow
- Chemotherapy that damages bone marrow
- Hypersplenism that destroys blood cells
- Congenital bone marrow depression or failure
- Autoimmune disorders that destroy neutrophils
- Overwhelming infections that destroy neutrophils
- Drugs that impair bone marrow production

■ = Independent   ▲ = Collaborative

Common Expected Outcome

Patient is at reduced risk for local or systemic infection, as evidenced by normal temperature and vital signs, chest x-ray film results within normal limits, negative results of blood and surveillance cultures, compliance with preventive measures, and prompt reporting of early signs of infection.

NOC Outcomes
Infection Status; Risk Control
NIC Interventions
Infection Protection; Infection Control; Self-Care Assistance; Home Maintenance Assistance; Support System Enhancement

Ongoing Assessment

Actions/Interventions	Rationales
▲ Monitor WBC with differential count (especially neutrophils and bands).	This is used to determine relative risk for bacterial infections associated with absolute neutrophil count (ANC). • Neutropenia: ANC less than 1500 cells/mm³ • Mild neutropenia: 1000 to 1500 cells/mm³ • Moderate neutropenia: 500 to 999 cells/mm³ • Severe neutropenia: less than 500 cells/mm³ The ANC can be calculated by using the following formula:

$$ANC = Total\ WBC \times \frac{\%\ Neutrophils}{100}$$
$$or$$
$$ANC = Total\ WBC \times \frac{(\%\ Segs + Bands)}{100}$$

Actions/Interventions	Rationales
■ Identify sources of low WBC count.	Several cytotoxic and immunosuppressive medications and therapies can potentially cause neutropenia (e.g., Tegretol, propylthiouracil, methimazole, Bactrim, Indocin, gold injections for rheumatoid arthritis, neoplastic agents).
■ Inspect body sites with high potential for infection (e.g., orifices, catheter sites, skin folds).	These are frequent sites for infection. Patients with neutropenia do not have the ability to fight infections.
■ Note abnormalities in color and character of sputum, urine, and stool that might indicate presence of infection.	Early detection facilitates prompt intervention for what could be a life-threatening infection.
■ Monitor for increased temperature, tachycardia, tachypnea, and hypotension.	Signs and symptoms are often subtle, with fever being the predominant warning sign.
■ Assess for local or systemic infection signs and symptoms (e.g., fever, chills, diaphoresis, local redness, warmth, pain, tenderness, excessive malaise, sore throat, dysphagia, retrosternal burning, cellulitis).	Fever and chills may be the initial presentation of infection because in the absence of granulocytes, locus of infection may develop without characteristic inflammation or pus formation. Lack of physical signs and symptoms does not exclude the possibility of infection.
■ Identify medication that the patient may have taken that would mask infection signs and symptoms (e.g., steroids, antipyretics).	Knowledge may lead to more aggressive assessments.
▲ Send and evaluate cultures as prescribed for temperature higher than 38.5° C (101.3° F).	These are required to determine the organism causing the infection and antibiotic sensitivity. In severely low counts, antibiotics are started before source of infection is known.

Therapeutic Interventions

Actions/Interventions	Rationales
■ Wash hands thoroughly with antimicrobial cleanser before physical contact with the patient.	Meticulous hand washing is a priority both in the hospital and in the home or ambulatory care setting. Hand washing removes transient and residual bacteria from hands and prevents transmission to the high-risk patient. Because microorganisms can also be transmitted from one site of infection to other portals of entry, thorough hand washing is also important between patient care activities (e.g., central line dressing change, mouth care, perineal care).
■ Encourage daily shower. Explain the need for perineal care (with soap and water) after urination and defecation.	The perineal area is a source of many pathogens and frequent portal of entry for microorganisms.
■ Apply lotion to body after bath and as needed.	The skin and mucous membranes are the first line of defense for the body; when this barrier is weakened or interrupted (e.g., dryness, cracking, abrasions), the site becomes a potential portal of entry for microorganisms and a source of infection.
■ Encourage meticulous oral hygiene before and after each meal and at bedtime.	Oral hygiene is important in prevention of periodontal disease as a locus of infection.
■ Encourage oral fluids.	Fluids assist in meeting hydration requirements (particularly during fever episodes).
■ Initiate low-bacterial diet (e.g., no fresh fruits or vegetables, only well-cooked foods).	This diet reduces the microbial level in foods, which could colonize and infect the gastrointestinal tract.
▲ Assist the patient in selection of high-protein, high-vitamin, high-calorie diet (refer to dietitian as needed).	This diet is for maintenance of optimal health status, which promotes improvement of host resistance and provides nutrients necessary to meet energy demands for bone marrow recovery and tissue repair.
▲ Administer stool softeners and high-fiber foods.	Stool softeners prevent constipation, which could traumatize the intestinal mucosa and increase the risk for perirectal abscess or fistula formation.
■ Avoid rectal temperatures, suppositories, and enemas.	These can traumatize the intestinal mucosa.
■ Encourage women to use sanitary napkins instead of tampons.	Napkins avoid trauma to vaginal mucosa.
■ Use sterile technique with dressing changes and catheter care.	This technique also applies to home health nurses and caregivers.
▲ Observe neutropenic protocol.	The neutropenic protocol protects the patient from exposure to environmental contagions.
■ Restrict contact with live plants.	Plants could harbor infective organisms.
■ Limit visitors. Discourage anyone with a current or recent infection from visiting either in the hospital or the home. Avoid contact with children of school age.	People with known infections are sources of opportunistic infections for the immunocompromised patient. Children are commonly exposed to sick playmates.
■ If hospitalized, avoid unnecessary invasive procedures. Limit intramuscular and subcutaneous injections.	This precaution minimizes risk for infection.
■ Initiate measures for fever control (e.g., cool sponge bath, cooling blanket, light covers, antipyretics).	Such measures promote comfort.
▲ Initiate intravenous broad-spectrum antibiotic therapy as prescribed, followed by culture-specific antibiotics.	Broad-spectrum therapy prevents early dissemination of suspected infection. Once the infection-causing organism is determined, antimicrobial therapy may be adjusted to the type of organism and infection and to the clinical response.
■ Instruct the patient regarding possible addition of granulocyte colony-stimulating factor (G-CSF) and granulocyte-macrophage colony-stimulating factor (GM-CSF) to the medical regimen.	These growth factors can enhance granulocyte recovery secondary to chemotherapy and potentiate the phagocytic activity of neutrophils. Typical medications include filgrastim, pegfilgrastim, and sargramostim.
■ Anticipate corticosteroid treatment.	Steroids are indicated to treat neutropenia caused by autoimmune reactions.

■ = Independent   ▲ = Collaborative

NANDA-I NDx **Deficient Knowledge**

Common Related Factor

Unfamiliarity with nature and treatment of condition.
Complexity of treatment
Misinterpretation of information
Lack of recall

Defining Characteristics

Questions to health care team
Verbalized inaccurate information

Common Expected Outcome

Patient or caregiver verbalizes understanding of medical diagnosis, treatment plan, safety measures, and follow-up care.

NOC Outcomes
Knowledge: Disease Process; Knowledge: Infection Control

NIC Interventions
Teaching: Disease Process; Teaching: Prescribed Medication; Infection Protection

Ongoing Assessment

Actions/Interventions	Rationales
■ Assess knowledge of neutropenia.	Understanding may vary among patients exhibiting their first episode versus patients who experience this side effect more routinely.

Therapeutic Interventions

Actions/Interventions	Rationales
■ Explain factors that contribute to low neutrophil count (e.g., chemotherapy, drug sensitivity).	Information enables the patient to understand the cause of the problem.
■ Explain that low neutrophil counts produce high susceptibility to infection.	Infection and sepsis in a neutropenic patient can be fatal. Patients must understand the significance of these counts and their own role in prevention.
■ Explain signs and symptoms of infection; instruct the patient to contact the appropriate health team member immediately if any signs or symptoms occur or are suspected.	Vigilant monitoring helps reduce consequences of infection.
■ Instruct the patient regarding: • Use of prescribed medications (indications, dosages, side effects)	Both antimicrobial medications and colony-stimulating factors are prescribed. Choice of antimicrobial depends on the type of infection present: viral, fungal, or bacterial. Colony-stimulating factors are growth factors that stimulate the bone marrow to produce granulocytes.
• Need for frequent blood draws	Blood draws are required to monitor neutrophil WBC status.
■ Instruct the patient regarding: • Importance of good hand washing • Importance of meticulous body and oral hygiene • Avoidance of shared drinking and eating utensils; need to wash food well • Avoidance of crowds and persons with current or recent infection	Patients must understand strategies and measures by which they can protect themselves during times of compromised defense. Most infections result from organisms residing in the local environment.
• Avoidance of contact with cat litter boxes, fish tanks, and human and animal excreta	These are possible sources of parasites that can cause infection in the immune-compromised person.

Actions/Interventions	Rationales

■ Instruct the patient regarding:
  • Avoidance of activities that may result in trauma to mucosa
  • Alternatives where appropriate (e.g., oral and axillary temperatures instead of rectal, electric razors instead of razor blades, sanitary napkins instead of tampons, tooth sponge instead of toothbrush); limited sexual intercourse if WBCs and platelets are low
	Trauma sites can easily become infected.
	These measures reduce the risk for injury and infection.

■ Instruct the patient to make routine dental visits when WBC counts are not compromised (e.g., before starting chemotherapy treatment or bone marrow transplantation).	Dental care reduces the opportunity for infection to begin in the oral cavity.

Related Care Plan

Impaired oral mucous membrane, p. 148

Organ Transplantation, Solid

Heart Transplantation; Lung Transplantation; Liver Transplantation; Kidney Transplantation; Living Kidney Donors

Solid organ transplantation is a treatment option for patients with end organ damage that has not responded to optimal medical therapy or alternative surgical strategies. Because of a limited supply of suitable organs for transplantation, candidates are carefully screened to ensure they meet selection criteria established by each transplant program. Comorbid conditions such as diabetes, vascular diseases, and malignancies are carefully evaluated to determine the added risk potential to an individual. Social support, psychosocial issues, and financial means are also carefully evaluated to maximize outcomes for patients and families. This care plan will present the nursing diagnoses, interventions, and outcomes across four types of solid organ transplantation: heart, lung, liver, and kidney. The organ-specific problems and interventions are presented first, followed at the end by presentation of three problems that relate to all types of transplantation.

Heart Transplantation

Candidate selection for heart transplantation is based on the consensus from the International Society for Heart and Lung Transplantation (ISHLT) reported in 2006. With the newer bicaval surgical approach to cardiac transplantation, there are fewer problems with junctional rhythm disturbances than are seen with the biatrial technique. Because of the increased number of immunosuppressive agents available, treatment can now be individualized for patients to diminish their risk for rejection episodes.

The most common diagnoses of patients referred for heart transplantation include ischemic cardiomyopathy and idiopathic dilated cardiomyopathy. Patients with New York Heart Association class 3 or 4 heart failure are often at risk for rhythm disturbances as well as for the development of biventricular failure. Many may have pacemakers and/or automatic internal cardiac defibrillators implanted to protect them from sudden death. Because of the shortage of suitable donor hearts, patients must be carefully screened to ensure that heart transplantation is the best and only option. Patients who have failed optimal medical therapy to control their heart failure are often candidates to be evaluated for transplantation. Mechanical circulatory assist devices can be used as a bridge to transplantation or as destination therapy in select cases.

In the United States there are about 2000 deceased donor heart transplants performed each year. Nursing care of patients during the immediate posttransplant period requires intravascular pressure monitoring, excellent clinical assessment skills, and a plan of care that addresses prevention of rejection, infection, and bleeding complications. Patient and family education is important in preparing recipients for self-care and for optimizing long-term outcomes.

■ = Independent   ▲ = Collaborative

NANDA-I NDx: Decreased Cardiac Output

Common Related Factors

Altered contractility (cold ischemic time; manipulation of heart)

Dysrhythmias (atrial fibrillation; ventricular ectopy)

Defining Characteristics

Rapid or weak pulse

Decrease in blood pressure (BP)

Shortness of breath

Crackles

Dizziness

Cool, clammy skin

Oliguria

Fatigue

Common Expected Outcome

Patient maintains optimal cardiac output as evidenced by regular cardiac rate and rhythm, strong peripheral pulses, blood pressure within acceptable limits, warm dry skin, clear breath sounds, and urine output greater than 30 mL/hr.

NOC Outcomes

Circulation Status; Cardiac Pump Effectiveness;

NIC Interventions

Hemodynamic Regulation; Dysrhythmia Management; Medication Administration; Electrolyte Management;

Ongoing Assessment

Actions/Interventions

■ Monitor electrocardiogram (ECG) continuously. Assess for tachycardia, bradycardia, and irregularity.

■ Assess for physical signs of decreased cardiac output: rapid or weak pulse; hypotension; dizziness; cool, clammy skin; shortness of breath; crackles; fatigue; decreased urine output.

▲ Monitor electrolytes.

■ Assess urine output.

Rationales

Many factors can contribute to the rhythm disturbances seen post heart transplantation. These are related to manipulation of the heart during procurement and transplantation, cold ischemic time during donor transport of donor graft (optimal time is less than 4 hours), electrolyte imbalance, and dysrhythmias associated with acute rejection.

During donor management and procurement of a heart there can be many factors affecting normal function of the heart. Many compensatory responses occur secondary to reduced cardiac output. The surgical technique for heart transplantation causes a denervation of the vagus nerve, resulting in a loss of its inhibitory mechanisms to slow the heart rate. Therefore heart recipients often have a higher-than-normal heart rate. The body must depend on circulating catecholamines to increase the heart rate during altered metabolic or physical requirements. A compensatory mechanism to situations such as hypovolemia or pump failure is usually not available.

Hypokalemia and hypomagnesemia are common causes of dysrhythmias and may be associated with a reduction in cardiac output.

Oliguria is a classic sign of decreased renal perfusion, secondary to low cardiac output.

Therapeutic Interventions

Actions/Interventions	Rationales
▲ Administer medication such as epinephrine, vasopressin, dobutamine, or theophylline as ordered. Avoid atropine.	Vasoactive medications increase heart rate and contractility, which enhance cardiac output. However, atropine is a parasympathetic blocking agent and is ineffective in the denervated heart.
▲ Use temporary epicardial pacing wires to maintain an adequate heart rate. Check rate, mode, milliamperes, and connections frequently.	Temporary pacing is used to support cardiac rhythm.
■ If life-threatening ventricular ectopy occurs, treat according to Advanced Cardiac Life Support (ACLS).	ACLS guidelines assist in defining treatment, except for the use of atropine.
▲ Administer electrolyte replacements as ordered.	Hypokalemia, hyperkalemia, and hypomagnesemia cause ventricular irritability and if severe and persistent, may result in a reduced cardiac output. Replacement therapy corrects deficiency.

NANDA-I NDx Risk for Decreased Cardiac Output: Right Ventricular Failure

Common Risk Factors

Right ventricular failure (secondary to preexisting pulmonary hypertension that can develop with congestive heart failure)

Reperfusion injury of the donor heart (with restoration of blood flow following the period of ischemia during procurement)

Acute rejection

Common Expected Outcome

Patient maintains optimal cardiac output, as evidenced by regular cardiac rate and rhythm, strong peripheral pulses, blood pressure within acceptable limits, warm dry skin, clear breath sounds, and urine output greater than 30 mL/hr.

NOC Outcome
Cardiac Pump Effectiveness; Circulation Status
NIC Interventions
Invasive Hemodynamic Monitoring: Hemodynamic Regulation; Shock Prevention

---

Ongoing Assessment

Actions/Interventions	Rationales
▲ Monitor cardiac output/cardiac index by thermodilution as needed.	Cardiac output measurements provide objective numbers to guide therapy.
▲ Assess *left heart function* by documenting hemodynamic parameters: pulmonary artery pressure (PAP), pulmonary capillary wedge pressure (PCWP), left atrial pressure, systemic vascular resistance.	Invasive hemodynamic monitoring provides information on pump function and fluid status. Left-sided heart failure can lead to or aggravate right-sided failure. PCWP provides important data on left heart function by reflecting left atrial pressures. Left ventricular failure causes a rise in left atrial pressures, which in normal conditions should be measured at 8 to 10 mm Hg. Elevations in left atrial pressures greater than 20 mm Hg are indicative of pulmonary edema. These measurements allow clinicians to titrate medications and optimize the patient's fluid status.

■ = Independent   ▲ = Collaborative

Actions/Interventions	**Rationales**
■ Assess for physical signs of left-sided heart failure: hypotension, crackles, shortness of breath, weak peripheral pulses, S_3-S_4 gallops.	Crackles and shortness of breath are signs of fluid overload from heart failure. Pulses are weak and BP low with reduced stroke volume and cardiac output. S_3 denotes reduced ventricular ejection. S_4 occurs with reduced compliance of the ventricle.
▲ Assess *right heart function* by documenting central venous pressure (CVP) readings.	CVP provides information on right heart filling pressures and fluid status. A normal CVP is between 2 and 6 mm Hg. Elevations indicate volume overload, whereas decreases indicate a dehydrated state.
■ Assess for physical signs of right heart failure: hepatomegaly, hepatojugular reflux, jugular vein distention, gastrointestinal upset, peripheral edema.	Right heart failure causes increased venous pressure and fluid congestion in hepatic and abdominal systems. Edema occurs when fluid accumulates in the extravascular spaces. Symmetrical peripheral edema is characteristic in heart failure.
■ Assess fluid balance (intake and output [I&O]) and weight gain.	Compromised regulatory mechanisms may result in fluid and sodium retention. Intake and output provides objective evidence of renal perfusion and fluid balance.
▲ Monitor laboratory values for renal and liver function.	Liver function provides evidence of right heart congestion or failure. Renal laboratory values provide evidence of function of the left heart.
■ Review echocardiogram results for right ventricular ejection fraction and dimensions of right ventricle.	An echocardiogram provides additional objective information on pump function.
■ Anticipate heart biopsy to verify possible rejection.	Heart biopsies are the gold standard for determining heart rejection. This is an invasive procedure that demonstrates lymphocyte/monocyte infiltrates that define rejection.

Therapeutic Interventions

Actions/Interventions	**Rationales**
▲ Administer parenteral fluids as ordered.	Increasing fluid volume may be required to maintain adequate filling pressures and to optimize cardiac output. PCWP and CVP readings should be used to guide interventions.
▲ Administer intravenous inotropes as ordered.	Inotropes increase myocardial contractility.
▲ Administer intravenous vasodilators as ordered, including inhaled nitric oxide.	Vasodilators help to decrease systemic vascular resistance, which reduces workload on the left ventricle. Nitric oxide is used to dilate the pulmonary vasculature in patients with pulmonary hypertension. This reduces the workload on the right ventricle.
▲ Maintain hemodynamic parameters at prescribed levels.	Close monitoring of these parameters guides titration of fluids and medications.
■ Maintain a quiet environment with the patient in semi-Fowler's position.	These measures reduce oxygen demands on the heart.
■ Maintain adequate oxygenation.	Oxygen optimizes cardiac function and reduces pulmonary vascular resistance through its vasodilator effect on the pulmonary vasculature.
▲ Prepare patient for possible surgical intervention with mechanical circulatory assist device to support left and right ventricles while awaiting heart transplantation.	There are several models and manufacturers of mechanical circulatory assist devices now available for patients with biventricular failure awaiting heart transplantation.

Risk for Bleeding/Hemorrhage

Common Risk Factors

Enlarged pericardial sac that can conceal active postoperative bleeding

Coagulopathies

Impaired liver function

Surgical side effects (elaborate suture lines and cannulation sites)

Treatment-related side effects (preoperative and intraoperative anticoagulation)

Common Expected Outcome

Patient does not exhibit signs of bleeding/hemorrhage, as evidenced by stable hemoglobin, hematocrit, and prothrombin time; BP and heart rate remain within normal limits.

NOC Outcomes
Blood Coagulation; Blood Loss Severity
NIC Interventions
Bleeding Precautions; Shock Prevention

Ongoing Assessment

Actions/Interventions	Rationales
■ Assess BP and hemodynamic measurements.	Hypotension and reduced CVP may signal hypovolemia secondary to bleeding.
■ Assess peripheral pulses, including capillary refill.	Pulses are weak with reduced stroke volume and cardiac output. Capillary refill is slow.
■ Monitor intake and output.	Oliguria is a compensatory response to reduced fluid volume.
■ Assess mediastinal chest tube drainage for significant decrease (tamponade) and/or increase (hemorrhage).	Greater than 100 mL/hr for 4 hours or abrupt decrease in drainage is significant. Note that patients with prior cardiomyopathy have an enlarged pericardial sac and over time the new smaller transplanted heart leaves a potential area to conceal postoperative bleeding.
▲ Monitor hemoglobin and hematocrit.	Drops in hemoglobin and hematocrit must be evaluated as an indication of blood loss. However, these laboratory values may also decrease as a result of a dilutional effect with administration of replacement fluids.
▲ Monitor prothrombin time (PT), partial thromboplastin time (PTT), and platelets.	The liver synthesizes many of the body's coagulation factors. Congestion in the liver because of heart failure may lead to elevations in PT and PTT, increasing the risk for hemorrhage. These tests help evaluate the ability of the blood to clot. Insufficient platelets will prevent adequate clotting.
■ Observe amplitude of ECG.	Decreased QRS voltage may indicate the development of cardiac tamponade.
■ Assess heart sounds.	Muffled heart sounds are a sign of tamponade.
▲ Review results of chest x-ray film for widening of mediastinal shadow.	A mediastinal shadow is seen with cardiac tamponade.

Therapeutic Interventions

Actions/Interventions	Rationales
■ Elevate head of bed to 30 degrees, and turn patient hourly.	This maneuver prevents impedance of mediastinal drainage.
■ Manipulate chest tubes, milking or stripping according to your hospital policies. Document the amount and type of drainage.	According to Cochrane Reviews, there are insufficient data from randomized clinical trials to determine the most effective methods for chest tube clearance.

■ = Independent   ▲ = Collaborative

Actions/Interventions

▲ Maintain suction to drainage tubes as ordered.

▲ Maintain current type and crossmatch to keep 2 units of cytomegalovirus (CMV)-negative packed red blood cells available at all times in the immediate postoperative period in the intensive care unit (ICU).

■ Use leukocyte-poor filters for all blood transfusions.

▲ Replace volume losses with colloids or crystalloids as ordered.

▲ If bleeding is persistent, prepare patient to return to the operating room.

Rationales

Suction facilitates effective drainage.

CMV-negative blood reduces the risk for transmitting infections to immunocompromised patients.

Leukocyte-poor filters provide an extra layer of protection.

Maintaining adequate circulating blood volume is a priority.

Emergency surgery may be required to correct bleeding problem.

NANDA-I NDx Ineffective Protection

Common Related Factors

Potential for acute heart rejection (characterized by perivascular and interstitial mononuclear cell infiltration, with potential for progression to necrosis)

Defining Characteristics

Fatigue/malaise
Increasing shortness of breath
Dysrhythmias
Positive endomyocardial biopsy results

Common Expected Outcomes

Patient and family verbalize understanding of signs and symptoms of rejection.

Patient and family verbalize understanding of the role of routine heart biopsies in detecting rejection.

NOC Outcome
Immune Status

NIC Interventions
Cardiac Care: Acute; Teaching: Disease Process

Ongoing Assessment

Actions/Interventions

■ Assess for signs of heart failure: increasing malaise/decreasing exercise tolerance, increased shortness of breath, hypotension, decreased urine output, peripheral edema, bradycardia.

▲ Review results of heart biopsy.

■ Evaluate ECG for conduction defects and dysrhythmias.

▲ Monitor immunosuppression levels of tacrolimus or cyclosporine.

▲ Monitor AlloMap levels.

Rationales

Fatigue and shortness of breath can be indicators of rejection. Signs and symptoms of heart failure may also be used as indicators of rejection.

There are no standardized clinical symptoms for detecting rejection, thus the heart biopsy remains the gold standard for detecting rejection. Biopsy results are graded according to the International Society for Heart and Lung Transplantation standards.

These ECG changes may represent signs of rejection.

Monitoring drug levels of immunosuppression is important to ensure that therapeutic levels are maintained.

In 2008 AlloMap testing was approved by the Food and Drug Administration (FDA) as an in vitro diagnostic test for determining the probability of heart rejection in stable patients. AlloMap testing helps to identify rejection in stable patients who are more than 2 months post transplantation. Initially this test was used with the heart biopsy to evaluate outcome correlation. This is a noninvasive, multigene expression test that has shown excellent correlation in multicenter studies.

Therapeutic Interventions

Actions/Interventions	Rationales
▲ Administer immunosuppressive agents daily as prescribed.	These agents reduce the risk for rejection. A variety of drugs with different mechanisms of actions are now available to allow clinicians to individualize immunosuppression.
■ Describe the procedure for the endomyocardial biopsy to the patient and family, including the environment in which the procedure will be performed and the use of local anesthesia and medication to relax the patient, if needed.	Routine endomyocardial biopsies are part of the posttransplant protocol. Biopsies are the standard by which rejection is confirmed. Most heart biopsies are performed in the cardiac catheterization laboratory, which can be intimidating to patients. Patients may require a mild sedative or relaxant before the biopsy. Some transplant centers use echo-guided biopsies.
■ Teach patient about signs and symptoms of acute rejection: increased fatigue, irregular pulse, lower-than-normal blood pressure, shortness of breath, peripheral edema.	Patients and families need to be able to describe signs and symptoms of rejection as part of the self-care initiative.
■ Educate patients and families about the requirements for heart biopsies, which are done at the transplant center according to protocol	Patients and families should be educated about this requirement before transplant as part of the informed consent process. It is important that they understand the rationale for biopsies and their role in detecting rejection.

Lung Transplantation

The first successful human single lung transplant was performed in 1983, followed by a successful double lung transplant in 1986. Less than 1500 lung transplants are performed annually in the United States with the majority of lungs being procured from deceased donors. Living lung transplants were performed for children with cystic fibrosis in the late 1990s and early 2000s. However, because of the risk to living donors, there were only three living donor lung transplants performed in 2007 and none in 2008. Lung transplantation is often complicated by infection.

The major diagnoses of patients requiring lung transplantation include emphysema, alpha$_1$-antitrypsin deficiency, interstitial pulmonary fibrosis, cystic fibrosis, and primary pulmonary hypertension. Because of the shortage of potential lungs for transplantation, patients are selected according to criteria described by the International Society of Heart and Lung Transplantation. Testing to determine candidacy for lung transplantation includes chest x-ray film, ventilation-perfusion ($\dot{V}/\dot{Q}$) scan, 6-minute walk, pulmonary function tests (PFTs), arterial blood gases, echocardiogram, and cardiac catheterization for patients over the age of 40.

Lung transplant recipients usually require intensive nursing care for the first 4 to 7 days immediately postoperatively. In this period complications include reperfusion injury, hemothorax, pneumothorax, pleural effusion, rejection, and infection.

Ineffective Airway Clearance

Common Related Factors	Defining Characteristics
Denervated lung following transplantation	Changes in respiratory rate or depth
Decreased energy and fatigue (ineffective cough)	Abnormal breath sounds (crackles, rhonchi, wheezes)
Copious and tenacious tracheobronchial secretions	Dyspnea
Pain	Ineffective cough
Impaired respiratory muscle function	Excessive secretions
	Hypoxemia/cyanosis
	Abnormal arterial blood gases

■ = Independent   ▲ = Collaborative

Common Expected Outcome

Patient will maintain clear open airways as evidenced by normal rate and depth of respiration, normal breath sounds, and ability to cough up secretions.

NOC Outcomes
Respiratory Status; Airway Patency
NIC Interventions
Airway Management; Airway Suctioning

Ongoing Assessment

Actions/Interventions	Rationales
■ Assess airway for patency.	Maintaining the airway is always the first priority. Patients require ventilator support for several days post transplantation. Potential complications of primary graft dysfunction, pleural effusion, and pneumothorax prolong the need for mechanical ventilation.
■ Auscultate lungs for decreased, absent, or adventitious breath sounds.	Diminished breath sounds or the presence of adventitious sounds (course crackles or wheezes) may indicate a mucous plug or other airway obstruction such as a pleural effusion.
■ Assess respirations; note quality, rate, rhythm, depth, dyspnea on exertion, and position for breathing.	Abnormality indicates respiratory compromise. An increase in respiratory rate and rhythm may be a compensatory response to airway obstruction.
■ Assess for subcutaneous air (also called subcutaneous emphysema).	Subcutaneous air is a sign of pneumothorax. Small air leaks are not uncommon post lung transplantation. This is sometimes associated with smaller-size donor lungs for the size of the recipient.
■ Palpate for decreased chest expansion on one side and for tracheal shift.	Pleural effusions can result in chest expansion decrease on the affected side along with a tracheal shift away from the affected side.
▲ Review chest x-ray film with physicians.	With a pleural effusion, the chest x-ray film will indicate fluid in the pleural spaces. Fluid may be serous, blood, pus, or chyle. The chest x-ray film may reveal a pneumothorax, which would indicate excessive air in spaces surrounding the lungs. In most cases a pneumothorax post lung transplant will clear within several days.
▲ Use pulse oximetry to monitor oxygen saturation; assess arterial blood gases.	Increasing $Paco_2$ levels and decreasing Pao_2 provide clinicians with information on respiratory needs of patients. Oxygen saturation should be kept at 90% or greater. Ventilator settings can be changed to meet the needs of a lung recipient.
■ Assess quality, color, odor, and amount of sputum being suctioned from endotracheal tube.	Abnormalities in sputum may be the result of infection and must be cultured and treated early to prevent sepsis.
▲ While patient is on mechanical ventilator, monitor for peak airway pressures and airway resistance.	Increases in these parameters signal accumulation of secretions or fluid and potential for ineffective ventilation.

Therapeutic Interventions

Actions/Interventions	Rationales
■ Maintain chest tubes until drainage has ceased and the new lung is inflated.	Chest tubes allow drainage of fluids around the lungs that is often found post lung transplantation. Once there is no sign of pneumothorax or drainage, the chest tubes may be discontinued.

Actions/Interventions

▲ Culture sputum if the color, consistency, or odor is suspicious.

■ Use suctioning for patients on mechanical ventilation.

■ Position patient in upright position (keep head of bed elevated).

▲ Coordinate optimal time for postural drainage and percussion.

Rationales

Early intervention for possible infection may prevent sepsis. Immunocompromised patients are at greater risk for serious infections.

Keeping the airway free of mucus is important because the patient's cough reflex may be diminished with presence of endotracheal tube.

This position promotes better lung expansion and improved air exchange.

Postural drainage should be performed every 4 to 6 hours and improves the removal of bronchial secretions.

Ineffective Protection Post Lung Transplantation

Common Related Factors

Possibility of acute allograft rejection
Chronic rejection
Acute infection

Defining Characteristics

Positive lung biopsy results
Shortness of breath
Fever
Leukocytosis
Nonproductive cough
Malaise
Hypoxemia
Oxygen desaturation

Common Expected Outcomes

Patient and family verbalize understanding of signs and symptoms of rejection.
Patient and family verbalize understanding of the role of routine lung biopsy in detecting rejection.

NOC Outcome
Immune Status
NIC Interventions
Teaching: Disease Process; Acute Care

Ongoing Assessment

Actions/Interventions

■ Assess patient for clinical features of rejection: dyspnea, malaise, fever, leukocytosis, nonproductive cough, hypoxemia, oxygen desaturation.

■ Review results of pulmonary function tests, biopsies, and sputum cultures to assist in differentiating between infection and rejection.

Rationales

Rejection symptoms are often nonspecific; diagnosis is often based on clinical symptoms, which must be differentiated from infection.

Signs and symptoms of lung rejection and infection can mimic one another and are difficult to differentiate. Lungs have a predisposition to infection because of their exposure to the external environment. To differentiate infection from rejection may require Gram-stained sputum cultures as well as transbronchial washings and biopsies. Biopsies can be performed via bronchoscopy, but results have yielded a poor sensitivity and accuracy. The best tissue samples come from a biopsy performed via thoracotomy. Perivascular infiltrates on biopsy are graded according to the International Society for Heart and Lung Transplantation standards.

■ = Independent   ▲ = Collaborative

Actions/Interventions	Rationales
▲ Review chest x-ray film with physicians.	Ischemia-reperfusion injury (also known as primary graft dysfunction [PGD]) following lung transplant continues to be a source of early death. Daily evaluation of the chest x-ray film provides the clinician with opportunities for early intervention. The recipient macrophages are believed to become activated during ischemia-reperfusion injury, which results in severe lung damage.
■ Monitor ECG for cardiac dysrhythmias: tachycardia, atrial dysrhythmias.	Tachycardia may be related to fluid loss, bleeding, pain, or catecholamine release with stress of surgery. Atrial dysrhythmias may be caused by inflammation near pulmonary vein and atrial cuff suture lines.

Therapeutic Interventions

Actions/Interventions	Rationales
▲ Maintain PAP within normal range, as ordered.	Normal PAP protects the anastomosis site and helps to prevent pulmonary edema in the early postoperative stage.
■ Maintain chest tubes inserted around new lung(s).	Two or more chest tubes are inserted to allow transplanted lung(s) to fully expand. Air, serous fluid, and blood can be drained via chest tubes.
▲ Begin positive pressure ventilation in cases of primary graft dysfunction or ischemia-reperfusion injury. Decrease tidal volumes, and maintain oxygen delivery.	Treatment options for PGD are similar to those used in acute respiratory distress syndrome (ARDS).
▲ Consult respiratory therapist for chest physiotherapy as needed.	Chest physiotherapy includes the techniques of postural drainage and chest percussion to loosen and mobilize secretions in smaller airways to keep the airways clear and prevent infection. This is especially used in treatment of PGD.
▲ Administer immunosuppressive agents as prescribed.	These agents reduce the risk for rejection. A variety of drugs with different mechanisms of actions are now available to allow clinicians to individualize immunosuppression.

Liver Transplantation

Liver transplantation is a treatment option for persons with end-stage liver disease for whom all possible modes of surgical and medical treatment have been exhausted.

The indications for liver transplantation can be either acute (fulminant) liver failure or chronic liver disease. The most common causes of chronic liver disease and cirrhosis are hepatitis C, alcohol, nonalcoholic steatohepatitis (NASH), primary biliary cirrhosis (PBC), and primary sclerosing cholangitis (PSC). Less-common causes are hepatitis B and metabolic diseases like hemochromatosis and Wilson's disease. Patients with hepatocellular carcinoma must meet certain criteria, called the Milan criteria, in order to be considered for liver transplant. Milan criteria state that there must be one single tumor less than 5 cm or no greater than three tumors each measuring less than 3 cm.

The absolute contraindications for liver transplant are active alcohol or substance abuse, severe cardiopulmonary or other comorbid conditions that would preclude meaningful recovery after transplant, active extrahepatic malignancy, hepatic malignancy with macrovascular or diffuse tumor invasion, active and uncontrolled infection, technical and/or anatomical barriers, psychological factors that would likely preclude recovery after liver transplantation, and brain death. Relative contraindications for liver transplant include advanced age, cholangiocarcinoma (can be considered under strict protocols), chronic or refractory infections, human immunodeficiency virus (HIV), previous malignancy within 5 years, portal vein thrombosis, active psychiatric illness, and poor social support.

A liver transplant evaluation is performed by a comprehensive team that reviews each individual's need and examines data from several imaging studies and a battery of laboratory tests. Patients are listed on the waiting list according to their blood type and Model of End-Stage Liver Disease (MELD) score, which is calculated by using the patient's international normalized ratio (INR), creatinine, and total bilirubin. This score ranges from as low as 6 to as high as 40. The surgical procedure entails the excision of both donor and recipient livers and transplantation of the donor liver into the recipient (orthotopically transplanted). Live donor liver transplantation involves removing a portion of the liver from a healthy donor who underwent extensive workup for suitability before the surgery.

Because of the chronic systemic problems resulting from end-stage liver disease and the technical complexity of the transplant procedure, postoperative recovery can be complicated. However, with ongoing compliance with medical therapy and adherence to lifestyle changes, the transplant patient can live an active and productive life.

 NANDA-I NDx **Risk for Bleeding/Hemorrhage**

Common Risk Factors

Coagulopathy (from preoperative splenomegaly, thrombocytopenia, and poor hepatic synthetic function from chronic liver disease)

Preoperative portal hypertension (with esophageal and gastric varices, increased risk for postoperative bleeding)

Common Expected Outcome

Patient does not exhibit signs of bleeding/hemorrhage, as evidenced by stable hemoglobin, hematocrit, and prothrombin time, and BP and HR within normal limits.

NOC Outcomes
Blood Coagulation; Blood Loss Severity
NIC Intervention
Bleeding Precautions

Ongoing Assessment

Actions/Interventions	Rationales
■ Monitor pulse, BP, and hemodynamic measures.	Hypotension and reduced CVP may signal hypovolemia secondary to bleeding.
■ Assess peripheral pulses, including capillary refill.	Pulses are weak with reduced stroke volume and cardiac output. Capillary refill is slow.
■ Monitor intake and output.	Oliguria is a compensatory response to reduced fluid volume.
■ Assess abdominal Jackson-Pratt (JP) drains for significant cessation (i.e., tamponade of a blood vessel) or increase (i.e., hemorrhage).	Greater than 100 mL/hour for 4 hours or abrupt decrease of drainage is significant.
▲ Monitor hemoglobin and hematocrit with serial laboratory studies.	Drops in hemoglobin or hematocrit must be evaluated as an indication of blood loss, although hematocrit may also decrease as fluids are administered because of dilution.
▲ Monitor PT/PTT and platelet count; check activated clotting time.	The liver is responsible for the synthesis of clotting factors. These tests help evaluate ability of blood to clot. Deficiencies guide ongoing treatment.
▲ Check results of abdominal computed tomography (CT) scan if indicated.	This test provides information about the liver, especially relating to source of any bleeding.

■ = Independent   ▲ = Collaborative

Therapeutic Interventions

Actions/Interventions	Rationales
■ Elevate head of bed to 30 degrees, and turn patient hourly.	This position facilitates proper tube drainage.
■ Empty Jackson-Pratt drains every 2 hours, and note amount and type of drainage. Document output.	Current practice is to not strip JPs unless they are clotted.
▲ Maintain current type and crossmatch to keep 2 units of packed red blood cells available at all times during the ICU stay. Use CMV-negative blood if the patient is CMV-negative.	Being prepared helps ensure early treatment and reduce potential complications. CMV-negative blood reduces the risk for transmitting infections to immunocompromised patients.
▲ Replace volume losses with colloids or crystalloids as ordered.	Maintaining adequate circulating blood volume is a priority.

Ineffective Protection

Common Related Factors

Potential for acute graft rejection
Chronic rejection

Defining Characteristics

Fatigue/malaise
Elevated liver function tests: alanine transaminase (ALT), aspartate transaminase (AST), total bilirubin
Abnormal coagulation studies
Changes in bile drainage from T-tube
Changes in stool color
Fever
Right upper quadrant pain

Common Expected Outcomes

Immediate postoperative period: Early detection of rejection is achieved through ongoing assessment of liver function, coagulation abnormalities, and changes in color of T-tube drainage.
Post discharge: Patient and family verbalize understanding of early signs of rejection.

NOC Outcomes
Immune Status
NIC Interventions
Acute Care; Teaching; Disease Process

Ongoing Assessment

Actions/Interventions	Rationales
▲ Assess for increasing liver function test results.	Elevation in liver function test results and coagulation abnormalities represent signs of rejection.
■ Assess T-tube drainage.	Changes in color or consistency should be reported to the physician. Bile should be golden brown. Lighter color or the presence of sludgelike drainage may indicate poor liver function.
▲ Monitor tacrolimus/sirolimus trough levels (drawn 1 hour before dose).	Nontherapeutic levels increase risk for rejection.

Therapeutic Interventions

Actions/Interventions	Rationales
▲ Administer immunosuppressive agents daily as prescribed.	These agents reduce risk for rejection. A variety of drugs with different mechanisms of actions are now available to allow clinicians to individualize immunosuppression.
■ Describe to the patient the procedure of an ultrasound-guided liver biopsy.	Protocol liver biopsies are performed if indicated. Biopsies are the gold standard and definitive procedure to confirm rejection.
■ Teach patient about the signs and symptoms of acute rejection.	By the time of patient discharge, it is vital for the patient and family to assume full responsibility for care.

Kidney Transplantation

Kidney Transplant Recipient

In 2008 there were 10,551 deceased-donor kidney transplants and 5,963 living-donor kidney transplants nationally. Over 78,000 individuals are currently awaiting a suitable kidney donor. Kidney transplant is viewed as the superior treatment for end-stage renal disease (ESRD). Receiving a kidney transplant entails an anterior surgical incision that may or may not remove the patient's own kidney, depending on the disease process that contributed to the development of ESRD. Most individuals will keep their native organ, and the new kidney will be placed in the abdomen with the donor ureter connected to the recipient's bladder. In the case of abscessed polycystic kidney disease, the affected native kidney will be removed to minimize the risk for abscess and infection development in the recipient.

The primary reasons for ESRD development include the following (in contributory order): diabetes mellitus (type 1 or 2), hypertension, glomerulonephritis, and polycystic kidney disease.

 NANDA-I NDx ## Risk for Ineffective Renal Perfusion

Common Risk Factors

Acute tubular necrosis (reperfusion injury of donor kidney before transplantation)
Rejection

Common Expected Outcome

Patient maintains optimal renal perfusion/function as evidenced by urinary output greater than 30 mL/hr, BP within normal limits for patient, normal blood urea nitrogen (BUN)/creatinine ratio, urinalysis within normal limits, and comparable intake and output.

NOC Outcomes

Kidney Function; Tissue Perfusion: Abdominal Organs; Urinary Elimination

NIC Interventions

T-Tube Care: Urinary; Urinary Elimination Management; Fluid/ Electrolyte Management; Hemodynamic Regulation

---

Ongoing Assessment

Actions/Interventions	Rationales
■ Monitor intake and urinary output by Foley catheter.	This provides information on glomerular function and fluid status.
■ Monitor urine specific gravity.	Specific gravity measures the ability of the kidneys to concentrate urine. The ability to concentrate is lost in intrarenal failure.
▲ Monitor blood and urine laboratory values for renal function (BUN, creatinine, potassium; urinalysis).	BUN, creatinine, and potassium levels are elevated in reduced renal function. The presence of protein or blood in the urine indicates an abnormal state. Urine sodium concentrations are high with renal damage yet low with prerenal causes.
■ Monitor daily weights.	Daily weights help to determine fluid balance.

■ = Independent   ▲ = Collaborative

Actions/Interventions

- Assess for signs of fluid overload: elevated CVP, jugular vein distention (JVD), peripheral edema, abdominal distention especially at surgical site, nausea, lung crackles upon auscultation.
- Monitor all output devices and drains as ordered.

▲ Assess laboratory values for immunosuppressant therapeutic values.

Rationales

Assessments are key to early detection of poor kidney function and fluid overload following transplantation. CVP between 6 and 12 cm H_2O prevents hypotension and hypoperfusion of the kidneys.

Negative-pressure drainage devices help direct patient healing process. Devices provide an early indicator of blood loss around renal capsule.

Monitoring drug levels of immunosuppression is important to ensure that therapeutic levels are maintained. Immunosuppressants are cleared through the renal system. Excessive blood levels may negatively impact renal and hepatic function. Therapeutic value ranges for tacrolimus (Prograf) for new kidney recipients must be closely monitored for their impact on BUN and creatinine. Therapeutic range and routine renal laboratory values are key to successful immunosuppressant therapy. Values MUST be drawn before dosing patient.

Therapeutic Interventions

Actions/Interventions

▲ Administer parenteral fluids and diuretics as ordered. Replace urine output milliliter for milliliter.

▲ Administer antihypertensives as ordered.

▲ Deliver and monitor oxygen as ordered to maintain saturation levels of 90% or better. Wean from supplemental oxygen when patient is able to achieve saturation levels of 90% or greater on room air.

▲ Administer immunosuppression as ordered.

- Provide education to renal transplant recipients with every medication administration.

Rationales

The kidney's ability to regulate fluid balance is lost with impaired renal function. Close fluid management is important. Volume replacement may be especially important in prerenal cases.

Altered renal function routinely disrupts blood pressure regulation.

Optimal oxygenation level maximizes hemodynamic status and improves renal blood flow.

These agents reduce the risk for rejection. A variety of drugs with different mechanisms of action are now available to allow clinicians to individualize immunosuppression.

Kidney recipients must receive adequate education and be encouraged to care for their graft at all stages of the transplant process. The most significant contributing factor to graft rejection in the first year is lack of compliance with medication regimen.

NANDA-I NDx Ineffective Protection for Transplanted Kidney

Common Related Factors

Possibility of acute allograft rejection (at cellular level kidney rejection demonstrates interstitial edema, tubulitis, and mononuclear infiltration)

Polyomavirus allograft neuropathy (PVAN)

Defining Characteristics

Positive ultrasound-guided kidney biopsy results
Decreased urine output
Fever
Pain over graft site
Elevated serum creatinine
Loss of graft function

Common Expected Outcomes

Patient and family verbalize understanding of early signs and symptoms of rejection.

Patient/family verbalize understanding of the role of routine kidney biopsy in detecting rejection.

NOC Outcome
Immune Status
NIC Intervention
Teaching: Disease Process

Ongoing Assessment

Actions/Interventions	**Rationales**
■ Monitor intake and output . Report output less than 30 mL/hr.	Decreased output indicates a potential problem with the transplanted kidney. Early intervention may prevent loss of the transplanted kidney.
▲ Monitor serum creatinine and report elevations.	Elevated serum creatinine can be an indicator of kidney rejection. Early intervention may prevent loss of the transplanted kidney.
▲ Monitor for therapeutic levels of immunosuppression.	Immunosuppressive medications help to decrease the risk for kidney rejection; however, toxic levels of the drugs may cause a rise in creatinine.
▲ Check polyomavirus test result.	Graft rejection and polyomavirus can be difficult to differentiate. Both can cause a nephropathy and loss of allograft function. Laboratory results will help differentiate etiology. Urine cytology may be able to detect polyomavirus; however, the gold standard for differentiating rejection and polyoma virus is the kidney biopsy. It is important to verify the diagnosis because treatment interventions are different.
■ Assess patient for clinical features of rejection: malaise, fever, edema, pain over graft site, increased weight, decreased urine output, microscopic hematuria.	Rejection symptoms are often nonspecific; diagnosis is based on clinical symptoms. The diagnosis must differentiate between rejection and polyomavirus.

Therapeutic Interventions

Actions/Interventions	**Rationales**
■ Describe the ultrasound-guided biopsy procedure to the patient.	Biopsies may be frightening to patients. Explaining the procedure and the environment of the room in which the procedure will be done helps to alleviate some of the fear.
■ Review results of ultrasound-guided needle biopsy to assist in differentiating cause of renal dysfunction.	Biopsies continue to be the gold standard for diagnosing acute rejection.
▲ Administer immunosuppressive agents as prescribed. Anticipate that patient may require increases in immunosuppression such as pulse steroids during rejection episodes.	Immunosuppressive agents reduce the risk for rejection. A variety of drugs with different mechanisms of action are now available to allow clinicians to individualize immunosuppression. Antithymocyte globulins and monoclonal antibodies may be used as immunosuppressive agents in the immediate postoperative periods because they do not affect renal function. Higher doses of steroids or other immunosuppressive agents may help combat the rejection episode.
■ Teach the patient and family about signs and symptoms of rejection.	Patients and families need to be able to identify early symptoms of rejection and to contact the transplant center with symptoms for early intervention.

■ = Independent   ▲ = Collaborative

Living Kidney Donors

The most frequently performed transplant procedure, kidney transplantation, also accounts for the largest majority of living donors and is associated with the highest patient and graft survival rates. Greater than 95% of living organ donations in 2008 were living kidney donations. Education and information are key to maximizing outcomes, and they minimize stress for living kidney donors. Living kidney donors experience a thorough evaluation by a special living-donor advocacy team, including: assessment of physical well-being; review of family history; review of past medical history of diabetes, hypertension, heart disease, and weight control; and a psychiatric evaluation by a designated psychiatrist who has a specialty in living organ donation. The living-donor team is composed of a separate group of health care professionals from the recipient transplant team and includes a social worker, living donor transplant coordinator, living donor advocate, psychiatrist, nephrologist, and surgeon.

Living kidney donors are healthy patients who experience a major abdominal surgery that will be painful, with a recovery expected to last 6 to 8 weeks. Care providers must be ready to manage the juxtaposition of this situation. Most hospitalized patients undergoing major surgery are very uncomfortable before a procedure with hope of improving their condition; in contrast, living organ donors are healthy people who will potentially feel much worse after their health care experience. This can be difficult to cope with for family and donors alike.

NANDA-I
NDx **Deficient Knowledge**

Common Related Factors
New procedure
Unfamiliarity with the preoperative routine, surgical procedure, potential complications, recovery

Defining Characteristics
Questioning health care team
Misconceptions

Common Expected Outcomes
Patient and significant others demonstrate understanding of the need for the kidney donation, the preoperative routine/evaluation, surgical procedure, potential complications, and recovery phase.

NOC Outcomes
Knowledge: Disease Process; Knowledge: Procedure

NIC Interventions
Teaching: Preoperative; Teaching: Procedure; Teaching: Activity

---

Ongoing Assessments

Actions/Interventions

■ Assess the donor's understanding of the need for living kidney donors—whether by family or friends.

Rationales

Donating a kidney is a major decision. The patient needs to be well-informed before consenting. Kidneys from living donors have better survival rates than those from deceased donors. Although kidneys donated from living relatives may be the best match, donations from friends as well as strangers now have high success rates.

Actions/Interventions	Rationales
■ Assess how comfortable the patient is in making the decision to donate.	Information provides a basis for discussion and education. Patients should not feel pressured to donate. This is a very individual decision. Although some people may be very enthusiastic, others may be scared and overwhelmed by what they feel they "should do."
■ Assess understanding of the preoperative evaluation, surgical procedure, potential complications, and recovery period.	The patient may be overwhelmed by making the "decision" to donate and may not have absorbed the specific information related to the donation procedure.
■ Provide information on testing for eligibility to donate along with the basic workup evaluation.	Donors are between the ages of 18 and 70. They should be in good general health, have normal kidney function, and have a compatible blood type/antigen match and crossmatch. The evaluation includes a physical examination, laboratory tests to verify that the kidneys (and other organs) are working normally, and a CT scan to verify that the kidneys are normal. Usually there is a meeting with the surgeon and a psychosocial evaluation to prepare for the emotional aspects of donating.
■ Provide information on any risks associated with donation.	The main risks for kidney donation are those associated with most surgeries: potential for bleeding and infection. Research supports that donors can live long healthy lives after donating a kidney. However, donors are told to avoid contact sports to reduce risk for trauma to remaining kidney.
■ Provide information on the surgical procedure: open or laparoscopic incision.	Type of surgery involved may help patient make decision to donate as well as prepare them for the procedure. Traditional "open" surgery has a longer abdominal incision, longer hospitalization/recovery period and is associated with greater amounts of postoperative pain compared with the newer laparoscopic surgery.
■ Explain the usual hospital recovery period, pain management, monitoring for complications (infection, bleeding), urinary catheter, monitoring kidney function and fluid status, progressive diet, early ambulation.	Patients are better able to ask questions when they have basic information on what to expect.
■ Provide instructions for discharge and home follow-up: to avoid heavy lifting, to expect some tiredness and need for rest, to return to work in 2 to 6 weeks depending on type of surgery/work, follow-up appointment with surgeon.	For successful recovery, the patient and family must know how to provide home care, how to identify problems, and what to do when problems arise. Abdominal discomfort and fatigue are the most common issues during recovery.

Problems Common to Solid Organ Transplant Recipients: Risk for Infection, Ineffective Coping, and Knowledge Deficit

 Risk for Infection

Common Risk Factors

Immunosuppressive drug therapy
Break in skin integrity with surgical procedure
Poor nutrition because of preoperative condition with end-organ failure

■ = Independent ▲ = Collaborative

Common Expected Outcomes

Patient, family, and staff caring for patient comply with strict infection control precautions.
Patient avoids hospital-associated infections during this admission.

NOC Outcomes
Immune Status; Risk Detection; Risk Control
NIC Intervention
Infection Protection

Ongoing Assessment

Actions/Interventions	Rationales
■ Observe all catheter sites and wound-healing process for drainage.	Infection is the leading cause of death after solid organ transplantation. Patients are at greater risk for infection because of recent surgical procedure, the high doses of immunosuppression required to prevent rejection, and pretransplant factors associated with end-organ diseases.
▲ Culture any suspicious drainage from wound sites.	Purulent or foul-smelling drainage may indicate infection. Laboratory cultures determine pathogens present and guide therapies. Bacterial infections are most frequently encountered in the intermediate postoperative period. Occasionally infections may be transmitted from the donor organ.
■ Monitor vital signs routinely. Monitor temperature every 2 hours if elevated.	A temperature greater than 37° C (98.6° F) may indicate systemic infection.

Therapeutic Interventions

Actions/Interventions	Rationales
■ Keep the patient in a private room until discharge.	Private rooms help to prevent cross-contamination and infection.
■ Maintain aseptic technique and strict hand washing.	The use of aseptic techniques for procedures helps to minimize pathogen contamination and decreases the risk for infection in this immunocompromised population.
■ Ensure adequate diet high in calories and protein.	Good nutrition supports the healing process after surgery.
■ Encourage coughing and deep breathing.	Coughing and deep-breathing exercises after surgery allow for lung expansion and a more optimal exchange of oxygen and carbon dioxide by the lungs. This also helps to minimize the development of pneumonias after surgery.
▲ Administer prophylactic antiinfective therapy as ordered: ganciclovir, sulfamethoxazole and trimethoprim (if not allergic to sulfa drugs), antibiotics.	Immunosuppression is often the highest in the immediate postoperative period; thus the patient is most susceptible to infection during this time. Because patients are not able to mount an immune response, prophylaxis against common infections is considered best practice.
■ Change all dressings, endotracheal tube tape, respiratory tubing, and other equipment daily.	Changing dressings decreases skin irritation and ensures closer monitoring of invasive line sites. The lungs are the most common site of infection. Replacing equipment daily decreases the incidence of contamination.
■ Control environmental traffic by limiting visitors and staff into the patient's room. Exclude personnel and visitors with colds and any infectious diseases from contact with patient.	Protective protocols help reduce the risk for infection. Limiting traffic into the patient's room reduces the risk for infection transmission.

Actions/Interventions

▲ Implement infection prevention strategies through bundles:
  - Elevation of the head of bed between 30 and 45 degrees
  - Daily sedation vacation and daily assessment of readiness to extubate
  - Oral care
  - Peptic ulcer disease prophylaxis
  - Deep vein thrombosis prophylaxis

Rationales

Bundles provide a structured guideline for improving patient outcomes. Health care–associated infections have been reduced through bundles recommended by the Institute for Healthcare Improvement (IHI). The development of pneumonia in hospitalized patients has been associated with bacteria from biofilm that are aspirated into the respiratory tract.

 Risk for Ineffective Coping

Common Risk Factors

Fear of dying
Stress of waiting for surgery
Perceived body image changes
Steroid-induced body changes
Sexual dysfunction
Guilt over donor's death
Fear of possibility of rejection of new organ following transplantation
Loss of role

Common Expected Outcomes

Patient displays feelings appropriate to initial stage of coping.
Patient displays acceptance of transplant process.
Patient displays beginning signs of effective coping: relaxed appearance, sleeping well, ability to concentrate, interest in surroundings and activities.

NOC Outcomes
Coping: Role Performance; Family Coping
NIC Intervention
Coping Enhancement

Ongoing Assessment

Actions/Interventions

■ Assess the patient's feelings about self and body.

■ Assess response to changes in appearance.

■ Assess the patient's usual coping mechanisms and their previous effectiveness.

■ Assess for signs of ineffective coping.

Rationales

Each individual reacts in a unique way. Perceptions should be assessed, not assumed.

Side effects of tacrolimus, sirolimus and steroid therapy can cause weight gain, increase or decrease in body and facial hair, moon face, and fragile skin.

Successful adjustment is influenced by previous coping success. Patients with history of maladaptive coping may need additional resources. Likewise, previously effective skills may be inadequate in the present situation.

Ineffective coping mechanisms must be identified to promote constructive behaviors.

Therapeutic Interventions

Actions/Interventions

■ Encourage patient and family to express feelings.

■ Establish open lines of communication.

Rationales

Verbalization of feelings and sharing of emotions facilitate effective coping.

The nurse is in an ideal position to guide the patient through this stressful period.

■ = Independent   ▲ = Collaborative

Actions/Interventions

▲ Involve social services and pastoral care for additional and ongoing support resources for the patient and significant others.

■ Suggest resource persons, such as social worker, team psychologist, and support groups.
■ Introduce new information using simple terms, and reinforce instructions or repeat if needed.
■ Refer to a support group.

Rationales

The patient and family may have long-term adjustments to make based on the change in the patient's health status. The patient who was chronically ill before transplant may have difficulty moving from the "sick role" to one of being well. The family may need additional support adapting to these changes in the patient's ability to participate in family responsibilities.
Specialty expertise may be required.

Depending on the degree of anxiety, the patient and family may not be able to absorb all information at one time.
Relationships with persons with common interests and goals can be beneficial. Sometimes it decreases anxiety to have a person who has had a transplant talk with the patient or family and answer questions.

NANDA-I NDx **Deficient Knowledge**

Common Related Factor
Unfamiliarity with surgical procedure and long-term care

Common Expected Outcome
Patient and significant others demonstrate understanding of disease state, surgical procedures, recovery phase, activities, medications and their side effects, and preventative care by discharge.

NOC Outcomes
Knowledge: Disease Process; Knowledge: Treatment Regimen

NIC Interventions
Teaching: Preoperative; Teaching: Procedure/Treatment; Teaching: Prescribed Medications; Teaching: Prescribed Diet; Teaching: Activity; Teaching: Disease Process

Ongoing Assessment

Actions/Interventions

■ Assess the patient or significant other's understanding of surgical procedure, follow-up care, diet, medications and their side effects, activity progression, special precautions for avoiding infections, and risk factor modification.

Rationales

Preoperative patients are usually critically ill and may have difficulty retaining information. Postoperative patients may be overwhelmed by the amount of important information for which they are responsible.

Therapeutic Interventions

Actions/Interventions

Preoperative:
■ Describe surgical procedure, including the ICU regimen and length of stay.
Before discharge:
■ Coordinate discharge teaching with transplant nursing staff, dietitian, occupational and physical therapists, social worker, pharmacist, and members of other significant departments.

Rationales

Patients are better able to ask questions when they have basic information about what to expect.

For successful recovery, patient and family must know how to provide home care, how to identify problems, and what to do when problems arise.

Actions/Interventions

- Inform the patient and family that the patient will have periodic diagnostic testing such as laboratory tests and biopsies.
- Instruct the patient in how to use a flowchart for the medications to be taken at home.
- Educate patient about the potential side effects of each medication.
- Discuss possibility of emotional lability and mood alteration.
- Instruct the patient to adhere to a diabetic diet with no concentrated sweets. Avoid grapefruit juice.

- Instruct the patient to expect some incisional pain for the first few weeks postoperatively; not to drive for at least 6 to 8 weeks and while taking pain medication; not to lift anything greater than 10 pounds for 6 to 8 weeks and avoid strenuous activity. Instruct patient that he or she may be able to return to work in approximately 3 to 6 months.
- Instruct in importance of practicing good hygiene measures.
- Review signs and symptoms of wound complications, including wound drainage, redness or swelling, or infection. Instruct abdominal transplant patients about wound dehiscence.
- Discuss modification of risk factors for diabetes and heart disease. Discuss primary prevention: cancer screening, dual-energy x-ray absorptiometry (DEXA) scans, ophthalmology, and dermatology.

Rationales

These evaluations provide important information on health status.

Medication regimen can be complicated for some types of transplants.

Corticosteroids present common problems that patients must be prepared to identify, prevent, and treat.

These are partly related to steroids and partly to the stress of surgery and the recovery phase.

A diabetic diet decreases the amount of steroid-induced hyperglycemia. Grapefruit and grapefruit juice interact with immunosuppressive agents as a result of binding to the same enzyme. This blocks processing of the drugs, resulting in higher and potentially toxic levels of the drugs.

Patients need to balance time for recovery with progressive activity to increase physical conditioning. Patients need appropriate self-monitoring skills to prevent injury.

Good hygiene decreases incidence of infection.

Instruction allows for prompt intervention in the event of a complication.

A variety of conditions can be exacerbated through immunosuppressive drugs and side effects.

Related Care Plans

Activity intolerance, p. 8
Acute pain, p. 151
Anxiety, p. 18
Deficient fluid volume, p. 72
Disturbed body image, p. 24
Impaired physical mobility, p. 133
Powerlessness, p. 162

Sickle Cell Disease

Vasoocclusive Crisis

Sickle cell disease is a severe genetic hemolytic anemia caused by mutations in the HBB gene resulting in a defective hemoglobin molecule (HbS). This disease is found in Africans, African Americans, and people from Mediterranean countries. The formation of sickle cells is increased by low oxygen partial pressure. Factors associated with sickling include hypoxia, dehydration, infection, acidosis, cold exposure, and exertion. This chronic disease can cause impaired renal, pulmonary, nervous system, and spleen function; increased susceptibility to infection; and ultimately decreased life span. Sickle cell pain crisis is defined as pain of sufficient severity to require medical attention and hospitalization. The severe pain, usually in

■ = Independent   ▲ = Collaborative

the extremities, is caused by the occlusion of small blood vessels by sickle-shaped red blood cells. Research continues in identifying effective antisickling agents and possible gene therapy to correct this defect. Bone marrow/stem cell transplant can cure sickle cell disease. These are difficult procedures currently reserved for children with minimal organ damage from the disease. This care plan focuses on the physical and emotional aspects of sickle cell disease.

NANDA-I NDx Risk for Ineffective Therapeutic Regimen Management

Common Risk Factors

Social support deficits
Family patterns of health care
Excessive demands on individual or family
Knowledge deficit
Decisional conflicts
Perceived powerlessness

Common Expected Outcomes

Patient verbalizes understanding of sickle cell disease, prevention of crisis, and appropriate treatment.
Patient identifies appropriate resources.
Patient verbalizes intention to follow prescribed regimen.
Patient demonstrates ongoing adherence to treatment plan.

NOC Outcomes
Knowledge: Disease Process; Knowledge: Health Behaviors
NIC Interventions
Teaching: Individual; Teaching: Disease Process; Support System Enhancement; Genetic Counseling

Ongoing Assessment

Actions/Interventions

- Assess pattern of crisis episodes and compliance with treatment plan.
- Assess for related factors that may negatively affect success in following the regimen.
- Assess the individual's perception of the health problem.

Rationales

Crises may occur as frequently as weekly or only sporadically, such as once a year. Treatment is supportive. There is no cure.
Knowledge of causative factors provides direction for subsequent intervention.
The patient may not understand the chronicity of this disease or his or her ability to control some of the precipitating factors.

Therapeutic Interventions

Actions/Interventions

- Explain causes of sickle cell disease and the pain of crisis.

- Inform the patient of the benefits of adhering to the prescribed lifestyle.

Rationales

Hypoxia is the primary stimulus for an acute pain crisis in sickle cell disease. With hypoxia, the erythrocyte containing the HbS hemoglobin changes shape from a biconcave disk to an elongated or crescent-shaped cell. The abnormally shaped erythrocyte can obstruct capillaries and contribute to hypoxemia, tissue ischemia, and pain.
Benefits may involve significantly less pain and hospitalization. Patients who believe in the efficacy of the recommended treatment to reduce crisis episodes are more likely to engage in it.

Actions/Interventions

- Instruct the patient in preventable and treatable situations that can precipitate crisis: decreased fluid intake, infection, strenuous exertion, emotional stress, smoking, alcohol ingestion, extreme fatigue, cold exposure, hypoxia, high altitudes, and trauma.
- Instruct the patient in the importance of the following:
  - Drinking at least 4 to 6 liters of fluid daily
  - Dressing appropriately in severe cold weather
  - Taking prescribed medications such as folic acid

  - Keeping follow-up appointments

- Instruct the patient in the necessity of contacting a health care provider at the first sign of infection.

- Inform the patient of high risk for leg ulcers, which are commonly seen around the ankle and shin area.
- Refer to support groups.

- Inform the patient of the need for genetic counseling in family planning.

Rationales

Patients with sickle cell disease can reduce the number of acute crisis episodes by avoiding situations that contribute to the development of hypoxia.

Fluids reduce blood viscosity.
Cold causes vasoconstriction and reduced blood flow.
Medications replace depleted folic acid stores in the bone marrow.
Sickle cell disease is a chronic condition, so ongoing evaluation is important in maintaining desired health status.
Sickle cell patients have functional asplenia (no spleen), which interferes with phagocytosis. Early assessment facilitates prompt treatment.
Because of altered circulation to the area, these lesions are difficult to treat and often become infected.
Groups that meet for mutual support and information can be beneficial, especially to patients coping with chronic illness.
Pregnancy has increased risks for women with sickle cell disease. Also, the sickle cell trait is genetically transmitted.

NANDA-I NDx **Acute Pain**

Common Related Factor

Pain from medical problem (vasoocclusive crisis hypoxia, which causes cells to become rigid and elongated, thus forming crescent shape)

Defining Characteristics

Patient reports pain
Guarding behavior
Self-focused
Facial mask of pain

Common Expected Outcomes

Patient reports satisfactory pain control at a level less than 3 to 4 on a 0 to 10 rating scale.
Patient implements a pain management plan that includes pharmacologic and non-pharmacologic strategies.
Patient exhibits increased comfort such as baseline levels for pulse and blood pressure, relaxed muscle tone or body posture.

NOC Outcomes

Medication Response; Pain Control; Comfort Status

NIC Interventions

Pain Management; Analgesic Administration; Distraction

Ongoing Assessment

Actions/Interventions

- Assess for pain characteristics:

  - Severity (use 0-10 scale)

Rationales

Pain of sickle cell crisis can be severe, requiring large doses of medication.
The lack of objective criteria by which sickle cell disease and even occurrence of crises can be judged makes evaluation difficult. However, the patient's report of pain should be believed and the patient treated appropriately.

■ = Independent ▲ = Collaborative

Actions/Interventions

- Location

- Type

- Duration

▲ Monitor laboratory values (e.g., hemoglobin [Hgb], electrophoresis for amount of sickling, and red blood cell [RBC] count).

Rationales

This usually described as bone or joint pain, less often as muscle pain. This may include abdominal or back pain.

The type of pain may be reported as tenderness or inability to move affected joint, swelling in area, warmth or redness.

Pain may persist for several days.

The hemoglobin level decreases even more during times of pain crisis. A severe decrease in functioning RBCs may indicate the need for replacement transfusion of packed RBCs.

Therapeutic Interventions

Actions/Interventions

▲ Administer pain medications as prescribed:

- Opioid analgesics (morphine sulfate, Dilaudid, or fentanyl by IV injection or via PCA pump)
- Nonsteroidal antiinflammatory drugs (NSAIDs) with narcotics

▲ As pain control is achieved, begin titration of medication, as prescribed.

▲ Administer prescribed oral or IV fluids (6 to 8 liters/day).

▲ Initiate transfusion or exchange transfusion of packed RBCs, as ordered.

■ Use additional comfort measures such as positioning devices, splints for joint discomfort, foam overlay mattresses, or moist heat and massage if preferred.

■ Use distraction devices such as television or movies, as well as relaxation techniques.

■ Provide rest periods.

▲ Administer oxygen as indicated.

▲ Administer hydroxyurea as prescribed.

Rationales

Initial sickle cell pain crisis requires parenteral intravenous (IV) administration on an around-the-clock schedule. Undertreatment of pain by health care providers is a common problem for patients with sickle cell pain crisis. Patients with sickle cell pain crisis have been shown to metabolize opioid and analgesics at a faster-than-normal rate. Larger-than-usual doses of analgesics may be needed to control the pain. The use of IV patient-controlled analgesia (PCA) may diminish the patient's need to make frequent requests for analgesics. Patients may develop opioid tolerance and physical dependence with prolonged use of these analgesics.

Morphine is the drug of choice. Medications should be given intravenously on a routine basis for acute pain.

NSAIDs work in peripheral tissue. Some block synthesis of prostaglandins that stimulate nociceptors. They are effective in managing mild to moderate pain. Oral doses are indicated for milder pain.

Both oral narcotics and NSAIDs may be prescribed for home care.

Fluids promote hemodilution, which reverses agglutination of sickled cells within the microcirculation. Hydration and reversal of viscous blood flow in small blood vessels work to reestablish blood flow so that tissue necrosis does not occur. Hydration may reduce the duration of the pain.

Transfusion of packed RBCs can restore the oxygen-carrying capacity or blood volume. Exchange transfusion can be used in emergencies and in chronic transfusions because of improved viscosity effects and to reduce iron overload potential.

Adjunct therapies can promote comfort. Heat and massage increase circulation to the area.

These heighten one's concentration upon nonpainful stimuli to decrease one's awareness and experience of pain.

Rest reduces tissue oxygen demand and helps reduce pain.

Hypoxia aggravates sickle cell disease.

The development and use of hydroxyurea in the treatment of SCD patients has been highly successful and has been proven effective in the prevention of painful episodes. It is recommended that patients with moderate to severe disease and who have experienced 3 or more acute pain crises in the previous uear should be considered for hydroxyurea treatment.

Risk for Ineffective Coping

Common Risk Factors

Inadequate level of perception of control
Inadequate support system
Inadequate level of confidence in ability to cope
Chronicity of disease

Common Expected Outcomes

Patient identifies own maladaptive coping behaviors.
Patient identifies available resources and support systems.
Patient describes and initiates alternative coping strategies.

NOC Outcomes
Coping; Social Support
NIC Interventions
Coping Enhancement; Support System Enhancement

Ongoing Assessment

Actions/Interventions	Rationales
■ Assess the patient's ability to openly express feelings about disease.	Patients may need assistance in sharing feelings, especially if they sense that health care providers are judging them or doubt the severity of their pain. Patients with SCD commonly experience depression that is often overlooked, misunderstood, or ignored. This problem can exacerbate the physical pain patient's experience as well as overall quality of life.
■ Assess the family's and significant others' support for disease management.	Although family and friends can be great allies, they sometimes may have trouble dealing with chronic illnesses.
■ Assess how often the patient goes to the emergency department for crisis management.	Frequency of emergency department visits provides information on the patient's ability to follow the prevention and treatment plan.
■ Assess the frequency of hospital admissions.	Patients frequently need to escalate their "controlling" behaviors to gain attention of health care providers, who may see the patient as "only seeking medication."
■ Assess for level of fatigue secondary to anemia.	Fatigue may compromise effective coping.

Therapeutic Interventions

Actions/Interventions	Rationales
■ Set aside time to talk with the patient when the pain is controlled.	During crisis, the patient is distracted by the pain and may not be receptive to counseling.
■ Assist the patient in understanding the chronicity of this disease and the need to follow the suggested treatment plan.	The patient may not understand his or her ability to control some of the precipitating factors.
■ Provide information on coping strategies.	Strategies that have worked in the past may no longer be effective.
■ Establish a working relationship with the patient through continuity of care.	An ongoing relationship facilitates trust and can assist with problem solving and successful coping.
▲ Involve social services, psychiatric liaison support groups, and/or pastoral care as additional and ongoing support resources.	The patient or family may need additional help to deal with chronic problems. Participation in support groups may allow the individual to realize that others have the same problem, and they may use this as a means to find alternative coping mechanisms.

■ = Independent ▲ = Collaborative

Actions/Interventions

- Avoid placing the patient in crisis in the same hospital room with another crisis patient.
- Inform the patient of community resources such as the Sickle Cell Disease Association of America.

Rationales

Contact with similar patients may only intensify behavior if the crisis is precipitated by maladaptive behavior.

Relationships with persons with common interests and goals can be beneficial.

Related Care Plans

Activity intolerance, p. 8
Risk for impaired skin integrity, p. 185
Risk for infection, p. 114

Systemic Lupus Erythematosus

SLE; Lupus

Systemic lupus erythematosus (SLE) is a chronic, autoimmune disease that causes a systemic inflammatory response in various parts of the body. The cause of SLE is unknown, but genetics and hormonal and environmental factors are involved. Under normal circumstances the body's immune system produces antibodies against invading disease antigens to protect itself. In individuals with SLE the body loses its ability to discriminate between antigens and its own cells and tissues. It produces antibodies against itself, called *autoantibodies,* and these antibodies react with the antigens and result in the development of immune complexes. Immune complexes proliferate in the tissues of the patient with SLE and result in inflammation, tissue damage, and pain. Mild disease can affect joints and skin. More severe disease can affect kidneys, heart, lung, blood vessels, central nervous system (CNS), joints, and skin.

There are three type of lupus. The discoid type is limited to the skin and only rarely involves other organs. Systemic lupus is more common and usually more severe than discoid; it can affect any organ system in the body. With systemic lupus there may be periods of remission and flares. The third type of lupus is drug induced. The drugs most commonly implicated in precipitating this condition are hydralazine, procainamide, isoniazid, D-penicillamine, and some antiseizure drugs. Symptoms usually do not present until after months or years of continued administration. The symptoms are usually abolished when the drugs are discontinued.

Women are affected by SLE nine times more often than men, most commonly between 10 and 50 years of age. It is also more common among African Americans and in Asians. That the symptoms occur more frequently in women, especially before menstrual periods and during pregnancy, may indicate that hormonal factors influence development and progression of the disease. For some individuals, the disease remains mild and affects only a few organ systems; for others, the disease can cause life-threatening complications that can result in death. This care plan addresses the nursing management of patients with systemic lupus in an ambulatory setting.

NANDA-I NDx Deficient Knowledge

Common Related Factors

New condition, treatment
Complexity of treatment
Misinterpretation of information
Emotional state affecting learning
Unfamiliarity with information resources

Defining Characteristics

Multiple questions
Verbalizing inaccurate information
Request for information
Inaccurate follow-through on instructions

Common Expected Outcome

Patient verbalizes understanding of disease process and its treatment.

NOC Outcomes
Knowledge: Disease Process; Knowledge: Medication; Knowledge: Treatment Regimen
NIC Interventions
Teaching: Disease Process; Teaching: Prescribed Medications

Ongoing Assessment

Actions/Interventions	Rationales
■ Assess knowledge of SLE and its treatment.	Lack of knowledge about SLE and its chronic and progressive nature can compromise the patient's ability to care for self and cope effectively.

Therapeutic Interventions

Actions/Interventions	Rationales
■ Introduce or reinforce disease process information: unknown cause, chronicity of SLE, processes of inflammation and fibrosis, remissions and exacerbations, control versus cure.	The goal of treatment is to reduce inflammation, minimize symptoms, and maintain normal body functions. The incidence of flares can be reduced by maintaining good nutrition and engaging in exercise habits.
■ Discuss common diagnostic tests.	A variety of immunologically based tests may be performed (e.g., antinuclear antibody [ANA], erythrocyte sedimentation rate [ESR], serum protein electrophoresis, rheumatoid factor, serum complement). Tests may also be indicated to assess for major organ or systemic involvement, such as kidney and liver assessments.
■ Introduce or reinforce information on drug therapy. Instruct the patient in potential effects of steroids, immunosuppressant medication, and other drugs used to treat SLE.	Patients are better able to ask questions when they have basic information about what to expect.
• Nonsteroidal antiinflammatory drugs and COX-2 inhibitors	These drugs are used for their antiinflammatory actions. These agents should never be administered on an empty stomach. Side effects include gastrointestinal distress.
• Antimalarials (hydroxychloroquine, chloroquine)	These medications are used in the treatment of skin and joint symptoms of SLE. Side effects are rare, but patients are cautioned to see their eye physician several times a year to rule out the development of irreversible retinopathy. Patients may also experience mild gastrointestinal disturbances.
• Corticosteroids	This classification of drugs is used for their antiinflammatory and immunoregulatory properties (they suppress the activity of the immune system). The dose is regulated to secure maximum benefits from the drug's administration with minimal side effects. Topical preparations are effective for skin problems. Oral-dose prednisone may be indicated for minor disease effects. Use lowest dose possible. Common side effects include facial puffiness, buffalo hump, diabetes mellitus, osteoporosis, avascular necrosis of the hip, increased appetite, increased infection risk, cataracts, and increased risk for infection.

■ = Independent ▲ = Collaborative

Actions/Interventions	Rationales
• Stress to the patient the importance of not altering the steroid dose or suddenly stopping the medication.	Steroids must be tapered slowly after high-dose or long-term use. The body produces the hormone cortisol in adrenal glands. After high-dose or long-term use of exogenous forms of steroids, the body no longer produces adequate cortisol levels. Increased cortisol levels are needed in times of stress. Without supplementation, a steroid-dependent person will enter addisonian crisis. The nurse must stress the importance of wearing a medical alert tag at all times that states the patient uses steroids and immunosuppressants.
• Immunosuppressants (azathioprine, cyclophosphamide, mycophenolate mofetil)	This classification of drug is used to suppress the activity of the immune system, thereby decreasing the proliferation of the disease, especially during severe flare and in renal or CNS involvement. Side effects include increased infection risk caused by bone marrow suppression, nausea and vomiting, sterility, hemorrhagic cystitis, and cancer.
■ Provide information on appropriate clinical trials.	New therapies for lupus are being researched all the time. Qualified patients may find hope and even relief from symptoms and complications.
■ Instruct the patient to monitor for signs of fever.	Fever is a common manifestation of SLE in the active phase of the disease. Patients should also report accompanying chills, shaking, and diaphoresis. Patients taking aspirin as an antipyretic should have frequent liver studies performed, because aspirin use by patients with SLE has been demonstrated to cause transient liver toxicity.
■ Instruct the patient about the possibility of developing organ system involvement:	
• Renal involvement	About 50% of patients develop some type of glomerulonephritis. This is the most common cause of death.
• Instruct the patient to report changes in urinary output, the presence of edema, elevations in blood pressure (BP), or sudden weight changes.	It is important to report subtle changes in an effort to prevent progression of renal damage through early identification of changing conditions.
• Cardiac involvement	Pericarditis, endocarditis, and myocarditis may occur, although sometimes without any manifestations. Accelerated atherosclerosis may also develop secondary to long-term steroid use.
• Instruct the patient to report tachycardia, shortness of breath, and chest pain.	
• Raynaud's phenomenon	Diminished blood flow to the fingers and toes in response to cold results in color changes that follow a prescribed pattern: blanching or white phase, cyanosis or blue phase, and erythema or red phase.
• Instruct patients to protect extremities from cold exposure, including using oven mitts or mittens when removing food from the refrigerator and avoiding placing feet on a cold floor.	
• Suggest that the patient wear multiple layers of clothing in a cold environment.	
• CNS involvement	Headache, transient ischemic attack, stroke, and depression may occur. Changes in level of consciousness have been reported in the early active stages of aggressive SLE. These changes are often accompanied by an increase in the activity of the disease in other organ systems.
• Pulmonary involvement	Pleuritis or pleural effusion may occur.
■ Instruct in opportunities for support groups in the community or on reputable Internet websites.	Members of groups that come together for specialized problems can be helpful to each other.
■ Instruct in lifestyle activities that can help reduce flare-ups: rest, avoiding sun exposure, engaging in regular exercise, and eating a balanced diet of grains, fruits, and vegetables.	A positive approach to useful therapies allows the patient to be an active partner in treating this chronic condition.

Impaired Skin Integrity

Common Related Factors

Inflammation
Vasoconstriction
Exacerbation of disease process
High-dose corticosteroid use
Use of immunosuppressant drugs

Defining Characteristics

Redness
Pain and tenderness
Itching
Skin breakdown
Oral and nasal ulcers
Skin rash
Diffuse areas of hair loss
Loss of discrete patches of scalp hair
Scalp hair loss possibly accompanied by lesions, scarring, or dry, scaling skin tissue

Common Expected Outcomes

Patient maintains optimal skin integrity, as evidenced by absence of rashes and skin lesions.
Skin lesions are identified early so that treatment can be implemented.
Patient verbalizes ability to cope with hair loss.
Patient identifies ways to conceal scalp loss as required by personal preference.

NOC Outcomes

Tissue Integrity: Skin and Mucous Membranes; Knowledge: Treatment Regimen; Body Image

NIC Interventions

Teaching: Disease Process; Skin Care: Topical Treatments; Skin Surveillance; Body Image Enhancement

---

Ongoing Assessment

Actions/Interventions	Rationales
■ Assess for erythematous rash, which may be present on the face, neck, or extremities.	The classic "butterfly" rash may appear across the bridge of the nose and on the cheeks and is characteristically displayed in the configuration of a butterfly. This is evident in about 50% of patients.
■ Assess skin for integrity.	Small lesions may appear on the oral and nasal mucous membranes. Disklike lesions that appear as a dense maculopapular rash may occur on the patient's face or chest.
■ Assess for photosensitivity.	Patients may respond violently to ultraviolet light or to sunlight. Disease flares or outbreaks of severe rash may occur in response to exposure.
■ Assess the patient's description of pain.	Gathering information about pain can guide treatment. Each individual may exhibit slightly different presentations.
■ Assess the degree to which symptoms interfere with patient's lifestyle and body image.	There is a broad range of behaviors associated with body image changes, ranging from totally ignoring the change to preoccupation with it.

Therapeutic Interventions

Actions/Interventions	Rationales
■ Instruct the patient to clean, dry, and moisturize intact skin; use warm (not hot) water, especially over bony prominences; use unscented lotion (e.g., Eucerin or Lubriderm). Use mild shampoo.	Scented lotions may contain alcohol, which dries skin. Prescribed solutions reduce dryness of the scalp and maintain skin integrity.
■ Encourage adequate nutrition and hydration.	These measures promote healthy skin and healing in the presence of wounds.
■ Recommend prophylactic pressure-relieving devices (e.g., special mattress, elbow pads).	Such devices aid in the prevention of skin breakdown.

■ = Independent   ▲ = Collaborative

Actions/Interventions	Rationales
■ Instruct the patient to avoid contact with harsh chemicals (e.g., household cleaners, detergents) and to wear appropriate protective gloves, as needed. Avoid hair dye, permanent solution, and curl relaxers.	Chemicals aggravate this condition.
For skin rash:	
■ Instruct the patient to:	
• Avoid ultraviolet light.	The sun can exacerbate skin rash or precipitate a disease flare. Special lotions, glasses, and other items may be required to protect skin from exposure to sunlight.
• Wear maximum protection sunscreen (SPF 15 or above) in the sun. Sunbathing is contraindicated.	
• Wear a wide-brimmed hat and carry an umbrella.	
• Wear protective eyewear.	
■ Introduce or reinforce information about use of hydroxychloroquine sulfate (Plaquenil).	This antimalarial drug is a slow-acting medicine used to relieve or reduce inflammation and rash. It may take 8 to 12 weeks for effect. A potential side effect is retinal toxicity. The patient must follow up with an ophthalmologist every 6 months. Topical cortisone medication may likewise be used.
■ Inform the patient of the availability of special makeup (at large department stores) to cover rashes, especially facial rash (e.g., Covermark [Lydia O'Leary], Dermablend, Marilyn Miglin).	These preparations are especially formulated to completely cover rashes, birthmarks, and darkly pigmented areas. This will help the patient who is having problems adjusting to body image changes.
For oral ulcers:	
■ Instruct the patient to rinse mouth with half-strength hydrogen peroxide three times a day.	Hydrogen peroxide helps keep oral ulcers clean.
■ Instruct the patient to avoid spicy or citric foods.	These foods might irritate fissures or ulcers in mucous membranes.
■ Instruct the patient to keep ulcerated skin clean and dry. Apply dressings as needed.	Skin care is necessary to prevent infection and promote healing.
■ Instruct the patient to apply topical ointments as prescribed.	Vitamins A and E may be useful in maintaining skin health.
For hair loss:	
■ Instruct the patient that scalp hair loss occurs during exacerbation of disease activity.	Scalp hair loss may be the first sign of impending disease exacerbation. Scalp hair loss may not be permanent. As disease activity subsides, scalp hair begins to regrow.
■ Instruct the patient that scalp hair loss may be caused by high-dose corticosteroids (prednisone) and/or immunosuppressant drugs.	Hair will regrow as dose decreases.
■ Encourage the patient to investigate ways (e.g., scarves, hats, wigs) to conceal hair loss.	Hair loss may interfere with lifestyle and self-image.

NDx Joint Pain/Stiffness

Common Related Factor

Inflammation associated with increased disease activity

Defining Characteristics

Verbalized complaint of joint pain or stiffness
Guarding on motion of affected joints
Facial mask of pain
Moaning or other pain-associated sounds

Common Expected Outcomes

Patient reports pain/stiffness at a level less than 3 or 4 on a 0 to 10 rating scale.
Patient implements a pain management plan that includes pharmacologic and nonpharmacologic strategies.
Patient is able to participate in self-care activities.

NOC Outcomes

Pain Control; Medication Response; Mobility

NIC Interventions

Analgesic Administration; Pain Management; Exercise: Joint Mobility

Ongoing Assessment

Actions/Interventions	Rationales
■ Assess for signs of joint inflammation (redness, warmth, swelling) or decreased motion.	Usual signs of inflammation may not be present with this disease.
■ Assess description of pain.	Patients with SLE often experience arthralgias of many joints with morning stiffness. Joint stiffness related to SLE may not be related to activity or overuse; it is instead a response to immune complexes proliferating and setting up an inflammatory response in that particular body part. Patients with SLE may also have arthritis; thus stiffness and discomfort are multifactorial.
■ Determine past measures used to alleviate pain.	Patients may not know of or may not have tried all currently available treatments. Pain management is directed at resolution of discomfort as it is presenting at that specific moment in time, because relief measures may change with the joints affected.
■ Assess the impact of pain or stiffness on the patient's ability to perform interpersonally, socially, and professionally.	SLE-related arthritis usually does not result in deformity as in rheumatoid arthritis, but physical activity may still be severely limited at times. Strategies may have to be developed so that the patient is able to maintain a maximum level of function in each of these areas.

Therapeutic Interventions

Actions/Interventions	Rationales
■ Instruct the patient to take antiinflammatory medication as prescribed. Explain the need for taking the first dose of the day as early in the morning as possible with a small snack.	The sooner the patient takes medication, the sooner stiffness will abate. Antiinflammatory drugs should not be taken on an empty stomach.
■ Suggest nonnarcotic analgesics as necessary.	Narcotic analgesia appears to work better on mechanical pain and is not particularly effective in dealing with pain associated with inflammation. Narcotics can be habit forming.
■ If the patient is hospitalized, ask about the normal home medication schedule and try to continue it.	Patients often develop effective regimens for dealing with their disease, and this should be respected.
■ Encourage the patient to assume an anatomically correct position with all joints. Suggest that the patient use a small flat pillow under the head and not use a knee gatch or pillow to prop the knee.	Such measures assist in preventing development of contractures.
■ Encourage use of ambulation aids when pain is related to weight bearing.	Crutches, walkers, and canes can be used to absorb some of the weight from the inflamed extremity.
■ Suggest that the patient apply a bed cradle.	Protective devices keep pressure of bed covers off inflamed lower extremities.
▲ Consult an occupational therapist for proper splinting of affected joints.	Specialty expertise may be required.
▲ Encourage the patient to wear splints, as ordered.	Splints provide rest to inflamed joints and may reduce muscle spasms
■ Encourage use of alternative methods of pain control such as relaxation, guided imagery, or distraction.	These measures may augment other medications used to diminish pain.
■ Encourage the patient to take a 15-minute warm shower or bath on arising.	Warmth reduces stiffness and relieves pain. Water should be warm. Excessive heat may promote skin breakdown.
■ Encourage the patient to perform range-of-motion exercises after the shower or bath, two repetitions per joint.	These exercises help reduce stiffness and maintain joint mobility.
■ Remind the patient to allow sufficient time for all activities.	Performing even simple activities in the presence of significant joint stiffness can take longer.
■ Remind the patient to avoid prolonged periods of inactivity.	Activity is required to prevent further stiffness and to prevent joints from freezing and muscles from becoming atrophied.

■ = Independent ▲ = Collaborative

Fatigue

Common Related Factors

Disease state
Anemia
Depression

Defining Characteristics

Lack of energy, listless, tired
Excessive sleeping
Compromised concentration
Decreased performance
Inability to maintain usual level of physical activity
Inability to restore energy even after sleep

Common Expected Outcomes

Patient verbalizes reduction in fatigue level, as evidenced by reports of increased energy and ability to perform desired activities.
Patient demonstrates use of energy-conservation principles.

NOC Outcomes

Activity Tolerance; Endurance; Energy Conservation; Sleep

NIC Interventions

Energy Management; Simple Relaxation Therapy

Ongoing Assessment

Actions/Interventions	Rationales
■ Assess the patient's description of fatigue: timing (afternoon or all day), relationship to activities, and aggravating and alleviating factors.	This information may be helpful in developing and organizing patterns of activity that optimize the times when the patient has the greatest energy reserve.
■ Determine nighttime sleep pattern.	The discomfort associated with SLE may obstruct sleep.
■ Determine whether fatigue is related to psychological factors (e.g., stress, depression).	Fatigue is best treated by determining the causative factor. Depression is a common problem for people suffering from chronic disease, especially when discomfort is an accompanying problem. Medications are available that are successful in treating clinical depression.

Therapeutic Interventions

Actions/Interventions	Rationales
■ Reinforce energy-conservation principles:	
• Pacing of activities (alternating activity with rest)	The patient often needs more energy than others to complete the same tasks.
• Adequate rest periods (throughout day and night)	Energy reserves may be depleted unless the patient respects the body's need for increased rest.
• Organization of activities and environment	Organization can help the patient conserve energy and reduce fatigue.
• Proper use of assistive and adaptive devices	Adequately used, these devices can support movement and activity, resulting in conservation of energy.
If fatigue is related to interrupted sleep:	
■ Encourage a warm shower or bath immediately before bedtime.	Warm water relaxes muscles, facilitating total body relaxation; excessive heat may promote skin breakdown.
■ Encourage gentle range-of-motion exercises (after shower or bath).	These exercises maximize the muscle-relaxing benefits of the warm shower or bath.
■ Encourage the patient to sleep in an anatomically correct position and not to prop up affected joints.	Good body alignment will result in muscle relaxation and comfort.
■ Encourage the patient to change position frequently during the night.	Repositioning promotes comfort.

Actions/Interventions

- Instruct the patient to avoid stimulating foods (caffeine) or activities before bedtime.
- Encourage the use of progressive muscle-relaxation techniques.
- ▲ Suggest nighttime analgesic and/or long-acting antiinflammatory drug as ordered.

Rationales

Environmental stimuli can inhibit relaxation, interrupt sleep, and contribute to fatigue.

These techniques promote relaxation and rest.

Relief of pain can facilitate rest and sleep.

Related Care Plans

Acute pain, p. 151
Chronic pain, p. 155
Disturbed body image, p. 24
Grieving, p. 82
Insomnia, p. 117
Ineffective coping, p. 49
Self-care deficit, p. 170

Hematolymphatic, Immunological and Oncological Care Plans

■ = Independent   ▲ = Collaborative

Renal and Urinary Tract Care Plans

Acute Renal Failure

Acute Tubular Necrosis (ATN); Renal Insufficiency

In acute renal failure (ARF), the kidneys are incapable of clearing the blood of the waste products of metabolism. This may occur as a single acute event, with return of normal renal function, or may result in chronic kidney disease or kidney failure. Renal failure can be divided into three major types: prerenal failure (resulting from a decrease in renal blood flow); postrenal failure (caused by an obstruction); and intrarenal failure (caused by a problem within the vascular system, the glomeruli, the interstitium, or the tubules of the kidney). Hospital-acquired renal failure is most likely a result of acute tubular necrosis (ATN), which results from nephrotoxins or an ischemic episode. Because of normal declines in renal function related to age, older patients are more at risk when receiving nephrotoxic agents such as intravenous (IV) contrast media or certain medications. During the period of loss of renal function, hemodialysis, peritoneal dialysis, or continuous renal replacement therapy may be required to clear the accumulated toxins from the blood. This care plan focuses on the patient with ARF during hospitalization.

NDx Impaired Renal Function

Common Related Factors

Severe renal ischemia secondary to sepsis, shock, or severe hypovolemia with hypotension (usually after surgery or trauma)

Nephrotoxic drugs (including antibiotics such as amphotericin B or aminoglycosides)

Renal vascular occlusion

Hemolytic blood transfusion reaction

Defining Characteristics

Increased blood urea nitrogen (BUN) and serum creatinine

Reduced creatinine clearance

Urine specific gravity fixed at or near 1.010

Hematuria, proteinuria

Urine output less than 400 mL/24 hr (in absence of inadequate fluid intake or fluid losses by other route)

Weight gain

Hyperkalemia, hyperphosphatemia, hypocalcemia, metabolic acidosis, hyponatremia, and hypermagnesemia

Decreased hemoglobin and hematocrit

Common Expected Outcome

Patient achieves optimal urinary elimination, as evidenced by the following: urine output greater than 30 mL/hr; electrolytes, BUN within or near normal levels; and normal specific gravity.

NOC Outcomes

Urinary Elimination; Fluid Balance; Vital Signs

NIC Interventions

Urinary Elimination Management; Fluid/Electrolyte Management

Ongoing Assessment

Actions/Interventions	Rationales
■ Monitor and record intake and output; include all fluid losses (e.g., stool, emesis, and wound drainage). Report output less than 30 mL/hr.	Patients may exhibit oliguria (less than 400 mL/day) or anuria (less than 100 mL/day) in the early phases of ARF. Their fluid status also changes as they move from an oliguric to diuretic phase. In the diuretic phase the patient is at risk for dehydration and hypokalemia. The diuretic phase of ARF indicates gradual return of glomerular function. Fluid replacement therapy is calculated to replace fluid losses from all sources.
■ Monitor urine specific gravity.	Specific gravity measures the ability of the kidneys to concentrate urine. The ability to concentrate urine is lost in intrarenal failure and remains low at 1.010.
■ Palpate suprapubic area for bladder distention.	Bladder distention indicates that the flow of urine is blocked. Urine backs up into the renal pelvis, resulting in hydronephrosis and anuria. This process is the leading cause of postrenal ARF.
▲ Monitor blood and urine laboratory tests as prescribed:	
• BUN, creatinine	Both BUN and creatinine are elevated in renal failure; however, creatinine is more specific and reliable because it is not affected by diet, blood in the gut, or metabolism.
• Sodium	Hyponatremia is caused by the dilutional effect of hypervolemia because water excretion is impaired.
• Potassium	Levels rise in ARF because the kidneys are unable to filter and excrete potassium.
• Calcium, phosphate	In ARF, the ability to excrete phosphate and to activate vitamin D needed for calcium absorption in the gut is impaired. The serum calcium level falls to less than 8.5 mg/100 mL and serum phosphate is increased to greater than 4.5 mg/100 mL.
• Magnesium	Hypermagnesemia occurs as a result of decreased excretion of magnesium due to the damage of the kidney.
• pH	Metabolic acidosis develops because acid cannot be excreted, and the production of bicarbonate and ammonia (to correct the acidosis) is decreased.
• Urinalysis (especially for protein and blood), urine sodium, creatinine clearance	The presence of protein or blood indicates an abnormal state. The 24-hour creatinine clearance test or outpatient spot urine testing provides evidence of the kidney's ability to clear creatinine. Older patients will normally have a somewhat reduced clearance. A creatinine clearance of less than 10 mL/min indicates kidney failure. Urine sodium concentrations are high with renal damage, yet low with prerenal causes.
• Hemoglobin/hematocrit	Anemia occurs as a result of insufficient erythropoietin production. Erythropoietin is a hormone produced by the kidney that promotes the formation of red blood cells.
■ Monitor daily weights.	Changes in daily body weight reflect changes in fluid balance. Sudden weight gains indicate fluid retention and not true weight gains.
■ Monitor for signs and symptoms of excess fluid volume:	
• Edema (degree and location)	When water excretion is impaired, fluid is retained and moves from the vascular space into interstitial spaces.
• Neck vein distention	Engorgement of neck veins with the head of the bed at 30 to 45 degrees indicates excess fluid volume.

■ = Independent   ▲ = Collaborative

Actions/Interventions	Rationales
• Hypertension	Excess circulatory volume contributes to an increase in blood pressure (BP).
• Crackles	Movement of fluid from pulmonary circulation into alveolar spaces causes adventitious lung sounds.
• Increased respiratory rate	Presence of fluid in the alveoli impairs gas exchange and causes a compensatory increase in respiratory rate.

Therapeutic Interventions

Actions/Interventions	Rationales
▲ Evaluate the cause of the renal failure: prerenal, intrarenal, postrenal.	Medical therapy is determined by the cause of renal failure.
▲ Maintain patency of Foley catheter. If urine output decreases, irrigate catheter with sterile saline solution to ensure patency.	Maintaining catheter patency excludes low urinary tract obstruction as a cause of decreased urine output.
▲ Administer fluids and diuretics as prescribed.	The kidney's ability to regulate fluid balance is lost in ARF, and hypervolemia can easily occur. Close fluid management is important. Volume replacement may be especially important in prerenal causes. Diuretics are used cautiously in ARF. Loop diuretics, such as furosemide, and osmotic diuretics are used most often.
▲ When administering medications (e.g., antibiotics) metabolized by kidneys, remember that excretion of these drugs may be altered. Dosages, frequency, or both may require adjustment.	Drug excretion will be affected by impaired renal function, and increased drug levels and toxicity can occur.
▲ Anticipate renal replacement therapy if conservative management is ineffective.	Hemodialysis is the most commonly used renal replacement therapy for the patient with ARF. Renal replacement therapies are used to clear excess fluid and waste products.

NANDA-I NDx **Excess Fluid Volume**

Common Related Factors
Compromised regulatory mechanisms
Excess fluid intake
Excess sodium intake

Defining Characteristics
Jugular vein distention (JVD), increased central venous pressure (CVP)
Increased BP
Tachycardia
Weight gain, edema
Presence of S_3 gallop
Crackles
Shortness of breath, dyspnea, tachypnea, orthopnea
Restlessness

Common Expected Outcome
Patient is normovolemic, as evidenced by urinary output greater than or equal to 30 mL/hr, balanced intake and output, stable weight, reduction of edema, heart rate (HR) less than 100 beats/min, and absence of pulmonary congestion.

NOC Outcome
Fluid Balance
NIC Intervention
Fluid Management; Fluid Monitoring

Renal and Urinary Tract Care Plans

Ongoing Assessment

Actions/Interventions	Rationales
■ Weigh the patient daily.	Patient weights are a good indicator of fluid status. Weight gains of 1-2 pounds in 24 hours are associated with fluid volume excess.
■ Monitor and record intake and output. Include all stools, emesis, and drainage.	Close monitoring of all fluid losses and urine output is necessary to determine adequate replacement needs and to prevent excessive administration of oral or IV fluids during decreased renal function.
■ Monitor heart rate, BP, and respiratory rate. Inspect jugular veins.	Fluid volume excess causes increased BP, tachycardia, and tachypnea. Jugular verins will be distended.
■ Auscultate breath sounds and heart sounds for signs of fluid overload.	The patient may have crackles and an S_3 gallop. The kidney's ability to regulate fluid balance is lost in ARF, and hypervolemia can easily occur, resulting in heart failure.

Therapeutic Interventions

Actions/Interventions	Rationales
▲ Administer IV medications in least amount of fluid possible.	Fluid intake needs to be reduced during periods of decreased renal function.
▲ Administer oral and IV fluids as prescribed.	If urine output remains high, volume replacement needs can be considerable. The diuretic phase of renal failure requires fluid replacement as well as close monitoring of sodium and potassium levels. With tubular patency partially restored, sodium and potassium losses may occur. The patient may still require renal replacement therapy during this phase for clearance of solutes and toxins.
▲ Administer medications (e.g., diuretics) as prescribed.	Diuretic therapy requires close supervision because reduced blood volume can result in inadequate renal perfusion. Furosemide can be nephrotoxic and may further nephron injury.
■ If peripheral edema is present, move the patient gently and reposition often.	Edematous skin is more susceptible to breakdown.
▲ Prepare the patient for renal replacement therapy if indicated.	Renal replacement therapies such as ultrafiltration or hemodialysis clear the body of excess fluid and waste products.

Risk for Decreased Cardiac Output

Common Risk Factors

Dysrhythmias caused by electrolyte imbalance from ARF:
- Decreased renal elimination of electrolytes: potassium, phosphate, magnesium, sodium
- Metabolic acidosis (present with ARF): exacerbates hyperkalemia by causing cellular shift of hydrogen and potassium; excess hydrogen ions are traded intracellularly with potassium ions, causing increased extracellular potassium
- Hyponatremia: results from excessive intracellular fluid (dilutional effect), edema, and restricted IV or dietary intake
- Hypocalcemia: may also occur; exact cause is unknown

Volume overload leading to heart failure
Pericarditis or pericardial effusion
Dehydration resulting from the diuretic stage of ARF

■ = Independent   ▲ = Collaborative

Common Expected Outcome

Patient maintains adequate cardiac output (CO), as evidenced by systolic BP within 20 mm Hg of baseline; HR 60 to 100 beats/min with regular rhythm; urine output greater than or equal to 30 mL/hr; strong peripheral pulses; warm, dry skin; eupnea with absence of pulmonary crackles; orientation to time, place, person.

NOC Outcomes

Circulation Status; Vital Signs; Electrolyte and Acid-Base Balance

NIC Interventions

Hemodynamic Regulation; Electrolyte Management

Ongoing Assessment

Actions/Interventions	Rationales
■ Assess for signs of decreased CO: change in BP, heart rate, CVP, peripheral pulses; JVD; decreased urine output; abnormal heart sounds; dysrhythmias; anxiety or restlessness.	These signs may indicate decreased CO. Fluid volume excess and electrolyte imbalances can reduce myocardial contractility and lead to decreased cardiac output, especially in older adults and patients with a history of cardiac disease.

▲ Monitor serum electrolytes as prescribed, assessing for electrolyte disturbances:
 Hyperkalemia (potassium greater than 5.5 mEq/liter):
 • Electrocardiogram changes:
   • Increased T waves
   • Widened QRS segment
   • Prolonged PR interval
 • Bradycardic dysrhythmias
 Hyponatremia (sodium less than 115 mEq/liter):
 • Nausea and vomiting
 • Lethargy, weakness
 • Seizures (with severe deficit)
 Hypocalcemia (calcium less than 6 mg/100 mL):
 • Perioral paresthesia
 • Twitching, tetany, seizures
 • Cardiac dysrhythmias
	Electrolyte imbalances can be caused by very high ultrafiltration rates seen in continuous renal replacement therapies (CRRTs). High clearances of small molecules such as sodium, potassium, and bicarbonate occur as a result. Inadequate replacement of fluids and electrolytes during CRRT may also contribute to electrolyte imbalances.

■ Monitor cardiac rhythm.	Hyperkalemia and hypocalcemia can cause life-threatening dysrhythmias. These dysrhythmias can cause serious decrease in cardiac output.
■ Auscultate heart sounds for the presence of a third heart sound (indicating heart failure) or a pericardial friction rub (indicating uremic pericarditis).	If either is present, the patient may require prompt renal replacement therapy. Pericarditis can occur with ARF and develop into a pericardial effusion and even result in cardiac tamponade. Pericarditis is thought to be caused by the presence of uremic toxins in the pericardial fluid.
▲ Monitor chest x-ray reports.	Enlargement of the cardiac silhouette on x-ray film may indicate early signs of heart failure from excess fluid volume.
▲ Monitor for signs and symptoms of metabolic acidosis: • Arterial blood pH less than 7.4 • Altered HCO_3^- (bicarbonate) levels • Plasma bicarbonate levels less than 22 mEq/liter	Decreasing arterial pH and bicarbonate levels indicate metabolic acidosis. In ARF, acidosis develops when the kidney is not able to synthesize ammonia and reabsorb bicarbonate. Acid production in ARF results in a significant decrease in serum bicarbonate. The renal tubular cells are unable to reabsorb bicarbonate ions.

Actions/Interventions

- Increased respiratory rate and depth, dyspnea

- Tachycardia, initially progressing to bradycardia as the acidosis worsens
- Hypotension

- Decreased level of consciousness

- Fatigue and malaise

- Nausea and vomiting

Rationales

The lungs increase the excretion of carbon dioxide in an attempt to decrease the levels of bicarbonate present in body fluids. This mechanism represents respiratory compensation for metabolic acidosis.

Electrolyte imbalances such as hyperkalemia that occur with acidosis can contribute to cardiac dysrhythmias.

At a pH of 7.2 or less, myocardial depression and vasodilation may produce hypotension.

Changes in cerebral blood flow in acidosis can alter neurotransmission.

Acidosis increases cellular resistance to insulin and decreases energy metabolism.

Nausea and vomiting occur as metabolic wastes accumulate in the circulatory system and tissues.

Therapeutic Interventions

Actions/Interventions

▲ Administer medications as prescribed:
- Sodium bicarbonate

- Calcium salts

- Glucose and/or insulin drip

- Potassium exchange resins

▲ Prepare the patient for renal replacement therapy when indicated.

▲ If dysrhythmias occur, treat as appropriate.

▲ Notify the physician of presence of pericardial friction rub.

▲ If signs of decreased CO are noted:
- Administer oral and IV fluids as prescribed. Note effects.

- Administer inotropic agent as prescribed.

Rationales

Sodium bicarbonate will temporarily shift potassium back into the cell. This action helps with the correction of acidosis or hyperkalemia. However, it can result in elevation of sodium and water retention from the sodium load.

Calcium salts treat hypocalcemia. Calcium salts may also be given to stabilize the cell membrane from depolarization in the hyperkalemic state.

Insulin is able to shift potassium back into the cells to correct hyperkalemia. The glucose is administered to prevent hypoglycemia from the effect of insulin.

Resins exchange potassium for sodium in the gastrointestinal tract, thereby decreasing serum potassium levels. The bound potassium is then excreted in the bowel movement. These resins are used to correct hyperkalemia. They may be administered orally or rectally. There is a risk for increasing sodium levels and fluid retention.

Hemodialysis is the most common renal replacement therapy used in ARF. This therapy removes excess fluid and corrects electrolyte imbalances. CRRT slowly removes water, electrolytes, and uremic toxins and is indicated for hemodynamically unstable patients not able to tolerate conventional hemodialysis.

Treating dysrhythmias helps reduce risk for decreased cardiac output.

If pericarditis is present, the patient will need to be started on steroids or nonsteroidal antiinflammatory drugs to reduce inflammation and discomfort. Also, heparin use should be limited to decrease the potential for bleeding into the pericardial space.

Administration of fluids will help increase CO by increasing circulating blood volume.

An increase in myocardial contractility will help increase CO through an increase in stroke volume.

■ = Independent ▲ = Collaborative

Imbalanced Nutrition: Less Than Body Requirements

Common Related Factors
Stomatitis
Anorexia, decreased appetite
Nausea, vomiting
Diarrhea
Constipation
Melena, hematemesis

Defining Characteristics
Loss of weight
Documented inadequate caloric intake
Caloric intake inadequate to keep pace with abnormal disease or metabolic state

Common Expected Outcomes
Patient or caregiver verbalizes and demonstrates selection of foods or meals that will achieve a cessation of weight loss.
Patient weighs within 10% of ideal body weight.

NOC Outcome
Nutritional Status: Nutrient Intake
NIC Intervention
Nutrition Management

Ongoing Assessment

Actions/Interventions	Rationales
■ Assess for possible cause of decreased appetite or gastrointestinal discomfort (e.g., stomatitis, anorexia, nausea and vomiting, diarrhea, constipation, melena, or hematemesis).	Uremia manifestations include gastrointestinal disturbances related to the accumulation of toxins and altered intestinal motility (increased or decreased).
■ Assess actual oral intake; obtain calorie counts as necessary.	This provides accurate measurement of nutritional intake.
▲ Monitor serum laboratory values (e.g., electrolytes, albumin level).	Serum albumin indicates degree of protein depletion (3.8 to 4.5 g/100 mL is normal).
■ Assess weight gain pattern.	Weight gain is often related to fluid retention. A weight increase of ½ to 1 pound a week is associated with increased nutritional intake.

Therapeutic Interventions

Actions/Interventions	Rationales
■ Administer small, frequent feedings as tolerated.	The patient with gastrointestinal symptoms will tolerate small meals better than large meals.
■ Make meals look appetizing; try to eliminate other procedures at mealtime if possible, and focus on eating.	Decreasing distractions at mealtime allows the patient to focus attention on eating. The patient needs to use available energy to increase nutritional intake.
■ Provide frequent oral hygiene.	Frequent oral hygiene will keep oral mucous membranes moist and stimulate saliva production, which can help increase the patient's oral intake.
■ Offer ice chips or hard candy if not contraindicated.	These decrease the discomfort of thirst.
▲ Consult a dietitian.	In general, a diet high in carbohydrates and low in protein is used to reduce catabolism and prevent additional elevations of BUN.
▲ Adjust potassium and phosphorus restriction as indicated.	In ARF, the kidney is unable to excrete potassium and phosphorus. Dietary restriction is needed to keep serum levels within normal limits.
▲ Administer enteral or parenteral feedings as prescribed.	Tube feedings or total parenteral nutrition (TPN) helps maintain optimal nourishment; however, patients are at increased risk for fluid volume overload.
▲ Offer antiemetics as prescribed.	Controlling nausea may improve the patient's appetite and food intake.

Actions/Interventions

▲ Administer antacids and H₂-receptor blocking agents.

▲ Provide renal replacement therapy as ordered.

Rationales

These drugs reduce gastric acidity and prevent mucosal ulceration. Antacids should not contain magnesium because the patient with ARF cannot excrete magnesium, and hypermagnesemia would develop.

Therapy removes uremic toxins and prevents the gastrointestinal complications that result from accumulation of uremic toxins.

Risk for Infection

Common Risk Factors

Uremia resulting in decreased immune response
Use of indwelling catheters, dual-lumen venous catheters, peripherally inserted central catheters, Foley catheters, and endotracheal (ET) tubes

Common Expected Outcomes

Patient remains free of infection, as evidenced by normal vital signs and absence of purulent drainage from wounds, incisions, and tubes.
Infection is recognized early to allow for prompt treatment.

NOC Outcomes
Risk Control; Risk Detection; Immune Status
NIC Intervention
Infection Protection

Ongoing Assessment

Actions/Interventions

■ Assess for potential sites of infection: urinary, pulmonary, wound, or IV line.

■ Monitor temperature.

▲ Monitor white blood cell (WBC) count.

■ Note signs of localized or systemic infection; report promptly.

▲ If infection is suspected, obtain specimens of blood, urine, and sputum for culture and sensitivity, as prescribed.

Rationales

Infection must be monitored closely because there is a tendency for development of infection with ARF. Infection increases the mortality associated with ARF, especially in older patients.

Because of a decreased immune response, an elevated temperature may not be present with infection in the patient with ARF.

The patient's WBC count will increase in the presence of infection.

Infection is the leading cause of death in ARF. Local signs of infection include redness, warmth, and swelling. Systemic signs of infection may include fever, elevated WBC, and fatigue.

Identifying the source of the infection is necessary to plan appropriate therapy.

Therapeutic Interventions

Actions/Interventions

■ Provide meticulous skin care.

■ Use aseptic technique during dressing changes, wound irrigations, catheter care, and suctioning.
■ Avoid use of indwelling catheters or IV lines whenever possible.

Rationales

Skin is the first line of defense against infection. Skin that is clean, dry, and free of prolonged pressure is resistant to breakdown and possible infection.

The patient's risk for infection is decreased when aseptic technique is used during care activity.

Invasive lines increase the patient's exposure to infectious agents.

■ = Independent   ▲ = Collaborative

Actions/Interventions

■ Protect the patient from exposure to other infected people.

▲ If infection is present, administer antibiotics, as prescribed.

Rationales

Visitors, family members, and other patients with obvious infections pose an infection risk to the patient in renal failure who may be immunocompromised.

Treatment of any infection with antibiotics is necessary to prevent further complications associated with infections.

NANDA-I NDx ## Deficient Knowledge

Common Related Factor

New condition

Defining Characteristics

Verbalized confusion about treatment
Lack of questions
Request for information

Common Expected Outcome

Patient and significant others verbalize understanding of ARF and associated treatments.

NOC Outcome
Knowledge: Disease Process
NIC Intervention
Teaching: Disease Process; Teaching: Procedure/Treatment

Ongoing Assessment

Actions/Interventions

■ Assess knowledge and understanding of ARF and its treatments.

Rationales

ARF occurs with an acute decline in renal function, and most patients have no prior exposure to or experience with the cause, treatment, or outcomes of ARF.

Therapeutic Interventions

Actions/Interventions

■ Explain all tests and procedures before they occur. Use terms the patient can understand; be clear and direct.

■ Explain the purpose of fluid restrictions.

■ Discuss the need for a reduced-protein diet.

■ Explain the need for renal replacement therapy as appropriate and what to expect during the procedure.
■ Discuss the need for follow-up visits after discharge.

▲ Encourage family conferences with members of the patient's health care team (e.g., physician, nurses, rehabilitation personnel, dietitians, social workers), as necessary.

Rationales

Patients are more likely to cooperate with care and experience less anxiety when they understand what is happening during tests and procedures.

As the patient moves from the oliguric to diuretic phase, fluid allowances will vary.

The reduced-protein diet helps prevent excessive elevations in BUN.

This therapy may involve hemodialysis, or CRRT.

Return of renal function may occur over a 12-month period, necessitating changes in medications, diet, and fluid restriction, as well as close medical supervision. Occasionally, renal function does not return and instead deteriorates to chronic renal failure.

Conferences facilitate family involvement in multidisciplinary planning. The patient may recover renal function or may need chronic dialysis if there is no return of kidney function.

Related Care Plans

Hemodialysis, p. 801
Ineffective coping, p. 49
Renal failure, chronic/End-stage renal disease, p. 818

Glomerulonephritis

Acute Poststreptococcal Glomerulonephritis; Acute Glomerulonephritis; Rapidly Progressive Glomerulonephritis; Chronic Glomerulonephritis

Glomerulonephritis, or inflammation of the glomeruli, is caused by an immune response to bacterial or viral infection, drugs or other chemicals, immunizations, or systemic disease such as systemic lupus erythematosus (SLE) and scleroderma. It is an autoimmune disease with either antiglomerular basement membrane antibodies or nonglomerular antigens reacting with antibodies and resulting in an immune reaction complement that becomes trapped with antibodies and antigens in the glomerular basement membrane. An inflammatory response occurs, resulting in decreased metabolic waste filtration and increased membrane permeability to large protein molecules. Tubular, interstitial, and vascular changes also occur. Another form of glomerulonephritis is rapidly progressive glomerulonephritis (RPGN). This form of the disease is precipitated by infection and chemicals and by Goodpasture's syndrome, an autoimmune disease that results in destruction of lung and renal tissue. RPGN is characterized by a sudden onset with rapid deterioration. In most cases, treatment requires dialysis and renal transplantation. Renal failure and chronic glomerulonephritis develop in about 50% of patients with RPGN. Chronic glomerulonephritis, which is often asymptomatic and undetected, can also result in renal failure and progress to end-stage renal disease. The more common acute glomerulonephritis (AGN) and acute poststreptococcal glomerulonephritis (APSGN) have less incidence in patients with renal failure (less than1%) or chronic glomerulonephritis (5% to 15%), with complete recovery occurring in most patients.

Excess Fluid Volume

Common Related Factors

Compromised regulatory mechanism (diminished glomerular filtration)
Increased sodium retention

Defining Characteristics

Periorbital edema
Generalized edema
Decreased output, oliguria
Hematuria
Proteinuria
Specific gravity greater than 1.020
Increased blood urea nitrogen (BUN) and creatinine
Mild or moderate hypertension

Common Expected Outcome

Patient is normovolemic as evidenced by absence of edema, urinary output greater than or equal to 30 mL/hr, balanced intake and output, stable weight, HR less than 100 beats/min, absence of pulmonary congestion.

NOC Outcomes
Fluid Balance; Electrolyte and Acid-Base Balance
NIC Interventions
Fluid/Electrolyte Management; Vital Sign Monitoring

■ = Independent　▲ = Collaborative

Ongoing Assessment

Actions/Interventions	Rationales
■ Determine history of illness: • When symptoms were first noticed • Exposure to drugs, recent immunizations • Exposure to other chemicals (hydrocarbons) • Exposure to or recent infection (viral or bacterial) • Known chronic diseases (SLE or scleroderma)	Known precipitants need to be treated or controlled.
■ Assess for edema.	Facial and periorbital edema occurs in the morning, whereas generalized edema appears later in the day and late in the course of the disease.
■ Measure intake and output.	The patient may become oliguric; persistent anuria or oliguria may indicate acute renal failure. A slight increase in output usually indicates increasing kidney function, with diuresis following in 3 to 4 days.
■ Evaluate heart rate (HR), respiration, and blood pressure (BP).	Moderate hypertension is expected; severe hypertension must be treated with antihypertensives. Changes in pulse and respiration may indicate cardiac decompensation from excess fluid volume.
■ Weigh daily.	Rapid weight increase with associated oliguria indicates diminishing renal function and fluid retention.
▲ Evaluate laboratory results: urinalysis, serum electrolytes, BUN, creatinine, erythrocyte sedimentation rate (ESR), and antistreptolysin O (ASO) titer.	Urinalysis may reveal 3+ to 4+ hematuria and proteinuria with increasing specific gravity. Serum electrolyte, especially sodium and potassium, and BUN or creatinine abnormalities reflect altered renal function. ESR reflects acute inflammation and can be used to follow the disease course. ASO titer can be used to detect streptococcal antibodies 4 to 6 weeks after infection.
▲ Review test results: magnetic resonance imaging, ultrasound, computed tomography, and/or possible renal biopsy.	Tests differentiate or confirm diagnosis of glomerulonephritis. Renal biopsy is not always necessary with good-quality radiography.
▲ Assess for hyperlipidemia, hypoalbuminemia, massive proteinuria, and fatty casts in the urine.	Presence indicates development of nephrotic syndrome, seen in approximately 20% of adult cases of glomerulonephritis.

Therapeutic Interventions

Actions/Interventions	Rationales
▲ Restrict fluid intake to equal urinary output and insensible loss.	Fluid intake from all sources (oral or IV) should be limited to replace fluid losses. Limiting fluid intake minimizes risks of pulmonary edema, hypertension, and cardiac failure.
■ Provide a no-added-salt diet.	Increased sodium will increase fluid retention.
▲ Restrict potassium only if the patient is oliguric.	Potassium is retained if the patient is oliguric. Hyperkalemia can cause cardiac dysrhythmias.
▲ Restrict protein if BUN is elevated, indicating increase in circulating nitrogenous wastes.	Increased circulating nitrogenous wastes pose risk for metabolic acidosis, especially if the patient is oliguric.
▲ Administer antihypertensives and, in severe cases, loop diuretics such as furosemide (Lasix), bumetanide (Bumex), or ethacrynic acid (Edecrin).	These medications control blood pressure and fluid volume.
■ Keep the patient on bed rest until hypertension, proteinuria, and hematuria are resolved.	Bed rest decreases metabolic demand and enhances diuresis.
▲ Prepare the patient for possible renal replacement therapies such as hemodialysis.	Patients at risk for significant complications and renal failure can benefit from early initiation of dialysis.

Deficient Knowledge

Common Related Factors

New diagnosis
Hospitalization
Treatment regimen

Common Expected Outcome

Patient verbalizes understanding of the disease process, treatment regimen, and follow-up care required.

Defining Characteristics

Verbalizes inaccurate information
Many questions
Inaccurate follow-through of instructions

NOC Outcomes
Knowledge: Disease Process; Knowledge: Treatment Regimen

NIC Interventions
Teaching: Disease Process; Teaching: Treatments, Procedures

Ongoing Assessment

Actions/Interventions

■ Assess for knowledge of disease process and current status.

Rationales

Most patients have no prior experience with glomerulonephritis.

Therapeutic Interventions

Actions/Interventions

■ Provide information about the course of disease and all treatments and procedures.

■ Explain home care measures: intake and output, BP measurement.
■ Explain the need for follow-up care.

Rationales

This information allows the patient to make informed decisions regarding care. Patients need to understand the importance of dietary and fluid restrictions as part of the treatment plan.

Once stabilized, patients are discharged from the hospital to recuperate at home.

Although most patients (70%) recover completely, there may be persistent hematuria and above-average BUN for some weeks. A small percentage of patients may progress to chronic glomerulonephritis or acute renal failure.

Related Care Plans

Acute renal failure, p. 790
Fatigue, p. 66

Hemodialysis

Internal Arteriovenous Fistula; Graft; Central Venous Catheter

Hemodialysis is the diffusion of solute molecules and fluids across a semipermeable membrane. Dialysis is often necessary to sustain life in persons with no or very little kidney function. Hemodialysis may also be used to remove drugs from the circulatory system as part of the treatment for drug overdoses. Dialysis may be a short-term therapy in situations such as ARF or long-term therapy for the patient with chronic renal failure. The purpose of dialysis is to remove excess fluids, toxins, and metabolic wastes from the blood. The primary mechanisms of dialysis are diffusion, osmosis, and ultrafiltration. The composition of the dialysis

■ = Independent ▲ = Collaborative

solution establishes a concentration and/or osmotic gradient to promote diffusion and osmosis of urea, creatinine, and electrolytes from the blood to the dialysate. Ultrafiltration is used to remove excess fluid by adjusting pressures in the blood compartment and the dialysate compartment. Rapid changes in vascular volume and electrolyte concentrations during hemodialysis can result in complications such as hypotension, muscle cramping, and cerebral edema. Hemodialysis increases the patient's risk for infection. The most common source for infection is through vascular access sites. The incidence of blood borne infections such as HIV and hepatitis B and C has decreased with improved screening of patients and use of dedicated equipment for patients with these infections.

Hemodialysis requires a vascular access. This can be accomplished by surgically creating an arteriovenous (AV) fistula or graft (synthetic material used to connect an artery and a vein); or by insertion of an external catheter into a large central vein. The internal AV fistula is made by surgically creating an anastomosis between an artery and a vein, thus allowing arterial blood to flow through the vein, causing engorgement and enlargement. Placement may be in either forearm, using the radial artery and cephalic vein or brachial artery and cephalic vein. The internal AV fistula is the preferred access for long-term hemodialysis and must heal and mature before it may be used for access in hemodialysis. The central venous catheter may be either single or double lumen. A single-lumen catheter serves as the arterial source, and the venous return is made through a peripheral vein or by the use of an alternating flow device. A double-lumen catheter is used for both the arterial source and the venous return. Because of their location and low durability, femoral catheters are usually used only with inpatients on a short-term basis. Central venous catheters can be used for weeks or even months on an outpatient basis. The use of the fistula, graft, or external catheter should be performed by a trained dialysis nurse.

NANDA-I NDx Risk for Decreased Cardiac Output

Common Risk Factors
Decreased fluid volume
Hypotension
Cardiac dysrhythmias
Anemia

Common Expected Outcome
Patient has adequate cardiac output, as evidenced by systolic BP within 20 mm Hg of baseline; heart rate 60 to 100 beats/min with regular rhythm; strong peripheral pulses; warm, dry skin; eupnea with absence of pulmonary crackles; and oriented to time, place, person.

NOC Outcomes
Cardiac Pump Effectiveness; Circulation Status
NIC Interventions
Cardiac Care; Hemodynamic Regulation

Ongoing Assessment

Actions/Interventions

Predialysis:

■ Assess blood pressure and heart rate.

Rationales

This assessment establishes a baseline for monitoring the patient's vital signs after dialysis. Sinus tachycardia and hypotension are indicators of decreased cardiac output post dialysis. Orthostatic hypotension is an early indicator of deficient fluid volume after dialysis. Rapid removal of fluid volume during dialysis leads to decreased circulatory volume and decreased cardiac output.

Actions/Interventions	Rationales
■ Assess body weight.	Change in body weight is an accurate indicator of fluid losses that are expected to occur during dialysis.
■ Assess level of consciousness; peripheral pulses; capillary refill; heart sounds; respiratory rate and rhythm; skin temperature, color, and moisture.	Establishing a baseline assessment provides for comparison with assessments when the patient completes dialysis. Restlessness, irritability, and decreased concentration occur with changes in cerebral perfusion after dialysis. Weak peripheral pulses with slow or absent capillary refill are indicators of decreased cardiac output. The patient may develop a gallop heart rhythm. Respirations may become rapid and shallow with reduced cardiac output. Cold, pale, clammy skin occurs as a secondary response to compensatory increases in sympathetic nervous system stimulation with decreased cardiac output.
■ Assess for signs of bleeding.	Use of heparin during dialysis increases the risk for bleeding, which can compromise cardiac output.

Therapeutic Interventions

Actions/Interventions	Rationales
▲ Consult with the physician about withholding medications before dialysis.	Vasoactive drugs may contribute to postdialysis hypotension if given before dialysis. These drugs include antihypertensives, antidysrhythmics, and vasodilators. The drugs are usually withheld before dialysis.
▲ Administer intravenous fluids as needed.	Fluid replacement therapy may be indicated to increase circulatory volume after dialysis.

NANDA-I
NDx **Risk for Infection**

Common Risk Factors

Hemodialysis access site
AV access cannulation

Common Expected Outcome

Patient is free of infection as evidenced by normal body temperature and white blood cell count, and no drainage, redness, or swelling at vascular access site.

NOC Outcomes
Infection Status; Risk Control
NIC Intervention
Infection Protection

Ongoing Assessment

Actions/Interventions	Rationales
■ Assess for signs and symptoms of infection: pain around the catheter site or over the access site; fever; red, swollen, warm area around catheter exit or access site; drainage from catheter exit or access site.	Temporary vascular accesses are at highest risk for infection.
▲ Obtain blood and catheter exit site culture if there is evidence of infection.	This culture allows for identification of the causative agent and allows for appropriate antibiotic therapy.
■ Visually inspect and palpate the areas around and over intact dressing for phlebitis, tenderness, inflammation, and infiltration.	Early assessment facilitates immediate recognition of problems that may be life-threatening.

■ = Independent   ▲ = Collaborative

Therapeutic Interventions

Actions/Interventions	Rationales
Central venous catheter:	
■ Maintain asepsis with the catheter during dialysis:	
• Clean area with antiseptic.	The antiseptics used for site care will vary and must be compatible with the catheter material. Commonly used antiseptics include povidone-iodine, chlorhexidine, and electrolyte chloroxidizers (e.g., ExSept).
• Use aseptic technique when initiating or discontinuing dialysis.	This method reduces introduction of pathogens via the access site.
• Disinfect catheter hub caps and blood line connections before separation.	Disinfectants used must be compatible with catheter materials; acceptable agents include povidone-iodine and electrolyte chloroxidizers. Catheter lumens and tips should never be left open to air to reduce the risk for contamination by airborne pathogens.
• Wear surgical masks for all connect and disconnect procedures and dressing changes.	It is important to prevent the spread of infectious droplets that may contaminate connection sites and catheter exit sites.
• Change the sterile dressing over the catheter exit site after each dialysis treatment.	Dialysis units develop policies on the sterile dressing changes.
• Restrict the use of the catheter for no other purpose but hemodialysis.	Use of the catheter for multiple purposes increases the risk for infection.
■ Instruct the patient to keep the dressing clean and dry at all times:	Meticulous care of the catheter site and maintenance of dry intact dressing lessens infection risk. The patient needs to recognize when to seek professional help to maintain the access site integrity.
• Protect the catheter dressing during bathing.	
• Advise against swimming.	
• If the dressing loosens, instruct the patient to reinforce with tape.	
• If the dressing comes off or becomes wet, instruct the patient to go to the dialysis unit, clinic, or emergency department, as appropriate, as soon as possible for aseptic catheter site care if he or she is incapable of performing such care at home.	
AV fistula or AV graft	
■ Maintain asepsis with AV fistula or graft during dialysis:	
• Wash access site with antibacterial soap and water before disinfection and cannulation.	Cleansing the skin first decreases the number of microorganisms present on the skin and increases the effectiveness of antiseptics.
• Disinfect the cannulation sites with antiseptic agent.	Commonly used antiseptics include povidone-iodine, alcohol, chlorhexidine, and electrolyte chloroxidizers.
• Cover cannulation sites with sterile dressings during treatment and after fistula needle removal.	Dressings can usually be removed 4 to 6 hours after dialysis.
• Allow only dialysis staff to cannulate AV access.	Only persons trained to perform venipuncture on a fistula or graft should do so. The access is the patient's lifeline and requires expert care and use.

Risk for Ineffective Peripheral Tissue Perfusion

Common Risk Factor
Interruption in AV access blood flow

Common Expected Outcome
Patient's AV access remains patent, as evidenced by palpable thrill, bruit on auscultation, and adequate color or temperature in extremity.

NOC Outcomes
Circulation Status; Tissue Perfusion: Peripheral
NIC Interventions
Circulatory Care; Skin Surveillance

Ongoing Assessment

Actions/Interventions	Rationales
■ Assess AV fistula or graft for presence of adequate blood flow:	
• Palpate for thrill.	Vibrations should be palpable. This sensation is often compared to that of a purring cat.
• Auscultate for bruit.	A "swishing" sound should be audible. When the artery is connected to the vein, blood is shunted from artery into vein, causing turbulence. This may be palpated above the venous side of the access for thrill or buzzing and is heard as a swishing or bruit with stethoscope auscultation.
• Assess capillary refill.	Refill greater than 6 seconds indicates impaired circulation.
• Check for mottling of skin and temperature of the affected limb.	A cool extremity denotes compromised perfusion.
• Assess for pain in the extremity distal to access.	Pain results from inadequate tissue perfusion.

Therapeutic Interventions

Actions/Interventions	Rationales
■ Instruct the patient to maintain proper positioning of the access limb. Consider elevating the limb postoperatively in an arm sling when the patient is ambulatory.	These actions reduce dependent edema.
■ As the access site heals, encourage normal use of the access limb.	This measure promotes healing and reduces edema.
■ Notify the physician when pain in the extremity is accompanied by decreased sensation and decreased temperature in the extremity with pallor or cyanosis.	These are symptoms of seriously inadequate perfusion that require surgical revision of the access to prevent permanent damage to the extremity's nerves and tissues.
■ Instruct the patient regarding the following preventive measures:	
• Do not allow blood pressure (BP) measurement in access limb.	Activities that constrict arterial blood increase the risk for obstruction of the vascular access.
• Do not allow blood to be drawn from the access limb.	Venipunctures increase the risk for compromised circulation.
■ Instruct the patient to avoid activities that endanger access patency, including the following:	Thrombosis is a common complication of vascular access. Causes include thrombi (caused by venipuncture), extrinsic pressure (BP cuff, tourniquet, sleeping on limb, or tight clothes), or trauma to the access limb (related to activities or sports that involve active use of limb).
• Sleeping on access limb	
• Wearing tight clothing over the limb with access	
• Carrying bags, purses, or packages over the access arm	
• Participating in activities or sports that involve active use of and/or trauma to the access limb	

■ = Independent ▲ = Collaborative

NANDA-I NDx Deficient Knowledge

Common Related Factors
New procedure
New diagnosis
Home management required

Common Expected Outcome
Patient and caregivers verbalize knowledge of hemodialysis and measures to prevent and manage complications.

Defining Characteristics
Questions
Confusion about treatment
Inability to comply with treatment
Lack of questions

NOC Outcome
Knowledge: Treatment Regimen
NIC Interventions
Teaching: Procedure/Treatment; Teaching: Prescribed Activity/Exercise

Ongoing Assessment

Actions/Interventions	Rationales
■ Assess knowledge of dialysis, vascular access, and complications.	Patients receiving hemodialysis in an outpatient center may feel dependent on nursing staff for all care and not realize their responsibility in maintaining the vascular access and preventing complications.

Therapeutic Interventions

Actions/Interventions	Rationales
■ Review the purpose of dialysis and rationale for the access device.	This information reinforces the need for the vascular access placement and maintenance. Patients need to understand that this is their lifeline.
■ Demonstrate and request return demonstration of access care before discharge. Recommend a home health nurse visit as appropriate.	This approach to teaching supports the patient's learning of new skills. The home health nurse can reinforce this learning.
■ Instruct the patient to inform dialysis staff immediately of any signs and symptoms of infection: pain over access site; fever; red, swollen, and warm access site; drainage from access; red streaks along access area.	Prompt intervention is necessary to prevent more serious complications.

■ Explain the importance of maintaining asepsis with the external catheter.
  • Protect catheter dressing while bathing (tub and sponge baths only); no swimming; no showers.
  • Apply dressing to the catheter exit site as ordered.
  • Secure the catheter to prevent tugging and pulling on catheter exit site.
	Infection is almost an inevitable complication of an external vascular device. Infection may be localized cellulitis, but septicemia can occur. Meticulous daily care and avoidance of trauma to the area can lessen the risk for infection.
	This measure prevents accidental dislodging of the catheter.

■ Teach the patient how to manage accidental separation or dislodgment of the external access connections or accidental removal of the central venous catheter.	Information given to the patient or caregiver will increase awareness of troubleshooting measures and reduce possible anxiety.
■ Instruct the patient or caregiver in care of dressings, if applicable.	This knowledge helps reduce the risk for infection.
■ Inform the patient with an AV fistula that maturation may be hastened by exercising: • Begin resistance exercises 10 to 14 days after surgery.	Exercises should be initiated only at the direction of the dialysis staff and physician. Resistance exercises cause vessels to stretch and engorge with blood.

Actions/Interventions

- Use light tourniquet to the upper arm. Be careful, however, not to occlude blood flow with the tourniquet; apply tightly enough to distend vessels.
- Instruct the patient to open and close his or her fist.
- Repeat exercises for 5 to 10 minutes, four or five times daily.
- ■ Teach the patient how to check for adequate blood flow through the fistula or graft:
  - Designate specific areas to feel for pulses and thrill.
  - Demonstrate how to feel for pulses and thrill.
- ■ Discuss dietary and fluid requirements and restrictions: low sodium, low potassium, low phosphorus, adequate protein, high calories, free fluids. Arrange dietary consultation if necessary.
- ■ Recommend medical alert bracelet.

Rationales

This method pumps arterial blood against venous resistance caused by the tourniquet. The patient's squeezing of rubber ball, tennis ball, hand grips, or a rolled-up pair of socks helps exert pressure.

Absence of a thrill may indicate clotting of access with the need to inform dialysis staff immediately. Waiting to de-clot access may result in inability to "save access" and may require surgery to establish new vascular access.

Patients receiving hemodialysis have stricter restrictions than peritoneal dialysis patients because of the intermittent provision of hemodialysis.

The vascular access is the patient's lifeline, which must be treated carefully and used only by a trained dialysis nurse.

Peritoneal Dialysis

Intermittent Peritoneal Dialysis; Continuous Ambulatory Peritoneal Dialysis; Continuous Cyclic Peritoneal Dialysis

Peritoneal dialysis is indicated for patients with kidney failure who have vascular access problems, who cannot tolerate the hemodynamic alterations of hemodialysis, or who prefer the independence of managing their own therapy in their home environment. A peritoneal catheter is placed through the anterior abdominal wall to achieve access into the peritoneum. During peritoneal dialysis, the peritoneum functions as the membrane by which molecules flow from the side of higher concentration to the side of lower concentration. This procedure removes excess fluid and waste products from the body. Peritoneal dialysis may be performed as intermittent peritoneal dialysis (IPD), continuous ambulatory peritoneal dialysis (CAPD), or continuous cyclic peritoneal dialysis (CCPD). Peritoneal dialysis provides more gradual physiological changes than hemodialysis and is appropriate for the older adult patient with diabetes and cardiovascular disease. It is contraindicated in patients with peritonitis, recent abdominal surgery, or respiratory insufficiency because the fluid in the peritoneum decreases lung volume. This care plan focuses on peritoneal dialysis in the acute care setting with teaching for the ambulatory and home care setting.

Excess Fluid Volume

Common Related Factors

Renal insufficiency
Increased peritoneal permeability to glucose, water, and protein

Defining Characteristics

Acute weight gain
Elevated blood pressure (BP)
Peripheral edema
Shortness of breath
Orthopnea
Crackles

■ = Independent ▲ = Collaborative

Common Expected Outcome

The patient is normovolemic, as evidenced by balanced intake and output, stable weight, absence or reduction in edema, heart rate less than 100 beats/min, absence of pulmonary congestion.

NOC Outcomes
Fluid Balance; Systemic Toxin Clearance: Dialysis
NIC Interventions
Fluid Management; Fluid Monitoring; Peritoneal Dialysis Therapy

Ongoing Assessment

Actions/Interventions	Rationales
■ Obtain baseline weight when peritoneal cavity is empty, then every day.	Weight gain can be caused by dialysate reabsorption or fluid excess.
■ Measure inflow and outflow of dialysate with each exchange, checking that the outflow is greater than or equal to inflow, and maintain a record of cumulative fluid balance.	The concentration of the dialysate fluid determines the rate and amount of fluid removal. An acutely ill hospitalized patient may receive 12 to 24 exchanges in 24 hours, whereas with CAPD the patient may only have 4 exchanges daily, with dwell times ranging from 4 to 10 hours.
■ Monitor BP and heart rate (HR).	Increased BP and HR may be an indication of fluid retention.
■ Check catheter for kinks, fibrin, or clots.	Obstruction of outflow of fluid from the catheter may result in retained fluid in the abdomen.
■ Assess work of breathing and for presence of tachypnea, retractions, nasal flaring, and orthopnea.	Patients already fluid-overloaded who receive 1 to 2 liters of additional fluid in the peritoneal space may be significantly compromised. If dialysate fluid is retained in the abdomen, it may cause pressure on the diaphragm, resulting in a decrease in lung expansion and possible respiratory distress.
■ Auscultate lung sounds.	Increased fluid absorption can lead to pulmonary congestion.
■ Check for sacral and peripheral edema from fluid excess or protein depletion from dialysis, especially with more hypertonic dialysates.	Edema may develop if adequate fluid volumes are not removed by the dialysis exchanges or the exchanges are resulting in removing protein that the patient is not nutritionally replacing.
▲ Monitor serum magnesium, potassium, calcium, and phosphorus levels.	Electrolyte imbalances may occur if a balanced concentration of dialysate is not used.

Therapeutic Interventions

Actions/Interventions	Rationales
■ Instruct the patient to change position frequently. Elevate head of bed at 45 degrees, and turn patient from side to side.	Position changes facilitate drainage and help prevent pulmonary complications by preventing an upward displacement of the diaphragm, which can result from inadequate drainage.
▲ Institute fluid restrictions as appropriate.	Fluid restrictions are individualized for peritoneal dialysis patients.
▲ Administer intravenous (IV) fluids via an infusion pump, if possible.	Use of infusion pumps reduces the risk for rapid infusion of fluids into the circulatory system.
■ Elevate edematous extremities.	Elevation of extremities increases venous return and lessens edema.
▲ Notify the physician if electrolyte imbalance is present.	Early intervention can reduce adverse effects from electrolyte imbalances.
▲ In the acute care setting, notify the physician and change the dialysate concentration when the patient reaches dry weight.	Modification of the dialysate concentration prevents dehydrating the patient by removing too much fluid.

Actions/Interventions

- Stop dialysis if drainage is less than infusion.

- Ensure proper functioning if using automatic cycler for the peritoneal dialysis exchanges.

- For home or ambulatory care: instruct in maintenance of fluid restriction and maintenance of a diary monitoring the cumulative record of dialysate inflow or outflow exchange. Also, instruct to obtain daily weights (dry weights) at the same time daily.

Rationales

Overinfusion causes pain, dyspnea, nausea, and electrolyte imbalance.

The cycler may be used to deliver CCPD, IPD, or nightly peritoneal dialysis. For nightly peritoneal dialysis, the machine cycles four to eight exchanges per night with alarms built into the system to make it safe for the patient to sleep at home.

The patient is responsible for monitoring fluid balance.

NDx Risk for Infection

Common Risk Factor

Possible contamination of peritoneal catheter entry site

Common Expected Outcomes

Patient remains free of infection, as evidenced by normal temperature and absence of purulent drainage from wounds, incisions, and tubes.

Infection is recognized early to allow for prompt treatment.

NOC Outcomes
Infection Status; Risk Control
NIC Interventions
Infection Protection; Peritoneal Dialysis Therapy

Ongoing Assessment

Actions/Interventions

- Assess the patient for signs or symptoms of infection: fever; generalized malaise; complaints of abdominal pain, tenderness, warm feeling, or chills; rigid abdominal wall; peritoneal catheter site reddened with discharge; cloudy returned dialysate; positive culture and sensitivity results; nausea; vomiting; or diarrhea.

- Assess peritoneal fluid drainage:
  - Cloudiness (normal is clear)

  - Volume

▲ If infection is suspected, collect effluent as appropriate for the following:
  - WBC count with differential

  - Culture or sensitivity with Gram stain

▲ Assess area around the catheter site. Evaluate purulent drainage by culture and sensitivity.

Rationales

Peritonitis carries a great risk for infection, and repeated occurrences may necessitate catheter removal with need for hemodialysis.

This change in color indicates increased white blood cell (WBC) count.

Decreased volume is noted with increased peritoneal permeability.

WBC count of 100 cells/mm^3 with 50% polymorphonucleocytes indicates peritonitis.

Identification of the specific microorganism is needed for appropriate antibiotic. Gram stain may reveal fungus, which takes 5 to 7 days to grow.

Area should be clean with no signs of inflammation. Culture and sensitivity testing will identify infecting pathogens and guide selection of appropriate antibiotics.

■ = Independent   ▲ = Collaborative

Actions/Interventions

- Auscultate bowel sounds.

- Monitor temperature.
- Instruct the patient in the need to notify the nephrologist, dialysis staff, or home health nurse for any signs of infection.

Rationales

Absent bowel sounds may indicate ileus from bacterial toxins that lead to infection.
An elevated temperature occurs with infection processes.
Treatment can be instituted quickly, and more serious complications can be prevented.

Therapeutic Interventions

Actions/Interventions

- Use strict aseptic technique, and apply a mask to the patient and each person in the room when setting up dialysis and connecting the patient to the peritoneal dialysis tubing set.

- Ensure aseptic handling of the peritoneal catheter and connections.
- Maintain drainage receptacle below the level of the peritoneum.
- Anchor connections and tubing securely.

▲ If peritonitis is suspected administer antibiotics intraperitoneally as prescribed, using shortened dwell periods for the first 24 hours.
▲ Perform exit site care according to unit or agency protocol.

Rationales

Improper technique during connection can lead to catheter site infection, the most common complication of peritoneal dialysis. It is critical to maintain aseptic technique in peritoneal dialysis. The patient should be thoroughly instructed in this technique for home use. Tubing connection devices are commercially available to help maintain an aseptic system.
"Touch contamination" of the catheter and connections increases the risk for infection.
Positioning to promote gravity drainage prevents backflow of dialysate.
Securing all connections and tubing prevents inadvertent disconnection and risk for infection. This also prevents pulling and pressure on the catheter exit site, which can cause skin breakdown and predispose to infection.
Peritoneal administration places medications at the source of infection. Shortened dwell periods are used so that dialysate reabsorption is decreased.
Exit sites are a potential source of infection. Cleansing the area and dressing changes at regular intervals reduce the risk for infection. Each unit has an established exit site care protocol.

NANDA-I NDx Acute Pain

Common Related Factors

Actual infusion of dialysate
Rapid infusion of dialysate
Distended abdomen
Peritonitis
Infusion of cold dialysate

Defining Characteristics

Patient reports pain in abdomen or scapula region
Abdominal guarding

Common Expected Outcomes

Patient reports satisfactory pain control at a level less than 3 to 4 on a 0 to 10 rating scale.
Patient uses pharmacological and nonpharmacological pain relief strategies.
Patient exhibits increased comfort such as baseline levels for pulse, blood pressure, respirations, and relaxed muscle tone or body posture.

NOC Outcome
Pain Control
NIC Interventions
Pain Management; Peritoneal Dialysis Therapy

Ongoing Assessment

Actions/Interventions	Rationales
■ Assess for signs of discomfort during dialysate instillation.	Infusion of larger amounts of dialysate, especially at a rapid rate, can cause abdominal pressure and discomfort or back discomfort from the additional weight. Fortunately, the use of newer cycling systems has significantly reduced this problem.
■ Assess for pain in the scapula region.	Referred pain to the scapula occurs with rapid infusion of dialysate or when air is inadvertently infused into the peritoneal cavity.

Therapeutic Interventions

Actions/Interventions	Rationales
■ For hospitalized patients, remain at the bedside during initiation of dialysis. Do not allow air inflow with the exchange; always use warm fluids.	Cool fluids can cause cramping.
■ Change the patient's position.	Changing position relieves discomfort during inflow.
■ If the patient experiences scapula pain, allow adequate drain time and position the patient on his or her side with knees to chest.	Retention of any air from the peritoneal cavity may cause pain. Positioning facilitates removal of dialysate and air.
■ Explain reasons for inflow pain.	Fluid with a lower pH than the body's causes discomfort until equilibration occurs; air in cavity causes discomfort; pressure on organs and diaphragm causes discomfort until the patient becomes accustomed to the procedure; cold or hot solution may be uncomfortable.
■ If discomfort is associated with flow rate, reduce rate as appropriate.	Rapid infusion rates may lead to abdominal cramping or pain.
■ If lower back pain is the problem, suggest use of an orthopedic binder and regular low back exercises.	These measures support back muscles.
▲ If peritonitis is the cause of pain, administer antibiotics as prescribed.	Antibiotics are required to treat the infectious process. Antibiotics will be adjusted based upon peritoneal fluid cultures.

NANDA-I NDx **Deficient Knowledge**

Common Related Factor

Unfamiliarity with peritoneal dialysis technique and its complications

Defining Characteristics

Verbalizes inaccurate information
Requests information
Expresses frustration and confusion when performing task
Performs task incorrectly
Acknowledges noncompliance

Common Expected Outcomes

Patient or caregiver becomes proficient at performing peritoneal dialysis.
Patient or caregiver is able to verbalize signs and symptoms indicating when to contact health care personnel.

NOC Outcome
Knowledge: Treatment Regimen
NIC Interventions
Teaching: Procedure/Treatment; Peritoneal Dialysis Therapy; Teaching: Psychomotor Skill

■ = Independent   ▲ = Collaborative

Ongoing Assessment

Actions/Interventions	Rationales
■ Assess knowledge of the purpose or goals of peritoneal dialysis.	Knowledge of the goals of therapy is the basis for training on procedural steps, complications, and fluid management goals.
■ Assess understanding of the types of peritoneal dialysis available for the home setting.	Automated cycler machines are most often used while the patient is sleeping at night. Ambulatory techniques requiring manual exchanges (CAPD) are also an option for independent patients.
■ Assess ability to perform tasks related to peritoneal dialysis.	The advantage of peritoneal dialysis over hemodialysis is the greater independence and greater mobility, especially during dialysis with CAPD. The major disadvantage is the possibility of developing peritonitis. The patient or a trained family member needs to be capable of performing the tasks of peritoneal dialysis to be allowed to do home dialysis. Training of the patient and/or family members is a structured process conducted by a peritoneal dialysis training nurse.

Therapeutic Interventions

Actions/Interventions	Rationales
■ Review patient diagnosis and need for peritoneal dialysis.	An understanding of the importance of performing the procedure as prescribed may increase patient compliance.
■ Discuss dietary or fluid requirements and restrictions: low sodium, low potassium, low phosphorus, adequate protein, high calories. Fluids are generally not restricted, but intake should not be excessive. Arrange dietary consultation if necessary.	As a rule, peritoneal dialysis patients have more liberal dietary allowances than hemodialysis patients because of the continuous nature of peritoneal dialysis and the loss of protein during the process.
■ Demonstrate and request return demonstration of peritoneal catheter care.	Catheter-related infection puts patient at great risk.
■ Demonstrate and have patient perform repeat demonstration of dialysis procedure. Emphasize how to adapt techniques to home environment: • Appropriate hand-washing techniques • Steps to peritoneal dialysis: • Ensuring a clean work area • Using appropriate supplies • Checking dialysate for expiration date, dextrose concentration, correct volume, pinhole leaks, and foreign particles • Wearing mask during the procedure • Clamping tubing; using sterile technique when spiking or unspiking from dialysate	Supervised practice of skills and positive feedback from the nurse will add to the patient's confidence about managing peritoneal dialysis at home.
■ When instructing in CAPD, review the use of commercially available devices that help maintain the sterility of the system during tubing connections.	It is of critical importance to maintain sterile technique to prevent infection.
■ Work collaboratively with the patient to fine-tune the length of dialysis, diet regulations, pain management, and diversion needs.	Careful planning helps the patient achieve optimum benefit of the treatment.
■ Provide information on securing materials for traveling and vacations.	Patients must plan ahead when scheduled to be away from home. Supplies may need to be shipped to the destination before travel.
■ Describe signs and symptoms of infection or peritonitis, including basis of occurrence and when to call the health care provider.	Early detection and treatment preserves peritoneal membrane functionality and decreases the loss of membrane surface area and function.

Actions/Interventions

■ Discuss return appointments, follow-up care, and emergency numbers.

■ Arrange for a home health nurse or a peritoneal dialysis training nurse visit, as appropriate.

▲ Arrange a social service consultation, if necessary.

Rationales

Ongoing care on an outpatient basis allows for laboratory monitoring, physical examination, and treatment management discussions.

Home care visits allow for assessment of procedures in the home environment and offer support in the environment where the procedure is conducted.

Patients may have financial needs related to long-term dialysis that can be addressed.

> ### Related Care Plan
> Ineffective therapeutic regimen management, p. 194

Renal Calculi

Kidney Stones; Urolithiasis; Nephrolithiasis; Staghorn Calculi

Renal stones are a common problem, affecting men more frequently than women, and whites more commonly than African Americans. People in warmer climates are more commonly affected, probably indicating that dehydration is a factor. Stones may form anywhere in the urinary tract but most often form in the kidney; they commonly move to other parts of the urinary tract, causing pain, infection, and obstruction. Approximately 90% of stones pass spontaneously. Stones may be treated medically, mechanically (by nephroscopic technique or by lithotripsy [use of shock waves to crush the stones]), or surgically (by pyelolithotomy or nephrolithotomy). Renal stones may be made up of calcium phosphate, calcium oxalate, uric acid, cystine, magnesium ammonium phosphate (so-called struvite stones), or combinations of these substances. Calculi develop in situations associated with decreased urine flow, urinary tract injury, and metabolic disorders that alter calcium balance. Changes in urine pH and side effects of some drugs may also contribute to stone formation. Staghorn calculi are large stones that fill and obstruct the renal pelvis. The process of stone formation begins with supersaturation of the urine by one or more salts. As the concentration of salts in the urine increases, the salts precipitate into a solid state. These solid-state salts form crystals that grow into a stone. This growth process is influenced by the pH of the urine, the patient's hydration status, the presence of other crystals and biological material in the kidney, structural changes in the urinary tract, and crystal growth–inhibiting substances. This care plan addresses management of the patient hospitalized with kidney stones; it also addresses postoperative and postlithotripsy care.

NANDA-I
NDx ## Deficient Knowledge

Common Related Factors

Unfamiliarity with factors related to development of urolithiasis
Unfamiliarity with potential courses of management
Need for long-term management
Need for prevention of recurrence of renal calculi

Defining Characteristics

Multiple questions
Lack of questions
Anxiety about management
Recurrence of urolithiasis

 = Independent ▲ = Collaborative

Common Expected Outcome

Patient verbalizes understanding of factors related to development and recurrence of renal calculi and verbalizes understanding of treatment options.

NOC Outcomes
Knowledge: Disease Process; Knowledge: Treatment Regimen

NIC Interventions
Teaching: Disease Process; Teaching: Prescribed Diet; Teaching: Prescribed Medication; Teaching: Procedure/Treatment

Ongoing Assessment

Actions/Interventions	Rationales
■ Assess knowledge of renal stone prevention.	Recurrence of renal stones may indicate knowledge deficit regarding prevention.
■ Assess for family history of kidney stones.	Incidence of stones is higher among individuals with positive family history.
■ Assess understanding about relationship of diet, fluid intake, activity, and climate to development or recurrence of renal stones.	Restriction of calcium intake may not prevent recurrence of calcium salt stones. Increased protein intake may be a more significant factor in calcium stone formation. Increased calium intake may decrease the formation of calcium salt stones. Studies suggest a relationship between intake of sucrose and sodium with increased stone formation. Persons in the southeastern and southwestern United States are more likely to develop calculi; this is thought to be a result of warmer weather, higher chance for dehydration, and more concentrated urine. Persons who have a sedentary lifestyle or limited mobility are at higher risk for development of calculi because of calcium loss from bones combined with urinary stasis.
■ Assess for history of medical factors that predispose to formation of renal stones.	Medical conditions that result in stasis of urine or calcium imbalance are associated with development of urolithiasis.

Therapeutic Interventions

Actions/Interventions	Rationales
■ Teach the patient about straining all urine.	This procedure detects passage of stone, stone fragments, or gravel. If the type of stone (i.e., composition) is unknown, the stone may be sent to a laboratory for analysis. This assists in planning therapy to prevent the recurrence of stones and for diet modification. Stone fragments may continue to pass for weeks after stone crushing or lithotripsy.
■ Teach the patient the following regarding diet:	
For patients with stones related to hypercalciuria:	
• Limit protein intake.	Diets high in protein are associated with calcium stone formation.
For patients with stones related to oxalate:	
• Foods containing oxalate should be restricted.	These sources of oxalate include green leafy vegetables, coffee, tea, chocolate, colas, peanuts, and peanut butter.
• Add cranberry juice to diet.	Cranberry juice has been shown to decrease the formation of oxalate stones.
For patients with stones related to uric acid:	
• An alkaline-ash diet should be followed.	Foods encouraged on an alkaline-ash diet include dairy products; fruits, except cranberries, plums, and prunes; vegetables, beans, and meats.

Actions/Interventions	**Rationales**
For patients with struvite stones:	
• An acid-ash diet is recommended.	Foods encouraged on an acid-ash diet include meat, eggs, poultry, fish, cereals, and most fruits and vegetables.
■ Teach the patient the importance of maintaining a fluid intake of 3000 to 4000 mL/day.	High-flow, low-solute (dilute) urine prevents stasis and flushes urine crystals from the kidney.
■ Teach the patient about medications used to prevent the recurrence of renal calculi:	
• Sodium cellulose phosphate	This drug binds calcium so that gastrointestinal absorption of calcium is decreased.
• Diuretic agents (thiazide)	These drugs increase tubular reabsorption of calcium, making it less available for calculi formation in the urinary tract.
• Cholestyramine	This drug binds oxalate and enhances gastrointestinal excretion.
• Allopurinol	This drug reduces uric acid production.
• Antibiotics	These drugs are used long-term to prevent chronic urinary tract infections that can be precursors to renal calculus formation.
■ Teach patients to increase activity.	Increased physical activity prevents stasis of urine in the bladder. In men, prostatic hyperplasia and resulting urine stasis may contribute to stone formation.
■ Teach the patient the following about possible courses of treatment:	
• Medical management	Ninety percent of stones pass spontaneously; there may be considerable pain, nausea, and vomiting. If it is thought that the stone is moving and will pass, management will consist of fluid therapy, pain management, and antibiotics to prevent or treat infection caused by stasis of urine and/or obstruction caused by the stone.
• Mechanical intervention	Percutaneous catheters may be used to instill chemicals to dissolve the stone. Nephroscopic procedures using a basket to catch and crush the stone may be used. Use of shock waves, either passed through percutaneous catheters or transmitted through a fluid medium from outside the body (extracorporeal shock wave lithotripsy), may be used to pulverize stones so that the fragments can pass.
• Surgical intervention	Surgical procedures include ureterolithotomy (an incision into a ureter to remove a stone), pyelolithotomy (incision into the renal pelvis to remove a stone), and nephrolithotomy (incision into the calyx of the kidney to remove a stone). Partial or complete nephrectomy may be done if damage or infection from the stone is severe.
■ Teach the patient to report signs of infection:	Early recognition of infection allows for prompt treatment.
• Pain not relieved by medication	
• Fever accompanied by nausea, vomiting, chills	
• Changes in appearance or odor of urine	

Acute Pain

Common Related Factors	**Defining Characteristics**
Irritation by presence of, obstruction by, or movement of the stone	Verbal reports of pain, usually severe
Obstruction of flow of urine caused by the stone	Restlessness
	Grimacing
	Sleeplessness
	Diaphoresis
	Nausea/Vomiting

■ = Independent   ▲ = Collaborative

Common Expected Outcomes

Patient reports satisfactory pain control at a level less than 3 to 4 on a 0 to 10 rating scale.

Patient uses pharmacological and nonpharmacological pain relief strategies.

Patient exhibits increased comfort such as baseline levels for pulse, blood pressure, respirations, and relaxed muscle tone or body posture.

NOC Outcome
Pain Control

NIC Interventions
Pain Management; Analgesic Administration

Ongoing Assessment

Actions/Interventions	Rationales
■ Assess location and duration of pain. Use a quantitative rating scale (0 to 10) to assess pain intensity.	Pain associated with kidney stones is typically located in the flank region and may radiate to the pelvic or abdominal area. The pain pattern is sometimes referred to as renal colic. Patients may report the pain as a 9 or 10 on a pain rating scale. Pain subsides when and if the stone passes into the bladder.
■ Assess symptoms related to severe pain.	Pain related to kidney stone obstruction or movement is commonly severe and may be associated with profuse diaphoresis, nausea, and vomiting.
■ Assess patency of drains or catheters in postoperative patients.	Obstructed flow of urine results in increased renal pressure and causes or intensifies pain.

Therapeutic Interventions

Actions/Interventions	Rationales
▲ Administer analgesics as prescribed; evaluate effectiveness.	These drugs promote comfort and prevent peak periods of pain. Patients may require opoid analgesics for severe pain.
■ Explore and use nonpharmacological pain management methods that have been successful for the patient in the past.	Positioning, distraction, and application of heat may relieve or ease pain and reduce amount of analgesic required. Patients with renal calculi typically assume a crouched, still position; motion may be associated with increased pain.

NANDA-I NDx **Risk for Infection**

Common Risk Factors

Obstructed flow of urine
Stasis
Instrumentation of urinary tract
Percutaneous punctures communicating with renal pelvis
Long-term use of collection devices
Incisions
Presence of gravel

Common Expected Outcome

Patient remains free of infection as evidenced by normal temperature, normal white blood cell (WBC) count, and clear urine.

NOC Outcomes
Infection Status; Risk Control; Risk Detection

NIC Interventions
Infection Protection; Tube Care: Urinary; Incision Site Care

Ongoing Assessment

Actions/Interventions	Rationales
■ Monitor urine output.	Desired urine output is 2000 to 3000 mL/24 hr. The more dilute and the higher the flow of urine, the less stasis there is; this lessens the possibility of further stone formation and increases the possibility that the stone will pass spontaneously.
■ Monitor urine for hematuria, cloudiness, and odor.	Hematuria results from trauma to the urinary tract as the stone moves. Urine cloudiness and foul odor are signs of infection.
■ Observe for the following changes in elimination pattern: • Dysuria • Frequency • Hesitancy • Retention	These symptoms are usually indicative of a urinary tract infection.
■ Monitor temperature.	Urinary tract infection can result in very high fever.
▲ Monitor WBC count.	Elevated WBC count is a sign of infection.
Postprocedure:	
■ Observe percutaneous sites and/or incisions for redness, swelling, and pain.	These manifestations may indicate infection.
▲ Obtain a culture of urine and drainage from around catheters (meatal or percutaneous).	Antibiotic therapy will be based on the specific microorganism causing the infection.
■ Check pH of urine.	Urine with a pH of 6.0 or greater (i.e., alkaline urine) is more susceptible to infection than acidic urine.

Therapeutic Interventions

Actions/Interventions	Rationales
■ Encourage fluid intake of 3000 to 4000 mL of fluid daily.	Increased fluid intake keeps urine diluted and the flow of urine high to prevent stasis and infection.
■ Clean and/or replace leg bags, gravity collection bags, and any other collection system daily.	This measure prevents accumulation of pathogens.
■ Teach and encourage meatal care every 8 hours for patients with indwelling catheters.	This measure reduces pathogens around catheter.
■ Encourage measures to acidify urine. Recommend vitamin C (ascorbic acid), 500 to 1000 mg/day; and cranberry juice, four to six 8-ounce glasses per day.	Acidic urine inhibits the growth of pathogenic bacteria. Cranberry juice yields hippuric acid as it metabolizes and is excreted.
▲ Administer antibiotics as prescribed.	Specific antibiotics will reduce pathogens and resolve infection.
■ If a catheter is removed, encourage the patient to continue drinking fluids; instruct the patient to notify the physician if the patient has not voided 6 hours after catheter removal.	Maintaining urine output is essential to prevent infection, even after the catheter is removed.
■ Instruct the patient to report worsening in pain, fever, or chills.	Patients need to report signs of infection early.
■ Following surgical procedures, teach the patient or caregiver to change dressings over percutaneous nephrostomy tubes and incisions as prescribed, using good handwashing and aseptic technique.	Patients and their caregivers can prevent infection through use of appropriate hygiene measures at home.

■ = Independent ▲ = Collaborative

Renal Failure, Chronic/End-Stage Renal Disease

Uremia

End-stage renal disease (ESRD) is defined as irreversible kidney disease, causing chronic abnormalities in the body's homeostasis and necessitating treatment with dialysis or renal transplantation for survival. ESRD is also called stage 5 chronic kidney disease (CKD). In this stage of CKD the glomerular filtration rate has decreased to less than 15 mL/min/1.73 m². African Americans have a higher incidence of ESRD than whites. Diabetes and hypertension are the most common causes. Uremia, or uremic syndrome, consists of the signs, symptoms, and physiological changes that occur in renal failure. These changes involve all body systems and are related to fluid and electrolyte abnormalities, accumulation of uremic toxins that cause physiological changes and altered function of various organs, and regulatory function disorders (e.g., hypertension, renal osteodystrophy, anemia, and metastatic calcifications). Patients with ESRD may be limited in their ability to carry out normal activities. This care plan may be used for the patient with ESRD in inpatient, outpatient, or at-home settings.

Excess Fluid Volume

Common Related Factors

Excess fluid intake
Excess sodium intake
Compromised regulatory mechanisms

Defining Characteristics

Edema
Blood pressure (BP) elevated (above patient's normal BP) before dialysis
Weight gain
Distended neck veins
Orthopnea
Tachycardia
Restlessness

Common Expected Outcome

Patient is normovolemic as evidenced by normotensive BP, weight gain less than 2 to 3 pounds between hemodialysis treatments, reduction of edema, heart rate (HR) less than 100 beats/min, and absence of pulmonary congestion.

NOC Outcomes
Fluid Balance; Electrolyte and Acid-Base Balance
NIC Intervention
Fluid/Electrolyte Management

Ongoing Assessment

Actions/Interventions	Rationales
■ Assess for signs of fluid volume excess: elevated BP, tachycardia, tachypnea, edema, weight gain, distended neck veins, and orthopnea.	The signs of fluid volume excess are the result of sodium retention and increased intracellular fluid volume.
■ Auscultate for crackles.	Crackles signify the presence of fluid in the small airways.
■ Assess the amount of peripheral edema by palpating area over the tibia, ankles, sacrum, and back and by assessing appearance of the face.	Dependent areas often exhibit signs of edema formation.

Actions/Interventions

- Assess the patient's compliance with dietary and fluid restrictions at home.
- Assess weight at every visit before and after dialysis (weight gain not to exceed 2 to 3 pounds between visits).

Rationales

Excess fluid and/or sodium intake can lead to fluid volume excess in the ESRD patient.

Changes in weight are a reliable measure of fluid gains and losses.

Therapeutic Interventions

Actions/Interventions

- Have the patient sit up if he or she complains of shortness of breath.
- Advise the patient to elevate his or her feet when sitting down.
- Instruct in administration of antihypertensive medications if prescribed.

- Instruct the patient regarding restricting fluid intake as required by the patient's condition.
- Instruct the patient regarding restricting dietary sodium.

- Instruct the patient in methods to relieve dry mouth and maintain fluid restriction:
  - Suggest taking ice chips, as needed.

  - Suggest using sugar-free hard candy or gum.

  - Suggest frequent mouth rinses using ½ cup of mouthwash mixed with ½ cup of ice water.
- ▲ Adjust dialysis therapy as indicated.

Rationales

This position promotes pooling of fluid in the lung bases and makes more lung tissue available for gas exchange.

This position reduces fluid accumulation in the lower extremities by increasing venous return.

Control of blood pressure helps preserve remaining nephron function and slows progression of ESRD. Common medications include calcium channel blockers and angiotensin-converting enzyme inhibitors. As a rule, hypertension management can be difficult in this population and may require multiple medications.

Patients on dialysis need to understand the importance of maintaining fluid balance between treatments.

Sodium intake produces a feeling of thirst. By restricting sodium intake, the amount of fluid a patient drinks can be reduced.

One cup of ice equals only ½ cup of water. Sucking a cup of ice takes much longer than drinking ½ cup of water; patient can attain more satisfaction.

Sucking on hard candy or chewing gum can stimulate saliva secretion and relieve dry mouth.

Rinses can produce freshness in the mouth and temporarily alleviate thirst.

Dialysis treatments are calculated to remove excess fluid and maintain a normovolemic state.

Risk for Decreased Cardiac Output

Common Risk Factors

Fluid volume excess
Electrolyte imbalances
Accumulated toxins
Pericarditis

Common Expected Outcome

Patient has adequate cardiac output as evidenced by systolic BP within 20 mm Hg of baseline; heart rate of 60 to 100 beats/min with regular rhythm; urine output greater than or equal to 30 mg/hr; strong peripheral pulses; warm, dry skin; eupnea with absence of pulmonary crackles; and orientation to person, time, and place.

NOC Outcomes

Circulation Status; Electrolyte and Acid-Base Balance

NIC Interventions

Hemodynamic Regulation; Hemodialysis Therapy; Electrolyte Management

■ = Independent   ▲ = Collaborative

Ongoing Assessment

Actions/Interventions	Rationales
■ Monitor BP and HR.	Hypertension is experienced by the majority of patients with renal failure. Tachycardia may occur as a compensatory response for decreasing cardiac output.
■ Assess skin warmth and peripheral pulses.	Peripheral vasoconstriction causes cool, pale, diaphoretic skin and diminished peripheral pulses.
■ Assess level of consciousness.	Early signs of cerebral hypoxia are restlessness and anxiety, leading to agitation and confusion.
■ Use pulse oximetry to monitor oxygen saturation; assess ABGs as ordered.	Pulse oximetry is a useful tool to detect changes in oxygenation. Oxygen saturation should be at 90% or greater.
■ Monitor for dysrhythmias.	Cardiac dysrhythmias may result from the low perfusion state, acidosis, hypoxia, hyperkalemia, or hypocalcemia.
▲ Monitor laboratory study findings for serum potassium, calcium, phosphorus, blood urea nitrogen (BUN), and creatinine.	These tests provide data on electrolyte imbalances and accumulated toxins. The BUN may also be increased from nonrenal causes such as dehydration; however, in those situations the creatinine will not be elevated. Hyperkalemia can cause the most serious life-threatening dysrhythmias.
■ Auscultate heart sounds for the presence of pericardial friction rub, distant or muffled heart sounds; assess for hypotension and jugular venous distention.	Chronic renal failure patients on dialysis are at high risk for development of pericarditis, increasing the risk for pericardial effusion and pericardial tamponade. Pericarditis is thought to be caused by the presence of uremic toxins in the pericardial fluid. Pericarditis can develop into a pericardial effusion and even result in cardiac tamponade.

Therapeutic Interventions

Actions/Interventions	Rationales
▲ Administer oral and intravenous (IV) fluids as prescribed. Use fluid restriction as appropriate.	Optimal fluid balance improves cardiac output.
▲ Administer medications as prescribed:	These medications temporarily equilibrate electrolyte disturbances and reduce the risk for dysrhythmias.
• Sodium bicarbonate	Sodium bicarbonate will temporarily shift potassium back into the cell to correct metabolic acidosis and hyperkalemia. However, it can result in elevation of sodium and water retention from the sodium load.
• Glucose and insulin drip	Insulin shifts potassium back into the cells to correct metabolic acidosis and hyperkalemia. Glucose is administered to prevent hypoglycemia from the effect of insulin.
• Potassium-exchange resins	These resins exchange potassium for sodium in the gastrointestinal tract, thereby decreasing serum potassium levels. The bound potassium is excreted in the bowel movement.
• Calcium salts	Calcium salts treat hypocalcemia. They may also be given to stabilize the cell membrane from depolarization in the hyperkalemic state.
▲ Administer oxygen as needed.	Oxygen improves arterial saturation.
▲ Treat dysrhythmias as appropriate.	Untreated dysrhythmias contribute to decreased cardiac output.
▲ Administer inotropic agents as prescribed.	These drugs increase myocardial contractility.
▲ Prepare the patient for dialysis when indicated.	Providing information allows the patient to ask questions, discuss fears and concerns, and develop a basic understanding of the treatment process and procedure.

Risk for Injury: Hypocalcemia

Common Risk Factors

Phosphorus retention (level greater than 5 mg/100 mL)
Bone resorption of calcium (demineralization)
Increased parathyroid hormone
Inadequate calcium absorption

Common Expected Outcomes

Patient's risk for hypocalcemia is diminished through ongoing assessment and early intervention.
Patient follows appropriate ambulation and safety measures.

NOC Outcomes

Electrolyte and Acid-Base Balance; Medication Response

NIC Interventions

Electrolyte Management: Hypocalcemia;
Electrolyte Management: Hyperphosphatemia

Ongoing Assessment

Actions/Interventions

- Assess for signs and symptoms of hypocalcemia: tingling sensations at the ends of fingers or around the mouth, muscle cramps and carpopedal spasms, tetany, convulsion.
- ▲ Monitor calcium and phosphorus levels regularly to determine whether the patient is at risk for metastatic calcification from high-calcium replacement and high-phosphate level.
- Assess for signs or symptoms of extremity pain and joint swelling.
- Observe the patient's gait, ambulation, and movement of extremities.
- Assess for history of tendency to fracture easily.

Rationales

The inability of the kidneys to excrete phosphorus leads to hyperphosphatemia with resultant hypocalcemia.

Hypercalcemia can result from the calcium binders used to decrease phosphate levels. Metastatic calcifications occur from calcium phosphate deposits in soft tissues of the body (e.g., blood vessels, joints, lungs, muscles, myocardium, and eyes).
Calcium phosphate deposits can be painful.

Hypocalcemia can lead to bone pain, neuromuscular irritability, and altered mobility.
The decreased blood calcium level causes a demineralization of the bones that makes them brittle, porous, painful, and thinner.

Therapeutic Interventions

Actions/Interventions

- Instruct the patient in the need to restrict dietary phosphorus intake.
- ▲ Administer or instruct the patient to take phosphate-binding medications (e.g., calcium acetate, sevelamer hydrochloride, calcium carbonate) as prescribed. Avoid magnesium antacids that may not be excreted by the impaired kidneys.
- ▲ Evaluate the need for or instruct the patient to take vitamin D analogs as ordered.
- Discuss needed safety measures: uncluttered room, orientation to surroundings, proper lighting.
- ▲ Refer to rehabilitation medicine or physical therapy as indicated for instruction in use of ambulation aids and safe transfer techniques.

Rationales

Phosphorus and calcium have an inverse relationship. Hyperphosphatemia worsens hypocalcemia.
The phosphate-binding medication acts to keep ingested phosphorus from being absorbed; instead, phosphorus can bind with medication and be excreted through bowel movement.

There are several vitamin D analogs that promote calcium absorption.
Bones become so fragile that they break easily, even from mild trauma.
Use of assistive devices for ambulation may reduce the risk for injury.

■ = Independent   ▲ = Collaborative

Renal and Urinary Tract Care Plans

NANDA-I NDx Ineffective Protection: Anemia/Thrombocytopenia

Common Related Factors

Bone marrow suppression secondary to insufficient renal production of erythropoietic factor

Increased hemolysis leading to decreased life span of red blood cells secondary to abnormal chemical environment in plasma

Nutritional deficiencies

Bleeding tendencies: decreased platelets and defective platelet cohesion, inhibition of certain clotting factors

Blood loss related to hemodialysis procedure

Defining Characteristics

Decreased hemoglobin (Hgb) and hematocrit (Hct)

Fatigue or pallor

Decreased platelet count

Increase in coagulation times

Bruising tendencies

Common Expected Outcome

Patient maintains near-normal Hgb and Hct levels and adequate platelet counts.

NOC Outcome
Blood Coagulation

NIC Interventions
Bleeding Precautions; Surveillance

Ongoing Assessment

Actions/Interventions	Rationales
■ Observe for signs of anemia: fatigue, pallor, decreased activity tolerance.	Anemia is associated with decreased oxygen-carrying capacity of red blood cells.
■ Observe for signs of thrombocytopenia: bruising tendencies, bleeding from puncture sites and incisions.	Uremia leads to coagulopathies and increases the patient's risk for bleeding.
■ Use pulse oximetry to monitor oxygen saturation; assess ABGs as ordered.	Pulse oximetry is a useful tool to detect changes in oxygenation. Oxygen saturation should be at 90% or greater.
▲ Monitor results of laboratory studies (Hgb, Hct, platelets, coagulation studies), as prescribed.	The Hct may be as low as 20% to 22% from the reduced secretion of erythropoietin by the kidney. Decreased platelet counts and alterations in clotting factors may occur with dialysis and use of anticoagulants.
■ Test stools and emesis for blood if Hct and Hgb drop.	Gastrointestinal bleeding may be identified by testing for the presence of occult blood.

Therapeutic Interventions

Actions/Interventions	Rationales
■ Instruct the patient in the signs and symptoms of gastrointestinal bleeding.	The patient needs to be alert for signs of bright red blood per rectum or for a change in feces to a black, tarry color and consistency. These changes are associated with gastrointestinal bleeding.
▲ Administer or instruct the patient in administration of epoetin alfa (Epogen), as prescribed.	This decreases the effects of the anemia and helps reduce the need for frequent blood transfusions by maintaining Hgb and Hct.
▲ Instruct the patient to take iron supplements as ordered.	Even with the use of epoetin alfa, functional iron stores may be low.
▲ Instruct the patient in the need for folic acid, as prescribed.	Folic acid corrects iron deficiency. Folic acid is lost during dialysis and must be given after treatments.

Actions/Interventions

▲ Administer oxygen as prescribed.

▲ Anticipate or administer blood transfusions if Hct falls below 20%.

■ For patients with thrombocytopenia, institute precautionary measures for patients with a tendency to bleed: avoid intramuscular injections, and monitor heparin administration closely.

■ Draw all laboratory specimens through an existing arterial or venous access line.

■ Instruct the patient in the use of soft toothbrush and electric razor and in avoiding constipation, forceful blowing of the nose, and contact sports.

■ Instruct the patient to avoid aspirin products.

■ Instruct the patient in the importance of wearing a medical alert bracelet.

Rationales

Supplemental oxygen improves oxygen saturation and arterial PO_2.

With recent advances in medical therapy (e.g., Epogen), blood transfusions are only required for severely compromised patients.

Any needle stick is a potential bleeding site. Heparin is used to decrease the risk for clotting in the extracorporeal circuit during hemodialysis. In patients at risk for bleeding, heparin doses may need to be reduced or discontinued.

Bleeding can occur easily because of platelet abnormalities. Precautionary measures need to be implemented.

These measures reduce the risk for bleeding.

Aspirin inhibits platelet aggregation and prolongs bleeding time.

It is critical to alert community members and health care workers to the patient's medical condition in case of emergency.

NANDA-I NDx **Risk for Situational Low Self-Esteem**

Common Risk Factors

Change in perceptions as autonomous and productive individual

Loss of organ function

Dependence on outpatient dialysis

Financial strain due to disability status or need to seek a less physically demanding job

Disturbed body image

Common Expected Outcome

Patient manifests more positive self-esteem as evidenced by verbalization of positive feelings about self.

NOC Outcomes
Self-Esteem; Coping
NIC Interventions
Self-Esteem Enhancement; Counseling; Support System Enhancement

---

Ongoing Assessment

Actions/Interventions

■ Assess for signs of low self-esteem: self-negating verbalizations, depression, expressed anger, withdrawal, expressions of shame or guilt, or evaluation of self as unable to deal with events.

Rationales

The long-term dialysis patient is faced with long-term changes in lifestyle, occupation, and financial status. The patient's future depends on medications, dietary restrictions, and dialysis. The patient may grieve this loss of autonomy.

■ = Independent   ▲ = Collaborative

Therapeutic Interventions

Actions/Interventions	Rationales
■ Assist the patient in identifying the major areas of concern related to altered self-esteem. Use a problem-solving technique with the patient.	The nurse-patient relationship can provide a strong basis for implementing other strategies to assist the patient and family with adaptation.
■ Assist the patient in incorporating changes in health status into activities of daily living (ADLs), social life, interpersonal relationships, and occupational activities.	As the patient's condition worsens with ESRD, it is more difficult to engage in even routine activities. The patient may have difficulty accepting the need to ask others for help with daily activities.
■ Talk with the patient, caregivers, and friends, if possible, about expectations regarding chronic dialysis or renal transplantation.	Survival depends on such treatments. The patient may resent such dependence.
■ Allow the patient time to voice concerns and express anger related to having a chronic condition.	Denial and anger are anticipated responses to the diagnosis of a chronic illness.
■ Encourage an attitude of realistic hope.	Hope provides a way of dealing with negative feelings.
▲ Use case managers, social workers, and clergy as necessary.	They can provide psychological support and assist in financial arrangements.
■ Provide or encourage discussions with other patients with ESRD.	Such patients can share their responses to illness.
■ Encourage use of support groups.	Groups that come together for mutual goals can be most helpful.
▲ Refer to psychiatric consultant as necessary.	Most dialysis patients experience some degree of emotional imbalance. With professional psychiatric consultation, most patients can gradually accept changed self-esteem.

NANDA-I
NDx # Risk for Impaired Skin Integrity

Common Risk Factors
Edema related to ESRD
Peripheral neuropathy from ESRD

Common Expected Outcomes
Patient's optimal skin integrity is maintained, as evidenced by the absence of breakdown.
Patient demonstrates self-care measures to reduce or treat pruritus.

NOC Outcome
Tissue Integrity: Skin and Mucous Membranes
NIC Interventions
Skin Surveillance; Skin Care: Topical Treatments

Ongoing Assessment

Actions/Interventions	Rationales
■ Assess skin integrity for pitting of extremities on manipulation and demarcation of clothing and shoes on the patient's body.	Chronic fluid excess can result in skin breakdown.
■ Assess for the presence of peripheral neuropathy.	Sensations such as paresthesias (burning), weakness, and twitching are common signs of neuropathy. Altered peripheral sensation reduces the patient's awareness of skin breakdown from prolonged pressure or trauma.
■ Assess for dry, scaling skin.	Uremic skin does not have the usual amount of oil because of decreased sweat and oil glands.
■ Assess for pruritus.	Pruritus can be caused by dry skin and/or calcium phosphate precipitation.

Therapeutic Interventions

Actions/Interventions	Rationales
■ Instruct the patient to wear loose-fitting clothing when edema is present.	Restrictive clothing can increase risk for skin breakdown.
■ Teach factors important to skin integrity: nutrition, mobility, hygiene, early recognition of skin breakdown.	Each factor plays a role in preventing skin breakdown or contributes to successful skin healing if breakdown has occurred.
■ Instruct the patient regarding dangers when heating or cooling devices are used.	The peripheral neuropathy can impair sensation, especially in the lower extremities.
▲ Encourage the patient to take prescribed medications to reduce altered phosphorus levels (phosphate binders).	Elevated phosphorus levels lead to pruritus and excoriation of the skin because of scratching.
■ Stress the importance of not scratching skin and of keeping fingernails short.	Scratching can cause lesions and open sores.
■ Suggest skin lotions or emollients for dry, scaling skin.	Lotions and emollients can provide lubrication and lipids to the skin and provide comfort.
■ Suggest use of tepid water for bathing.	Increased warmth can increase the itch.
▲ Instruct the patient to take medications to reduce pruritus (antihistamines).	Antihistamines can relieve itching.

Risk for Ineffective Therapeutic Regimen Management

Common Risk Factors

Knowledge deficit
Lack of resources
Side effects of treatment, diet, and medications
Poor relationship with health care team
Denial of full extent of disease process and treatment needed

Common Expected Outcomes

Patient demonstrates adherence to treatment plan.
Patient verbalizes intention to follow prescribed regimen.

NOC Outcomes
Compliance Behavior; Participation: Health Care Decisions; Knowledge: Treatment Regimen
NIC Intervention
Self-Modification Assistance; Teaching: Individual

Ongoing Assessment

Actions/Interventions	Rationales
■ Assess for signs of noncompliance: missed appointments, excessive fluid gains between dialysis treatments, unused medications, abnormal laboratory values, acknowledgment of noncompliance, and early treatment termination.	The presence of these factors indicates that the patient is not following the therapeutic regimen.
■ Assess the patient's understanding of the treatment regimen, including dialysis and diet.	The extent of the patient's understanding determines whether an added knowledge base will help decrease the noncompliance.
■ Explore with the patient his or her feelings about illness and treatment.	According to the Health Belief Model, the patient's perceived susceptibility to and perceived seriousness and threat of disease affect compliance.
■ Determine additional factors that may contribute to noncompliance: coping difficulties, medication side effects, financial limitations, transportation problems.	Knowledge of causative factors provides direction for subsequent intervention.

■ = Independent   ▲ = Collaborative

Therapeutic Interventions

Actions/Interventions	Rationales
■ Promote decision making and management of treatment plan; use social support systems.	Social support has been closely linked to compliance with dialysis; it is necessary to manage the role demands of daily living, and it is especially important in coping with stressful life events and transitions.
▲ Explore alternatives with the health care team.	Collaborative planning that includes the patient and family with other members of the health care team can increase the patient's ability to follow a treatment program.
■ Contract with the patient for behavioral changes by establishing goals with the patient.	This method will help encourage cooperation and willingness to follow the established program.
■ If the patient lacks adequate support in following the treatment plan, initiate referral to a support group.	Groups that come together for mutual support and information can be beneficial.

 NANDA-I NDx

Ineffective Sexuality Patterns

Common Related Factors

Effects of uremia on the endocrine system: amenorrhea, failure to ovulate, and decreased libido in females; azoospermia, atrophy of testicles, impotence, decreased libido, and gynecomastia in males

Psychosocial effects of renal failure and its treatment

Defining Characteristics

Verbalization of concern about altered or reduced sexual function

Expressed decrease in sexual satisfaction

Reported change in relationship with partner

Common Expected Outcomes

Patient or couple verbalizes satisfaction with the way they express physical intimacy.

Both members of the couple exhibit behavior that is acceptable to his or her partner.

NOC Outcomes
Sexual Functioning; Self-Esteem
NIC Intervention
Sexual Counseling

Ongoing Assessment

Actions/Interventions	Rationales
■ Assess the patient's perception of change in or lack of sexual function.	Both genders characteristically experience infertility and a decreased libido.
■ Assess the impact of changes in sexual function on the patient.	Changes in sexual function can lead to depression, low self-esteem, and impaired interpersonal relationships.
■ Explore the meaning of sexuality with the patient.	The patient's perception of sexuality provides for a realistic approach to care planning.
■ Assess the need for counseling related to the need for contraception.	With the use of Epogen and with improvement in the female patient's Hgb and Hct levels, menses is often restored and the possibility of pregnancy increases. The patient may need help deciding about becoming pregnant. The outcomes for women on dialysis who become pregnant and the fetus are not positive.

Therapeutic Interventions

Actions/Interventions	Rationales
■ Encourage the patient to verbalize feelings about the change in or lack of sexual function.	Respecting the patient and treating his or her concerns as normal and important may foster greater self-acceptance.

Actions/Interventions

- Discuss alternate methods of sexual expression with the patient or significant others. Emphasize the importance of giving and receiving love and affection, as opposed to "performing."
- ▲ Confer with the physician about medical treatments and procedures that may alleviate some sexual dysfunction. Discuss the possibility of a penile implant or medications. If the patient has low zinc levels, discuss possible replacement therapy for male patients.

Rationales

Patients need to understand that intercourse is not the only method for a satisfying sexual relationship.

Patients may experience restoration of sexual function through use of a variety of therapeutic methods.

Deficient Knowledge

Common Related Factors

Lack of interest in learning
Unfamiliarity with disease process or treatment
Information misinterpretation

Common Expected Outcome

The patient verbalizes understanding of chronic renal failure, prevention of complications, medication therapy, and necessary dietary restrictions.

Defining Characteristics

Questions
Request for information
Verbalized confusion about treatment

NOC Outcomes

Knowledge: Disease Process; Knowledge: Treatment Regimen

NIC Interventions

Teaching: Disease Process; Teaching: Prescribed Diet

Ongoing Assessment

Actions/Interventions

- Assess understanding of ESRD.

Rationales

An understanding of ESRD will help with compliance with the needed treatment.

Therapeutic Interventions

Actions/Interventions

- Discuss end-stage renal failure with the patient, including the need for dialysis or renal transplantation for survival.
- Instruct the patient in dietary restrictions.

- Involve significant others in instruction sessions on special diets and fluid restrictions.
- Discuss the need for reading food labels for sodium, potassium, and other mineral content before using.
- Discuss the importance of taking prescribed medications. Discuss thoroughly dosages and side effects.

Rationales

Patients need information about treatment options in order to make informed decisions.

Diet needs to be individualized according to the impairment of renal function. In general, diets are high in carbohydrates (unless contraindicated by the diagnosis of diabetes mellitus) and within allotted sodium, potassium, phosphorus, and protein limits. Actual daily requirements depend on the type of dialysis treatment used (hemodialysis versus peritoneal dialysis).

Significant others may be the people who buy and/or prepare the patient's food.

Many processed foods contain high levels of sodium. The sodium may be in forms other than salt or sodium chloride.

Patients are better able to manage the complexity of their medications with sufficient knowledge.

■ = Independent   ▲ = Collaborative

Actions/Interventions

- Instruct the patient to notify health care personnel of any questions or concerns regarding over-the-counter medications and food or herbal supplements.
- Instruct the patient in recognition of complications such as fluid volume excess and electrolyte imbalances.

Rationales

This measure helps prevent complications from medications or other substances used inappropriately.

Changes in fluid and electrolyte balance may indicate the need for adjustments in the treatment plan. The patient and caregivers at home need to know early signs and symptoms to report to their health care provider such as headache, swelling of the hands and feet, weight gain of 1 to 2 pounds in 24 hours, or paresthesias.

Related Care Plans

Activity intolerance, p. 8
Disturbed body image, p. 24
Powerlessness, p. 162
Risk for infection, p. 114

Urinary Diversion

Bladder Cancer; Ileal Conduit; Koch Pouch; Nephrostomy; Sigmoidostomy; Ureterostomy; Vesicostomy

Urinary diversion is the surgical diversion of urinary flow from its usual path through the urinary tract. Urinary diversion procedures may be performed as a result of obstruction of the urinary tract; destruction of normal urinary structures by trauma; neurogenic bladder caused by disease or injury; and cancer, usually of the bladder. Bladder cancer occurs more often in older men than in women. When the tumors are superficial in the bladder wall, a variety of surgical procedures can be performed to remove the tumor and maintain normal urinary tract function. These procedures include transurethral resection, laser photocoagulation, and segmental cystectomy. If the bladder tumor is invasive and involves the trigone area, the preferred treatment is total cystectomy with a urinary diversion to maintain outflow of urine. Some procedures result in incontinence and necessitate the wearing of a collection system or pouch. Other procedures reroute the urinary flow to another structure (e.g., a surgically created internal reservoir, colon) from which the urine is eventually excreted (often called continent procedures). Nephrostomy may be performed under fluoroscopic control as an outpatient procedure. Other diversions require open abdominal surgery, and the patient is typically hospitalized for 4 to 7 days. This care plan addresses nursing care for new postoperative patients, as well as for individuals who have undergone urinary diversion at some point in the past.

NANDA-I NDx Deficient Knowledge: Preoperative

Common Related Factor

Lack of previous surgical experience

Defining Characteristics

Questions
Lack of questions
Verbalized misconceptions

Common Expected Outcome

Patient verbalizes understanding of proposed surgical procedure, including permanent loss of urinary continence and postoperative need for a collection system.

NOC Outcome
Knowledge: Treatment Procedures
NIC Interventions
Teaching: Preoperative; Teaching: Procedure/ Treatment

Ongoing Assessment

Actions/Interventions	Rationales
■ Assess the patient's understanding of the proposed surgical procedure:	Options depend on the nature of disease or disorder that makes the urinary diversion necessary.
• Ileal conduit (or ileal loop)	This procedure is the most common type of urinary diversion performed. It uses a piece ("loop") of small intestine as a conduit to which the ureters are attached. One end of the conduit is brought to the anterior abdominal surface as a stoma, over which a pouch must always be worn. An ileal conduit is usually done with cystectomy (removal of the bladder) for bladder cancer.
• Nephrostomy	Percutaneous catheterization of one or both kidneys is usually done when the urinary path is obstructed distally. Nephrostomy may be performed when the patient is not a candidate (e.g., a terminally ill cancer patient or a very poor surgical risk) for more permanent diversion. This necessitates wearing one or two leg bags for collection of urine.
• Sigmoidostomy	The ureters are anastomosed to the sigmoid colon. Urine is excreted with bowel elimination. The patient may experience bowel incontinence. The patient will not have an abdominal stoma.
• Ureterostomy (unilateral or bilateral)	This procedure is implantation of one or both ureters to the anterior abdominal wall as small stomas and is usually done when reestablishment of normal urinary flow is anticipated.
• Vesicostomy	This procedure is usually a temporary urinary diversion performed when the lower urinary tract must be bypassed (e.g., in urethral trauma). An opening is made into the bladder wall, which is attached to the lower anterior abdomen. A pouch must be worn over the vesicostomy stoma to collect the urine. This procedure may also be used to create a continent diversion by using a valve to prevent urine leakage at the stoma.
• Continent urinary diversions (e.g., Koch, Mainz, Indiana, or Florida pouch)	A continent urinary diversion uses a portion of the bowel to surgically create a reservoir that collects urine within the abdominal cavity. A stoma is created on the surface of the abdominal wall. The patient inserts a catheter through the stoma to drain urine from the reservoir.
■ Assess the patient's understanding of the proposed surgical procedure and its relationship to urinary continence.	It is important that the patient understand that the proposed surgical procedure will make him or her incontinent of urine. This incontinence necessitates wearing and maintaining an external collection device. Postoperative adaptation will require management of the collection system and incorporation of the altered function and the collection system into the body image or self-concept of the person.

■ = Independent ▲ = Collaborative

Renal and Urinary Tract
Care Plans

Actions/Interventions

- Assess the patient's knowledge about whether the urinary diversion proposed is temporary or permanent.

- Ask whether the patient has had contact with another person who has a urinary diversion.

Rationales

The patient's ability to cope with changes in activities of daily living necessitated by wearing an external collection device is facilitated when the patient understands that the diversion is permanent. Patients having temporary diversion may decline involvement in self-care and defer care to a family member or outside caregiver.

Previous contact, either positive or negative, influences the patient's perception of what his or her experience will be.

Therapeutic Interventions

Actions/Interventions

- Reinforce and reexplain the proposed procedure.

- Use diagrams, pictures, and models to explain anatomy and physiology of the genitourinary tract, pathophysiology necessitating urinary diversion, and proposed location of stoma:
  - Ileal conduit

  - Nephrostomy
  - Ureterostomy

  - Vesicostomy

- Show the patient the pouch or collection system that will be used postoperatively.

- Offer the patient a visit with a rehabilitated ostomate.

Rationales

Preoperative anxiety often makes it necessary to repeat instructions or explanations several times for the patient to comprehend.

Teaching methods need to be adapted to the patient's learning preferences.

This type of stoma is usually located in the lower right quadrant of the abdomen.

Tubes exit on one or both flanks, just below the costal margin.

This type of stoma is anywhere on the anterior abdominal surface, preferably below the waistline.

This type of stoma is on the anterior abdomen, suprapubic area.

Allowing the patient to wear the pouch or collection device is also helpful and may identify the need for relocation of the proposed stoma.

Sometimes contact with another individual who has experience with the condition is more beneficial than factual information given by a health professional.

NANDA-I NDx Risk for Self-Care Deficit: Toileting

Common Risk Factors

Presence of new stoma
Presence of poorly placed stoma
Presence of pouch
Poor hand-eye coordination

Common Expected Outcome

Patient performs self-care (emptying or changing pouch) independently.

NOC Outcome

Self-Care: Toileting

NIC Intervention

Ostomy Care

Ongoing Assessment

Actions/Interventions

- Assess for the following: presence of old abdominal scars, presence of bony prominences on anterior abdomen, presence of creases or skinfolds on abdomen, extreme obesity, scaphoid abdomen, pendulous breasts, ability to see and handle equipment.

- Assess for patient concerns about caring for stoma and collection pouch.

Rationales

Stoma placement is facilitated by a flat abdomen that has no scars, bony prominences, or extremes of weight. When these factors are present, the stoma site selection may need to be altered to locate the stoma where the patient can see and reach it and where a relatively flat surface for pouching exists.

Patients have many concerns that will influence their ability to successfully manage changes in toileting self-care associated with a stoma. These concerns may include the visibility of the stoma and collection pouch, handling the urine-filled pouch, or a noticeable smell.

Therapeutic Interventions

Actions/Interventions

- ▲ Consult an enterostomal therapy nurse or surgeon to mark the proposed stoma site indelibly in an area that the patient can easily see and reach; where scars, bony prominences, and skinfolds are avoided; and where hip flexion does not change contour.

- If possible, have the patient wear a collection device over the proposed site before surgery; evaluate effectiveness in terms of the patient's ability to see and handle equipment and to wear normal clothing.

Rationales

It is best to determine site selection with the patient in a sitting position. The patient needs to be included in the final decision for stoma placement.

Stoma location is a key factor in self-care. A poorly located stoma can delay or preclude self-care abilities. The patient can be shown how the collection bag works and how it can be covered by clothing.

Risk for Disturbed Body Image

Common Risk Factors

Presence of stoma
Presence of pouch or collection system
Loss of urinary continence
Fear of offensive odor or leakage
Fear of appearing different

Common Expected Outcome

Patient demonstrates enhanced body image and self-esteem, as evidenced by ability to look at, touch, talk about, and care for stoma and collection device.

NOC Outcomes
Body Image; Psychological Adjustment; Life Change

NIC Intervention
Body Image Enhancement; Ostomy Management

■ = Independent   ▲ = Collaborative

Ongoing Assessment

Actions/Interventions	Rationales
■ Assess the perceived impact of change in body structure and function.	The patient's response to real or perceived changes in body structure and/or function is related to the importance the patient places on the structure or function (e.g., a fastidious person may experience the presence of a urine-filled pouch on the anterior abdomen as intolerable, or a person who works out or swims may find the presence of visible tubes protruding from flanks as intolerable). However, some patients will express that such changes are "a small price to pay" for absence of disease.
■ Note verbal and nonverbal references to the stoma.	Patients often "name" stomas as an attempt to separate the stoma from themselves. Others may look away or totally deny the presence of the stoma until they are able to cope.
■ Note the patient's ability or readiness to look at, touch, and care for the stoma and ostomy equipment.	Often the first sign of a patient's readiness to participate in stoma care is when he or she looks at the stoma.

Therapeutic Interventions

Actions/Interventions	Rationales
■ Acknowledge the appropriateness of the emotional response to actual and perceived changes in body structure and function.	Because control of elimination is a skill or task of early childhood and a socially private function, loss of control precipitates a body image change and possible self-concept change.
■ Assist the patient in looking at, touching, and caring for the stoma when ready.	Patients look for reactions, both positive and negative, from caregivers. Positive reactions by the nurse, such as, "The stoma looks pink and healthy," or "The urine is clear and yellow, as it should be," helps the patient develop a sense of normalcy about the change in his or her elimination.
■ Assist patients in identifying specific actions that could be helpful in managing their perceived loss or problems related to their stoma.	Leakage of contents from the pouch, with resultant embarrassment about odor and loss of control, is a major concern. Emptying the collection device when it is about half full reduces the risk of the device leaking. A full device can pull away from the stoma because of the weight of the urine. Assuring the patient that skill will develop and that accidents are preventable will go a long way in helping him or her adapt to the altered structure or function.

NDx Risk for Ineffective Stoma Tissue Perfusion

Common Risk Factors

Surgical manipulation of small intestine (ileal conduit), bladder (vesicostomy), ureters (ureterostomy)
Poorly fitting faceplate

Common Expected Outcome

Patient's stoma remains pink and moist.

NOC Outcome
Tissue Perfusion: Abdominal Organs
NIC Interventions
Surveillance; Ostomy Care

Ongoing Assessment

Actions/Interventions	Rationales
■ Assess the stoma for adequate arterial tissue perfusion at least every 4 hours for the first 24 hours postoperatively:	
• Color of ileal conduit stoma	The ileal conduit stoma is a piece of rerouted small intestine with attached mesentery (blood supply). It should appear pink and moist if perfusion is adequate. Some postoperative edema is expected and will subside over a period of 2 to 6 weeks. When edema becomes severe, venous congestion, evidenced by a purplish discoloration of the stoma, may occur.
• Appearance of ureterostomy stoma	Because the ureters have a small diameter, manipulation at surgery or edema of surrounding tissue can compress the ureters at the skin line and compromise perfusion. Ureteral stomas should appear pink and moist if perfusion is adequate.
• Vesicostomy stoma	This stoma is constructed of inverted bladder that has been surgically sewn to abdominal skin; normal appearance is pink and moist. This stoma is least susceptible to impaired tissue perfusion.

Therapeutic Interventions

Actions/Interventions	Rationales
■ Ensure that the faceplate of the pouch is correctly fitted.	A faceplate that is tightly fitted to the stoma can reduce blood flow to the stoma and impede venous drainage, resulting in further edema and increasing the risk for ischemia.
■ Remove the faceplate, and notify the surgeon immediately if the stoma appears dusky blue, black, or dry.	A stoma that is dusky blue, black, or dry is receiving inadequate blood supply; usually the patient returns to surgery for stoma revision. Although this is primarily a concern during the first 24 to 48 hours postoperatively, patients should be taught to examine stoma color each time they perform a pouch change.

 NANDA-I NDx **Risk for Infection**

Common Risk Factors

Surgical incision
Small bowel anastomosis (ileal conduit)
Anastomosis of ureters to small bowel (ileal conduit), abdominal wall (ureterostomy)
Percutaneous access to renal pelvis (nephrostomy)
Direct opening into bladder (vesicostomy)

Common Expected Outcome

Patient remains free of infection as evidenced by normal temperature, normal white blood cell (WBC) count, absence of signs of local wound infection, and absence of purulent drainage from around nephrostomy tubes and all incision sites.

NOC Outcomes
Infection Status; Wound Healing: Primary Intention

NIC Interventions
Wound Care; Tube Care: Urinary; Ostomy Care; Infection Protection

■ = Independent ▲ = Collaborative

Ongoing Assessment

Actions/Interventions	Rationales
■ Assess surgical incisions and areas around percutaneous nephrostomies for redness, swelling, and suspicious drainage.	These changes may indicate wound infection.
■ Monitor temperature.	Temperature above 38.5° C (101.3° F) after the third postoperative day is an indication of infection.
■ Assess for signs of infection. Possible sites of infection in patients who have had urinary diversion surgeries include the following:	
• Anastomosis of ureters to small bowel • Area where ureters are attached to the abdomen	As the ileal conduit is fashioned, ureters are anastomosed into the segment of small bowel designated for the conduit; breakdown of these anastomoses results in peritonitis because urine spills into the peritoneal cavity instead of traveling to the conduit and out through the stoma. The patient may report abdominal pain and distention.
• Percutaneous puncture sites	These sites are where nephrostomy tubes have been placed.
• Bladder	In patients with a vesicostomy, the bladder communicates with the outside.
■ Monitor urine output.	Diminishing amounts of urine output in patients with an ileal conduit may indicate spillage of urine into the peritoneal cavity.
▲ Send any suspicious drainage from surgically placed drains to the laboratory.	Drainage is analyzed to determine if an internal urine leak is the cause of infection.
▲ Monitor WBCs.	Elevated WBC count is a sign of infection.
▲ Obtain culture of urine.	Laboratory culture determines pathogens present and guides antimicrobial therapy.
■ Check pH of urine.	Urine with a pH above 6.0 (i.e., alkaline urine) is more susceptible to infection than acidic urine.

Therapeutic Interventions

Actions/Interventions	Rationales
▲ Provide wound care to incisions and areas around percutaneous sites, vesicostomy outlet, and ureterostomies, as prescribed, using aseptic technique.	Standard precautions with dressing changes reduce the risk for wound infections.
■ Wash hands before handling any tubes or drains.	Hand washing combined with standard precautions reduces pathogens.
■ Maintain closed drainage systems, and change leg bags, gravity collection bags, and any other collection systems to prevent accumulation of pathogens.	Most patients can expect to wear a single collection device for up to 5 days; keeping the system closed reduces the risk for contamination. Collection devices should be emptied at least every 8 hours to prevent urine being reintroduced into the stoma.
▲ Encourage measures to acidify urine: • Vitamin C (ascorbic acid) 500 to 1000 mg/day	Acidic urine inhibits the growth of pathogenic bacteria.
• Cranberry juice, four to six 8-ounce glasses per day	Cranberry juice yields hippuric acid as it is metabolized and excreted.
▲ Encourage fluid intake of 3000 to 4000 mL daily.	Adequate fluid intake keeps urine diluted and flushes out bacteria.
■ Instruct the patient to report pain, fever, and chills.	Early recognition and reporting of signs of infection allows for prompt treatment.
▲ Administer antibiotics and antipyretics as prescribed.	These drugs eliminate infection and lower fever.

Deficient Knowledge: Stoma Care

NANDA-I NDx

Common Related Factors

Presence of new stoma
Presence of ureterostomy
Presence of percutaneous nephrostomy
Presence of vesicostomy

Defining Characteristics

Demonstrated inability to empty and change pouch
Verbalized need for information about diet, ordor, activity, hygiene, clothing, interpersonal relationships, equipment purchase, or financial concerns

Common Expected Outcome

Patient demonstrates ability to provide care for ostomy, nephrostomy tubes, and/or skin.

NOC Outcomes

Coping; Knowledge: Treatment Regimen; Social Support

NIC Interventions

Home Maintenance Assistance; Teaching: Psychomotor Skill; Support System Enhancement; Ostomy Care

Ongoing Assessment

Actions/Interventions	**Rationales**
■ Assess the patient's perception of ability to care for self at time of discharge.	Preexisting poor eyesight or lack of manual dexterity can be real problems for patients providing self-care.
■ Assess resources (family member, friend, other caregiver) who may be available and willing to assist the patient with care after discharge.	With shorter hospitalizations and same-day surgeries, patients often do not have adequate time for learning and returning demonstration before assuming full responsibility for self-care. Also, concerned others, in addition to assisting with or providing care, are often comforted by being able "to help somehow."
■ Assess the patient's ability to empty and change pouch (ileal conduit, vesicostomy).	Some patients will be independent in emptying their pouch by time of discharge; many will still need assistance and may require outpatient follow-up or in-home care.
■ Assess the patient's ability to care for peristomal skin.	Care of peristomal skin is important to promote skin integrity and reduce the risk for fungal skin infections.
■ Assess the patient's ability to identify peristomal skin problems:	
• Excoriation	This problem appears as a sore, reddened area, most typically the result of a poorly fitted faceplate that allows urine to contact the skin, too frequent changing of the pouch, or frequent accidents in which urine comes into contact with the skin.
• Crystal formation	A collection of white crystals around the stoma or on skin around the stoma or tubes forms when urine is highly alkaline.
• Yeast infection	This type of infection acts as an abrasive, resulting in excoriation, and appears as a beefy-red, itchy area around the stoma or tubes. Infection tends to spread by "satellite," small round extensions at the perimeter of the main area of redness.
• Contact dermatitis	This problem is usually the result of allergy to some product in use around the stoma or tubes and appears as a continuous reddened area; it may itch and feel painful. Contact dermatitis can develop even after years of successful use of products. It is characterized by its size and shape, which approximate the area of contact with the offending product.

■ = Independent   ▲ = Collaborative

Actions/Interventions

- Assess the patient's knowledge about the following:
  - Diet

  - Activity

Rationales

Patients with urinary diversion are instructed to drink 3000 to 4000 mL of fluid per day to prevent stasis and infection. This amount may need to be adjusted for persons with diminished cardiovascular, renal, or pulmonary function.

Patients may bathe or shower with the pouch on or off; patients with nephrostomy tubes should always cover gauze dressings with waterproof dressing (e.g., OpSite, Tegaderm) or with waterproof tape. Other activities are governed by the patient's desire and energy level. Patients may be afraid to engage in usual activities, such as sports or sex. The lack of confidence in abilities usually diminishes as the patient gains control over management of the urinary diversion and fear of an "accident" diminishes.

Therapeutic Interventions

Actions/Interventions

- Provide teaching during the first and subsequent pouch changes or during opportunities to care for nephrostomy tubes.
- Include one or more caregivers as appropriate or desired by the patient.

- Gradually transfer responsibility for care to the patient or family.

- Allow at least one opportunity for supervised return demonstration of a pouch change before discharge from the hospital, or arrange for home nursing care.

- Teach the patient how to care for peristomal skin or skin around the nephrostomy tube:
  - Wash and dry skin around the stoma and tubes using soap and water.
  - Apply a liquid barrier film (Bard Protective Barrier Film, Skin Prep).
  - Change the pouch every 3 to 6 days.

- Discuss odor control, and acknowledge that odor (or fear of odor) can impair social functioning.

- Discuss availability of ostomy support groups.

Rationales

Even before patients are able to participate actively, they can observe and discuss ostomy care.

It is beneficial to teach others alongside the patient, as long as all realize that the goal is for the patient to become independent in self-ostomy care. Patients with nephrostomy tubes cannot reach the flank and will need to rely on another person to provide care.

The patient and caregivers need to gain confidence in their ability to care for the urinary diversion before discharge.

Self-ostomy care requires both cognitive and psychomotor skills; postoperatively, learning ability may be decreased, requiring repetition and opportunity for return demonstration. Teaching in the patient's home setting helps the patient fit the routine and equipment management into his or her own setting. Problem solving small but important issues assists the patient toward adaptation.

Initial cleaning of the skin removes pathogens and skin oils that can reduce adherence of pouching adhesives.

These products protect skin from moisture and any adhesives used in the area.

More frequent changing strips away epithelial cells and can led to excoriation.

Odor control is best achieved by attention to pouch hygiene; urinary equipment can be rinsed with a half-and-half solution of water and vinegar to reduce urinary odor. Certain foods (e.g., asparagus, coffee) cause a disagreeable urinary odor and can be eliminated from the diet to control odor. Patients should not be given "absolutes," but rather assisted in deciding what is worth eliminating versus what is really important or enjoyed.

Ongoing peer support helps the patient gain confidence with long-term ostomy care.

Actions/Interventions

- Instruct the patient to maintain contact with an enterostomal therapy nurse.
- For patients who travel, provide local enterostomal therapy resources and phone numbers.

Rationales

These contacts help the patient with follow-up care and problem solving.

Travel away from home poses special concerns in terms of buying equipment, managing emergencies, and adjusting to different surroundings. Having a resource to call upon often eases these concerns.

Urinary Tract Infection

UTI; Pyelonephritis; Cystitis; Urethritis; Nephritis

Urinary tract infection (UTI) is an invasion of all or part of the urinary tract (kidneys, bladder, urethra) by pathogens. UTIs are usually caused by bacteria, most typically *Escherichia coli,* although viral and fungal organisms may also cause UTI. UTIs may begin as pathogens from the perineum and ascend through the urethra to the urinary bladder. UTIs are common nosocomial infections and often result following instrumentation (e.g., catheterization or diagnostic procedures of the genitourinary tract). The Centers for Disease Control and Prevention (CDC) has prepared guidelines for prevention of catheter-associated urinary tract infections (CAUTI). These guidelines include recommendations for appropriate use of urinary catheters in hospital and long-term care settings, and alternatives to indwelling urinary catheters for management of patient problems with urination. UTIs are more common in women than men, particularly in sexually active, younger women. UTIs, which can be chronic and recurring, can lead to systemic infection such as urosepsis, which can be life-threatening. In older patients, diagnosis and treatment of UTIs may be delayed because patients may be asymptomatic or demonstrate only subtle cognitive changes and urinary incontinence rather than the typical complaints of urgency, frequency, burning, and pain upon urination. If infections of the urinary tract are not treated effectively, renal damage and loss of renal function can occur. The focus of this care plan is care of any individual with a UTI in any setting.

NDx Infection

Common Related Factors

Instrumentation or catheterization
Indwelling catheter
Improper toileting
Pregnancy
Chronically alkaline urine
Stasis (urinary retention)

Defining Characteristics

Burning on urination
Frequency of urination
Foul-smelling urine
Fever/chills
Suprapubic tenderness
Elevated white blood cell (WBC) count
Hematuria
Bacteriuria
Low back pain or flank pain
Fatigue
Anorexia
Incontinence (older adults)
Cognitive changes (older adults)

■ = Independent   ▲ = Collaborative

Common Expected Outcome

Patient is free of UTI as evidenced by clear, non–foul-smelling urine; pain-free urination; normal WBC count; and absence of fever, chills, flank pain, and/ or suprapubic pain.

NOC Outcomes

Infection Status; Medication Response; Urinary Elimination

NIC Interventions

Urinary Elimination Management; Teaching: Prescribed Medication; Fluid Management

Ongoing Assessment

Actions/Interventions

■ Assess for any history that would predispose the person to UTI.

■ Assess for signs and symptoms of UTI: frequency, urgency, and burning or pain on urination, cloudy or bloody urine, complaints of lower abdominal pain or suprapubic pain. Assess for signs that kidneys are involved: flank or back pain.

▲ Assess laboratory data:
  • Urinalysis: hematuria (presence of blood in the urine), pyuria (presence of pus [WBCs] in the urine)
  • Bacteria count in urine

  • Urine culture and sensitivity

  • WBC count

Rationales

History of UTIs, instrumentation, sexual activity, history of sexually transmitted infections, previous surgeries of the genitourinary tract that may have resulted in scarring, and/or recent antibiotic therapy may all place the individual at increased risk for developing UTI.

Frequency of urination, a sensation of urgency, and burning or pain on urination are classic signs of UTI. It is important to note that patients with UTI may be asymptomatic, especially those with recurrent infection; in older patients who may not be cognitively capable of describing symptoms, a general change in behavior or decline in overall functional ability often heralds a UTI. Confusion and incontinence are often the only signs of UTI in the older adult.

The inflammatory response associated with infection leads to red blood cells and white blood cells in the urine.

Bacterial counts of 10^5 are usually considered diagnostic for UTI, although lower counts may also indicate UTI.

Identification of the causative organism is necessary for selecting the most effective antibiotic.

Leukocytosis is a systemic response to infection.

Therapeutic Interventions

Actions/Interventions

■ Encourage the patient to drink extra fluid.

■ Instruct the patient to void often (every 2 to 3 hours during the day) and to empty the bladder completely.

■ Suggest cranberry or prune juice, or vitamin C, 500 mg to 1000 mg/day.

■ Encourage the patient to finish all prescribed antibiotics; note effectiveness.

■ Limit use of indwelling bladder catheters to manage incontinence.

Rationales

Fluid promotes urine production, and flushes bacteria from the urinary tract; minimum fluid intake is 2 to 3 L/day.

A regular pattern of urination enhances bacterial clearance, reduces urine stasis, and prevents reinfection; voiding in an upright position can facilitate bladder emptying.

These measures acidify urine; bacteria grow poorly in an acidic environment. Ideal urine pH is around 5. Cranberry juice has been shown to decrease bacterial adherence to the bladder wall. The juice may take several weeks to produce a therapeutic result.

Drugs may be used in combination (i.e., more than one antimicrobial at a time) to reduce development of bacterial resistance. The usual length of antibiotic therapy is 5 to 10 days; patients with pyelonephritis typically require a 3- or 4-day course of parenteral antibiotics to prevent bacteremia and sepsis. Long-term antibiotic therapy may be prescribed for patients with chronic UTIs.

Catheters increase the risk for infection. Other measures such as regular toileting can prevent infection.

Acte Pain

Common Related Factor
Infection

Defining Characteristics
Burning on urination
Cramps or spasm in lower back and bladder area
Facial mask of pain
Guarding behavior
Protective decreased physical activity

Common Expected Outcomes
Patient reports satisfactory pain control at a level less than 3 to 4 on a 0 to 10 rating scale.
Patient uses pharmacological and nonpharmacological pain relief strategies.
Patient exhibits increased comfort such as baseline levels for pulse, blood pressure, respirations, and relaxed muscle tone or body posture.

NOC Outcome
Pain Control
NIC Interventions
Heat/Cold Application; Pain Management

Ongoing Assessment

Actions/Interventions

■ Assess the patient's description of pain. Inquire as to the quality, nature, and severity of pain.

Rationales

Typically, pain associated with UTI is described as burning on urination. Patients may also experience lower abdominal or suprapubic pain. Patients with renal involvement (i.e., pyelonephritis) will have back or flank pain. Some patients are asymptomatic.

Therapeutic Interventions

Actions/Interventions

■ Apply a heating pad to the suprapubic area or lower back.
■ Instruct the patient in use of a sitz bath.
▲ Encourage use of analgesics (e.g., acetaminophen) and/or antispasmodics (e.g., phenazopyridine), as prescribed.
■ Use distraction and relaxation techniques whenever appropriate.

Rationales

This measure relieves pain.
Sitz baths may reduce perineal discomfort and pain.
These drugs relieve pain and bladder spasms caused by UTI.

Complementary and alternative therapies provide nonpharmacological approaches to pain management.

 Deficient Knowledge

Common Related Factor
Unfamiliarity with nature and treatment of UTI

Defining Characteristics
Verbalizing inaccurate information
Multiple questions
Lack of questions
Recurrent UTI

Common Expected Outcome
Patient verbalizes knowledge of causes and treatment of UTI, controls risk factors, and completes medical treatment of UTI.

NOC Outcome
Knowledge: Treatment Regimen
NIC Interventions
Teaching: Disease Process; Teaching: Prescribed Medication

■ = Independent   ▲ = Collaborative

Ongoing Assessment

Actions/Interventions	Rationales
■ Assess knowledge of UTI risk factors, prevention, and treatment.	Frequent recurrences of UTI may indicate that the patient does not understand risk factors or medical management of UTI.

Therapeutic Interventions

Actions/Interventions	Rationales
■ Provide health teaching. Teach the patient:	The goal of patient teaching is to resolve the current infection and prevent recurrence.
• Need for follow-up urine cultures	Periodic urine cultures determine effectiveness of the antimicrobial therapy.
• Need for frequent bladder emptying	Voiding at first urge prevents stasis of urine in the bladder and minimizes the opportunity for bacterial growth.
• Hygienic measures; showering is preferable to tub bathing	Good hygiene decreases concentration of pathogens.
• Wiping from front to back	This technique prevents the introduction of enteric pathogens into the urethra.
• Need for changing underpants daily and wearing well-ventilated clothing (e.g., cotton underpants, cotton-crotched pantyhose) and avoidance of tight or constricting underwear or pants.	Synthetic materials harbor moisture and provide a medium for perineal bacterial growth.
■ Teach the patient to complete full course of antibiotic medication, even if symptoms resolve.	Urinary symptoms of burning, frequency, and urgency often resolve in the first few days of antibiotic therapy. Patients may discontinue drug therapy because they feel better. If the full course of drug therapy is not completed, the bacterial colony will grow and cause recurrent infection.
■ Encourage reporting of signs and symptoms of recurrence.	One to 2 weeks after completion of a course of antimicrobial therapy is a common time frame for signs and symptoms to recur.

Related Care Plans

Acute pain, p. 151
Risk for infection, p. 114

Men's Health Care Plans

Benign Prostatic Hyperplasia (BPH)

Benign prostatic hyperplasia (BPH) is a common urological disorder in men, and its incidence is age related. The prevalence rises from approximately 20% in men 41 to 50 years of age to 50% in men 51 to 60 years of age, then to more than 90% in men 80 years of age and older. BPH is an overgrowth of muscle and connective tissue (hyperplasia) of the prostate gland. As the glandular tissue enlarges, it causes obstruction of the urethra. Severity of symptoms may be ranked according to the American Urological Symptom Index. Early diagnosis and staging have improved with the availability of prostate ultrasound technology. Treatment options include medications that cause either regression of overgrown tissue or relaxation of the urethral muscle tissue; nonsurgical treatment, including direct heat application, dilatation, laser, or placement of stents to allow drainage; and surgical treatment to remove prostate tissue. The focus of this care plan is the patient with newly diagnosed BPH.

 NANDA-I NDx **Urinary Retention**

Common Related Factor

Urethral blockage

Defining Characteristics

Obstructive symptoms:
- Hesitancy
- Straining to start void
- Bladder distention
- Weak or narrowed stream
- Increased residual urine volume

Irritative symptoms:
- Frequency
- Urgency
- Nocturia

Common Expected Outcome

Patient has unobstructed flow of urine and empties bladder completely, either by medications, catheterization, after medical or noninvasive therapies, or after surgical removal of hyperplastic prostatic tissue.

NOC Outcome
Urinary Elimination

NIC Interventions
Urinary Catheterization; Urinary Elimination Management

Ongoing Assessment

Actions/Interventions	Rationales
■ Assess urinary elimination; inquire about obstructive symptoms, which include hesitancy, difficulty starting a stream, dribbling at the end of a void, straining to void, weak or narrow stream, and irritative symptoms such as frequency, urgency, and nocturia.	The male urethra is surrounded by the prostate gland. When the prostate gland is enlarged as a result of prostatic hyperplasia, the urethra is compressed; symptoms are a result of the decreased caliber of the urethra. Irritative symptoms occur because of obstruction that causes a hypersensitivity of the bladder.
■ Assess history of urinary tract infections (UTIs).	Because the flow of urine is chronically obstructed, stasis of urine occurs and infections are common.
■ Assess the symptom severity of BPH according to the American Urological Association's Symptom Score for BPH (Table 10-1).	This tool provides serial objective measurements of symptom severity.
■ Assess for pain or discomfort.	Pain may be related to concurrent urinary tract infection, residual urine, or bladder distention.
■ Assess for any over-the-counter (OTC) medication use.	OTC decongestants and antihistamines can slow urinary flow and increase symptoms.
■ Percuss and palpate the abdomen for distended bladder.	The lower abdomen becomes distended as the urine volume increases in the bladder. Urinary retention is a key symptom.
■ Assess postvoid residual urine (PVU).	Data aid in detection of urinary stasis and impaired detrusor function. PVU can be assessed by postvoid catheterization, x-ray films, or most simply by ultrasound.
■ Assess intake and output, noting the amount and frequency of voids.	Data give clues to completion of bladder emptying.
■ Assess for hematuria.	Hematuria can result from distention of the bladder with resultant rupture of small blood vessels.
▲ Review x-ray films or ultrasound findings.	Hydroureters (distended ureters) and hydronephrosis (enlarged, overdistended kidneys) may result from longstanding obstruction caused by prostatic disease.

Therapeutic Interventions

Actions/Interventions	Rationales
■ Encourage oral fluids for adequate hydration, but do not push fluids or overhydrate.	Rapid filling of the bladder can precipitate complete urinary retention. Overhydration can aggravate problem of residual urine and bladder distention. Coffee and other caffeinated beverages can increase urine amount and urgency.
▲ Prepare the patient for the possible need for an indwelling catheter to restore flow of urine. NOTE: Special catheters with curved or firm tips may be needed to accomplish catheterization in the patient with an enlarged prostate.	Indwelling catheterization is used to allow free drainage of the bladder. Chronic urinary obstruction can result in severe damage to the kidneys and, ultimately, renal failure.
■ Encourage the patient to take medications to reduce prostate size and improve urinary flow.	Prostate size can be reduced with a 5α-reductase inhibitor such as finasteride and dutasteride. These drugs inhibit production of the hormone dihydrotestosterone (DHT), which enhances prostate growth. A class of α-blocking agents—terazosin, doxazosin, tamsulosin, silodosin, and alfuzosin—all relax musculature within the bladder neck and improve urinary flow. Using both classes of drugs together alleviates more symptoms and prevents the progression of BPH.
■ Encourage therapeutic lifestyle modifications.	These modifications may have a mild effect and include limiting fluids before bed, reducing caffeine and alcohol intake, and double voiding before bed.
■ Encourage the patient to take antibiotics as prescribed.	Medication may be indicated to treat or prevent UTI resulting from obstruction and stasis.

TABLE 10-1   The American Urological Association's Symptom Score for Benign Prostatic Hyperplasia (BPH)

	Not at all	Less than 1 time in 5 times	Less than half of the time	About half of the time	More than half of the time	Almost always
During the past month or so, how often did you have the feeling of not having completely emptied your bladder after urinating?	0	1	2	3	4	5
During the past month or so, how often did you have to urinate again less than 2 hours after you finished urinating?	0	1	2	3	4	5
During the past month or so, how often did you have to stop and start the urinary stream several times while urinating?	0	1	2	3	4	5
During the past month or so, how often did you find it difficult to delay urination?	0	1	2	3	4	5
During the past month or so, how often did you find that your urinary stream was weak?	0	1	2	3	4	5
During the past month or so, how often did you have to push or strain to begin urinating?	0	1	2	3	4	5
Frequency of Waking Up to Urinate						
During the past month or so, how often did you typically get up to urinate between going to bed in the evening and waking up in the morning?	0	1 (one time)	2 (two times)	3 (three times)	4 (four times)	5 (five times)

Modified from Barry MJ, Fowler FJ, O'Leary MP, et al. The American Urological Association Symptom Index for benign prostatic hyperplasia. *J Urol* 148:1549, 1992.
Score key:
Mild = 0 to 7 points; moderate = 8 to 9 points; severe = 20 to 35 points.

NANDA-I NDx   Deficient Knowledge

Common Related Factor
Newly diagnosed prostate disorder

Common Expected Outcome
Patient demonstrates understanding of diagnostic procedures and treatment options for BPH.

Defining Characteristics
Questions to health care team
Stated misconceptions or confusion regarding diagnosis and treatment options

NOC Outcomes
Knowledge: Disease Process; Knowledge: Treatment Regimen

NIC Interventions
Teaching: Disease Process; Teaching: Procedures/Treatment

■ = Independent   ▲ = Collaborative

Ongoing Assessment

Actions/Interventions	Rationales
■ Assess the patient's understanding of prostate disorders and the following commonly performed diagnostic procedures for prostate disorders:	Men are often embarrassed or hesitant to discuss prostate problems and often delay seeking attention for symptoms for which onset is typically gradual.
• Digital rectal examination (DRE)	The American Urological Association recommends that men older than 50 years of age should have an annual DRE for the purpose of prostate palpation.
• Uroflowmetry	Urodynamic flow studies include determination of flow rate and evaluation of residual urine.
• Cystourethroscopy	Visualization of the bladder and urethra through a fiberoptic scope allows the physician to see the extent of enlargement and consequent obstruction.
• Urinalysis	Examination of the urine for presence of blood, white blood cells (WBCs), and/or bacteria is useful in the identification of UTI, which often accompanies obstruction that causes stasis of urine.
• Laboratory studies: blood urea nitrogen (BUN) and creatinine; prostate-specific antigen (PSA)	BUN and creatinine determine renal function, which can be impaired as a result of long-standing obstructive uropathy. PSA is used to differentiate BPH from prostate enlargement caused by cancer. PSA can also be increased in prostatic infection, irritation, and after recent ejaculation. It can be measured in total or free portions and generally is viewed over time and evaluated with other portions of the examination. An elevated PSA alone is not diagnostic of prostate cancer.
• Prostate ultrasound	This ultrasound is performed rectally using a wand type of ultrasound to examine the prostate gland for enlargement.
■ Assess the patient's understanding of the following treatment options for prostate disorders: *Medical management:*	
• Medications	Medications may include hormone manipulation or use of smooth muscle relaxers that relax the prostatic urethra. Drugs that block androgens (e.g., finasteride, dutasteride) and α-adrenergic blockers, which relax the urethra (doxazosin, terazosin, alfuzosin, tamsulosin, and silodosin) may be used. More recent medications block α-receptors, which are localized in the prostate and bladder neck; these result in an increase in urinary flow with fewer side effects.
Minimally invasive therapies for BPH:	
• Dilatation of the urethra	Dilatation enhances urine flow. This procedure may need to be repeated periodically.
• Placement of urethral stents	Stents are small tubes that allow for drainage of urine by pushing back the prostatic urethra. They were used in the past for poor-operative-risk patients but are infrequently used now because of secondary obstruction over time.
• Transurethral vaporization of the prostate	This vaporization procedure has reduced bleeding complications and has shorter recovery times but has greater risk for urinary retention, necessitating further treatment.
• Transurethral microwave therapy	Several techniques can be employed to heat and destroy excess prostatic tissue and reduce compression of the urethra.
• Transurethral needle ablation	Low-level radio frequency energy using needles is delivered to burn away designated areas of the enlarged prostate. This procedure is used in patients with comorbidities and provides sustained clinical improvement in most men.

Actions/Interventions	**Rationales**
Surgical management for BPH:	Several surgical approaches are available.
• Transurethral resection of the prostate (TURP)	This "closed" procedure is widely used to treat BPH and remains the gold standard for evaluating newer therapies. The surgeon removes the prostate by inserting a resectoscope through the urethra to remove obstructing tissue. The TURP is significantly less traumatic than open forms of surgery.
• Suprapubic prostatectomy • Retropubic prostatectomy • Perineal prostatectomy	These three procedures are "open" surgical procedures using a variety of approaches. They are used when the prostatic tissue is very enlarged or when the bladder needs repair.
• Laser-assisted surgery	This newer procedure uses a laser to make the incision into the prostate.
• Robotic surgery	This is a new, minimally invasive surgery completed with the aid of the da Vinci robotic platform to decrease surgical side effects and increase return to sexual function and full continence.

Therapeutic Interventions

Actions/Interventions	**Rationales**
■ Discuss with the patient the advantages and disadvantages of medical and surgical treatment options.	Many factors affect selection of optimal treatment, including severity of symptoms, ability to tolerate medication side effects, medical contraindications to surgery, and concern for postoperative erectile dysfunction. Specific rates of sexual function, continence issues and postsurgical complications should be referred to the surgeon.
■ Provide the patient with postprocedure instructions about signs and symptoms to be reported, including:	Early assessment of complications facilitates prompt treatment.
• Hematuria	In the first few weeks after TURP, some bleeding is expected. However, thick red urine or clots must be reported.
• Infection	Urinary instrumentation and surgical incisions carry risk for sepsis.
• Unresolved incontinence or retention	Temporary incontinence is common until healing has occurred. Retention is also common after urethral catheterization.
■ Discuss PSA testing.	Controversies exist over routine PSA testing because of the number of false-positive results. Rising levels of PSA can be an indication of an enlarging prostate or prostate cancer.
■ Teach about the need for annual prostate examination.	Existing prostatic tissue could become cancerous. One treatment does not reduce future risk for prostate disease.
■ Teach about behavioral methods to reduce symptom severity or reduce occurrence or aggravation of symptoms: • Limit fluid intake after dinner.	Reducing fluids can help avoid nocturia and interrupted sleep.
• Avoid medications known to worsen urinary symptoms such as cold preparations, diuretics, antispasmodics, antihistamines, and some antidepressants.	These medications may precipitate acute urinary retention or worsen existing symptoms.
■ Discuss any prior experience in taking over-the-counter herbs such as saw palmetto extract to relieve symptoms.	This extract has the most evidence to date for use in treating symptoms in men with mild disease. Further research is ongoing. Other herbal therapies include African star grass and pygeum bark.
■ Provide Internet resources for further education.	The National Cancer Institute and the National Kidney and Urologic Diseases Information Clearinghouse offer excellent materials.

■ = Independent   ▲ = Collaborative

Risk for Deficient Fluid Volume

Common Risk Factors

Postoperative hemorrhage from transurethral resection of the prostate

Inadequate fluid intake (to reduce symptoms)

Common Expected Outcome

Patient is normovolemic, as evidenced by stable blood pressure (BP) and heart rate (HR) and absence of gross hematuria.

NOC Outcomes
Urinary Elimination; Fluid Balance
NIC Interventions
Bladder Irrigation; Bleeding Reduction; Tube Care: Urinary

Ongoing Assessment

Actions/Interventions	**Rationales**
■ Monitor for decreased BP, orthostatic BP, and increased HR.	Reduction in circulatory blood volume can cause hypotension and tachycardia. Postural hypotension, especially in the elderly, is a common manifestation of fluid deficit.
■ Monitor intake and output.	Intake and output should include careful record of any irrigation fluid instilled.
▲ Monitor BUN and creatinine clearance.	Elevated BUN and creatinine suggest fluid deficit.
■ Monitor amount and severity of hematuria and clots in the urine.	Bright red blood in the urine is expected over the first 24 hours after transurethral resection but should irrigate to clear pink without clots during that period.
▲ Monitor hemoglobin and hematocrit.	Decreases indicate significant blood loss, contributing to fluid status problem.

Therapeutic Interventions

Actions/Interventions	**Rationales**
■ Encourage oral fluids as prescribed or tolerated by the patient. IV fluids may be ordered.	Oral fluid replacement is indicated for mild fluid deficit and is a cost-effective method for replacement treatment. Older patients have a decreased sense of thirst and may need ongoing reminders.

Related Care Plans

Ineffective sexuality patterns, p. 182
Insomnia, p. 117
Urinary retention p. 202
Risk for infection, p. 114

Prostate Cancer

Radical Prostatectomy; Localized Prostate Cancer

Prostate cancer is the most common non–skin cancer among males in the United States. There has been a significant increase in prostate cancer findings since the introduction of the recommended blood screening of prostate-specific antigen (PSA). Annual health screenings including digital rectal examination and PSA test are recommended for all men older than 50 years and younger high-risk men. More than 70% of prostate cancers are diagnosed in men older than 65 years of age. African Americans have a higher risk for this cancer. With prostate cancer, the patient is generally asymptomatic until obstructive symptoms of the urinary tract appear. Transrectal ultrasound is used to detect nonpalpable tumors and stage localized cancers. Biopsy is needed to confirm diagnosis. Medical and surgical options depend on the stage of the cancer, symptoms, and response to other therapies. Treatment may include the traditional radical prostatectomy, newer laparoscopic nerve-sparing procedures for more localized cancers, radiation (external beam or seed implant), hormonal therapy, and chemotherapy. There are two approaches for a radical prostatectomy for cancer: retropubic and perineal. The approach depends on several factors, such as coexisting bladder abnormalities, size of the prostate, and the degree of risk of the surgical candidate. Each procedure has its advantages and disadvantages. Patients presenting with early-stage cancer in which only a small amount of cancer is noted on biopsy may be considered for active surveillance (watchful waiting) as an alternative to more aggressive therapies. In addition, many clinical trials are available for patients needing additional treatments. The focus of this care plan is on the patient undergoing a radical prostatectomy.

NANDA-I NDx Fear

Common Related Factors

Lack of knowledge about diagnosis, treatment, and prognosis
Treatment by active surveillance (watchful waiting)
Treatments and invasive procedures
Threat of death
Anticipated or perceived physical threat

Defining Characteristics

Identifies fearful feelings or object of fear
Tension
Apprehension
Alertness

Common Expected Outcomes

Patient uses effective coping behaviors to reduce fear response.
Patient verbalizes a reduction or absence of fear.

NOC Outcomes

Fear Self-Control; Coping

NIC Interventions

Anxiety Reduction; Presence; Calming Techniques; Emotional Support

Ongoing Assessment

Actions/Interventions	Rationales
■ Determine what patient is fearful of by careful questioning.	The external source of fear can be identified, and current responses can be assessed.
■ Assess level of fear as mild, moderate, or severe.	The threat to health, life, and role function resulting from cancer can predispose the patient to fear/anxiety.

■ = Independent   ▲ = Collaborative

Actions/Interventions

- Determine factors affecting fear.

- Determine the patient's support systems.

- Determine the patient's coping methods.

Rationales

Many misconceptions exist regarding prognosis, treatments, and potential complications such as sexual dysfunction. Patients with small, localized tumors treated by active surveillance may find "watching" over time to be more stressful than anticipated. Accurate assessment data about the source of the patient's concern guide appropriate treatments and supportive coping strategies.

In some cases, there may be no readily available resources. Evaluation of supportive persons from the past may provide the assistance required at this time.

These determine the effectiveness of coping strategies currently used by the patient.

Therapeutic Interventions

Actions/Interventions

- Give the patient opportunity to ask questions or verbalize concerns.

- Provide education about diagnosis and treatment plan.
- Provide information about resources for coping with the diagnosis.

- Assist in identifying strategies used in the past to deal with fearful situations.

▲ Instruct in the use of physician-ordered antianxiety medications.

Rationales

Men's concerns may include fear of death, feelings of loss of control, questions regarding determination of appropriate treatment, and how diagnosis and treatment may affect relationships with significant other.

Education decreases anxiety and promotes cooperation.

The increased public awareness of prostate cancer has resulted in a variety of lay and professional books and Internet sites for information. Social services, support groups, and community agencies can help the patient cope with his illness and treatments.

This helps patient focus on fear as a real and natural part of life that has been and can continue to be dealt with successfully.

Short-term use of antianxiety medications can relieve unpleasant feelings.

Risk for Sexual Dysfunction

Common Risk Factors

Injury to perineal nerves during surgery
Presence of indwelling urinary catheter
Dribbling and long-term incontinence
Decreased libido
Radiation side effects

Common Expected Outcomes

Patient or significant other is able to discuss concerns about sexual functioning.
Patient or significant other expresses improved satisfaction in sexual activity.
Patient adapts sexual therapies as needed to enhance performance.

NOC Outcomes
Sexual Functioning; Knowledge: Disease Process

NIC Interventions
Sexual Counseling; Teaching: Disease Process

Ongoing Assessment

Actions/Interventions	Rationales
■ Assess the patient's and significant other's expectations for sexual function.	Although many men undergoing prostatectomy are older, do not assume that sexual functioning is unimportant.
■ Assess the patient's and significant other's understanding of the potential impact that surgery may have had on sexual functioning.	A discussion of the possible negative impact of prostatectomy on sexual functioning should occur preoperatively, but often the patient is too anxious or preoccupied with other information (e.g., fear about surgery, prognosis with cancer diagnosis) to comprehend fully. If this is the case, the patient may benefit from postoperative discussion. Not all patients who have had prostatectomy have sexual dysfunction. Perineal resection carries the highest risk for sexual dysfunction. Newer nerve-sparing surgical procedures are becoming available and may be an option for some men. Radiation therapy side effects may include erectile dysfunction (ED). Overall, most men will experience some sexual dysfunction in the first few months after treatment.
■ Assess whether the patient and significant other need or want information during the postoperative period or if they prefer to wait a few weeks.	Timing of patient readiness to learn should guide the teaching plan. At a minimum, written materials can be given to the patient.
■ Assess for urinary incontinence after removal of the catheter.	The psychological impact of urinary incontinence can negatively impact the patient's perceived ability to perform sexually. Dribbling may occur for as long as a few months after prostatectomy and catheter removal.

Therapeutic Interventions

Actions/Interventions	Rationales
■ Teach the patient which nerves are necessary for erection and ejaculation; distinguish between sterility and impotence. Clarify all language; use diagrams and models as needed, depending on the patient's learning style.	Patients may be embarrassed to ask questions that highlight a limited knowledge base; however, many misconceptions may exist.
■ Offer the patient and significant other suggestions for alternatives to usual sexual practices during the postoperative period.	Usual sexual activity can be resumed 4 to 6 weeks after surgery.
■ Explain medications and mechanical devices available to patient to enhance erection.	Medications such as 5-phosphodiesterase inhibitors (e.g., sildenafil) may be prescribed to maintain blood flow to the corpora cavernosa during recovery or for long-term follow-up. Mechanical devices (vacuum devices or penile prostheses) may be tried to create an erection.
■ Inform the patient that retrograde ejaculation often occurs after prostatectomy.	Retrograde ejaculation means that ejaculate goes into the bladder rather than into the urethra; this is harmless and results in a cloudy discoloration of the urine. This is of no consequence in terms of sexual performance or satisfaction.
■ Discuss urinary incontinence as a consequence of prostatectomy; teach Kegel exercises.	Dribbling may occur for months and then resolve. Kegel exercises will increase sphincter tone needed to achieve continence. They should be performed at each time of urination and several times throughout the day. Occasionally, incontinence after prostatectomy is permanent.
▲ Refer for sexual counseling as indicated.	Specialty therapy may be indicated for some patients. Changes in sexual function may have adverse effects on the couple's relationship.

■ = Independent   ▲ = Collaborative

NANDA-I NDx **Deficient Knowledge, Postoperative**

Common Related Factors

Need for home management
New condition, procedure, treatment
Misinterpretation of information

Defining Characteristics

Questions to health care team
Verbalized inaccurate information

Common Expected Outcome

Patient verbalizes understanding of need for follow-up care, wound care, and management of incontinence and/or erectile dysfunction.

NOC Outcomes

Knowledge: Disease Process; Knowledge: Treatment Procedures

NIC Interventions

Wound Care; Teaching: Disease Process

Ongoing Assessment

Actions/Interventions	Rationales
■ Assess understanding of need for further treatment (e.g., chemotherapy, radiation therapy) that may be required in patients who have had surgery to remove prostatic cancer.	These treatments are part of the overall management to eliminate cancer cells that were not removed at surgery.
■ Assess ability to care for surgical wounds.	Infection is a common complication. Assessment provides basis for further education.
■ Assess understanding of potential dribbling and methods for improving and dealing with incontinence.	The extent of the problem depends on the type of resection performed.
■ Assess knowledge of resources for ED.	ED may occur as a complication of prostate surgery. ED may not have been a problem in the past; thus the patient may be unaware of available resources.

Therapeutic Interventions

Actions/Interventions	Rationales
■ Teach wound care:	Accurate, clear information provides rationale for assuming responsibility for self-care at home.
• Retropubic wounds	Stitches or staples are usually removed 7 to 10 days postoperatively. Daily cleaning of the wounds with soap and water is sufficient.
• Perineal wounds	Stitches or staples are usually removed 7 to 10 days postoperatively; these wounds, however, remain tender longer than abdominal wounds because of their location. They are also at higher risk for infection because of proximity to the anus. Warm sitz baths or tub baths once or twice daily are recommended until the wound has healed completely and soreness is gone.
■ Teach the patient the following about incontinence: • Remind the patient that urinary incontinence may resolve up to 1 year postoperatively.	This knowledge may reduce anxiety and may help the patient with decision making about management of urinary elimination.
• Encourage use of Kegel exercises.	These exercises improve perineal musculature and control over the urinary stream. They need to be performed several times throughout the day.
• Refer the patient to a self-help incontinence group if incontinence is a problem.	Relationships with persons with common issues can be beneficial.

Actions/Interventions

- Instruct the patient regarding self-care and temporary use of an indwelling catheter, if needed.

■ Teach the patient to report any of the following:
  - Signs of infection: fever; unusual drainage from incisions; unusual drainage from the urethra, especially in patients having transurethral resection
  - Signs of urinary tract infection (cloudy, foul-smelling urine; frequency)
  - Hematuria
  - Unresolved incontinence

Rationales

Some patients are discharged with an indwelling catheter still in place. They are better able to ask questions when they have basic information about what to expect.

For successful recovery the patient must know how to identify problems and what to do when problems occur. Early assessment facilitates prompt treatment.

Related Care Plans

Erectile dysfunction (see the **Evolve** website)
Ineffective coping, p. 49
Acute pain, p. 151
Risk for infection, p. 114
Stress urinary incontinence, p. 110

Sexually Transmitted Infections (STIs)

Sexually transmitted infections (STIs) are infections that occur as a result of sexual contact with an infected person. Although most cases of STI are associated with oral or genital sexual activity, some can be transmitted through contact with infected blood, such as hepatitis B. The incidence of specific STIs has changed over time. Some infections have reached epidemic proportions among specific cohorts of populations, and variance occurs among regions and countries. This content will address the United States. Many factors have contributed to the rise in types of STIs and number of people infected in the United States. These include ease of travel; increased population mobility; changes in cultural and social norms regarding sexual activity, marriage, and women's roles; more explicit sexual content in popular media; and decreased use of barrier methods of contraception, such as condoms. Research indicates a strong correlation between the incidence of STI and drug abuse. Many drug abusers, especially women, trade sex for drugs. Many times, STIs coexist with other STIs. That is, when a patient presents with one STI, there is a higher risk that he or she will have others and should be screened for them. This care plan describes the most common STIs: chlamydia, gonorrhea, syphilis, genital herpes, genital warts, trichomoniasis, and chancroid.

See also Human Immunodeficiency Virus (HIV), *p. 715.*

NANDA-I Deficient Knowledge

Common Related Factors

New diagnosis of STI
Information misinformation, or misinterpretation of diagnosis
Lack of exposure
Fear of acquired immunodeficiency syndrome (AIDS)
Embarrassment about topic, shame, fear

Defining Characteristics

Multiple questions
Lack of questions
Inaccurate follow-through of previous instruction
Inappropriate or exaggerated behaviors (e.g., hysteria, hostility, agitation, or apathy)

■ = Independent   ▲ = Collaborative

Common Expected Outcome

Patient verbalizes understanding of the disease process, transmission, prevention strategies, complications, and treatment modalities.

NOC Outcomes
Knowledge: Disease Process; Knowledge: Treatment Regimen
NIC Interventions
Crisis Intervention; Learning Facilitation; Teaching: Individual

Ongoing Assessment

Actions/Interventions	Rationales
■ Assess barriers to learning.	While patients may have their own personal barriers (e.g., guilt, embarrassment), health care professionals may themselves be uncomfortable in eliciting key information or in providing required information. Repetition of information may be necessary at a follow-up meeting to solidify learning.
■ Determine the patient's previous knowledge of the disease process, routes of transmission, complications, and treatment modalities.	Information is assimilated into previous assumptions and facts. Patients may have misconceptions about disease transmission and treatment. Patients may not be knowledgeable about the long-term risks and effects of STIs.
■ Determine the patient's understanding of medical terminology as well as slang or lay terms.	It is important to speak in terms the patient understands. Accurate information about sex and STIs is not always easily available to younger patients. Material must be presented at the educational and developmental level of each individual.
■ Determine sexual orientation, number of sexual partners, and recent sexual activities in a nonjudgmental manner.	STIs are spread during homosexual and heterosexual activity. Risks increase with the number of lifetime sexual partners. Judgmental attitudes may preclude patients from following through with a treatment plan. Frequently health care providers are unsure of what language to use in facilitating this discussion. It is best to approach this in a factual, matter-of-fact manner. Examples of questions include: "Are you or have you been sexually active?" "How many partners have you had in your life?" "Were they male, female, or both?" "Do you use condoms?" For men who have sex with men (MSM), it is necessary to ask if they participate in anal insertive sex and if a condom is used.

Therapeutic Interventions

Actions/Interventions	Rationales
■ Teach the medication regimen, which includes the name of the drug, dosage, administration, side effects, and action of the prescribed medication.	Effective treatment requires that the patient complete prescribed medications to prevent reinfection.
■ Review basic hygiene before topical administration of drugs (e.g., wash lesions with soap and water, keep area dry, wear loose-fitting cotton undergarments).	Basic hygiene of lesions helps prevent further contamination. Cotton products decrease perspiration.
■ Discuss the importance of notifying all sexual partners.	It may be necessary for patients to identify their other sexual contacts to decrease disease spread in the community. This decreases the chance of reinfection and of further spread of the disease. In most states, STIs are reportable diseases. Public health workers will contact sexual partners for testing and treatment.
■ Instruct the patient about scheduling appointments and treatments.	Follow-up testing is necessary to prove eradication of certain STIs.

Actions/Interventions

- Instruct the female patient regarding the importance of yearly gynecological examinations with Papanicolaou (Pap) smears. Encourage male patients to have yearly testicular examinations.
- Instruct patients in safe methods of preventing STI transmission:
  - Kissing
  - Touching
  - Mutual masturbation
  - Oral sex with latex condom
- Instruct in use of latex male condom.

- Discuss the benefits of monogamous relationships.

Rationales

These are excellent screening tools and provide a wonderful opportunity for education.

These methods are considered "safe" in preventing STIs because there is no exchange of infected body fluids between sexual partners.

Latex male condoms, when used consistently and correctly, can reduce the risk for transmission of most STIs.

The surest way to avoid transmission of STIs is to abstain from sexual contact or to be in a long-term mutually monogamous relationship with a partner who has been tested and is known to be uninfected.

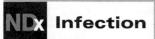

NDx Infection

Common Related Factors

Inadequate primary defenses
Tissue destruction
Extension of infection
Sexual exposure
Insufficient knowledge to avoid exposure

Defining Characteristics

Urethral discharge
Genital lesions
Fever
Malaise
Dysuria
Enlarged lymph nodes

Common Expected Outcome

Patient has a decrease in or complete resolution of symptoms of infection.

NOC Outcome
Infection Status
NIC Interventions
Infection Control; Infection Protection

Ongoing Assessment

Actions/Interventions

- Assess for signs and symptoms associated with specific STIs:
  - Vaginal or penile discharge
  - Dysuria
  - Genital lesions
  - Abdominal pain
- Assess for general signs and symptoms of infection:
  - Fever
  - Malaise
  - Lymphadenopathy
- Identify those at risk (e.g., sexual partners, persons who share drug needles).
- Assess individual risk factors for reactivation of disease process.

Rationales

Urethral inflammation is a common symptom in men with STI. The discharge may be purulent. Men will often complain of pain and burning with urination. In women, yeast infections such as trichomoniasis usually present with malodorous vaginal discharge and vulvar itching. The characteristics of genital lesions vary with specific STIs.

Some STIs, such as genital herpes or primary HIV infection, may be associated with general symptoms of infection. Enlarged lymph nodes may occur in the inguinal area with many of the STIs.

Those exposed may require treatment to prevent the spread or development of the infection.

Recurrence of genital warts or genital herpes is common.

■ = Independent   ▲ = Collaborative

Therapeutic Interventions

Actions/Interventions	Rationales
■ Provide information about the pertinent STI	There is a wide range of STIs that can confuse the public. Each has its own infective organism and pattern of symptoms. Diagnosis varies depending on the specific STI. Diagnostic aids include history, physical examination, Pap smears, serology testing, and tissue cultures and stains. Both gonorrhea and chlamydia may be diagnosed in men by nucleic acid amplification tests ordered on a spot urine sample. This is the most sensitive testing available and is painless for the patient. For many infections the definitive diagnostic test has yet to be developed. Treatment is based on Centers for Disease Control and Prevention (CDC) guidelines.
• Chlamydia Trachomatis	*Chlamydia trachomatis* infection is the most common STI. Symptoms range from none to dysuria, to purulent vaginal or penile discharge, to pelvic inflammatory disease (PID) in women. Treatment includes course of antibiotic therapy. Latex male condoms may prevent transmission. Sexual partners must be notified and treated. This is a mandatory reportable STI.
• Gonorrhea	Gonorrhea is caused by the *Neisseria gonorrhoeae* organism, which produces vaginal discharge, abnormal uterine bleeding, and PID. If the infection is acquired during menstruation, the risk for dissemination increases. It can affect joints and skin, causing arthralgias and skin lesions. Treatment includes a course of antibiotics, partner notification with treatment, as well as mandatory reporting to the state. Prevention may be acquired through consistent and correct condom usage.
• Syphilis	Syphilis is caused by *Treponema pallidum.* Sexual transmission occurs only in the presence of mucocutaneous lesions. Syphilis is easy to cure in its early stages, with penicillin being the treatment of choice. Diagnosis of syphilis can be made by several methods. The most common is through blood testing. Screening is usually completed with the Venereal Disease Research Laboratory (VDRL) test or the rapid plasma reagin (RPR) test.
• Genital herpes	Genital herpes is an incurable and recurrent viral infection caused by the herpes simplex virus (HSV). HSV causes painful genital lesions that start as papules or vesicles. Diagnosis of genital herpes may be made by viral culture of an actual lesion or by serology testing. Treatment includes systemic antiviral therapy, which may control the signs and symptoms but does not cure the disease. Genital herpes may be transmitted even when no lesions are present, contrary to previously held beliefs. Even though condoms may help prevent some disease transmission, they are not fail-safe because of the location of the lesions.
• Genital warts	Genital warts are caused by human papillomavirus (HPV) infection. There are many strains of HPV, some of which are associated with cervical dysplasia. Visible genital warts are dominated by HPV strains 6 and 11. Clinically, genital warts are nonpainful and asymptomatic. Treatment consists of using antimitotic gels or immune-enhancing cream for removal. Even though treatments may eliminate the warts, it does not erase infectivity. Sometimes HPV will clear on its own.

Men's Health Care Plans

Actions/Interventions	Rationales
• Trichomoniasis	Although trichomoniasis occurs in both men and women, it is one of the most common STIs in women, characterized by malodorous vaginal discharge and vulvar irritation and/or itching. Often it is asymptomatic in men, or a transient dysuria or mild discharge may occur from urethritis. Polymerase chain reaction (PCR) testing on a urine sample is the only reliable means of testing for trichomoniasis, and this is limited by its availability. More rarely, prostatitis or even infertility can result. Although trichomoniasis in men can be transient and clear on its own, to avoid reinfection concurrent therapy and abstinence from sexual activity are advised until treatment of both partners has been completed. The offending organism is *Trichomonas vaginalis,* which responds to treatment with oral metronidazole. Persons taking this drug must be cautioned against alcohol intake during and several days after treatment.
• Chancroid	Chancroid is an acute ulcerative disease caused by *Haemophilus ducreyi,* a gram-negative bacillus. Some patients with chancroid are also infected with *T. pallidum* or HSV. These infections are associated with an increased rate of human immunodeficiency virus (HIV) transmission. Diagnosis of chancroid is challenging, and often presumptive diagnosis is made. Recommended treatment is with azithromycin or ceftriaxone.
■ Teach about use of antiinfective agents as indicated:	Extended therapy may be indicated for reactivation of disease process, or in the presence of other medical diseases such as HIV infection. The reader is referred to the CDC website for the most current treatment guidelines for STIs.
• Acyclovir, famciclovir, valacyclovir	These antivirals are the primary treatment for genital herpes. They may be given orally or be used topically for mild disease. Intravenous administration is recommended for severe disease and recurrent lesions. Long-term use at lower dosages is suggested to reduce transmission to partners.
• Penicillin	Penicillin is the treatment of choice for syphilis. It can be given as a single intramuscular injection in the early stages of the disease. In the later stages, multiple injections may be used, or the drug may be given intravenously.
• Doxycycline, erythromycin, tetracycline, ceftriaxone, azithromycin	These agents are used alone or in combination for the treatment of chancroid, chlamydia, and gonorrhea. Treatment regimens, combinations, and length of therapy differ and change according to antimicrobial resistance patterns, stages of disease, or if the patient is co-infected with HIV. Updated treatment guidelines may be obtained from www.cdc.gov/std.
• Metronidazole	This drug is the treatment of choice for trichomoniasis.
• Antimitotic gels or immune-enhancing cream	These agents are effective in treating genital warts.
■ Teach the patient to complete the prescribed treatment and take all medications.	Recurrence and transmission of infection can occur if the patient does not take all of the medication. Patients often stop treatment prematurely when symptoms disappear.

■ = Independent   ▲ = Collaborative

Actions/Interventions	Rationales
■ Teach about recurrence and/or reinfection.	Have the patient abstain from sexual activity during treatment and for the prescribed number of days afterward. Partners should be evaluated and treated to prevent reinfection of the patient. Persons with herpes should abstain from sexual activity with unaffected partners when lesions or other symptoms of herpes are present, and they should understand that about 70% of new cases are transmitted through silent viral shedding.
■ Provide the patient with information and education obtained from the latest guidelines.	The National Guideline Clearinghouse and the CDC are two excellent Internet resources.
■ Notify the local health department.	In most states, STIs must be reported to local health departments for case finding. Laws and regulations regarding which STIs are reportable vary by state.
■ Teach about prevention.	Condoms can reduce transmission of HPV if lesions are on the penis or in the urethra. Some centers are beginning to vaccinate men having sex with men patients with Gardasil vaccine to reduce risk for rectal cancer caused by HPV.

NANDA-I NDx **Disturbed Body Image**

Common Related Factors
Lesions
Urethral discharge
Odiferous discharge
Topical medications

Defining Characteristics
Verbalizes fear, anger, anxiety
Verbalizes feelings of inadequacy and low self-worth
Discusses difficulty with coping with diagnosis of STI
Actual change in body
Change in social behavior (withdrawal, isolation)
Refusal to discuss infection

Common Expected Outcome
Patient demonstrates enhanced body image and self-esteem as evidenced by the ability to look at, talk about, and care for the altered body part.

NOC Outcomes
Body Image; Self-Esteem
NIC Intervention
Self-Esteem Enhancement

Ongoing Assessment

Actions/Interventions	Rationales
■ Assess and validate feelings about changes in appearance and body function.	The value or importance the patient places on the body part is more important than its actual value.
■ Note the patient's withdrawal from social situations.	STIs are associated with a social stigma. Withdrawal may indicate feelings of social isolation or fear of rejection by others.
■ Assess the impact of body image disturbance in relation to patient's developmental stage.	Early experience with STIs and its "social stigma" may affect developmental changes at a time when fostering social and intimate relationships is particularly important.
■ Assess coping mechanisms that the patient has used in the past.	Previous coping strategies may not be adequate to support patient adjustment.

Therapeutic Interventions

Actions/Interventions	Rationales
■ Encourage verbalization of positive or negative feelings about body changes.	It is worthwhile to encourage the patient to separate feelings about changes in the body from feelings of self-worth.

Actions/Interventions

- Assist the patient in identifying the extent of changes in appearance.
- Provide hope within the parameters of the disease process. Do not give false reassurance.
- Encourage the patient and significant other to interact.

- Refer to support groups.

▲ Refer for sexual counseling to help cope with sexuality issues.

Rationales

This helps begin the process of looking toward the future and how sexual activity will be different.

Hope promotes a positive attitude and provides an opportunity to plan for the future. Many STIs can be cured.

This maintains an open line of communication. One's partner has a key role in treatment and follow-up.

Lay persons in similar situations offer a different type of support, which is perceived as helpful.

The patient may need professional assistance to deal with issues and accept self.

Related Care Plans

Anxiety, p. 18
Noncompliance, p. 139

Testicular Cancer

Malignant tumors of the testes are rare, accounting for only 1% of all the cancers in men reported in the United States each year. It is one of the most curable solid tumor cancers. Although the cause of testicular cancer is unknown, both congenital and acquired factors are associated with tumor development. The most common risk factors for testicular cancer are undescended testicles, family history of this cancer, and previous cancer of one testicle.

Classification by histological types of tumors as well as clinical staging determines the treatment. Classification by histology is divided into two major divisions: (1) seminoma and (2) nonseminomatous germ tumors, which include embryonal, teratoma, choriocarcinoma, and mixed tumors.

The most common clinical staging system categorizes testicular cancer as stage I, a lesion confined to the testes. Stage II involves regional lymph node spread in the abdomen, and stage III is spread beyond the retroperitoneal lymph nodes. Reflecting the improvement and refinement of combination chemotherapy, survival in testicular cancer has dramatically improved, with a cure rate of more than 95% according to the American Cancer Society.

NDx Health-Seeking Behaviors: Technique for Monthly Testicular Self-Examination (TSE)

Common Related Factor

Lack of knowledge about regular testicular self-examination (TSE)

Common Expected Outcome

Patient correctly performs TSE.

Defining Characteristics

Desire for increased control of health
Expresses concern about current health status

NOC Outcome

Knowledge: Health Promotion

NIC Interventions

Self-Modification Assistance; Health Education: TSE

■ = Independent   ▲ = Collaborative

Ongoing Assessment

Actions/Interventions	Rationales
■ Assess the patient's knowledge of TSE.	Patients learn material most important to them. Patients recovering from unilateral testicular cancer need to be aware that they are at increased risk for cancer in the other testicle.
■ Assess the patient's confidence in his ability to perform TSE.	According to self-efficacy theory, positive conviction that one can perform a behavior is correlated with performance and successful outcome.
■ Be alert to signs of avoidance (e.g., changing the subject or becoming withdrawn).	Denial is a defense mechanism that can block learning and the assimilation of information.

Therapeutic Interventions

Actions/Interventions	Rationales
■ Present method of TSE using audiovisual aids or tapes, then allow for question-and-answer period.	Different people take in information in different ways. Multiple learning methods may enhance retention of the TSE information.
■ Identify known risk factors: • Family history of testicular cancer • Cryptorchid testes (undescended testicle) • Cancer of one testicle	These nonmodifiable risk factors need to be recognized by men, especially white males 20 to 40 years of age who are at highest risk.
■ Instruct in warning signs of testicular cancer: • Lump on testes that is small, hard, and painless • Pain/discomfort in the testes • Heaviness in testes or scrotum • Discomfort in lower abdomen or groin	Malignant tumors of the testes are rare but are the most common malignancy in males 20 to 40 years of age. Being aware of signs facilitates early diagnosis and treatment, and saves lives.
■ Instruct in procedure of TSE: • Examine testicles monthly immediately after a shower or bath. • Examine each testicle separately by gently rolling it between thumb and fingers. • Report any lump or swelling or any changes in size, shape, or consistency of the testes to the health care provider as soon as possible.	Patients must be given accurate information. The warmth from the water relaxes the scrotal sac. Testicular tumors tend to appear deep in the center of the testicle. Early detection of changes facilitates treatment and can affect the cure.

NDx Deficient Knowledge

Common Related Factors

New condition/procedure/treatments
Misinterpretation of information
Emotional state affecting learning
Unfamiliarity with information resources

Defining Characteristics

Verbalizes inaccurate information
Questioning health care team

Common Expected Outcome

Patient demonstrates an understanding of the risk for and causes of testicular cancer, common diagnostic procedures, and treatment options.

NOC Outcomes

Knowledge: Disease Process; Knowledge: Treatment Regimen

NIC Interventions

Teaching: Disease Process; Teaching: Preoperative; Teaching: Procedure/Treatment

Ongoing Assessment

Actions/Interventions	**Rationales**
■ Assess knowledge of the diagnosis and treatment options.	This information provides the starting point for an educational session. This topic is difficult for many men to discuss. Men may not realize how curable testicular cancer has become.

Therapeutic Interventions

Actions/Interventions	**Rationales**
■ Encourage questions about the diagnosis of testicular cancer and proposed treatment regimen.	Questions facilitate open communication between patient and health care team and allow verification of understanding of given information and the opportunity to correct misconceptions. Often patients are embarrassed about asking questions and may need permission to ask them.
■ Provide information on diagnostic testing:	
• Review of TSE results	Most commonly men note a lump that is painless but uncomfortable, or they may note swelling.
• Physical examination of testes, lymph nodes, and abdomen	Testes are evaluated for lumps and swelling. Other organs are evaluated for potential metastatic disease.
• Laboratory tests: tumor markers such as alpha fetoprotein (AFP) and beta-human chorionic gonadotropin (β-HCG), lactate dehydrogenase (LDH)	These markers are used to diagnose types of cancer as well as response to treatment.
• Diagnostic tests:	
• Ultrasound	Ultrasound aids in determining solid versus fluid-filled masses and benign versus malignant tumor.
• Computed tomography and magnetic resonance imaging	These scans detect metastatic lesions.
• Chest x-ray film and bone scan	These detect metastatic lesions.
• Radical inguinal orchiectomy (removal of one or both testes)	This procedure is used both for biopsy diagnosis and for treatment. The interval between discovery of a scrotal lump in the testes and radical orchiectomy is often within 1 week.
■ Provide preoperative teaching about orchiectomy.	This is a relatively uncomplicated procedure to remove the testicle. The procedure may be a same-day surgery or may require an overnight hospital stay.
■ Provide preoperative teaching about retroperitoneal lymph node dissection (RPLND).	Lymph node dissection is used for tumor staging. Treatment modalities depend on this staging process. RPLND is more commonly seen with embryonic cancer because of its high rate of metastasis.
■ Instruct in potential for infertility and option for semen storage.	Removal of only one testicle does not interfere with a normal erection and ability to produce sperm. However, more complete surgery (RPLND) and follow-up treatments may render the man infertile. The patient may feel secure knowing there is the potential for semen storage and future access to his sperm.
■ Explain the need to consult with both an oncologist and radiologist regarding chemotherapy and/or radiation therapy.	Both radiation and chemotherapy are generally coordinated by the medical oncologist. The nurse serves as the advocate by offering support, providing information, and coordinating follow-up appointments with the urologist.
■ Provide information on follow-up therapy:	Men must realize that testicular cancer is not a death sentence. Many modalities are available to treat advanced disease.
• Chemotherapy	Chemotherapy is indicated for nonseminomatous tumors or for metastatic disease. Many effective therapies are available, including cisplatin, ifosfamide, etoposide, vinblastine, and bleomycin.

■ = Independent   ▲ = Collaborative

Actions/Interventions

- Radiation therapy

■ Provide referral to the National Cancer Institute, the American Cancer Society, or the Lance Armstrong Foundation.

Rationales

Radiation beam therapy is indicated for patients with pure seminoma, because this tumor is radiosensitive.

Patients may be unaware of services available for questions or problem solving. Referral provides the patient and family with additional helpful resources, including support groups.

Ineffective Sexuality Patterns

Common Related Factors

Lack of knowledge about alternative responses to change in sexual response
Recent orchiectomy
Infertility

Defining Characteristics

Reported changes in sexual activities
Actual or perceived limitations secondary to orchiectomy

Common Expected Outcome

Patient or couple verbalizes satisfaction with the way they express physical intimacy.

NOC Outcomes
Sexual Identity: Acceptance; Self-Esteem
NIC Interventions
Sexual Counseling: Anticipatory Guidance;
Teaching: Sexuality

Ongoing Assessment

Actions/Interventions

■ Assess type of surgical/medical treatment received.

■ Explore current and past sexual patterns, practices, and degree of satisfaction.
■ Identify level of comfort in discussion of patient and/or significant other.

■ Assess the patient's or couple's prior plans for conceiving children.

Rationales

This information guides instruction. Unilateral orchiectomy does not interfere with ejaculation and fertility, though patients with testicular cancer often have reduced sperm counts independent of treatment. Also, prior medical or psychological conditions or more advanced cancer treatment may affect sexual performance.

This information aids in developing a realistic approach to care planning.

It is important for the nurse to create an environment wherein the patient and/or couple feel safe and comfortable in discussing their feelings.

Inability to conceive after surgery or treatment (unless sperm was banked) can affect the individual or couple in many ways, threatening their self-esteem, gender roles, and interactions.

Therapeutic Interventions

Actions/Interventions

■ Explore awareness of and comfort with a range of sexual expression and activities (not just sexual intercourse).

Rationales

Patients and couples may have limited knowledge of ways to express their sexuality. The patient may be unaware of potential options.

Men's Health Care Plans

Actions/Interventions

- Discuss the effect of an orchiectomy on future fertility.

- ▲ Refer to a reproductive specialist about sperm banking.

- Encourage discussion of feelings regarding alternative methods for reproduction.

- Refer to support groups.

Rationales

Removal of only one testicle does not interfere with ejaculation and fertility. Removal of lymph nodes (RPLND) can cause infertility. Removal of both testes does cause infertility. Cancer treatments can also affect sexual function. It is important to provide accurate information to relieve unnecessary fears. Failure to conceive can affect the individual or couple in many ways, threatening their self-esteem, gender roles, and sexual interactions.

If fathering a child is an important role for the patient, and sperm banking is not an option, discuss other options such as donor insemination and adoption.

Removing one testicle does not affect fertility or sexual function. Newer "nerve-sparing" surgical procedures are improving fertility rates.

Support and self-help groups are unique sources of information and empathy. With the high cure rate among patients with advanced disease, a growing number of survivors are serving as role models and political advocates.

Disturbed Body Image

Common Related Factors

Orchiectomy
Permanent alterations in structure/function

Defining Characteristics

Focusing behavior on changed body part or function
Refusal to look at, touch, or care for scrotal sac
Change in social behavior (withdrawal or isolation)
Actual change in structure/function

Common Expected Outcome

Patient demonstrates enhanced body image as evidenced by the ability to look at, care for, and talk about the altered appearance of the scrotal sac.

NOC Outcomes

Body Image; Self-Esteem

NIC Interventions

Body Image Enhancement; Grief Work Facilitation; Coping Enhancement

---

Ongoing Assessment

Actions/Interventions

- Assess and validate feelings about changes in appearance.

- Assess perceived impact on social behavior or personal relationships.

- Assess previous coping strategies.

Rationales

The extent of the response is related more to the value or importance the patient places on the body part than to the actual value or importance.

Young adult men may be particularly affected by changes in the structure or function of their bodies at a time when they are developing social and intimate relationships.

This helps the patient identify ways of coping that were successful in the past, although prior coping skills may not be adequate at this time.

■ = Independent ▲ = Collaborative

Men's Health Care Plans

Therapeutic Interventions

Actions/Interventions	Rationales
■ Acknowledge normalcy of emotional response to actual or perceived change in body structure and function.	Acknowledging the patient's emotional response enables the patient to move through the grieving process.
■ Teach the patient self-care activities related to body image.	These enable adaptation to the changes in body image.
■ Reinforce any attempts to care for the scrotum.	Positive reinforcement allows the patient to feel good about accomplishments and gain confidence.
■ Provide information about institutional, Internet-based, political, and community resources for coping with testicular cancer.	Social services, support groups, and community agencies can help the patient cope with this illness and treatments. As more men are being cured of this cancer, there is a growing body of "survivors" serving as role models and advocates, for example, The Lance Armstrong Foundation.

Related Care Plans

Cancer chemotherapy, p. 681
Cancer radiation therapy, p. 694

Women's Health Care Plans

Breast cancer is the most commonly occurring cancer in American women (except skin cancer). It is the second leading cause of cancer death in women; lung cancer remains the most fatal of all cancers for both men and women. A woman has a one-in-eight lifetime risk for developing this highly treatable disease. Despite its common occurrence, most women with breast cancer will not succumb to the disease; the 10-year survival rate is approximately 90% with about 2.5 million breast cancer survivors in the United States. Complete sequencing of the human genome has lead to the identification of two genes associated with the development of breast cancer and ovarian cancer. Women who carry a mutation in the BRCA1 or BRCA2 gene are known to be at increased risk for the development of breast cancer, and these cancers often develop at a much younger age than usual (age 45 or younger). The lifetime breast cancer risk for women with hereditary cancer (defined as having an inherited mutation in the BRCA1 or BRCA2 gene) is 56% to 85%. Hereditary breast cancer, however, accounts for only 5% to 10% of all breast cancer cases. The remainder of all breast cancers (85%) do not have an identified hereditary component. In other words, most women who get breast cancer have a noninherited form. In these women the incidence of the disease increases with age, with most occurring in women over 50 years of age.

Two other risk factors are associated with an increased risk for breast cancer: exposure to radiation (e.g., women who have received chest irradiation as prior treatment for other malignancies such as Hodgkin lymphoma) and the period of time that the body makes estrogen. The earlier a woman begins to menstruate and the later she has her first pregnancy, or following prolonged hormone replacement therapy, the higher her risk for breast cancer. The later menopause occurs in a woman, the higher her postmenopausal risk for breast cancer. Another significant risk factor is cigarette smoking. Research suggests that some women have a slow-acting form of a liver enzyme that normally detoxifies carcinogens, permitting the carcinogens present in tobacco to remain in the body longer.

With the use of breast self-examination and screening mammography, most breast cancer is successfully diagnosed at an early stage. Treatment recommendations are made according to the disease stage and may include surgery, radiation, and/or chemotherapy. Prognosis is related to the stage and type of tumor. Adjuvant chemohormonal therapy has decreased recurrence and has improved survival rates in most subgroups of patients. Even though the treatment modalities have lengthened the survival time for metastatic breast cancer, stage IV or metastatic disease is not curable.

Surgical management of breast cancer includes two major approaches: (1) breast conservation therapy, often referred to as a lumpectomy, or (2) removal of the entire breast, which is called a modified radical or radical mastectomy. Both of these surgical approaches may also include examination of the axillary lymph nodes for evidence of micrometastatic disease, usually through sentinel lymph node (SLN) biopsy. The presence or absence of disease in the lymph nodes determines prognosis (and subsequent treatment) and is referred to as nodal status. Women with node-negative disease generally have a better prognosis than women with node-positive disease. Women undergoing mastectomy have several options for breast reconstruction, including immediate or delayed reconstruction. The timing depends on several factors, including cancer treatment protocol, other medical problems, and the woman's preference. Breast-conserving therapy (lumpectomy) with adjuvant chemotherapy and/or radiation therapy is considered a treatment that is medically equivalent to mastectomy.

Specialized breast cancer treatment centers are available, providing a multidisciplinary treatment approach (e.g., medical and surgical oncologists, gynecologists, radiation oncologists, clinical nurse specialists, nurses, and social workers). This care plan addresses the surgical management of breast cancer. Follow-up care and adjunct treatment would be performed in the ambulatory care setting.

NANDA-I NDx Deficient Knowledge: Preoperative

Common Related Factors
Unfamiliarity with proposed treatment plan and procedures
Uncertainty about treatment options
Misinterpretation of information
Decisional conflict
Emotional state affecting learning

Defining Characteristics
Asks questions about diagnostic tests and treatment options
Verbalizes inaccurate information

Common Expected Outcome
Patient verbalizes understanding of breast cancer, its diagnosis, treatment options, and prognosis.

NOC Outcomes
Knowledge: Disease Process; Knowledge: Treatment Regimen
NIC Interventions
Teaching: Disease Process; Teaching: Procedures/Treatment

Ongoing Assessment

Actions/Interventions	Rationales
■ Assess understanding of diagnostic testing.	Thorough understanding of indications for testing is necessary for informed consent to be given.
■ Assess understanding of relationship between disease stage and prognosis and treatment.	Tumor size, spread to lymph nodes, and metastasis to distant organs are staged from 0 to IV. The lower the number the less the cancer has spread. Tumor staging classification is helpful to determine extent of disease and the optimal treatment plan.
■ Assess understanding of treatment modalities: • Surgery • Radiation • Chemotherapy • Hormonal therapy • Clinical trials	Most women want a collaborative relationship in disease management and require information about treatment rationales. They may have a preference for specific treatment plan, but decision-making capacity may be challenged because of stress of disease.

Therapeutic Interventions

Actions/Interventions	Rationales
■ Explain rationale for diagnostic procedures: • Clinical examination of breast	Lesion (lump) usually occurs in the upper outer quadrant of the breast. It is typically hard, irregularly shaped, nonmobile, and poorly delineated.

Actions/Interventions	Rationales
• Mammography	Mammography is used to locate the position and extent of a known tumor and to screen for the presence of other abnormalities not detected by clinical examination. Newer techniques such as digital mammograms and computer-aided detection and diagnosis have helped identify suspicious changes on mammograms.
• Breast biopsy	Biopsy is performed via fine-needle aspiration, needle core biopsy, excisional biopsy or lumpectomy, or needle localization for microscopic examination to confirm benign or malignant tissue diagnosis.
• Lymph node dissection and sentinel lymph node biopsy	A the presence or absence of disease in the lymph nodes determines prognosis (and subsequent treatment). Women with node-negative disease generally have a better prognosis.
• Breast ultrasound	The ultrasound can determine whether the lesion is solid or cystic (fluid-filled). Lesions larger than 1 cm can be evaluated.
• Tumor tissue testing (hormone receptor assays, DNA, and protein markers with diagnostic and prognostic value)	Estrogen and progesterone are female hormones affecting breast and other cancer tissues. The level of hormone receptors present in the tumor indicates the tumor's dependence on these hormones. Tumors are classified as estrogen receptor or progesterone receptor (ER/PR) positive or negative according to the amount of receptor protein present. This classification suggests tumor growth and treatment options. Tumors with positive receptors (more prevalent in postmenopausal women) are associated with better prognosis and longer survival.
• Complete physical examination	It is important to screen for signs of cancer in other locations.
• Liver function tests and scans	These tests aid in identifying possible liver metastasis.
• Genetic markers (e.g., HER2/neu)	This test of the biopsy sample aids in determining prognosis and monitoring the course of disease. The HER2/neu gene is associated with breast cancer; an overexpression gives the patient a poorer prognosis. The best prognosis is ER/PR-positive, HER2/neu-negative; the worst prognosis is ER/PR-negative, HER2/neu-positive.
• Bone scan	Bone scan is used in ruling out bone metastasis.
• Computed tomography (CT) scan/magnetic resonance imaging (MRI)	These scans are used in evaluating for tumors and distant sites of metastasis.
■ Explain rationale for suggested treatment based on site, type, and stage of tumor:	
• The TNM classification system	This system is used to stage breast cancer according to the extent of the primary tumor (T), regional lymph node metastasis (N), distant metastasis (M).
• Clinical stages	The clinical stages range from stage 0 to IV. Stage 0 implies in situ (localized) cancer; stage IV implies extensive metastasis. Sentinel lymph node biopsy has replaced axillary lymph node dissection as the first-line biopsy procedure for most women.
• *Stage 0:* Treated by lumpectomy with radiation or mastectomy	
• *Stages I and II:* Treated with lumpectomy or mastectomy, with sentinel lymph node biopsy. The use of adjuvant radiation, chemotherapy, or hormonal or biological therapy is dependent on a number of prognostic indicators (e.g., tumor size, nodal status, hormone receptor status, age, menopausal status).	
• *Stages III and IV:* Mastectomy and systemic chemotherapy; other adjuvant therapies (radiation, hormonal or biological therapy) are dependent on prognostic indicators as listed previously.	

■ = Independent   ▲ = Collaborative

Actions/Interventions	Rationales
• Chemoprevention	This is the prophylactic use of antiestrogen agents (e.g., tamoxifen) in women at high risk for development of breast cancer.
• Prophylactic mastectomy	This preventive surgery consists of a total mastectomy in high-risk women with immediate breast reconstruction.
■ Explain new treatment approaches: • Hormonal therapy	ER/PR-positive tumors respond to hormonal treatment with antiestrogens. A number of different antiestrogen therapies are available depending on the menopausal status of the woman, including tamoxifen and anastrozole.
• Biological (trastuzumab [Herceptin])	Trastuzumab (Herceptin) is a monoclonal antibody that targets the HER2/neu protein expressed on the surface of breast cells. Approximately 20% of all women with breast cancer overexpress this protein, which leads to unregulated cell growth. The use of Herceptin can slow the growth of cancer cells.
• Angiogenesis inhibitors (bevacizumab)	New monoclonal antibody drugs target growth factors that normally optimize enhanced blood vessel development. When these drugs stop this growth, the tumors cannot grow.
■ Explain the choices for breast reconstruction: • Timing: • Immediate—can be preferred option because it avoids a second surgery and reduces trauma of mastectomy. Permanent implant procedure is most commonly used. • Delayed—often advised if immediate cancer therapies are to be started, thus avoiding delay of incisional healing post reconstruction. • Procedures: • Permanent implant—uses tissue expander (balloon inserted below the pectoral muscle to gradually stretch the skin with weekly saline injection before inserting the permanent implant). Indicated for smaller-breasted women, because it does not result in the typical "sag" of the natural breast. • Skin flap using woman's own tissue—abdominal or back muscle or other flap is rotated to surgical site to create a mound to simulate a breast. It results in a more natural breast shape and feel but requires a more extensive surgical procedure. • Construction of nipple (areola). This is a secondary procedure to design a projecting nipple.	Women vary in their response to mastectomy. Breast reconstruction is performed to provide symmetry to the breasts. It does not interfere with cancer treatments or increase the risk for future cancer. Some women may prefer to use external padding to accomplish this. More recently breast reconstruction has gained in popularity because of improved plastic surgery techniques. It is considered reconstructive, not cosmetic surgery.
■ Provide teaching materials (e.g., videos, slides, reliable Internet websites, and printed information). Contact the National Cancer Institute in Bethesda, Maryland (1-[800]-4-CANCER) for additional materials.	Providing the patient with information in different formats allows her to choose the format that best suits her learning style and needs.

Acute Pain

Common Related Factors

Contraction of tissue resulting from surgery and healing process
Intraoperative arm position
Possible injury to brachial plexus
Lymphedema
Infection and phlebitis

Common Expected Outcomes

Patient reports satisfactory pain control at a level of 3 to 4 on a 0 to 10 rating scale.
Patient appears comfortable.
Patient performs range-of-motion (ROM) exercises with minimal discomfort.

Defining Characteristics

Verbalizes pain or discomfort
Guarding behavior
Restlessness and irritability
Appearance of discomfort

NOC Outcomes

Circulation Status; Pain Level; Pain Status; Medication Response

NIC Interventions

Circulatory Precautions; Circulatory Care; Pain Management; Positioning

Ongoing Assessment

Actions/Interventions	Rationales
■ Note subjective reports of pain and discomfort.	Pain assessment is the basis for an individualized approach to pain management.
■ Assess for probable cause of pain.	Different etiological factors respond better to different therapies.
■ Assess neurovascular status of affected arm immediately after surgery and at regular intervals.	This assessment detects possible brachial plexus injury.
■ Measure biceps 2 inches above elbow of affected arm immediately after surgery and every shift.	An increase in arm circumference may indicate impaired lymphatic drainage.
■ Evaluate ROM of affected arm.	Woman may refrain from certain movements to reduce pain.
■ Assess for signs of infection or phlebitis in the affected arm (e.g., pain, redness, warmth, and swelling).	Early identification of complications allows for early intervention.

Therapeutic Interventions

Actions/Interventions	Rationales
■ Keep arm elevated on two pillows while the patient is in bed (mastectomy).	This maneuver decreases edema and promotes lymph drainage.
■ Avoid constriction of the affected arm.	This prevents circulatory impairment and subsequent discomfort.
■ Protect affected arm from injury. Ensure that no procedures are performed on the affected arm (e.g., blood pressure, blood drawing, intravenous injections). Post notice at the bedside.	Mastectomy procedures remove lymph nodes and lymphatic vessels that drain the arm on the involved side of the body, increasing the risk for injury and infection in the involved arm.
■ Instruct regarding postoperative exercises: • Straight arm extension and abduction • Straight elbow raises • Wall climbing • Repeated 5 to 10 times per hour as tolerated	These exercises increase ROM progressively in the affected arm and relieve discomfort from possible tissue contraction.
■ Administer analgesics for pain as required (e.g., before ROM exercises are performed).	Patients have a right to effective pain relief.

■ = Independent   ▲ = Collaborative

Risk for Situational Low Self-Esteem/Disturbed Body Image

Common Risk Factors

Permanent alterations in structure/function
- Excision of breast and adjacent tissue
- Beginning scar tissue
- Asymmetrical breasts caused by implant or prosthesis fit or by lumpectomy

Diagnosis of cancer

History of sexual problems

Common Expected Outcome

Patient demonstrates enhanced body image, as evidenced by use of positive coping strategies, use of available resources, and absence of or decreased number of self-deprecating remarks.

NOC Outcomes
Body Image; Self-Esteem; Social Support

NIC Interventions
Body Image Enhancement; Self-Esteem Enhancement; Support System Enhancement

Ongoing Assessment

Actions/Interventions	Rationales
■ Assess and validate feelings about changes in appearance.	The extent of the response is related more to the value or importance the patient places on the breast than the actual value.
■ Assess perceived impact on social behavior or personal relationships.	Younger women may be particularly affected by changes in their body, although elderly women may likewise be strongly affected.
■ Assess for changes in the patient's self-perceptions following surgery (e.g., preoccupation with altered body part, concerns about loss of femininity and sexual identity, and negative feelings about body image).	The psychological impact of surgery may be devastating to self-esteem. Cultural and societal values about a woman's breast will influence the patient's response to surgery.
■ Assess for previous problems with self-esteem, body image, or sexual relations and how they were resolved.	Patients with a history of coping difficulties may need additional resources. Likewise, previously successful coping skills may be inadequate in the present situation.

Therapeutic Interventions

Actions/Interventions	Rationales
■ Encourage the patient to look at the wound and help care for it.	Looking at the wound is often the first indication that the patient is ready to participate in self-care.
■ Encourage the patient to verbalize feelings about effects of surgery on the ability to function as a woman, a sexual partner, and a worker.	It is worthwhile to encourage women to separate feelings about changes in body structures and/or function from feelings about self-worth.
■ Assist the patient with wearing a prosthetic insert at discharge.	Wearing a prosthesis can provide a feeling of normalcy.
■ Provide information on shops specializing in prostheses; arrange an in-hospital consultation if possible.	Community resources provide support for the woman who is adjusting to changes in her body.
■ Encourage the family (especially significant others) to provide positive input (i.e., feelings of being loved and needed).	Limited or impaired social supports cause adjustment difficulties.

Actions/Interventions

- Refer the patient to community support resources (e.g., Reach to Recovery).

- Provide the patient with information about reconstructive options.

Rationales

Interactions with women who have successfully dealt with breast surgery can help with adjustment to the changed body.

Increased effectiveness of reconstructive surgical techniques can restore body contours in women who do not want to wear external prostheses. Some women may opt to have this procedure done during initial mastectomy surgery. Although plastic surgery procedures have made great advances, the woman must understand that the artificial breast will not be exactly like the other breast.

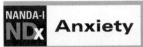

Anxiety

Common Related Factors

Diagnosis of cancer
Uncertain prognosis

Defining Characteristics

Restlessness
Expressed concern about health
Focus on self
Difficulty concentrating

Common Expected Outcomes

Patient uses effective coping mechanisms.
Patient describes a reduction in the level of anxiety expressed.

NOC Outcomes
Anxiety Self-Control; Social Support; Coping
NIC Interventions
Anxiety Reduction; Support System
   Enhancement

Ongoing Assessment

Actions/Interventions

- Assess for signs of anxiety (e.g., withdrawal, crying, restlessness, or inability to focus).
- Assess previous successful coping strategies.

Rationales

The threats accompanying a diagnosis of cancer can cause anxiety about health and continued productivity.
These strategies may be useful in dealing with the current crisis.

Therapeutic Interventions

Actions/Interventions

- Encourage verbalizations about feelings of grief, anger, fear, and anxiety.

- Reassure the patient that these feelings are normal.

- Provide accurate information about the future with breast cancer.

- Assist in use of previously successful coping measures.

Rationales

Verbalization of actual or perceived threats can help reduce anxiety. Initial focus may be on the threat of dying rather than on reactions to the mastectomy.
Stages of fear and grief over change or loss of a body part are normal.
Most women have experience with women who have died of breast cancer. Misinformation should be corrected, and new treatment options and prognosis explained.
This helps patient focus on anxiety as a real and natural part of life that has been and can continue to be dealt with successfully. Modification may be necessary for this specific problem.

■ = Independent   ▲ = Collaborative

Actions/Interventions

▲ Work collaboratively with other health care providers as indicated (social worker, psychologist, chaplain).

■ Support realistic assessment; avoid false reassurances.

▲ Administer antianxiety medications as ordered and indicated.

Rationales

An interdisciplinary approach to patient care provides the patient with diverse support and resources.

This approach assists the patient in dealing with the current crisis and in gaining control over the situation. False reassurances are never helpful to the patient and only serve to relieve the discomfort of the care provider.

Short-term use of medications can relieve unpleasant feelings.

NANDA-I NDx **Deficient Knowledge: Postoperative**

Common Related Factors

Need for home management
New condition and treatment
Misinterpretation of information
Unfamiliarity with existing informational resources

Defining Characteristics

Questions to health care team
Verbalized inaccurate information

Common Expected Outcome

Patient verbalizes understanding of proper wound care and need for follow-up care.

NOC Outcomes

Knowledge: Disease Process; Knowledge: Treatment Regimen

NIC Interventions

Teaching: Disease Process; Teaching: Procedures/Treatment; Wound Care

---

Ongoing Assessment

Actions/Interventions

■ Assess knowledge level of home care and required health maintenance.

Rationales

The patient may be unaware of important self-care procedures. For successful recovery the patient must know how to provide home care, how to identify problems, and what to do should problems arise.

Therapeutic Interventions

Actions/Interventions

■ Educate about wound care and arm care (if applicable):

• Check wound drain (if in place) for color of drainage, amount of output, and suction pressure. Empty drainage device as needed and compress and recap.

• Expect that the arm will be stiff and uncomfortable.

• Continue ROM exercises for at least 1 month.

Rationales

Information enables the woman to assume responsibility for self-care recovery at home.

Wound drainage will normally decrease in volume, and can be removed by surgeon when less than 30 mL in 24 hours. Color will change from red/pink to clear. Fluid accumulation can be a source of infection. Wound drainage malfunction requires immediate intervention.

Exercise decreases stiffness, but numbness may remain for a prolonged time if nodes were dissected.

Exercise eases tension in the arm and shoulder, maintains muscle tone, and improves lymph and blood circulation on the affected side.

Actions/Interventions

- Notify the health care provider regarding fever, swelling, wound drainage, or injury.
- Protect the arm from injury and infection.

- Use an electric razor when shaving, gloves when gardening or doing dishes, and mitts when handling hot dishes.
- Avoid blood draws, intravenous lines, and injections or blood pressure measurement in the operative arm during subsequent medical treatments.
- Carry heavy packages or handbags with the opposite arm.
- Massage the incision site gently with cocoa butter and vitamin E cream.
- Wear temporary prosthesis or brassiere at least occasionally.
- ■ Instruct about activity guidelines:
  - Resume all routine activities as tolerated (e.g., driving).
  - Resume sexual activity as tolerated
- ■ Instruct about required follow-up care:
  - Monthly breast self-examination (BSE)

  - Annual mammogram (or more often)

  - Reconstructive surgery (if desired)

  - Importance of large-breasted women being fitted with weighted prosthesis as soon as possible
- ■ Instruct about possible family needs:
  - All women older than 20 years of age should perform monthly BSE.
  - Women older than 40 years of age should have an annual mammogram.
- ■ Instruct in follow-up consultations with medical and radiation specialists if required because of nodal status.
- ■ Provide appropriate educational materials from the American Cancer Society, the National Cancer Institute, the Susan G. Komen Breast Cancer Foundation, or YWCA's ENCORE program.

Rationales

Prompt assessment facilitates early intervention.

The operative arm will remain vulnerable to lymphedema after axillary lymph node dissection.
The woman needs to learn to protect the operative arm from any type of injury for the rest of her life.
These measures reduce the risk for injury to the blood and lymphatic vessels in the operative arm.

This measure reduces the risk for muscle and joint strain in the operative arm.
These products promote healing and skin softness and minimize scar formation.
These help adjustment to recent loss of breast.

Each woman will progress at her own rate based on the extent of surgical intervention and related treatment regimen.

Women may hesitate to perform BSE because of difficulty viewing or touching the surgical site on the chest or fear of finding another lump.
There is increased risk for cancer in the opposite breast. Mammography can identify breast tumors before they are palpable.
Reconstructive surgery does not influence survival rates but may improve the quality of life. It may be contraindicated in locally advanced, progressively metastatic, or inflammatory cancer.
This measure provides balance for proper posture.

Risk is increased in daughters or sisters of women with breast cancer and is further increased in daughters or sisters of women with premenopausal bilateral breast cancer or if more than one relative has cancer.

Ongoing evaluation is necessary for the development of lymphedema, metastasis, and recurrence of cancer.
Information from specialty organizations can enhance learning and compliance. Although family and friends can be great allies, often a formal support group or communication with a cancer survivor is most helpful.

Related Care Plans

Cancer chemotherapy, p. 681
Cancer radiation therapy, p. 694
Ineffective peripheral tissue perfusion, p. 199
Ineffective sexuality patterns, p. 182

■ = Independent   ▲ = Collaborative

Cervical Cancer

Cancer of the cervix is one of the most common cancers affecting women's reproductive organs, occurring between 35 and 55 years of age. It is more commonly seen in the African American and Hispanic populations. Although the number of cases and deaths have significantly declined over the past 20 years, it remains a serious health risk. Several factors increase one's risk for cervical cancer, including human papillomavirus (HPV) infection, lack of regular Papanicolaou (Pap) smear screening, many sexual partners, early sexual activity, history of sexually transmitted infections, long-term use of birth control pills, having many children, weakened immune systems, and smoking habit. At least 95% of the cases are reported to be related to sexual exposure to HPV. A vaccine approved by the Food and Drug Administration for HPV is recommended for girls as young as 9 to 12 years of age and for women 13 to 26 years of age.

The death rate from cervical cancer has significantly dropped as a result of Pap tests. When diagnosed at an early, preinvasive stage, the survival rate is nearly 100%. According to the American Cancer Society, invasive cancer that is diagnosed while still confined to the cervix has a 5-year survival rate of around 91%. Treatment options depend on the tumor stage at diagnosis. Treatment may consist of conization, LEEP (loop electrosurgical excision procedure), cryosurgery, cauterization, laser surgery, hysterectomy, radiation, chemotherapy, or biological therapy.

NANDA-I NDx Deficient Knowledge

Common Related Factors
Unfamiliarity with disease and treatment
New condition, procedure, treatment
Complexity of treatment
Emotional state affecting learning

Defining Characteristics
Multiple questions to health care team
Verbalizes inaccurate information

Common Expected Outcome
Patient verbalizes understanding of the risk factors and diagnosis and treatment procedures for cervical cancer.

NOC Outcomes
Knowledge: Disease Process; Knowledge: Treatment Regimen

NIC Interventions
Teaching: Disease Process; Teaching: Procedure/Treatment

Ongoing Assessment

Actions/Interventions

- Assess understanding of cervical cancer. Identify any existing misconceptions.

Rationales

Women may have misinformation about types of female cancers and their causes, treatments, and prognoses. Previous experience with other women being treated for cancer or who have died of cancer will influence beliefs; some of these may be negative or incorrect.

Therapeutic Interventions	
Actions/Interventions	**Rationales**
■ Explain that the cause of cervical cancer is unknown, although several risk factors have been identified: • Exposure to HPV and other sexually transmitted infections • Many sexual partners • Early sexual activity (before 18 years of age) • Smoking history • Chronic cervical infections • Weakened immune systems • Long-term use of birth control pills • Multiparity	Various strains of the sexually transmitted HPV account for 95% of diagnosed cases. Persistence of HPV infection in the body without treatment is what puts a woman at risk. Sexually transmitted infection (STI) viruses have been linked to atypical cell transformations that eventually convert to cancerous cells. However, not all women with HPV infections develop cancer. Studies have demonstrated higher incidences in women who have early and varied sexual habits. The mechanism between cigarette smoking and cervical cancer is unclear, although it is proposed that smoking affects the immune system's ability to respond to strains of viruses. Its effects increase with the number of cigarettes smoked daily and with pack-years of smoking. Women with weakened immune systems from human immunodeficiency virus (HIV) or immunosuppressant agents are also at higher risk.
■ Explain signs and symptoms of cervical cancer.	Early cancer usually has no specific signs and is not identified without a screening Pap test. However, as the cancer progresses, abnormal bleeding is the major sign (e.g., from the vagina after intercourse, between periods, or after menopause). An increased watery, bloody vaginal discharge may also be noted.
■ Discuss common diagnostic procedures: • Pelvic examination and Pap test	The Pap test allows for detection of abnormal cells. It is only a screening test, not for diagnosis. Newer Pap smear collection procedures have enhanced diagnostic ability. Women should avoid douching or using spermicidal foams or creams for about 2 days before testing to avoid altering any abnormal cells.
• Colposcopy	Colposcopy uses a lighted magnifying instrument to examine the vagina and cervix for epithelial abnormalities.
• Biopsy	Biopsy may include a simple "punch" technique using forceps to pinch off a small piece of tissue. Another method is termed *LEEP* (loop electrosurgical excision procedure), in which an electric wire loop slices off a thin, round area of tissue. These biopsies are performed under local anesthesia.
• Conization (cone biopsy)	Conization is surgery to remove a cone-shaped piece of tissue from the cervix as well as the cervical canal. It can be used for diagnosis as well as treatment.
■ Discuss the treatment options for precancerous and cancerous conditions. *Precancerous* • Conization/LEEP • Cryosurgery (freezing) • Laser surgery • Hysterectomy	Many factors determine the optimal treatment for precancerous lesions. These depend on the severity of the lesion (grade), whether the woman wants to have children in the future, the age of the woman, and her general health. Like conization and LEEP procedure, laser therapy can be performed as an office procedure in which energy from the light beam destroys the abnormal cells it comes in contact with. Cryosurgery is a treatment that freezes a section of cervix to destroy abnormal cells. Hysterectomy may be indicated if abnormal cells are found inside the cervical opening and the woman is not interested in having children.

■ = Independent   ▲ = Collaborative

Actions/Interventions

Cancer of cervix
- Surgery (hysterectomy)
- Radiation therapy (external/internal)
- Chemotherapy
- Biological therapy

■ Discuss common side effects related to treatments.

Rationales

Treatment for cervical cancer often requires a radical hysterectomy or radiation therapy or both. If the tumor is small, surgery may be sufficient treatment. Radiation is more effective for larger tumors or for tumors that have spread outside the cervical area but are confined to the pelvic area. The radiation may come from external sources or from an internal implant. Platinum-based chemotherapy with concurrent radiation is recommended for systemic treatment. Chemotherapy involves systemic treatment. Biological therapy uses substances to boost the body's immune system (e.g., interferon). Most women will benefit from seeking a second opinion to guide optimal therapy.

Minor surgery causes pelvic cramping, bleeding, or a watery discharge. Hysterectomy involves pain in the lower abdomen, some difficulty voiding or having bowel movements, and fatigue. If the uterus was removed, women will no longer have menstrual periods and may experience a change in their sexuality. Patients having external radiation therapy may experience local hair loss and drying and reddening of skin. Patients with internal implants must avoid intercourse. Both types of radiation can cause diarrhea and uncomfortable voiding. Chemotherapy effects vary with the agent used and the patient's response to it.

NANDA-I NDx Risk for Ineffective Coping

Common Risk Factors

Threat of malignancy
Situational crisis
Inadequate support system
Inadequate coping methods
Lack of knowledge related to disease process

Common Expected Outcome

Patient uses available resources and support systems.
Patient describes and initiates effective coping strategies.
Patient describes positive results from new behavior.

NOC Outcomes
Coping; Anxiety Self-Control; Decision Making
NIC Interventions
Coping Enhancement; Decision-Making Support; Anxiety Reduction; Emotional Support

Ongoing Assessment

Actions/Interventions

■ Assess patient's knowledge of disease and treatment.

■ Assess for coping mechanisms used in previous illnesses or prior personal problems.

Rationales

Patients may hear the word "cancer" or even the words "precancerous tumor" and expect to die. Realistic information about the high survival rates with cervical cancer needs to be conveyed.

Successful coping is influenced by previous successes. Patients with a history of maladaptive coping may need additional resources. Likewise, previously successful coping skills may be inadequate in the present situation.

Actions/Interventions

- Evaluate resources and support systems available to the patient at home and in the community.

Rationales

With diagnosis of a precancerous tumor, the patient may need only short-term support to get through the initial diagnosis and treatment period. For women with advanced disease requiring more radical surgery, radiation, or chemotherapy treatment, ongoing support will be required. Available support systems may change over time.

Therapeutic Interventions

Actions/Interventions

- Establish a working relationship with the patient through continuation of care.

- Provide opportunities for the patient or significant other to openly express feelings, fears, and concerns. Avoid false reassurances.

- Assist the patient with becoming involved as comanager of her treatment plan.

- Provide information the patient wants and needs. Do not provide more than the patient can handle.
- Encourage the patient to communicate feelings with significant others.
- Encourage participation in self-help groups as available.

Rationales

An ongoing relationship establishes trust, reduces the feeling of isolation, and may facilitate coping. The nurse is in an ideal position to guide women through this stressful period.

Verbalization of actual or perceived threats can help reduce anxiety. Patients receiving radiation implant therapy may express a sense of social isolation while hospitalized, especially with staff required to limit presence in the room and restrict visitors. False assurances are never helpful to the patient and only serve to relieve the discomfort of the care provider.

This provides a way for the patient to gain some control over the situation. Many patients with advanced disease become quite educated about their treatment plan and possible side effects.

People who are coping ineffectively have reduced ability to assimilate information.

Unexpressed feelings can increase stress.

Relationships with women with common interests and experiences can be beneficial. Women need to help spread the word that this cancer is easily treated if diagnosed early.

Related Care Plans

Acute pain, p. 151
Cancer chemotherapy, p. 681
Cancer radiation therapy, p. 694
Disturbed body image, p. 24
Hysterectomy, p. 875
Ineffective sexuality patterns, p. 182

Hysterectomy

Salpingectomy; Oophorectomy; Total Abdominal Hysterectomy; Cervical Cancer

Hysterectomy is a surgical procedure that involves the removal of the uterus with or without removal of the cervix. The surgery may also include removal of the ovaries (oophorectomy) and the fallopian tubes (salpingectomy). Indications for the surgery include endometriosis, uterine fibroids, cancer, uterine prolapse or bleeding, and ectopic pregnancy. Although other, less-invasive treatments can be considered for most of these problems, hysterectomy might be the only option for cancer. Hysterectomy is the second most common surgical procedure in women, with approximately 600,000 hysterectomies performed each year in the United States. Hysterectomy with oophorectomy results in surgically induced menopause.

■ = Independent   ▲ = Collaborative

The woman may experience symptoms of menopause more severely than normal menopause because of the sudden loss of hormones.

Every attempt is usually undertaken to retain the reproductive function of women who are still of childbearing age; however, certain clinical situations, such as aggressive forms of cancer, may require aggressive surgery. A hysterectomy can be performed using an abdominal, vaginal, or laparoscopic approach. The surgical approach used is dependent on the surgeon and patient, as well as on the amount of visualization and area of manipulation required. The bulk of recovery takes place at home with patients gaining full function within 2 weeks if the vaginal approach was used for the procedure, and 4 to 6 weeks if the abdominal approach was used.

NANDA-I NDx Deficient Knowledge: Surgical Treatment

Common Related Factors
Unfamiliarity with anatomy and physiology, surgical procedure, recovery process, and menopausal process
Misinterpretation of information
Fear and anxiety
Emotional state affecting learning

Defining Characteristics
Verbalized inaccurate information
Inaccurate follow-through of instructions
Inability to concentrate or focus on information presented
Questioning members of health care team

Common Expected Outcomes
Patient verbalizes understanding of the reason for hysterectomy, surgical procedures anticipated, postoperative recovery, discharge instructions, and follow-up care.
Patient actively participates in planning of care.

NOC Outcomes
Knowledge: Disease Process; Knowledge: Treatment Regimen

NIC Interventions
Teaching: Disease Process; Teaching: Procedure/Treatment; Teaching: Prescribed Activity/Exercise

Ongoing Assessment

Actions/Interventions
■ Assess the patient's understanding of the indications for surgery.

Indications include the following:
- Severe endometriosis
- Fibroids or nonmalignant tumors of the reproductive tract that are symptomatic
  - Unresponsive to medical management
  - Painful pelvic and abdominal adhesions
- Malignant tumors, including cervical, endometrial, ovarian, or vaginal

Elective indications include the following:
- Family history of reproductive malignancies
- Menstrual irregularities
- Severe dysmenorrhea or premenstrual syndrome
- Termination of reproductive potential

Rationales
Thorough understanding of indications for the procedure is necessary for informed consent to be given. This information provides the starting base for education. Teaching standardized content that the patient already knows wastes valuable time and hinders learning.

Actions/Interventions	Rationales
■ Assess the patient's and family's understanding of immediate and long-term postsurgical recovery period.	The postsurgical recovery period may be difficult and more prolonged than expected. For successful recovery, the patient must know how to provide home care, how to identify problems, and what to do when problems arise.
■ Assess the patient's understanding of ongoing gynecological needs following hysterectomy.	Patients may assume that the need for yearly or regular gynecological care ceases after hysterectomy.

Therapeutic Interventions

Actions/Interventions	Rationales
■ Provide preoperative instruction, including rationale for planned surgical approach, explanation of procedures, activity restrictions, and recovery process.	A variety of surgical approaches can be performed, with abdominal hysterectomy performed most frequently. Each approach has its own protocol that may vary among institutions. Patients are better able to ask questions when they have basic information about what to expect.
■ Provide discharge instructions:	Accurate, clear information provides rationale for treatment/follow-up care and assists the patient in assuming responsibility for care. For successful recovery, the patient must know how to provide home care, how to identify problems, and what to do when problems arise.
• Abdominal support may be helpful.	This support prevents strain on the incision line.
• Avoid lifting heavy objects for about 2 months.	This reduces strain on the abdominal muscles and surgical incisions.
• Place nothing in the vagina; no penetrating intercourse is permitted for 4 to 6 weeks.	These restrictions facilitate healing.
• Showers, sponge bathing, light activity, and exercise are permitted.	Showers are preferred over tub baths to reduce risk for infection. Gradual increase in exercise is encouraged within limits of fatigue.
• Notify the physician of any of the following: increased bleeding, pain, foul-smelling discharge, or symptoms of thrombophlebitis (e.g., leg pain; swelling of calf during ambulation; swollen, red, hot area behind calf).	Early assessment facilitates prompt treatment.
■ Instruct the patient about resuming home activities: • Plan brief periods of graduated activity. • Minimize or limit climbing stairs.	Fatigue is common after most surgeries and limits ability to maintain usual household and work activities. Patient may need to consider use of a bedside commode if living in a two-story house with one bathroom.
■ Instruct about the need for removal of sutures or staples at postsurgical checkup.	Understanding increases cooperation with routine follow-up procedures.
■ Stress the need to continue with routine gynecological examinations.	Periodic examination of the breasts and ovaries and Papanicolaou (Pap) tests are still recommended in case cervical cancer should ever recur. Patients on hormone therapy (HT) may be evaluated more often.

NANDA-I NDx Deficient Knowledge: Surgical Menopause

Common Related Factors	Defining Characteristics
Unfamiliarity with surgical menopause Unfamiliarity with hormone therapy	Requests information about the expected symptoms of menopause Questions about the use of HT

■ = Independent ▲ = Collaborative

Common Expected Outcome

Patient verbalizes knowledge of the effects of surgical menopause and the advantages and disadvantages of HT.

NOC Outcome
Knowledge: Medication
NIC Interventions
Teaching: Disease Process; Teaching: Prescribed Medication

Ongoing Assessment

Actions/Interventions	Rationales
■ Assess understanding of menopause.	Women who have both uterus and ovaries removed undergo a menopause. Most women have some minimal information about the female climacteric, but few women understand the entire surgical process or the effects of surgical menopause.
■ Assess knowledge about HT.	Individual evaluation is required to determine appropriateness of HT. All women must be given enough information to make an informed choice. Risks are present with and without the use of HT. After hysterectomy, progesterone is no longer required to offset the risk for uterine cancer.

Therapeutic Interventions

Actions/Interventions	Rationales
■ Describe surgical menopause.	With removal of the uterus or removal of the uterus, tubes, and even one ovary, the remaining ovary will continue to function until menopause, when follicular development ceases and the female body goes through a series of changes resulting from estrogen withdrawal. Removal of both ovaries (surgical menopause) results in a sudden, precipitous decrease in hormone levels. The changes that occur are more rapid. Hot flashes begin 1 to 2 days after surgery. Changes in skin and hair occur more rapidly, within months rather than over years.

■ Discuss the benefits and risks associated with estrogen therapy (ET).
Benefits
• Immediate:
  • Reduces hot flashes
  • Relieves vaginal dryness
  • Improves urinary tract symptoms (incontinence and infection)
  • Maintains skin thickness and elasticity
  • Improves sleep
  • Reduces mood swings
• Long-term:
  • Reduces bone resorption
Risks
• Immediate:
  • Menstrual symptoms of breast swelling, mood swings
  • Fluid retention
  • Aggravation of migraines
	The decision to take estrogen is based on each woman's personal profile. If surgical menopause results from the hysterectomy/oophorectomy, ET may be prescribed to relieve menopausal symptoms. Usually these symptoms are short-lived, and many women do not require therapy. However, there are significant risks also associated with this therapy. Only short-term therapy may be needed if the outcome is symptom management with the lowest effective dose. Although ET can reduce the risk for osteoporosis fractures, other therapies should be considered given its associated risks.
	
	About two-thirds of women who start on HT stop secondary to unpleasant side effects.

Actions/Interventions	Rationales
• Long-term:	Evidence from the Women's Health Initiative (the largest, randomized controlled trial) reports that HT should not be taken for the primary prevention of coronary heart disease, stroke, or dementia. In fact, starting HT may be associated with an increased risk for cardiovascular events for some women. If HT is taken for more than 5 years, there is also an increased risk for breast cancer.
• Increased risk for cardiovascular problems	
• Increased risk for breast cancer	
• Increased risk for blood clotting	
• Increased risk for gallbladder disease	
	Each woman needs to evaluate the risks/benefits of treatment based on her personal health history.
Relative contraindications:	
• History of breast cancer	
• History of hormone-sensitive cancer	
• Liver disease	
• History of blood clotting disorders	
• History of cardiovascular disease	
■ Describe common HT regimens:	HT needs to be "customized" to the woman, her goals, and any experienced side effects.
• Cyclic hormone therapy versus continuous combined	
• Systemic versus local	
■ Describe the role of selective estrogen receptor modulators (SERMs).	SERMs (e.g., tamoxifen and raloxifene) exert tissue-specific effects. They exhibit some of estrogen's beneficial effects on lipid levels and bone metabolism but do not exhibit the adverse effects on breast tissue. Likewise, raloxifene has an adverse effect on endometrial tissue (i.e., cancer) and is the first SERM to be approved for osteoporosis prevention (although its effect is weaker than that of estrogen). The SERMs do increase the risk for thromboembolic events and do not relieve hot flashes (actually, they may intensify them).
■ Counsel the patient to discuss potential ET questions with her health care professional. Examples include the following:	Women need to be comanagers of their health. Only with proper information can they make an informed decision.
• "Is estrogen right for me?"	
• "How will it benefit my body?"	
• "What risk might I encounter?"	
• "What type of regimen is best for me?"	
• "How long should I take it?"	
• "What side effects can I expect?"	
• "Will I be compliant?"	

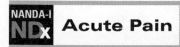

NANDA-I NDx   Acute Pain

Common Related Factors	Defining Characteristics
Incision(s)	Verbal complaint of pain
Intraoperative positioning	Guarding behaviors
Manipulation of intraabdominal contents	Self-focusing and narrowed focus
Gas pains	Distraction behavior
	Facial mask of pain
	Alteration of muscle tone
	Autonomic responses

■ = Independent   ▲ = Collaborative

Common Expected Outcomes

Patient reports satisfactory pain control at a level less than 3 to 4 on a 0 to 10 rating scale.

Patient uses pharmacological and nonpharmalogical pain-relief measures.

Patient is able to perform self-care activities and ambulate with progressive effectiveness.

NOC Outcome
Pain Control
NIC Interventions
Analgesic Administration; Pain Management; Patient-Controlled Analgesia (PCA)

Ongoing Assessment

Actions/Interventions

- Assess cause of pain:

  - Intraoperative position

  - Manipulation of intraabdominal contents.

  - Extreme gas pains

- Assess level of pain, patient's expectations for pain relief, and response to medications.

- Assess effectiveness of other pain-relief measures:
  - Position change
  - Back rub
  - Heat application
  - Relaxation and breathing modifications
  - Biofeedback

Rationales

Postsurgical pain may be a result of the incision and manipulation at the surgical site, carbon dioxide remaining in the abdominal cavity following laparoscopy, or other factors. Correct diagnosis of the cause of the pain guides the selection of an appropriate intervention.

Intraoperative positioning may result in intense shoulder pain. This pain responds well to a heating pad or massage.

Manipulation of the intraabdominal contents required to visualize the uterus may cause internal pain related to organ and bowel manipulation in addition to the incisional pain. This may be alleviated with postoperative analgesia, positioning, and abdominal splinting.

These gas pains occur from intraoperative manipulation of bowel and from intraoperative and postoperative medications.

The Joint Commission (TJC) mandates frequent, regular assessment of pain. Some patients may be content to have pain decreased; others will expect complete elimination of pain. This affects their perceptions of the effectiveness of the treatment modality. Patients have a right to effective pain relief.

Chemical analgesia may not be effective in relieving pain; other methods may be needed. Some patients may be unaware of the effectiveness of nonpharmacological methods.

Therapeutic Interventions

Actions/Interventions

▲ Administer pain medications every 3 to 4 hours as ordered. Ask the patient to rate her comfort level and what she feels is necessary.

- Anticipate periods of mobility, and administer an analgesic 20 to 30 minutes before.
- Consider patient-controlled analgesia (PCA) via the epidural or intravenous routes.

Rationales

TJC mandates frequent, regular assessment and treatment of pain. Patients have a right to effective pain relief. Pain medications are absorbed and metabolized differently by patients, so their effectiveness must be evaluated individually by the patient. Around-the-clock administration of analgesics on a regular schedule keeps the patient's pain level within a comfortable range.

Decreasing pain levels permits ambulation and improves healing.

Individual patients react to pain and analgesia differently. Epidural morphine reduces or eliminates incisional pain for 18 to 24 hours. This facilitates early ambulation and prevents many postsurgical complications. PCA provides a continuous basal dose of analgesia while allowing the patient to self-medicate up to a preprogrammed maximum dose/bolus.

Actions/Interventions

- Initiate comfort measures:
  - Position in correct anatomical alignment. Support position with pillows or wedges.
  - Use abdominal splinting during movement.

  - Apply heat or ice as needed.

  - Encourage relaxation and breathing modification.

Rationales

This position reduces pain and muscle tension.

Splinting supports incision and abdominal muscles, reducing discomfort.

Heat reduces pain through improved blood flow to the area and through reduction of pain reflexes. Cold reduces pain, inflammation, and muscle spasticity by decreasing the release of pain-inducing chemicals and slowing conduction of pain impulses.

These techniques are used to bring about a state of physical and mental awareness and tranquility.

 NANDA-I NDx **Disturbed Body Image**

Common Related Factors

Fears of loss of sexual identity or femininity
Loss of childbearing capacity
Effects of surgical menopause on ability to be sexually satisfied
Permanent alterations in function (removal of uterus)

Common Expected Outcomes

Patient verbalizes positive statements about body and self.
Patient identifies available resources to aid in coping.

Defining Characteristics

Self-deprecating remarks
Verbalized negative feelings about surgically altered body
Decreased attention to grooming
Refusal to discuss or acknowledge change

NOC Outcomes
Body Image; Grief Resolution; Psychosocial Adjustment: Life Change
NIC Interventions
Body Image Enhancement; Grief Work Facilitation; Coping Enhancement; Teaching: Sexuality

---

Ongoing Assessment

Actions/Interventions

- Assess knowledge level about loss of reproductive function.

- Assess feelings about self and body.

Rationales

Many persons have misconceptions about reproduction. After hysterectomy, pregnancy cannot occur because the patient no longer has a uterus to house a developing embryo/fetus. If a woman has a whole or partial ovary remaining, ovulation continues. Reproductive ability may be maintained through cryopreservation of ova or embryos for later transplantation in a surrogate. This must be done before surgery.

Loss of reproductive ability may result in lowered feelings of femininity and sexuality. These feelings may be exaggerated by the physical and emotional changes accompanying surgical menopause. Body image changes are affected by age; reason for surgery; religious, cultural, and childbearing expectations; previous childbearing discomfort; history of dysmenorrhea; and previous unpleasant physical or emotional experiences accompanying menstrual cycle.

■ = Independent   ▲ = Collaborative

Actions/Interventions

- Determine ability and comfort in discussing effect of surgery on personal relationships.

- Assess understanding of the effect of hysterectomy on sexuality and sexual desire and functioning.

- Note the frequency of self-critical remarks.

Rationales

It is important for the nurse to create an environment where the couple feels safe and comfortable in discussing feelings. Open discussion of these issues with partners corrects misconceptions about potential changes in personal relationships. It also identifies specific problem areas to be addressed before and after surgery.

Physical and psychological effects of hysterectomy may alter sexual relations after the 4- to 6-week abstinence required by surgery. Exploration of these feelings promotes more normal adaptation.

Negative statements about the affected body part indicate limited ability to integrate the change into the patient's self-concept.

Therapeutic Interventions

Actions/Interventions

- Provide accurate information about the effect of hysterectomy on reproductive ability, anatomy/physiology, surgical menopause, and cryopreservation of ova or embryos if desired.

- Encourage the patient and significant others to express feelings, ask questions, and correct misconceptions.

- Provide anticipatory guidance on management of symptoms and physical changes resulting from surgery.
- Explore physiological and emotional influences on sexual functioning:
  - Explain discomforts and fatigue.
  - Explain process of sexual functioning and response.
  - Encourage support from spouse or significant other.
  - Make appropriate referrals for treatments or counseling.

Rationales

It is important not to make assumptions about a woman's acceptance or willingness to permanently end her reproductive ability. Information enables the woman to take control of her life following surgery and elicits her cooperation in decision making and postoperative treatments.

Explanations of surgical menopause may be clarified by comparisons with naturally occurring menopause. Exploration of the most current treatment options to decrease or alleviate symptoms enables the woman to select the options most acceptable to her and her lifestyle.

This guidance helps the woman gain control over the situation.

A woman's response to hysterectomy may range from relief that pregnancy is no longer possible (leading to more enjoyable sexual activity) to sexual difficulties such as difficulty achieving orgasm, painful intercourse (dyspareunia), and conflicts regarding sexual identity. HT and individual or family counseling may provide relief of these symptoms.

Related Care Plans

Constipation, p. 46
Fatigue, p. 66
Urinary retention, p. 202
Ineffective coping, p. 49
Menopause, p. 882

Menopause

Perimenopause; Hormone Therapy

Menopause is the point in a woman's life when menstruation stops, as does the ability to reproduce. It is usually confirmed when a woman does not have a menstrual period for 12 consecutive months, in the absence of any biological or physiological causes. It occurs naturally as a part of the aging process. The mean or median age of natural menopause ranges from 48 to 52 years of age. Cancer chemotherapy, cigarette smoking, and surgical trauma to the ovarian blood supply may contribute to the onset of menopause. There may also be a link between heredity and age at menopause.

The 2 to 8 years preceding menopause and 1 year after the final menses is often referred to as the perimenopause. Perimenopause begins with the onset of endocrinological, biological, and clinical changes often associated with menopause. Subtle hormonal changes often begin in a woman's 30s. During perimenopause, a woman's oocytes undergo accelerated depletion, which results in cessation of ovulation and changes in serum and hormone levels. The pituitary gland increases the secretion of follicle-stimulating hormone (FSH) to increase ovarian secretion of estrogen, a hormone that decreases during the perimenopause. FSH levels can fluctuate during the perimenopause and may require stopping the use of oral contraceptives before a diagnosis of menopause can be made. Estradiol levels decrease, resulting in insufficient levels to maintain the endometrial lining. Menstrual cycles may become irregular, and the intervals between menses may become shorter. This irregularity may result in an unplanned pregnancy until amenorrhea has been present more than 1 year. Abnormal uterine bleeding may result from anovulation, uterine fibroids, abnormalities in the uterine lining, cancer, and blood clotting problems. Pathology must be ruled out before a diagnosis of menopause can be made.

Symptoms during the perimenopause include vasomotor symptoms (e.g., hot flashes or flushes, palpitations, anxiety, and sleep disturbances) and genitourinary effects (e.g., vulvovaginal atrophy and urinary tract conditions). The role of hormone therapy (HT), which encompasses both estrogen therapy (ET) and combined estrogen-progestogen therapy (EPT) in treating these symptoms, is well accepted. Evidence from the Women's Health Initiative, the largest randomized, controlled trial, reports that HT should not be taken for the primary prevention of coronary heart disease, stroke, or dementia. In fact, starting HT may be associated with an increased risk for cardiovascular events for some women. If EPT is taken for more than 5 years, there is also an increased risk for breast cancer. Finally, although HT can reduce the risk for osteoporosis fracture, other therapies should be considered given its associated risks.

 Deficient Knowledge

Common Related Factors
Unfamiliarity with treatment plans
Uncertainty about treatment options
Misinterpretation of information
Decisional conflict

Defining Characteristics
Asks questions about diagnostic tests and treatment options
Makes statements indicating misinformation
Expresses inability to make choice about treatment options

Common Expected Outcome
Patient verbalizes understanding of the process of menopause, its diagnosis, and its treatment options.

NOC Outcomes
Knowledge: Disease Process; Knowledge: Treatment Regimen
NIC Interventions
Teaching: Disease Process; Teaching: Procedure/Treatment

Ongoing Assessment

Actions/Interventions	Rationales
■ Assess understanding of perimenopausal symptoms.	Diagnosis is facilitated by complete reporting of symptoms.
■ Assess understanding of the relationship between the normal process of aging and perimenopausal symptoms.	It may be important to emphasize that symptoms are related to "biological" aging, not emotional or attitudinal age.

■ = Independent ▲ = Collaborative

Actions/Interventions

- Assess understanding of treatment options:
  - Hormone therapy (ET/EPT)
  - Complementary therapies

Rationales

Most women want a collaborative relationship in the management of this normal biological process and require information about preference for specific treatment options.

Therapeutic Interventions

Actions/Interventions

- Explain the physiological process of menopause:
  - Cessation of ovulation
  - Hormonal fluctuations
  - Expected symptoms

- Explain diagnostic tests commonly performed:
  - Blood test for hormone levels

  - Complete physical and pelvic examination
- Discuss the benefits and risks associated with hormone therapy (ET/EPT).

  Benefits
  - Immediate:
    - Reduces hot flashes
    - Relieves vaginal dryness
    - Improves urinary tract symptoms (incontinence/infection)
    - Maintains skin thickness and elasticity
    - Improves sleep
    - Reduces mood swings
  - Long-term:
    - Reduces bone resorption

  Risks
  - Immediate:
    - Irregular bleeding
    - Menstrual symptoms of breast swelling, mood swings
    - Fluid retention
    - Aggravation of migraines
  - Long-term:
    - Increased risk for uterine cancer
    - Increased risk for endometrial cancer

    - Increased risk for heart problems
    - Increased blood clotting
    - Increased risk for breast cancer

Rationales

Women should have accurate information about menopause before its onset. Negative images about menopause have been reinforced by the general public and in the popular media. Women need to understand the physiological process of menopause, its effect on sexuality and reproduction, methods to manage symptoms, and treatment options to promote health and prevent postmenopausal problems such as osteoporosis and heart disease.

This test can determine level of hormonal fluctuations for FSH and estrogen. The North American Menopause Society (NAMS), however, does not recommend hormone testing, because menopausal hormone levels fluctuate throughout the day, as well as day to day.

An examination rules out pathology.

The decision to take ET/EPT is based on each woman's personal profile. The primary indication for hormone therapy (ET/EPT) is for relief of menopausal symptoms; however, there are significant risks also associated with this therapy.

Only short-term therapy may be needed if the outcome is symptom management.

Although ET can reduce the risk for osteoporosis fracture, other therapies should be considered given its associated risks.

About two-thirds of women who start on HT stop secondary to unpleasant side effects.

Estrogen therapy increases the risk for endometrial and uterine cancer in women with an intact uterus; however, if combined with progestogen the risk is reduced.

Evidence from the Women's Health Initiative reports that hormone therapy should not be taken for the primary prevention of coronary heart disease, stroke, or dementia. In fact, starting hormone therapy may be associated with an increased risk for cardiovascular events for some women. If EPT is taken for more than 5 years, there is also an increased risk for breast cancer.

Actions/Interventions

Relative contraindications:
- Known or suspected pregnancy
- History of breast cancer
- History of hormone-sensitive cancer
- Unexplained uterine bleeding
- Liver disease
- History of blood clotting disorders
- History of cardiovascular disease

■ Describe common HT regimens:
- Estrogen-progestogen therapy
  - Cyclic versus continuous versus intermittent

- Estrogen therapy
  - Systemic versus local

- Progestogen therapy

■ Describe the role of selective estrogen receptor modulators (SERMs).

■ Counsel the patient to discuss potential HT questions with her health care professional. Examples include the following:
- "Is HT right for me?"
- "How will it benefit my body?"
- "What risk might I encounter?"
- "What type of regimen is best for me?"
- "How long should I take it?"
- "What side effects can I expect?"
- "Will I be compliant?"

■ Describe some nonpharmacological therapies important for maintaining health and reducing menopausal symptoms:
- Proper diet (low fat; increased fruits and vegetables, high fiber)
- Weight control

Rationales

Hormone therapy increases the risk for serious adverse effects in these situations.

ET/EPT needs to be "customized" to the woman, her goals, and any experienced side effects. A woman with an intact uterus needs to take progestogen with estrogen to prevent uterine cancer. Monthly bleeding differs with type of therapy. The current recommendation is the lowest effective dose for the shortest duration to provide symptom relief.

With systemic ET, patch delivers estrogen directly through the skin into the blood, bypassing the liver. This helps reduce problems with blood clots and gallbladder disease. Vaginal creams and rings work locally, yet a small amount of estrogen can circulate in the body. Vaginal ET will not relieve hot flashes, and the risks associated with it are unclear. ET is generally prescribed for women without a uterus.

This therapy may be indicated during perimenopause for symptomatic women with high estrogen levels.

SERMs (e.g., tamoxifen and raloxifene) exert tissue-specific effects. They exhibit some of estrogen's beneficial effects on lipid levels and bone metabolism but do not exhibit the adverse effects on breast tissue. Likewise, raloxifene has an adverse effect on endometrial tissue (i.e., cancer) and is the first SERM to be approved for osteoporosis prevention (although its effect is weaker than that of estrogen). The SERMs do increase the risk for thromboembolic events and do not relieve hot flashes (actually, they may intensify them).

Women need to be comanagers of their health. Only with proper information can they make informed decisions.

Menopause is not a medical disease. Regular positive health habits may be adequate to promote good health.

As the body's metabolism slows down and estrogen levels reduce, women are prone to gain weight gradually over the following years. Thus it is important to reduce daily caloric intake by 200 to 400 kcal and increase exercise.

■ = Independent   ▲ = Collaborative

Women's Health Care Plans

Actions/Interventions

- Adequate calcium intake
- Exercise

- Smoking cessation

- Other therapies

■ Describe other pharmacological therapies used for reducing menopausal symptoms.

Rationales

Intake of 1200 to 1500 mg daily is required.

Weight-bearing exercise helps stimulate bone growth. Aerobic, strength training, and stretching exercises on a regular basis are all important.

Cessation helps reduce hot flashes and improve high-density lipoprotein (HDL) profile, as well as reduce risks from blood clotting.

Clinical trials are currently evaluating the effectiveness of phytoestrogens (plant estrogens) for treatment of menopausal symptoms, primarily hot flashes. Recently, soy-derived isoflavones have been shown to reduce hot flashes for some women, depending on the product. Isoflavones derived from red clover have not been proven effective in the reduction of hot flashes. The evidence for the use of black cohosh is not strong, suggesting that it may be somewhat helpful with mild symptoms. The evidence for the use of vitamin E for symptom relief suggests that it may be a reasonable option for a trial, but the dose should be kept at 400 IU or less. The use of therapies such as dong quai, evening primrose oil, and ginseng is not recommended by NAMS.

Low-dose antidepressants such as venlafaxine (Effexor), paroxetine (Paxil), fluoxetine (Prozac), citalopram (Celexa), and sertraline (Zoloft) are recommended for hot flashes for women who are not candidates for HT, including breast cancer survivors. Nausea and sexual dysfunctions are side effects. Gabapentin (Neurontin) is also recommended by NAMS as a treatment option for hot flashes. Finally, some antihypertensives (e.g., clonidine) have demonstrated moderate efficacy with high adverse effects for treatment of symptoms.

NANDA-I NDx **Ineffective Coping**

Common Related Factors

Maturational crisis (changing body image)
Inadequate level of confidence in ability to cope
Inadequate social support

Defining Characteristics

Restlessness and irritability
Verbalizes fear of losing femininity
Sleep disturbances
Verbalization of inability to ask for help

Common Expected Outcomes

Patient uses available resources and support systems.
Patient describes and initiates effective coping strategies.
Patient describes positive results from new behaviors.

NOC Outcomes

Anxiety Self-Control; Coping; Social Support

NIC Interventions

Anxiety Reduction; Coping Enhancement; Decision-Making Support; Support System Enhancement

Ongoing Assessment

Actions/Interventions	Rationales
■ Assess for symptoms of ineffective coping.	As women progress through menopause, they may experience mood swings, emotional upset, and irritability, which may be attributed only to hormonal fluctuations when other factors (e.g., insomnia and other life stresses) may be the cause. Although menopause itself does not cause depression, women who have a history of psychological disorders (e.g., depression) are vulnerable to recurrent episodes at this time.
■ Assess understanding of relationship between hormone fluctuations and normal process of perimenopause and menopause.	Some women may feel incapacitated by the thought of hormonal changes, buying into the "raging hormone" stereotype. Women need to understand that this is a natural process. In some countries, women are revered as they go through this stage.
■ Assess for feelings of optimism and value of self in future.	Not all women view menopause as a loss of sexuality. Many feel excited about their future.
■ Assess for resources and support systems available.	Resources may include family, other women, health care provider, community groups, and spiritual counseling.
■ Assess for impaired memory.	Fatigue and labile hormone levels may disrupt ability to remember small details, causing further frustration.

Therapeutic Interventions

Actions/Interventions	Rationales
■ Provide opportunities for the patient to express fears and concerns.	Verbalization of actual or perceived fears can help reduce anxiety and enhance coping ability.
■ Encourage the patient to identify her own coping strengths and abilities.	Most women, by the time of menopause, have dealt successfully with many complex problems. During situational crises patients may be unable to recognize their strengths. Opportunities to highlight one's past coping skills can be useful.
■ Identify community resources and support groups (especially women's groups).	Most women rely on one another for both information and understanding. Use of support group networks can be a great source of strength. In addition, such groups can reduce any sense of isolation the woman may experience.

Ineffective Sexuality Patterns

Common Related Factors
Knowledge of altered body function
Lack of knowledge about alternative responses to changes in sexual response related to menopause
Skill deficit related to health-related transitions

Defining Characteristics
Reported changes in sexual activities
Reported difficulties in sexual activities (e.g., painful intercourse)

Common Expected Outcomes
Patient verbalizes relief of symptoms with correct treatment.
Patient or couple verbalizes satisfaction with the way they express physical intimacy.

NOC Outcomes
Sexual Functioning; Knowledge: Sexual Functioning
NIC Interventions
Sexual Counseling; Teaching: Sexuality

■ = Independent   ▲ = Collaborative

Ongoing Assessment

Actions/Interventions	Rationales
■ Assess understanding of perimenopausal symptoms.	Understanding increases comfort with one's perimenopausal body.
■ Assess severity of physical symptoms.	Some women may just lose interest in sexual performance, whereas others may experience painful intercourse.
■ Assess understanding of possible causes of altered sexuality.	Fluctuating hormone levels contribute to vaginal dryness, sex drive changes, thinning of the vaginal mucosa, and alkalinity of the vaginal secretions. As a result of these changes, a woman may experience dyspareunia, perineal burning and itching, and an increase in vaginal infections. The woman may have concerns about her femininity, sexual attractiveness, and ability to have a satisfying sexual relationship.

Therapeutic Interventions

Actions/Interventions	Rationales
■ Explain physiological changes impacting sexuality: • Dryness of vaginal mucosa • Hormonal fluctuations causing hot flashes	Knowledge *normalizes* the process and reduces anxiety. As estrogen levels decline, tissues become thinner, drier, and less elastic.
■ Explain treatments to reduce vaginal dryness.	Vaginal lubricants such as K-Y Jelly and Astroglide or moisturizers such as Vagisil or Replens may facilitate intercourse. Vaginal estrogen can be administered locally using a vaginal tablet, ring, or cream to reduce vaginal dryness. Regular intercourse, likewise, promotes lubrication.
■ Assist in talking with the woman's partner about personal concerns and feelings.	Menopause is a natural process. Sexuality is not tied to intercourse. Starting out with other ways to show intimacy may be helpful.
■ Explain the need to discuss with the partner her slower arousal time and need for longer foreplay.	Longer foreplay is often satisfying to women, and it promotes lubrication. The patient should give herself appropriate time to be aroused.
■ Explore the use of complementary techniques.	These may include Lachesis for anxiety, sepia for vaginal dryness, and Natrum Mur for emotional well-being. Supplementation with soy products has been studied, because soy contains high levels of phytoestrogens that bind to estrogen receptors. Positive results have been demonstrated in several studies, but additional research is necessary. Quality and standardization guidelines have not been established.

NANDA-I NDx Insomnia

Common Related Factor
Gender-related hormonal shifts

Defining Characteristics
Patient reports difficulty staying asleep
Patient reports lack of restorative sleep
Observed/reported lack of energy

Common Expected Outcome
Patient achieves optimal amounts of sleep, as evidenced by rested appearance, verbalization of feeling rested, and improvement in sleep pattern.

NOC Outcome
Sleep
NIC Intervention
Sleep Enhancement

Ongoing Assessment

Actions/Interventions

■ Assess severity of sleep deprivation.

■ Determine frequency and severity of night sweats.

■ Assess additional factors contributing to sleep loss.

■ Assess routines occurring before sleep.

■ Assess methods used to alleviate symptoms and their level of effectiveness.

Rationales

Most adult women need 6 to 9 hours of sleep at night. Sleep deprivation is positively correlated with increase in other symptoms. Hot flashes and night sweats can disrupt the usual sleep cycle. This can cause many women to be unable to concentrate at work, further aggravating their response to menopause.

Night sweats are often a consequence of hot flashes. Women commonly awaken with soaking sweats followed by chills.

Environmental temperatures, stresses, caffeinated beverages, and vigorous exercise immediately before sleep can aggravate the situation.

Sleep patterns are unique to each individual and knowledge may guide intervention.

Information can guide future interventions.

Therapeutic Interventions

Actions/Interventions

■ Explain physiological processes resulting in sleep disruption.

■ Suggest methods for improving environment and routines to facilitate sleep.

■ Provide tips for dealing with night sweats.

■ Discuss role of hormone therapy (ET/EPT).

Rationales

Understanding reduces anxiety and fear and helps to normalize the experience.

Avoiding alcohol and caffeine and emotional interactions before sleep enhances the environment and is conducive to satisfactory sleep patterns. Maintaining a regular sleep schedule and cooler room temperatures may improve sleep cycles.

Wearing cool cotton clothing to bed and changing bedclothes during the night may be helpful.

HT successfully relieves vasomotor symptoms during menopause.

Related Care Plans

Hysterectomy, p. 875
Osteoporosis, p. 670

Ovarian Cancer

The cause of ovarian cancer remains unknown. It has been linked to the presence of mutations in the BRCA1 and BRCA2 genes. If mutations are present, a woman's risk for ovarian cancer is 40% greater than for a woman without the genes. About 90% of ovarian cancers develop in the epithelial layer covering the ovaries, most commonly in postmenopausal women and more commonly in white women. Eighty percent of ovarian cancers are first diagnosed in stage III or IV because the early stages are often asymptomatic; this explains the high mortality rate. Increased awareness of early, nonspecific symptoms (abdominal swelling and digestive and bladder problems) can lead to earlier detection and treatment. Later signs of ovarian cancer include increased abdominal girth caused by the tumor size or ascites; abdominal, pelvic, or low back pain; urinary urgency and frequency; and constipation. Treatment depends on the stage at diagnosis. Early stages are treated with surgical removal of the uterus, ovaries, and fallopian tubes, together with the tumor. Later stages are treated with radiation therapy and chemotherapy. A late diagnosis is associated with a poor prognosis. This care plan does not address surgical management.

■ = Independent   ▲ = Collaborative

Deficient Knowledge

Common Related Factors

Unfamiliarity with disease and treatment plan
Complexity of treatment
Emotional state affecting learning

Common Expected Outcomes

Patient verbalizes understanding of the diagnosis and treatment procedures for ovarian cancer.
Patient freely discusses treatment options.

Defining Characteristics

Multiple questions to health care team
Verbalized inaccurate information

NOC Outcomes

Knowledge: Disease Process; Knowledge: Treatment Regimen

NIC Interventions

Teaching: Disease Process; Teaching: Procedure/Treatment

Ongoing Assessment

Actions/Interventions	Rationales
■ Assess understanding of ovarian cancer and treatment options. Identify any existing misconceptions.	Women may have misinformation about types of female cancers. Previous experience with other women being treated for cancer, or who have died of it, will influence beliefs, some of which may be negative or misconceived. Ovarian cancer has a high mortality rate because of its advanced stage at diagnosis.

Therapeutic Interventions

Actions/Interventions	Rationales
■ Explain that the cause of ovarian cancer is unknown.	While the cause is unknown, there are some possible risk factors that women need to be informed of. These include family history, advanced age, infertility, ovarian dysfunction, obesity, and mutations of the BRCA genes.
■ Discuss clinical manifestations.	No specific symptoms are recognized until the advanced stage, then abdominal swelling and/or pain, bloating and/or feeling of fullness, vague but persistent gastrointestinal complaints, and bowel and bladder dysfunction manifest. Many of these symptoms also occur earlier, but women tend to attribute them to other causes. Increased awareness of possible symptomatology is key to early detection.
■ Discuss common diagnostic procedures: • Pelvic examination • CA-125 blood test • Pelvic ultrasound • Computed tomography (CT) scan/magnetic resonance imaging (MRI) • Laparoscopy and biopsy	Unlike the Papanicolaou (Pap) test for cervical cancer, there is no specific screening test for ovarian cancer. A woman at high risk is recommended to have a pelvic examination, a CA-125 blood test, and an ultrasound performed twice a year beginning at 30 years of age and continuing for the rest of her life or until her ovaries are removed. Pelvic examination is used to assess for masses and growths. This examination can be challenging in obese women. CA-125 is a tumor marker for ovarian cancer; however, many false-positive results are possible. Pelvic ultrasound evaluates shape and size of ovaries. CT scans and MRI provide detailed cross-sectional images. Laparoscopy and biopsy are used to determine the stage and extent of disease, guiding therapy.

Actions/Interventions

- Discuss staging of ovarian cancer:
  - I—Confined to one or both ovaries
  - II—Spread to other areas within pelvic area
  - III—Spread to lining of abdomen or to lymph nodes within abdomen
  - IV—Spread to organs beyond abdomen
- Discuss common treatment approaches:
  - Total abdominal hysterectomy and bilateral salpingo-oophorectomy
  - Chemotherapy
  - Radiation therapy (external and/or implanted)
  - Clinical trials

Rationales

Staging guides treatment options. Stage III is the most common stage at diagnosis.

Treatment depends on the stage and extent of disease. For stage I, the usual treatment is total hysterectomy to remove (debulk) as much tumor as possible. In addition, chemotherapy or intraperitoneal radiation implants are usually included. At stage II, external (teletherapy) or internal (brachytherapy) radiation or systemic chemotherapy is used after tumor debulking. Stages III and IV are usually treated with chemotherapy. Common drugs include carboplatin, cisplatin, docetaxel, and paclitaxel. Overall, combination therapy is required to treat this malignant disease. Intraperitoneal chemotherapy is also used. Women are encouraged to participate in available trials either researching new treatments or comparing different treatments. Such participation will provide knowledge about the best way to treat this cancer.

 Acute Pain

Common Related Factors

Pain resulting from medical problems (increased abdominal pressure caused by tumor or metastasis to abdominal structures)
Pain resulting from surgical/medical treatments

Defining Characteristics

Patient reports pain
Guarding of abdominal region
Self-focused
Relief or distraction behavior (moaning, crying, restlessness)
Alteration in muscle tone

Common Expected Outcomes

Patient reports satisfactory pain control at a level less than 3 to 4 on a 0 to 10 rating scale.
Patient uses pharmacological and nonpharmacological pain-relief strategies.

NOC Outcomes

Pain Control; Pain Status; Medication Response

NIC Interventions

Pain Management; Positioning; Distraction; Relaxation

Ongoing Assessment

Actions/Interventions

- Assess severity, quality, and location of pain.

- Assess the effect of psychological factors on pain.

Rationales

Pain is typically abdominal but may radiate to the pelvic or low back area. Pain is caused by pressure on abdominal structures as the tumor enlarges, or related to surgical intervention.

Pain is accentuated when the patient feels loss of control and when self-concept or role is threatened. The poor prognosis associated with ovarian cancer may cause grieving in anticipation of death.

■ = Independent   ▲ = Collaborative

Actions/Interventions

■ Assess the patient's expectations for pain relief.

■ Assess the effect of pain on performance of activities of daily living (ADLs) and activities perceived as meaningful by the patient.

Rationales

Some patients may be content to have pain decreased; others expect complete elimination of pain. This affects their perceptions of the effectiveness of the treatment modality and their willingness to participate in additional treatments.

Fatigue, anxiety, or depression associated with pain can limit the person's ability to complete self-care activities and fulfill role responsibilities.

Therapeutic Interventions

Actions/Interventions

■ Suggest positions for comfort.

■ Teach alternative techniques to reduce pain:
  • Imagery

  • Distraction techniques

  • Relaxation exercises

  • Massage of back and shoulders

▲ Administer analgesics as prescribed; develop a schedule for giving pain medications. Evaluate effectiveness.

Rationales

The following positions are helpful in reducing pain related to pressure: side-lying with knees bent and Fowler's position.

The use of a mental picture or an imagined event involving the five senses can distract oneself from painful stimuli.

These techniques heighten one's concentration on nonpainful stimuli to decrease one's awareness and experience of pain. Some methods are breathing modifications and nerve stimulation.

Techniques using physical and mental awareness increase muscle relaxation and reduce tension and pain.

Massage interrupts pain transmission, increases endorphin levels, and decreases tissue edema. This intervention may require another person to provide the massage.

Ongoing medication alleviates peak pain periods. Pain medications are absorbed and metabolized differently by patients, so their effectiveness must be evaluated individually by the patient.

NANDA-I NDx # Risk for Ineffective Breathing Pattern

Common Risk Factors

Presence of ascites (collection of protein-rich fluid in peritoneal cavity)

Pleural effusions

Common Expected Outcome

Patient maintains an effective breathing pattern, as evidenced by relaxed breathing at normal rate and depth and absence of dyspnea.

NOC Outcome

Respiratory Status: Ventilation

NIC Interventions

Respiratory Monitoring; Positioning; Medication Administration

Ongoing Assessment

Actions/Interventions

■ Assess for presence of ascites:

  • Measure abdominal girth, taking care to measure at the same point consistently.

Rationales

Ascites is a thord-spacing collection of protein rich fluid in the peritoneal cavity. Its volume can be severe enough to impair respiratory function.

This technique provides objective data regarding progression of ascites.

Actions/Interventions

- • Percuss the abdomen
- • Check for ballottement.
- ■ Assess breathing pattern, and the position that the patient assumes for easiest breathing.

- ■ Monitor effect of ineffective breathing pattern on ability to perform ADLs.
- ■ Assess for signs of pleural effusion: decreased or absent breath sounds, flat sound on percussion.

Rationales

Percussion over the abdomen sounds dull when fluid is present. This fluid is a fluid wave caused by shifting of ascetic fluid.

Severe ascites secondary to ovarian cancer can impair breathing by limiting full excursion of the diaphragm. Compromised breathing may present as tachypnea, shallow breathing and complaints of dyspnea. An upright position facilitates breathing because ascetic fluid assumes a gravity-dependent position, relieving pressure on the thoracic cavity.

Ineffective breathing reduces gas exchange and contributes to fatigue and activity intolerance.

Pleural effusions similarly compromise breathing, resulting in shortness of breath. They are confirmed by chest x-ray film.

Therapeutic Interventions

Actions/Interventions

- ■ Instruct about pacing activities.

- ■ Assist to Fowler's position.

- ▲ Assist with paracentesis.

- ▲ Facilitate shunt (LeVeen shunt, Denver shunt) function for patients with chronic ascites.

  - • Apply abdominal binder.

  - • Encourage use of an incentive spirometer.

  - • Administer diuretics as prescribed (for patients with a peritoneovenous shunt).
- ▲ Assist with thoracentesis.

- ▲ Administer oxygen as prescribed.

Rationales

Pacing activities reduces episodes of dyspnea from fatigue and excessive oxygen demand.

This position relieves pressure from the ascitic abdomen on the thoracic cavity.

Paracentesis is a bedside procedure to remove ascitic fluid from the peritoneal cavity. A trocar catheter is inserted into the abdomen using sterile technique. The procedure is done to relieve abdominal pressure.

Fluid reaccumulates rapidly following paracentesis. Peritoneovenous shunting returns ascitic fluid to vascular space and provides continuous relief of ascites.

This binder increases intraperitoneal pressure, causing the valve in the shunt to return fluid into the vascular space.

Inspiring against pressure causes the valve in the shunt to open and shunt ascitic fluid into the vascular space.

Diuretics facilitate excretion of excess fluid especially in patients with a peritovenous shunt.

Thoracentesis (removal of pleural fluid by needle) drains fluid from the pleural space to relieve dyspnea.

Supplemental oxygen will maximize oxygen saturation which should be 90% or greater.

Risk for Imbalanced Nutrition: Less Than Body Requirements

Common Risk Factors

Poor appetite secondary to disease, side effects of therapies, and pressure from ascites

Depression

Fear

Common Expected Outcome

Patient maintains an adequate nutritional intake, as evidenced by calorie intake of at least 1800 kcal/day.

NOC Outcome
Nutritional Status: Food and Fluid Intake
NIC Interventions
Nutrition Therapy; Nutrition Monitoring

■ = Independent   ▲ = Collaborative

Ongoing Assessment

Actions/Interventions

- Evaluate weight history and current weight.

- Determine body weight distribution, checking limbs for wasting.
- Assess appetite and factors considered by the patient to influence appetite.

- Assess caloric intake.

Rationales

Ascites may cause a significant increase in overall body weight, although the body is actually cachectic.
Weight loss may appear insignificant until the weight of the ascitic abdomen is considered.
Appetite is a complex phenomenon involving physiological well-being and psychological, psychosocial, and environmental factors. Anorexia may result from disease, treatment modalities, complications, and/or emotional turmoil of coping with a potentially terminal disease.
Caloric counts quantify nourishment intake to provide accurate assessment.

Therapeutic Interventions

Actions/Interventions

- Involve the patient and caregiver in selection of calorie-dense, high-protein, high-fiber meal plans.

- ▲ Consult a dietitian for dietary selections palatable to the patient.
- Encourage small, frequent, nutrient-dense meals (at least six per day).
- Encourage activity or exercise as tolerated.
- Suggest mealtime companions and maintenance of a pleasant environment.
- ▲ Give antiemetics as prescribed.
- Educate about oral hygiene.

Rationales

Involving patients in their own nutritional care has been found to raise their intake of protein and energy levels. Calories and protein are necessary for strength and healing; fiber combats constipation resulting from inactivity and increased intraabdominal pressure.
Dietitians have a greater understanding of the nutritional value of foods and may be helpful.
Small feedings reduce the work of digestion.

Activity enhances appetite by stimulating peristalsis.
Attention to the social aspects of eating is important in both the hospital and the home setting.
Antiemetics prevent or alleviate nausea and vomiting.
A clean, moist mouth and mucous membranes may make food more palatable.

Related Care Plans

Cancer chemotherapy, p. 681
Constipation, p. 46
Grieving, p. 82
Hysterectomy, p. 875
Ineffective coping, p. 49

Pelvic Inflammatory Disease (PID)

Sexually Transmitted Infection (STI); Salpingitis; Oophoritis

Pelvic inflammatory disease (PID) is an infective process involving the uterus, fallopian tubes, and ovaries, as well as the peritoneum, pelvic veins, and connective tissue. Untreated PID can become a chronic condition; tissue destruction and scarring can cause the formation of abdominal and reproductive adhesions, resulting in infertility or ectopic pregnancy. Treatment includes cultures, diagnosis of infectious agent, and parenteral or intravenous (IV) antibiotics, usually on an outpatient basis. Both the patient and her sexual partner or partners must be treated. Treatment of this problem is complicated by the increasing prevalence of major pathogens such as *Chlamydia* and *Neisseria gonorrhoeae*, plus syphilis, human papillomavirus (HPV), and human immunodeficiency virus (HIV). Sexually transmitted infections (STIs) have reached epidemic levels, with some pathogens developing antibiotic-resistant strains. There is a positive correlation between the number of sexual partners and the risk for developing PID. Women who use an intrauterine device (IUD) for birth control may be at increased risk for infection because pathogens may ascend via the locator string into the uterine cavity. Women who have recently given birth or had an abortion have an entry portal for infectious agents at the placental site. When other STIs are present, PID must be ruled out. Condoms may be helpful in reducing the incidence of STIs, although research indicates that the microscopic openings in condoms may be larger than some of the infectious organisms. Vaginal spermicides used alone can reduce the risk for cervical gonorrhea and chlamydia. The most effective way to prevent the transmission of STIs is to avoid sexual intercourse with an infected partner. The Centers for Disease Control and Prevention (CDC) recommends yearly *Chlamydia* testing of all sexually active women age 25 years or younger, pregnant women, and older women with multiple sex partners.

Deficient Knowledge

Common Related Factors

New diagnosis
Misinterpretation of information
Cognitive limitations
Unfamiliarity with cause of disease, medical management, or prevention
Embarrassment about topic, shame, fear
Emotional response

Common Expected Outcome

Patient verbalizes an understanding of PID infection, potential complications, medical treatment, and prevention of recurrence.

Defining Characteristics

Multiple questions
Inaccurate follow-through of instructions
Inappropriate or exaggerated behaviors
Lack of attention to teaching, changing subject

NOC Outcomes

Knowledge: Disease Process; Knowledge: Treatment Regimen

NIC Interventions

Teaching: Disease Process; Teaching: Prescribed Medications

Ongoing Assessment

Actions/Interventions	Rationales
■ Assess knowledge of PID.	Although PID is a frequently encountered infection in women, health care providers cannot assume that all women are knowledgeable.
■ Assess knowledge of the consequences of PID.	Infertility is a major complication. Frequent PID can result in ectopic pregnancy, cervical pathology, and resistance of organisms to antibiotics.
■ Assess past experience with STIs.	Women with gonorrhea or chlamydial infections are at higher risk for PID.
■ Obtain a sexual history.	Incidence of PID increases with multiple sex partners, risky sexual behaviors, and contact with an infected partner.

■ = Independent ▲ = Collaborative

Therapeutic Interventions

Actions/Interventions	Rationales
■ Remain supportive and nonjudgmental.	The moral stigma of an STI may be an obstacle for those seeking care for a real or suspected STI. Vaginal infections often result in emotional distress. Seeking medical care must not result in a negative response.
■ Explain transmission of PID.	Acute or chronic PID is transmitted during or soon after sexual intercourse or pelvic surgery (e.g., abortion or childbirth). Infections may occur secondary to the use of an IUD. The use of condoms with spermicide reduces the infection rate.

■ Teach the signs and symptoms of PID:
• Early, acute case symptoms include the following:
  • Excessive menstrual cramping
  • Bleeding or spotting outside of the regular menses
  • Painful urination and sexual intercourse
  • Dull abdominal pain or backache
  • Constipation
  • Low-grade fever
  • General malaise
• Late symptoms include the following:
  • Pelvic pain
  • Copious, foul-smelling vaginal discharge
  • Nausea and vomiting
	Symptoms may be absent in women until late in the course of the illness. Symptoms may mimic ectopic pregnancy or appendicitis.

■ Explain common diagnostic tests. • Physical examination • Gynecological examination • Laboratory testing • Pregnancy testing • Pelvic ultrasound • Laparoscopy	Information alleviates apprehension and promotes cooperation. Lower abdominal tenderness or pain is a cardinal symptom. Laboratory testing may include erythrocyte sedimentation rate (ESR), C-reactive protein, white blood cell count, and cultures. Ectopic pregnancy mimics PID. Therefore pregnancy status must be determined before treatment with antibiotics. Pelvic ultrasound is used to rule out other etiologies such as appendicitis. Laparoscopy permits an optimal view of abdominal and pelvic organs and facilitates culture testing.
■ Explain treatment regimens. • Outpatient antibiotic therapy—most common	Antibiotic treatment options are guided by culture and antibiotic sensitivity results. Most patients can manage their treatment at home.
• Inpatient antibiotic therapy for high risk	Hospitalization may be required for patients who are pregnant, have severe symptoms, or are not responding to oral medications.
• Treatment of sex partner(s); abstinence from sexual intercourse	The patient can be easily reinfected by the sexual partner, who may be infected but asymptomatic. Sexual partners must be notified and treated. This is a mandatory reportable STI. Abstenance during treatment is important to prevent spread of infection.

NDx Infection

Common Related Factors

Gram-positive cocci
- *Chlamydia trachomatis*
- *N. gonorrhoeae*
- Streptococcus

Gram-negative cocci
- *Escherichia coli*
- *Haemophilus influenzae*

Anaerobes
- *Gardnerella vaginalis*
- *Bacteroides*

Common Expected Outcome

Patient manifests signs of treated infection as evidenced by absence of fever, absence of pain, absence of vaginal discharge, and negative culture results.

Defining Characteristics

Edematous vaginal mucosa
Copious, malodorous, greenish-yellow vaginal discharge
Fever
Positive culture or screening test results
Formation of an abscess
Progression to peritonitis

NOC Outcomes

Infection Status; Medication Response

NIC Interventions

Infection Control; Fertility Preservation;
Teaching: Prescribed Medication

Ongoing Assessment

Actions/Interventions

▲ Assess for presence of minimum criteria for diagnosis of PID:
- Lower abdominal tenderness on palpation
- Adnexal tenderness
- Cervical motion tenderness

▲ Assess for additional criteria to increase specificity of diagnosis:
- Elevated temperature (greater than 38.3° C [101° F])
- Abnormal cervical or vaginal discharge
- Elevated ESR and/or C-reactive protein
- Positive culture of cervical infection with *N. gonorrhoeae* or *C. trachomatis*

■ Assess pregnancy status
- History of last menstrual period
- Abnormal menses

■ Assess past STI history.

▲ Monitor culture results.

Rationales

The CDC recommends using a low threshold and minimal criteria to maximize diagnosis of PID because of its potential for serious reproductive damage to women. Treatment is thus instituted on the basis of these criteria after other competing diagnoses are ruled out.

According to the CDC, presence of these additional criteria increases specificity of the diagnosis.

The patient's pregnancy status must be known before antibiotics are administered. Certain antibiotics are not safe during pregnancy.

More than one STI may be present at the same time. The presence of a titer elevation may represent an old or a new infection. Serial titers may be required.

Some antibiotic regimens will be implemented before culture and sensitivity results are received. Culture reports must be checked to ensure that organisms are sensitive to the current antibiotic regimen.

■ = Independent   ▲ = Collaborative

Therapeutic Interventions

Actions/Interventions	Rationales
▲ Institute drug treatment as ordered. These drugs may include: • Cefoxitin • Probenecid • Ceftriaxone • Doxycycline • Tetracycline • Cefotetan	All patients with PID require oral or IV antibiotics, depending on severity of illness. Unlike specific STI organisms wherein a single treatment regimen is known, PID represents a complex syndrome that can be caused by a variety of organisms. Thus no single regimen of choice exists for PID. Therefore CDC guidelines are designed to provide broad-spectrum coverage for the most common pathogens, using at least two antibiotics.
■ Teach importance of proper administration of medications and completion of course of treatment.	This will prevent ineffective treatment, recurrence of symptoms, and the development of antibiotic-resistant organisms.
■ Stress importance of notifying sexual contacts.	Treatment of partners prevents transmission or reinfection. This is a mandatory reportable STI.
■ Maintain blood and body fluid precautions. If the patient is hospitalized, maintain infection precautions: • Dispose of soiled items according to infection control policy. • Maintain strict hand washing for all persons in contact with the patient. • Cleanse all equipment with disinfectant. • Use utensils or gloves when handling soiled materials.	These precautions reduce the risk for transmitting infection to others.
■ Discourage continuous use of perineal pads. Instruct to avoid use of tampons.	This reduces the risk for reinfection from exudates on the pad. Tampons can be a medium for further bacterial growth and may inhibit drainage of pelvic exudates.
■ Explain importance of abstaining from sexual intercourse until after follow-up visit.	The patient can be easily reinfected by the sexual partner, who may be infected but asymptomatic. Sexual partners also must be treated.
■ Discuss contraceptive use. • The CDC makes the following recommendations about the proper use of male condoms: • Use a new condom with each act of sexual intercourse. • Carefully handle the condom to avoid damaging it with fingernails, teeth, or other sharp objects. • Put the condom on after the penis is erect and before genital contact with the partner. • Ensure that no air is trapped in the tip of the condom. • Ensure that adequate lubrication exists during intercourse, possibly requiring the use of exogenous lubricants. • Use only water-based lubricants with latex condoms. Oil-based lubricants can weaken latex. • Hold the condom firmly against the base of the penis during withdrawal, and withdraw while the penis is still erect to prevent slippage.	Condoms may reduce the transmission of certain STIs. Spermicide-coated condoms have been associated with *E. coli* urinary tract infection. Consistent use of condoms, with or without spermicidal lubricant or vaginal application of spermicide, is recommended.
• The female condom—a lubricated polyurethane sheath or pouch with a ring on each end that is inserted into the vagina.	The female condom is an effective mechanical barrier to viruses, including HIV.
■ Instruct the patient to notify the physician of the following: • Reappearance of severe symptoms • Lack of menstruation • Nonmenstrual bleeding • Severe abdominal cramps • Presence of purulent, malodorous vaginal discharge	Early assessment facilitates prompt treatment.
■ Refer to an STI clinic and/or social worker as indicated.	Risky sexual behaviors may require the implementation of a regular surveillance program (every 4 to 6 weeks or more often).

Women's Health Care Plans

NANDA-I NDx Acute Pain

Common Related Factors
Pelvic cavity inflammation
Excoriated perineal area
Development of abdominal adhesions

Defining Characteristics
Report of pain
Self- or narrowed focus
Distraction behaviors
Alteration in muscle tone
Autonomic responses

Common Expected Outcomes
Patient reports satisfactory pain control at a level less than 3 to 4 on a 0 to 10 rating scale.
Patient uses pharmacological and nonpharmacological pain-relief measures.

NOC Outcome
Pain Control
NIC Interventions
Pain Management; Analgesic Administration

Ongoing Assessment

Actions/Interventions	Rationales
■ Assess for pain characteristics.	Pain may be continuous and crampy; bilateral, lower abdominal or back pain; or increasing when uterus is moved (e.g., during vaginal examination). Pain may increase with activity.
■ Assess bowel sounds.	Cessation of bowel sounds may indicate progression to peritonitis.
■ Assess response to medication effects and side effects.	Antibiotics are the treatment of choice to reduce inflammation caused by the infection. Analgesics can be added as needed.

Therapeutic Interventions

Actions/Interventions	Rationales
▲ Administer or instruct patients in how to self-medicate with antibiotics and oral and topical analgesics, as prescribed.	Effective antibiotic management will eventually treat causative factors, subsequently relieving pain. The patient may experience extreme discomfort requiring narcotic analgesia. However, aggressive antibiotic therapy may prevent tubal damage that would otherwise predispose the patient to ectopic pregnancy or infertility.
■ Teach comfort measures: • Heat (dry or moist) • Positioning with extra pillows • Perineal care	These measures enhance the effect of pharmacological analgesia and promote comfort.
■ Encourage a semi-Fowler's position as often as possible.	This position promotes drainage of pelvic exudates and prevents development of pelvic abscesses.

Related Care Plans
Disturbed body image, p. 24
Ineffective coping, p. 49
Ineffective sexuality patterns, p. 182

■ = Independent   ▲ = Collaborative

Pelvic Relaxation Disorder

Pelvic Floor Disorders; Uterine Prolapse; Enterocele; Cystocele; Rectocele

Pelvic relaxation disorder (PRD) is the symptomatic expression of involuntary urinary incontinence, pelvic fullness, and or fecal incontinence. It is a quality-of-life issue that affects patients in personal, social, and relationship areas. Symptoms may be mild to severe but are a result of the relaxation of the pelvic floor and the surrounding structures. This is a common symptom of aging adults; thus the condition will become of greater concern to health care providers. However, it is rarely discussed by patients because of personal embarrassment. Testing must initially rule out pelvic masses. Initial treatment may be conservative, such as pelvic floor exercises (Kegel exercises), medications, and pessary. Those with more severe symptoms may require laparoscopic or abdominal/pelvic surgery.

NANDA-I NDx Deficient Knowledge

Common Related Factors

New diagnosis
Misinterpretation of information
Unfamiliarity with cause of disease, medical management
Embarrassment about topic

Defining Characteristics

Requests for information
Inaccurate follow-through of instructions

Common Expected Outcome

Patient verbalizes an understanding of causes of pelvic relaxation disorder, diagnostic procedures, preventive factors to control symptoms, and available medical/surgical treatments.

NOC Outcomes
Knowledge: Disease Process; Knowledge: Treatment Procedure(s)

NIC Interventions
Teaching: Disease Process; Teaching: Prescribed Activity/Exercise; Teaching: Prescribed Diet

Ongoing Assessment

Actions/Interventions	Rationales
■ Assess knowledge of causes of PRD.	Although PRD is common (1 out of 4 women and some men experience these symptoms), patients may not talk about it to others. Health care professionals cannot assume that all women are knowledgeable about PRD.
■ Assess the patient's history of signs and symptoms. Ask about vaginal protrusions or fullness in lower abdominal area.	Women can experience a variety of symptoms, most commonly urinary incontinence, bowel incontinence, impaired sexual functioning, prolapsed bladder or uterus, and body image issues. Nurses need to be aware of sensitive nature of subject because of fears of embarrassment and isolation.
■ Assess understanding of diagnostic testing.	Disorders may be detected during routine physical examination. Pelvic masses need to be ruled out. Urodynamic testing and magnetic resonance imaging (MRI) will help determine specific areas of weakness.

Actions/Interventions

- Assess level of urinary versus fecal incontinence.
- Assess understanding of treatment options.

Rationales

Urinary incontinence is the more common symptom of PRD.
Most women want a collaborative relationship in the management of this common condition and require information about preference for specific treatment options.

Therapeutic Interventions

Actions/Interventions

- Provide information on the patient's predisposing factors.

- Differentiate between cystocele (sagging bladder or urethra), rectocele (relaxed, sagging rectal mucosa), enterocele (protrusion of intestinal wall into the vagina), and uterine prolapse (relaxed uterus).
- Discuss self-care issues that can reduce symptoms:
  - Avoiding straining from constipation (use of mild laxatives) and from heavy lifting
  - Benefits of weight loss
  - Avoidance of caffeine, alcohol, and carbonated drinks.

- Instruct regarding good perineal hygiene. Explain that internal and external collection devices are available for both female and males. Suggest use of undergarments, diapers, absorbent pads, and waterproof linen.

- Encourage use of clothing that can be easily and quickly removed.
- Instruct in treating existing perineal skin excoriation with a vitamin-enriched cream, followed by a moisture barrier.
- Instruct the patient in the importance of muscle retraining through performing Kegel exercises.

- Instruct in methods for manual reduction of prolapsed uterus (gently pushing uterus into vagina).
- Describe the benefits of pessary devices.

- Explain common medications used to treat urinary incontinence.
- For problems related to fecal incontinence, provide gentle rectal hygiene and minimal manipulation. Do not take rectal temperature.

Rationales

Loss of muscle tone causes protrusion of bladder or uterus. Pressure adds to loss of urine or fecal control. Common causes include previous history of birth trauma, multiple births, connective tissue disorders, aging process, hormone deficiency, congenital defects, previous pelvic surgery, anal intercourse, and conditions that chronically raise intraabdominal pressure (e.g., constipation and obesity).

The specific symptoms experienced are related to the medical diagnosis.

Straining when defecating hard stool is a common cause of exacerbation of urinary and fecal symptoms. Excessive body weight causes increased abdominal pressure and puts added strain on the pelvic floor muscles. Prolonged standing can aggravate this. High-volume intake of stimulants contributes to bladder irritation and adds to bladder urge or stress incontinence.

Consistent hygiene practices reduce irritation of perineal tissue. Patients may not be aware of the variety of products available for incontinence. Making suggestions for preparation of items that need to be discreetly carried for accidents can help reduce embarrassment during "accidents."

Clothing can be a factor in functional incontinence if it takes time to remove before defecating.

Moisture-barrier ointments are useful in protecting perineal skin from urine scalds.

In the early stages of disease, these exercise help strengthen the weakened muscles of the pelvic floor. They are performed by "tightening" the vaginal muscles and anal sphincter for about 10 seconds, then relaxing for 10 seconds. They can be repeated 30 to 80 times a day for best effects. These exercises can benefit incontinence and enhance sensations during sexual intercourse.

This technique may reduce discomfort and facilitate voiding.

A pessary is a ring- or donut-shaped device made of silicone or plastic and individually fitted for each patient. It is inserted into the vagina to support pelvic structures, relieve pressure on the bladder, and reduce prolapse. It is usually removed one to two times a week overnight then reinserted.

A variety of medications are available and are discussed in: Stress Urinary Incontinence care plan below.

These measures prevent tearing the thin rectal tissue.

■ = Independent ▲ = Collaborative

Actions/Interventions

- For fecal incontinence problems, suggest use of natural bulking agents such as banana, rice, and yogurt, or bulk-forming agents (e.g., Metamucil) to increase stool bulk.
- Provide information on possible surgical procedures: laparoscopic and/or abdominal/pelvic surgery.
- On discharge, provide the patient with a follow-up appointment and important telephone numbers.

Rationales

These foods/agents help provide bulk to the stool by absorbing fluids from the stool.

Accurate knowledge of the planned procedure and care routines can help reduce anxiety and fear of the unknown.
For successful recovery, the patient needs to know who to contact when problems arise.

Stress Urinary Incontinence

Common Related Factors

Weak pelvic muscles (prolapse of tissue)
Obesity—high intraabdominal pressure
Multiple vaginal deliveries
Hypoestrogen (aging)
Prior pelvic surgery

Defining Characteristic

Observed/reported involuntary leakage of urine on exertion; with coughing, laughing, sneezing.

Common Expected Outcomes

Patient is continent of urine or verbalizes satisfactory management.
Patient implements activities to increase pelvic floor muscle tone.
Patient uses available products to reduce incontinence problems.

NOC Outcomes

Urinary Continence; Urinary Elimination; Self-Care: Toileting

NIC Intervention

Urinary Incontinence Care

Ongoing Assessment

Actions/Interventions

Preoperative care:

- Obtain history of bladder habits and frequency of past episodes of incontinence. Assess whether urine is lost involuntarily during coughing, sneezing, lifting, or exercise.

- Examine the perineal area for skin breakdown, infection, and number of pads.

Postoperative care:

- Record voiding habits, and assess bladder for complete emptying
- ▲ Notify the physician of large blood loss and/or vital sign changes.

Rationales

Stress urinary incontinence is associated with physical activity and exertion. Whenever intraabdominal pressure increases, relaxed pelvic floor muscles allow urine to escape involuntarily. Symptoms occur when there is poor muscle support of the pelvic floor and ineffective closure mechanisms of the bladder neck and the urethral sphincter.
Urine leakage may cause odor, bacteria, and infection. Patients need good skin care to avoid infection and further irritation.

Pain medication may cause retention. Swelling may prevent complete emptying.
Significant blood loss can lead to hypovolemic shock and requires immediate intervention.

Therapeutic Interventions

Actions/Interventions

Preoperative care:

- Encourage weight loss if obese.

- Encourage patient to maintain adequate fluid intake.

Rationales

Obesity is associated with increased pressure on the urinary bladder.
Patients often restrict fluid to reduce incontinence episodes.

Actions/Interventions	Rationales
■ Instruct in commonly prescribed medications: • Darifenacin (Enablex) • Oxybutynin (Ditropan) • Tolterodine (Detrol) • Topical vaginal estrogens	According to patient degree of symptoms with the absence of pathology, treatment with medications has been found to be beneficial. Anticholinergic medications such as Enablex, Ditropan and Detrol are commonly prescribed. They relax the muscles in the bladder that improves the ability to control urination. Topical estrogens may be used rather than systemic oral medications. A trial of at least 12 weeks is necessary to determine effectiveness.
■ Teach the patient to perform Kegel exercises.	Kegel exercises are used to strengthen the muscles of the pelvic floor and can be practiced with a minimum of exertion.
■ Teach women patients the use of a vaginal pessary (device reserved for nonsurgical candidates).	This device works by elevating the bladder neck, thereby increasing urethral resistance. Problems from pessaries include vaginal discharge, odor, and vaginal erosion.
■ For patients who are not responsive to medical procedures, prepare for workup for possible surgery.	Urodynamics, imaging, and cystoscopy are necessary to exclude pathology, especially in elderly patients with an overactive bladder. Newer surgical interventions should be offered after careful consideration of the risk-benefit ratio for each woman and the amount of evidence currently available.
■ Prepare the patient for surgery as indicated, explaining the specifics of selected procedure: • Burch's colposuspension • Marshall-Marchetti • Slings • Mesh kits	Many types of procedures are used to control stress incontinence and selection is determined by individualized patient needs. The most commonly performed are Burch's colposuspension (considered the gold standard), Marshall-Marchetti, and sling procedures. There are a variety of sling procedures, each using similar principles but different products with biomechanical properties. Because midurethral slings have demonstrated success, newer "mesh kits" have been introduced to replace or reinforce vaginal tissue. Safety and efficacy remain to be seen from these newly employed procedures.
■ Refer to stress urinary incontinence website: www.nafc.org.	This website provides additional resources, support, and information.

Postoperative care:

■ Provide routine postoperative assessments and care, especially noting completeness and frequency of urine output.	Intake and output are key determinants of efficiency of bladder emptying.
■ Instruct to continue with Kegel exercises.	These exercises can continue to improve muscle strength.
■ Instruct patient to consult physician as to when to resume sexual intercourse and other key activities.	Each patient recovers at his or her own pace, especially depending on age and comorbid conditions.

Disturbed Body Image

Common Related Factors

Alterations in function (bladder/rectal sphincter/vagina)
Sudden, unpredictable, chronic urinary incontinence
Sudden, unpredictable, chronic fecal incontinence
Fears of loss of sexual abilities/identity

Defining Characteristics

Verbalization about altered structure of a body part
Verbalized negative feelings about body
Change in social behavior: avoidance of social activities and/or sexual relations
Refusal to discuss or acknowledge change
Embarrassment about topic
Self-deprecating remarks

■ = Independent   ▲ = Collaborative

Common Expected Outcomes

Patient begins to accept problem and verbalize positive statements about body and self.

Patient identifies available resources to aid in coping.

Patient accurately describes effects of treatment on improving functional abilities.

NOC Outcomes
Body Image; Self-Esteem; Psychosocial Adjustment

NIC Interventions
Body Image Enhancement; Coping Enhancement; Self-Esteem Enhancement; Teaching: Sexuality

Ongoing Assessment

Actions/Interventions	Rationales
■ Note the frequency of the patient's self-critical remarks.	Negative statements about the affected body part indicate limited ability to integrate the change into the patient's self-concept.
■ Determine specific situations in which patient may have had an "accident" that caused significant embarrassment.	Knowledge of the specifics can help in determining a coping strategy.
■ Determine the patient's behavior such as avoidance of social activities and avoidance of sexual activity.	There is a broad range of behaviors associated with disturbed body image. Sexual dysfunction is a common consequence of PRD.
■ Assess information about the nature, onset, duration, and course of any sexual problems.	Problems with sexuality may be long-standing or recently associated with PRD.
■ Use questionnaire if available to identify level of partner support or understanding.	Information provides basis for care planning.

Therapeutic Interventions

Actions/Interventions	Rationales
■ Acknowledge normalcy of emotional responses to medical problem.	Experiencing frustration and negative feelings over loss of function of one's body is normal and typically involves some length of time. Expression of feelings can enhance person's coping strategies.
■ Use a relaxed, accepting manner in discussing sexual issues.	Patients are often hesitant to report such concerns or difficulties because sexuality remains a private matter for many within our culture. An honest relationship facilitates problem solving and successful coping.
■ Teach the patient adaptive behavior (e.g., use of diapers, absorbent pads, and waterproof linen, concealing clothing).	This compensates for the actual change in body function.
■ Discuss regular routine of bladder and bowel emptying early in the day if sexual relations are to occur at night.	Simple steps to deal with the problem may help the patient gain some control over the situation.
■ Provide information for hygienic improvement before and after sexual relations.	These strategies may help patients feel better about themselves.
■ Explore awareness of and comfort with a range of sexual expression and activities (not just sexual intercourse).	Patients and couples may have limited knowledge of ways to express their sexuality.
■ Refer the patient to support groups composed of individuals with similar problems.	Use of lay groups or individuals may help patient to recognize ways to cope with body changes and offer a different type of support that is perceived as helpful.

CHAPTER

12

Endocrine and Metabolic Care Plans

Cushing's Syndrome

Hypercortisolism; Cushing's Disease; Adrenocortical Hyperfunction

Cushing's syndrome reflects an excess of glucocorticoids. Depending on the cause of the syndrome, mineralocorticoids and androgens may also be secreted in increased amounts. The syndrome may be primary (an intrinsic adrenocortical disorder, e.g., neoplasm), secondary (from pituitary or hypothalamic dysfunction with increased adrenocorticotrophic hormone [ACTH] secretion resulting in glucocorticoid excess), or iatrogenic (from prolonged or excessive administration of corticosteroids). The syndrome results in fluid and electrolyte disturbances, suppressed immune response, altered fat distribution, and disturbances in protein metabolism. Changes in physical appearance that occur with Cushing's syndrome can have significant influence on the patient's body image and emotional well-being. The focus of this care plan is on the ambulatory patient with Cushing's syndrome.

Deficient Knowledge

Common Related Factor

Lack of experience with Cushing's syndrome

Common Expected Outcomes

Patient verbalizes an understanding of Cushing's syndrome and guidelines for therapy.
Patient implements appropriate therapy.

Defining Characteristics

Questioning, especially if repetitive
Verbalized misconceptions
Repeated hospital admissions for complications

NOC Outcomes

Knowledge: Disease Process; Knowledge: Treatment Regimen; Knowledge: Infection Control

NIC Interventions

Teaching: Disease Process; Teaching: Prescribed Diet; Infection Protection

Ongoing Assessment

Actions/Interventions	Rationales
■ Assess level of knowledge of Cushing's syndrome and the guidelines for therapy.	An individualized teaching plan begins with assessment of the patient's previous knowledge and understanding of the disorder. The patient or family must understand the disease process and receive specific instructions related to treatment, methods to control symptoms, signs of infections, complications, and indicators of when to notify the physician. Cushing's syndrome may cause alterations in level of consciousness because of the effects of cortisol on hippocampal neurons. The patient may have impaired memory. This change may limit the patient's ability to learn new information.

Therapeutic Interventions

Actions/Interventions	Rationales
■ Explain all tests to the patient:	The patient may undergo a variety of diagnostic tests for Cushing's syndrome. Many of the tests require patient co-operation in collecting urine specimens over an extended time period.
• Urine free cortisol, 17-hydroxycorticosteroids (17-OHCS), 17-ketosteroids (17-KS)	To begin the urine collection, the patient is instructed to void and discard this specimen. Then, the patient needs to save all urine for 24 hours. Medications may need to be withheld for several days before urine collection. In Cushing's syndrome, urine free cortisol is elevated. Levels of 17-OHCS (metabolites of cortisol) and 17-KS (metabolites of androgens) are elevated in Cushing's syndrome.
• Dexamethasone suppression tests	These tests require a combination of urine collections, blood specimens, and administration of dexamethasone. The overnight test is done as an initial screening and does not require urine collection. A prolonged version of the test may be done over 3 days or 6 days. The results help determine the cause of the patient's Cushing's syndrome.
• Computed tomography, magnetic resonance imaging, and selected arteriography	These diagnostic studies are used to identify lesions of the adrenal gland, pituitary gland, or other body organs (lungs, gastrointestinal [GI] tract, pancreas) that are associated with stimulation of cortisol secretion.
■ Anticipate the need to discuss or reinforce the probable treatment in correcting the hypersecretion of hormone:	
• If an intrinsic adrenocortical disorder: probable surgery for removal of the adenoma, tumor, or adrenal glands.	Adrenalectomy is the treatment of choice for the patient with an adrenal tumor or adrenal hyperplasia that is causing Cushing's syndrome.
• If a disorder secondary to pituitary hypersecretion: trans-sphenoidal pituitary tumor resection or irradiation.	Treatment of pituitary tumors is indicated for patients when the Cushing's syndrome is secondary to ACTH hypersecretion. Surgical therapy usually involves a transsphenoidal hypophysectomy. Radiation therapy may be used as part of the management of these patients.
• If iatrogenic: gradual discontinuation of excessive administration of corticosteroids as the patient's condition permits.	When Cushing's syndrome is secondary to prolonged administration of glucocorticoids, treatment is focused on discontinuing the medication. This approach requires gradual lowering of the dose over time to decrease the risk for adrenal insufficiency if the drug is stopped suddenly. If the patient's condition does not allow for discontinuing glucocorticoids, attempts will be made to adjust the dose and frequency of administration to minimize suppression of the normal hypothalamic-pituitary-adrenal function.

Actions/Interventions

- Instruct the patient to report signs of localized or systemic infection.

- Instruct the patient to report areas of skin breakdown and inadequate wound healing.

- Teach the patient about regular evaluation of serum glucose levels.

- Reinforce dietary instructions. Instruct the patient in a high-calcium diet.

- Instruct the patient regarding signs of osteoporosis such as fractures, kyphosis, or height loss.

- Instruct the patient regarding fat distribution.

- Explain how to obtain a medical identification tag and the importance of wearing it.

Rationales

Increase in glucocorticoids inhibits the immune response with a suppression of allergic response, as well as inhibition of inflammation. An elevated temperature may not be present with infection because of the decreased immune response.

Wound healing is prolonged in Cushing's syndrome. This change occurs because of impaired protein synthesis from increased cortisol levels.

Increased cortisol levels contribute to impaired glucose metabolism. Hyperglycemia is a common effect. The patient may develop disease-induced diabetes mellitus.

Cushing's syndrome results in weight gain and calcium and protein loss. A high-calcium diet prevents worsening of osteoporosis.

Muscle wasting, fatigue, weakness, and osteoporosis are associated with excess glucocorticoids. These changes put the patient at risk for fractures. Kyphosis and a decrease in height occur with spinal compression fractures.

Chronic cortisol hypersecretion redistributes body fat, with increased fat deposited on the back, shoulder, trunk, and abdomen.

The tag can inform others of the patient's condition as a warning so that appropriate treatment will occur in an emergency situation.

NANDA-I NDx **Disturbed Body Image**

Common Related Factors

Increased production of androgens (giving rise to virilism in women; hirsutism [abnormal growth of hair])

Disturbed protein metabolism resulting in muscle wasting, capillary fragility, and wasting of bone matrix: ecchymosis, osteoporosis, slender limbs, striae (usually purple)

Abnormal fat distribution along with edema resulting in moon face, cervicodorsal fat (buffalo hump), trunk obesity

Defining Characteristics

Verbal identification of feeling about altered body structure

Verbal preoccupation with changed body

Refusal to discuss or acknowledge change

Change in social behavior (withdrawal, isolation, flamboyancy)

Compensatory use of concealing clothing

Common Expected Outcome

Patient demonstrates enhanced body image and self esteem as evidenced by ability to look at, touch, talk about, and care for actual and perceived altered body parts and functions.

NOC Outcomes
Body Image; Self-Esteem
NIC Intervention
Body Image Enhancement

Ongoing Assessment

Actions/Interventions

- Assess for changes in personal appearance caused by the glucocorticoid excess.

Rationales

These changes may include obesity, thin extremities with muscle atrophy, moon face, red cheeks, buffalo hump, increased body and facial hair. Hyperpigmentation of skin, hair, and mucous membranes occurs as a result of increased levels of melanocyte-stimulating hormones and ACTH. Acne may result from adrenal androgen excess.

■ = Independent   ▲ = Collaborative

Actions/Interventions

■ Assess the patient's feelings about changed appearance and coping mechanisms.

■ Assess use of coping mechanisms.

Rationales

Negative statements about changes in appearance indicate disturbed body image. The patient may withdraw from social interaction. Depression may occur.

Previously successful coping skills may be inadequate in the present situation.

Therapeutic Interventions

Actions/Interventions

■ Encourage expression of feelings about changes in appearance.

■ Reassure the patient that the physical changes are a result of the elevated hormone levels and most will resolve when those levels return to normal.

■ Promote coping methods to deal with the patient's change in appearance (e.g., adequate grooming, flattering clothes).

■ Refer to or identify local support groups.

■ Provide an atmosphere of acceptance and positive caring.

Rationales

It is worthwhile to encourage the patient to separate feelings about changes in body structure and/or function from feelings about self-worth. Expression of feelings can enhance the person's coping strategies.

Information helps the patient develop realistic expectations about the changes in physical appearance.

Learning methods to compensate for changes in appearance enhances the patient's self-esteem. Helping patients remember how they managed body image issues in the past may facilitate adjustment to the current issue.

Talking with people who have experienced similar situations provides social support. Members of a support group offer coping strategies that have proven successful.

Patients look to others for feedback about their appearance. When the nurse responds to the patient in an accepting manner, it supports the patient's adjustment to his or her appearance.

NANDA-I NDx Risk for Injury

Common Risk Factors
Poor wound healing
Decreased bone density
Increased capillary fragility

Common Expected Outcome
Patient implements measures to prevent injury.

NOC Outcomes
Knowledge: Fall Prevention; Knowledge: Personal Safety; Risk Control; Fall Prevention Behavior

NIC Interventions
Fall Prevention; Surveillance; Environmental Management: Safety; Bleeding Precautions

Ongoing Assessment

Actions/Interventions

■ Assess skin for signs of bruising and feces for occult blood.

Rationales

Patients with Cushing's syndrome will experience loss of collagen tissue that supports the superficial small blood vessels and capillaries. This change makes these blood vessels more susceptible to rupture with minimal trauma. The patient may experience easy bruising and GI bleeding.

Actions/Interventions

- Assess skin for signs of breakdown.

- Ask the patient about problems with slow wound healing.

- Assess the patient for decreased height and kyphosis.

▲ Prepare the patient for bone density evaluation.

Rationales

Cushing's syndrome causes thinning of the skin because of loss of collagen and stretching from increased fat deposits. The skin is more easily damaged, with resulting skin breakdown.

Increased cortisol levels increase catabolism of peripheral tissues. Impaired nitrogen metabolism associated with Cushing's syndrome contributes to impaired protein synthesis and delayed wound healing.

Hypercortisolism that occurs with Cushing's syndrome causes increased bone resorption, decreased bone formation, increased renal calcium excretion, and decreased calcium absorption from the intestines. These changes lead to decreased bone density and development of osteoporosis. Spinal compression fractures result in decreased height and an exaggerated anterior-posterior curvature of the thoracic spine (kyphosis).

This diagnostic procedure provides information about the loss of bone density.

Therapeutic Interventions

Actions/Interventions

- Instruct the patient in activities to decrease the risk for bleeding:
  - Use a soft toothbrush.
  - Use an electric razor.

  - Eat a high-fiber diet with adequate fluid intake.

- Apply direct pressure over venipuncture sites, injection sites, or wounds for at least 1 minute or longer.

- Instruct the patient about keeping the skin clean and moisturized.
- Encourage the patient to increase dietary intake of calcium and vitamin D.

▲ Administer calcium and vitamin D supplements.

- Discuss with the patient safety measures for ambulation and daily activities.

Rationales

This device decreases trauma to the gums.
This type of razor reduces the risk for cutting the skin when shaving.
These measures decrease the risk for developing constipation, which can result in lower GI bleeding.
Because of capillary fragility, the patient will bleed more easily. Direct pressure helps control bleeding and reduce bruising.
Excessive dryness or excessive moisture increases the risk for skin breakdown.
The patient can add generous amounts of low-fat dairy products and green leafy vegetables to increase calcium intake. Vitamin D is necessary for absorption of calcium from the intestine.
Supplemental calcium and vitamin D are indicated if dietary sources are not adequate.
The patient needs to take precautions with daily activities to reduce trauma that can result in skin trauma, bruising, or bleeding. Cushing's syndrome is associated with loss of bone density and development of osteoporosis. The patient is at risk for pathological fractures as a result of minor stress on the weaker bones. The patient needs to assess the home and work environment for hazards that would contribute to falls. These hazards include loose rugs, highly waxed or wet floors, and stairs with poor lighting or inadequate handrails.

■ = Independent   ▲ = Collaborative

Endocrine and Metabolic Care Plans

Risk for Excess Fluid Volume

Common Risk Factors

Retention of sodium and water caused by glucocorticoid excess

Marked sodium and water retention if mineralocorticoids are also in excess

Common Expected Outcome

Patient is normovolemic as evidenced by urinary output greater than or equal to 30 mL/hr, balanced intake and output, stable weight (or loss attributed to fluid loss), absence or reduction of edema, heart rate less than 100 beats/min, absence of pulmonary congestion (crackles).

NOC Outcomes
Fluid Balance; Electrolyte and Acid-Base Balance
NIC Interventions
Fluid Monitoring; Fluid Management; Electrolyte Management

Ongoing Assessment

Actions/Interventions	Rationales
■ Assess heart rate and BP.	Cushing's syndrome may result in hypertension caused by expanded fluid volume with sodium and water retention. Tachycardia occurs as a compensatory response to circulatory overload.
■ Assess for signs of circulatory overload: weight gain, edema, jugular vein distention, crackles, shortness of breath, dyspnea.	Documentation of circulatory overload directs prompt intervention. Excessive glucocorticoid and mineralocorticoid secretion predisposes the patient to fluid and sodium retention.
▲ Monitor laboratory results (especially potassium and sodium).	Excessive glucocorticoids cause sodium and water retention, edema, and hypokalemia. Mineralocorticoids regulate sodium and potassium secretion, and excess levels cause marked sodium and water retention as well as marked hypokalemia.
■ Assess for cardiac dysrhythmias.	Hypokalemia is associated with excessive glucocorticoids, which can result in cardiac dysrhythmias.

Therapeutic Interventions

Actions/Interventions	Rationales
■ Encourage a diet low in sodium with ample potassium.	These dietary changes help control development of edema and hypokalemia.
■ Instruct the patient to reduce fluid intake as prescribed.	Regulating fluid intake is necessary to prevent circulatory overload.
▲ Administer or instruct the patient to take diuretics as prescribed.	Diuretics promote sodium and water excretion. Potassium-sparing diuretics may be prescribed to prevent further loss of potassium.
■ Advise the patient to elevate his or her feet when sitting down.	This position reduces fluid accumulation in the lower extremities.
▲ Administer or instruct the patient to take antihypertensive medications as prescribed.	Mineralocorticoid excess causes hypertension due to sodium and water retention.

Related Care Plans

Activity intolerance, p. 8
Diabetes mellitus, p. 911
Ineffective coping, p. 49
Risk for impaired skin integrity, p. 185

Diabetes Mellitus

Type 1; Type 2

Diabetes mellitus is a disorder of metabolism in which carbohydrates, fats, and proteins cannot be used for energy. Insulin, a hormone secreted by islet cells of the pancreas, is required to facilitate movement of glucose across cell membranes. Once inside the cell, glucose is the primary metabolic fuel. Type 1 diabetes occurs when the pancreas is no longer able to secrete insulin. This condition occurs as a result of an autoimmune process with destruction of pancreatic beta cells and is usually a condition of children or young adults. The autoimmune process is triggered by a combination of genetic predisposition and environmental stimuli such as a virus. The result of the insulin deficiency is hyperglycemia. Its onset is abrupt. It represents 5% to 10% of the cases of diabetes. Type 2 diabetes results because of resistance of peripheral tissue receptors to the effects of insulin. This type of diabetes also has a genetic predisposition for insulin resistance in skeletal muscles, fat cells, and liver cells. Type 2 diabetes is characterized by hyperinsulinemia and hyperglycemia. Over time the beta cells of the pancreas fail to produce sufficient insulin. Its onset is slow and gradual, with many individuals having had the disease 10 years before diagnosis. It represents 90% to 95% of the cases of diabetes. This is usually a condition of middle-aged to older individuals, although a recent increase in the incidence of type 2 diabetes has occurred in children. Obesity is a major factor in the development of type 2 diabetes. Current studies relate waist circumference of 40 inches for men and 35 inches for women to increased risk for this form of diabetes.

Diabetes is a major public health problem; more than 16 million individuals, or 6.5% of the population, have the disease. Diabetes causes significant morbidity and mortality. Seventy percent of diabetes-related deaths are from cardiovascular disease. The severity of dyslipidemia and hypertension is higher in the person with type 2 diabetes. Diabetes is the most common single cause of end-stage renal disease in the United States. Diabetic retinopathy is the most frequent cause of new cases of blindness among adults 20 to 74 years of age. Diabetes is the leading cause of nontraumatic lower extremity amputations in the United States. This care plan concentrates on the care of individuals with type 2 diabetes.

NANDA-I NDx Risk for Unstable Blood Glucose Level

Common Risk Factors

Insulin deficiency with inability to utilize nutrients
Excessive intake in relation to metabolic needs
Sedentary activity level

Common Expected Outcome

Patient maintains blood glucose and glycosolated hemoglobin levels within defined target ranges.

NOC Outcomes

Blood Glucose Level; Knowledge: Medication, Diet, Prescribed Activity; Knowledge: Diabetes Management

NIC Interventions

Hyperglycemia Management; Teaching: Prescribed Activity/Exercise; Teaching: Prescribed Diet; Teaching: Prescribed Medication

 = Independent   ▲ = Collaborative

Ongoing Assessment

Actions/Interventions	**Rationales**
■ Assess for signs of hyperglycemia.	Hyperglycemia results when inadequate insulin is present to use glucose. Excess glucose in the bloodstream creates an osmotic effect that results in increased thirst, increased hunger, and increased urination. The patient may also report nonspecific symptoms of fatigue and blurred vision.
▲ Monitor blood glucose levels at each office visit, and review blood glucose history.	Changes in blood glucose levels, as recorded by the patient, will indicate the patient's success in managing his or her diabetes.
▲ Monitor HbA$_{1c}$-glycosylated hemoglobin.	HbA$_{1c}$ is a measure of blood glucose over the previous 2 to 3 months. Current recommendations are to have HbA$_{1c}$ measured four times each year. The desired goal is to have HbA$_{1c}$ levels less than 6.5% to 7%.
▲ Monitor serum insulin levels.	Hyperinsulinemia occurs early in the development of type 2 diabetes. Obesity and insulin receptor dysfunction in peripheral tissues stimulates insulin secretion from the pancreas. Over many years pancreatic cells fail to secrete sufficient insulin leading to hyperglycemia.
■ Assess current knowledge and understanding of prescribed diet.	Nonadherence to dietary guidelines can result in hyperglycemia. Current guidelines from the American Diabetes Association recommend an individualized plan that promotes healthy eating.
■ Assess pattern of physical activity.	Physical activity has an insulin-like effect and helps lower blood glucose levels. Regular exercise is an important part of diabetes management and reduces the risk for cardiovascular complications.

Therapeutic Interventions

Actions/Interventions	**Rationales**
▲ Establish goals with the patient for weight loss; glucose, lipids and HbA$_{1c}$ measurements; and exercise.	*Weight:* Moderate weight loss of 10 to 20 pounds has been shown to improve hyperglycemia, dyslipidemia, and hypertension. *Glucose:* For intensive control, range should be between 80 and 120 mg/dL before meals. *HbA$_{1c}$:* Level should be less than 7%. *Exercise:* Patient should perform 30 minutes of moderate physical activity on most days of the week.
■ Review progress toward goals on each subsequent visit.	Patient involvement in the treatment plan enhances adherence to treatment regimens. Interest in learning new health behaviors increases when the patient helps set the agenda for change and feels like an active participant.
■ Assist the patient in identifying eating patterns that need changing.	This information provides the basis for individualized dietary instruction.
▲ Refer to a registered dietitian for individualized diet instruction.	An individualized meal plan based on body weight; blood glucose, and lipid patterns should be developed for each patient. Protein intake is recommended to be 15% to 20% of total calories. Fats are recommended to be no more than 20% of total caloric intake. Saturated fats should be less than 10% of total fat intake. The remaining calories will come from carbohydrates. The type of carbohydrate (sugar or starch) is less important than total carbohydrate intake. Dietary fiber of 20 to 35 g/day is associated with improved glycemic control.

Endocrine and Metabolic Care Plans

Actions/Interventions	Rationales
■ Instruct the patient to take oral hypoglycemic medications as directed:	Each category of oral agent acts on a different site of glucose metabolism. Hypoglycemia occurs less frequently with oral agents; however, episodes of hypoglycemia can occur in patients who do not have regular eating habits.
• Second-generation sulfonylureas: glipizide (Glucotrol), glyburide (DiaBeta), glimepiride (Amaryl)	These drugs stimulate insulin secretion by the pancreas.
• Meglitinides: repaglinide (Prandin)	These drugs stimulate insulin secretion by the pancreas.
• D-Phenylalanine derivatives: nateglinide (Starlix)	These stimulate rapid insulin secretion to reduce increases in blood glucose that occur soon after eating.
• Biguanides: metformin (Glucophage)	These drugs decrease the amount of glucose produced by the liver and improve insulin sensitivity.
• α-Glucosidase inhibitors: acarbose (Precose), miglitol (Glyset)	These drugs delay absorption of glucose into the blood from the intestine.
• Thiazolidinediones: pioglitazone (Actos), rosiglitazone (Avandia)	These drugs decrease insulin resistance.
• Incretin modifier: sitagliptin phosphate (Januvia)	This drug increases insulin secretion and decreases glucagon secretion to reduce the production of glucose.
■ Instruct the patient to take insulin medications as directed:	Insulin is required for individuals with type 1 diabetes and for many with type 2 diabetes who develop insulin deficiency over time. Beta cells begin to fail about 10 to 20 years after development of type 2 diabetes.
• Rapid-acting insulin analogs: lispro insulin (Humalog), insulin aspart	Duration of action is 2 to 3 hours for Humalog and 3 to 5 hours for aspart.
• Short-acting insulin: regular	Duration of action is 4 to 8 hours.
• Intermediate-acting insulin: neutral protamine Hagedorn (NPH), insulin zinc suspension (Lente)	Duration of action is 18 to 26 hours.
• Intermediate and rapid: 70% NPH/30% regular	Premixed concentration has a duration of action similar to that of intermediate-acting insulins.
• Long-acting insulin: Ultralente, insulin glargine (Lantus)	Duration of action for Ultralente is 36 hours and for glargine is at least 24 hours.
■ Instruct the patient to prepare and administer insulin with accuracy.	Inconsistencies in technique of insulin preparation and administration can result in elevated blood glucose levels.
• Injection procedures	Absorption of insulin is more consistent when insulin is always injected in the same anatomical site. Absorption is fastest in the abdomen, followed by arms, thighs, and buttocks. The current American Diabetes Association recommendation is to administer insulin into the subcutaneous tissue of the abdomen.
• Rotation of injection within one anatomical site	Injection of insulin in the same site over time will result in lipoatrophy and lipohypertrophy with reduced insulin absorption.
• Storage of insulin	Insulin should be refrigerated at 2° to 8° C (36° to 46° F). Unopened vials may be stored until expiration date. To prevent irritation from injection of cold insulin, vials of insulin may be stored at temperatures of 15° to 30° C (59° to 86° F) for 1 month. Opened vials should be discarded after that time.
• Mixing of insulins: consult manufacturer's guidelines	Mixing of two insulins in one syringe is technically difficult for some patients. Accuracy with this technique is essential. Some insulin products cannot be mixed (glargine) or should be administered shortly after preparation (rapid-acting and Ultralente, and rapid-acting and intermediate).

■ = Independent   ▲ = Collaborative

Actions/Interventions

- Instruct the patient in using continuous subcutaneous insulin infusion (CSII) pump.

 Instruct the patient to exercise.

- Refer the patient to an exercise physiologist, physical therapist or cardiac rehabilitation nurse for specific exercise instructions.
- Thirty to 60 minutes with warm-up and cool-down periods
- Three to four times a week for glycemic control
- Five to 7 days a week for weight loss
- Instruct in methods to maintain hydration and avoid hypoglycemia during exercise.

Rationales

A CSII is a portable insulin pump that allows for a continuous subcutaneous infusion of a basal insulin dose. The patient can increase doses for mealtime. Adjustments in the dose of rapid-acting insulin in the pump reservoir are based on regular capillary blood glucose monitoring results. This insulin delivery system allows the patient more flexibility in timing insulin administration to mealtimes. Insulin infusion devices provide for improved outcomes of blood glucose control compared with multiple daily injections. Use of insulin pumps requires a highly motivated patient to learn how to manage the pump.

Exercise improves glucose levels patterns and assists with weight loss.

Specific exercises can be prescribed based on any physical limitations the diabetic individual may have.

Warm-ups before exercise and stretching after exercise help prevent muscle injury. Studies have shown sustained improvement in glucose control when a regular exercise program is maintained.

Dehydration can hasten hypoglycemia, especially in hot weather. Patients may need to add a snack before exercise if they experience hypoglycemia.

NANDA-I NDx Risk for Ineffective Therapeutic Regimen Management

Common Risk Factors

New-onset diabetes
Complex medical regimen
Insufficient knowledge about diabetes and its treatment

Common Expected Outcome

Patient demonstrates knowledge of diabetes self-care measures.

NOC Outcomes

Knowledge: Diabetes Management; Blood Glucose Level; Diabetes Self-Management

NIC Interventions

Mutual Goal Setting; Teaching: Disease Process; Teaching: Individual; Teaching: Prescribed Diet

Ongoing Assessment

Actions/Interventions	**Rationales**
■ Assess the patient's prior efforts to manage diabetes care regimen.	This knowledge provides an important starting point in understanding any complexities the patient perceives in implementation of diabetes management regimen. The patient may report past experiences of feeling overwhelmed by attempts to manage medications, diet, exercise, blood glucose monitoring, and other measures to treat diabetes and prevent complications.
■ Evaluate self-management skills, including ability to perform procedures for blood glucose monitoring.	Self-management skills determine the amount and type of education that needs to be provided.
■ Assess for factors that may negatively affect success with following the regimen.	Limited vision may impair the patient's ability to prepare and administer insulin accurately. Limited mobility and loss of fine motor control can interfere with skills needed for insulin administration and blood glucose monitoring. This assessment can lead to appropriate referrals for adaptive equipment.
■ Assess financial resources for health care.	The cost of medications and supplies for blood glucose monitoring may become barriers to the patient with limited financial resources.

Therapeutic Interventions

Actions/Interventions	**Rationales**
■ Ensure that the patient has knowledge about symptoms, causes, treatment, and prevention of hyperglycemia.	Elevated blood glucose levels in individuals with previously diagnosed diabetes indicate the need to evaluate diabetes management.
• Symptoms: polyuria, polydipsia, polyphagia, weight loss, elevated blood glucose levels, fatigue, blurred vision, poor wound healing	The buildup of glucose in the body results in symptoms that can be identified by the patient. Ensure that the patient has been educated regarding these symptoms.
• Causes: increased food intake, decreased medications, infection, illness, stress	Increased food intake or decreased medication use for diabetes causes increased blood glucose levels. Illness, infection, and increased stress increases counterregulatory hormones that elevate blood glucose levels.
• Treatment: increased fluid intake, medications to reduce blood glucose levels, identification and treatment of cause	Dehydration causes many of the symptoms related to hyperglycemia. The patient may receive insulin to reduce blood glucose and prevent diabetic ketoacidosis (DKA).
• Prevention: adherence to dietary guidelines and medical regimen; blood glucose monitoring conducted on a regular basis permits early treatment of hyperglycemia	Nonadherence to medical regimen is frequently a cause of hyperglycemia. Effective long-term management of blood glucose levels reduces the risk for vascular complications of diabetes mellitus. These complications include nephropathy, neuropathy, retinopathy, cerebrovascular disease, and coronary artery disease.
■ Ensure that the patient has knowledge about symptoms, causes, treatment, and prevention of hypoglycemia.	Frequent episodes of hypoglycemia in individuals with previously diagnosed diabetes indicate the need to evaluate diabetes management.
• Symptoms: *autonomic*—trembling, shaking, sweating, pounding heart rate, fast pulse, tingling in extremities, heavy breathing; *neuroglycopenic*—slow thinking, blurred vision, slurred speech, trouble concentrating, fatigue or sleepiness	Autonomic symptoms represent the action of counterregulatory hormones, initially epinephrine, to the effects of lowered blood glucose levels. Neuroglycopenic symptoms occur because of depletion of glucose in the central nervous system.

■ = Independent ▲ = Collaborative

Actions/Interventions	Rationales
• Causes: *meals*—delayed or missed meals or snacks, irregular timing of meals, irregular carbohydrate content of meals; *medications*—increased dose, medication taken at the wrong time; *activity*—increased physical activity without additional carbohydrate intake.	All cases of hypoglycemia are caused by excess insulin in relation to available nutrients.
• Treatment: 10 to 15 g of carbohydrate for blood glucose levels less than 70 mg/dL; 30 g may be needed for levels less than 50 mg/dL. Examples of 10-g sources include 3 to 4 glucose tablets, 8 to 10 Lifesavers candies, and 4 to 6 ounces of fruit juice.	Ten to 15 g of carbohydrate should raise blood glucose levels 30 to 45 mg/dL. Glucose-containing products will produce faster results than those containing fat or protein.
• Prevention: adherence to medication and dietary guidelines, regular self-monitoring of blood glucose, accurate medication-taking practices.	Hypoglycemia can largely be prevented by appropriate self-management behaviors.
▲ Refer to social services for help with financial resources.	Nonadherence to a treatment plan may occur because of limited resources for purchasing medications and blood glucose monitoring supplies. Some costs may not be covered by health insurance.
■ Review current dietary goals for type 2 diabetes with the patient and family: normalize blood glucose and lipid values, improve eating habits, restrict caloric intake, achieve moderate weight loss, maintain consistent carbohydrate intake at meals and snacks, and decrease fat intake.	Successful outcomes for nutritional management require not only active participation by the patient but also participation by family members. The person responsible for meal planning and preparation needs to have a good understanding of nutritional management for diabetes.
■ Review blood glucose monitoring results on each contact with the patient.	This measures progress to achieving previously set blood glucose goals. Positive feedback on goal attainment helps motivate the patient to continue with health behaviors for effective diabetes management.
■ Instruct the patient in how to use blood glucose results in overall diabetes management: review basics of pattern management.	Instruction allows the patient to identify when therapy adjustments need to be made in diabetes treatment. Using blood glucose monitoring results allows the patient to make adjustments in food intake, exercise, and medication dosage in order to maintain therapeutic outcomes for blood glucose levels. Monitoring allows the patient to identify the onset of side effects of therapy or the onset of complications of the disease.
■ Evaluate effectiveness of previous instruction.	Evaluation provides opportunity to correct any errors in technique. Education is an ongoing process that requires reinforcement over time.
■ Instruct the patient in diabetes management during illness.	
• Instruct the patient to take all diabetes medications.	Insulin requirements increase with illness. Secretion of catecholamines, cortisol, and growth hormone in response to the stress of illness results in increased blood glucose levels.
• Self-monitor blood glucose every 2 to 4 hours.	Increased frequency of blood glucose testing provides information on response of blood glucose to therapy.
• Test urine for ketones every 3 to 4 hours if blood glucose is consistently greater than 300 mg/dL in the presence of abdominal pain, nausea, and/or vomiting.	Testing provides for early detection of DKA.
• Drink 8 ounces of fluids every 4 hours: sugar-free drinks are recommended when the patient is able to maintain normal carbohydrate intake. Substitute drinks containing sugar when the individual is unable to eat solid food due to anorexia.	Sufficient fluid intake is needed to prevent dehydration that occurs with hyperglycemia.
■ Instruct the patient in how and when to take additional rapid- or short-acting insulin as directed.	Supplements of rapid-acting insulin may be required every 2 to 3 hours to treat hyperglycemia.

Actions/Interventions

- Instruct when to contact the primary care provider: blood glucose levels greater than 300 mg/dL, vomiting for more than 2 to 4 hours, failure of urinary ketones to clear within 12 hours, symptoms of dehydration, or symptoms suggesting development of DKA or hyperglycemic hyperosmolar nonketotic syndrome (HHNS).

- Instruct the patient to carry medical identification at all times.

- Instruct the patient about planning for diabetes management when traveling such as putting medications in carry-on luggage.

Rationales

Early treatment of hyperglycemia can prevent the occurrence of DKA or HHNS.

It is important for medical personnel to be able to identify the patient as having diabetes to provide appropriate care in an emergency.

Some travel may involve time changes that can disrupt the patient's usual routines.

 NANDA-I NDx

Risk for Injury: Feet

Common Risk Factors

Hyperglycemia
Peripheral sensory neuropathy
Autonomic neuropathy
Immune system deficits
Vascular insufficiency

Common Expected Outcome

Patient is free of injury to feet.

NOC Outcomes
Tissue Integrity: Skin and Mucous Membranes; Self-Care: Hygiene; Knowledge: Treatment Regimen

NIC Interventions
Foot Care; Skin Surveillance; Nail Care; Teaching: Individual

---

Ongoing Assessment

Actions/Interventions

- Assess the general appearance of the foot. Note hygiene.

- Assess the status of the nails.

- Assess skin integrity. Note color of skin, presence or absence of ulceration, moisture, quality of the skin, and presence of dermatitis.

Rationales

Foot lesions and associated wound infections are the most common reason for hospitalization of the patient with diabetes. The patient's feet should be inspected at every visit. The patient may be unaware of injuries to the feet as a result of decreased sensation from peripheral neuropathy.

Fungal infections in nails serve as a port of entrance for bacteria. The person with diabetes has an increased risk for infection because of impaired immunity. Individuals with thickened, deformed, or ingrown nails should be referred to their primary care provider for appropriate treatment.

Autonomic neuropathy leads to decreased perspiration, causing excessive dryness and fissuring of the skin. Skin breakdown predisposes the patient to infection.

■ = Independent ▲ = Collaborative

Endocrine and Metabolic Care Plans

Actions/Interventions

- Note the presence or absence of callus formation or corns.

- Assess the circulatory status of the foot by palpation of peripheral pulses. A Doppler ultrasound transducer can be used when pulses are no longer palpable.
  - Dorsalis pedis
  - Posterior tibial
- Assess for evidence of infection. Local symptoms include redness, drainage, and swelling. Systemic symptoms include fever and malaise, and loss of blood glucose control.
- Assess for edema.

- Assess protective sensation with 5.07 monofilament.

- Examine hosiery and shoes for condition and fit.

- Assess the patient's ability to reach his or her feet and perform self-examination and nail care.

Rationales

Pressure over bony prominences leads to callus formation. This condition can lead to the development of skin breakdown.

The foot is extremely vulnerable to circulatory changes from macrovascular complications of diabetes mellitus. The development of atherosclerosis is accelerated in the patient with diabetes as a result of alterations in lipid metabolism.

Infection may be the initiating event for eventual amputation. Symptoms of pain and tenderness may be absent because of neuropathy.

Edema is a major predisposing factor to ulcerations. Autonomic neuropathy results in loss of vasomotor reflexes and swelling in the foot.

The absence of protective sensation places the patient at high risk for foot injury.

Localized redness over bony prominences indicates the shoe is too tight.

This provides basis for future patient education.

Therapeutic Interventions

Actions/Interventions

- Instruct the patient in principles of hygiene: wash feet daily in warm water using mild soap, but avoid soaking the feet. Dry carefully and gently, especially between the toes. Encourage use of moisturizing lotion at least once daily. Avoid area between the toes.
- Teach the patient to inspect feet daily for cuts, scratches, and blisters. Use a mirror if necessary to examine the bottom of the foot. Instruct the patient to use both visual inspection and touch.
- Report signs of infection immediately to the primary care provider:
  - Area of skin breakdown
  - Increase in temperature as compared with the same location on the opposite foot
  - Discharge that develops an odor
- Teach the patient to inspect shoes daily by feeling the inside of the shoe for irregularities in the lining, sharp objects in the sole of the shoe, or foreign bodies in the shoe.
- ▲ Instruct the patient in appropriate footwear. Have the foot size measured, and try shoes on before purchase. Refer patients with hammertoes to a podiatrist or foot care specialist for extra-depth or custom-molded footwear.

- Instruct the patient to wear clean, well-fitting stockings made from soft cotton, synthetic blend, or wool.
- Teach the patient to avoid thermal injuries by:
  - Testing the temperature of bathwater with the elbow, wrist, or thermometer
  - Avoiding use of heating pads, hot water bottles, or electric blankets
  - Maintaining a safe distance from heat sources such as the fireplace or space heater

Rationales

Maceration between the toes predisposes the patient to infection. The use of lotion replaces moisturizing effects lost by autonomic neuropathy. Select lotion with low alcohol content to prevent further drying of the skin.

All surfaces of the foot need to be examined, including skin between the toes. Touch will identify skin surface alterations that are not evident by sight.

Early treatment is essential in prevention of amputation. Clinical studies on amputations have found that as many as 85% of patients have foot ulcers before amputation.

Careful daily assessment reduces risk for injury to the foot. Peripheral neuropathy and loss of protective sensation limits the ability of the patient to feel irregularities that could precipitate an injury to the foot.

Width: The widest part of the shoe must accommodate the widest part of the foot. *Length:* There should be 1½ inches of space between the longest toe and the end of the shoe. *Toe box:* The toe box should be high with a rounded toe. *Heel height:* This should be less than 2 inches.

Soft cotton or wool absorbs moisture from perspiration and discourages an environment in which fungus can thrive.

Sensory neuropathy may result in loss of normal pain and temperature sensation. These changes increase risk for burns.

Actions/Interventions

- Instruct patients to always wear protective footwear; never go barefoot.
- Instruct the patient to trim nails straight across and to file sharp corners to match contour of the toe. Suggest that a family member or podiatrist trim the nails when the patient cannot see well or has difficulty reaching his or her feet.
- Instruct the patient to avoid self-treatment:
  - Do not use adhesive tape, wart treatments, corn plasters, or strong antiseptics.
  - Do not use over-the-counter fungal products without approval of the primary care provider.
  - Avoid "bathroom surgery."

- Stress the importance of maintaining normal blood glucose levels.

- Encourage the patient to stop smoking.

Rationales

Keeping the feet covered prevents injury to the foot.

This technique avoids injury to the toes when self-care cannot be provided.

Many over-the-counter agents contain salicylic acid, which can cause ulceration in the diabetic foot.
Over-the-counter products may increase microbial resistance when they are used inappropriately.
Cutting away corns and calluses increases the risk for further foot injury and infection.
Elevated blood glucose or glycosylated hemoglobin levels are associated with risk for foot ulcers. Hyperglycemia impairs wound healing.
Chronic vasoconstriction, caused by smoking, reduces the ability of tissues to heal.

Related Care Plans

Chronic pain, p. 155
Deficient knowledge, p. 122
Diabetic ketoacidosis (see the **Evolve** website)
Ineffective sexuality pattern, p. 182
Risk for infection, p. 114
Risk for impaired skin integrity, p. 185

Hyperthyroidism

Graves' Disease

Hyperthyroidism occurs as a result of increased circulating levels of thyroid hormones. Women are affected more often than men. The peak age for diagnosis of the disorder is 20 to 40 years. The most common cause is Graves' disease. This form of hyperthyroidism is an autoimmune disorder that contributes to a failure of the normal regulation of thyroid hormone secretion. Other causes of hyperthyroidism include toxic multinodular goiter, thyroid gland tumors, and pituitary gland tumors. The clinical manifestations of hyperthyroidism develop as a result of the hypermetabolic effects of increased thyroid hormones on all body systems. These manifestations include heat intolerance, irritability, restlessness, goiter, tachycardia, palpitations, increased blood pressure, diaphoresis, weight loss, increased appetite, diarrhea, visual changes, menstrual irregularities and changes in libido. Thyrotoxic crisis or thyroid storm is a rare but severe form of hyperthyroidism that develops suddenly in response to excessive stress or poorly controlled hormone levels. The management of hyperthyroidism includes drug therapy, radioactive iodine therapy, and surgical removal of all or part of the thyroid gland.

■ = Independent   ▲ = Collaborative

NANDA-I NDx **Deficient Knowledge**

Common Related Factors
New diagnosis of hyperthyroidism
Unfamiliarity with information
Hyperactivity, fatigue, and emotional instability affecting
learning

Common Expected Outcome
Patient and family verbalize correct information about
hyperthyroidism and its treatment.

Defining Characteristics
Multiple questions
Lack of questions
Decreased attention span and concentration
Inaccurate information

NOC Outcomes
Knowledge: Disease Process; Knowledge:
Medication; Information Processing
NIC Interventions
Learning Facilitation; Teaching: Individual

Ongoing Assessment

Actions/Interventions	Rationales
■ Assess the patient's current knowledge of hyperthyroidism.	Patient teaching begins with what the patient and family members already know about the disease and its treatment.

Therapeutic Interventions

Actions/Interventions	Rationales
■ Teach the patient and family about hyperthyroidism.	Knowledge of the disease process and its manifestations helps the patient and family understand treatment options. This information aids the patient in assuming responsibility for care at a later time. The family may be more supportive with new understandings of the disease and its manifestations.
■ Provide a quiet, calm atmosphere without interruptions.	The patient with hyperthyroidism experiences a hypermetabolic state that leads to hyperactivity with fatigue, and cyclic changes in mood. These manifestations may contribute to a decreased attention span and impaired concentration. Teaching sessions may need to be short and planned at times when the patient can concentrate and pay attention. Learning new information requires using energy that may aggravate fatigue.
■ Teach the patient and family measures to manage symptoms, conserve energy, and promote comfort: • Environmental control • Frequent rest periods • Delegation of activities, especially those requiring fine motor control	Until hormone levels are reduced with drug or radiation therapy, the patient and family need to know how to manage symptoms associated with increased metabolic activity. The patient will complain of heat intolerance and diaphoresis. A cool environment with dim lighting will promote comfort and encourage rest. The patient may be hyperactive and experience fine motor tremors that interfere with activities requiring fine motor control. The family needs to support the patient by helping with these activities. Balancing periods of rest with periods of hyperactivity will help conserve the patient's energy.
■ Reinforce information the patient has received about treatment options for hyperthyroidism:	Information provided by the physician may need to be repeated frequently. Written information needs to be available to reinforce verbal instructions.

Endocrine and Metabolic Care Plans

Actions/Interventions	Rationales
• Antithyroid medications such as propylthiouracil (PTU)	These medications work by blocking iodide binding in the thyroid gland. This action decreases production of thyroid hormones. PTU also interferes with conversion of T_4 to T_3, the more potent of the two hormones. The patient needs to learn the importance of taking the drug at evenly spaced intervals during the day to achieve the maximum therapeutic benefit. Because of the chance of liver toxicity the patient needs information about appropriate symptoms to report and follow-up care for laboratory studies of liver function.
• Iodine preparations	Iodine is given most often before surgery and for a very short term of therapy. It acts to decrease the vascularity of the thyroid gland and promote storage of hormone in the gland. The patient needs to understand that iodine may cause a metallic taste.
• Radioactive iodine (^{131}I)	Radioactive iodine is taken up by the cells of the thyroid gland. This therapy is a form of local radiation that destroys a portion of the thyroid gland and thereby reduces hormone production. The therapy takes several weeks to provide the patient with significant symptom relief, so other antithyroid drugs may be given early in the therapy. The patient and family need to understand that the level of radioactivity is low and quickly clears from the body. Special safety precautions are not needed. Most patients achieve therapeutic benefit after one treatment. The patient may develop hypothyroidism after treatment depending of the amount of gland tissue destroyed. Thyroid replacement therapy may be required.
• β-Adrenergic antagonists	β-Blockers inhibit the increased sympathetic nervous system activity associated with hyperthyroidism. The drugs are given to aid in management of symptoms such as tachycardia, palpitations, and tremors. This class of drugs has no direct effect on the thyroid gland or its hormones.
• Surgical removal of all or part of the thyroid.	Surgery is reserved usually for patients who develop a large goiter that impairs breathing or swallowing.

NANDA-I NDx

Imbalanced Nutrition: Less Than Body Requirements

Common Related Factor

Intake less than metabolic needs

Defining Characteristics

Weight loss
Increased physical activity
Increased appetite

Common Expected Outcomes

Patient gains weight and maintains stable weight.
Patient takes in sufficient calories and essential nutrients to support metabolic activity.

NOC Outcomes

Nutritional Status: Nutrient Intake;
 Knowledge: Diet

NIC Interventions

Nutritional Monitoring; Nutrition Management;
 Teaching: Diet

■ = Independent ▲ = Collaborative

Ongoing Assessment

Actions/Interventions	Rationales
■ Assess weight.	The patient with hyperthyroidism will experience a decrease in body weight because of an increased basal metabolic rate.
■ Assess appetite.	The patient is likely to report experiencing a significant increase in appetite and sensations of hunger. This inverse relationship between the person's increased appetite and decreasing weight is a characteristic finding in hyperthyroidism.
■ Assess the patient's typical food intake through a 24-hour recall.	Determining the patient's typical intake provides a basis for an individualized plan of nutrition support for the patient's increased metabolic needs.

Therapeutic Interventions

Actions/Interventions	Rationales
■ Help the patient select foods that provide a balanced diet with increased calories in the form of carbohydrates and proteins.	The high T_3 and T_4 levels create an increased demand for calories to support the high metabolic rate of cells. The patient may need more than 3000 calories/day to support metabolic activity. Protein catabolism exceeds protein anabolism in hyperthyroidism, creating a state of negative nitrogen balance.
■ Provide increased fluid intake.	Additional fluid intake is necessary to support the increased metabolic activity. Increased diaphoresis is a common manifestation of hyperthyroidism.
■ Encourage the patient to eat small, frequent meals and snacks.	Eating five to six small meals throughout the day requires less energy than eating three larger meals. This approach will help the patient increase caloric intake without adding to fatigue.
■ Encourage the patient and family to have foods available that are easy to eat such as sandwiches and other "finger foods."	The patient may be too restless and hyperactive to sit down for regular meals. Foods that can be eaten while the patient is moving around will help support increased nutritional intake.
■ Teach the patient to limit foods that increase peristaltic activity.	Diarrhea is a common manifestation of hyperthyroidism. Foods that are highly seasoned or have high insoluble fiber content are more likely to aggravate the diarrhea.
■ Provide supplemental vitamins and minerals.	The higher basal metabolic rate increases the need for additional vitamins and minerals. Supplements will correct preexisting deficiencies and prevent their reoccurrence.
▲ Refer the patient and family to a registered dietitian.	The dietitian can provide the patient and family with resources to increase nutritional intake.

NANDA-I NDx Disturbed Body Image

Common Related Factors	Defining Characteristics
Goiter	Enlarged neck from goiter
Exophthalmos	Bulging eyes from exophthalmos
	Verbalization about change in appearance of face and neck
	Refusal to talk about change in appearance
	Wears dark glasses and/or clothing to conceal bulging eyes and goiter

Common Expected Outcome

Patient demonstrates enhanced body image and self-esteem as evidenced by ability to talk positively about changes in appearance.

NOC Outcomes
Body Image; Self-Esteem
NIC Interventions
Body Image Enhancement; Grief Work Facilitation; Coping Enhancement

Ongoing Assessment

Actions/Interventions	Rationales
■ Assess the patient's perception of changes in appearance related to goiter or exophthalmos.	A change in appearance that is highly visible to the patient and others may create more of a threat to the patient's body image.
■ Assess the patient's current behavior related to goiter and exophthalmos.	The patient may ignore the changes in appearance or be preoccupied with hiding or covering the changes. The patient may use dark glasses to cover the eyes and scarves or high-necked shirts to cover the goiter. The patient may avoid public gatherings because of embarrassment.
■ Note the frequency of the patient's comments about his or her appearance related to an enlarged neck or bulging eyes.	Negative statements by the patient about changes in appearance indicate limited ability to integrate the change into the patient's self-concept.

Therapeutic Interventions

Actions/Interventions	Rationales
■ Provide the patient with information about goiter and exophthalmos.	Accurate information about these changes in physical appearance will support the patient's cognitive appraisal of the changes. Goiter develops from hypertrophy and hyperplasia of the thyroid tissue as a result of increased hormone levels. The gland may be three to four times its normal size. Exophthalmos develops as a result of proptosis, eyelid retraction, muscle swelling, and orbital tissue edema. The patient has a wide-eyed stare with protruding eyes. Although goiter may regress with hyperthyroidism therapy, exophthalmos may not regress.
■ Encourage verbalization of feelings about the changes in appearance.	Expressions of positive and negative feelings may enhance the patient's coping strategies.
■ Help the patient identify ways of coping that have been effective in the past.	Patients have experienced body image changes in the past as part of normal growth and development or other illnesses or injury. Coping strategies that were effective then may be effective in this situation.
■ Maintain appropriate eye contact and positive caring when interacting with the patient.	Health care providers represent a microcosm of society, and their actions and behaviors are scrutinized as the patient develops coping strategies.
■ Assist the patient with adaptive behaviors.	Wearing dark glasses not only promotes visual comfort for the patient with exophthalmos but also conceals the bulging eyes and startled appearance. Clothing and accessories may help cover the enlarged neck or distract attention to other parts of the body.

■ = Independent   ▲ = Collaborative

Risk for Hyperthermia

Common Risk Factors

Increased basal metabolic rate
Heat intolerance

Common Expected Outcome

The patient maintains body temperature below 39° C (102.2° F)

NOC Outcomes
Thermoregulation; Vital Signs
NIC Interventions
Temperature Regulation; Fever Treatment

Ongoing Assessment

Actions/Interventions	Rationales
■ Assess body temperature.	Tympanic or rectal temperature measurement provides the most accurate indication of core body temperature.
■ Assess for precipitating factors.	Hyperthermia is a manifestation of thyroid storm or thyroid crisis. This condition occurs with poorly controlled hyperthyroidism or during periods of extreme physical or emotional stress.

Therapeutic Interventions

Actions/Interventions	Rationales
■ Maintain a cool environmental temperature.	Heat intolerance is a common manifestation of hyperthyroidism because of the increased basal metabolic rate. Cooler room temperatures promote patient comfort and assist in reducing stress.
■ Encourage the patient to wear light, loose clothing. Use an electric fan to circulate room air.	These measures promote evaporative cooling of the body.
■ Provide increased fluid intake.	Diaphoresis is a common manifestation of hyperthyroidism. Increased fluid losses contribute to elevated body temperature.
■ Encourage frequent bathing with tepid water.	This measure not only promotes evaporative cooling of the body but also promotes patient comfort.
■ Monitor the patient's adherence to therapy for hyperthyroidism.	Patients who are inconsistent taking prescribed antithyroid medications increase the risk for developing thyroid crisis and hyperthermia.

Related Care Plans

Anxiety, p. 18
Diarrhea, p. 54
Fatigue, p. 66
Insomnia, p. 117
Thyroidectomy, p. 928

Hypothyroidism

Myxedema; Goiter

Hypothyroidism occurs because of a deficiency in thyroid hormone. Almost every system in the body is affected through a general slowing of metabolic processes. The disorder is common, especially among women older than 30 years of age. In the older adult, hypothyroidism may be overlooked because many of the manifestations are related to changes associated with the normal aging process (constipation, intolerance to cold, decreased activity tolerance, weight gain, lethargy, decreased short-term memory, depression). The most common cause of hypothyroidism is an autoimmune inflammation (Hashimoto's thyroiditis) of the thyroid gland with resulting atrophy of glandular tissue. Hypothyroidism may also develop after a thyroidectomy. Myxedema occurs in hypothyroidism as a result of hyaluronic acid accumulation in tissues. Fluid binds to the hyaluronic acid, producing skin puffiness most noticeable around and below the eyes. Myxedema also causes enlargement of the tongue, which contributes to the impaired speech patterns of the patient with hypothyroidism. When hypothyroidism goes undiagnosed or undertreated, the patient may develop myocardial hypotonic function and ventricular dilation. The patient is at risk for developing decreased cardiac output and systemic tissue and organ hypoxia. This situation is a rare occurrence called myxedema coma and is considered life threatening. Goiter, enlargement of the thyroid gland, may occur when hypothyroidism is the result of decreased hormone synthesis. When hormone production is reduced, thyroid-secreting hormone (TSH) secretion increases owing to lack of negative feedback. The size of the thyroid gland increases as a result of TSH stimulation.

NANDA-I NDx

Imbalanced Nutrition: More Than Body Requirements

Common Related Factor

Intake greater than metabolic needs

Defining Characteristics

Weight gain
Decreased appetite
Sedentary activity level

Common Expected Outcome

Patient maintains stable weight and takes in essential nutrients.

NOC Outcomes
Nutritional Status: Nutrient Intake; Knowledge: Disease Process

NIC Interventions
Nutritional Monitoring; Nutrition Management; Teaching: Disease Process

Ongoing Assessment

Actions/Interventions	Rationales
■ Assess weight.	Patients with hypothyroidism experience weight gain related to slowing of metabolic processes and excess fluid volume.
■ Assess appetite.	Patients with hypothyroidism experience decreased appetite. This inverse relationship between decreased appetite and increasing weight is a characteristic finding in hypothyroidism.
■ Assess the patient's typical food intake through a 24-hour recall.	Determining the patient's typical intake provides a basis for an individualized plan of nutrition support for the patient's changing metabolic needs.

■ = Independent   ▲ = Collaborative

Therapeutic Interventions

Actions/Interventions

- Teach the patient to follow a low-calorie, low-cholesterol, low-saturated-fat diet.

- Teach the patient and family about the effect of hypothyroidism on body weight.

▲ Consult with a dietitian to determine the patient's caloric needs.
- Provide assistance and encouragement as needed at mealtime.
- Encourage the patient to eat six small meals throughout the day.
- Teach the patient about sources of dietary fiber.

Rationales

Because of the decreased metabolic rate, the patient requires fewer calories to support metabolic activity. The patient with hypothyroidism tends to have higher cholesterol levels.

The patient and family need to understand the inverse relationship between weight gain and appetite in hypothyroidism. When thyroid hormone replacement therapy is initiated, the patient may experience weight loss. However, appetite may increase. This change may require a calorie-controlled diet to prevent additional weight gain.

The dietitian can calculate appropriate caloric requirements to maintain nutrient intake and achieve a stable weight.

Because of decreased energy levels, the patient may need help with eating to ensure adequate intake of essential nutrients.

This approach to eating may promote adequate intake of nutrients in the patient with decreased energy levels.

Constipation is a common manifestation of hypothyroidism. Dietary fiber attracts water into the fecal mass to keep it soft and easier to pass.

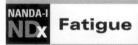 **Fatigue**

Common Related Factor

Hypometabolic state

Defining Characteristics

Increased rest requirements
Lethargic
Verbalization of overwhelming lack of energy
Unable to complete desired activities

Common Expected Outcome

Patient verbalizes reduction of fatigue and increased ability to complete desired activities.

NOC Outcomes

Activity Tolerance; Endurance; Energy Conservation; Self-Care: Activities of Daily Living

NIC Interventions

Activity Therapy; Energy Management

Ongoing Assessment

Actions/Interventions

- Assess patient's ability to perform activities of daily living.

- Assess the patient's energy level and muscle strength and tone.

Rationales

Fatigue can limit the person's ability to participate in self-care and perform his or her role responsibilities.

Slowing of metabolism results in decreased energy levels. Muscles may be weaker and joints stiffer because of mucin deposits in joints and interstitial spaces. This type of cellular edema may contribute to delayed muscle contraction and relaxation. The patient may report generalized weakness and muscle aches.

Therapeutic Interventions

Actions/Interventions	Rationales
■ Help the patient identify desired activities and responsibilities.	Activities that are important to the patient should be planned during those times of the day when the patient usually has the most energy.
■ Encourage the patient to keep a daily log of energy levels and activities for at least 1 week.	A record of energy levels and activities will help the patient identify periods of peak energy.
■ Teach the patient to alternate periods of rest with periods of activity.	Frequent rest periods will promote energy conservation.
■ Encourage the patient to ask for assistance with activities.	This energy conservation technique will help the patient participate in and complete desired activities.
■ Teach the patient that activity tolerance and endurance will improve in response to thyroid medication.	Thyroid hormone supplements will gradually increase cellular metabolism, with a resulting increased energy level. In patients with preexisting cardiac disease, increases in metabolic rate may precipitate angina because of increased demands on the heart.

NANDA-I NDx   Deficient Knowledge

Common Related Factors
Lack of exposure to hypothyroidism
Unfamiliarity with information resources
New disease process

Defining Characteristics
Verbalizes lack of information about hypothyroidism and its treatment
Limited questioning about hypothyroidism and taking thyroid hormone supplements

Common Expected Outcome
Patient and family members verbalize correct information about hypothyroidism and taking thyroid hormone supplements.

NOC Outcomes
Knowledge: Disease Process; Knowledge: Medication
NIC Interventions
Teaching: Disease Process; Teaching: Prescribed Medication

Ongoing Assessment

Actions/Interventions	Rationales
■ Assess the patient's current knowledge of hypothyroidism and thyroid hormone replacement therapy.	Patient teaching should begin with what the patient and family members already know about the disease and its treatment.

Therapeutic Interventions

Actions/Interventions	Rationales
■ Teach the patient and family about hypothyroidism.	The patient with hypothyroidism may experience impaired memory, decreased attention span, hearing loss, and confusion. These neurological changes can interfere with learning new information. Teaching sessions should be planned at times when the patient is best able to concentrate. Information may need to be repeated to facilitate learning. Written information reinforces verbal presentations.

■ = Independent   ▲ = Collaborative

Actions/Interventions	Rationales
■ Teach the patient and family about taking thyroid hormones. • Review expected benefits and possible side effects. • Encourage the patient to keep follow-up appointments for blood work. • Instruct the patient to take dose in the morning to reduce chances of insomnia.	Levothyroxine sodium (Synthroid) is a synthetic thyroid hormone used most often for hormone replacement therapy. Thyroid hormone should be taken on a regular schedule to achieve hormone balance. It may take several weeks or longer for a full therapeutic benefit to be noticed. The patient is usually started on a small dose that is gradually increased until a euthyroid state is achieved. As thyroid hormone levels increase, the patient may experience weight losss and insomnia. The patient needs to report symptoms such as palpitations or chest pain. These symptoms may occur as metabolic and oxygen consumption increase. Hormone replacement therapy is usually a lifelong commitment.
■ Encourage the patient to have medical identification about hormone therapy and to inform all health care providers.	Medical identification provides other health care providers with information to guide decisions about care. Levothyroxine is highly protein bound in circulation. This drug characteristic contributes to may drug interactions. The patient needs to notify all health care providers about taking this drug.

Related Care Plans

Constipation, p. 46
Disturbed body image, p. 24
Hypothermia, p. 103

Thyroidectomy

Hyperthyroidism; Thyrotoxicosis; Thyroid Storm

Thyroidectomy is the surgical removal of the thyroid gland performed for benign or malignant tumor, hyperthyroidism, thyrotoxicosis, or thyroiditis in patients with very large goiters, or for patients unable to be treated with radioiodine or thioamides. The surgical procedure may be a total thyroidectomy or subtotal, which is partial removal of the thyroid gland. This care plan focuses on the postoperative management of a patient undergoing a thyroidectomy.

NANDA-I NDx **Risk for Ineffective Breathing Pattern**

Common Risk Factors

Hematoma
Laryngeal edema
Vocal cord paralysis
Diminished ability to clear secretions

Common Expected Outcome

Patient will maintain an effective breathing pattern, as evidenced by relaxed breathing at normal rate and depth and absence of dyspnea.

NOC Outcome
Respiratory Status: Ventilation
NIC Interventions
Respiratory Monitoring; Airway Management; Oxygen Therapy

Ongoing Assessment

Actions/Interventions	**Rationales**
■ Assess respiratory rate and rhythm.	Increase in respiratory rate is an early sign of postoperative edema or hematoma formation in the upper airways.
■ Assess for work of breathing, presence of dyspnea, stridor, or intercostal rib retractions.	This information aids in determining the onset of respiratory distress. Stridor is an upper airway sound that occurs when laryngeal edema is present.
■ Note voice quality.	Edema may result in changes in voice quality, such as hoarseness, for 3 to 4 days after surgery. However, paralysis of the vocal cord may result from recurrent laryngeal nerve damage, which could result in closure of the glottis and the need for emergency tracheostomy.
■ Observe neck for swelling.	These changes may be indicative of edema and/or internal bleeding or hematoma formation. The patient may complain of feeling full at the incision site.
■ Assess wound drains for amount of drainage.	Decreased drainage in the first 24 hours may indicate obstruction of the wound drain. Accumulation of fluid in the wound contributes to edema and possible airway and breathing compromise.
■ Examine the wound for evidence of hematoma or oozing. Assess dressing, both anterior and posterior, and assess behind the neck for pooling.	Gravity tends to pull the drainage posteriorly. The neck dressing may be dry but bleeding may pool behind the neck when the patient is in a supine or semi-Fowler's position in bed.

Therapeutic Interventions

Actions/Interventions	**Rationales**
■ Keep head of bed elevated to 45 degrees.	Elevation limits formation of edema at the surgical site.
▲ Use an ice collar as appropriate.	Cold decreases edema formation.
■ Encourage deep breathing and use of an incentive spirometer every hour.	Deep breathing and use of an incentive spirometer keeps alveoli open and promotes effective breathing.
■ Instruct the patient to cough only as needed.	Coughing clears secretions. It can irritate the incisional area, so it is used only to clear secretions and not as a routine.
■ Suction as needed.	Suctioning clears secretions if the patient is unable to clear the airway.
■ Administer humidified air as needed.	Humidified air may help with the postoperative hoarseness experienced from intubation and postoperative edema. Increased humidification of inspired air promotes easier breathing and thinner secretions.

Risk for Injury: Hypocalcemia

Common Risk Factors

Inadvertent surgical removal of parathyroid glands or trauma to parathyroid glands (hypoparathyroidism)
Damaged blood supply to parathyroid glands (usually temporary but may be permanent)

Common Expected Outcome

Patient's risk for injury is decreased, as evidenced by serum calcium level in normal range and absence of signs of hypocalcemia.

NOC Outcome
Electrolyte and Acid-Base Balance
NIC Intervention
Electrolyte Management: Hypocalcemia

■ = Independent   ▲ = Collaborative

Ongoing Assessment

Actions/Interventions	Rationales
▲ Monitor serum ionized calcium level. Notify the physician if ionized calcium level is less than 2.1 mEq/liter.	Postoperative hypocalcemia may occur as a result of inadvertent surgical removal of or trauma to the parathyroid glands. Ionized calcium is the only form of calcium used by the body for muscle contraction, cardiac function, neuron transmission, and blood clotting. In the laboratory, ionized calcium levels are adjusted based on the pH of the blood sample. The venous specimen may be drawn in the same syringe used for arterial blood gases. Normal values for ionized calcium are 2.1 to 2.6 mEq/liter.
■ Assess for presence of circumoral and peripheral (fingers and toes) paresthesia. Instruct the patient to report development of these signs immediately.	Neuromuscular irritability is an early indicator of hypocalcemia. In addition to paresthesias, the patient may experience muscle twitching (tetany), facial grimacing, nausea, vomiting, abdominal cramping, hypotension, and mental confusion. Seizures may occur in severe hypocalcemia.
■ Observe for tremors in extremities and any seizure activity.	These changes indicate neuromuscular irritability from hypocalcemia.
■ Assess for lethargy, headache, and confusion.	These findings are additional signs of hypocalcemia.
■ Check for presence of Chvostek's sign.	This assessment technique is performed by tapping the cheek over the facial nerve; a positive sign results in a twitch of the lip or facial muscles that is indicative of hypocalcemia.
■ Check for Trousseau's sign.	Carpal spasm is induced by inflation of the blood pressure (BP) cuff 20 mm Hg above the patient's systolic BP for 3 minutes; it is also indicative of hypocalcemia.
■ Assess for laryngeal stridor.	Stridor may result from hypocalcemia.
▲ Monitor serum potassium and magnesium levels.	Hyperkalemia and hypomagnesemia potentiate cardiac and neuromuscular irritability in the presence of hypocalcemia.

Therapeutic Interventions

Actions/Interventions	Rationales
▲ Administer calcium gluconate IV, as prescribed.	Calcium gluconate is given IV when ionized calcium levels are dangerously low or the patient shows signs of hypocalcemia.
▲ Administer oral calcium and vitamin D, as prescribed. Use caution in patients receiving digitalis preparations.	Oral calcium is administered to maintain ionized calcium levels within a normal range. This drug may be used if calcium levels are low but the patient has no signs of hypocalcemia. Vitamin D enhances intestinal calcium absorption. Calcium enhances the toxic effects of digitalis.
■ Institute seizure precautions as appropriate.	This safety measure prevents injury during seizure activity. These precautions may include side rails padded and bed in low position. Suction equipment should be available at the bedside.

Risk for Injury: Thyroid Storm, Hyperthyroidism

Common Risk Factors

Inadequate preoperative preparation (euthyroid state not achieved)
Increased release of thyroid hormone

Endocrine and Metabolic Care Plans

Common Expected Outcome

Patient is free of thyroid storm, as evidenced by vital signs within normal limits and no decrease in level of consciousness (LOC).

NOC Outcome
Electrolyte and Acid-Base Balance
NIC Intervention
Electrolyte Management: Hypercalcemia

Ongoing Assessment

Actions/Interventions	Rationales
■ Assess HR, temperature, and BP.	Any increase in temperature, systolic BP and heart rate without a specific known cause should be considered thyroid storm. Thyroid storm can occur postoperatively as the result of increased hormone release from manipulation of the gland intraoperatively. This condition precipitates a hypermetabolic state similar to hyperthyroidism.
■ Assess for presence of heat intolerance.	Heat intolerance is a clinical symptom of thyroid storm.
■ Assess for gastrointestinal (GI) distress.	Elevated thyroid hormone level increases GI tract motility, possibly resulting in diarrhea.
■ Assess for restlessness and changes in LOC.	As thyroid storm progresses, LOC decreases and the patient may become comatose.

Therapeutic Interventions

Actions/Interventions	Rationales
▲ Maintain intravenous infusion for hydration and electrolyte balance.	The hypermetabolic state increases fluid needs.
▲ Protect the patient from adverse effects of excess thyroid hormone.	
• Lower temperature by keeping covers off; use hypothermia blanket; administer nonsalicylate antipyretic agents; give sponge bath.	It is important to use nonsalicylate antipyretics, because salicylates increase free thyroid hormone levels, which would worsen the condition.
• Administer antithyroid drug (iodine).	This drug inhibits thyroid hormone release.
• Administer β-receptor blocking agent.	This drug decreases the cardiovascular and neuromuscular effects associated with increased hormone levels.
• Administer adrenal corticosteroid as indicated.	This drug blocks thyroid hormone secretion.

Deficient Knowledge

Common Related Factors
New condition
Lack of familiarity with surgical treatment and medications

Defining Characteristics
Multiple questions
Lack of questions
Expressed need for further information

Common Expected Outcome
Patient and caregiver verbalize understanding of postoperative care for thyroidectomy.

NOC Outcomes
Knowledge: Disease Process; Knowledge: Treatment Regimen
NIC Interventions
Teaching: Disease Process; Teaching: Prescribed Medications

■ = Independent   ▲ = Collaborative

Endocrine and Metabolic Care Plans

Ongoing Assessment

Actions/Interventions	Rationales
■ Assess knowledge of thyroidectomy and postoperative care.	Building on current knowledge prepares for future compliance.

Therapeutic Interventions

Actions/Interventions	Rationales
■ Instruct the patient to inform the physician if any of the following develop:	
• Circumoral or peripheral paresthesia; tremors	These findings may result from a low serum calcium level. Infection may develop 7 to 10 days after surgery.
• Signs of infection: excessive or continual drainage from the incisional line, incision open and/or red	
• Signs of hematoma or increase in edema formation: difficulty in breathing, alteration in voice, sensation of pressure, tightness, fullness in neck	These symptoms require prompt intervention to decrease the risk of airway obstruction.
• Signs and symptoms of thyroid storm: temperature greater than 37.7° C (100° F), agitation and anxiety, hot and flushed skin, tachycardia, abdominal pain, nausea and vomiting, diarrhea, anorexia, or systolic hypertension	Thyroid storm is a life-threating condition and requires prompt intervention.
■ Instruct the patient to avoid abrupt head and neck movements until the suture line heals.	Abrupt movement of the head may cause wound dehiscence.
■ Instruct the patient in dosage, schedule, desired effects, and side effects of the medications sent home.	If a total thyroidectomy was done, the patient must develop a basic understanding of the long-term need for thyroid replacement therapy and the consequences of failure to take the medication.
■ Instruct in wound care:	
• Incisional care: cleansing; dressings as needed for drainage; keeping wound dry; patient may shower when approved by physician	These measures promote wound healing and decrease infection risk.
• Scar appearance and resolution over time: use of scarves and high collars	These modifications camouflage the scar until normal healing occurs. The patient needs to know that the scar will fade in appearance over several months.
■ Instruct the patient in range-of-motion (ROM) exercises for the neck.	Exercises strengthen the neck, return full ROM, and aid in the healing process.
■ Instruct the patient to avoid temperature extremes.	Exposure to extreme hot and cold temperatures promotes thyroid hyperplasia and increases the thyroid levels.
■ Instruct the patient who has undergone a partial thyroidectomy in dietary measures.	
• Maintain a low-calorie diet.	During the hypothyroid period, the patient should reduce caloric intake to prevent weight gain.
• Avoid foods that contain thyroid-inhibiting substances (goitrogens): turnips, rutabagas, soybeans.	These foods inhibit the return of thyroid activity.

Related Care Plans

Ineffective airway clearance, p. 11
Risk for infection, p. 114

Integumentary Care Plans

Skin Loss—Partial-Thickness/Full-Thickness; Carbon Monoxide Poisoning; Smoke Inhalation

Although the incidence of burn injury is on the decline, more than 500,000 burns still occur in the United States annually. Half of these require hospitalization in one of the specialized burn centers across the country. Thirty-five percent of all burn injuries occur in children. Mortality has improved over the years because of Advanced Burn Life Support, regional burn care, and early excision; overall mortality is around 6%. The most common mechanism of injury is thermal, which can be from a flame, scald, or direct contact, but injuries also present because of chemical, electrical, and radiation sources. The pediatric and geriatric populations are most vulnerable because of integumentary and immunological risks. Burn care ranges from major to minor, and care ranges from the emergent through the rehabilitative phase of injury.

NANDA-I NDx Impaired Skin Integrity

Common Related Factors

Major burn
Minor burn

Defining Characteristics

Blanching of skin
Redness
Leathery appearance
Skin color changes: brown to black
Blistering, weeping skin
Pain or absence of pain
Skin loss

Common Expected Outcomes

Patient receives appropriate wound care for degree of burn.
Patient exhibits satisfactory wound healing at burn sites.
Unburned skin remains intact and free of infection.

NOC Outcomes

Tissue Integrity: Skin and Mucous Membranes;
    Wound Healing: Secondary Intention

NIC Interventions

Wound Care; Wound Irrigation

Ongoing Assessment

Actions/Interventions	Rationales
■ Assess the percentage of body surface burned. Use the Lund-Browder chart (age-appropriate body surface chart).	Assessment is commonly used to determine total body surface area (TBSA) involved. TBSA estimation should include only partial- and full-thickness injury, not superficial. For quick assessment, the "rule of nines" is commonly used to estimate the extent of burn. Another method is that the patient's palm represents 1% TBSA, which is a helpful measuring tool when burns are scattered. Accurate calculation of TBSA is critical in determining fluid replacement therapy.
■ Identify and document the location of burns.	Treatment is determined by TBSA involved and location of burn.
■ Assess the depth of the wounds: • Epidermal/superficial: painful, pink, not blistered • Partial-thickness: painful, red/pink, often blistered • Full-thickness: anesthetic (not painful because of destruction of nerves), charred, gray, white	The deeper the wound, the greater the risk for infection, complications, and wound contractures.
■ Note areas where the skin is intact.	These areas must be cared for and preserved; they may serve as graft donor sites later.
■ Assess the degree of pain.	Full-thickness burns are anesthetic (painless) as a result of nerve destruction. Partial-thickness burns can cause severe pain because of exposed nerve endings. The patient may have deeper pain sensations from muscle ischemia.
■ Assess for adherent debris or hair.	Wound debris and any remaining surface hair can be sources of contamination. Epithelial migration in the healing wound is delayed if the wound is not clear of devitalized tissue.

Therapeutic Interventions

Actions/Interventions	Rationales
Major burns: ■ Provide a clean sheet.	The burn wound is not a sterile wound, so a sterile field is not required.
▲ Clean the burn wound with antimicrobial soap and water.	The wound must be cleansed with antibacterial soap to remove nonviable skin and rinsed thoroughly with water after cleansing to remove soap. This reduces risk for infection.
▲ Use hydrotherapy as prescribed.	Hydrotherapy aids in cleansing and loosening slough, exudate, and eschar. Wound debridement is necessary to provide a clean area for healing. A shower cart is often used to assist with this procedure.
▲ Apply topical bacteriostatic substances (e.g., silver sulfadiazine if the patient is not allergic to sulfa, bacitracin, Neosporin, silver-coated dressings, Sulfamylon), as ordered.	Topicals may be applied directly to the wound or impregnated into the bandage. These substances prevent removal of granulating skin and reduce the risk for infection. Topical agents provide some protection to the wound surface. This is a closed method that provides comfort and prevents wound desiccation. If an open method of wound care is used, the area is left open to air after ointment application. The risk with this method is increased heat loss.
■ Elevate extremities, if possible.	Elevation reduces swelling.
■ Dress wounds.	Dressings prevent burn-to-burn contact. The closed method of wound care uses gauze dressings to cover burn surfaces. The dressings may be soaked with antimicrobial solutions.

Actions/Interventions	Rationales
■ Keep body and limbs in correct anatomical position.	Correct positioning prevents contractures.
▲ Administer analgesics before wound care, debridement, or dressing changes.	Patient comfort and cooperation with wound care are promoted with administration of analgesics. Patients must have procedural, background, and breakthrough pain medication.
▲ Treat facial wounds as ordered.	Facial burns may require an open or closed dressing depending on the depth of burn (more superficial burns may be left open to air). Use caution when wrapping over ears to minimize pressure. Place dry gauze in the ear to prevent accumulation of topical agents. Avoid placing undue pressure on ears; do not put a pillow under the head of a person with ear burns.
Minor burns:	
■ Clean the burn wound with antimicrobial soap and water.	This removes debris and reduces the risk for infection. The wound must be cleansed with antibacterial soap to remove nonviable skin and rinsed thoroughly with water after cleansing to remove soap. This reduces risk for infection.
▲ Apply topical bacteriostatic and antimicrobial medications as ordered. Cover the wound with dry, sterile dressing.	Topical applications prevent removal of granulating skin and reduce risk for infection.
▲ Treat blisters as ordered.	If blisters are located on an area that is not limiting mobility and not at risk for breaking, leave intact; otherwise, debride the wound because blister fluid can be an excellent medium for bacteria.
■ Instruct the patient and caregiver in necessary medical follow-up care.	Healing of burn wounds varies depending upon depth of burn. A partial-thickness burn takes 3 to 4 weeks for healing. Full-thickness burns require surgical intervention for healing. Scar maturation occurs during the rehabilitative phase, which is 1 year post injury in adults and 2 years post injury in children.
■ Teach the patient and caregiver about the appearance of a clean, noninfected burn wound. Any deviation from this should be reported to the health care provider.	Clean, noninfected burn wounds are pink and moist; produce clear yellow (serous) drainage; and are odor-free.

NANDA-I
NDx **Risk for Infection**

Common Risk Factors

Impaired skin integrity
Damage to respiratory mucosa
Presence of dead skin
Poor nutrition

Common Expected Outcome

Patient remains free of infection, as evidenced by normal temperature, normal white blood cell (WBC) count, and healing wounds.

NOC Outcomes
Risk Control; Risk Detection; Immune Status
NIC Interventions
Environmental Management; Surveillance; Infection Protection

■ = Independent   ▲ = Collaborative

Ongoing Assessment

Actions/Interventions	Rationales
■ Monitor temperature, and notify the physician if temperature exceeds 38.5° C (101.3° F).	Patients with burn injury are at increased risk for infection due to wounds and compromised immune function. Elevated temperature should arouse suspicion of infection.
▲ With each dressing change, monitor the wound for erythema surrounding the burn, change in exudate color or amount, or presence of odor from the dressing. Obtain a wound culture, and notify the physician if a change is noted.	The burn patient is at risk for infection. Appropriate topical and/or systemic agents can be customized after culture results are obtained.
▲ Monitor white blood count.	An increasing WBC indicates the body's efforts to combat pathogens. However, in older patients, infection can be present without an increased WBC count.
▲ On ventilated patients, elevate head of bed 30 degrees, provide oral care, and administer H_2 blockers and antacids, as ordered. Suction without the use of instilled saline.	More compromised patients requiring mechanical ventilation offer additional infection risks. The Centers for Disease Control and Prevention provide these guidelines for the prevention of nosocomial pneumonia.
■ Monitor endotracheal secretions, and obtain a bronchial alveolar lavage specimen if the patient is febrile.	This technique provides the optimal specimen for culture analysis.
▲ Monitor all invasive lines; use antimicrobial-coated catheters when appropriate. When catheters are removed, send the tips for culture if the patient is febrile.	Indwelling catheters represent a break in the body's normal first line of defense, are a source of infection and require meticulous care.
▲ Monitor the effectiveness of the topical agent by culturing the wound, as prescribed.	Vigilant monitoring helps reduce consequences of infection.

Therapeutic Interventions

Actions/Interventions	Rationales
■ Maintain aseptic technique in caring for wounds.	To prevent nosocomial contamination, the nurse should wear protective coverings when caring for the patient. Gowns, gloves, masks, shoe covers, and hair covers may be needed.
■ Trim or shave hair around the wound (except eyebrows, because this area never grows back).	Hair removal decreases contamination.
▲ Treat blisters as ordered.	Blisters are left intact if they are not impairing mobility and have little risk for breaking. Blister fluid acts as a natural barrier and facilitates healing. However, when a blister is broken, blister fluid is an excellent medium for bacterial growth.
▲ Apply topical agent (e.g., silver sulfadiazine, bacitracin, Neosporin, Sulfamylon, silver-coated dressing), as prescribed.	Topical agents provide some protection to the wound surface.
■ Implement isolation precautions if needed.	Strict isolation may be necessary to prevent infection in the immunocompromised burn patient. Staff may wear scrubs because they can be changed easily when they become soiled. Gowns, gloves, and masks should be worn. Methicillin-resistant *Staphylococcus aureus* (MRSA) surveillance screening should be performed upon admission for all patients and appropriate isolation instituted as needed.
▲ Administer intravenous (IV) antibiotics, which may be prescribed prophylactically but which should be specific to the cultured organism when identified.	IV antibiotics may be useful in treating systemic infection. However, wound infections, especially those near eschar, may be treated more easily with topical agents and debridement.
■ Provide frequent perineal care, using diversion catheters as needed.	A Foley catheter or a bowel management system (e.g., Zassi) may be required to divert fecal material for large body surface area burns. Contamination of wounds can lead to infection and impaired wound healing.

Actions/Interventions	Rationales
▲ Cover wounds with graft material or dressings as prescribed:	Covering burn wounds reduces fluid loss and protects the wound from invasion by bacteria. Early excision and grafting are desirable. Infection is the greatest threat to survival for the burned patient; covering wounds decreases the opportunity for contamination and therefore decreases risk for infection.
• Xenografts	Xenografts are temporary grafts and generally are skin from another species, typically porcine (pig) skin.
• Homograft	Homograft is skin from another human, typically cadaver skin or banked frozen skin. This temporary skin is used to provide coverage in preparation for autograft.
• Amnion	Amnion can be used as graft material for 48 hours per application.
• Synthetic dressings	Synthetic dressings are temporary dressings to cover wounds. Many products are available for use on partial-thickness burns or as temporary skin substitutes for full-thickness burns.
• Autograft	Healthy skin is taken from elsewhere on the patient's body; grafting is carried out in an operating room.
■ Before discharge, teach the patient or caregiver to monitor wound appearance and drainage.	A change in drainage color or amount may indicate infection. Patients need to be able to recognize important signs and changes in their condition so early treatment can be initiated.
■ Before discharge, teach the patient or caregiver to monitor body temperature.	Temperature greater than 38.5° C (101.5° F) may indicate infection.

Risk for Deficient Fluid Volume

Common Risk Factors

Inflammatory response to burn with protein and fluid shifts
Massive fluid shifting and circulating volume loss
Hemorrhage; stress ulcer (Curling's ulcer)
Extremes of age

Common Expected Outcomes

Patient maintains normal fluid volume, as evidenced by systolic blood pressure (BP) greater than or equal to 90 mm Hg (or patient's baseline), urine output greater than 30 mL/hr, and heart rate (HR) 60 to 100 beats/min.
Burn shock is prevented.

NOC Outcomes
Fluid Balance; Hydration; Electrolyte and Acid-Base Balance

NIC Interventions
Intravenous (IV) Insertion; Fluid/Electrolyte Management; Electrolyte Management: Hyperkalemia; Shock Prevention; Medication Administration

Integumentary Care Plans

■ = Independent   ▲ = Collaborative

Ongoing Assessment

Actions/Interventions	Rationales
■ Assess for signs and symptoms of fluid volume deficit.	Fluid shifts from the intravascular to extravascular space because of increased capillary permeability; the first 24 to 48 hours are most critical. Also, insensible loss from areas of lost skin are dramatically increased, adding to fluid volume deficit. NOTE: Restlessness, tachycardia, hypotension, thirst (thirst is a sensitive indicator of fluid deficit and hemoconcentration), pale and cool skin, oliguria (urine output less than 30 mL/hr, indicating inadequate renal perfusion), and hypoxia (as interstitial spaces fill with fluid, alveolar oxygen exchange is impaired) are common symptoms. Fluid volume deficit is directly proportional to the extent and depth of the burn injury.
▲ Monitor laboratory results for alteration in acid-base balance, catabolism (outpouring of potassium and nitrogen), and altered electrolyte levels.	Decreased tissue perfusion leads to a buildup of lactic acid and metabolic acidosis. Tissue destruction initially causes hyperkalemia. When capillary integrity is restored, excess potassium is eliminated and may lead to hypokalemia.
■ Monitor urine specific gravity every 4 hours.	Very concentrated urine (specific gravity greater than 1.020) indicates fluid volume deficit; a urine output of 30 to 50 mL/hr indicates adequate perfusion.
▲ Evaluate hemoglobin and hematocrit.	Elevated hemoglobin and hematocrit occur with fluid volume deficit and hemoconcentration.
■ Weigh the patient daily, taking care to use the same scale and bedding.	Changes in body weight may be better indicators of fluid balance than intake and output records.

Therapeutic Interventions

Actions/Interventions	Rationales
▲ Assist with IV and central line placements.	These IV lines are used for rapid fluid resuscitation to prevent circulatory collapse. Multiple large-bore lines or a central line may be required.
▲ Administer crystalloid solutions as prescribed.	Amount and rate are calculated on the basis of TBSA and depth of wound, using the Parkland formula. Over the first 24 hours according to the Parkland formula, give 4 mL of lactated Ringer's solution per percentage TBSA burn per kilogram body weight as follows: half in first 8 hours, one fourth in second 8 hours, and one fourth in third 8 hours. The Parkland formula is a resuscitation guideline. Patients may require more or less fluid based upon response to resuscitation. Patients with delayed presentation, dehydration, full-thickness injury and inhalation injury may require more fluid than the Parkland formula.
▲ Administer colloid solutions as prescribed.	As capillary permeability is decreased, colloid solutions may be used to restore and maintain vascular volume and correct sodium imbalances.
▲ Administer tube feeding.	Feedings minimize the potential for gastric bleeding and paralytic ileus, which can further add to fluid volume deficit.

Risk for Ineffective Breathing Pattern

Common Risk Factors

Burns to head and neck
Circumferential chest burns
Massive edema
Inhalation of smoke or heated air

Common Expected Outcome

Patient maintains an effective breathing pattern, as evidenced by relaxed breathing at normal rate and depth, absence of dyspnea, and normal arterial blood gases (ABGs).

NOC Outcome
Respiratory Status: Ventilation
NIC Interventions
Airway Management; Respiratory Monitoring

Ongoing Assessment

Actions/Interventions	Rationales
■ Assess for presence of burns to face and neck.	Facial burns may indicate that smoke inhalation and possible airway injury have occurred.
■ Assess for edema of the head, face, and neck.	As fluid shift begins to occur, the oral airway and trachea become constricted, decreasing the patient's ability to breathe.
■ Assess for history and evidence of smoke inhalation.	Inhalation injury usually occurs when the fire was in a closed space. It can lead to respiratory failure and/or carbon monoxide poisoning (see Risk for Poisoning: Carbon Monoxide, p. 941.
■ Assess respiratory rate, rhythm, and depth; assess breath sounds.	Respiratory rate and rhythm changes are early warning signs of impending respiratory difficulties. Crackles may be heard if fluid is accumulating from direct burn injury or as a result of fluid shifts associated with fluid resuscitation.
■ Assess for dyspnea, shortness of breath, use of accessory muscles, cough, and presence of cyanosis.	As moving air in and out of the lungs becomes more difficult, the breathing pattern alters to include use of accessory muscles to move the air. These manifestations suggest progressive hypoxia.
▲ Monitor ABGs.	The combined effect of airway edema and accumulation of interstitial fluid results in decreased alveolar ventilation. The patient may be hypoxemic (decreased Po_2) or have metabolic and/or respiratory acidosis.
▲ Use pulse oximetry to monitor oxygen saturation.	Pulse oximetry is a useful tool to detect changes in oxygenation. Oxygen saturation should be at 90% or greater.
■ Assess for changes in level of consciousness.	Restlessness, confusion and/or irritability can be early signs indicative of hypoxia. Lethargy and somnolence are late signs of hypoxia.
▲ Review chest x-ray study results.	Chest x-ray studies will reflect changing lung status.

Therapeutic Interventions

Actions/Interventions	Rationales
■ Raise head of bed, and maintain good body alignment.	This position promotes optimal diaphragmatic and lung excursion and chest expansion to facilitate breathing efforts.
▲ Maintain humidified oxygen delivery system.	Initially patients may receive 100% oxygen to maintain oxygen saturation. Humidity decreases viscosity of secretions.

■ = Independent ▲ = Collaborative

Integumentary Care Plans

Actions/Interventions

▲ Provide chest physical therapy if burns are not to the chest.
■ Encourage use of incentive spirometer.

▲ Be prepared for intubation and mechanical ventilation.

▲ Be prepared for escharotomy.

Rationales

Chest physical therapy loosens secretions caused by stasis.
Incentive spirometry promotes deep inspiration, which increases oxygenation and prevents alveolar collapse.
When edema is severe, an artificial airway may be the only means of ventilating the severely burned patient.
Burns of the chest may cause restriction and constriction that decreases chest expansion; escharotomy (cutting through or removing eschar) will be needed to alleviate constricted movement.

NANDA-I NDx

Risk for Ineffective Peripheral Tissue Perfusion

Common Risk Factors

Blockage of microcirculation
Blood loss
Compartment syndrome (edema restricting circulation)
Circumferential eschar

Common Expected Outcome

Patient maintains optimal tissue perfusion to extremities, as evidenced by strong palpable pulses, reduction in absence of pain, warm dry extremities, and normal sensation in extremity.

NOC Outcomes
Circulation Status; Tissue Perfusion: Peripheral
NIC Interventions
Circulatory Care; Vital Signs Monitoring

Ongoing Assessment

Actions/Interventions

■ Check pulses of all extremities; use Doppler if necessary. Notify physician immediately of noted alteration in perfusion.
■ Monitor BP and HR for abrupt changes.

■ Assess color and temperature of extremities.

■ Check for pain, numbness, or swelling of extremities.

Rationales

Weak, thready pulses may not be palpable. Also, feeling pulses through extremely edematous tissue or skin covered with eschar may be difficult.
Stable blood pressure is necessary to maintain adequate tissue perfusion. Abrupt drop in BP and change in HR can indicate decreased blood flow secondary to severe third spacing (movement of fluid into spaces normally without fluid), which impedes venous return.
Cool, discolored extremities indicate compromised tissue perfusion. This situation, if untreated, can result in limb loss.
Circumferential burns with eschar are most likely to cause altered tissue perfusion to extremities, because as fluid shift occurs and eschar cannot stretch, pressure is exerted on tissue, vessels, and nerves.

Therapeutic Interventions

Actions/Interventions

■ Maintain good alignment of extremities. Elevate extremities on pillows or in a specially made sling.
▲ Apply sequential compression device on nonburned extremities.

Rationales

Careful positioning allows adequate blood flow without compression on arteries, also reducing edema.
Compression devices improve venous return.

Actions/Interventions

■ Perform passive range of motion if needed.

▲ Prepare for and assist with fasciotomy or escharotomy to treat full thickness circumferential burns.

Rationales

Exercise reduces venous stasis and further circulatory compromise.

Escharotomy (incision through the burn crust) or fasciotomy (incision through eschar and fascia) are indicated when the circulation is compromised due to increased pressure in the burned limb. This procedure relieves compression of nerves or blood vessels.

Risk for Poisoning: Carbon Monoxide

Common Risk Factor

Smoke inhalation

Common Expected Outcome

Patient maintains normal oxygen and carboxyhemoglobin levels.

NOC Outcome
Respiratory Status: Gas Exchange
NIC Intervention
Oxygen Therapy

Ongoing Assessment

Actions/Interventions

■ Monitor for carbon monoxide poisoning in any burn patient.
▲ Measure carboxyhemoglobin levels on admission to the emergency department.

■ Monitor for dyspnea, headache, and confusion, which may accompany carbon monoxide poisoning.

Rationales

Poisoning is seen especially in patients with other signs and symptoms of smoke inhalation or facial burns.

Carbon monoxide has a high affinity for the hemoglobin molecule; when hemoglobin molecules are bound to carbon monoxide, they are not available to transport oxygen.

At low carboxyhemoglobin levels (less than 10%), the patient may be asymptomatic or complain of a headache. Dizziness, nausea, and syncope occur at carboxyhemoglobin levels above 20%. Seizures and coma develop in patients with carboxyhemoglobin levels above 40%.

Therapeutic Interventions

Actions/Interventions

▲ Administer 100% humidified oxygen. Anticipate administration of hyperbaric oxygen in some cases.

Rationales

The patient may require airway intubation and mechanical ventilation to support an effective airway and gas exchange. According to the American Burn Association's clinical practice guidelines, hyperbaric oxygen is indicated if carbon monoxide poisoning is the only injury, because increasing the delivery of 100% oxygen at increased pressure is theorized to reduce the half-life of carboxyhemoglobin.

Risk for Imbalanced Nutrition: Less Than Body Requirements

Common Risk Factors

Prolonged interference in ability to ingest or digest food
Increased basal metabolic rate
Loss of protein from dermal wounds

■ = Independent   ▲ = Collaborative

Common Expected Outcome

Patient maintains an adequate nutritional intake, as evidenced by stable weight.

NOC Outcomes
Nutritional Status: Biochemical Measures;
Nutritional Status: Food and Fluid Intake
NIC Interventions
Nutrition Therapy; Nutrition Monitoring

Ongoing Assessment

Actions/Interventions	Rationales
■ Obtain base weight; weigh daily if possible, using same scale and linens.	Such consistency facilitates accurate measurement and evaluation.
■ Measure fluid intake and output, including oral and intravenous intake.	Changes in fluid balance can be reflected in daily weight changes. All snacks, foods from home, and items that are liquid at room temperature (gelatin, sherbet) should be included as oral intake.
■ Closely monitor caloric intake.	Patients with major burns may require 40% to 100% increase in calorie intake to keep up with hypermetabolic state and wound protein loss.
▲ Monitor skin test results for cellular immunity.	Anergic patients (those unable to muster a cellular immune response) are seriously nutritionally depleted.
▲ Monitor serum albumin levels.	Serum albumin gives an indication of protein reserve. Levels less than 2.5 g/dL indicate serious protein depletion and are linked to morbidity and mortality.
■ Check for bowel sounds, and monitor residuals of enteral feeding.	Early enteral feeding may be started upon admission to prevent paralytic ileus.
▲ Monitor nitrogen balance.	If nitrogen output is greater than nitrogen intake, the patient will become nutritionally depleted.
■ Determine environmental or situational factors (pain, odors, unpleasant sounds) that may affect eating.	These factors can diminish appetite.

Therapeutic Interventions

Actions/Interventions	Rationales
▲ Consult a dietitian to assist in meeting nutritional needs.	Dieticians have a greater expertise in calculating caloric needs. The Curreri formula is used to calculate the caloric needs for the burn patient to support homeostasis and wound healing: (25 kcal × Usual body weight [in kg]) + (40 kcal × %TBSA) = Calories. The patient may need 1.5 to 3 g/kg/day of protein to maintain nitrogen balance.
▲ Provide nutritional supplementation and replacement as needed.	Multivitamins, zinc, vitamin C, phosphorus, magnesium, and calcium are often provided daily or as needed based on laboratory results. Such supplements can be used to optimize balanced nutritional intake.
■ Plan dressing changes or other unpleasant situations away from mealtime.	Comfort enhances interest in eating.
■ Involve the patient in selection of menu to the extent possible.	Involving patients in their own nutritional care has been found to raise intake of protein and energy levels.
▲ Administer tube feeding as ordered.	The gastrointestinal tract is the most efficacious route for absorption and use of nutrients. Feedings may be continuous or intermittent.

Acute Pain

Common Related Factor

Burn injury

Defining Characteristics

Reports of pain
Increased restlessness
Alterations in sleep pattern
Irritability
Facial mask of pain
Guarding behavior, protecting body part
Self-focused
Narrowed focus
Autonomic responses (change in BP, HR, RR)

Common Expected Outcomes

Patient reports satisfactory pain control at a level less than 3 to 4 on a 0 to 10 rating scale.
Patient uses pharmacological and nonpharmacological pain relief strategies.
Patient exhibits increased comfort such as relaxed muscle tone and baseline levels for pulse, BP, and respirations.

NOC Outcomes

Comfort Status; Medication Response; Pain Control

NIC Interventions

Analgesic Administration; Pain Management; Simple Relaxation Therapy; Patient-Controlled Analgesia; Distraction

Ongoing Assessment

Actions/Interventions	Rationales
■ Assess type, location, quality, and severity of pain/discomfort.	The pain experience varies with extent of the burn injury. As wound healing begins, patient may complain of pruritus. Relief of this discomfort is important because scratching can disrupt fragile new skin or grafts.
■ Assess factors that may contribute to an increased perception of pain (e.g., anxiety, fear).	Knowing different etiological factors can guide effective therapies.
■ Monitor HR, BP, restlessness, and ability to focus.	Increasing pain can cause transient increases in respiratory and cardiac rates and blood pressure. Attention to associated signs may help the nurse in evaluating pain.
■ Evaluate and document effectiveness of chosen pain control methods.	Changing effectiveness of pain treatments is expected. Partial-thickness burns are very painful; pain will decrease over time and with healing. Full-thickness burns do not cause pain because of nerve destruction, but as nerves regenerate, pain will increase.

Therapeutic Interventions

Actions/Interventions	Rationales
▲ Administer sedatives and analgesics prescribed for pain.	Intravenous morphine is the drug of choice. Adjuvant drugs such as psychotropics may be added.
■ Provide background, procedural, and breakthrough pain control.	Burn patients have pain all the time, so they require three types of control.
▲ Consider use of patient-controlled analgesia.	This method of analgesic administration allows the patient to manage pain relief within prescribed limits and increases the patient's sense of control over pain.
■ Avoid pressure on injured tissues; use a bed cradle.	Bed cradle keeps linen off the legs.

■ = Independent ▲ = Collaborative

Actions/Interventions

- Alleviate all unnecessary stressors or sources of discomfort.
- Allay fears and anxiety.
- Turn the patient; obtain a pressure-relieving mattress or bed, as needed.
- ▲ Premedicate the patient for dressing changes; allow sufficient time for the medication to take effect.
- Moisten dressing with water to allow for trauma-free removal of dressing.
- Use distraction and relaxation techniques as indicated.

Rationales

A quiet, relaxed environment aids in promoting comfort.
Fear may intensify perception of pain.
These interventions help relieve pressure points and improve circulation to painful areas.
Manipulation of burn surfaces increases the patient's pain.

This technique eases dressing removal by loosening adherents and decreasing pain.
These complementary therapies can be effective. Distraction heightens one's concentration upon nonpainful stimuli to reduce awareness and experience of pain. Relaxation techniques bring about a state of physical and mental awareness and tranquility.

NANDA-I NDx Deficient Knowledge

Common Related Factors
Unfamiliarity with follow-up care
Need for long-term rehabilitation, follow-up care

Defining Characteristics
Questions to health care team
Verbalized misconceptions
Potential for failure to continue needed care or treatment

Common Expected Outcome
Patient or caregiver verbalizes understanding and ability to care for wound, mobilize resources, get follow-up care, and report signs of complication.

NOC Outcomes
Knowledge: Treatment Regimen; Coping; Family Participation in Professional Care

NIC Interventions
Discharge Planning; Support System Enhancement; Teaching: Disease Process; Teaching: Prescribed Activity/ Exercise; Teaching: Psychomotor Skill

Ongoing Assessment

Actions/Interventions

- Assess the need for ongoing wound or graft site care.

- Assess the need for continued rehabilitation (occupational therapy [OT], physical therapy [PT], psychosocial support).

- Assess the patient's perceived ability to care for self after discharge.

- Assess resources (environmental and human) in the home that can be tapped for assistance.

Rationales

Grafted skin is delicate and at continued risk for breakdown and infection. Patients must have a comprehensive understanding of the physical care required after discharge.
A variety of factors (e.g., inability to cope with body image changes; guilt about the injury, or the cause of fire or accident; need for further reconstructive surgery; use of scar prevention garments) may require care for months beyond hospital discharge.
Patients will be responsible for evaluating their condition on a daily basis to make determinations about preventive strategies and therapeutic interventions. This information may give some perspective on home care needs.
Although family and friends can be great allies, they sometimes may have trouble dealing with the complexities of long-term follow-up.

Therapeutic Interventions

Actions/Interventions	Rationales
▲ Involve a social worker or case manager early in the course of hospitalization.	Discharge planning may be a complicated process requiring a long period of planning.
■ Instruct the patient or caregiver in wound care of graft sites and donor sites: continue to use aseptic technique until the wound is completely healed; cover open wounds with gauze; keep wounds clean and moisturized with a lanolin-based cream; avoid sun exposure of newly grafted skin.	Careful wound care is essential because infection and contractures can occur during the rehabilitative phase of burn recovery.
■ Instruct the patient in care and use of scar-prevention garments, which are usually worn at all times (removed for bathing and wound care) up to 18 months after injury.	These may need to be replaced often to maintain elasticity sufficient for their purpose. The use of pressure garments and dressings can control development of hypertrophic scarring.
■ Instruct the patient or caregiver to report any of the following: signs or symptoms of wound infection (redness, swelling, pain, unusual drainage); limitation of movement, which can result from delayed contracture formation; inability to cope with disfigurement, role change.	Early identification of signs of infection or contractures facilitates needed treatment. Difficulty adjusting to home and loss after a burn injury is common. Additional support with coping will be necessary with integration back into society during the rehabilitative phase.
■ Instruct patient in pruritus, which is commonly present during the rehabilitative phase.	Patients can manage pruritus better if they are educated. Antihistamines, increased lotion, and oatmeal baths may help alleviate symptoms. Patients should avoid caffeine, nicotine, and chocolate because they can increases pruritus.
■ Encourage the patient or caregiver to maintain a follow-up schedule with the physician, registered nurse, PT, and OT, as well as social services.	Patients who become comanagers of their care have a greater stake in achieving a positive outcome.

NANDA-I NDx Disturbed Body Image

Common Related Factors

Massive edema
Visible burns
Dressings
Loss of function secondary to burns or burn treatment
Scarring or contractures
Loss of normal skin color
Use of scar-prevention garments

Defining Characteristics

Refusal to look at or care for altered body part
Verbal identification of feeling about altered structure or function of body part
Refusal to discuss change
Focusing behavior on changed body part

Common Expected Outcome

Patient demonstrates enhanced body image, as evidenced by ability to verbalize feelings, participate in self-care, and reintegrate into activities of daily living (ADLs) as capable.

NOC Outcomes

Body Image; Social Involvement; Social Support

NIC Interventions

Grief Work Facilitation; Body Image Enhancement; Coping Enhancement; Active Listening; Presence

■ = Independent   ▲ = Collaborative

Ongoing Assessment

Actions/Interventions	Rationales
■ Note the patient's ability to look at burns or dressings and his or her reactions to them.	Denial, looking away, or refusing to participate may indicate body image disturbance or may represent a normal stage of the grieving process.
■ Note the frequency and tone of critical remarks directed toward self regarding appearance and/or function.	The extent or severity of response is highly related to value placed on a body part or function affected. Negative statements about the affected body part indicate limited ability to integrate the change into the patient's self-concept.
■ Assess the perceived impact of actual change on ADLs, social behavior, personal relationships, and/or occupational activities.	This may give some perspective on any perceived misconceptions that could affect recovery.

Therapeutic Interventions

Actions/Interventions	Rationales
■ Demonstrate positive caring in routine activities.	Professional caregivers are a "testing ground" for societal reaction to appearance; a supportive relationship facilitates coping with body image disturbance.
■ Acknowledge the normalcy of the patient's emotional response to the actual or perceived change in body structure or function.	Experiencing stages of grief over change/loss of a body part or function is normal. The length of time varies between individuals.
■ Encourage verbalization of feelings about changed body.	It is worthwhile to encourage the patient to separate feelings about changes in body from feelings of self-worth. Expression of feelings can enhance the person's coping strategies.
■ Help the patient identify actual changes.	Patients may perceive changes that are not actually present. Scar maturation may take up to 2 years. Skin appearance may continue to improve during that time.
■ Assist the patient in identifying frightening or worrisome potential situations; role-play responses.	This technique gives the patient "practice" in responding to staring, questions, unwanted sympathy, and thoughtless behaviors that he or she may encounter.
■ Encourage attendance at a support group.	Participation in support groups may allow the patient to realize that others have the same problem and that he or she may use this as a means to find suggestions for specific care challenges.

Related Care Plans

Deficient fluid volume, p. 72
Gastrointestinal bleeding, p. 589
Ineffective coping, p. 49

Pressure Ulcers (Impaired Skin Integrity)

Pressure Sores; Decubitus Ulcers; Bedsores

Pressure ulcers are a major health problem. Nurses play a key role in prevention and successful treatment. The National Pressure Ulcer Advisory Panel (NPUAP) redefined pressure ulcer as "a localized injury to the skin and/or underlying tissue usually over a bony prominence, as a result of pressure or pressure in combination with shear and/or friction." Prolonged pressure occurs when tissue is between a bony prominence and a hard surface such as a mattress. The pressure compresses small blood vessels and leads to ineffective tissue perfusion. Loss of perfusion causes tissue hypoxia and eventually cellular death. In addition to prolonged pressure, friction and shearing force contribute to the development of pressure ulcers. These forces are present when a patient slides down in bed and is pulled up against the surface of the mattress. Pressure ulcers are usually staged to classify the degree of tissue damage observed.* Pressure ulcers stage I through III can heal with aggressive local wound treatment and proper nutritional support; stage IV pressure ulcers often require surgical intervention (e.g., flap closure, plastic surgery). Pressure ulcers affect persons, regardless of age, who are immobile, are malnourished, or have contributing conditions (e.g., incontinence, decreased level of consciousness). Wound care remains a challenge for nurses and the health care team. More research in wound healing is needed. This care plan is based on recommendations from the NPUAP, the National Guideline Clearinghouse, and the Agency for Healthcare Research and Quality (AHRQ) Pressure Ulcer Prevention Guidelines. This care plan addresses care issues in hospital, long-term care, or home settings.

*Panel for the Treatment of Pressure Ulcers. (1994). *Treatment of pressure ulcers: Clinical practice guideline, No. 15* (AHCPR Pub No. 95-0652). Rockville, MD: Agency for Health Care Policy and Research, Public Health Service, U.S. Department of Health and Human Services.

Impaired Skin Integrity

Common Related Factors

Extremes of age
Immobility
Imbalanced nutritional state
Mechanical factors (friction, shear, pressure)
Pronounced bony prominences
Impaired circulation
Impaired sensation
Incontinence
Moisture
Radiation
Hyperthermia or hypothermia
Chronic disease state
Immunological deficit
Impaired cognition

Defining Characteristics

Destruction of skin layers
Disruption of skin surfaces
Invasion of body structures
Pressure ulcer stages
- Deep tissue injury (new stage):
  - Purple or maroon localized area of intact skin or blood-filled blister due to pressure damage of underlying soft tissue
- Stage I:
  - Epidermis intact
  - Nonblanchable redness of a localized area usually over a bony prominence; area may be painful, firm, soft, warmer or cooler than adjacent tissue
- Stage II:
  - Partial-thickness skin loss of dermis
  - Shallow, open ulcer with a red-pink wound but without slough; may have an intact or open/ruptured serum-filled blister
- Stage III:
  - Full-thickness tissue loss
  - Subcutaneous fat may be visible
  - Bone, tendon, or muscle is not exposed
  - Slough may be present; may include undermining and tunneling
- Stage IV:
  - Full-thickness tissue loss with exposed muscle, bone, joint, and/or body cavity
  - Usually has adherent necrotic material (slough)
  - Undermining and tunneling may develop
- Unstageable:
  - Full-thickness tissue loss in which actual depth of ulcer is completely obstructed by slough and/or eschar in the wound bed

■ = Independent   ▲ = Collaborative

Common Expected Outcomes

Patient receives stage-appropriate wound care, experiences pressure reduction, and has controlled risk factors for prevention of additional ulcers.

Patient experiences healing of pressure ulcers.

NOC Outcomes

Wound Healing: Secondary Intention; Tissue Integrity: Skin and Mucous Membranes

NIC Interventions

Pressure Ulcer Prevention; Pressure Ulcer Care; Positioning; Pressure Management

Ongoing Assessment

Actions/Interventions	Rationales
■ Use objective tool for pressure ulcer risk assessment: • Braden scale • Norton scale	These are validated tools for risk assessment. The Braden scale is the most widely used. It consists of six subscales: sensory perception, moisture, activity, mobility, nutrition, and friction/shear. *Acute care:* Assessment should be carried out on all patients on admission and every 24 to 48 hours or sooner if the patient's condition changes. *Long-term care:* Assess on admission, weekly for 4 weeks, then quarterly and whenever resident's condition changes (www.NPUAP.org).
■ Assess specific risk factors for pressure ulcers:	Even patients who already have a pressure ulcer continue to be at risk for further injury. Centers for Medicare and Medicaid Services (CMS) recommends that nurses consider all potential risk factors for pressure ulcers beyond those noted on standard tools.
• Determine the patient's age and general condition of the skin.	Skin of older patients is less elastic, has less padding and moisture, and has thinning of the epidermis, making for higher risk for skin impairment.
• Specifically assess skin over bony prominences (sacrum, trochanters, scapulae, elbows, heels, inner and outer malleolus, inner and outer knees, back of head).	These areas are at highest risk for breakdown due to tissue ischemia from compression against a hard surface.
• Assess the patient's awareness of the sensation of pressure.	Normally individuals shift their weight off pressure areas every few minutes; this occurs more or less automatically, even during sleep. Patients with decreased sensation are unaware of unpleasant stimuli (pressure) and do not shift weight, thereby exposing skin to excessive pressure.
• Assess the patient's ability to move (shift weight while sitting, turn over in bed, move from bed to chair).	Immobility is the major risk factor in skin breakdown.
• Assess the patient's nutritional status, including weight, weight loss, and serum albumin levels, if ordered.	Albumin level less than 2.5 g/dL is a grave sign, indicating severe protein depletion.
• Assess for history of radiation therapy.	Irradiated skin becomes thin and friable, may have less blood supply, and is at higher risk for breakdown.
• Assess for fecal and/or urinary incontinence.	The urea in urine turns into ammonia within minutes and is caustic to the skin. Stool may contain enzymes that cause skin breakdown. Diapers and incontinence pads with plastic liners trap moisture and hasten breakdown.
• Assess for environmental moisture (wound drainage, excessive perspiration, high humidity).	Moisture may contribute to skin maceration.
• Assess the surface that the patient spends a majority of time on (mattress for bedridden patient, cushion for persons in wheelchairs).	Patients who spend the majority of time on one surface need a pressure reduction or pressure relief device to lessen the risk for breakdown.

Actions/Interventions

- Assess the amount of shear (pressure exerted laterally) and friction (rubbing) on the patient's skin.

- Assess skin on admission and daily for increasing number of risk factors.
- Assess for history of preexisting chronic diseases (e.g., diabetes, malignancy, acquired immunodeficiency syndrome [AIDS], or peripheral and/or cardiovascular disease).
- ■ Assess and stage pressure ulcers (see Defining Characteristics on p. 947).

- ■ Measure the size of the ulcer, and note the presence of undermining.

- ■ Describe the condition of the wound or wound bed:
  - Color

  - Odor

  - Presence of necrotic tissue

  - Visibility of bone, muscle, or joints

- ■ Assess for wound exudate.

- ■ Assess the condition of wound edges and surrounding tissue.

- ■ Assess ulcer healing, using pressure ulcer scale for healing (PUSH) tool.

- ■ Assess pain level, especially related to dressing changes and procedures.

Rationales

Shearing forces are most commonly noted on the sacrum, scapulae, heels, and elbows from skin-sheet friction, from semi-Fowler's positioning and repositioning, and from lift sheets.

The incidence of skin breakdown is directly related to the number of risk factors present.

Patients with chronic diseases typically manifest multiple risk factors (see above) that predispose them to pressure ulceration. These include poor nutrition, poor hydration, incontinence, and immobility.

Staging is important because it determines the treatment plan. Staging should be assessed at each dressing stage. It reflects whether the epidermis, dermis, fat, muscle, bone, or joint is exposed. If the ulcer is covered with necrotic tissue (eschar), it cannot be accurately staged. Stage I ulcers are difficult to detect in darkly pigmented skin. Use of mirrors/penlight may be helpful.

The ulcer dimensions include length, width, and depth. An ulcer begins in the deepest tissue layers before the skin breaks down. Therefore the opening of the skin's surface may not represent the true size of the ulcer.

Color of tissue is an indication of tissue viability and oxygenation. White, gray, or yellow eschar may be present in stage II and III ulcers. Eschar may be black in stage IV ulcers.

Odor may arise from infection present in the wound; it may also arise from necrotic tissue. Some local wound care products may create or intensify odors and should be distinguished from wound or exudate odors.

Necrotic tissue is tissue that is dead and eventually must be removed before healing can take place. Necrotic tissue exhibits a wide range of appearances: thin, white, shiny, brown, tough, leathery, black, hard.

In stage IV pressure ulcers, these may be apparent at the base of the ulcer. Wounds may demonstrate multiple stages or characteristics in a single wound (i.e., healthy tissue with granulation may be present along with necrotic tissue).

Exudate is a normal part of wound physiology and must be differentiated from pus, which is an indication of infection. Exudate may contain serum, blood, and white blood cells and may appear clear, cloudy, or blood-tinged. The amount may vary from a few cubic centimeters, which are easily managed with dressings, to copious amounts not easily managed. Drainage is considered "excessive" when dressing changes are needed more often than every 6 hours.

Surrounding tissue may be healthy or may have various degrees of impairment. Healthy tissue is necessary for use of local wound care products requiring adhesion to the skin. Presence of healthy tissue demarcates the boundaries of the pressure ulcer.

This tool provides standardization in measurement of wound healing. It quantifies surface area, exudate, and type of wound tissue. It is located at the National Pressure Ulcer Advisory Panel website (www.NPUAP.org).

The Joint Commission mandates frequent and regular assessment of pain. Prophylactic medications may be indicated.

■ = Independent   ▲ = Collaborative

Therapeutic Interventions

Actions/Interventions	Rationales
■ Change the patient's position frequently: bed-bound persons every 2 hours and chair-bound every hour.	Position changes relieve pressure, restore blood flow, and promote skin integrity.
■ Use pressure-redistributing beds, mattress overlays, and chair cushions.	These devices redistribute pressure when frequent position changes are not possible. Avoid using doughnut type of devices and sheepskin for accomplishing redistribution goals.
▲ Clean ulcer with a nontoxic solution such as normal saline (0.9%).	Cleansing the ulcer removes debris and bacteria, which promotes healing.
▲ Provide local wound care as follows: *Stage I*	The goal is to prevent further damage and shearing away of the epidermis.
• Apply a flexible hydrocolloid dressing (e.g., DuoDerm, Sween-A-Peel) or a vapor-permeable membrane dressing (e.g., OpSite, Tegaderm).	These dressings prevent friction and shear.
• Apply vitamin-enriched emollient to skin every shift.	Emollient moisturizes skin.
• Apply topical vasodilator (e.g., Proderm, Granulex). *Stage II*	A topical vasodilator increases circulation to skin. The goal is to prevent further damage and shearing away of the epidermis. A moist environment can aid wound healing.
• Hydrogels (Aqua Skin, Carrasyn V)	Hydrogels are used for shallow ulcers without exudates and promote wound debridement and healing.
• Hydrocolloids or vapor-permeable membrane dressing	Hydrocolloids promote wound debridement and healing. Do not use with heavy exudate–producing wounds.
• Alginates (Kalginate, Kaltostat, Sorbsan)	Alginates are used for ulcers with exudates or moderate drainage. Avoid in both dry and heavily bleeding ulcers. They can be used in Stage II to IV ulcers.
• Gauze with sodium chloride solution	This maintains a moist environment but requires multiple dressing changes. Dressings must be removed *while still wet.* Dressings absorb small amounts of drainage.
Stage III and IV • Consult a plastic surgeon to perform sharp debridement (surgical removal of eschar)	This surgical procedure removes any necrotic thick eschar to promote future healing.
• Gauze with sodium chloride solution	This maintains a moist environment but requires multiple dressing changes as described for stage II.
• Foams	Foams reduce odor and repel bacteria and water. They can be used with moderate to heavy drainage. They may macerate surrounding skin.
• Wound fillers	Wound fillers are used in conjunction with other dressings. They absorb exudates, fill the wound, and cause autolytic debridement.
• Debridement	Debridement is an important step in overall management of ulcers. See Other therapies below.
• Negative pressure wound therapy	See Other therapies below.
• Palliative wound care *Other therapies* • Sharp debridement	See Other therapies below. Sharp debridement uses a scalpel or laser to remove devitalized tissue. It is very effective, especially when cellulitis or sepsis is involved.
• Mechanical debridement	Mechanical debridement uses a physical method for removing necrotic tissue, such as wet-to-dry gauze, which adheres to tissue and is later removed. Unfortunately, often healthy granulation tissue is also removed.

Actions/Interventions	Rationales
• Autolytic debridement	Autolytic debridement uses enzymes already present in the wound to dissolve the necrotic tissue, usually with a hydrocolloid or hydrogel.
• Enzymatic debridement (collagenase, chlorophyll, papain)	Enzymatic debridement uses proteolytic enzymes to remove necrotic tissues. These agents work by selectively digesting the collagen portion of the necrotic tissue. Care should be taken to prevent damage to surrounding healthy tissues.
• Biosurgery	Biosurgery uses maggots for quick debridement.
• Negative pressure wound therapy	Negative pressure wound therapy involves a device for draining stage III and IV wounds that would require frequent dressing changes. It decompresses the interstitial fluid in the wound, thus improving blood flow, promoting granulation tissue, and increasing fibroblasts. There is growing evidence of its benefits.
• Topical growth factors	Colony-stimulating factors, fibroblast growth factors, and nerve growth factors are currently under study for pressure ulcers, though they have been found to be effective in diabetic and venous ulcers.
• Electrical stimulation	Stimulation of many cellular processes enhances healing.
• Palliative wound care	Palliative wound care may be an option for a patient with a chronic, nonhealing wound. These wounds occur in patients with preexisting debilitating disease. This option requires a comprehensive history as well as evaluation of the patient's goals for comfort and independence. Goals include control of symptoms, control of caregiver strain, and reduction of stress in the patient and family. Education must be conveyed that while the wound is nonhealing and remains open indefinitely, it can remain stable. These cases may require referral to a wound specialist.

NANDA-I NDx   Risk for Infection

Common Risk Factors

Open pressure ulcer
Poor nutritional status
Proximity of sacral wounds to perineum

Common Expected Outcomes

Patient remains free of local or systemic infection, as evidenced by absence of copious, foul-smelling wound exudate.
Patient maintains normal body temperature.

NOC Outcomes
Infection Status; Nutritional Status: Food and Fluid Intake
NIC Interventions
Infection Protection; Wound Care; Nutrition Management

■ = Independent   ▲ = Collaborative

Ongoing Assessment

Actions/Interventions	Rationales
■ Assess pressure ulcers for drainage, color of tissue, and odor.	All wounds produce exudate; the presence of exudate that is clear-to-straw-colored is normal. Purulent green or yellow drainage in large amounts typically indicates an infection, as does foul-smelling drainage. Infected tissue usually has a gray-yellow appearance without evidence of pink granulation tissue.
▲ Obtain wound cultures, if available.	All pressure ulcers are colonized (i.e., will culture out bacteria) because skin normally has flora that will be found in an open skin lesion; however, all pressure ulcers are not infected. Infection is present when there is copious, foul-smelling, purulent drainage and the patient has other symptoms of infection (fever, increased pain) and a bacteria count greater than 10^5. Swab cultures are not recommended. Rather, tissue biopsy should be used to quantify and qualify the aerobic and anaerobic organisms present.
■ Assess the patient for unexplained sepsis.	When septic workup is done, the pressure ulcer must be considered a possible cause.
■ Assess nutritional status.	Patients who are seriously nutritionally depleted (e.g., serum albumin less than 2.5 mg/dL) are at risk for developing infection produced by a pressure ulcer. In addition, patients with pressure ulcers lose tremendous amounts of protein in wound exudate and may require 4000 kcal/day or more to remain anabolic.
■ Assess for urinary and/or fecal incontinence.	Sacral wounds, because of their proximity to the perineum, are at highest risk for infection caused by urine and/or fecal contamination. It is sometimes difficult to isolate the wound from the perineal area.
■ Monitor temperature.	Fever may indicate infection, unless the patient is immunocompromised or diabetic.
▲ Monitor white blood cell (WBC) count.	Elevated WBC count may indicate infection, although in very old individuals, WBC count may rise only slightly during an infection, indicating a diminished marrow reserve.

Therapeutic Interventions

Actions/Interventions	Rationales
▲ Provide local wound care as prescribed (see pp. 950).	The type and level of wound treatment depends on the staging of the ulcer and the type of infection present.
■ Provide thorough perineal hygiene after each episode of incontinence.	This minimizes pathogens in the area of sacral pressure ulcers.
▲ Consult the dietitian for assistance with a high-calorie, high-protein diet.	These patients, because of their overall condition, often require enteral or parenteral nutrition to meet nutritional needs.
▲ Administer antibiotics as prescribed.	Complicated wounds may develop cellulitis or sepsis, requiring antibiotic therapy. Oral antibiotics or topical silver sulfadiazine can be effective.
▲ Provide hydrotherapy if available.	Hydrotherapy is needed to achieve wound cleansing and to promote circulation.

Risk for Ineffective Health Maintenance

Common Risk Factors

Need for long-term pressure ulcer management
Lack of previous similar experience
Possible need for special equipment
Impaired functional status

Common Expected Outcome

Patient and caregiver verbalize understanding of the following aspects of home care: pressure relief, wound care, nutrition, and incontinence management.

NOC Outcomes
Knowledge: Treatment Regimen; Decision Making; Coping; Family Functioning

NIC Interventions
Discharge Planning; Family Support; Decision-Making Support; Teaching: Prescribed Activity/Exercise; Teaching: Prescribed Diet

Ongoing Assessment

Actions/Interventions	Rationales
■ Assess the patient's and caregiver's understanding of the long-term nature of wound healing of pressure ulcers and palliative wound care.	Pressure ulcers may take weeks to months to heal, even under ideal circumstances. Wounds heal from the base of the ulcer up, and from the edges of the ulcer toward the center. Palliative wound care may be appropriate for clean, chronic, nonhealing wounds.
■ Assess the patient's and caregiver's knowledge of and ability to provide local wound care.	Patients are no longer kept hospitalized until pressure ulcers have healed. The need for local wound care may continue for weeks to months.
■ Assess for the availability of pressure reduction or pressure-relief surface.	Patients may take thick, dense foam mattresses home from the hospital to place on their own bed. Rental provision of low–air-loss beds (e.g., Flexicare, KinAir) and air-fluidized therapy beds (e.g., Clinitron, Skytron, FluidAir) may be arranged but often pose financial difficulty because few payer sources will cover the cost of these beds in the home.
■ Assess understanding of and ability to provide high-calorie, high-protein diet throughout the course of wound healing.	Patients may require enteral feeding (through gastronomy tube, nasogastric feeding tubes, or the oral route), which requires knowledge of preparation and use of special equipment (e.g., feeding pumps and administration sets).
■ Assess the patient's and caregiver's understanding of the relationship between incontinence and further skin breakdown or complications of healing.	Managing incontinence may be the most difficult aspect of home management and is often the reason decisions for nursing home placement are made.
■ Assess the patient's and caregiver's understanding of the prevention of further pressure ulcer development.	Patients who are incapable of independent movement will need frequent repositioning to reduce risk for breakdown in those areas that are intact.

Therapeutic Interventions

Actions/Interventions	Rationales
■ Teach the patient and caregiver local wound care, and provide an opportunity for return demonstration.	This allows the learner to use new information immediately, thus enhancing retention. Immediate feedback allows the learner to make corrections, rather than practice the skill incorrectly.

■ = Independent　▲ = Collaborative

Actions/Interventions	Rationales
■ Teach the patient and caregiver to report the following signs indicating wound infection: purulent drainage, odor, fever, malaise.	Early assessment prompts early intervention.
■ Provide written instructions with listed resources.	Long-term management requires specific written plans to enhance adherence to treatment. Several Internet resources provide lay education.
▲ Involve a social worker or case manager.	Referral helps the patient and family determine whether placement in an extended care facility is needed. Because many patients with pressure ulcers are older, it is often an older spouse who is available to provide care; as a result of the intensive nursing care needs of these patients, discharge to home is often unrealistic.
■ Consider or discuss with the patient and caregiver the need for in-home nursing care or homemaker services.	These provide all or part of the patient's care and can be less costly to the patient. In addition, keeping the patient in his or her own environment (if possible) reduces the risk for nosocomial infection and keeps the patient in familiar surroundings.
■ Consider or discuss with the patient and caregiver the possible need for respite care.	Long-term responsibility for patient care in the home is taxing; those providing the care may need help to understand that their own needs for relaxation are essential to the maintenance of health and should not be viewed as "shirking responsibility."
■ Teach the patient and caregiver the importance of pressure reduction and relief: • Use of specialty surface; if provision of specialty beds is a problem because of reimbursement issues, a water bed may be a reasonable alternative • Use of pressure reduction and relief surface where the patient sits • Turning schedule that does not compromise other body areas	Information can foster enhanced adherence to pressure ulcer treatment guidelines.
▲ Consult a wound specialist to evaluate care in the home.	Besides evaluating ability to deliver care, the specialist may be useful in securing specialty equipment.
▲ Include a dietitian in teaching how to plan high-calorie, high-protein meals, or how to supplement regular meals with dietary supplements.	Specialty expertise may be required.
■ Teach the patient and caregiver how to manage incontinence: • Use of external catheters • Care of indwelling catheters if no other option is feasible • Use of underpads or linen protectors • Use of moisture barrier ointments	Teaching proper techniques can prevent leakage and skin problems. Reusable products such as underpads or linen protectors made of cloth with a waterproof lining are better for the patient's skin and are more economical but require laundering. Moisture barrier ointments protect intact skin from excoriation.

Related Care Plans

Caregiver role strain, p. 36
Enteral tube feeding, p. 584
Imbalanced nutrition: less than body requirements, p. 142
Plastic surgery for wound closure (see the **Evolve** website)

Psoriasis

Psoriasis is a noninfectious common inflammatory skin disorder that results in an overproduction of epidermal cells that are evident as red, dry, itchy patches of thickened skin that may be associated with silvery scales. Symptoms vary from person to person. Patches are usually found on the arms, legs, trunk, or scalp but can occur anywhere, most commonly on the knees or elbows and usually in a symmetrical, bilateral pattern. Though the specific cause is not known, it seems to be related to an immunological process in which T cells malfunction, causing increased production of both normal skin cells and T cells that compete for space. The newly formed cells are shunted to the outer layer of skin while the older cells have yet to be removed. These combinations result in accumulation of thick patches on the skin's surface. Specific triggers have been identified, including infections, stress, injury to the skin, smoking, and cold weather.

Psoriasis is a chronic disease for which most people experience recurrent periods of flare-ups and remissions. There is no cure, but for most individuals the symptoms are more of an inconvenience; however, the more severe cases can be disabling when associated with psoriatic arthritis. Treatment is geared to disrupting the overproduction of cells and removing the dry scales to smoothen the skin. Therapy consists of combinations of topical medications, light therapy, and a variety of oral medications. This care plan focuses on nursing care in the outpatient setting.

NANDA-I NDx Knowledge Deficit

Related Factors
New condition/treatment
Unfamiliarity with treatment regimen
Lack of recall

Defining Characteristics
Questioning health care team
Verbalized inaccurate information
Inaccurate follow-through of previous instructions

Common Expected Outcome
Patient verbalizes understanding of disease process, preventive care, and treatment plan.

NOC Outcomes
Knowledge: Disease Process; Knowledge: Medication; Knowledge: Treatment Regimen

NIC Interventions
Teaching: Disease Process; Teaching: Prescribed Medications

Ongoing Assessment

Actions/Interventions	Rationales
■ Assess the patient's level of knowledge of psoriasis and its treatment.	Patients will be responsible for evaluating their condition on a daily basis to make determinations about preventive strategies and therapeutic intervention.
■ Assess how long psoriasis has been a problem and any patterns of remission and exacerbation, as well as any associated factors.	Information provides data as to how the patient may have handled flare-ups in the past or whether he or she has engaged in preventive measures that were successful.

■ = Independent   ▲ = Collaborative

Therapeutic Interventions

Actions/Interventions	Rationales

Actions/Interventions

- Introduce or reinforce information about diagnosis, disease process, chronicity of skin disease, symptoms, remissions, and exacerbations:
  - Diagnosed by presentation of typical skin patches (plaque psoriasis) such as red, raised patches with silvery scales or peeling; can be itchy. Plaques tend to appear bilaterally on the same area of the body.
  - Chronic condition with periods of exacerbation then remission. For some this condition can be disabling. May develop psoriatic arthritis causing joint pain/stiffness.
- Provide information about preventive home care strategies:
  - Maintain moisturized skin.
  - Soak in bathwater with oil or bath salts to moisturize skin, remove scales, and reduce inflammation.
  - Bath with coal tar or similar agents to remove scales.
  - Avoid irritating cosmetics and soaps.
  - Consider light therapy such as daily exposure of skin to natural sunlight (helps many but may exacerbate condition in others).
  - Avoid exposure to triggers such as:
    - Stress, smoking, infections, local injury to skin, intense sun exposure
- Provide information about common medical treatments:
  Topical agents
  - Corticosteroids—antiinflammatory medications that slow cell turnover
  - Coal tar—reduces itching and slows production of excess skin cells; this is probably the oldest treatment
  - Anthralin—tree bark extract found to be very effective; it acts by normalizing DNA activity in skin cells
  - Retinoids—normalize DNA activity, reduce redness of skin and size of patches
  - Vitamin D_3 (calcipotriene)—slows production of excess skin cells
  - General moisturizers—help reduce scaling and itching, though they do not heal psoriasis
  Systemic medications
  - Psoralens—drugs that make the skin more sensitive to light; must be combined with ultraviolet light therapy (PUVA) for effectiveness
  - Methotrexate— suppresses immune system and slows production of skin cells
  - Cyclosporine—suppresses immune system and slows production of skin cells
  - Biologics (immunomodulators); for example:
  - Alefacept—given as weekly injection to suppress immune system and slow production of skin cells
  - Etanercept—used for psoriatic arthritis to reduce inflammation
  Phototherapy
  - UVB ultraviolet light, which is usually combined with other medical therapies; newer narrow band UVB may be more effective
  - Psoralen plus ultraviolet A (PUVA)
  - Excimer laser—treats only the involved skin area

Rationales

Patients must have a comprehensive understanding of the disease to actively participate in their own care.

Many home measures can help reduce flare-ups, treat symptoms, and improve appearance of damaged skin.

The choice of which drug for one's condition depends on many factors. Guidelines recommend starting with the mildest treatments such as topical creams and light therapy. There is not one drug that will work most effectively for all patients. Patients often rotate medications or combine them as needed. Some medications such as the biologics are expensive, costing several thousand dollars per year.

Actions/Interventions

- Stress the importance of long-term follow-up.

- Encourage the patient to discuss new or over-the-counter treatments with health care workers.

- Suggest referral to an arthritis specialist for optimal treatment of psoriatic arthritis.

Rationales

Psoriasis is a chronic condition so far with no cure. Ongoing research may find better treatments and possible cure in the future.

The patient may be vulnerable to fads or advertisements claiming curative effects of high-dose vitamins, special health foods, or similar unproven therapies.

This practitioner may be in the best position to understand the nuances of an individual's disease and be aware of the latest treatment regimens.

Risk for Disturbed Body Image

Common Risk Factors

Visible skin plaques
Psoriatic arthritis with joint deformity

Common Expected Outcomes

Patient verbalizes enhanced adaptation to changes in appearance, as evidenced by ability to look at, talk about, and care for skin lesions.
Patient verbalizes ways to conceal skin plaques as required by personal preference.

NOC Outcome
Body Image
NIC Interventions
Body Image Enhancement; Coping Enhancement

Ongoing Assessment

Actions/Interventions

- Assess perception of changed appearance.

- Assess the patient's behavior related to appearance.

Rationales

Mild outbreaks of psoriasis may not affect one's appearance and resultant body image. However, more severe or chronic cases with flare-ups lasting weeks or months may significantly affect how patients view their appearance to others. The peeling and itching of the skin or the joint problems with related arthritis can be overwhelming for some, causing a preoccupation with their skin condition.

Patients with potential body image issues may reduce their socialization based on fear about reactions of others.

Therapeutic Interventions

Actions/Interventions

- Assist the patient in articulating responses to questions from others regarding skin plaques and infectious risk.

- Allow patients to verbalize feelings regarding their skin condition.
- Instruct the patient to avoid contact with harsh chemicals and triggers for psoriasis as well as to use materials such as moisturizers that can reduce scaling and further inflammation (see Knowledge Deficit above).

Rationales

Patients may need some guidance in determining what to say to people who comment about the appearance of their skin. Psoriasis is not a contagious skin condition.

Through talking, the patient can be guided to separate physical appearance from feelings of personal worth.

Patient needs to be aware of therapies to reduce symptoms.

■ = Independent   ▲ = Collaborative

Actions/Interventions

■ Assist the patient in identifying ways to enhance appearance.

■ Suggest referral to psoriasis support group.

Rationales

Clothing, cosmetics, and accessories may direct attention away from the skin lesions. Careful use of concealing clothing may help the patient who is having problems adjusting to body image changes.

Groups that come together for mutual goals can be supportive and often provide helpful information.

NANDA-I NDx Impaired Skin Integrity

Common Related Factor

Disease process

Defining Characteristics

Inflammation
Dry, scaly skin
Erosions, fissures
Pruritus, pain

Common Expected Outcome

Patient maintains optimal skin integrity within limits of the disease, as evidenced by intact skin.

NOC Outcomes
Knowledge: Treatment Regimen; Tissue Integrity: Skin and Mucous Membranes
NIC Interventions
Skin Care: Topical Treatments; Skin Surveillance

Ongoing Assessment

Actions/Interventions

■ Assess skin, noting areas affected by color changes, any raised areas with scaling and patches, along with any plaques.

■ Assess the skin systematically.

■ Identify signs of itching and scratching.

Rationales

Psoriasis has characteristic patterns of skin changes and lesions.

Patches are usually found on the arms, legs, trunk, or scalp but can occur anywhere. Knees and elbows are most common. Psoriasis has a characteristic bilateral component.

The patient who scratches the skin to relieve intense itching may cause open skin lesions with an increased risk for infection.

Therapeutic Interventions

Actions/Interventions

▲ Encourage the patient to adopt skin care routines to decrease skin irritation:
 • Bathe or shower using lukewarm water and bath salts or oils.

 • After bathing, allow the skin to air dry or gently pat the skin dry. Avoid rubbing or brisk drying.
 • Apply topical lubricants immediately after bathing.

Rationales

One of the first steps in the management of psoriasis is to prevent further drying of the skin.

Long bathing or showering in hot water causes drying of the skin and can aggravate itching through vasodilation. Bath oils and salts help moisturize the skin to reduce further cracking of plaque.

Rubbing the skin with a towel can irritate the skin and exacerbate the itch-scratch cycle.

Lubrication with fragrance-free creams or ointments serves as a barrier to prevent further drying of the skin through evaporation. Moisturizing is the cornerstone of treatment.

Actions/Interventions

▲ Apply topical steroid creams or ointments.

■ Encourage the patient to avoid aggravating factors: long sun exposure, smoking, stress.

Rationales

These drugs reduce inflammation and promote healing of the skin. These are discussed under Knowledge Deficit above. Some change in lifestyle may be indicated to reduce triggers.

Related Care Plan

Chronic pain, p. 155

Shingles

Herpes Zoster

After chickenpox infection, the varicella zoster virus (VZV) lays dormant in the ganglia of the spinal nerve tracts. Shingles is an infectious viral condition caused by a reactivation of this latent VZV. Reactivation usually occurs in individuals with impaired immunity; it is common among older adults. Approximately 20% of people who have had chickenpox will develop herpes zoster. VZV produces painful vesicular eruptions along the peripheral distribution of nerves from posterior ganglia and is usually unilateral and characteristically occurs in a linear distribution, abruptly stopping at the midline both posteriorly and anteriorly. Although VZV typically affects the trunk of the body, the virus may also be noted on the buttocks or face. With facial involvement there is concern about involvement of the eye and cornea, potentially resulting in permanent loss of vision. Secondary infection resulting from scratching the lesions is common. An individual with an outbreak of VZV is infectious for the first 2 to 3 days after eruption. The incubation period ranges from 7 to 21 days. The total course of the disease is 10 days to 5 weeks from onset to full recovery. Some individuals may experience painful postherpetic neuralgia long after the lesions heal. Shingles is characterized by burning, pain, and neuralgia. VZV infection can lead to central nervous system (CNS) involvement; pneumonia develops in about 15% of cases. This disease is routinely treated on an outpatient basis unless CNS involvement or pneumonia occurs. A herpes zoster vaccination is now available for older adults.

NANDA-I NDx **Risk for Infection**

Common Risk Factors

Skin lesions (papules, vesicles, pustules)
Crusted-over lesions
Itching and scratching

Common Expected Outcomes

Patient remains free of secondary infection, as evidenced by intact skin without redness or lesions.
Risk for disease transmission is minimized through use of universal precautions.

NOC Outcomes

Knowledge: Infection Control; Risk Control; Risk Detection; Tissue Integrity: Skin and Mucous Membranes

NIC Interventions

Infection Protection; Wound Care

■ = Independent   ▲ = Collaborative

Integumentary Care Plans

Ongoing Assessment

Actions/Interventions	Rationales
■ Assess for presence and location of skin lesions.	Lesions are fluid-filled, becoming yellow, and finally crusting over, on one side of the trunk or buttock. Lesions follow the path of dermatomes and occur in bandlike strips. Lesions may occur also on the face, arms, and legs if nerves for these areas are involved. As lesions rupture and crust, they take on the appearance of the lesions associated with chickenpox.
■ Assess for lesions around the eye or ear.	Particular attention needs to be given to assessing lesions near the eyes and ears because the virus may cause serious damage to the eyes and ears. This can cause blindness or hearing difficulties. To detect lesions on the cornea, the physician or nurse practitioner will stain the cornea in the office with fluorescein stain and view the typical lesions under a Wood's lamp.
■ Assess for pruritus or irritation from lesions, and amount of scratching. Assess for signs of localized infection: redness and drainage from lesions.	Secondary infection can occur because scratching opens pustules and introduces bacteria.
▲ Obtain culture and sensitivity test of suspected infected lesions, as ordered.	Culture and sensitivity test provides an indication for appropriate antibiotic therapy.
▲ Obtain additional cultures and blood work, as ordered.	Viral cultures, Tzanck smear, or viral smear may be required for diagnosis. Serological diagnoses may also be obtained.
■ Assess the patient and family immunization status and past history of chickenpox.	Patients with shingles are contagious to others who have not had chickenpox. Those who have had varicella vaccine are considered immune but should have varicella titers to confirm immunity.

Therapeutic Interventions

Actions/Interventions	Rationales
■ Discourage scratching of lesions. Encourage the patient to trim fingernails.	These measures prevent inadvertent opening of lesions, cross-contamination, and bacterial infection.
■ Suggest use of gauze to separate lesions in skin folds.	This reduces irritation, itching, and cross-contamination.
■ Teach contact isolation.	VZV is spread by contact with fluid from lesions containing viruses.
■ Instruct the patient in the use of systemic steroids, if ordered, for antiinflammatory effect.	Use of steroids is controversial; they are most commonly used for severe cases.
■ Instruct the patient in the use of antiviral agents, as ordered.	Antiviral agents are most effective during the first 72 hours of an outbreak, when viruses are proliferating. Drugs of choice are acyclovir, famciclovir, or valacyclovir.
■ Use universal precautions in caring for the patient to prevent transmission of the disease to self or other patients.	VZV can be transmitted to others and cause chickenpox in the person who has not previously had the disease.
■ Instruct the patient to avoid contact with pregnant women and immunosuppressed individuals.	Active lesions can be infectious, and immunosuppressed individuals are more susceptible.

NANDA-I NDx Acute/Chronic Pain

Common Related Factor	Defining Characteristics
Nerve pain, most commonly thoracic (55%), cervical (20%), lumbar and sacral (15%), ophthalmic division of trigeminal nerve	Complaints of pain localized to affected nerve Complaints of sharp, burning, or dull pain Facial mask of pain Alteration in muscle tone

Common Expected Outcomes

Patient is comfortable, as evidenced by an ability to rest.
Patient reports satisfactory pain control at levels less than 3
to 4 on a 0 to 10 rating scale.

NOC Outcomes
Pain Status; Pain Control
NIC Interventions
Pain Management; Teaching: Prescribed
Treatment

Ongoing Assessment

Actions/Interventions

■ Assess the patient's description of pain or discomfort:
quality, severity, location, onset, duration, precipitating or
relieving factors.

■ Assess for nonverbal signs of pain or discomfort.

Rationales

The patient may describe the pain as a tingling sensation, a
burning pain, or extreme hyperesthesia in one area of the
skin. These sensations usually precede the development of
skin lesions by several days. Postherpetic neuralgia is a
chronic pain syndrome that may continue after the skin
lesions have healed. The patient may have constant pain or
intermittent episodes of pain.

Each individual has his or her own pain threshold and
ways to express pain or discomfort. Some individuals
may deny the experience of pain when it is present.
Attention to associated signs may help the nurse evaluate pain.

Therapeutic Interventions

Actions/Interventions

■ Instruct the patient to do the following:
  • Apply cool, moist dressings to pruritic lesions with or
    without Burrow's solution several times a day. Discon-
    tinue once lesions have dried.
  • Use topical steroids (antiinflammatory effect), antihista-
    mines (antiitching effect, particularly useful at bedtime),
    and analgesics.
  • Avoid rubbing or scratching the skin or lesion.

  • Avoid temperature extremes, in both the air and
    bathwater.
  • Wear loose, nonrestrictive clothing made of cotton.

▲ Administer medications as prescribed.

Rationales

This provides relief and reduces risk for secondary infection.

A variety of medications may be required to provide relief.

Scratching stimulates the skin, which in turn increases
itchiness. It also can increase the possibility of secondary
infection.
Tepid water causes the least itching and burning.

Constrictive, nonbreathing garments may rub lesions and
aggravate skin irritation. Cotton clothing allows evaporation of moisture.
Oral narcotic analgesics (hydrocodone, codeine) are typically prescribed during the acute phase. Analgesics, antidepressants, and antiepileptic medications may be used
in the management of postherpetic neuralgia. Topical
preparations for postherpetic neuralgia include capsa-
icin cream (Zostrix) and lidocaine-prilocaine cream
(EMLA).

■ = Independent   ▲ = Collaborative

Risk for Disturbed Body Image

Common Risk Factors

Visible skin lesions
Preoccupation with changed body part

Common Expected Outcomes

Patient demonstrates positive body image, as evidenced by
ability to look at, talk about, and care for lesions.
Patient verbalizes feelings about lesions and continues
daily activities.

NOC Outcome
Body Image
NIC Interventions
Body Image Enhancement; Coping
Enhancement

Ongoing Assessment

Actions/Interventions	Rationales
■ Assess perception of changed appearance.	Because the course of an outbreak may span several weeks, patients typically need to work and/or carry out their usual routine; they may require assistance coping with changes in appearance.
■ Note verbal references to skin lesions.	Scarring may occur with repeated outbreaks or if lesions are infected.

Therapeutic Interventions

Actions/Interventions	Rationales
■ Assist the patient in articulating responses to questions from others regarding lesions and infectious risk.	Rehearsal of set responses to anticipated questions may provide some reassurance.
■ Suggest use of concealing clothing when lesions can be easily covered.	This may help the patient who is having problems adjusting to body image changes.

 Deficient Knowledge

Common Related Factors

Herpes zoster outbreak
New condition and procedures
Complexity of treatment
Emotional state affecting learning

Defining Characteristics

Questioning members of health care team
Verbalizing inaccurate information
Inadequate follow-up of instruction

Common Expected Outcome

Patient or caregiver verbalizes needed information about
disease, treatment, and possible complications of herpes
zoster.

NOC Outcomes
Knowledge: Disease Process; Knowledge:
Treatment Regimen
NIC Interventions
Teaching: Disease Process; Teaching: Individual;
Teaching: Prescribed Medication

Ongoing Assessment

Actions/Interventions

- Determine the patient's and caregiver's understanding of the disease process, complications, and treatment.

- Because of potential infectivity, determine whether the patient's caregiver or family has had chickenpox, varicella vaccine, or is immunocompromised.

Rationales

It is necessary for patients and caregivers to understand that an occult disease may have weakened the patient and allowed expression of the herpes zoster.

Even though varicella vaccine does not confer immunity to shingles, it is less common in varicella-vaccinated adults than those who have had chickenpox.

Therapeutic Interventions

Actions/Interventions

- Provide necessary information to the patient and caregiver, including written information:

  - Description of herpes zoster, including how disease is spread
  - Explanation of need for isolation
  - Need to notify health professionals of signs of CNS inflammation (changes in level consciousness)
- Encourage herpes zoster vaccination (Zostavax).

Rationales

Patients may confuse terminology and confuse herpes zoster with genial herpes. Because the patient may be reluctant to ask, clarify this point for the patient. Patients must have a comprehensive understanding of their disease to actively participate in their own care.

Fluid from lesions contains viruses, which are spread by direct contact.

Patient should isolate clothing and linen, including towels.

Early assessment facilitates prompt treatment of complications.

This vaccination is recommended for individuals 60 years or older. It is not recommended for pregnant women or those with primary or acquired immunodeficiencies or any allergy to its components. A 50% decrease in future outbreaks and greater than 60% reduction in postherpetic neuralgia have been reported.

Skin Cancer

Basal Cell Carcinoma; Squamous Cell Carcinoma; Malignant Melanoma

Tumors of the skin may be benign, premalignant, or malignant. Malignant tumors are categorized as either nonmelanoma cancers (basal cell carcinoma and squamous cell carcinoma) or melanoma. Prolonged exposure to sunlight is the primary cause of all forms of skin cancer. It has been estimated that more than 1 million cases of skin cancer are diagnosed each year. Basal cell carcinoma is the most common form of skin cancer followed by squamous cell cancer. Both of these forms of skin cancer can be cured with early detection and intervention. They rarely metastasize to other parts of the body. Malignant melanoma is the most serious form of skin cancer and is ranked as the seventh most common cancer in the United States. It is estimated that 1 in 50 people will develop melanoma in their lifetime. The risk for melanoma has quadrupled in the last 25 years. The 5-year localized survival rate is 98%, and the overall 5-year survival rate is 91%. Melanomas can metastasize to regional lymph nodes or to visceral organs if not diagnosed in the early stages. It is estimated that in the next few years there will be 62,000 new cases of invasive melanoma and 54,000 cases of melanoma in situ.

Premalignant skin conditions include actinic keratosis, solar keratosis, and actinic cheilitis. Most premalignant lesions later develop into squamous cell carcinoma. Actinic keratosis occurs most often in older adults. The skin lesions are usually rough, scaly raised growths that range in color from brown to red. The lesions of actinic cheilitis occur on the lower lip, causing dryness, and scaling.

■ = Independent   ▲ = Collaborative

Impaired Skin Integrity

Common Related Factor

Tumors

Common Expected Outcome

Patient maintains optimal skin integrity within limits of the disease.

Defining Characteristics

Erosions of the skin with drainage or bleeding
Destruction of the epidermis

NOC Outcome

Tissue Integrity: Skin and Mucous Membranes

NIC Interventions

Skin Surveillance; Chemotherapy Management; Incision Site Care; Wound Care

---

Ongoing Assessment

Actions/Interventions	**Rationales**
■ Assess skin lesions for change in shape, size, color, bleeding, or exudates. *Basal cell carcinoma:* • An open sore that bleeds, oozes, or crusts and does not heal after 3 weeks • A persistent reddish patch on the chest, shoulders, arms, or legs that may crust or itch • A shiny nodule that is pearly or translucent and different in color than the surrounding skin • A pink growth with elevated borders and a crusted center; blood vessels may be prominent as the growth enlarges *Squamous cell carcinoma:* • A wartlike growth that crusts and bleeds • A persistent, scaly red patch with irregular borders that crusts or bleeds • An elevated growth with a central depression that may bleed and grows rapidly	Regular inspection of skin that is chronically exposed to the sun is important to identify skin cancers in their earliest stages. Any change in the skin with development of a new growth or an open sore that fails to heal may be a precursor to skin cancer. Some skin cancers may resemble psoriasis or eczema in the early stages. These conditions need prompt referral to a physician for further evaluation and diagnosis.
Malignant melanoma: • Evaluate for changes in existing moles or development of a new pigmented skin lesion paying specific attention to: *Asymmetry:* Most early melanomas are asymmetrical. A line through the middle does not create matched halves. *Border:* Borders may be uneven or scalloped. *Color variability:* Normal moles are an even brown color. Melanomas may have many colors (brown, black, red, blue, pink). *Diameter:* Moles greater than 6 mm should be evaluated for removal. This is larger than the eraser on a pencil. *Evolution:* Melanomas change in color, shape, or size over a short period of time. Any changing moles need to be evaluated by a dermatologist.	Risk for malignant melanoma is increased in persons with a previous personal or family history of melanoma or in persons with more than 50 larger or atypical (dysplastic) moles.
▲ Assist with tissue biopsy.	Biopsy of any skin growth is necessary to determine the type of cancer.

Therapeutic Interventions

Actions/Interventions	Rationales
▲ Anticipate and prepare the patient for surgical therapy:	Many of the surgical procedures used in the treatment of skin cancer can be done using local or regional anesthesia in an outpatient setting.
• Cryosurgery	With cryosurgery liquid nitrogen is used to destroy the tumor by freezing. This is a bloodless procedure. Redness, swelling, blistering, and crusting may occur in the treatment area. This is primarily used for premalignant lesions.
• Mohs microscopic surgery used in nonmelanoma skin cancer	The surgeon removes a very thin layer of tissue. Each layer is examined under a microscope. Repeated layers are removed and examined until the area is free of tumor cells. This procedure is used in areas of recurring tumors or in areas on the face because it preserves the greatest amount of healthy tissue.
• Excisional surgery	The entire growth is removed with a surrounding border of normal tissue. The incision is closed with sutures.

• Reexcision and sentinel lymph node dissection (SLND)
  • The surgical margins for reexcision are determined by the depth of invasion of the original biopsy.
  • 0.5-cm margin—in situ melanoma
  • 1-cm margin—melanoma less than 1 mm
  • 2-cm margin—melanoma 1.1 to 4 mm
  • Lymphoscintigraphy and SLND are recommended for patients with tumors greater than 1.1 mm. Complete lymph node dissection is indicated for patients with positive sentinel lymph nodes or palpable lymph nodes.
	Lymphoscintigraphy is used to map lymph system drainage and locate the sentinel nodes that are the first one or two nodes that are closest to the tumor. These can be removed and evaluated to detect early micrometastatic disease. Accurate staging and identification of early micrometastasis is important in identifying patients who would benefit from complete lymph node dissection and those eligible for adjuvant immunotherapy.

▲ Administer immunotherapy (α-interferon, interleukin) or chemotherapy in the adjuvant or metastatic melanoma patient.	For patients diagnosed with stage III or IV melanoma, chemotherapy, immunotherapy, or vaccine therapy may be indicated. These treatments are often used in combination, and patients may participate in clinical drug trials. These treatments are rigorous, and patient teaching and nursing and medical support during treatment are critical. Patients often require inpatient hospitalization.
▲ Assist with application of topical chemotherapeutic agents.	Topical application of fluorouracil (5-FU) in a cream or lotion is effective in treating actinic keratosis and cancers that involve only the superficial layers of the skin. Intense inflammation may occur during treatment, but scarring afterward is rare.
▲ Anticipate and prepare the patient for radiation therapy.	Radiation therapy is indicated for patients who are not candidates for surgery because of preexisting health problems. A series of treatments is usually given over several weeks. Permanent changes in skin color and texture may develop in the treatment area.

NANDA-I NDx **Disturbed Body Image**

Common Related Factor	Defining Characteristics
Alterations in structure: • Visible tumor • Surgical scars and grafts	Verbalizes feelings about changes in physical appearance and reactions of others Negative statements about physical appearance Refusal to discuss or acknowledge change Focusing behavior on changed appearance Change in social behavior (withdrawal)

■ = Independent　▲ = Collaborative

Common Expected Outcome

Patient demonstrates enhanced body image as evidenced by ability to look at, touch, talk about, and care for altered body part.

NOC Outcomes
Body Image; Coping; Social Interaction

NIC Intervention
Body Image Enhancement

Ongoing Assessment

Actions/Interventions	Rationales
■ Assess the patient's perception of alteration in appearance.	The nurse needs to understand the patient's attitudes about visible changes in the appearance of the skin that occur with skin cancer and its treatment. The extent of the response is more related to the value or importance the patient places on the appearance of the skin.
■ Assess the patient's behavior related to appearance.	There is a broad range of behavior associated with body image disturbance ranging from totally ignoring the alteration to preoccupation with it. Patients with body image issues may try to hide or camouflage their lesions. Their socialization may decrease based on their anxiety or fear about the reactions of others.

Therapeutic Interventions

Actions/Interventions	Rationales
■ Allow the patient to verbalize feelings regarding skin condition.	Through talking, the patient can be guided to separate physical appearance from feelings of personal worth.
■ Assist the patient in identifying ways to enhance appearance.	Clothing, cosmetics, and accessories may direct attention away from skin lesions and scars. The patient should not aggravate skin lesions or healing surgical sites.
■ Assist the patient in articulating responses to questions from others regarding lesions.	Patients may need guidance in determining what to say to people who comment about the appearance of their skin.
■ Assist the patient with referral for plastic and reconstructive surgery.	Surgical excision of skin cancer of the head and neck may require removal of extensive amounts of tissue. The patient may be a candidate for skin grafting and reconstructive surgery.

NANDA-I NDx Deficient Knowledge

Common Related Factors

New diagnosis of skin cancer
Lack of information about prevention and sun safety
Unfamiliarity with treatment options
Complexity of treatment
Misinterpretation of information
Lack of recall

Defining Characteristics

Questions regarding prognosis and risk for metastasis
Verbalizing inaccurate information
Inaccurate follow-through of information

Common Expected Outcome

The patient verbalizes knowledge about skin cancer prevention and treatment.

NOC Outcomes
Knowledge: Disease Process; Knowledge: Health Behaviors; Tissue Integrity: Skin and Mucous Membranes

NIC Interventions
Teaching: Disease Process; Teaching: Procedure/Treatment; Skin Surveillance; Skin Care: Topical Treatment

Ongoing Assessment

Actions/Interventions	Rationales
■ Assess knowledge of diagnosis and treatment options.	The patient needs information about skin cancer and treatment options to make informed decisions about care.
■ Assess knowledge of skin cancer prevention and sun safety behaviors.	Skin cancers can recur, and the patient needs to know about methods to reduce exposure to ultraviolet light.

Therapeutic Interventions

Actions/Interventions	Rationales
■ Provide information about methods to decrease skin exposure to ultraviolet light. • Avoid exposure to artificial sources of ultraviolet light such as sunlamps and tanning booths. • Practice sun protection and avoidance every day. • Limit sun exposure during midday hours (10 AM to 4 PM), when the sun's rays are most intense. • Apply sunscreen with an SPF (sun protection factor) of 15 or higher with UVA and UVB protection. Apply liberally to all sun-exposed areas, and reapply every 2 hours and after swimming or perspiring. • Wear sunglasses for eye protection. • Wear sun-protective clothing with tightly woven fabrics and wide-brimmed hats.	Ultraviolet light from natural and artificial sources is the contributing or primary cause of skin cancer. Reducing exposure can prevent recurrence of tumors and development of new lesions.
■ Teach the patient and a family member to do monthly skin self-examinations. • Do examination in a well-lighted room using a full-length mirror and a hand-held mirror. • Become familiar with all birthmarks, moles, and skin blemishes. Look for changes in size, shape, or color. • Monitor all skin sores that do not show signs of healing after 3 weeks. • Look at all body surfaces in the mirror, including the front and back of the body, both right and left sides, scalp, between fingers and toes, nail beds, and between skin folds. • Give special attention to all skin surfaces exposed to the sun. • Use a comb or blow dryer to move hair on the scalp for better visualization. • Ask a family member to examine skin in hard-to-see areas.	Early diagnosis of skin cancer is associated with better chances for cure and less disfigurement from surgical interventions. The best time for skin self-examinations is after bathing or showering.

■ = Independent   ▲ = Collaborative

Actions/Interventions	Rationales
■ Provide information regarding importance of annual skin examination by a physician.	Patients who have had a malignant melanoma are seen on a regular follow-up schedule with a physician at 3-, 6-, and 12-month intervals for a complete skin examination and lymph node examination and for additional diagnostic studies, if indicated.
■ Educate regarding websites with information for health care professionals and patients: • Skin Cancer Foundation: www.skincancer.org • American Cancer Society: www.cancer.org • American Academy of Dermatology: www.aad.org • National Institutes of Health: www.nih.gov • Melanoma Research Foundation: www.melanoma.org • Oncology Nursing Society: www.ons.org	Several Internet resources provide useful lay education. Patients must have a comprehensive understanding of the disease to actively participate in their own care.

Psychosocial Care Plans

Dying is part of living. It is an active process, but it is rare when we are able to mark the beginning or the middle of an individual's dying. The end, of course, is death. There are individuals who report having come back from death and who have shared their memories of their experiences, but no one has been able to report on the state of actual death. Because death remains an unknown, it is a source of great mystery and endless speculation. Assisting patients and their families with making quality-of-life and end-of-life decisions to achieve a peaceful death is a daunting task for the health care professional in the context of the twenty-first century.

Still, much is known about dying. The process has been observed from time immemorial. Each person dies in his or her own way. This process is influenced by cultural norms, family traditions, and the people and setting among which a person's death takes place. The patient at the end of life may experience both actual and anticipatory losses. Pain, diminished abilities, fear, discomfort, massive dysfunction of organ systems (with or without the application of ever more complicated measures to prolong life), and the resounding implications his or her death will have on others require the patient to integrate enormous amounts of information and undergo extraordinarily complicated emotions.

Health professionals who understand the inevitability of a patient's death may seek to provide patients with an opportunity for a "good death," or a positive dying experience. Although the characteristics of a good death will vary, most providers agree that patients should be allowed to die with dignity, surrounded by loved ones and free of pain, with everything having been done that could have been done. A good death includes much more, but this care plan guide addresses the emotional aspects of death and dying. This care plan has been written in accordance with the Hospice and Palliative Nurses Association's Statement on the Scope and Standards of Hospice and Palliative Nursing Practice.

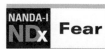 **Fear**

Common Related Factors	Defining Characteristics
Threat of death	Expressions of fear and mixed emotions
Pain and anticipation of pain	Rapid respirations and heart rate
Anticipation or perceived threat of danger	Wide-eyed appearance
Unfamiliar environment	Tension, jitteriness, and irritability
Environmental stressors	Impulsive behavior
Separation from support system	Hyperalertness and preoccupation
Treatments and invasive procedures	
Sensory impairment	
Phobias and anxieties	
Concern about future ability of survivors to manage	
Dependence on others	

Common Expected Outcomes

Patient identifies source of fear related to dying.
Patient implements a positive coping mechanism.
Patient verbalizes reduction and absence of fear.

NOC Outcomes

Fear Control; Coping

NIC Interventions

Presence; Active Listening; Security Enhancement; Spiritual Support; Support System Enhancement

Ongoing Assessment

Actions/Interventions	Rationales
■ Help the patient express his or her fears by careful, thoughtful questioning and active listening.	Do not assume that because a patient is dying that his or her fears are limited to death. Fears are patient-specific. Patients may have fears over leaving dependents behind to fend for themselves or fear of embarrassment. Sometimes a fear can be resolved through a specific intervention; at other times the fear simply remains a concern. Being present and being silent are powerful communication techniques. It is also important for the nurse to acknowledge his or her own fears.
■ Assess the nature of the patient's fear and the methods that the patient uses to cope with that fear.	Fear ranges from a paralyzing, overwhelming feeling to mild, nagging concern. Some fears can be resolved by providing the patient with information (reassurance that the patient will have pain medications available and will not suffer intractable pain); other fears can be managed through talking and sharing. The patient's philosophy about death may influence his or her ability to cope.
■ Document verbal and nonverbal expressions of fear.	Documenting expressions of fear gives care providers the information they need to provide support to the patient. Physiological symptoms and/or complaints will intensify as the level of fear increases. Fear differs from anxiety in that fear is a response to a recognized threat. However, symptoms of fear are similar to those of anxiety.

Therapeutic Interventions

Actions/Interventions	Rationales
■ Confirm your awareness of the patient's fear. Validate the feelings the patient is having, and communicate an acceptance of those feelings.	In Western culture, there is a great reluctance to discuss death. Loved ones may think that the patient who is dying should be protected from the knowledge that his or her condition is terminal, or the patient may deny death as a possibility until the final moment. This limits the patient's ability to work through emotions.
■ Spend time with the patient.	Care providers may feel they need a reason to be with the dying patient or that they need to be performing a clinical task to justify their presence in the patient's room. However, the simple act of being present can have profound significance. This presence may involve talking or touching, ministering to a physical need, or simply sitting near the bedside.

Actions/Interventions	Rationales
■ Reframe hope to alleviate fear.	Patients may fear impending hopelessness or abandonment and need reassurance and validation that comfort (palliation) is obtainable.
■ Encourage reminiscing.	Reminiscing provides reassurance that one's life has meaning and eases the intensity of the present reality.
■ While interacting with the patient, maintain a calm and accepting manner that expresses care and concern.	Patients who are talking about real feelings do not want false reassurances. They do need to feel safe in discussing troubling matters. Some of the social isolation that dying patients feel is the result of trying to protect intimate friends and family members from their need to talk about their impending death and what it means to them.
■ Be aware of the subjects that are difficult for you to discuss. Acknowledge your difficulty to the patient.	Patients may sense the care provider's discomfort and confuse the provider's behavior with the withholding of information or a lack of candor. Professional sensitivity to personal or cultural issues will help demonstrate integrity and truthfulness.
■ Provide continuity of care.	An ongoing relationship establishes trust and is a basis for communicating fearful feelings. The need for continuity of care increases in direct proportion to the intensity of the emotional material on which the patient is working. Patients rarely select a single individual to work on all of their emotional concerns. Rather, patients will share their fears with certain individuals, while sharing anger with others. The care provider will use behavioral and verbal cues from the patient to determine the patient's readiness to begin work on an issue. Continuity in care providers creates an environment in which this can best be accomplished.
■ Confirm that fear is a normal and appropriate response to situations when pain, danger, or loss of control is anticipated or experienced.	This reassurance places fear within the scope of normal human experiences.
■ As the patient's fears wax and wane, encourage him or her to explore specific events preceding the onset of specific fears.	It is sometimes helpful to recognize what factors precipitate a fear response. This information may be useful in helping the patient cope with her or his feelings.
■ Assist the patient in identifying coping and comfort strategies that were helpful in the past.	Identifying these strategies helps the patient focus on fear as a real and natural part of life that has been and can continue to be dealt with successfully.
■ Include family members in care activities.	Involvement of family in the care of the dying patient may assist in their sense of worth and decrease their sense of fear and helplessness in the dying process.
■ Assess sensory stimulation preferences. Remove unnecessary threatening equipment.	Fear may escalate with overstimulation or understimulation. Although staff are comfortable around high-technology medical equipment, many patients are not.
■ Encourage rest and relaxation.	Rest builds inner coping resources. The health care team will need to pace activities (especially for older adults) in order to conserve the patient's energy and offset fatigue.
■ Instruct the patient in the performance of self-calming measures:	These measures reduce fear or make it more manageable.
• Breathing exercises	These exercises reduce the physiological response to fear (i.e., increased blood pressure, pulse, respiration).
• Relaxation, meditation, or guided imagery exercises	These exercises promote relaxation and relieve distress.
• Affirmations and calming self-talk exercises	These exercises enhance the patient's self-confidence.

■ = Independent   ▲ = Collaborative

Grieving

Common Related Factor
Impending death

Defining Characteristics
Expressed feelings regarding potential loss of own life
Expressed feelings regarding potential loss of significant others
Expressed feelings regarding potential loss of possessions
Expressions of guilt, anger, sorrow, or anxiety
Suppressed feelings
Changes in sleep, eating habits, libido, level of activity

Common Expected Outcomes
Patient verbalizes feelings regarding impending death.
Patient has functional support systems to aid in his or her grieving process.

NOC Outcomes
Grief Resolution; Coping; Caregiver Emotional Health

NIC Interventions
Grief Work Facilitation; Dying Care; Presence; Anticipatory Guidance

Ongoing Assessment

Actions/Interventions	Rationales
■ Identify the patient's grieving process.	Patients will express grief in varied and personal ways. Although the process of grieving has been described as clearly defined phases, grief rarely manifests in a prescribed sequencing of feelings and experiences. Patients and their families revisit the phases of the grief process repeatedly. Grief helps make inevitable loss tolerable.
■ Consistently reassess the phase of grieving being experienced by the patient or significant others.	This reassessment allows the care provider to place the patient and family's feelings, which are often turbulent and contradictory, within a framework that is sometimes more understandable.
■ Assess whether the patient and significant others are in different phases of grieving.	When appropriate, share this assessment with patients or family members. This may assist their understanding of conflicts or differences in expectations.
▲ Identify available support systems: family, peer support, primary physician, consulting physician, nursing staff, social worker, clergy, therapist, counselor, and professional or lay support group.	Multiple options for help broaden the opportunities for patients and families to personalize their methods of problem resolution.
▲ Evaluate the need for referral to hospice, home health, social services, legal consultants, or support groups.	As more and more patients die in their homes while receiving services from community resources, families are assuming more responsibility for end-of-life care. Although there are compelling financial reasons why this is so, there also seems to be a philosophical shift among consumers to reject extraordinary means to extend life when death is inevitable.

Therapeutic Interventions

Actions/Interventions	Rationales
■ Establish a comfortable connection with the patient and significant others. Listen and encourage the patient and significant others to verbalize feelings.	This connection opens lines of communication and facilitates successful resolution of grief. The patient and family need to complete unfinished business in their relationships through open communication and shared feelings.

Actions/Interventions

- Provide a safe space for the expression of grief.

- Maximize privacy.

- Anticipate strong emotions.

- Help significant others to understand that a patient's verbalizations of anger should not be perceived as personal attacks.

- Provide information about the patient's health status without false reassurances or taking away all hope.

- Encourage the patient and family to engage in meaningful dialogue.

- Encourage family members to talk with a patient who may be unresponsive.

- Facilitate conversations with the patient and significant others on "final arrangements" (e.g., burial, autopsy, organ donation, funeral).

- Encourage the patient and significant others to share their wishes regarding who should be present at the time of death.
- Confirm for significant others that not being present at the time of death does not indicate lack of love or caring.

- ▲ Follow unit policies to identify the patient's critical status (e.g., color-coded door marker).

- ▲ Identify needs for additional support systems (e.g., peer support, groups, clergy).

- ▲ Foster continuity of end-of-life care across settings (e.g., home care, residential care, hospice care).

- Facilitate understanding of the nearing death awareness. Attentively and sensitively listen to the patient, and affirm the experience.

Rationales

The environment needs to support the patient's expressions of grief (e.g., the ability to see a man cry, to see mourners make wide gestures with their hands and bodies, to listen to loud vocalizations and crying). Expressions of feelings is more likely to occur in a private setting.

Privacy facilitates the patient's or family's expression of their feelings and communication without interruption.

Patients whose emotional responses to life have been fairly predictable in the past may experience turbulent and disrupting grief. The use of a bereavement specialist may prove helpful in working through this phase.

It is important for the family to understand that the dying patient is processing a large amount of highly emotional information. Help them understand that anger is part of the process of accepting death.

Hope is a basic survival instinct. Because no one knows the future, allow patients and their families to remain hopeful until death is imminent. After being informed of a poor prognosis, many patients and their families experience a defensive retreat from the shock of what they have been told. During this time, patients may engage in denial and wishful thinking. They may become unwilling to participate in self-care or may become indifferent about it.

Exploring potential reality issues in a nonthreatening manner will lead to informed decision making and assist the patient and family in verbalization of the anticipated loss.

Encouraging family members to talk and visit with the patient, even if the patient is unresponsive, instills hope. It has been shown that the patient is well aware of his or her surroundings (especially audible) beyond the point of responsiveness.

A clear understanding of the patient's and family's belief systems and cultural differences will help in advocating and facilitating open and honest communication regarding difficult subject matter. This provides a clear communication framework for building patient safety and assurance.

Families and significant others think about this but may feel uncomfortable discussing this issue together.

The moment of death cannot be predicted. It is important to remember that individual needs of each of the bereaved are different yet essential to the process of grieving.

This identification informs all staff of the patient's status and ensures that staff members do not act or respond inappropriately when encountering the patient or family.

Patients and families often become immersed in their grief and forget to access the resources available to them. Others may require expert help in negotiating grief. In either case, the care provider may be able to offer the observation that additional help is available.

The hospice concept offers an interdisciplinary approach and adds a unique dimension to end-of-life care for both patients and families.

The families and significant others may need assurance and education on the phenomenon of transition from this life.

■ = Independent   ▲ = Collaborative

NANDA-I NDx Powerlessness

Common Related Factors

Terminal illness
Irreversible physical decline
Loss of independence
Invasive health care services

Defining Characteristics

Verbal expressions of having lost control or influence over life
Reluctance to participate in decision making
Diminished patient-initiated activities
Submissiveness, apathy
Withdrawal, depression
Aggressive behavior, acting out, irritability
Decreased interest in activities of daily living

Common Expected Outcomes

Patient participates in care decisions.
Patient makes important end-of-life decisions.

NOC Outcome

Participation: Health Care Decisions

NIC Interventions

Presence; Decision-Making Support

Ongoing Assessment

Actions/Interventions	Rationales
■ Assess the patient's need for power and control.	Patients can identify those aspects of self-governance that are most important to them. Actively listen so the patient truly feels heard (e.g., offer your presence).
■ Assess for feelings of hopelessness, depression, and apathy.	These feelings may be components of grief. There may be a tremendous guilt associated with any loss of control. Subsequent interventions will be critical to facilitating feelings of well-being and empowerment, especially in older adults.
■ Identify situations and/or interactions that may increase the patient's feelings of powerlessness.	Many medical routines are superimposed on patients without ever receiving the patient's permission. This can foster a sense of powerlessness in patients. It is important for care providers to recognize the patient's right to refuse procedures. Unresolved loss may trigger feelings of powerlessness and even persist over time.
■ Assess the patient's decision-making energy level and ability.	Powerlessness is not the same as the inability to make a decision. It is the feeling that one has lost the implicit power for self-governance. Energy conservation will help reduce or relieve fatigue so the patient will be better able to use available energy for appropriate decision making.
■ Recognize the patient's wishes for information about end-of-life decisions.	This recognition may help differentiate powerlessness from knowledge deficit. Realistic expectations actually decrease distress and worry, once again enhancing the patient's decision making (i.e., empowerment). A patient simply experiencing a knowledge deficit may be mobilized to act in his or her own best interest after information is given and options are explored. The act of providing information may heighten a patient's sense of autonomy.

Actions/Interventions	Rationales
■ Determine whether the patient has an advance directive, a durable power of attorney for health care, or a living will.	
• Advance directive	An advance directive is a legal document that expresses the patient's wishes and desires for his or her health care treatment in case he or she becomes terminally ill and unable to articulate wishes and desires. These directives will act in the place of the patient's verbal requests and serve as assurance that the patient's end-of-life decisions will be honored.
• Durable power of attorney for health care	This document allows the patient to designate another person to make health care decisions on the patient's behalf. The durable power of attorney for health care becomes effective if the patient becomes unable, either temporarily or permanently, to make his or her own health care decisions. Implicit in this is the fact that the patient has discussed his or her desires with this appointed individual. If the patient becomes able to resume making his or her own decisions, then the durable power of attorney for health care is no longer in effect.
• Living will declaration	This document contains instructions that a patient be allowed to die if he or she becomes terminally ill and unable to communicate to the extent required by law. It recognizes the patient's desire not to be kept alive artificially and sets parameters on the limits to which health care providers are to go.

Therapeutic Interventions

Actions/Interventions	Rationales
■ Support the patient's sense of autonomy by involving the patient in decision making, by giving and accepting information, and by assisting the patient with controlling the environment as appropriate.	The ultimate decision-making authority lies within the patient. However, the goal of the health care professional is to assist patients in identifying and verbalizing their preferences in making authentic choices.
■ Assist the patient with developing an advance directive.	An advance directive allows patients to make decisions about their lives even after they are unable to express their own needs and desires.
■ Implement personalized methods of providing hygiene, diet, and sleep. Enhance basic care by offering food, drink, comfort, and security.	Allowing or helping the patient decide when and how these things are to be accomplished will increase the patient's sense of autonomy.
■ Encourage comfortable furnishings and surroundings.	Having comfortable surroundings will enhance the patient's sense of autonomy and acknowledges the patient's right to have dominion over controllable aspects of his or her own life. This gives some normalcy to life during the dying process.
■ Provide the patient with acceptable opportunities for expressing feelings of anger, anxiety, and powerlessness.	Verbalizing these feelings may diminish or diffuse the patient's sense of powerlessness. The care provider may need to make a special effort to maintain a careful sense of timing and compassion to alleviate the patient's feelings of loneliness or abandonment.
■ Offer continuity of a support network.	Encourage personal control by offering continuity in staffing and sustained involvement of significant others.

■ = Independent   ▲ = Collaborative

NANDA-I NDx Spiritual Distress

Common Related Factors

Terminal illness
Separation from loved ones
Separation from religious and cultural ties
Challenged belief and value system
Pain and suffering

Common Expected Outcome

Patient expresses value and comfort in his or her personal belief system.

Defining Characteristics

Questions meaning of life and death and/or belief system
Seeks spiritual assistance
Voices guilt, loss of hope, spiritual emptiness, or feeling of being alone
Appears anxious, depressed, discouraged, fearful, or angry

NOC Outcomes
Dignified Dying; Spiritual Well-Being
NIC Interventions
Spiritual Support; Presence

Ongoing Assessment

Actions/Interventions	Rationales
■ Assess history of religious affiliation.	Information regarding specific religion and importance of rituals or practices may improve understanding of the patient's needs while dying.
■ Assess spiritual beliefs.	Individuals may have other important beliefs in addition to those from religion that provide strength and inspiration at the end of life.
■ Assess the spiritual meaning of illness and death. • "What is the meaning of your illness?" • "How does grief affect your relationship with God, your beliefs, or other sources of strength?" • "Do your illness and grief interfere with expressing your spiritual beliefs?"	These questions provide a basis for understanding the patient's distress. The patient's process of introspection will assist him or her in the process of comprehending the loss.
■ Assess whether patients need help with unfinished business.	Patients may not find peace or acceptance until important affairs are in order. The health care team can provide guidance to patients while assisting in identifying strengths and values pertinent to their system.

Therapeutic Interventions

Actions/Interventions	Rationales
■ Provide understanding and acceptance. Support crying by offering caring touch.	Sharing concerns and understanding of the end-of-life journey the patient and family are experiencing will reveal the integrity and professionalism that the care provider holds in helping them through the dying process.
■ Encourage verbalization of feelings of anger or loneliness.	Patients need the opportunity to express feelings associated with fear of abandonment.
▲ When requested by the patient, arrange for clergy, religious rituals, or the display of religious objects.	Patients may derive comfort and solace from these intimate spiritual experiences.
■ If requested, sit with the patient who wishes to pray, and arrange for clergy at time of death as requested by the patient.	Being open to cultural and religious differences will allow the patient's traditions and rituals to be a part of their care while providing comfort and compassion to both the patient and family.
■ Do not provide intellectual solutions for spiritual problems.	Spiritual beliefs are based on faith and are independent of logic.

Actions/Interventions

- Encourage the patient to continue to search for truth by continuing to examine beliefs.

- Offer opportunities to share feelings verbally, in writing, through art, or through taping (audio or video).

FINAL NOTE:

- Acknowledge that nurses experience loss too.

Rationales

Reconstitution and reorganization of beliefs often follow times of questioning a philosophical and spiritual construct.

Leaving a historical legacy can help bring meaning to one's life.

Caring for patients and their families/significant others at the end of life is the essence of nursing. Nurses experience a rich opportunity to observe the grace and goodness of the human spirit within those final hours. In order to be totally present for the patients, the nurse must also take the time for self-care of emotional and spiritual needs.

Related Care Plans

Acute pain, p. 151
Caregiver role strain, p. 36
Chronic pain, p. 155
Impaired physical mobility, p. 133
Ineffective coping, p. 49

Substance Abuse and Dependence

Alcohol and Drug Abuse/Dependency and Withdrawal

Substance abuse is a pattern of problem substance use. This pattern includes a single behavior or constellation of behaviors within a 12-month period: failure to fulfill major role obligations (e.g., at work or within family); substance use in dangerous situations (e.g., while driving or operating heavy equipment); substance use that results in legal problems (e.g., arrest for driving under the influence); and social and interpersonal problems (e.g., arguments, domestic violence). Substances that may be abused include alcohol, prescription drugs, and illegal drugs.

Substance dependence is a pattern of substance use that results in biochemical, psychological, and behavioral changes. This pattern includes at least three of the following maladaptive behaviors within a 12-month period: (1) tolerance (the need for increased amounts of the substance to achieve the desired effect or a diminished effect from use of the same amount of the substance); (2) withdrawal (symptoms occur when the substance is withheld or the substance must be used in specific amounts to prevent withdrawal symptoms); (3) need for greater amounts of the substance over longer periods than was originally intended; (4) failure of efforts to stop substance use; (5) increased time spent in activities that support obtaining, using, and recovering from the substance (drug-seeking behavior); (6) abandonment of activities that were once important (e.g., sports, school) because of substance use; (7) continued substance use despite realization that problems are made worse by the substance use.

The problem of substance abuse and dependence crosses all gender, age, racial, social, and economic boundaries; it truly is an equal-opportunity killer. The patterns of substance abuse and dependence begin with a voluntary choice to use the substance. With continued use of the substance the person loses the ability to choose not to use it. Their behavior becomes marked by a compulsive need to find and consume the drug or alcohol. This change in behavior is related to prolonged exposure to the substance and its effect on brain function. Substance abuse and dependence is a multi-dimensional problem. Effective treatment programs

■ = Independent   ▲ = Collaborative

address these complex dimensions and their consequences. Substance disorders may be part of a dual diagnosis in which substance disorder is the primary or secondary problem. Both problems require treatment. A patient may be hospitalized during the initial withdrawal phase of treatment, but treatment must continue on an outpatient basis. Because substance disorders are relapsing disorders, remission and recovery require continuous treatments.

 NANDA-I NDx **Deficient Knowledge**

Common Related Factors
Denial of abuse/dependence
Lack of substance abuse education
Cognitive impairment
Apathy

Defining Characteristics
Lack of questions
Lack of recall
Information misinterpretation
Lack of insight

Common Expected Outcome
Patient verbalizes understanding of substance abuse and dependence and accepts treatment.

NOC Outcome
Disease Process
NIC Intervention
Teaching: Disease Process

Ongoing Assessment

Actions/Interventions

- Assess substance abuse history including type of substances used, amount used, routes of administration, and most recent episode of use.

- Assess for consequences of substance use such as financial, social, or family problems.

- Identify the patient's supportive relationships.

- Assess knowledge of behavioral, physical, and psychological effects of substance abuse and dependence.

Rationales

This information provides the foundation for individualizing a teaching plan based on the patient's abuse of specific substances. Many patients abuse and are dependent on more than one substance. The type of substances abused by the patient may have changed over time. Substance abuse may coexist with other psychiatric, developmental, or cognitive problems that result in a dual diagnosis. A variety of assessment tools are available to gather information about a patient's substance abuse and dependence. These tools include Addiction Severity Index, Alcohol Use Disorders Identification Test (AUDIT), CAGE, Drug Abuse Screening Test (DAST), and Substance Abuse Subtle Screening Inventory (SASSI).

Substance abuse presents the patient with problems that pervade virtually every aspect of his or her life. Significant economic resources are needed to support substance abuse over a prolonged period. The patient may have experienced problems maintaining employment, loss of financial savings, loss of friendships, and loss of stable family relationships. The patient may have a history with the criminal justice system related to substance abuse.

All relationships are affected by the substance use behavior; significant others who are affected by the substance use also need support and information.

Many patients have accurate information regarding their substance abuse, yet substance use takes place despite this knowledge.

Therapeutic Interventions

Actions/Interventions	Rationales
■ Provide accurate information about substance abuse and treatment: • Medically assisted detoxification.	It is critical that patients have current and accurate information regarding substance abuse and dependence. Detoxification and withdrawal is the first step in the treatment process for a patient with substance abuse and dependence problems. Patients who abuse drugs and/or alcohol may avoid seeking treatment because of fears and misconceptions about withdrawal and detoxification. Medically assisted detoxification provides the patient with medications to reduce the severity of withdrawal symptoms.
• Behavioral therapy such as individual or group counseling and 12-step programs.	Cognitive-behavioral and motivational therapies support the patient's readiness to begin treatment and make behavior changes, help the patient recognize and cope with situations that stimulate substance abuse, and abstain from drugs and/or alcohol. These treatment approaches may involve individual or group counseling in out-patient or residential treatment settings. Twelve-step programs such as Alcoholics Anonymous (AA) provide guiding principles for the process of recovery from substance abuse. These 12 principles have been adapted to a variety of recovery programs for other types of substance abuse and compulsive behavior problems.
• Medications for opioid and alcohol dependence.	Medications are used in the treatment of substance abuse to reestablish normal brain function, reduce withdrawal symptoms, diminish cravings, and help prevent relapse. For patients with opioid abuse, drugs such as methadone, buprenorphine, and naltrexone act on the same brain receptors as the opiates being abused by the patient. Drugs for alcohol dependence include naltrexone, acamprosate, and disulfiram. Naltrexone blocks brain receptors associated with the rewarding effects of drinking and diminishes the craving for alcohol. Acamprosate is used to ease symptoms of alcohol withdrawal. Disulfiram blocks metabolism of alcohol and leads to extremely unpleasant symptoms when the patient drinks alcohol.

■ Teach patient and family about health risks associated with substance abuse:
  • Blood borne infections
  • Liver disease
  • Cardiovascular and cerebralvascular disease
	Patients and families need to understand the health risks associated with substance abuse. Patients who use the intravenous route for substance abuse and share needles with others are at very high risk for transmission of blood-borne infections such as HIV and hepatitis B. The toxic effects of alcohol are associated with the development of cirrhosis and cancer of the liver. Patients who abuse drugs and/or alcohol have a high risk for developing hypertension and stroke. Cocaine abuse is associated with increased incidence of hemorrhagic stroke in otherwise healthy individuals.

■ = Independent   ▲ = Collaborative

Actions/Interventions

■ Refer family members to support groups and counseling.

■ Instruct in what symptoms to bring to the attention of the health care provider (e.g., withdrawal symptoms, delirium tremens, paranoid feelings, seeing or hearing things that are not there).

Rationales

Family members may need additional information, support, and counseling to cope with the effects of the patient's substance abuse. Family members may experience feelings of guilt, despair, and hopelessness. They may have a history of attempts to change the behavior of the patient with little or no success. Many treatment programs offer separate counseling and support sessions for family members. AA offers programs (Al Anon/Alateen) for family members and friends of alcohol abusers.

Acute symptoms of withdrawal, cravings, or intoxication may signal life-threatening events that require professional care.

NANDA-I NDx Noncompliance With Treatment Program

Common Related Factors

Denial of substance abuse and dependency
Rationalization of substance abuse and dependency
Treatment dropout
New financial, social, personal, and legal problems
Impaired functioning abilities
Blaming attitudes

Defining Characteristics

Behavior indicative of continued substance use
Objective tests, physiological measurement, detection of markers
Evidence of relapse
Failure to keep appointments
Failure to progress
Inability to set or maintain mutual goals

Common Expected Outcomes

Patient follows treatment plan.
Patient substance screens remain negative.
Patient returns to treatment after relapse.

NOC Outcomes

Adherence Behavior; Compliance Behavior; Treatment Behavior: Illness or Injury

NIC Interventions

Self-Responsibility Facilitation; Family Involvement; Therapy: Individual; Therapy Group; Counseling

Ongoing Assessment

Actions/Interventions

■ Assess the patient's use of denial, rationalization, and blame to sustain his or her habit.

■ Assess any secondary gains from substance abuse.

▲ Perform random substance screens.

Rationales

Substance users have an enormous capacity to explain the behaviors they use to support substance use. Rationalization and denial may obstruct a patient's ability to be honest with care providers.

Perceived gains (e.g., friends, income) promote relapse.

Support and rewards for compliance are important to recovery.

Therapeutic Interventions

Actions/Interventions	Rationales
■ Support the patient's growing awareness of substance abuse behaviors.	Positive support may encourage the patient to work toward greater understanding of his or her own behavior. Keep in mind that insight is only the first step toward recovery and that insight without action is meaningless.
■ Identify the patient's effort to blame or explain and reject change.	Allowing rationalizations to be unchallenged sanctions behavior. Patients must take responsibility for their own behavior.
■ Promote participation in support groups for recovery.	Professional and self-help programs have been shown to provide immediate help and effective lifelong support for patients recovering from substance abuse and dependence.
■ Plan for small, steady improvements.	It is realistic to expect patients to refrain from alcohol and drugs one day at a time. However, recovery from substance abuse is marked by relapses.
■ Help the patient learn to identify difficult feelings.	Articulating thoughts and feelings sometimes helps discharge emotions.
■ Reward positive actions.	Rewarding positive actions may help sustain them. Success promotes more success.
■ Spend time with the patient, but avoid reinforcing an already low self-esteem.	These patients experience a sense of pervasive worthlessness, helplessness, and hopelessness. It is important to be realistic about the negative, maladaptive behaviors they have used to support their substance use while still being able to affirm their worth as human beings and their individual value to themselves and others.

Related Care Plans

Caregiver role strain, p. 36
Common mood disorders: depression and bipolar
    disorder (see the **Evolve** website)
Ineffective coping, p. 49
Imbalanced nutrition: less than body requirements,
    p. 142
Ineffective health maintenance, p. 92
Impaired home maintenance, p. 95
Interrupted family processes, p. 64
Powerlessness, p. 162

■ = Independent   ▲ = Collaborative

Page numbers followed by *f* indicate figures; *t*, tables; *b*, boxes.

Alex
Alexandra
Ale

A Alexandra

Alexandra

Alexandra

Alexandra